Complications following Surgery

9

02

Classification of complications

Classically, complications can be divided into the cause
(specific to the surgery performed or general to any surgery) and the time period in which they arise (immediate,
early and late) (Table 9.1). Many of the complications
have specific investigations and treatments (see section
Common or important problems). This approach to
classification provides a useful way of ensuring important
complications are not forgotten but does not often help

when faced by real clinical problems in actual patients.
Several of these common clinical presentations are discussed below.

Common clinical presentations

Low urine output (oligo-anuria)

Urine output is of prime concern in the postoperative
management of patients and several points should be
borne in mind when assessing the rate of urine formation
in a given patient.
● Urine output is used as a reflection of glomerular filtration rate (GFR), which is itself a reflection of renal blood
flow (RBF) and hence the overall hydration status of the
patient.
● Surgery produces the 'stress response' and hence tends
to lower urine volume below the normal rate for a given
patient.
● Many factors other than RBF may affect GFR and hence
urine output.
● Urine output (and GFR) should be corrected for body
weight.
● As a rule of thumb, a minimum acceptable urine output is 0.5 mL/kg per h.
   When assessing a patient with a low or apparently
zero urine output it is important to be methodical;
one approach is given in Fig. 9.1. It is important to act

Table 9.1 Complications of a bowel resection for colon cancer.

	Immediate	Early	Late
Specific to the operation	Intraoperative haemorrhage	Wound infection Anastomotic breakdown Intra-abdominal abscess	Adhesion-related problems Anastomotic stricture Wound hernia
General to the anaesthesia	Perioperative myocardial infarction Anaphylactic reaction	Pulmonary collapse Deep vein thrombosis Cannula phlebitis Urinary tract infection	Pulmonary embolism

02

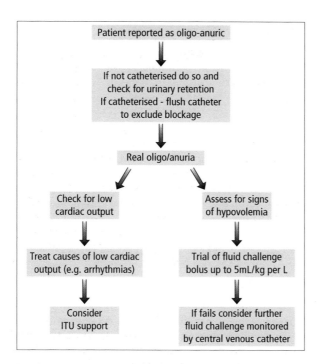

Figure 9.1 Diagnostic algorithm for oligo-anuria.

promptly on a genuinely low or absent urine output; prolonged problems with poor renal perfusion can rapidly lead to acute tubular damage and necrosis and eventually to established acute renal failure.

Fluid challenges in oliguria

The role of a fluid challenge is to assess whether the oliguria is due to simple hypovolemia. The principles of a fluid challenge are:

● that it should reflect the volume of fluid by which the circulation is anticipated to be depleted;

● the fluid should be given over a short period of time and the response assessed over the next hour or so;

● the fluid used is less important than choosing the correct volume and giving it over the correct time span — normal saline is as good as any other fluid for a challenge. Great care should be taken when deciding to give a fluid challenge. An assessment needs to be made of the cardiac function of the patient. Those with poor cardiac output or cardiac reserve (such as those with known ischaemic heart disease, known pulmonary hypertension or the elderly) are much more likely to develop acute pulmonary oedema with a prompt fluid challenge. Do not repeat a fluid challenge unless there is good reason to believe the patient is grossly hypovolaemic. If it is felt that further challenges are appropriate, monitoring of the central

venous pressure (CVP) response to the challenges may be necessary.

Advanced therapies

Furosemide

High-ceiling loop diuretics such as furosemide may have a role in preventing the establishment of renal damage in oligo-anuria. They work not only by reducing sodium reabsorption and so causing a diuresis but also have an effect on RBF by promoting increased flow in the renal cortex. Provided a patient has a properly restored circulating fluid volume, doses of furosemide may help promote the re-establishment of urine flow. High-dose furosemide infusions are usually reserved for the intensive care setting or with specialist advice.

Dopamine

The kidney contains dopaminergic receptors and it has been suggested that low-dose dopamine infusions would activate these receptors to increase RBF without affecting other systems. It is more likely that dopamine infusions promote RBF through a general stimulation of the cardiovascular system (inotropic and chronotropic effects) rather than an isolated renal effect. Their role is to support renal function in established acute or prerenal failure.

Renal support

In cases where renal function does not improve with prompt restoration of the circulating volume and attempts to restore renal function by diuretics or inotropes, it may be necessary to provide renal support until renal function returns spontaneously (which may be prolonged). Methods to replace or support renal function include haemofiltration, haemodialysis and haemodiafiltration. The main indications for providing renal support are:

● failure to excrete water causing fluid overload;

● failure to excrete potassium causing hyperkalaemia;

● rising serum urea to toxic levels;

● failure to autoregulate acid–base balance.

Confusion

Confusion is common on surgical wards. As patients get older and are admitted nearer to the time of surgery, simply being in hospital and waking up following a major operation and anaesthetic are causes for confusion, especially in the elderly. However, confusion should never be treated as a simple matter of disorientation until the major causes have been considered and eliminated. These causes can be remembered by the acronym 'DAM Hypos' (Table 9.2).

Never treat confusion with sedatives unless the cause is certain, however appealing it may be to have the patient

Table 9.2 Common causes of confusion in the postoperative patient.

Drugs
Anaesthetic agents
Analgesics (opiates)
Normal drugs being given
Normal drugs *not* being given

Acute systemic infections
Wound infections
Anastomotic leak
Chest infection

Metabolic disturbances
Hypokalaemia/hyperkalaemia
Hyponatraemia/hypernatraemia
Hypoglycaemia/hyperglycaemia
Fluid overload
Alcohol withdrawal

Hypotension
Occult haemorrhage
Inadequate fluid infusion
Low cardiac output (arrhythmias, myocardial ischaemia, pulmonary embolism)

Hypoxia

---

quiet and undisturbed for the benefit of other patients, the nurses and the doctors. A simple guide is 'Check the vitals, check the bloods, check the drug chart and check the abdomen'.

Pyrexia

A raised temperature is the single most common finding on a surgical ward. A mildly raised temperature is a normal part of the early postoperative response to major surgery. However, the development of a temperature following surgery should always be cause for concern.

The likely cause varies according to when the temperature appears. The most common causes are shown in Fig. 9.2. The form of the temperature chart can also give important clues as to the cause (Fig. 9.3). As ever, a high swinging temperature suggests a collection of pus, either in a body cavity (e.g. pelvic abscess, subphrenic abscess or empyema) or within a body organ (e.g. gallbladder empyema, pyometria, renal abscess). A low-grade 'grumbling' temperature suggests a low-grade infective or inflammatory process (e.g. deep vein thrombosis or cannula-related sepsis).

Management of postoperative pyrexia

A thorough assessment of the patient, including a brief history and physical examination, is necessary. If a likely source is identified, then specimens should be taken wherever possible to identify the causative organism (e.g. wound swabs for a wound infection). If the patient is not unwell and the cause is a minor infection, it may be appropriate to withhold antibiotics until the cause is known. If the patient is unwell or the cause is considered potentially serious, antibiotics (oral or intravenous) should be started using a 'best guess' as to the likely causative organism (e.g.

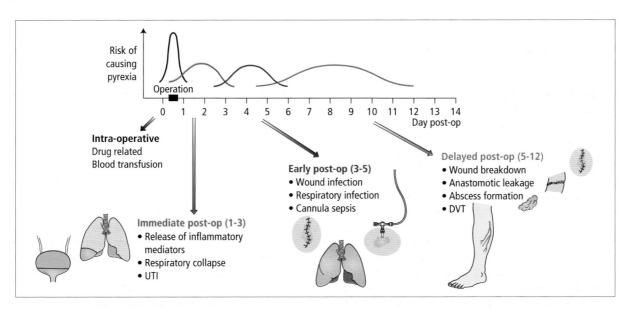

Figure 9.2 Causes of postoperative pyrexia according to time of appearance.

02

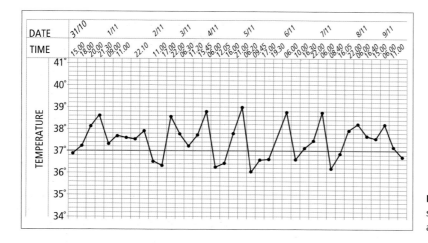

Figure 9.3 Patient observation chart showing pyrexia caused by an intra-abdominal abscess.

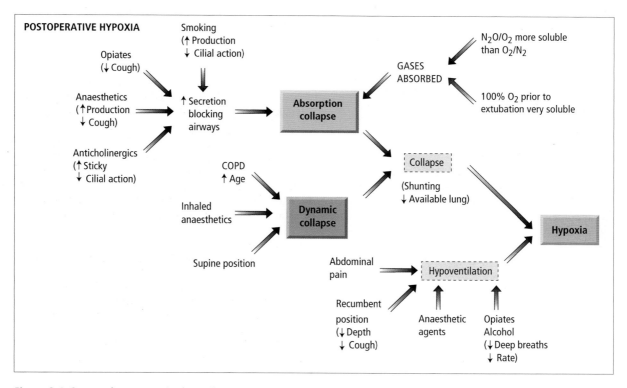

Figure 9.4 Causes of postoperative hypoxia.

an antistaphylococcal antibiotic for significant cannula-related sepsis).

If the cause is unclear, it is usual to collect a 'septic screen' from the patient. This includes a urine sample, sputum sample, swabs of any suspicious wounds or cannulae, chest X-ray and blood cultures. For patients who have had recent abdominal surgery where an intra-abdominal cause is suspected, contrast-enhanced com-

puted tomography (CT) of the abdomen is often requested urgently. If the patient is unwell and the cause is unknown, then it is best to start broad-spectrum intravenous antibiotics with a view to refining treatment once the results of the screen are known. If the diagnosis appears to be deep venous thrombosis, anticoagulation should be discussed with the surgical team.

A good guide is to remember that intra-abdominal

complications may first manifest only with pyrexia and a high index of suspicion should be maintained for complications of the surgery itself.

Hypoxia

Postoperative hypoxia is more common than documented, especially in patients who have had major thoracic or abdominal surgery. The cause may be multifactorial (Fig. 9.4). There are two key factors in the management of postoperative hypoxia.

1 Have a low index of suspicion. Mild confusion, mild hypotension and slight tachycardia may be the only signs of quite profound hypoxia. If in doubt, check for hypoxia and treat it.

2 Concentrate on the mechanics and basic physiology of ventilation first. Adequate analgesia, proper patient positioning, humidified oxygen and physiotherapy (active and passive) are the mainstays of treatment.

Chest radiography and antibiotics

Both chest radiography and antibiotics for 'chest infection' have a limited role in the management of postoperative hypoxia. The patchy small airway collapse that is a common cause after major surgery is rarely visualized on the chest radiograph and there may be frank consolidation present that is not seen. Chest X-ray is useful where pneumothorax or pleural effusions are suspected as contributory factors.

Most postoperative respiratory problems are not due to classical 'pneumonia' of any type. Provided the collapse and hypoventilation that underlies many problems is treated, any infectious element usually resolves spontaneously. Systemic antibiotics should be reserved for cases where there is a strong suspicion of established lobar consolidation or where the patient shows signs of systemic sepsis.

02

Complications following surgery at a glance

Definitions

Complication: an additional disorder or problem arising in the course, or as a result, of a disease, injury or abnormality

Oliguria: an abnormally small amount of urine (< 400 mL/day)

Anuria: no urine passed in a day

Confusion: a state of disorientation arising from loss of contact with reality, disturbance of memory, hallucination or dementia

Pyrexia (fever): an elevation of the body temperature, taken in the mouth, above 37 °C

Hypoxia: a deficiency of oxygen in the tissues

Common presentations indicating a postoperative complication

Low urinary output (see also Chapter 14)
● Minimal acceptable urinary output is 0.5 mL/kg per h (30 mL/h for most adults)
● Low urine output reflects GFR, which reflects RBF, which reflects arterial blood pressure and general level of hydration

Management
● Low urinary output: catheterize patient to confirm. True oliguria tested by fluid challenge (5 mL/kg per h)
● Signs of hypovolaemia present (tachycardia, low blood pressure): tested by fluid challenge (5 mL/kg per h)
● No response to fluid challenge: place central line to monitor CVP ± transfer to HDU/ICU
● May need diuretics, inotropes or renal support (haemofiltration, haemodialysis, haemodiafiltration)

02

Confusion
Common after surgery particularly in the elderly. Seek and treat cause. Don't just give sedation!
- Drugs
  (a) Anaesthetic agents
  (b) Analgesics especially opiates
  (c) Normal drugs: administered/not being administered
  (d) Alcohol withdrawal
- Metabolic
  (a) Hypokalaemia/hyperkalaemia
  (b) Hyponatraemia/hypernatraemia
  (c) Hypoglycaemia/hyperglycaemia
  (d) Fluid overload
- Hypoxia
- Infections
  (a) Chest
  (b) Wounds
  (c) Intra-abdominal
  (d) Urine
- Hypotension
  (a) Haemorrhage
  (b) Dehydration
  (c) Low cardiac output (arrhythmias, myocardial infarction, pulmonary embolism)

Assessment of a confused patient
- Check vitals
- Check chest
- Check abdomen
- Check drugs
- Check urine
- Check bloods

Pyrexia (see also Chapter 7)
- Pyrexia is a common sign of infection
- A mildly raised temperature is normal in the early postoperative period, indicating response to major surgery
- If pyrexia develops follow 'Note, Check, Do, Give, Treat' scheme outlined in Chapter 7

Hypoxia (see also Chapter 11)
- Common after surgery, especially thoracic or upper abdominal surgery
- Mild confusion, mild hypotension and slight tachycardia may be only clinical features
- Check and monitor hypoxia with pulse oximetry
- Treatment should concentrate on restoring normal ventilation:
  (a) Adequate analgesia
  (b) Proper patient positioning
  (c) Humidified oxygen
  (d) Physiotherapy (active and passive)
- Chest X-ray and antibiotics have a limited role

Common or important problems

Postoperative complications involving some common problems are covered in other chapters (blood transfusion, Chapter 6; surgical infections, Chapter 7).

Anastomotic leak

Leakage from any kind of intestinal, biliary or urinary anastomosis is a relatively rare but potentially life-threatening complication. The possibility of the presence of a leak should be borne in mind in all patients who have an anastomosis and in whom progress is not as expected or who show signs of sepsis not otherwise explained.

A leak may manifest in several distinct clinical scenarios and may occur at any time following surgery, although most often it is diagnosed between days 4 and 14 postoperatively.

Peritonitis

When a leak occurs at an intra-abdominal anastomosis and there is failure to control the spread of leaking contents by surrounding tissues or omental fat, peritonitis usually ensues. The clinical picture is typically one of a patient becoming rapidly unwell, with a rising tachycardia, fever, hypotension and increasing abdominal pain. The abdomen may be difficult to assess, particularly if the patient is in the early postoperative period when abdominal examination is uncomfortable (other than patients having epidural analgesia). The absence of obvious clinical peritonitis should *not* dissuade the surgeon from the diagnosis of a leaking anastomosis.

Free gas on the chest radiograph may be an unreliable sign in the early period because gas is usually seen up to 3 days after laparotomy; however, a large volume of free gas appearing much later than this is often diagnostic of a major problem. On investigation, neutrophilia and

metabolic acidosis are typically, but not necessarily, present.

Management

The principles of management are as follows.

● Stabilize the patient and maintain the cardiovascular and respiratory systems. Patients should have good intravenous access established and usually require fluid resuscitation to support the cardiovascular system. High-dose oxygen and monitoring of vital signs, urine output and oxygen saturation should be started.

● Begin treatment for presumed systemic sepsis. High-dose intravenous antibiotics are usually given on the basis of 'most likely organism'. In the case of bowel surgery, this must include antibiotics active against Gram-negative and anaerobic organisms.

● Reoperate to control the leak in the quickest, most effective way. Once the patient is stable, urgent surgery is required for definitive treatment of the leak. This usually means control of the leak by exteriorizing the ends of the anastomosis, insertion of a drain or, rarely, repair of the leak.

Once a leaking anastomosis and peritonitis have been diagnosed, treatment must be begun immediately, if necessary with the help of the intensive care unit, as peritonitis carries one of the highest rates of morbidity and mortality of any complication.

Intra-abdominal abscess

Frequently, a small leak may be contained by the surrounding body tissues or the adherence of the omentum to the site. This prevents widespread contamination by the leak but may result in the formation of a local abscess. The abscess is commonly, but not always, found in the region of the anastomosis (e.g. pelvic abscess following surgery on the rectum).

The clinical picture tends to be one of a high swinging fever and associated variable tachycardia, localized abdominal pain and poor postoperative progress. The location of the abscess may also give rise to symptoms (e.g. rectal pain and mucous discharge with a pelvic abscess, chest and shoulder tip pain with a subphrenic abscess).

Neutrophilia and metabolic acidosis are also frequent findings on investigation. The chest radiograph may occasionally show an air–fluid level in a subphrenic abscess. Where an intra-abdominal abscess is suspected, the investigation of choice is contrast-enhanced CT.

Management

The management of the patient depends on the clinical picture. If the patient is very unwell and the degree of sepsis caused by the abscess is severe, then treatment should be the same as for patients with a leak and peritonitis. If the degree of sepsis is not severe, most abscesses will resolve with percutaneous drainage and antibiotic treatment. The most common method of drainage is CT- or ultrasound-guided drain insertion under local anaesthetic.

Occasionally, open surgical drainage may be necessary where the abscess is surrounded by other organs or is inaccessible. In the case of a pelvic abscess, drainage can sometimes be made through the wall of the rectum or through the anastomosis, avoiding an external drain of any kind.

Enteric fistula

A leak may occasionally present with the formation of a fistula (usually between the leaking point and the surgical wound or drain hole). This most often represents a small leak and abscess formation that has escaped detection and which 'points' through the tissue planes opened up by the surgery as the 'path of least resistance'.

The clinical picture is typically the development of an erythematous, apparently infected area of wound or drain site that begins to discharge pus and then bowel contents, bile or urine. On close review the patient is often seen to have had a low-grade temperature and signs of infection prior to the development of the fistula. Patients who develop a fistula are rarely severely septic. Although it signifies a leak, this is almost always contained by the body tissues directing the fistula outwards.

Management

If the patient shows signs of peritonitis or gross sepsis, then management should be as for peritonitis. If not, the principles of management of a postoperative fistula are as follows.

● Drain any associated abscesses that will prevent healing of the fistula. Where these are present, CT- or ultrasound-guided drainage is employed.

● Ensure the fistula can drain properly at the exit point, i.e. the wound is draining freely (e.g. into a stoma bag).

● Maintain fluid balance and nutrition during the healing. Initially this means support with intravenous fluids but may also mean intravenous nutrition if the fistula is large or slow to heal.

● Provided that there is no obstruction to the bowel or source of the fistula, the fistula will close spontaneously.

Wound complications

Wound infection

Superficial wound infection may occur after any sort of surgery, the risk of infection being related to many factors. An increase in wound infection rates is seen with

increasing length of time spent in hospital prior to surgery, emergency or urgent surgery vs. elective surgery, malnutrition or immunosuppression of the patient, and surgery that involves opening body viscera (e.g. bowel or biliary tract) or surgery for septic indications (e.g. acute diverticulitis).

The most common source of infection is the skin flora of the patient (e.g. *Staphylococcus aureus*). Another common cause is contamination with organisms from the site of surgery (e.g. *Escherichia coli* from bowel cases).

The infection usually presents with a low-grade temperature and a painful erythematous wound with a purulent discharge. It can often be managed by simply allowing the infection to drain freely by opening the infected area of the wound and cleaning the site with antiseptic solution. Only for large or deep infections are antibiotics required. A wound infection is nowadays categorized as a superficial surgical site infection.

Wound dehiscence

Breakdown of the deeper layers (fascia and muscle) of a wound may be due to infection but may also represent problems with poor healing and/or poor surgical suturing technique. Nowadays, abdominal wounds rarely dehisce. This complication is more common in the elderly and the chronically ill or malnourished patient.

The first sign is often a high volume of clear, straw-coloured, serous discharge from the wound, indicating that the deeper tissue layers are no longer in close contact and this allows peritoneal fluid to leak out. If the skin and subcutaneous layers also break down, the patient is left with omentum or loops of bowel protruding into the wound. Although this is often a dramatic and very distressing occurrence for the patient, it is actually not particularly dangerous. Provided there is no strangulation of the bowel loops in the wound, repair can be left until the next suitable operating slot. The wound should be dressed with soft swabs and an occlusive dressing to prevent excessive fluid losses from the exposed bowel.

Wound breakdown after thoracic, neck or limb surgery is much less common and rarely needs a return visit to theatre for repair.

Wound hernia

A late complication of abdominal surgery is the development of incisional wound hernia. This may be the consequence of early partial wound dehiscence but is more often the result of chronic failure of the tissues of the scar. It is more common in the obese patient or patients with risk factors for other hernias such as chronic cough (see Chapter 24).

Other infections (see also Chapter 7)

Cannula-related sepsis

Cannula-related sepsis is the most common complication suffered by patients on surgical wards. Although the majority of infections are trivial, a proportion can develop a nasty local cellulitis and a small proportion go on to develop septicaemia as a result. In the UK every year patients die from septicaemia, infective endocarditis and metastatic abscesses originating from cannula-related infections. Most of these infections can be prevented by simple measures related to good hygiene and sensible practice.
- Cannulae should be inserted under clean conditions and properly dressed to avoid contamination.
- Intravenous infusions should be changed only as necessary to reduce the risk of contamination of the cannula.
- Cannulae should be changed regularly rather than waiting for signs of sepsis to develop in a cannula that has been present for many days.

Urinary infection

The urinary tract is often instrumented or catheterized in surgical patients. The urethral orifices are notoriously rich in bacterial flora and, once introduced, the lower urinary tract in particular is prone to the development of infection in a short period of time. Ascending infection involving the upper renal tract and kidney is uncommon but can cause major complications.

As a rule, catheters should be used only when strictly necessary, inserted as aseptically as possible and removed at the first suitable opportunity. As soon as signs of urinary infection are present, any catheter should be removed if possible and the patient treated by promotion of an active diuresis as well as oral antibiotics that are concentrated in the urine.

Intestinal obstruction (see also Chapter 23)

Mechanical

Mechanical intestinal obstruction is uncommon as an early complication following surgery. Certain procedures have a particular risk of mechanical obstruction (e.g. after intestinal stoma formation, following abdominoperineal excision of the rectum), although most mechanical intestinal obstruction following surgery occurs as a late complication due to adhesions (see later).

The majority of postoperative mechanical obstructions resolve spontaneously, although reoperation is occasionally required when a loop of bowel is trapped in a suture.

Paralytic

Paralysis of the gastrointestinal tract, particularly the small bowel, may occur after any operation, not just those involving opening of the abdomen. Many factors may contribute to the development of postoperative ileus, including handling of the bowel, procedures on the bowel itself, anaesthetic drugs (especially epidural anaesthetics), analgesics such as opiates, electrolyte imbalances and underlying endocrine abnormalities such as thyroid disease.

The principles of management are:
• maintain adequate fluid and electrolyte balance, correcting any initial abnormalities that might be contributing to the cause;
• rest the gastrointestinal tract with nil-by-mouth or the insertion of a nasogastric tube if the patient is vomiting;
• remove any drugs that might be contributing to the cause;
• maintain the nutritional requirements of the patient by parenteral methods only when the ileus is persistent or when prolonged periods without oral nutrition are expected.
Most cases of postoperative paralysis resolve spontaneously and there is little role for drugs that promote gastrointestinal motility.

Fluid and electrolyte imbalance
(see also Chapter 13)

Fluid and electrolyte disturbances following surgery may occur for several reasons.
• Inappropriate administration of fluid replacement therapy by the medical staff, causing excessive or insufficient infusion of sodium, potassium or water.
• Excessive losses of electrolytes, particularly sodium and potassium, due to nasogastric tubes, high intestinal stoma outputs, intestinal fistulae, diuretics or other drugs.
• Intrinsic renal disease exacerbated by surgery or administered drugs.

The consequences of imbalances can include paralytic ileus, persisting nausea and vomiting, metabolic acidosis or alkalosis, confusion or even convulsions (especially in the susceptible such as the elderly and very young).

Thromboembolic disease

Deep vein thrombosis

Up to 20% of patients undergoing major surgery and in hospital longer than 7 days may develop deep vein thrombosis (DVT). The risk is highest in women using the contraceptive pill and those undergoing major pelvic surgery. The majority of these will not be clinically apparent and only 1% or so of patients will develop life-threatening complications such as pulmonary embolism. Prophylaxis for DVT is now a recognized part of routine preoperative care for most patients undergoing emergency or major surgery (see Chapter 5).

Postoperatively, the signs of DVT (see Chapter 28) may be masked, especially in patients undergoing major lower limb orthopaedic surgery, and it is necessary to have a high index of suspicion. The diagnosis is usually made postoperatively by a combination of duplex ultrasound scanning of the above-knee venous system, serum D-dimer FDP levels and occasionally venography. Patients in whom anticoagulation is not contraindicated because of their surgery should receive standard full anticoagulation, initially with heparin.

Pulmonary embolism

Postoperative pulmonary embolism may present as chest pain, dyspnoea, hypoxia, confusion or even an unexplained persistent tachycardia or pyrexia. The classic signs of haemoptysis and sudden-onset dyspnoea together with electrocardiographic changes are present in only a few patients postoperatively. The chest X-ray is usually unhelpful and a ventilation–perfusion scan often inappropriate. Recent advances in scanning technology make CT pulmonary angiography a very sensitive and specific test where the diagnosis is seriously considered.

Adhesions

Adhesions may form in body cavities (pleura and peritoneum) normally lubricated by only a thin film of serous fluid. Any inflammatory insult may provoke a reaction in the mesothelial lining of the cavity, with formation of a fibrinous membrane that tends to stick the mesothelial surfaces together. These thin, 'filmy', fibrinous adhesions are common after any insult such as infection (e.g. underlying pneumonia or appendicitis) or surgical transgression of the cavity (e.g. after pneumonectomy or uncomplicated bowel surgery). Fibrinous adhesions usually resolve with no lasting effect after 6–8 weeks.

A proportion of patients have an apparent underlying predisposition for these adhesions to heal by organization and fibrosis, with the result that much more dense fibrotic adhesions form between mesothelial layers. In the abdomen these bands of tissue may form between or over loops of small bowel in particular. In some cases, despite the presence of fibrous adhesions, there are no clinical symptoms. In others they may lead to 'kinking' or compression of small-bowel loops, causing obstruction and even infarction of the blood supply. Such complications may occur shortly after the adhesions form, within months of surgery, or many years after.

02

Factors related to the formation of adhesions include:
- unknown patient genetic factors;
- presence of infection or gross inflammation at the time of surgery;
- use of powdered (starch) surgical gloves;
- use of biological suture materials (which provoke a strong tissue reaction);
- cooling of intestinal loops.

Management of adhesional obstruction
(see also Chapters 15, 31)

The principles of management of adhesional obstruction are the same as for any other cause, namely:
- maintenance of fluid and electrolyte balance;
- rest of the gastrointestinal tract;
- prevention of complications;
- surgery when appropriate.

The diagnosis of obstruction caused by adhesions is one of exclusion and even in patients with previous abdominal surgery, other causes of mechanical obstruction should be considered before assuming adhesions as the cause. Surgery for adhesions should generally be avoided, since in those patients prone to their formation, adhesions are likely following any operation for their division and the surgery may be prolonged and fraught with complications. Surgery is generally indicated only where complications have developed (e.g. intestinal ischaemia is suspected) or the obstruction is failing to resolve with a reasonable period of conservative management.

Key points

- Oligo-anuria is an acute surgical emergency: work methodically to identify the cause and treat it promptly
- Confusion should never be treated by sedatives until all major causes have been excluded
- In postoperative infections, target antibiotics to the cause whenever possible and use broad-spectrum treatment as a last resort
- Suspect occult hypoxia in patients following abdominal and thoracic surgery and treat them with simple measures aimed at restoring normal physiology
- Suspected peritonitis due to anastomotic leak is a surgical emergency and requires urgent resuscitation and treatment
- Most anastomotic leaks that result in intra-abdominal abscesses can be managed non-operatively
- Cannula-related sepsis is a very common complication that is potentially serious and, occasionally, life-threatening
- Postoperative obstruction is usually paralytic and rarely needs surgery
- Beware electrolyte imbalances in patients with nasogastric tubes or intestinal stomas
- All patients on a surgical ward are at risk of deep vein thrombosis

Common surgical complications at a glance

Definitions

Wound dehiscence: a process where the deep layers of an abdominal wound burst and viscera protrude on to the abdomen

Paralytic (adynamic ileus): temporary failure of gut peristalsis, resulting in failure of onward movement of bowel content, vomiting, distension and absent bowel sounds

Adhesions: Abnormal fibrous bands found in the pleuroperitoneal cavities that develop following an inflammatory insult, resulting in an abnormal connection between bodily parts that are normally separate

Anastomotic leak
- Leakage from any anastomosis (intestinal, biliary or urinary) is rare but potentially life-threatening
- Usually occurs 4–14 days postoperatively

Presentations
- Peritonitis: resuscitate and reoperate
- Intra-abdominal abscess: drain abscess either radiologically or surgically
- Enteric fistula: control; may close spontaneously

Wound problems (wound infection, see Chapter 7)
Superficial wound infection
- Common
- Treatment: drainage (open the wound), culture the pus and give antibiotics

Wound dehiscence
- Uncommon
- Treatment: reassure patient, occlusive dressing, resuture wound

Wound (incisional) hernia
- Late failure of wound
- May need surgical repair

Other infections
Cannula-related sepsis
- Careful aseptic technique for insertion of cannulae
- Change infusions only as necessary
- Re-site cannulae regularly

Urinary infection
- Only use catheters when strictly necessary
- Aseptic technique for insertion
- Remove at earliest opportunity

Intestinal obstruction
Mechanical
- Uncommon in early postoperative period
- Usually due to adhesions and appears during first 2 years after surgery

Paralytic (adynamic) ileus
Occurs immediately postoperatively

Predisposing factors
- Bowel handling
- Bowel operations
- Anaesthetic agents (epidural drugs)
- Analgesics (opiates)
- Electrolyte imbalance (low K^+, Ca^{2+}, Mg^{2+})
- Endocrine abnormality (thyroid disease)
- Infection shock injury

Management
- Maintain fluid and electrolyte balance
- 'Rest' gastrointestinal tract: nil-by-mouth or nasogastric tube
- Discontinue potentially exacerbating drugs
- If prolonged, give parenteral nutrition

Adhesions
- Any inflammatory process in the pleuroperitoneal cavity causes a fibrinous membrane to develop that sticks two mesothelial surfaces together (e.g. pleura to lung, peritoneum to bowel, bowel to bowel)
- They are common and develop after any surgery to the pleuroperitoneal cavity. In some people they develop into dense fibrous bands and may lead to obstruction or gangrene by ensnaring the bowel
- Problems occur in about 10% of patients after abdominal surgery
- Adhesions are the most common cause of intestinal obstruction

Factors related to adhesion formation
- Genetic (unknown)
- Infection/inflammation at time of surgery
- Use of powdered (starch) surgical gloves
- Use of biological suture materials

Management
Non-operative
- 'Rest' gastrointestinal tract: nasogastric tube
- Maintain fluid and electrolyte balance
- Exclude other causes of obstruction

Surgery (avoid if possible as it creates more adhesions)
- If obstruction not resolving after a few days
- If peritonism develops

Fluid and electrolyte imbalance (see also Chapter 15)
Causes
- Inappropriate (too much or too little) administration of water, Na^+ or K^+
- Excessive losses of electrolytes from nasogastric tubes, high intestinal fistula, diuretics
- Renal disease

Consequences
- Nausea and vomiting
- Paralytic ileus
- Metabolic acidosis or alkalosis
- Confusion
- Convulsions

Thromboembolic disease (see Chapter 29)
Deep vein thrombosis
- May develop in up to 20% of patients undergoing major surgery and in hospital for > 7 days
- Risk highest in women on contraceptive pill and patients having pelvic surgery
- Prophylaxis mandatory for patients undergoing major surgery (see Chapter 5)
- Full anticoagulation with low-molecular-weight heparin initially and warfarin for 6 months

Pulmonary embolism
- Chest pain, dyspnoea, hypoxia, confusion, unexplained tachycardia or pyrexia
- Full anticoagulation with low-molecular-weight heparin initially and warfarin for 6 months

02

Evidence-based medicine

Royal College of Surgeons of England *Care of the Critically Ill Surgical Patient*, course manual.

http://www.rcoa.ac.uk/publications.htm   Royal College of Anaesthetists audit publications

02

Must know Must do

Must know

Principles underlying rehabilitation of patients after recovery from disease, operation or injury

Must do

Attend physiotherapy department

Attend prosthetic/orthotic department

Talk with stoma therapist

Attend multidisciplinary meeting concerned with rehabilitation/continued care of a patient known to you

Introduction

Rehabilitation is the process whereby a patient is actively helped to return to a maximum potential lifestyle — physical, mental and social — after illness, accident or surgery. All patients undergoing surgery or suffering illness need some form of rehabilitation. The vast majority conduct this process themselves with no specific help from the medical/surgical/paramedical team, e.g. a young car mechanic following appendicectomy for acute appendicitis will gradually reintroduce himself to work and his leisure activities. For other patients, the need for rehabilitation is more obvious and is critical for their ability to achieve an optimum level of 'lifestyle'.

The work of rehabilitation is carried out by all members of the medical, nursing and paramedical team and may include specialists in both the hospital and the community. Initially rehabilitation starts in hospital but rapidly progresses to rehabilitation in the community. Ultimately, rehabilitation takes place in an environment most suited to the patient, preferably at home. Rehabilitation may be carried out by individual medical or surgical specialties. However, specialists in rehabilitation medicine provide a professional and cost-effective approach and may save time and effort through their expertise.

Principles of rehabilitation

Rehabilitation should begin as soon as possible and potential disabilities should be anticipated. Disability may be either:

- *primary*, i.e. directly due to the disease or injury (e.g. direct trauma, amputation, stroke); or
- *secondary*, i.e. as a complication of the disease or injury (e.g. muscle atrophy, joint contractures, decubitus ulcers, depression).

For patients undergoing elective treatment, planning for the potential rehabilitation needs of the patient should ideally form part of the pretreatment assessment so that the correct specialists can be involved in the patient's care as soon as appropriate.

Rehabilitation is a team effort and often demands the services and enthusiasm of many groups and individuals to be effective (Fig. 10.1). The aim of the team must be to prepare a plan of action culminating not in the patient's discharge from hospital but in the restoration of as normal a lifestyle as practical. However, rehabilitation should not be overly ambitious and limitations set by disability must be appreciated. The setting of unrealistic and overoptimistic goals is as counterproductive as setting no goals at all.

Physiotherapy

Physiotherapists use a variety of techniques to prevent patients developing complications, to relieve pain and to enhance physical activity. These techniques include the following.

- Chest physiotherapy: deep-breathing exercises, incentive spirometry, coughing, chest percussion.
- Muscle exercise and re-education: active and passive exercises, stretching, joint movements. Electrotherapy may be used to stimulate denervated muscles.
- Walking: teaching patients to stand and walk, initially with support (physiotherapists, parallel bars, walker frames, crutches, stick) and then without support, progressing to walking up stairs.

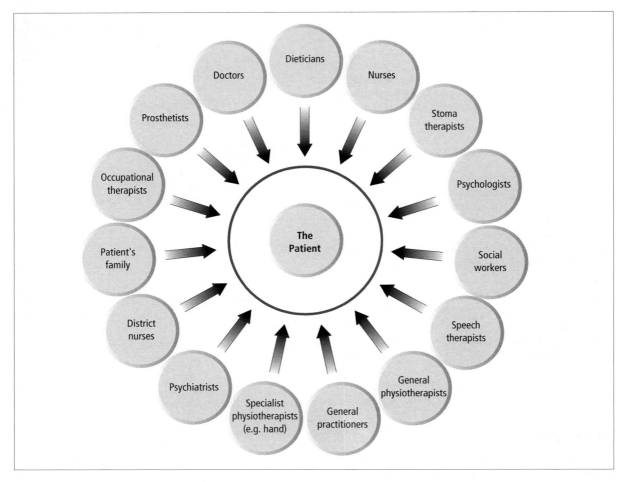

Figure 10.1 Contributors to the rehabilitation process.

● Pain relief: both heat (superficial and deep) and cold are used to relieve pain. Transcutaneous electrical nerve stimulation (TENS) is also commonly used in the management of chronic pain. Massage may be combined with heat to reduce oedema and relax muscle tension.
● Ultraviolet therapy: some decubitus ulcers (pressure sores) respond favourably to ultraviolet light.
● Hydrotherapy: helps to relieve pain, reduce muscle spasm and induce relaxation.

Occupational therapy

The aims of occupational therapy are to:
● assist in increasing the physical rehabilitation of the patient;
● assess and maximize the patient's ability to perform daily activities, including self-care, mobility and communication, known as *activities of daily living* (ADL);

● provide splints and other prostheses to facilitate independent daily living;
● give emotional and motivational support to patients during rehabilitation.

Social services

The social services should be contacted as early as possible so that the particular care required for a given patient will be available when the patient is ready for discharge from hospital. The social worker will:
● inform the patient what services are available;
● evaluate which services are appropriate for a patient, e.g. whether the patient should go home and be provided with meals on wheels, home help and district nursing or be offered supervised accommodation;
● coordinate the provision of services for the patient; and
● maximize financial benefits for the patient.

02

Rehabilitation in general at a glance

Definition

Rehabilitation: the process whereby a patient is actively helped to return to a maximum potential lifestyle (physical, mental and social) after illness, accident or surgery

General points

- All patients undergoing surgery or suffering illness need some form of rehabilitation
- Rehabilitation is carried out by doctors, nurses and paramedics in both the hospital and the community
- Rehabilitation takes place in an environment most suited to the patient, preferably at home
- Specialists in rehabilitation medicine provide a professional and cost-effective approach and may save time and effort through their expertise

Principles of rehabilitation

- Planning for the potential rehabilitation needs to start early, preferably before treatment
- Potential disabilities should be anticipated:
  - (a) Primary disability: due to the disease or injury
  - (b) Secondary disability: due to a complication of the disease or injury
- Rehabilitation is a team effort
- Prepare a plan of action culminating in the restoration to as normal a lifestyle as practical
- Setting unrealistic or overoptimistic goals is as counterproductive as setting no goals at all

Physiotherapy

- Prevents complications
- Relieves pain
- Enhances physical activity

Techniques

- Chest physiotherapy
- Muscle exercise and re-education
- Electrotherapy to stimulate denervated muscles
- Standing and walking
- Pain relief: heat, cold, electrical stimulation (TENS), massage
- Ultraviolet light (for some decubitus ulcers)
- Hydrotherapy

Occupational therapy

- Assist in increasing the physical rehabilitation of the patient
- Assess and maximize the patient's ability to perform ADL
- Provide splints and other prostheses to facilitate independent daily living
- Give emotional and motivational support to patients during rehabilitation

Social services

- Inform the patient what services are available
- Evaluate which services will be appropriate for the patient
- Coordinate the provision of services for the patient
- Maximize financial benefits for the patient

Specific problems of rehabilitation

Musculoskeletal disorders

Rehabilitation of the musculoskeletal system may be viewed as the recovery from trauma caused by chance accident or surgery. In both cases the needs of the whole patient and family must be catered for and must, if possible, span the whole of the subject's lifestyle, including pastimes and work.

Isolated injuries

Whatever the cause (trauma, musculoskeletal disease or surgery), the principles of isolated musculoskeletal rehabilitation are the same:

- pain relief to allow early mobilization;
- active and passive physiotherapy to preserve/regain range of movement;
- occupational therapy to encourage adaptation of function.

Generally, patients are taught simple exercises that they can perform at home, with supervision at outpatient follow-up. While in hospital an attitude of progress towards recovery must be engendered from the first day, otherwise regression to a dependent state rapidly becomes established. Specialist physiotherapy is particularly important in areas such as hand and upper limb injury/surgery, as loss of function is both rapid and debilitating but can be reversed by appropriate therapy.

Multiple injuries

Multiple injuries are more problematic and often associated with head injury so that rehabilitation needs to be instituted as soon as medical and surgical management permits. In these cases commitment of large resources may be required to ensure optimal recovery. For example, following a head injury that may have involved many months in bed, vigorous physiotherapy will be required to re-establish motor function, speech therapy may be required to re-establish the patient's ability to speak and

occupational therapy to help the patient back to independent living. Careful psychological examination is also essential because the presence of psychological disturbance is often underestimated unless a full assessment is performed. The long-term effects of head injury can be one of the most difficult areas in rehabilitation as behaviour and personality changes may make reintegration into the community very difficult.

Gastrointestinal disorders

Intestinal stomas

Patients in whom stomas have been created have specific concerns and needs and require expert advice concerning the management of the stoma. Patients are often concerned about leakage, odour and, in the case of colostomies, noisy expulsion of gas. Ileostomies may also be associated with skin irritation and preventive measures need to be taken to avoid dermatitis. Particularly for young patients, the psychosexual implications of even a temporary stoma are extremely important and should be addressed with care. Meeting other young people with a stoma may be an excellent way of allaying fears about their 'body image' and self-esteem.

If the stoma is created electively, then the skin can be marked preoperatively and the stoma placed in the optimal site for the patient. Postoperatively, the patient should be encouraged to take charge of stoma care as soon as practicable. Most hospitals now have a stoma nurse or therapist dedicated to dealing with patients who have stomas. A wide variety of appliances are now available that attach securely to the abdominal wall, do not leak and do not allow any malodorous gas to escape (Fig. 10.2). The stoma therapist will help the patient choose the most suitable appliance and give dietary advice. A number of 'ostomy' support groups also exist that provide assistance to patients with stomas. Most patients learn to manage their stoma very efficiently and live 'normal' lives.

Neurological disorders

Following head injury, stroke, paraplegia or extensive neurological deficits, patients require intensive rehabilitation to allow them to achieve their maximum potential. They often require extensive early and late rehabilitation, such as:
- chest care (to avoid infection);
- protection of pressure areas;
- assistance with bladder and bowel function;
- assistance with or modification of feeding;
- assistance with mobilization (including active and passive physiotherapy);
- speech therapy.

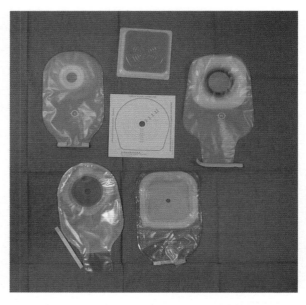

Figure 10.2 Range of stoma appliances available.

Patients and their relatives also need constant support and encouragement.

Cardiovascular disorders

Peripheral arterial disease

Rehabilitation for peripheral arterial disease and its surgery begins almost immediately after diagnosis. Common areas where rehabilitation can be of considerable importance include:
- provision of mobility aids;
- alteration of home layout to avoid the necessity of climbing many flights of stairs repeatedly;
- exercise classes and exercise programmes;
- smoking cessation programmes.

Following reconstructive surgery or surgery for arterial ulcers, early physiotherapy and mobilization may be undertaken in hospital in order to maximize the benefit of increased exercise capacity.

Venous disease

One area where early rehabilitation and physiotherapy can be of great assistance in minimizing the effects of disease is following deep vein thrombosis (DVT), particularly extensive iliofemoral thrombosis. Active mobilization and physiotherapy can reduce the effects of leg swelling and stiffness associated with extensive DVT and may help reduce the risk of development of long-term postphlebitic limb syndrome.

02

Transplantation

Transplant recipients have to come to terms with a life-long commitment to continued medical care and intervention. Early after transplantation the problems of the continuing medical care and drug therapy may be balanced by the euphoria of a successful transplant, and psychological support of the patient may need to include balancing unrealistic expectations of future progress. Encouraging an independent lifestyle is important, particularly taking responsibility for ongoing drug treatment and medical follow-up.

Long-term rehabilitation may include support for the patient during reintroduction to work. Psychological rehabilitation may also be necessary for those patients in whom the transplant fails. Profound grief, anger and resentment may occur that can interfere with the patient's recovery.

Malignancy

Rehabilitation following surgery for malignancy may involve many aspects.

Psychological

A diagnosis of malignancy often precipitates a profound reaction that can be a mixture of grief, anger, resentment and helplessness. After the initial diagnosis and medical problems have been addressed, this reaction can greatly affect the patient's ability to recover from the effects of treatment and achieve a 'normal' lifestyle. Support from nurses, specialist nurses, general practitioners, palliative care specialists and psychologists may all be necessary to help the patient come to terms with the diagnosis.

Physical

Depending on the site of the primary or secondary tumour(s) and the nature of any surgery performed, there may be many physical limitations for which rehabilitation is important.

● Feeding and nutrition, e.g. following oesophageal or gastric surgery the patient requires the advice of dieticians, speech therapists, stoma therapists.
● Mobility and ADL, e.g. general debility and limitations imposed by systemic malignancy requiring alterations to the home environment, home aids, social support.
● Chest physiotherapy: following pulmonary or intra-thoracic oesophageal surgery.
● Speech therapy: following laryngeal or upper oeso-phageal surgery.
● Stoma therapy: following some types of surgery for abdominal malignancy.

Amputation

Following amputation, patients have to cope with very specific problems; this group of patients presents an ideal model to illustrate all aspects of rehabilitation.

The trauma of the surgery has profound psychological effects on the individual concerned. For the *traumatic amputee* there has been no warning or preparation prior to limb loss. The majority of these patients are young and following the accident there may be considerable anguish, disbelief and despair at the amputation and the perceived problems that may follow. The initial postoperative period requires considerable care and understanding and should be handled by experienced staff. Full explanations must include realistic consideration of likely outcome and description of the rehabilitation process that is to follow.

In contrast, the elderly *vascular amputee* has usually had a period of pain and suffering prior to surgery. The patient will have often chosen amputation as a means of relieving the severe pain of an ischaemic limb. Counselling patients preoperatively is extremely valuable and should wherever possible be undertaken by experienced staff. In addition, relatives need to be included in these discussions as their understanding and reassurance can help the patient overcome the natural fear of the future.

The expertise of the rehabilitation team and the facilities at its disposal can affect the ultimate success of the rehabilitation process. The rehabilitation team caring for the amputee (of whatever age) must be a closely integrated group of professionals who work together.
● *Nursing staff*: provide day-to-day care of the patient, with particular attention to pressure areas and care of the stump.
● *Physiotherapist*: provides assessment of early mobilization of the patient:
      (a) chest physiotherapy to avoid chest infections;
      (b) early mobility to avoid DVT, including use of early walking aids;
      (c) mobility with a prosthesis.
● *Prosthetist*: manufacture, fitting and maintenance of artificial limbs.
● *Occupational therapist*: teaching aids to daily living skills and assessment of home circumstances, including domiciliary visits at home with the patient.
● *Social workers*: arrange domiciliary services (e.g. home help, meals-on-wheels) and may help with financial matters.
● *General practitioner*: continuing care once discharge has occurred.
● *District nurses*: nursing in a home situation.

The whole team should meet regularly to discuss the patient's progress and decide on realistic goals that the patient can achieve. Patients should be involved in the discussion so that they are aware of what is to be achieved.

Family members also need to be kept aware of progress and of problems as they arise. As the rehabilitation process proceeds, the goals may need to be modified in the light of progress.

Work

In the case of a young amputee, the return to work can be an important issue. The social worker and occupational therapist can give initial guidelines and discussion with the employer can be helpful. In a situation where return to the former work is not possible, the patient is referred to the *disablement employment adviser*, who has a statutory responsibility to advise on retraining programmes and potential employers. Local charitable organizations may also offer employment advice.

Social reintegration

The amputee may initially feel isolated and handicapped by surgery. Family and friends play a vital role in encour-aging the patient to reintegrate. A range of clubs and societies (e.g. National Association for Limbless Disabled) exist to help amputees. To encourage this reintegration, rapid discharge home is important but should only be undertaken once prosthetic fitting has been completed and the occupational therapist has assessed the patient's home. If discharged too early, demoralization of both patients and relatives can reduce the ability to achieve full potential.

Follow-up

The patient needs to remain in lifelong contact with a limb-fitting centre for the maintenance and provision of prostheses. Regular reviews are initially necessary as the stump matures and the patient adapts to the new situation. The review clinics act as both a stump and prosthetic review but also as an opportunity for open discussion on how the patient is managing at home. In this way, shortfalls in service provision and the identification of areas in which help can be provided are assessed.

02

Specific problems of rehabilitation at a glance

Musculoskeletal disorders
Isolated injuries
- Pain relief to allow early mobilization
- Active and passive physiotherapy to preserve/regain range of movement
- Occupational therapy to encourage adaptation of function

Multiple injuries
- Rehabilitation needs to be instituted as soon as medical and surgical management permits
- Commitment of large resources may be required to ensure optimal recovery

Gastrointestinal disorders
Intestinal stomas
Patient concerns
- Leakage
- Odour
- Noisy expulsion of gas
- Skin irritation
- Psychosexual concerns
- Body image issues

Management
- Create stoma in optimal site
- Patient should be encouraged to take charge of stoma care

- Stoma therapist
- Choose the most suitable appliance
- Give dietary advice
- 'Ostomy' support groups

Neurological disorders
- Chest care (to avoid infection)
- Protection of pressure areas
- Assistance with bladder and bowel function
- Assistance with or modification of feeding
- Assistance with mobilization (including active and passive physiotherapy)
- Speech therapy
- Constant support and encouragement for patient and family

Cardiovascular disorders
Peripheral arterial disease
- Smoking cessation programmes
- Exercise classes and exercise programmes
- Mobility aids/alteration of home layout

Venous disease
- Active mobilization and physiotherapy after DVT
- Bandaging, mobilization and active ankle exercises with venous ulcers

02

Amputation

Traumatic amputee
- No warning prior to limb loss
- Young patients
- Anguish, disbelief and despair

Vascular amputee
- Pain and suffering prior to amputation
- Elderly patients
- Amputation may be a great relief

Malignancy

Psychological
- Grief, anger, resentment and helplessness

Physical
- Feeding and nutrition
- Chest physiotherapy
- Speech therapy
- Stoma therapy
- Mobility and ADL

Transplantation
- Psychological support:
  (a) Deal with unrealistic expectations of future progress
  (b) Graft failure may lead to grief, anger and resentment
- Encourage an independent lifestyle
- Encourage responsibility for continuing drug treatment and medical follow-up

Hypoxic States and Airway Obstruction

Must know Must do

Must know

Cause and management of acute hypoxia
Immediate and supportive management of the hypoxic patient
Clinical features and diagnosis of acute hypoxia
Principles and practicalities of airway control
Oxygen therapy
Indications for mechanical ventilation

Must do

Visit the intensive care unit to learn about types of ventilatory support
Become familiar with the various oxygen masks, humidifiers, and pulse oximetry equipment
Observe endotracheal intubation
Observe percutaneous tracheostomy
Assist/observe patients undergoing CPR

Table 11.1 Causes of hypoxia.

Hypoxic hypoxia
Decreased Po_2 in inspired air (high altitude)
Hypoventilation
   Depression of respiratory centre (head injuries, opiates, cerebrovascular accident)
   Shallow respirations due to pain (after chest or upper abdominal surgery, pleurisy)
   Airway obstruction (foreign body, aspiration)
   Increased airway resistance (asthma, emphysema)
   Large pneumothorax (trauma, rupture of emphysematous bulla)
Alveolar–capillary diffusion block
   Decreased alveolar membrane area (pneumonia, pulmonary congestion)
   Fibrosis of alveolar or pulmonary capillary walls (pulmonary fibrosis)
Abnormal ventilation–perfusion ratio
   Perfusion of unventilated alveoli (atelectasis)
   Ventilation of underperfused alveoli (pulmonary embolism)
   Shunting of venous blood into arterial circulation (cyanotic congenital heart disease)

Anaemic hypoxia
Anaemias (hypoxia is worse on exercise)
Carbon monoxide poisoning (binds to haemoglobin to produce carboxyhaemoglobin, which cannot release oxygen)

Stagnant hypoxia
During shock, slow circulation to the tissues produces hypoxia and damage (e.g. renal failure)

Histotoxic hypoxia
Inhibition of the cytochrome oxidase system in the tissues (cyanide poisoning)

Introduction

The general term for lack of oxygen is *hypoxia* while the specific term for lack of oxygen in the arterial blood is *hypoxaemia*. Hypoxia may be acute or chronic. Acute hypoxia is immediately life-threatening if left uncorrected for more than a few minutes. Acute hypoxia causes cardiac arrest and severe cerebral impairment, leading to brain death or gross permanent mental disability should the patient survive. Thus acute hypoxia is seldom seen in isolation and usually requires cardiopulmonary resuscitation (CPR). Chronic hypoxia is seen in chronic obstructive or restrictive lung disease (see also Chapter 38). The causes of hypoxia are listed in Table 11.1.

Causes of acute hypoxia

The two most important causes of sudden hypoxia are impaired level of consciousness and aspiration.

Impaired level of consciousness

Impaired level of consciousness from any cause (e.g. head injury, sedation, cerebrovascular accident) can be accompanied by depression of the respiratory centre

03

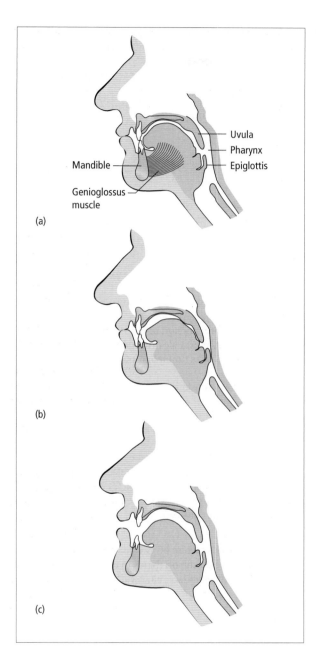

Figure 11.1 Upper-airway obstruction. (a) The tongue is normally lifted forwards in the mouth by the action of the genioglossi muscles, which are attached to the inner surface of the symphysis of the mandible. (b) If the patient is unconscious or has a fracture of the mandible, the tongue may fall back into the pharynx and cause airway obstruction. Flexion of the head causes more narrowing of the pharynx, exacerbating the situation. (c) The triple-airway manoeuvre is used to correct the resulting airway obstruction: the neck is extended, the mandible is displaced forwards and the mouth opened.

(diminished ventilatory drive). Loss of consciousness is also accompanied by loss of the protective gag and cough reflexes such that aspiration of foreign material into the bronchopulmonary tree is likely. In addition, the tongue musculature is relaxed and the neck muscles fail to lift the base of the tongue from the posterior pharyngeal wall. If the patient's head is in the flexed or mid-position, acute obstruction of the upper airway supervenes. Hypopharyngeal obstruction by this mechanism is the commonest cause of hypoxia encountered in clinical practice. This type of upper-airway obstruction is commonly seen after head injuries with loss of consciousness (Fig. 11.1).

Aspiration

Aspiration of blood, vomit or gastric juice will result in severe laryngospasm in the stuporous or lightly comatose patient. In addition, and irrespective of the degree of coma, it causes lower-airway obstruction by a combination of bronchospasm, excessive bronchial secretions and mucosal oedema. If the aspirated fluid is irritant (e.g. gastric juice), it often progresses to pulmonary oedema and acute respiratory distress syndrome (ARDS; see Fig. 38.21). Aspiration syndromes are discussed fully in Chapter 38.

Acute cardiorespiratory disease

● Community-acquired pneumonia and hospital-acquired/ventilator-associated pneumonia (see Chapter 38).
● Imbalance between alveolar ventilation and perfusion, i.e. there is a mismatch of blood and airflow to the lungs (e.g. pulmonary collapse and pulmonary embolism).
● Right-to-left shunting (blood returns to the left heart without being oxygenated).
● Impairment of gaseous diffusion due to thickening of the alveolar–capillary interface between blood and inspired air.
● Defective extrapulmonary ventilation due to diminished central (cerebral) ventilatory drive or disease/trauma limiting effective chest wall and diaphragmatic movement.
● Important medical disorders accompanied by hypoxaemia are heart failure, severe lobar pneumonia and status asthmaticus.

Traumatic chest injuries

These include certain types of pneumothorax and injuries to the pulmonary parenchyma (see Chapter 38).

Facial fractures

Occlusion of the laryngeal orifice by the prolapsed tongue is particularly prone to occur in patients with fractures of the body of the mandible. The upper airway may also be compromised directly by fractures of the middle third of the face, when the maxillae are driven backwards over the laryngeal orifice.

Extrinsic upper-airway compression

Thyroid disease

Extrinsic compression of the upper airway in patients with thyroid disease may occur in several ways. Bleeding inside a thyroid nodule may result in rapid enlargement with compression of the trachea, especially if it occurs in a retrosternal thyroid, as the rigid boundary of the thoracic inlet cannot accommodate the sudden increase in volume. Tracheal compression is also encountered in advanced thyroid cancer (especially of the anaplastic variety), in the late stages of Reidel's thyroiditis (due to fibrous contracture) and after thyroidectomy (due to postoperative bleeding with clot compression underneath the strap muscles). If, as rarely happens nowadays, both recurrent laryngeal nerves are damaged during thyroid surgery, severe asphyxia is encountered when the endotracheal tube is removed because the paralysed vocal cords become opposed in the midline and occlude the laryngeal orifice.

Malignancy

Extrinsic compression from secondary tumour deposits or lymphomas in the mediastinum is usually part of the superior vena cava compression syndrome. In addition to the respiratory difficulties, there is marked congestion of the upper half of the body. When due to lymphomas, rapid relief is obtained by appropriate urgent therapy with chemotherapy and radiotherapy. Endovascular stents are also used to relieve superior vena cava compression syndrome.

Clinical features of hypoxia

Symptoms

If the patient is *unconscious*, the only reliable clinical manifestations of hypoxia are central cyanosis, abnormal respiration (rapid, slow, apnoea, gasping) and hypotension. Complete airway obstruction leads to asphyxia and cardiac arrest within 5–10 min. Incomplete airway obstruction in the unconscious patient is noisy (rattling, stridor).

The *conscious* hypoxic patient is cyanosed, anxious, restless, sweating and often confused. Accessory muscles of respiration are recruited, with indrawing of the supraclavicular spaces. Stridor is an inspiratory whooping sound that indicates partial obstruction of the trachea (intrinsic or extrinsic).

Apnoea (defined as cessation of breathing in the expiratory position) is the most serious clinical situation and demands immediate active intervention (see below).

Physical examination

1 Examine the patient and ensure that there is no obstruction to the airway.
2 Determine the presence or absence of pulse (femoral or carotid). If the patient is apnoeic and there is no pulse, full CPR should be instituted immediately (see below).
3 If spontaneous respiration is present, the essential physical examination is assessment of the respiratory system (see Chapter 11). Briefly, this should include:
   (a) inspection of the chest wall: for injuries, expansion and paradoxical movement, i.e. chest wall moves in with inspiration and out with expiration;
   (b) auscultation of both lung fields: for air entry to both lungs, abnormal breath sounds (crepitations, bronchial breathing);
   (c) percussion: if air entry is absent, this will determine whether the affected hemithorax is hyperresonant (air in pleural cavity), dull (pneumonic consolidation) or stony dull (fluid).

Investigations

The most important immediate investigation is blood gas analysis of a femoral arterial blood sample. With respiratory failure the blood gases will indicate respiratory acidosis, but if there has been significant anoxia to the tissues (e.g. cardiac arrest) there will also be a metabolic acidosis due to accumulation of lactic acid (see Chapter 13).

A portable chest radiograph should also be obtained. It is imperative that the hypoxic patient is never sent to the radiological department for the chest X-ray. Other investigations such as portable electrocardiography (ECG) are needed in the event of cardiac arrest.

Principles of treatment of the hypoxic patient

The principles underlying basic life support in the immediate management of the acutely hypoxic patient are:
A airway control;
B breathing support;
C circulatory support;
D determine the cause.
Once the critical situation has been controlled, the underlying cause must be treated.

03

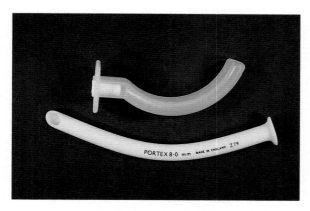

Figure 11.2 Oropharyngeal and nasopharyngeal airways.

Airway control

The first measure is to correct hypopharyngeal obstruction. This is achieved by the triple-airway manoeuvre:
1 extension of the neck;
2 forwards displacement of the mandible;
3 opening the mouth (see Fig. 11.1c).

Next, any secretions or fluid (vomit, blood) in the mouth or pharynx are removed by suction, intraoral foreign bodies including dentures are removed, and a nasopharyngeal or oropharyngeal airway (Fig. 11.2) is inserted if the patient is unconscious. If the upper airway is blocked, a laryngoscopic examination is performed to clear the pharynx and rapidly assess the situation. Then an endotracheal tube is passed or, if this fails, a cricothyroidotomy or minitracheostomy is performed (Fig. 11.3). Usually senior staff are available for this contingency.

The *Heimlich manoeuvre* is a first-aid procedure used to relieve upper-airway obstruction caused classically by inhalation of a bolus of food, the so-called café coronary syndrome. Standing behind the patient, place your arms around the patient's upper abdomen and, clasping your hands together, firmly force upwards under the ribs. In this way the air in the chest is compressed and, with luck, the foreign body will be expelled from the upper airway.

Breathing support

Mouth-to-mouth breathing support

Expired air contains 16–18% oxygen and, when delivered adequately to the apnoeic patient via mouth-to-mouth or mouth-to-nose ventilation, achieves an arterial Po_2 (Pao_2) of 10 kPa or 75 mmHg (normal 13.3 kPa or 100 mmHg) if the patient's lungs are normal. Mouth-to-mouth breathing is commenced immediately and continued until oxygen delivery systems can be brought to the scene. The practical sequence is to tilt the patient's head backwards and inflate the lung by mouth-to-mouth ventilation. If this meets with an obstruction, the patient's mouth is closed and mouth-to-nose ventilation is tried. After an airway has been introduced one can change to mouth-to-airway ventilation.

Self-refilling bag-valve unit (Fig. 11.4)

In the non-intubated patient, experience is required for the efficient use of this equipment with a mask. Once the patient has been intubated, the bag-valve unit is particularly effective for maintaining oxygenation. It permits respiration during both spontaneous and artificial ventilation. The unit consists of a self-refilling bag with an inlet valve to which an oxygen cylinder is attached, and has a non-rebreathing valve at the mask or endotracheal tube.

Circulatory support

Circulatory support involves external cardiac massage for cardiac arrest and the insertion of adequate intravenous lines for volume replacement and drug administration. For external cardiac massage the patient is placed supine on a hard surface. The aim is to compress the heart between the sternum and the spine, thereby forcing blood from the heart and producing a circulation. It is important to feel the femoral or carotid pulse during CPR to ensure that an adequate circulation is being produced. External cardiac massage is performed by placing the heel of one hand, with the other hand on top, over the lower half of the sternum. With the arms extended the sternum is pressed down and then released at a rate of about 60 times per minute. Excessive force should be avoided, as there is a risk of fracturing the ribs. External cardiac massage must be coordinated with ventilation, with one respiration being given for every five compressions. CPR must not be interrupted for more than 10 s. An algorithm for the use of drugs and defibrillation during CPR is given in Fig. 11.5.

Correction of underlying abnormality

Having resuscitated the patient, the specific condition that led to the hypoxic arrest must be treated, e.g. correction of maxillary fractures, pharmacological treatment of heart failure or asthma, antibiotics for pneumonia, etc. If the apnoea is thought to result from opioid-induced depression of the respiratory centre, naloxone hydrochloride is administered intravenously. In patients who aspirate gastrointestinal contents, acid damage to the lung with the development of ARDS is likely (see Chapter 38). These patients are given antibiotics and vigorous physiotherapy. If ARDS develops, the patient will require ventilation.

03

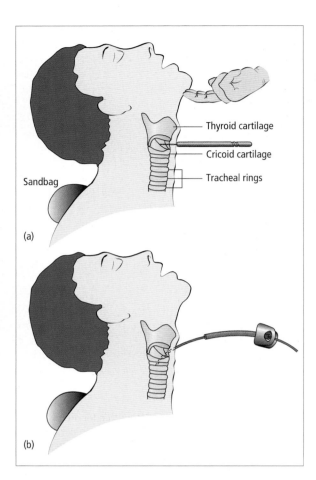

(a)

Thyroid cartilage

Cricoid cartilage

Tracheal rings

Sandbag

(b)

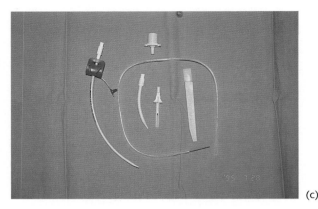

(c)

Figure 11.3 Minitracheostomy. (a) The head is extended and a small sandbag placed between the shoulder blades. The cricothyroid membrane is identified between the thyroid and cricoid cartilages. The overlying skin and cricothyroid membrane are infiltrated with local anaesthetic and a few drops of anaesthetic are flushed into the trachea. A transverse stab incision is made through the skin and subcutaneous tissue and the cricothyroid membrane is punctured. (b) An introducer is then passed through the wound into the trachea and over this the minitracheostomy tube (internal diameter 4 mm) is passed. The introducer is removed and the minitracheostomy tube is secured. A minitracheostomy allows for very effective aspiration of sputum in postoperative patients and may obviate the need for intubation and ventilation. (c) The equipment required to perform a minitracheostomy.

Oxygen therapy

Oxygen is often administered by mask to patients who are hypoxic but breathing spontaneously. A number of different types of mask are available.

● Oxygen is usually administered via masks that do not deliver a constant known percentage of oxygen to the patient; this is due to the variable dilution of oxygen in the mask by inspired air. Examples of these types of mask are the Mary Catteral (MC) and the Hudson, which administer oxygen concentrations ranging from 35 to 60%. Unless there is additional lung pathology, 35% oxygen is adequate for ensuring normal Pao_2 and oxygen toxicity is unlikely if less than 60% oxygen is administered.

● When more accurate oxygen administration is needed, a high-airflow oxygen enrichment (HAFLOE) mask such as the Ventimask is used (Fig. 11.6). Several models are available that are capable of administering oxygen in defined concentrations ranging from 24 to 60%.

● Accurate masks delivering low inspired oxygen concentrations are essential for patients with chronic lung

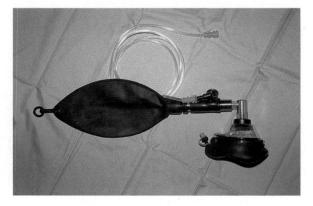

Figure 11.4 Self-refilling bag-valve unit consists of a self-refilling bag with an inlet valve to which an oxygen cylinder is attached and a non-rebreathing valve at the mask or endotracheal tube.

disease who have lost normal ventilatory control and depend on moderate hypoxaemia to stimulate the respiratory centre. Such patients require enough oxygen to avoid serious hypoxaemia but not so much that the Pao_2 reaches

03

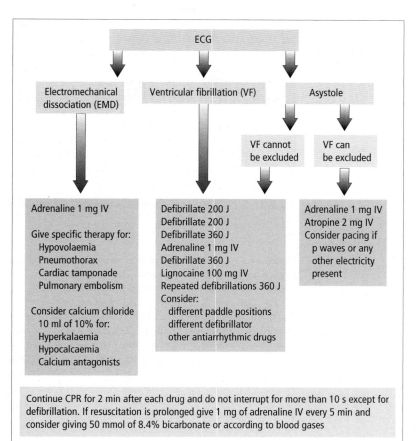

ECG

Electromechanical dissociation (EMD)

Ventricular fibrillation (VF)

Asystole

VF cannot be excluded

VF can be excluded

Adrenaline 1 mg IV

Give specific therapy for:
Hypovolaemia
Pneumothorax
Cardiac tamponade
Pulmonary embolism

Consider calcium chloride
10 ml of 10% for:
Hyperkalaemia
Hypocalcaemia
Calcium antagonists

Defibrillate 200 J
Defibrillate 200 J
Defibrillate 360 J
Adrenaline 1 mg IV
Defibrillate 360 J
Lignocaine 100 mg IV
Repeated defibrillations 360 J
Consider:
different paddle positions
different defibrillator
other antiarrhythmic drugs

Adrenaline 1 mg IV
Atropine 2 mg IV
Consider pacing if
p waves or any
other electricity
present

Continue CPR for 2 min after each drug and do not interrupt for more than 10 s except for defibrillation. If resuscitation is prolonged give 1 mg of adrenaline IV every 5 min and consider giving 50 mmol of 8.4% bicarbonate or according to blood gases

Figure 11.5 Algorithm for drug therapy and the use of defibrillation during cardiopulmonary resuscitation (CPR).

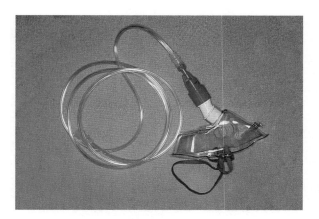

Figure 11.6 Ventimask.

the normal range, as this would result in apnoea due to loss of the respiratory drive.
● When longer oxygen therapy is needed, humidification is necessary, especially in patients who are mouth-breathers or who have sputum retention. Otherwise, tracheal secretions become inspissated by the cold dry inspired air–oxygen mixture. In addition, ciliary activity is lost. This further exacerbates the retention of bronchial secretions. Humidification is best achieved by blower humidifiers of the heated water or ultrasonic type.
● When oxygen is administered in very high concentrations, oxygen toxicity may occur. In practice this is only seen in ventilated patients breathing > 60% oxygen for more than 24 h. The manifestations of oxygen toxicity are lung damage, blindness from retrolental fibroplasia (seen in premature babies) and epilepsy.

Mechanical ventilation

The decision to perform tracheal intubation and ventilation is based on the clinical criteria shown in Table 11.2. Ventilatory support usually involves the application of intermittent positive pressure via an endotracheal tube or tracheostomy. Regular aspiration of secretions and physiotherapy is required. The underlying condition needs to be treated while the lung is supported. The endotracheal tube acts as a conduit for infection, and ventilator-associated pneumonia is a common problem.

Table 11.2 Clinical indications for tracheal intubation and mechanical ventilation.

Sao_2 < 90% on > 60% oxygen
Respiratory arrest or rate < 8/min
Tachypnoea > 35/min
Fatigue
Agitation, confusion, refusal of oxygen mask
Diminished conscious level
Airway obstruction or impairment
Rising $Paco_2$
Worsening respiratory acidosis

Types of mechanical ventilation

● *Controlled mandatory ventilation (CMV)*: this is the classic form of ventilation and the most basic. A preset tidal volume is delivered at a preset rate, regardless of any patient effort. The patient may 'fight the ventilator' and require deep sedation or muscle relaxation. Traditionally, tidal volumes of 10 mL/kg are used and patients are ventilated to normocarbia. There is now an increasing awareness of the potential of ventilator damage to the lung (barotrauma) in those patients with severe respiratory failure (see below).

● *Synchronized intermittent mandatory ventilation (SIMV)*: a preset tidal volume is delivered synchronized with the patient's respiratory effort. In the absence of effort, the breath is given after a set time lapse known as the SIMV period. Between mandatory breaths the patient is free to breathe through the ventilator circuit.

● *Pressure support*: when patient effort is detected, the machine applies a preset pressure to the airway thus assisting inspiration. As the lungs fill, the flow decreases and the inspiratory phase is terminated. In the absence of patient effort no ventilation occurs; thus it is only suitable for patients with adequate respiratory drive.

● *Pressure-control ventilation*: positive airway pressure is applied at a fixed rate. Patient effort is not required or sensed. The tidal volume depends on the resistance and compliance of the tubing, airways and lungs. Pressure-control ventilation is used in paediatric practice to compensate for variable leaks around uncuffed endotracheal tubes and in severe respiratory failure to limit barotrauma.

● *Positive end-expiratory pressure (PEEP)*: this is an adjunct to positive pressure ventilation. The airway pressure is never allowed to fall to zero, thus splinting the alveoli open in expiration. This aids recruitment of lung and improves matching of ventilation and perfusion. This is useful in any condition where the alveoli are prone to collapse, as in ARDS. Excessive PEEP can reduce cardiac output and blood pressure by raising intrathoracic pressure.

● *Continuous positive airways pressure (CPAP)*: this is effectively PEEP without positive pressure ventilation. The patient breathes spontaneously without assistance, but gains the benefit of airway splinting. It is used either via an endotracheal tube when the patient has been weaned from ventilatory support but is not ready for extubation or through a tight-fitting facemask as an alternative or precursor to intubation and ventilation.

When the patient recovers from respiratory failure, the functional inspired oxygen concentration (Fio_2) can be reduced. When it is below 50%, weaning from ventilation can be considered. Any muscle relaxants are stopped and sedation is reduced to encourage respiratory effort. After a short period of ventilation it may be possible to rapidly convert to spontaneous breathing and extubate the patient, but usually a process of weaning is required. Respiratory support is gradually reduced until the patient is performing the work of breathing.

Pulse oximetry

Pulse oximetry is a method for continuously measuring oxygen saturation. A small device placed on a digit estimates arterial oxygen saturation (Sao_2) by calculating relative absorption of light from two light-emitting diodes at different wavelengths. The process is repeated many times a second, and the non-pulsatile (non-arterial) component subtracted. The Sao_2 is displayed on a screen (Fig. 11.7).

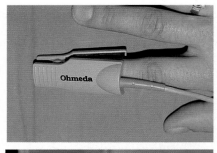
(a)

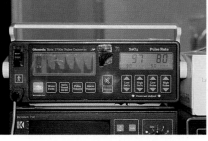
(b)

Figure 11.7 Pulse oximeter: (a) a small device placed on a digit detects blood flow by transillumination and plethysmography; (b) oxygen saturation and pulse rate are displayed continuously on a small screen.

Pulse oximetry is very useful in detecting hypoxic episodes during intubation and extubation, during the recovery period after surgery, especially in elderly and obese patients prone to hypoxaemia, and during gastrointestinal endoscopy. However, movement, peripheral vasoconstriction and the presence of carboxyhaemoglobin can produce inaccurate readings.

Hypoxia at a glance

Definitions

Hypoxia: lack of oxygen (usually meaning lack of oxygen delivery to tissues or cells)

Hypoxaemia: lack of oxygen in arterial blood

Apnoea: cessation of breathing in expiration

Common causes of hypoxia
Acute hypoxia
● Impaired level of consciousness
● Aspiration

Postoperative causes
● CNS depression, e.g. post anaesthesia
● Airway obstruction, e.g. aspiration of blood or vomit
● Poor ventilation, e.g. abdominal pain, mechanical disruption to ventilation
● Loss of functioning lung, e.g. ventilation–perfusion mismatch (pulmonary embolism, pneumothorax, collapse/consolidation)

General causes
● CNS depression, e.g. opiates, cerebrovascular accident, head injury
● Airway obstruction, e.g. facial fractures, aspiration of blood or vomit, thyroid disease or cervical malignancy
● Poor ventilation, e.g. pleural effusions, neuromuscular failure
● Loss of functioning lung, e.g. ventilation–perfusion mismatch (pulmonary embolism, pneumothorax, collapse/consolidation), right-to-left pulmonary shunt, traumatic chest injury

Key points
● During the first 48 h following upper abdominal surgery, 80% of patients are hypoxic. Have a high index of suspicion and treat prophylactically
● Adequate analgesia is more important than the sedative effects of opiates: ensure good analgesia in all postoperative patients
● Ensure the dynamics of respiration are adequate: upright position, abdominal support, humidified oxygen
● Acutely confused (elderly) patients on a surgical ward are hypoxic until proven otherwise
● Pulse oximetry Sao_2 values < 85% equate to Pao_2 < 8 kPa and are unreliable in patients with poor peripheral perfusion

Clinical features
In the unconscious patient
● Central cyanosis
● Abnormal respirations
● Hypotension

In the conscious patient
● Central cyanosis
● Anxiety, restlessness and confusion
● Tachypnoea
● Tachycardia, arrhythmias, atrial fibrillation (AF) and hypotension

Investigations
● Pulse oximetry: Sao_2 guide to arterial oxygenation
● Arterial blood gases (Pco_2, Po_2); pH and base excess for respiratory acidosis, metabolic acidosis later
● Chest radiograph: collapse/pneumothorax/consolidation/pleural effusion
● ECG: atrial fibrillation

Essential management
Airway control
● Triple-airway manoeuvre, suction secretions, clear oropharynx
● Consider endotracheal intubation in CNS depression/exhausted patients (rising Pco_2), neuromuscular failure
● Consider surgical airway (cricothyroidotomy/minitracheostomy) in facial trauma, upper-airway obstruction

Breathing
● Position patient upright
● Adequate analgesia
● Supplemental oxygen: mask/bag/ventilation
● Support respiratory physiology: physiotherapy, humidified gases, encourage coughing, bronchodilators

Circulatory support
● Maintain cardiac output
● Ensure adequate fluid resuscitation

Determine and treat the cause
Oxygen therapy
● Mask that delivers 30–60% oxygen diluted with inspired air (MC or Hudson mask)
● HAFLOE delivers oxygen in defined concentrations from 24 to 60%

- Humidification required for longer-term therapy
- Beware of toxicity in ventilated patients breathing > 60% oxygen for 24 h

Mechanical ventilation
- CMV: ventilator delivers a preset tidal volume at a preset rate regardless of what the patient does
- SIMV: ventilator delivers a preset volume synchronous with the patient's respiratory effort. If the patient does not attempt to breathe, a breath is given after a set time lapse
- Pressure support ventilator applies a preset pressure to the airway, assisting patient-generated inspiration
- Pressure-control ventilation: positive airway pressure is applied with a fixed rate regardless of patient. Used in

paediatrics to compensate for leaks around uncuffed endotracheal tubes
- PEEP: ventilator never allows airway pressure to fall to zero, thus keeping the alveoli open in expiration
- CPAP: this is PEEP without positive pressure ventilation. Airway pressure is maintained above zero but the patient breathes spontaneously. It is often given via a tight-fitting mask around the mouth and nose

Pulse oximetry
A method of continuous measurement of Sao_2 based on calculating relative absorption of light from two light-emitting diodes at different wavelengths

Evidence-based medicine

Copeland, G.P., Jones, D. & Walters, M. (1991) POSSUM: a scoring system for surgical audit. *Br J Surg* **78**, 356–360.

Knaus, W.A., Draper, E.A., Wagner, D.P. & Zimmerman, J.E. (1985) APACHE II: a severity of disease classification system. *Crit Care Med* **13**, 818–829.

03

Haemorrhage, Hypovolaemia and Shock

12

03

Must know Must do

Must know

Clinical features and management of the various types of shock

Assessment and monitoring of patients in shock

Complications of shock and their management

Causes and management of upper gastrointestinal haemorrhage

Causes and management of lower gastrointestinal haemorrhage

Must do

See and follow patients admitted with upper gastrointestinal bleeding

Help in the resuscitation of patients with hypovolaemic shock

Observe and follow patients admitted with lower gastrointestinal bleeding

Observe upper gastrointestinal endoscopy performed to stop bleeding peptic ulcer

Observe a flexible sigmoidoscopy

Observe a colonoscopy

Observe an emergency coeliac axis/mesenteric angiogram

Perform faecal occult blood in patients with hypochromic microcytic anaemia

Become familiar with the interpretation of small bowel enema and colonic barium enema

If possible, observe an enteroscopy

Introduction

Shock may be defined as acute circulatory failure with inadequate or inappropriate perfusion resulting in generalized cellular hypoxia. Inadequate tissue perfusion for whatever reason causes cellular hypoxia, thereby precipitating a number of intracellular reactions and a cytokine cascade, culminating in a metabolic acidosis. The latter, by altering vascular permeability, creates a vicious circle: there are increasing plasma losses from the circulation with reducing cardiac output (CO) and further acidosis, so that the state of shock becomes irreversible.

Classification of shock

The pathophysiological changes that occur in shock are summarized in Fig. 12.1.

Hypovolaemic shock

Hypovolaemia is defined as a reduced circulating blood volume (CBV = 70 mL/kg in an adult; 80 mL/kg in infants) and can be either *true* or *apparent*. True hypovolaemia results from contraction of CBV as a result of:
- loss of blood due to haemorrhage;
- loss of plasma due to burns;
- dehydration from deficits of water and saline.

Apparent hypovolaemia ensues because of increased vascular capacity, usually due to loss of peripheral resistance in the muscular arterioles (sepsis, adrenal insufficiency, anaphylaxis, neurogenic factors). However, in some of these conditions (e.g. sepsis) the situation is more complex as the increased capillary permeability induces intravascular fluid losses into the interstitial space.

Response to hypovolaemia

The adverse effects of hypovolaemia are the result of inadequate CO and hence inadequate cellular perfusion. Overall CO is determined by stroke volume (SV) and heart rate (HR): $CO = SV \times HR$. In a young fit adult at rest, each ventricle fills during diastole to reach an end-diastolic volume of 120 mL. With each ventricular contraction (systole), 70 mL is ejected from each ventricle. This amount is known as the ejection fraction, which is normally 60% of the volume present in each ventricle at the end of diastole. In accordance with Starling's law, the more the heart fills during diastole, the greater the volume expelled with each beat (SR), although the ejection fraction remains fairly constant. CO is then determined by the following factors.

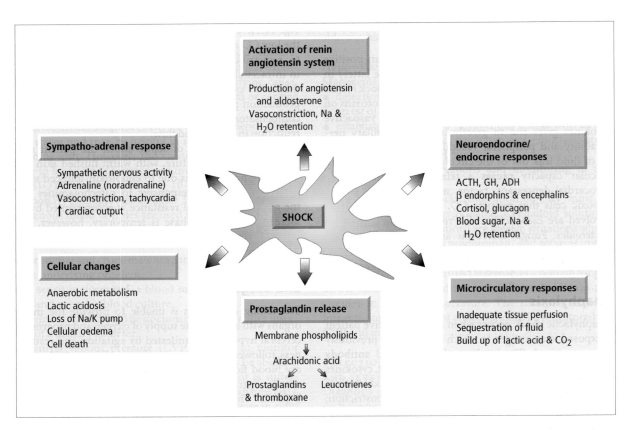

Figure 12.1 Shock, regardless of cause, initiates a series of pathophysiological changes aimed at protecting the organism and preserving its vital functions.

- *Preload* (i.e. venous filling/venous return) is reduced significantly in hypovolaemia.
- *Cardiac contractility*: diminished in hypovolaemia because of reduced end-diastolic filling/volume of the ventricles (and thus stretch of the cardiac muscle fibres).
- *Afterload* (i.e. peripheral arterial resistance) acts as an impediment to cardiac ejection; thus a reduced afterload tends to favour an increase in CO but only in the presence of an adequate CBV. In the hypovolaemic patient, peripheral resistance is initially increased (sympathetic and adrenal response) so that the percentage fall in blood pressure is always an underestimate of the drop in CO.
- *Heart rate*: within limits, tachycardia increases CO, although extreme heart rates reduce output by diminishing ventricular filling and coronary artery nutrient blood flow to the myocardium.

The response of an individual to blood loss varies considerably. Indeed there are young healthy individuals who, by virtue of the intense vasoconstriction they can mount in response to volume deficits, can lose as much as 25% of CBV without any significant change in arterial blood pressure. The response is influenced by age, dura-

tion and severity of injury, pre-existing myocardial disease, anaemia, and associated trauma. In the accident victim, the additional trauma alters the neuroendocrine and metabolic response. Thus trauma victims with mild to moderate hypovolaemia may have a normal or even elevated CO, and may be normotensive or even hypertensive after the accident.

Cardiogenic shock

Cardiogenic shock signifies central pump failure. It is most commonly seen after major myocardial infarction but is also encountered in ventricular arrhythmias (pump action ineffective), interruption of ventricular outflow by massive pulmonary embolus, and cardiac tamponade usually caused by direct penetrating injuries to the myocardium, where subsequent haemorrhage into the pericardial sac prevents adequate filling of the ventricles during diastole. Cardiogenic shock is characterized by profound hypotension and distended neck veins. It carries a high mortality even with prompt and energetic treatment.

03

whether the patient is still hypovolaemic (CVP remains unchanged or may even drop as the vasoconstriction subsides) or is likely to be overloaded (sharp elevation of CVP).

- Hourly urine output: an output > 30 mL/h indicates adequate renal perfusion.
- Pulse oximetry: preferably one that also displays the pulse plethysmogram in addition to percentage oxygen saturation.

More intensive monitoring is required in cardiovascularly unstable patients, including those who sustain major trauma. This includes the following (in addition to the above).

- Insertion of radial artery cannula for continuous monitoring of arterial pressure and to obtain samples for blood gas analysis.
- Core–peripheral temperature gradient: useful non-invasive indicator of peripheral perfusion.
- Insertion of pulmonary artery flotation catheter (Swan–Ganz catheter) allows monitoring of right atrial pressure, pulmonary artery pressure, pulmonary capillary wedge pressure, measurement of CO (by thermodilution), and sampling of mixed venous blood for oxygen saturation ($S\bar{v}o_2$). A number of important derived variables can be obtained from these measurements in conjunction with the results of blood gas analysis, including pulmonary vascular resistance, systemic vascular resistance, oxygen extraction ratio and systemic oxygen consumption.

Cardiogenic shock

The aim of treatment is to improve CO without increasing excessively the workload on the heart, which might further compromise the coronary circulation. Patients should have complete bedrest and be monitored in a coronary care unit. Pain relief should be achieved with diamorphine or morphine. If the patient has had a myocardial infarction, thrombolytic therapy in the form of streptokinase or recombinant tissue plasminogen activator should be administered as well as aspirin. If the patient is in heart failure, diuretics (e.g. furosemide 40 mg), nitrates, angiotensin-converting enzyme inhibitors, cardiac glycosides and dopexamine may be indicated. Arrhythmias must be avoided and controlled (Table 12.2).

Septicaemic shock

Septicaemic shock is commonly seen in surgical practice. The source of infection may arise *de novo* from a perforated viscus or may be due to postoperative complications (e.g. abscess, leaking anastomosis). Treatment is aimed at controlling infection and improving the hypovolaemic state caused by endotoxin-induced peripheral vasodilata-

Table 12.2 Management of common arrhythmias seen after myocardial infarction.

Arrhythmia	Treatment
Supraventricular tachycardia	Carotid massage Adenosine DC cardioversion
Atrial flutter or fibrillation	Digoxin Verapamil Amiodarone DC cardioversion
Complete heart block	Atropine Cardiac pacing
Ventricular arrhythmias	Lidocaine infusion Bretylium
Ventricular tachycardia	CPR DC cardioversion

CPR, cardiopulmonary resuscitation; DC, direct current.

tion. The latter is improved by the administration of colloid solutions, the volume of which is monitored by CVP and urine output. Blood cultures should always be carried out before antibiotic administration so that the sensitivity of the responsible organisms may be determined. In the interim a combination of penicillin, aminoglycoside and metronidazole should be effective against the most common organisms. The use of inotropes is often indicated in severely ill septic patients to maintain CO and preserve vital functions. The most frequently used inotropes are listed in Table 12.3. These drugs are very potent, however, and should only be used in an intensive care setting and in conjunction with the treatment of abnormalities that may impair cardiac performance, e.g. hypoxia, acidosis, hypocalcaemia. Intravenous hydrocortisone has been advocated in the treatment of septic shock but its use is controversial.

Anaphylactic shock

Anaphylactic shock may be precipitated as a response to an antigen to which the individual has been previously sensitized. The release of histamine and other vasoactive amines causes widespread vasodilatation, with increased capillary permeability. Bronchoconstriction is also a prominent feature that further exacerbates the tissue anoxia. The common causes of anaphylactic shock in hospital practice are the administration of radiological contrast media and intravenous drugs, e.g. penicillin. While most insect bites produce no more than a mild local hypersensi-

Table 12.3 Inotropic agents frequently used in patients with shock.

Dopamine
Low-dose: peripheral resistance falls secondary to dilatation of splanchnic and renal vasculature. Renal and hepatic blood flow increase. Renal-protective effect
High-dose: causes noradrenaline release, leading to vasoconstriction and loss of renal-protective effect

Dobutamine
Reduces systemic resistance and improves cardiac performance. Possibly has better inotropic effect than dopamine

Dopexamine
β_2-Adrenergic agonist and dopamine receptor agonist:
  Increased heart rate
  Increased cardiac index
  Increased cardiac output
  Decreased peripheral resistance
  No vasoconstriction

Adrenaline
Low-dose: β_2-adrenergic agonist effects
High-dose: α-adrenergic agonist effects:
  Vasoconstriction
  Decreased renal blood flow
  Peripheral gangrene

Noradrenaline
α-Adrenergic agonist effects

---

tivity, wasp and bee stings may produce full-blown anaphylactic shock with circulatory collapse in some people. Treatment consists of:
- intravenous fluids to compensate for the relative hypovolaemia produced by widespread capillary vasodilatation;
- intramuscular administration of adrenaline to improve CO and induce vasoconstriction;
- antihistamines to block the histamine receptors (for details see Chapter 6).
Specific treatment such as penicillinase is used if the anaphylactic reaction is due to penicillin.

Complications of shock

Apart from the profound effects on the cardiovascular system, shock may precipitate acute respiratory failure, acute renal failure, disseminated intravascular coagulation (DIC) or, more rarely, hepatic failure. Severely ill patients may develop systemic inflammatory response syndrome, which often results in multiple system organ failure (also known as multiple organ dysfunction syndrome) and, ultimately, death (see Chapter 16).

Disseminated intravascular coagulation

DIC is a major complication of septic shock. In this condition the various factors involved in the clotting mechanism are activated and widespread intravascular coagulation takes place, with consequent depletion of clotting factors, including platelets. Profuse spontaneous haemorrhage is then paradoxically produced and bleeding from operation sites may be uncontrollable. If the condition is suspected, diagnosis is confirmed by the high level of fibrin degradation products present in the serum. Intravenous heparin is administered to control the coagulation and the normal clotting factors are restored by giving fresh frozen plasma and platelets.

Stress ulceration

Severe haemorrhage may occur from multiple gastric erosions in critically ill patients. The erosions are secondary to mucosal ischaemia, which is caused by hypotension or the effects of endotoxin. Alteration in mucosal permeability allows back-diffusion of H^+, which stimulates excess acid secretion. Administration of antacids to raise the gastric pH to 7 may be of help; H_2-receptor antagonists have also been used, although their efficacy remains unproven. However, the elevation of pH may allow bacterial colonization of the stomach from the oropharynx, where Gram-negative colonization is common in seriously ill patients. To avoid bacterial overgrowth, cytoprotection with sucralfate has been used as an alternative to raising the pH.

Acute respiratory failure

Severe respiratory problems may develop after successful resuscitation of the shocked patient. The so-called shock lung syndrome may be associated with a variety of abnormalities, including sepsis, fat embolism, massive blood transfusion, oxygen toxicity and DIC. The varied aetiology has prompted the term 'acute respiratory distress syndrome' (ARDS) to cover all these conditions. Increasing evidence implicates activated white cells (e.g. by endotoxin via the complement system in the case of Gram-negative septicaemia) as the mediators of ARDS. The activated white blood cells release free radicals and hydrolytic enzymes that damage the endothelium of lung capillaries. The result is that the lungs become very oedematous; fibrin and microaggregates collect in the

03

interstitial spaces around the alveoli and capillaries, thus reducing efficient gas exchange (see also Chapter 38).

Clinically, respiration becomes more rapid, the Pao_2 falls significantly, even when the patient is breathing high concentrations of oxygen, and the increased respiration lowers the Pco_2, producing a respiratory alkalosis. Chest radiographs may change from normal to complete 'white-out' over a 24-h period. Treatment is mainly supportive and aimed at preserving adequate Pao_2. Intermittent positive-pressure ventilation is necessary if Pao_2 falls below 8 kPa. If intermittent positive-pressure ventilation fails to maintain adequate oxygenation, positive end-expiratory pressure of between 5 and 15 cm H_2O is used (see Chapter 11). Other measures to reduce oedema (e.g. maintaining plasma osmotic pressure by gastrointestinal or intravenous feeding and the administration of intravenous albumin, and the judicious use of diuretics) are important. Steroids and antibiotics are of doubtful value.

Acute renal failure

The commonest cause of acute renal failure in the surgical patient is a fall in GFR as a consequence of hypovolaemic shock. This is clinically manifest as oliguria with a daily urine output of between 400 and 700 mL, i.e. less than 20 mL/h.

When oliguria becomes established, fluid intake must be severely restricted and electrolyte concentrations carefully monitored. The blood urea will rise rapidly and serum K^+ tends to rise to dangerous levels, which can cause cardiac arrhythmias or cardiac arrest. A severe metabolic acidosis develops (see Chapter 13).

Fluid administration is restricted to 400 mL/day plus known losses. A rising K^+ may be controlled by giving intravenous glucose and insulin, calcium gluconate or ion-exchange resins. Sodium bicarbonate is used to control the metabolic acidosis. In most cases of acute renal failure some form of dialysis is necessary during the acute tubular necrosis phase. Peritoneal dialysis has the advantage of being a simple technique but haemodialysis is more efficient. At the end of the oliguric phase, assuming that acute tubular necrosis rather than acute cortical necrosis is the problem, the diuretic phase commences, during which large quantities of unconcentrated urine are passed and very high losses of Na^+ and K^+ may occur, which need careful management (see Chapter 14).

Acute hepatic failure

Rarely, severe shock may bring about acute hepatic failure. Encephalopathy, jaundice and coagulation disorders may supervene, with progressive coma and respiratory failure. Treatment is mainly supportive and the mortality is very high. Hepatic failure is discussed fully in Chapter 27.

Prognosis

The prognosis of patients with two or more system failures is poor. Each organ failure carries a mortality of about 30%. However, these mortality rates are additive, so that patients with three or more system failures have mortality rates of 90–95%.

Gastrointestinal haemorrhage

This is one of the most common clinical presentations in gastroenterological and general surgical wards. The causes, by topographical site in the gut, are outlined in Table 12.4. From a clinical standpoint, patients present with:
- iron-deficiency anaemia due to chronic occult blood loss with positive faecal occult blood, e.g. gastric cancer, right colon cancer;
- minor episodes of blood loss, e.g. rectal tumours, inflammatory bowel disease, etc.;
- acute gastrointestinal bleeding with hypovolaemic shock;
- recurrent obscure gastrointestinal bleeding.

Acute upper gastrointestinal bleeding

There are marked regional differences in the incidence even within a country. Thus in the UK, Aberdeen has a much higher incidence (116 per 100 000) compared with Oxford (47 per 100 000). The causes of upper gastrointestinal bleeding in descending order of frequency are outlined in Table 12.5. In 20%, the diagnosis is not clear despite upper gastrointestinal endoscopy at presentation because:
- there is too much blood in the stomach to permit adequate inspection;
- the lesion is missed;
- the lesion has healed;
- the source of bleeding is outwith the stomach and proximal duodenum.

Bleeding due to aspirin and non-steroidal anti-inflammatory drugs

All these drugs cause peptic ulcers in the stomach and duodenum. Aspirin increases the risks for both gastric and duodenal ulcers two to four times and accounts for 1 in 10 ulcer bleeds in patients aged over 60 years. The non-aspirin non-steroidal anti-inflammatory drugs (NSAIDs), such as fenbufen, benoxaprofen, indomethacin, ibuprofen and piroxicam, carry a higher risk of peptic ulceration

Table 12.4 Causes of gastrointestinal bleeding by site.

Foregut
Ulcers: usually drug induced
Oesophageal varices
Gastritis
Peptic ulcer: duodenal, gastric
Tumours: adenoma, smooth muscle, lymphoma
Vascular anomalies
Hereditary telangiectasia
Anastomotic suture line: postoperative
Mallory–Weiss syndrome
Trauma: including iatrogenic
Haemobilia
Chronic pancreatitis: aneurysms, sectorial portal
   hypertension

Midgut
Colorectal tumours/polyps
Small bowel tumours
Vascular anomalies: right colon and small bowel
Hereditary telangiectasia
Peutz–Jeghers polyps
Jejunal diverticula
Meckel's diverticulum: infants and children
Aorto-enteric fistula: patients with aortic grafts
Crohn's disease
Anastomotic suture line: postoperative
Portal hypertension: includes bleeding from stomal varices

Hindgut
Inflammatory bowel disease
Diverticular disease
Angiodysplasia
Ischaemic colitis
Trauma
Endometriosis
Anastomotic suture line: postoperative
Portal hypertension
Haemorrhoids

Table 12.5 Causes of upper gastrointestinal bleeding.

Disease category	Frequency (%)
Duodenal ulcer	29
Gastric ulcer	22
Oesophagitis and ulcer	12
Acute gastric lesions	7
Mallory–Weiss syndrome	7
Oesophageal varices	5
Gastric cancer	2
Diagnosis unclear	15

than aspirin and account for 20% of all bleeding ulcers in patients aged over 60 years. In the UK, 12 000 emergency upper gastrointestinal hospital admissions per annum (perforation, bleeding, acute pain) are caused by NSAIDs, with 2230 deaths. Overall, 30% of ulcer bleeds in patients above 60 years of age are due to aspirin or non-aspirin NSAIDs.

Aspirin and the NSAIDs act by inhibiting cyclooxygenase (COX) and thus the synthesis of prostaglandins. There are two isoforms of COX: COX-1 and COX-2. COX-1 is always present and is responsible for most of the physiological prostaglandin production involved in cytoprotection, especially of the gastric mucosa. In contrast, COX-2 is involved in the synthesis of prostaglandins that mediate the inflammatory response (including joint inflammation). Thus specific inhibitors of COX-2 suppress the inflammatory response while preserving the cytoprotective function of COX-1. COX-2 inhibitors such as meloxicam have decreased gastrointestinal toxicity but are less effective in pain relief.

Clinical presentation

The majority of patients are admitted as emergencies with:
- haematemesis (blood in vomit), which may be bright red or altered to look like 'coffee grounds' because of HCl digestion; or
- melaena (blood in stool), usually altered foul-smelling blood; or
- both.

Severity of upper gastrointestinal bleeding determines the presence and extent of hypovolaemia.
- Mild: no significant hypovolaemia (includes anaemic patients).
- Moderate: hypovolaemia that responds to volume replacement (crystalloids and blood); thereafter the patient remains stable.
- Severe: active continued major bleeding that renders resuscitation with transfused blood difficult, or recurrent major bleeding after successful resuscitation from the initial bleed.

Although this classification is useful in dictating management, the category can change after initial assessment from mild to severe. Thus complacency must be avoided and repeat clinical monitoring is essential even in patients with mild upper gastrointestinal haemorrhage. This situation is best exemplified by the patient who develops an aorto-enteric fistula after aortic replacement by prosthetic graft. The initial (secondary) bleeds may appear trivial yet are warning manifestations of an impending catastrophic haemorrhage that is often fatal. Persistent bleeding is diagnosed when the patient requires 8 units (> 60 years) or 12 units (< 60 years) or more over a 48-h period to

03

Table 12.6 Techniques for endoscopic control of upper gastrointestinal bleeding.

Injection therapy: vasopressors, sclerosants, thrombin, mixtures

Banding: alternative to injection sclerotherapy for oesophageal varices

H-F electrocoagulation: unipolar, bipolar, argon ion plasma coagulation

Heater probe

Photocoagulation (gas vapour lasers, diode array lasers)
  Non-contact (laser beam)
  Contact (with sapphire tip)

---

maintain the haemoglobin at 10 g/dL. In addition to the severity of the bleed, the patient must be examined for stigmata of chronic liver disease, which may indicate variceal haemorrhage. Examination of the cardiovascular and respiratory systems is necessary with appropriate investigations (chest X-ray and ECG). Significant cardiac and respiratory disease are important determinants of morbidity and mortality and influence the approach used to control bleeding.

Management

Diagnosis is based on upper gastrointestinal endoscopy carried out within 24 h of admission in haemodynamically stable patients and following resuscitation. All patients with acute upper gastrointestinal haemorrhage should have a joint consultation by a surgeon and gastroenterologist soon after admission. Patients with severe continued bleeding require surgery concomitantly with volume replacement through two large infusion cannulae. The hypovolaemia is corrected with blood and colloids/crystalloids and a catheter is inserted in the urinary bladder for hourly measurement of the urine output. A Salem sump nasogastric tube is inserted and hourly clinical observations commenced:
- pulse, blood pressure, CVP;
- pulse oximetry;
- urine output.

Endoscopic treatment
Control of bleeding in the majority of patients is achieved by interventional flexible endoscopic techniques carried out in a dedicated endoscopy suite with the necessary cardiovascular monitoring. The endoscopic techniques used for visible vessels and active bleeding are classified as thermal, electrocoagulation, photocoagulation and injection therapy (Table 12.6). Sometimes, a combination of tech-

niques, e.g. adrenaline injection therapy plus electrocoagulation or photocoagulation, is used and is reported to be beneficial by allowing a clearer target for the endoscopist and reducing the heat-sink effect when thermal energy is applied.

Indications for surgical treatment
- Patients with exsanguinating haemorrhage.
- Elderly patients (> 60 years): if more than 4 units of blood are necessary during the initial resuscitation on admission, patient has one recurrence of bleeding after initial endoscopic control of bleeding, and persistent bleeding requires 8 units of blood within 48 h.
- Younger patients (< 60 years): if 8 or more units of blood are required during the initial resuscitation and persistent bleeding requires 12 units of blood over a 48-h period.

Lower gastrointestinal bleeding

Unlike upper gastrointestinal bleeding, the vast majority of patients present electively, and only a minority are admitted as emergencies for massive bleeding and signs of hypovolaemia. In many cases such bleeding stops spontaneously; if it does not, it requires emergency treatment. The commonest cause of massive rectal bleeding is diverticular disease, although the bleeding may originate from vascular lesions of the colon or small bowel *and* from more proximal lesions, especially posterior duodenal ulcers.

Management

In massive rectal bleeding the priority is resuscitation, but investigation must proceed promptly during the resuscitation. The first step must be to exclude bleeding haemorrhoids by means of proctoscopy, and this should be followed by upper gastrointestinal endoscopy. If these are negative, urgent mesenteric angiography may locate the bleeding point. For intermittent bleeding with negative angiography, radionuclide-labelled red cell scanning may be used. The patient's own red cells are labelled with ^{51}Cr and reinjected so that a gamma-camera can be used to localize pooling of blood in the intestine. Surgical treatment is usually required for massive rectal bleeding, with resection of the appropriate segment of colon or small bowel after attempts at preoperative localization. Occasionally, it is necessary to proceed to laparotomy because of the severity of the bleeding. In this case, intraoperative colonoscopy with on-table antegrade colonic lavage is performed to locate the bleeding lesion. If this proves unsuccessful, colectomy and ileostomy are performed, preserving the rectal stump for later reanastomosis.

Haemorrhage, hypovolaemia and shock at a glance

Definition

Shock: a state of acute inadequate or inappropriate tissue perfusion resulting in generalized cellular hypoxia and dysfunction

Classification of shock
Hypovolaemic
True hypovolaemia is due to contraction of circulating blood volume:
- Blood loss (ruptured abdominal aortic aneurysm, upper gastrointestinal bleed, multiple fractures, etc.)
- Plasma loss (burns, pancreatitis)
- Extracellular fluid losses (vomiting, diarrhoea, intestinal fistula)

Apparent hypovolaemia is a result of increased vascular capacity due to loss of peripheral resistance in muscular arterioles:
- Sepsis
- Adrenal insufficiency
- Anaphylaxis
- Neurogenic

Cardiogenic
- Myocardial infarction
- Arrhythmias (atrial fibrillation, ventricular tachycardia, atrial flutter)
- Pulmonary embolus
- Cardiac tamponade
- Valve disease

Septic
- Gram-negative, less often Gram-positive, infections

Anaphylactic/distributive
- Release of vasoactive substances when a sensitized individual is exposed to the appropriate antigen

Pathophysiological response to shock
Regardless of cause, shock produces a series of changes aimed at protecting the organism and preserving its vital functions

Sympathoadrenal response	Sympathetic discharge	Vasoconstriction
	(Nor)adrenaline release	Tachycardia, increased CO
Activation of renin–angiotensin system	Angiotensin	Vasoconstriction
	Aldosterone	Na^+ and H_2O retention
Neuroendocrine response	Adrenocorticotrophic hormone, growth hormone	Na^+ and H_2O retention
	β-endorphins	Pain relief
	Cortisol, glucagon	Elevated blood sugar
Microcirculatory response	Inadequate perfusion	Fluid sequestered, acidosis
Cellular phospholipid injury	Arachidonic acid	
	Prostaglandins	Increased permeability
	Leukotrienes	Neutrophil activation
Cellular changes	Anaerobic metabolism	Lactic acidosis
		Loss of Na^+/K^+ pump
		Cellular oedema and death

Clinical features
Hypovolaemic and cardiogenic shock
- Pallor, coldness, sweating and restlessness
- Tachycardia, weak pulse, low blood pressure and oliguria

Septic shock
- Initially, warm flushed skin and bounding pulse
- Later, confusion and low-output picture

Investigation and management
Principles of management
- Identify the cause early and begin treatment quickly

- Shock in surgical patients is often overlooked: unwell, confused, restless patients may well be shocked
- Unless a cardiogenic cause is obvious, treat shock with urgent fluid resuscitation
- Worsening clinical status despite adequate volume replacement suggests the need for intensive care

Details of management
- Resuscitate patient, ABC, give 100% O_2 via mask
- Establish good i.v. access and set up CVP line (possibly Swan–Ganz catheter as well)
- Start i.v. infusion, usually crystalloid initially

03

- Monitor pulse, blood pressure, temperature, respiratory rate and hourly urinary output via catheter
- ECG, cardiac enzymes, echocardiography
- Haemoglobin, haematocrit, urea and electrolytes, creatinine
- Group and cross-match blood: haemorrhage
- Arterial blood gases
- Blood cultures: sepsis

Complications
- Acute renal failure (acute tubular necrosis)
- ARDS
- DIC
- Systemic inflammatory response syndrome (may ensue if shock not corrected)
- Acute hepatic failure
- Stress ulceration

Summary of management
- Airway and breathing: give 100% O_2, position patient upright, consider ventilatory support if necessary
- Circulation: ensure good i.v. access, urinary catheter, monitor cardiac rate and rhythm
- Deal with the cause of the shock, e.g. stop the bleeding, drain the abscess, remove the source of the anaphylactic antigen, etc.

Gastrointestinal haemorrhage
Definitions
Gastrointestinal haemorrhage is defined as loss of blood (which may be acute or chronic) from the gastrointestinal tract anywhere from the mouth to the anus

Anaphylactic	Cardiogenic	Septic	Hypovolaemic
i.v. fluids i.v. adrenaline i.v. antihistamines i.v. hydrocortisone	Optimize rate and rhythm (e.g. cardioversion, drugs) Optimize preload (e.g. adequate volume, diuretics) Optimize afterload (e.g. vasoconstrictors/dilators) Optimize cardiac function (e.g. thrombolytic therapy, inotropes, assist devices)	Fluids to restore circulating volume Antibiotics or surgery Support cardiac function (e.g. inotropes)	Identify and arrest losses (may include surgery) Restore circulating volume (crystalloids, colloids or blood) Support cardiac function

Causes

Anatomical site	Pathology
Mouth and pharynx	Carcinoma, trauma
Oesophagus	Oesophagitis, varices, peptic ulcer disease (PUD), Mallory–Weiss syndrome, carcinoma
Stomach	Gastritis, PUD, carcinoma (leiomyoma, lymphoma, Dieulafoy lesion, hereditary telangiectasia)
Duodenum	PUD (periampullary carcinoma, aortoduodenal fistula, haemobilia)
Small bowel	Meckel's diverticulum, intussusception, enteritis (infection, radiation, Crohn's), ischaemia, tumours
Colon	Angiodysplasia, polyps/carcinoma, diverticular disease, inflammatory bowel disease, ischaemia
Rectum	Polyps/carcinoma, proctitis, solitary rectal ulcer, trauma
Anus	Haemorrhoids, fissure-in-ano, carcinoma, perianal Crohn's disease

Aspirin and the NSAIDS
Aspirin and the NSAIDs inhibit the enzyme cyclooxygenase (COX). COX exists as two isoforms: COX-1 (responsible for physiological prostaglandin production) and COX-2 (mediates production of prostaglandins involved in inflammation). Specific COX-2 inhibitors suppress inflammation while preserving cytoprotective function of COX-1

- Aspirin use is the cause of 10% of all peptic ulcers in patients aged 60 years and over
- NSAID use is the cause of 20% of all peptic ulcers in patients aged 60 years and over
- In the UK, 12 000 patients are admitted with upper gastrointestinal pathology related to NSAID use annually
- Of these patients, 2230 (18.5%) die

Presentations
- Iron-deficiency anaemia due to chronic blood loss, e.g. gastric or caecal carcinoma
- Minor episodes of blood loss, e.g. rectal tumours, ulcerative colitis
- Acute major gastrointestinal bleeding (haematemesis or rectal bleeding) with hypovolaemic shock, e.g. duodenal ulcer, angiodysplasia
- Recurrent obscure bleeding, e.g. Meckel's diverticulum

Management
Upper gastrointestinal haemorrhage (heamatemesis, melaena or both)
- Secure airway, breathing and circulation, insert two large-bore i.v. cannulae, insert urinary catheter
- Send bloods for group and cross-match, full blood count, urea and electrolytes, creatinine
- Give i.v. fluids: crystalloids to begin and then blood if necessary
- Monitor pulse, blood pressure (CVP if patient is shocked), pulse oximetry, urinary output
- Assess severity:
  (a) Mild: no hypovolaemia
  (b) Moderate: hypovolaemia that responds to volume replacement, patient remains stable
  (c) Severe: active continued major bleeding requiring continuous resuscitation or recurrent major bleed
- Arrange diagnostic upper gastrointestinal endoscopy (see table below) within 24 h (sooner if bleed is severe)

Indications for surgery
- Exsanguinating haemorrhage
- > 60 years:
  (a) ≥ 4 units on initial resuscitation
  (b) one recurrent bleed after initial endoscopic control
  (c) persistent bleeding requiring 8 units in 48 h
- < 60 years
  (a) ≥ 8 units on initial resuscitation
  (b) persistent bleeding requiring 12 units in 48 h

Lower gastrointestinal haemorrhage (rectal bleeding)
- Most patients are elderly, bleeding is usually not severe and frequently stops spontaneously

- Massive haemorrhage with hypovolaemia: initial resuscitation is the same as for upper gastrointestinal haemorrhage. Investigation proceeds with resuscitation:
  (a) Proctoscopy: exclude haemorrhoids
  (b) Colonoscopy: often difficult to see anything because of blood
  (c) Upper gastrointestinal endoscopy: bleeding may be from a duodenal ulcer
  (d) Mesenteric angiography
  (e) Radiolabelled red blood cell scanning

Indications for surgery: continued bleeding
- Remove segment of bowel containing 'bleeder' if known from preoperative investigation
- If source unknown, perform laparotomy with intraoperative colonoscopy to try and identify 'bleeder'. If source still cannot be found, a total colectomy may be needed

Iron-deficient anaemia and obscure haemorrhage
These need to be investigated thoroughly to find the cause. Examination may include upper and lower gastrointestinal endoscopy, contrast studies of the whole bowel, nuclear medicine studies, laparoscopy with or without laparotomy

---

Should be performed within 24 h in appropriately equipped unit

Will give the diagnosis in 80% of patients

Will miss the diagnosis in 20% because:
  Large amounts of blood in stomach obscure the view
  Lesion is missed
  Lesion has healed
  Source of bleeding is more distal than the duodenum

Can be used to control the bleeding by:
  Injection therapy: vasopressors, sclerosants, thrombin, mixtures
  Banding: oesophageal varices
  H-F electrocoagulation
  Heater probe
  Photocoagulation

03

Fluids, Electrolytes, pH Balance and Nutrition

13

Must know Must do

Must know

Composition and distribution of fluids and electrolytes
in healthy subjects

Clinical features, diagnosis and management of fluid
and electrolyte disorders

Clinical features, diagnosis and management of
disorders of acid–base balance

Clinical features, diagnosis and management of
nutritional disorders

Common crystalloid and colloid solutions used in
surgical wards

At least one enteral feeding regimen

Core knowledge of parenteral feeding and its
complications

Must do

Participate in the fluid and electrolyte management of
patients after major surgery

Undertake clinical nutritional assessment of patients

Calculate the body mass index of patients

Observe and follow patients on parenteral nutrition

Observe and follow patients on enteral nutrition

Introduction

Surgical illness and operative intervention disrupt homeostasis and lead to changes in fluid, electrolyte and acid–
base balance. A grasp of the surgical physiology involved is
vital for understanding the principles of preoperative and
postoperative care. The monitoring and alteration of fluid
and acid–base status comprise the principal aspects of the
care of surgical patients.

Fluid and electrolytes

Distribution

Water constitutes approximately 70% of lean tissue mass,
the value varying with age, sex and patient circumstances.
In general, fluid distribution in a patient can be considered

to comprise three spaces: the intracellular and extracellular spaces, which are physiological; and the 'third space',
representing fluid accumulation in disease leading to
dehydration, which is pathological (Fig. 13.1). The intracellular compartment is the largest fluid compartment,
with a volume of 22–30 L. The extracellular compartment
is composed of the plasma or intravascular compartment
(3 L) and the interstitial space (10–12 L). Normally, there
is a continuous bidirectional movement of water between
the plasma and the interstitial fluid across the capillary
bed. This movement is governed by the hydrostatic pressure at the arteriolar end of the capillary and the oncotic
pressure of plasma at the venular extremity. The exchange
of fluid across the capillary membrane is, of course, essential for the supply of nutrients and oxygen to the tissues
and the elimination of waste products of metabolism.

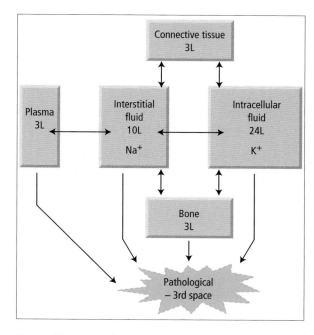

Figure 13.1 Extracellular and intracellular compartments of
the body in a 70-kg man.

Table 13.1 Daily requirements of a normal 70-kg man.

Input	Volume (mL)	Output	Volume (mL)
Oral liquids	1500	Urine	1500
Water in food	1000	Stool	300
Water of oxidation	300	Lungs	500
		Skin	500
Total	2800		2800

The osmolality (total particle concentration) is the same in all the fluid compartments and is normally 280–295 mosmol/kg H_2O. In contrast, the electrolyte composition of the intracellular compartment is very different from that of plasma and interstitial fluid. The main cation [positively charged atom attracted to a negative electrode (cathode)] in the plasma is Na^+ and the accompanying anions [negatively charged atoms attracted to a positive electrode (anode)] are Cl^- and HCO_3^-. In the normal state, plasma electrolytes account for the majority of plasma osmolality and there is a good correlation between the plasma concentration of Na^+ and plasma osmolality, i.e. a high plasma Na^+ signifies hyperosmolality and vice versa. In certain pathological states, the osmolality may also be elevated by the accumulation of large amounts of organic solutes, e.g. excess urea in renal failure and excess glucose in uncontrolled diabetes mellitus.

Fluid and electrolyte balance

Table 13.1 shows the inputs and outputs of 70-kg man in homeostasis. As a rule of thumb, the daily (24-h) requirements of an average subject are 100 mmol (2 mmol/kg) Na^+ and 60 mmol (1 mmol/kg) K^+.

Intravenous fluid therapy

During your time on the wards you will always see patients on drips; when you are a house officer, you will be responsible for siting the drip and managing the fluids from day to day. Intravenous fluid therapy is used extensively in surgery; indeed it is of vital importance that patients are adequately resuscitated prior to surgery, especially in the emergency situation.

The indications for fluid therapy are as follows.
● Preoperative resuscitation, e.g. before emergency surgery, elective surgery in a jaundiced patient.
● Replacement of abnormal losses, e.g. vomiting, diarrhoea, ileostomy bags.
● Provision of normal daily requirements if patient is nil by mouth.

● Postoperative resuscitation.
● Electrolyte disorders.
Thus patients not eating or drinking must be provided with their daily requirements, i.e. 2.5–3 L of water, 100 mmol Na^+ and 60 mmol K^+.

Types of fluids

Crystalloids
Normal saline
Dextrose saline
Hartmann's solution

Colloids
Natural, e.g. blood, albumin
Synthetic, e.g. gelatin-based infusions

On the wards you will mainly use crystalloids to provide the normal daily requirement and replace additional losses. Three major types of fluid are used: 0.9% sodium chloride, dextrose saline and 5% dextrose. The composition of these fluids is shown below.
● 1 L 0.9% sodium chloride contains 153 mmol NaCl.
● 1 L dextrose saline contains 31 mmol NaCl + 40 g dextrose.
● 1 L 5% dextrose contains 50 g dextrose.
Potassium can be added to these solutions in the form of potassium chloride (KCl).

Fluid replacement regimens

There are two major regimens used (Fig. 13.2a,b). If the patient is also losing additional fluid (e.g. vomiting, nasogastric tube, ileostomy), then this volume must also be measured and replaced over and above the normal requirements using normal saline.

Fluid status is judged by examination of the patient every day:
● check for signs of dehydration;
● check blood pressure and pulse;
● examine the abdomen and chest;
● check the ankles for oedema.
The fluid balance chart should be examined to determine the patient's fluid input and output. The hourly urine output is a good guide to fluid status; urine output should not fall below 30 mL/h. In most cases, the urine output falls because the patient is volume depleted.

Other fluids encountered in practice

● Hartmann's solution is the replacement fluid favoured by anaesthetists because it is a physiological mixture of

03

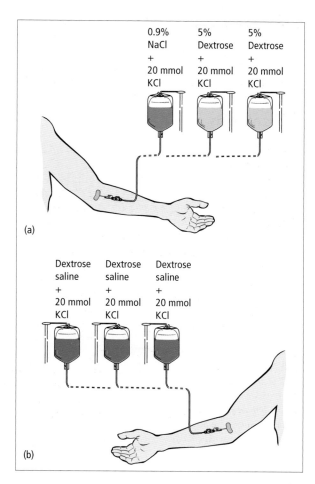

Figure 13.2 (a) Regimen for the normal daily fluid requirement that includes 1 L of 0.9% sodium chloride and 2 L of 5% dextrose with KCl added to each bag. (b) An alternative prescription of the normal daily fluid requirement in the form of 3 L of dextrose-saline with added KCl.

ions and water: 1 L Hartmann's solution contains 2 mmol Ca^{2+}, 5 mmol K^+, 29 mmol HCO_3^-, 110 mmol Cl^- and 131 mmol Na^+.

• All the solutions described so far have been crystalloids and are not confined to the intravascular compartment. On occasions, for example if a patient is shocked due to haemorrhage, fluid replacement of the intravascular compartment is essential. In these circumstances, gelatin colloid solutions are used. These are solutions of saline and gelatin: 1 L synthetic colloid contains 35 g gelatin, 6.25 mmol Ca^{2+}, 145 mmol Cl^- and 145 mmol Na^+. Because gelatin has a high molecular weight, it is confined to the intravascular compartment and thus acts as a plasma expander.

Assessment of adequacy of resuscitation

• Clinical history and observations: pulse, blood pressure, skin turgor.
• Urine output: oliguria defined as < 0.5 mL/kg per h
• Central venous pressure (CVP) or pulmonary capillary wedge pressure.
• Response of urine output or CVP to fluid challenge:
  (a) 200–250 mL bolus of colloid administered as quickly as possible;
  (b) response in CVP or urine output should be seen within minutes;
  (c) size and duration of the CVP response rather than actual value recorded is more important.

Fluid and electrolyte disturbances

Water

Water intoxication

This condition is rare and is caused by the administration of excessive amounts of 5% dextrose, especially in the presence of impaired renal function. Occasionally, it is associated with excessive secretion of antidiuretic hormone (ADH). There is an expansion of the intracellular and extracellular fluid compartments, a low serum Na^+ and widespread oedema. Irritability, drowsiness, convulsions and coma may occur. Treatment is by water restriction and sometimes administration of hypertonic saline.

Water depletion

Inadequate intake of water leads to dehydration and raised plasma Na^+ (hypernatraemia), with a rise in the osmolality of body fluids. Despite increased reabsorption of water by the kidneys, there is contraction of both the extracellular and intracellular fluid compartments. Clinically there is thirst, drowsiness and coma. Treatment consists of slow intravenous replacement with hypotonic saline solution. Rapid intravenous infusion with 5% dextrose is contraindicated as it will cause water intoxication with coma and convulsions.

Sodium

Hypernatraemia

Hypernatraemia may be due to excessive administration of Na^+ (usually iatrogenic from infusion of excessive amounts of Na^+ in intravenous fluids) or dehydration due to decreased fluid intake or water loss. The osmotic pressure of the extracellular fluid rises and the clinical picture is similar to that of water depletion (see above). Rarely, hypernatraemia is caused by primary hyperaldosteronism (Conn's syndrome, see Chapter 34). If the serum Na^+ rises above 160 mmol/L, hypernatraemic encephalopathy may

Table 13.2 Inappropriate antidiuretic hormone secretion.

Cranial
Head injury, e.g. base of skull fracture
Cerebral metastases

Peripheral
Carcinoma of the lung
Bronchial carcinoid
Tuberculosis
Pneumonia
Prostatic carcinoma
Pancreatic carcinoma
Lymphomas

occur. Treatment of hypernatraemia is by slow intravenous replacement with hypotonic saline solution.

Hyponatraemia

Deficiency of Na^+ is the most common acute biochemical disturbance encountered in surgical practice. The common causes of hyponatraemia (i.e. serum $Na^+ < 130$ mmol/L) are listed below.
- Na^+-rich losses from the gastrointestinal tract, e.g. vomiting, diarrhoea, intestinal obstruction.
- Renal Na^+ loss, e.g. Addison's disease.
- Diuretic use, particularly those that promote natriuresis, e.g. furosemide and the thiazide diuretics.
- Prolonged infusion of dextrose 5% alone.
- Transurethral resection of the prostate (TURP).
- Cardiac failure and cirrhosis of the liver.
- Inappropriate ADH secretion (Table 13.2).

In its most usual mild form, hyponatraemia is asymptomatic. When plasma Na^+ falls below 120 mmol/L patients become confused. There is severe contraction of the extracellular fluid compartment, with hypovolaemia, poor venous filling, oliguria, dry skin with loss of turgor

and sunken eyeballs. If Na^+ levels decrease below 110 mmol/L, convulsions and coma may ensue. Therapy for hyponatraemia is directed at the underlying cause. Losses of Na^+ can be replaced by increasing Na^+ intake without increasing daily fluid intake (e.g. giving normal saline continuously); water retention should be treated by fluid restriction.

Potassium

Hyperkalaemia

An elevated serum K^+ is encountered in acidotic, hypoxic and ischaemic states. In these conditions K^+ is released from cells. However, the most common cause of hyperkalaemia is K^+ retention due to renal failure. Clinically, hyperkalaemia is associated with diarrhoea, colicky abdominal pain and peaked T waves on the electrocardiogram (ECG) (Fig. 13.3). Irrespective of cause, a serum K^+ concentration above 6 mmol/L may precipitate a cardiac arrest (usually ventricular fibrillation). The treatment of hyperkalaemia entails correction of the underlying cause, together with measures designed to reduce the level of plasma K^+:
- administration of intravenous calcium gluconate or sodium bicarbonate or insulin and glucose (the latter two act by promoting the movement of K^+ into cells);
- administration of the cation-exchange resin calcium resonium by mouth or as an enema is also effective in removing excess body K^+;
- severe hyperkalaemia associated with renal failure is an indication for dialysis.

Hypokalaemia

A low serum K^+ is encountered in pyloric stenosis, high jejunal obstructions, liver failure and diarrhoea from any cause. Rarely, hypokalaemia is caused by primary hyperaldosteronism (Conn's syndrome). Clinically, hypokalaemia is characterized by lethargy, muscle weakness,

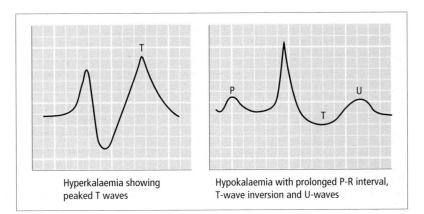

Figure 13.3 Typical ECG changes associated with hyperkalaemia and hypokalaemia.

Hyperkalaemia showing peaked T waves

Hypokalaemia with prolonged P-R interval, T-wave inversion and U-waves

03

adynamic ileus and life-threatening ventricular arrhythmias that may progress to cardiac arrest in asystole. The ECG shows a prolonged PR interval, T-wave inversion and classical U waves. Hypokalaemia is always accompanied by a metabolic alkalosis (see later). This is due to increased reabsorption of HCO_3^- and excretion of H^+ from the proximal tubules of the kidney. The correction of hypokalaemia has to be done gradually. If hypokalaemia is severe, intravenous KCl in a concentration of not more than 40 mmol/L may be administered. Such therapy should be monitored by ECG as severe cardiac arrhythmias may be encountered and require temporary interruption of the infusion.

Calcium

The normal range of total calcium concentration is 2.2–2.6 mmol/L. Calcium is usually bound to albumin, and the levels of both calcium and albumin should be measured together. (To correct for low serum albumin, 0.025 should be added to the serum calcium for every 1 g/L that the albumin is lower than 40 g/L.) The box below summarizes the common causes of hypocalcaemia and hypercalcaemia.

Hypercalcaemia

Hypercalcaemia is usually asymptomatic below a serum concentration of 3.5 mmol/L. Above this level, clinical features include muscle weakness, lassitude, drowsiness and hyperreflexia. Anxiety and mania may develop, with coma as a terminal event. Polyuria and polydipsia indicate impaired renal concentration. Nausea, vomiting, constipation and peptic ulceration may also occur. Treatment is directed at dealing with the underlying cause, although rapid reduction of serum calcium levels can be achieved by hydration with saline, calciuresis with diuretics (furosemide), steroids and specific drugs, e.g. mithramycin, calcitonin, ethylenediaminetetraacetic acid (EDTA) and bisphosphonates.

Hypocalcaemia

Hypocalcaemia (serum Ca^{2+} < 2 mmol/L) results in a dramatic clinical picture characterized by tetany. In its mildest form, there may be paraesthesiae and muscle cramps. The full-blown picture is characterized by hyperexcitability of the nervous system, most commonly expressed as carpopedal spasm. This consists of severe tonic contractions of the muscles of the hand; the fingers are bunched together and flexed at the metacarpophalangeal joints and the wrist is acutely flexed (*main d'accoucheur*). Similarly, the toes are flexed and the ankle joint acutely plantar flexed. Latent tetany may be demonstrated by Chvostek's sign (tapping over the facial nerve induces twitching of the facial muscles) and Trousseau's sign (carpal spasm induced by inflating a sphygmomanometer cuff above systolic pressure). Acute hypocalcaemia is treated by slow intravenous infusion of calcium gluconate (10% solution).

Acid–base balance

The pH is the negative logarithm of the hydrogen ion (H^+) concentration in the body fluids. Maintenance of a blood pH between 7.37 and 7.42 is essential for normal metabolic activity. As normal metabolism results in the generation of acids (e.g. lactic acid), particularly during physical exertion, efficient compensatory mechanisms are invoked to prevent any significant deviations in the pH. These compensatory mechanisms include those listed below.
- Buffer systems: intracellular buffers are proteins and phosphates while blood buffers are bicarbonate and haemoglobin.
- Lungs: overall regulation of pH consists of immediate buffering of acid metabolites, followed by pulmonary excretion of H^+ as water and carbon dioxide (CO_2).
- Kidneys: renal regulation of pH is achieved mostly by retention or excretion of HCO_3^-.

The lungs and kidneys act in concert such that in the presence of mild renal impairment, increased acid removal is achieved by the lungs and vice versa.

Common causes of hypocalcaemia and hypercalcaemia

Hypercalcaemia	Hypocalcaemia
Absorption induced	Hypoproteinaemia
Vitamin D excess	Vitamin D deficiency
Milk alkali syndrome	Parathyroidectomy
Sarcoidosis	Acute pancreatitis
Drugs, e.g. thiazides	Medullary carcinoma of thyroid
	Idiopathic

Bone disease
Secondary tumour deposits
Myeloma
Lymphoma
Paget's disease

Endocrine
Hyperparathyroidism
Ectopic parathyroid hormone (PTH) production
Thyrotoxicosis
Addison's disease

Fluid and electrolytes at a glance

Definitions

Homeostasis: the self-regulating feedback process that maintains internal stability in biological systems such as the human body

Mole: the amount of a substance that contains the same number of elementary particles (atom, ion, molecule) as there are atoms in 0.012 kg of carbon 12

Osmole: the standard unit of osmotic pressure (= molecular weight of dissolved substance in grams divided by number of particles into which the molecule dissociates in solution). *Serum osmolality* indicates the concentration of solutes in the serum and is expressed as milliosmoles per kilogram of water. The normal osmolality of body fluids is 280–295 mosmol/kg H_2O

Ion: an electrically charged atom. A cation is a positively charged atom that has lost an electron, e.g. Na^+, K^+. An anion is a negatively charged ion that has gained an electron, e.g. Cl^-, HCO_3^-

Fluid and electrolyte distribution and daily requirements

Fluid compartment	Volume (L)	Main cation
Extracellular		
Intravascular	3	Na^+
Interstitial	10–12	Na^+
Intracellular	22–30	K^+

Daily requirements
Water: 2.5–3 L
Na^+: 2 mmol /kg (~ 100 mmol)
K^+: 1 mmol/kg (~ 60 mmol)

Fluid therapy

Indications	Types of fluid	Composition (per L)
Preoperative resuscitation	*Crystalloids*	
Replacement of abnormal losses	Normal saline	153 mmol NaCl
Provide normal daily requirements	Dextrose 5%	50 g glucose
Correct electrolyte disorders	Dextrose-saline	31 mmol NaCl + 40 g glucose
	Sodium lactate (Hartmann's solution)	131 mmol Na^+ + 5 mmol K^+ + 2 mmol Ca^{2+} + 29 mmol HCO_3^- (as lactate) + 111 mmol Cl^-
	Colloids	
	Natural: blood, albumin	
	Synthetic (Gelofusine, Haemaccel)	35 g gelatin + 145 mmol Na^+ + 145 mmol Cl^- + 6.25 mmol Ca^{2+}

Typical daily fluid replacement regimens
Regimen 1
● 1 L 0.9% NaCl + 20 mmol K^+ over 8 h *plus*

● 2 L 5% dextrose + 40 mmol K^+ each litre over 8 h
Regimen 2
● 3 L dextrose-saline + 60 mmol K^+ over 8 h

Fluid and electrolyte disturbances

Disturbance	Cause	Findings	Treatment
Water intoxication	Excess administration of 5% dextrose Excess secretion of ADH	Oedema, confusion, coma, convulsions, low serum Na^+	Water restriction Rarely hypertonic saline is given
Water depletion	Inadequate intake of water	Thirst, drowsiness, coma, oliguria Raised serum Na^+, urea and haematocrit	Slow i.v. replacement with hypotonic saline solution

03

Disturbance	Cause	Findings	Treatment
Hypernatraemia	Dehydration Iatrogenic: excess i.v. saline Primary hyperaldosteronism (Conn's syndrome)	Similar to water depletion Serum $Na^+ > 160$ mmol/L causes hypernatraemic encephalopathy	Slow i.v. replacement with hypotonic saline solution
Hyponatraemia (most common disturbance seen in surgical practice)	GI: vomiting, diarrhoea Renal: Addison's disease Diuretics: furosemide Excess i.v. 5% dextrose TURP Cardiac failure, cirrhosis Inappropriate ADH secretion	$Na^+ < 130$ mmol/L: asymptomatic $Na^+ < 120$ mmol/L: confusion, contraction of ECF space, oliguria, hypovolaemia, dry skin, loss of turgor, sunken eyeballs $Na^+ < 110$ mmol: convulsions, coma	Treat the cause Give daily fluid requirement as i.v. normal saline Rarely hypertonic saline is given Water retention treated by fluid restriction
Hyperkalaemia	Renal failure Acidosis, hypoxia, ischaemia	Diarrhoea, colicky abdominal pain, peaked T waves on ECG $K^+ > 6$ mmol/L: cardiac arrest (VF)	Treat the cause Give i.v. calcium gluconate or $NaHCO_3$, i.v. insulin and dextrose Give calcium resonium p.o. or p.r. Dialysis
Hypokalaemia	Pyloric stenosis High jejunal obstruction Liver failure Diarrhoea Primary hyperaldosteronism (Conn's syndrome)	Lethargy, muscle weakness, ileus Prolonged PR interval, T-wave inversion, U waves on ECG Cardiac arrest (asystole) Metabolic alkalosis	Replace K^+ gradually If severe give KCl i.v. (≤ 40 mmol/L) Monitor ECG for arrhythmias during therapy
Hypercalcaemia	*Absorption induced* Excess vitamin D, sarcoidosis, milk alkali syndrome, drugs *Bone disease* Bony metastases, myeloma, lymphoma, Paget's disease *Endocrine* Hyperparathyroidism, ectopic PTH production, Addison's disease, thyrotoxicosis	Muscle weakness, lassitude, drowsiness, hyperreflexia Polydipsia, polyuria Nausea, vomiting, peptic ulceration Anxiety, mania, coma (terminal)	Treat the cause Hydration with saline Calciuresis (furosemide) Steroids Specific drugs, e.g. mithramycin, EDTA, calcitonin, bisphosphonates
Hypocalcaemia	Hypoproteinaemia Vitamin D deficiency Parathyroidectomy Acute pancreatitis Thyroid medullary carcinoma Idiopathic	Tetany: paraesthesiae, muscle cramps, carpopedal spasm, Chvostek's (face) and Trousseau's (hand/foot) signs	Slow i.v. infusion of 10% calcium gluconate solution

ECF, extracellular fluid; GI, gastrointestinal; VF, ventricular fibrillation.

Acidosis/alkalosis

Certain disease states overwhelm these homeostatic mechanisms and result in significant accumulation of acid or base, with corresponding deviations from normal pH. *Acidaemia* occurs when the pH falls below 7.36 and *alkalaemia* when the pH exceeds 7.44. Acidaemia, which signifies an excess of unbuffered H^+ in the blood and body fluids, is the more common disorder of acid–base balance. The compensatory mechanisms of the body try to normalize the pH in these situations and are reflected in changes in the blood gas analysis, from which the diagnosis of acidosis (tendency to low pH) and alkalosis (tendency to high pH) is made (see box below).

Common causes of acidosis and alkalosis and the blood gas findings typical of each abnormality

Metabolic acidosis
Causes
Hypoxic causes
Lactic acidosis
Non-hypoxic causes
Ketoacidosis
Excess HCO_3^- loss
Renal failure
Drugs (e.g. salicylates)

Blood gas picture
pH < 7.36 (H^+ > 44 nmol/L)
$Paco_2$ < 4.7 kPa
HCO_3^- < 18 mmol/L
Base excess < −5 mmol/L

Metabolic alkalosis
Causes
Excess H^+ loss
Nasogastric suction
Vomiting
Hypokalaemia
Excess alkali
$NaHCO_3$ ingestion
Diuretics
Excess citrate

Blood gas picture
pH > 7.44 (H^+ < 36 nmol/L)
$Paco_2$ > 6.0 kPa
HCO_3^- > 32 mmol/L
Base excess > +5 mmol/L

Respiratory acidosis
Causes
Decreased CO_2 excretion
Hypoventilation
Ventilation–perfusion
  mismatch
Airway obstruction
Increased CO_2 excretion
Hypermetabolism

Blood gas picture
pH < 7.38 (H^+ > 44 nmol/L)
$Paco_2$ > 5.7 kPa
HCO_3^- 22 mmol/L
Base excess −2 mmol/L

Respiratory alkalosis
Causes
Hyperventilation
Apprehension
Hysteria
CNS injury
Mechanical ventilation

Blood gas picture
pH > 7.42 (H^+ < 36 nmol/L)
$Paco_2$ < 5.3 kPa
HCO_3^- 22 mmol/L
Base excess +2 mmol/L

Blood gas changes

The blood gas analysis also provides the clinician with information about the metabolic or respiratory origin of the acid–base disturbance in an individual patient. This distinction is based on the relationship between the changes in pH and $Paco_2$. When the pH change occurs in the opposite direction to $Paco_2$ (i.e. pH down and $Paco_2$ up), the underlying cause is respiratory impairment. In contrast, in metabolic disturbances, the pH change occurs in the same direction as the $Paco_2$ (alkalosis, both up; acidosis, both down). The base excess is derived from the difference between the patient's standard bicarbonate and the normal mean and is a good indicator of metabolic disturbances. A base deficit of −5 to −10 mmol/L is present with metabolic acidosis (this is sometimes confusingly expressed as a 'base excess of −5 to −10 mmol/L'). With metabolic alkalosis, there is a base excess of +5 to +10 mmol/L. Thus from the blood gas analysis it is possible to calculate whether the patient is acidotic or alkalotic and whether the abnormality is metabolic or respiratory.

Nutrition

Malnutrition is recognized as an important factor affecting the outcome of many surgical patients. A malnourished patient has a significantly impaired immune system, delayed wound healing and reduced strength that manifests itself as decreased ventilatory function. Modern management of surgical patients places increasing importance on adequate nutrition. The current areas of intense discussion are when and how nutrition should be administered and how it changes outcome.

Nutritional assessment of the surgical patient (Fig. 13.4)

Previously, the assessment of nutritional status was performed from the end of the bed by observing the patient's general condition. This may still be useful, although there are more objective assessment parameters that can be used.
1 Clinical findings: history and examination, regular weights, body mass index.
2 Anthropometric measurements: skinfold thickness (e.g. triceps, iliac crest), arm circumference, grip strength.
3 Blood tests: serum albumin, serum transferrin, lymphocyte count.

Nutritional requirements

As with fluid requirements, the nutritional status and the requirements of the patient will change according to the state of health. In the surgical patient the aim is to prevent

03

pH balance at a glance

Definitions

pH: negative logarithm to the base of 10 of the free hydrogen ion concentration [H^+] in moles per litre ($pH = -\log[H^+]$). It is expressed as a positive number that describes the acidity or alkalinity of a chemical solution on a scale of 0 (acidic) to 14 (alkaline). The normal pH of body fluids is maintained between 7.3 and 7.5

Acidosis: accumulation of H^+ ions in the extracellular fluid resulting in a fall of pH below 7.36

Alkalosis: accumulation of base in the extracellular fluid resulting in an elevation of pH above 7.44

Buffer system: one that keeps the concentration of H^+ relatively constant. Intracellular H^+ buffers are proteins and phosphates; H^+ buffers in blood are HCO_3^- and haemoglobin. The lungs (by excreting H^+ as H_2O and CO_2) and the kidneys (by retaining or excreting HCO_3^-) also control H^+ levels and thereby the pH

Acid–base disturbance

	Causes	Blood gas picture	Treatment
Metabolic acidosis	Lactic acidosis Ketoacidosis Excess HCO_3^- loss Renal failure Drugs	$pH < 7.36$ $Pa_{CO_2} < 4.7$ kPa $HCO_3^- < 18$ mmol/L Base excess < -5 mmol/L	Treat underlying cause Sodium bicarbonate
Metabolic alkalosis	*H^+ loss* Nasogastric suction Vomiting Hypokalaemia *Excess alkali* $NaHCO_3$ ingestion Diuretics Excess citrate	$pH > 7.44$ $Pa_{CO_2} > 6.0$ kPa $HCO_3^- > 32$ mmol/L Base excess $> +5$ mmol/L	Treat underlying cause Isotonic sodium chloride i.v. and correction of hypokalaemia if present
Respiratory acidosis	Hypoventilation Ventilation–perfusion mismatch Airway obstruction Hypermetabolism	$pH < 7.38$ $Pa_{CO_2} < 5.7$ kPa HCO_3^- 22 mmol/L Base excess -2 mmol/L	Treat underlying cause
Respiratory alkalosis	*Hyperventilation* Apprehension Hysteria CNS injury Rapid-rate mechanical ventilation	$pH > 7.42$ $Pa_{CO_2} > 5.3$ kPa HCO_3^- 22 mmol/L Base excess $+2$ mmol/L	Treat underlying cause

depletion of protein stores as a result of increased catabolism, which can lead to a negative nitrogen balance. The average carbohydrate stores are depleted in 24 h, while protein and fat stores are depleted over the following month.

The daily calorie requirement for an adult is approximately 25–35 kcal/kg (105–147 kJ/kg); younger patients require higher calories per kilogram than older ones. However in some patients, e.g. those with severe burns, calorie requirements may increase by 100% above basal resting values. The protein requirement for an adult is 1–1.5 g/kg daily; since 6.25 g of protein provide 1 g of nitrogen, the average nitrogen requirement is approximately 12 g/day.

Delivery of nutritional therapy

Enteral nutrition

Enteral nutrition is preferred for the patient unable to maintain an adequate oral intake but who has a functioning gastrointestinal tract that can be used safely. Early

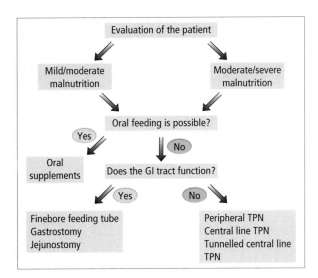

Figure 13.4 Overview of surgical nutrition.

enteral nutrition has been advocated in order to preserve intestinal structure and the role of the intestine in immune function. The absence of enteral feeding is related to villous and cellular atrophy.

Enteral feeding can be done initially by providing supplement drinks. If this is not sufficient, then an elemental diet can be given through a fine-bore nasogastric tube placed directly into the stomach or small bowel. These types of feeds (e.g. Osmolite) provide approximately 1912 kcal (8000 kJ) of energy plus about 70 g of protein in 2–3 L.

Types of feed

Polymeric (near-normal composition). These contain intact proteins, starches and long-chain fatty acids. They are useful in patients who have a functioning stomach and normal digestive capacity.

Disease specific. These are feeds tailored to meet the requirements of specific diseases, e.g. feeds for patients with liver disease are deficient in branched-chain amino acids, which can exacerbate encephaolopathy.

Elemental. These are chemically defined feeds that contain simple amino acids, oligosaccharides and monosaccharides. These require minimal digestion and are useful in patients with intestinal fistulae but are far from palatable.

Methods of administration

Apart from oral supplementation, enteral feed can be delivered through enteral tubes. Enteral nutrition can also be given via:
- gastrostomy: surgical or endoscopic (percutaneous endoscopic gastrostomy);
- jejunostomy: surgical.

Indications
- Long-term feeding
- Dysphagia, e.g. stricture, stroke
- Chronic disease, e.g. neoplasia
- Malnutrition
- Sepsis
- Burns
- Major surgery
- Coma/ICU

Complications
- Diarrhoea and vomiting
- Malposition or blocking of tube
- Feed intolerance
- Electrolyte imbalance
- Aspiration

Total parenteral nutrition

Total parenteral nutrition (TPN) can be given via a large peripheral vein or a central venous channel.

Indications
- Severe malnutrition
- Inability to swallow, e.g. oesophageal tumour
- Prolonged obstruction, high-output fistula
- Sepsis
- Burns where upper gastrointestinal tract is severely damaged
- Severe pancreatitis
- Prolonged ileus
- Short bowel syndrome
- Severe Crohn's disease

Complications
- Pneumothorax/haemothorax
- Cardiac tamponade
- Sepsis, e.g. *Staphylococcus epidermidis*, *Candida*, *Pseudomonas*
- Mineral overload
- Reactive hypoglycaemia
- Vitamin and mineral deficiencies

03

Nutrition at a glance

Definitions

Nutrition: the process of utilizing exogenous substances for the production of energy and the synthesis of new tissue

Food: any substance that can be used by the body to produce energy or some essential nutrient

Adverse surgical effects of poor nutrition
- Impaired immunity
- Delayed wound healing
- Decreased respiratory function
- Reduced muscle strength

Methods of assessing nutritional status
Clinical
- History and examination

- Weight measurement
- Body mass index

Anthropomorphic
- Skinfold thickness
- Arm circumference
- Grip strength

Blood tests
- Serum albumin
- Serum transferrin
- Lymphocyte count

Daily nutritional requirements
- Calories 25–35 kcal/kg (105–147 kJ/kg)
- Protein 1–1.5 g/kg
- Nitrogen 12 g

Delivery of nutrition

Type	Administration	Indications	Complications
Enteral Polymeric: near-normal Disease specific: tailored for patients with specific diseases Elemental: requires minimal digestion	Orally Gastrostomy Jejunostomy	Long-term feeding Dysphagia: stricture, stroke Chronic disease: neoplasia Malnutrition Sepsis/burns/major surgery Coma/ICU	Diarrhoea and vomiting Malposition or blocking of feeding tube Intolerance to feed Electrolyte imbalance Aspiration ± pneumonia
Total parenteral nutrition	Central line via internal jugular or subclavian vein	Severe malnutrition Inability to swallow Prolonged intestinal obstruction/ileus High-output intestinal fistula Sepsis Burns involving upper gastrointestinal tract Severe pancreatitis Short bowel syndrome Severe Crohn's disease	Pneumothorax Haemothorax Cardiac tamponade Line sepsis Mineral overload Reactive hypoglycaemia Vitamin deficiency Mineral deficiency

Evidence-based medicine

Halperin, M.L. & Goldstein, M.B. (1999) *Fluid, Electrolyte and Acid–Base Physiology: A Problem-based Approach*, 3rd edn. W.B. Saunders.

Lefever Kee, J. & Paulanka, B.J. (1999) *Fluids and Electrolytes with Clinical Applications: A Programmed Approach*. Thompson Learning.

Pestana, C. (2000) *Fluids and Electrolytes in the Surgical Patient*. Lippincott, Williams & Wilkins.
http://www.virtual-anaesthesia-textbook.com
http://www.medstudents.com.br
http://www.family.georgetown.edu
http://www.familypracticenotebook.com

03

Acute Renal Failure

14

03

Must know Must do

Must know

Causes, types and management of ARF
List of commonly used drugs, including antibiotics and
    analgesics, known to cause renal damage
Principles of renal replacement therapy

Must do

Clerk patients with chronic renal disease/failure
Follow patients being treated for ARF
Become familiar with the biochemistry of renal failure
Become proficient in catheterizing male and female
    patients
Observe patients undergoing haemodialysis and
    haemofiltration
Observe cadaveric-donor and living-donor-related
    renal transplantation

Introduction

Acute renal failure (ARF) is defined as the rapid onset of renal impairment resulting in the accumulation of nitrogenous waste products, i.e. urea and creatinine, within the body. The process may become irreversible because of:
- pre-existing renal damage (acute-on-chronic renal failure);
- irreversible damage;
- delays in treatment.

Acute tubular necrosis (ATN) is used to denote ARF where there is intrinsic but reversible damage to the kidney. ARF commonly presents with sudden anuria (no urine) or oliguria (< 400 mL/day). However, non-oliguric renal failure may also occur and is recognized by a persistently rising serum creatinine level in the presence of normal output of urine.

Classification

Renal failure may be classified into *prerenal*, *intrinsic* and *postrenal* (Fig. 14.1). Prerenal oliguria and ATN are the types of renal failure usually encountered following surgery. The causes of prerenal ARF are shown in Table 14.1. Prerenal ARF can progress to ATN (intrinsic ARF) if the underlying cause is not reversed promptly, although instrinsic ARF may arise directly from other causes (shown in Table 14.2).

Postrenal failure, which results from obstruction to urinary flow, is categorized as obstructive uropathy (see Chapter 39). When the kidney is obstructed, glomerular function does not cease completely because the filtrate is reabsorbed by the renal lymphatics and veins. Unrelieved, obstruction leads to ischaemic renal damage mediated by vasoactive hormones including renin, angiotensin, endothelin, etc. Return to useful function depends on duration/degree of obstruction and the presence/absence of infection above the obstruction. Following relief of obstruction, recovery of tubular function lags behind restoration of glomerular filtration rate (GFR), resulting in a diuresis.

Pathophysiology

ARF may occur as a consequence of shock. The reduction in circulating blood volume produces a significant decrease in renal blood flow, which may fall to one-third of its normal level. The GFR is correspondingly reduced and the patient becomes oliguric, producing only 400–700 mL of urine per 24 h, or less than 20 mL/h. When oligaemic states cause a reduction in renal blood flow, additional changes take place. There is a diversion of blood from the renal cortex and this exacerbates the situation by causing a further reduction in GFR. If the impairment in renal blood flow is of brief duration and blood volume is restored rapidly, the condition can be reversed and normal urine output resumed, although sometimes there is a lapse of some hours before this takes place. A more prolonged ischaemic insult causes ATN, with oliguria persisting for 1 to 3 or 4 weeks, followed by a period of diuresis when large volumes of dilute urine are passed each day. More profound ischaemia gives rise to cortical necrosis, an irreversible condition requiring renal dialysis and eventually renal transplant.

03

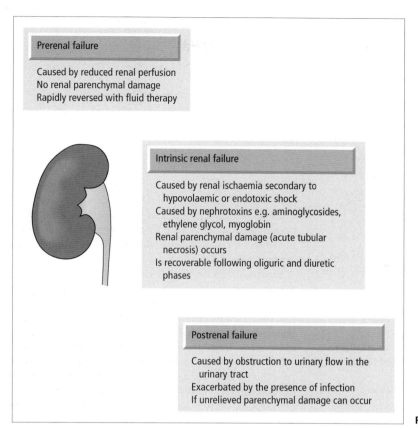

Prerenal failure

Caused by reduced renal perfusion
No renal parenchymal damage
Rapidly reversed with fluid therapy

Intrinsic renal failure

Caused by renal ischaemia secondary to
    hypovolaemic or endotoxic shock
Caused by nephrotoxins e.g. aminoglycosides,
    ethylene glycol, myoglobin
Renal parenchymal damage (acute tubular
    necrosis) occurs
Is recoverable following oliguric and diuretic
    phases

Postrenal failure

Caused by obstruction to urinary flow in the
    urinary tract
Exacerbated by the presence of infection
If unrelieved parenchymal damage can occur

Figure 14.1 Classification of renal failure.

Table 14.1 Aetiology of prerenal acute renal failure.

Reduced cardiac output
Acute myocardial infarction
Cardiac arrest
Cardiac failure
Significant valvular disease
Cardiac tamponade

Depleted circulating volume
Sepsis
Haemorrhage
Hypoalbuminaemia

Depleted extracellular fluid volume
Loss from gastrointestinal tract with diarrhoea, vomiting
Loss from urinary tract due to excessive diuresis
Loss from skin/body surface associated with sweating and
    burns

Vascular disease
Renal artery thrombosis/embolism

Once ARF becomes established, serious water and electrolyte disturbances occur. During the oliguric phase, water retention with a relatively low Na^+ may precipitate cardiac failure, accompanied by pulmonary and systemic oedema. The degree of dyspnoea may be sufficiently severe to warrant ventilatory support. Inability to excrete K^+ leads to dangerously high plasma levels, which may give rise to arrhythmias and, if uncontrolled, to cardiac arrest. Retention of H^+ ions precipitates metabolic acidosis. At first, hyperventilation and respiratory alkalosis compensate for this but these mechanisms eventually fail and the pH of the blood falls rapidly. This phase may be exacerbated by respiratory failure and a developing lactic acidosis. Both the blood urea and serum creatinine levels progressively increase and calcium levels may fall.

Clinical features

● Dyspnoea is a frequent problem and in some patients respiratory failure may require intermittent positive-pressure ventilation (see Chapter 38). The respiratory problems are due to fluid retention, with fluid overload giving rise to pulmonary as well as systemic oedema.

Table 14.2 Aetiology of intrinsic acute renal failure.

Inadequate/delayed treatment of prerenal acute renal failure
Most common cause in surgical practice

Ischaemia and toxin
Hypercalcaemia
Hepatorenal syndrome

Toxins
Aminoglycosides, cephalosporins, paracetamol, salicylates,
  paraquat, etc.

Tubular obstruction
Light-chain deposition in myeloma
Myoglobinuria (muscle injury, snake bite, heroin,
  barbiturates)
Haemoglobinuria (mismatched blood, nitrofurantoin)

Acute interstitial nephritis
Antibiotics: penicillin, cephalosporins, co-trimoxazole,
  vancomycin, rifampicin
NSAIDs: mefenamic acid, indomethacin, ibuprofen
Diuretics: thiazides, furosemide
Other drugs: sulfasalazine, allopurinol, gold, phenytoin
Infections: infectious mononucleosis, measles, Legionnaire's
  disease, etc.

Vascular (endothelial damage)
Vasculitis
Haemolytic–uraemic syndrome
Disseminated intravascular coagulation
Accelerated hypertension

Primary glomerulonephritis

Renal involvement secondary to systemic disease
Infection: bacterial endocarditis
Shunt nephritis: associated with ventriculoatrial shunts
Hepatitis B-associated nephritis
Diabetes
Vasculitis: Henoch–Schönlein purpura, systemic lupus
  erythematosus, polyarteritis nodosa, etc.

NSAIDs, non-steroidal anti-inflammatory drugs.

Metabolic acidosis (see Chapter 13) and pulmonary infection may contribute further to the respiratory difficulties.
● Hypertension may also be a consequence of fluid overload and retention of K^+ may give rise to arrhythmias.
● Gastrointestinal symptoms range from nausea and vomiting due to water intoxication to hiccups and diarrhoea, which frequently accompany uraemia. Stress ulceration and gastric erosions are common with ARF following shock, and gastrointestinal haemorrhage may be severe.
● Cerebral oedema and toxic metabolites cause confusion, drowsiness and eventually coma.

● A progressive anaemia may develop and coagulation defects may occur. Disseminated intravascular coagulation is a not uncommon development.
● Finally, there is a generalized impairment of the immune system, increasing the risk of serious infection, which is probably the commonest cause of death in ARF. The indiscriminate use of antibiotics exacerbates this risk by promoting the development of resistant strains of pathogenic bacteria.

Management

Prevention

ARF may be prevented by careful attention to preoperative fluid balance, proper monitoring of the patient peroperatively and avoidance of hypotension and sepsis. Patients at risk of developing renal failure, e.g. those with obstructive jaundice, should have an intravenous infusion established the night before surgery so that they are well hydrated. Remember that patients are starved prior to surgery and will not be allowed oral fluids for about 12 h (but often longer) before surgery. Patients undergoing major surgery should have a urinary catheter for hourly measurement of urine ouput during surgery and in the postoperative period. A central venous line and arterial line are usually inserted by the anaesthetist for haemodynamic monitoring.

Some drugs may help to avoid renal failure in certain situations. *Dopamine*, which at low doses (< 5 µg/kg per min) induces vasodilatation and increased renal perfusion, is frequently given to at-risk patients in an attempt to preserve renal function. *Mannitol*, an osmotic diuretic, may also protect renal function in some patients, such as those with obstructive jaundice or those at risk of rhabdomyolysis (e.g. following arterial embolectomy). Patients receiving known nephrotoxic drugs should have their renal function monitored regularly. In the case of aminoglycosides, plasma concentrations should be measured 1 h after intramuscular or intravenous administration and just prior to the administration of the next dose. This ensures that excessive and subtherapeutic doses are avoided. For gentamicin, the peak level should not exceed 10 mg/L, while the trough level should be less than 2 mg/L.

Conservative treatment

Identification and correction/removal of the cause is essential and any sepsis treated with a third-generation cephalosporin in the first instance. In oliguric patients with adequate circulating volume, intravenous diuretic is administered and may promote a diuresis. Removal of obstruction is necessary in obstructive anuria. The

03

Table 14.3 Treatment of hyperkalaemia.

---

1 10–20 mL of 10% calcium gluconate or chloride i.v.: has no effect on the serum potassium concentration but stabilizes the myocardial membrane

2 50 mL of 50% dextrose i.v. with 10 units of soluble insulin: drives potassium into the cells and should be started directly after step 1

3 200–300 mL of 1.4% sodium bicarbonate i.v.: drives potassium into cells and helps to correct the acidosis of acute renal failure. However, the fluid load necessary makes use of this agent less desirable in hyperkalaemic acute renal failure

4 Calcium resonium 15 g three times daily orally or by enema: binds potassium in the gut and releases calcium in exchange. Unlike the other actions listed this can control the serum potassium for hours to days

5 Dialysis: should be implemented if there is severe hyperkalaemia and/or the patient requires dialysis for other reasons, e.g. fluid overload

---

conservative management of intrinsic renal failure is only possible when the patient's condition is not so severe as to warrant immediate renal replacement therapy (RRT). Conservative management consists of:

- restriction of fluid intake to cover daily estimated losses (insensible perspiration and stools);
- restriction of first-class protein to 30 g/day to reduce nausea and anorexia;
- restriction of potassium intake to 20 mmol/day to minimize risk of hyperkalaemia;
- correction of biochemical abnormalities;
- maintenance of adequate nutrition, including parenteral nutrition (if required).

Hyperkalaemia is the most serious biochemical abnormality since it can cause cardiac arrhythmias and sudden death. Prompt detection and treatment are thus essential (Table 14.3).

Renal replacement therapy

Abnormalities of potassium, calcium and phosphate can be corrected by the various forms of RRT using dialysate or replacement solutions. The indications for RRT are:

- uraemia (significant retention of nitrogenous waste products with associated clinical signs);
- metabolic acidosis;
- hyperkalaemia;
- significant fluid overload.

Type of therapy

Treatment for the majority of patients with ARF requires adequate vascular access, most commonly achieved using the internal jugular vein with subclavian or femoral vein as lesser alternatives. The use of the subclavian route carries an increased risk of pneumothorax and venous stenosis. The femoral route is only suitable for short periods because of the high infection rate. Temporary lines may have a single, double or triple lumen. Double- and triple-lumen lines are associated with improved clearance of uraemic toxins, and the triple-lumen line allows administration of intravenous therapy without interfering with RRT. The choice is between the following.

- Haemodialysis: efficient small-molecule and volume removal.
- Haemofiltration: removes large molecules and volume by convection.
- Haemodiafiltration: combination of haemodialysis and haemofiltration.

Haemofiltration uses a highly permeable synthetic membrane and negative pressure in the dialysate compartment of the dialyser without dialysate flowing such that up to 80 L of fluid are removed from the patient in a 4-h session. Solute removal is by 'convection', or passive flow of solute with water. The desired proportion of the filtrate is replaced by infusion usually from preprepared sterile bags of replacement fluid. Convection allows greater removal of solutes in the 'middle molecular' range (110–500 Da) but is less efficient at the smaller end of the molecular spectrum, which contains most of the life-threatening compounds (Fig. 14.2).

Haemodialysis is based on diffusion across a semipermeable membrane porous to molecules under 500 Da. It thus exhibits high efficiency with regard to small-molecule and volume removal and is cost-effective but relies on well-trained personnel (Fig. 14.3). The combination of these two techniques is called *haemodiafiltration*. With this modality, the benefits of diffusion and convection are combined in a dialysis circuit similar to that used for haemofiltration but with dialysis fluid being pumped round the dialysate circuit.

Venovenous haemofiltration requires at least a double-lumen venous line and relies on a pumped system to create a gradient across the filter and hence a filtrate from the patient. If the patient is normotensive, it is possible to use an arterial and venous line to create the pressure gradient across the filter line (arteriovenous haemofiltration), thus removing the need for a pump in the circuit.

The choice between these types of support is normally decided by the renal physician and intensivist. All three modalities of RRT can be performed on an intermittent or continuous basis. Haemofiltration and haemodiafiltration are of great value in unstable patients with ARF and in the elderly with cardiac failure and severe arteriosclerosis. Patients with uncomplicated ARF whose cardiovascular system is stable are usually treated with intermittent

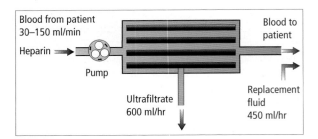

Figure 14.2 Haemofiltration. In a haemofiltration circuit, blood passes across a filtration membrane. Ultrafiltration rates of 600 mL/h are usual, removing toxins and fluid with a clearance of 10 mL/h. In the intensive care unit, many patients with acute renal failure are managed with continuous venovenous haemofiltration, which requires the use of a pump.

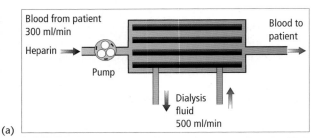

(a)

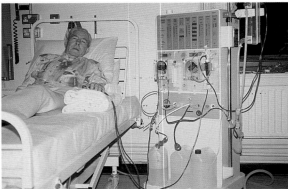

(b)

Figure 14.3 (a) Haemodialysis. In a haemodialysis circuit, blood and dialysis fluid circulate in a countercurrent fashion separated by a semipermeable membrane. Blood flow rates of 100–300 mL/min are usual and patients undergo haemodialysis for 3–5 h three times per week. Creatinine clearances are 100–150 mL/min during dialysis or 5–10 mL/min when calculated for a week. (b) Patient undergoing haemodialysis.

techniques, whereas more unstable patients, in whom fluid removal is more difficult, benefit from continuous therapies. Continuous treatment is especially useful for patients with cerebral oedema or hypoxia. Intermittent haemodialysis is the treatment of choice when there is a need for rapid removal of water-soluble substances such as potassium, myoglobin and drugs.

Nutritional management

Nutrition for patients with ARF is extremely important. All patients with dialysis-dependent ARF have higher nutritional requirements than normal, especially if the ARF arises as a complication of other severe illness. These patients have a relative insulin-resistant state, low triiodothyronine, decreased testosterone and increased energy expenditure above expected resting levels. Hyperglycaemia (insulin resistance) is not uncommon and glucose oxidation forms a smaller component of total energy consumption. Lipid and protein metabolism is also disturbed, with increased plasma triglycerides and increased protein catabolism. RRT adds a further strain. Whilst the glucose in haemofiltration fluids provides a large number of calories, amino acids are lost during RRT. The haemodynamic state of the patient may restrict the ability to supply the patient's nutritional requirements. Patients with ARF have the same daily requirements as other acutely sick patients, i.e. a caloric intake of 35 kcal/kg (147 kJ/kg) body weight and nitrogen 1.2 g/kg body weight, with the ratio between glucose and lipid in the non-protein part of the diet being 70/30.

Diuretic phase

As ARF resolves there is often a diuretic phase. This occurs because although filtration is restored, the concentrating ability of the recovering tubules has not. During this phase there is a risk of dehydration. The excessive fluid loss (as much as 20 L/day) must be replaced intravenously until the tubules are able to concentrate the urine. High urinary volumes such as these are unlikely to persist for more than a few days. The diuretic phase of renal failure may last several weeks to months but is usually shorter if patients do not become anuric or severely oliguric.

Prognosis

The prognosis of ARF depends on the underlying aetiology. The overall mortality has not changed materially during the past three decades and averages 50%. However, the mortality rate associated with certain categories of ARF has improved, e.g. ARF associated with trauma and obstetric disorders. Comorbid disease influences the outcome: ARF in patients nursed in intensive care units has an overall mortality of 70%. For all patients if there is associated failure of one other system the overall patient survival is less than 30% and failure of two systems reduces survival further to less than 10%. Increasing age also impacts adversely on survival.

03

Acute renal failure at a glance

Definitions

Acute renal failure: a sudden deterioration in renal function such that neither kidney is capable of excreting the waste products (e.g. urea, creatinine, potassium) that accumulate in the blood. It is fatal unless treated

Anuria: no urine passed

Oliguria: urine levels of < 0.5 mL/kg per h passed. Non-oliguric renal failure is characterized by a persistently rising serum creatinine level in the presence of normal output of urine

Classification
Prerenal failure (failure to perfuse kidney with blood)
● Reduced cardiac output: acute myocardial infarction, cardiac arrest, significant valvular heart disease, cardiac tamponade
● Depleted circulating volume: haemorrhage, sepsis, hypoalbuminaemia
● Depleted extracellular fluid volume:
   (a) Gastrointestinal loss: diarrhoea, vomiting
   (b) Genitourinary loss: diuresis
   (c) Loss from skin, body surface, peritoneum: sweating/burns/peritonitis
● Vascular disease: renal artery thrombosis or embolism

Intrinsic renal failure (damage to parenchyma of kidney)
● Inadequate/delayed treatment of prerenal failure leading to acute tubular necrosis. (commonest surgical cause)
● Ischaemia and toxin: hypercalcaemia, hepatorenal syndrome
● Nephrotoxins: aminoglycosides, cephalosporins, paracetamol, salicylates, paraquat
● Tubular obstruction: myeloma (light-chain deposition), myoglobinuria, haemoglobinuria
● Nephritis: acute glomerulonephritis, pyelonephritis, drugs (antibiotics, NSAIDs, diuretics, sulfasalazine, allopurinol, gold), diabetes mellitus
● Vascular endothelial damage: vasculitis, haemolytic–uraemic syndrome, disseminated intravascular coagulation, accelerated hypertension

Postrenal failure (obstruction to outflow of urine from kidney)
● Urinary tract obstruction, e.g. prostatic hypertrophy
● Obstructing renal calculi

Pathophysiology
Shock → reduction in circulating blood volume → decreased renal blood flow by 60% → decreased GFR → shunting of blood from renal cortex → oliguria

Outcome
Depends on duration of renal impairment:
● Short: full recovery
● Intermediate: ATN (oliguric phase for 1–3 weeks followed by diuretic phase)
● Prolonged: no recovery; requires long-term dialysis and/or renal transplantation

Fluid and electrolyte imbalance
● Water retention may precipitate congestive cardiac failure with pulmonary and systemic oedema
● K^+ retention causes hyperkalaemia, leading to arrhythmias and cardiac arrest
● H^+ retention causes metabolic acidosis. Serum urea and creatinine levels rise, Ca^{2+} falls

Clinical features
Specific to the cause
● Hypovolaemia: cool peripheries, tachycardia, confusion, restlessness, dry mucous membranes

Oliguric phase (may last hours/days/weeks)
● Oliguria
● Uraemia:
   (a) dyspnoea, confusion, drowsiness, coma
   (b) nausea, vomiting, hiccups, diarrhoea
   (c) anaemia, coagulopathy, gastrointestinal haemorrhage
● Fluid retention: hypervolaemia, hypertension
● Hyperkalaemia: arrhythmias
● Acidosis: metabolic
● Anaemia

Polyuric (recovery) phase (may last days/weeks)
● Polyuria: hypovolaemia, hypotension
● Hyponatraemia
● Hypokalaemia

Investigations
● Urinalysis
● Urea and electrolytes (especially K^+)
● Creatinine
● ECG/chest X-ray
● Arterial blood gases:
   (a) Normal Po_2
   (b) Low pH: metabolic acidosis
   (c) Low Pco_2: compensatory respiratory alkalosis
   (d) High base deficit: metabolic acidosis

Management
General
● Oliguria in a surgical patient is an emergency and the cause must be identified and treated promptly

- Prompt correction of prerenal causes may prevent the development of established renal failure
- Ensure the oliguric patient is normovolaemic as far as possible before starting diuretics or other therapies
- Do not use large blind fluid challenges, especially in the elderly; if necessary use a CVP line
- Established renal failure requires specialist support as electrolyte and fluid imbalances can be rapid in onset and difficult to manage

Prevention
- Keep at-risk patients (e.g. obstructive jaundice) well hydrated preoperatively and peroperatively
- Protect renal function in selected patients with drugs such as dopamine and mannitol
- Monitor renal function regularly in patients on nephrotoxic drugs (e.g. gentamicin)

Identification
- Exclude urinary retention as a cause of anuria by catheterization
- Correct hypovolaemia as far as possible. Use appropriate fluid boluses, if necessary guided by CVP
- A trial of bolus high-dose loop diuretics may be appropriate in a normovolaemic patient
- Dopamine infusions may be necessary but suggest the need for HDU or ITU care

Treatment of established renal failure
Conservative
- Maintain fluid and electrolyte balance:
  (a) Water intake: 400 mL/day plus measured losses
  (b) Na+ intake: limited to replace loss only
  (c) K+ intake: nil (dextrose and insulin and/or ion-exchange resins required to control hyperkalaemia)
  (d) Diet: high calorie, low protein (30 g/day) in a small volume of fluid
  (e) Acidosis: sodium bicarbonate
- Treat any infection

Renal replacement therapy (requires placement of double- or triple-lumen central venous line)
- Indications: hyperkalaemia, uraemia, metabolic acidosis, fluid overload
- Types of RRT
  (a) Haemofiltration: removes large molecules and volume by convection
  (b) Haemodialysis: efficient small-molecule and volume removal
  (c) Haemodiafiltration: combination of haemofiltration and haemodialysis
- Nutrition: patients with ARF have the same requirements as other sick patients:
  (a) Calories: 35 kcal/kg (147 kJ/kg) body weight daily
  (b) Nitrogen: 1.2 g/kg body weight daily
  (c) Glucose : lipid ratio 70/30

Diuretic phase
- Replace fluid losses (up to 20 L/day) until renal tubules are able to concentrate the urine

Treatment of hyperkalaemia
- 10–20 mL calcium gluconate or calcium chloride i.v.: stabilizes myocardial membrane
- 50 mL 50% dextrose + 10 units soluble insulin i.v.: promotes migration of K+ into cells
- 200–300 mL NaHCO$_3$ i.v.: promotes migration of K+ into cells and helps to correct metabolic acidosis
- Calcium resonium 15 g t.d.s. orally or by enema: binds K+ in the gut, releases calcium in exchange
- Dialysis: implement if hyperkalaemia is severe.

Evidence-based medicine

Renal Association (1997) *Treatment of Adult Patients with Renal Failure. Recommended Standards and Audit Measures*, 2nd edn. Royal College of Physicians, London.

Scottish Intercollegiate Guidelines Network (SIGN) (1997) *Investigation of Asymptomatic Microscopic Haematuria in Adults*. SIGN publication 17, Edinburgh.

Scottish Intercollegiate Guidelines Network (SIGN) (1997) *Investigation of Asymptomatic Proteinuria in Adults*. SIGN publication 18, Edinburgh.

The Acute Abdomen

Must know Must do

Must know

Clinical features of patients with acute abdomen

Clinical features and management of patients with acute appendicitis

Clinical features and management of patients with primary and secondary peritonitis

Causes, types, clinical features and management of intestinal obstruction

Complications that develop in patients with acute abdomen

Must do

See patients with acute abdomen and generalized peritonitis and follow their management

See patients with small and large bowel obstruction and follow their management

Familiarize yourself with the antibiotic policy used in the management of patients with acute abdomen

Learn to detect free gas under the diaphragm on the PA chest film in patients with gastrointestinal perforation

Insert a nasogastric tube in a patient with intestinal obstruction

Learn to examine hernial orifices to exclude strangulated external abdominal herniae

Observe an emergency appendicectomy

Observe an emergency laparotomy for acute abdomen

Introduction

The collective term *acute abdomen* is used to describe a group of acute life-threatening intra-abdominal conditions (including pelvic) that require emergency hospital admission and often emergency surgical intervention. Early recognition, adequate resuscitation and prompt treatment are necessary for recovery of these patients from potentially fatal conditions.

Aetiology (see Table 15.1)

The causes of an acute abdomen fall into four main categories:
- inflammatory;
- traumatic;
- obstructive;
- vascular.

Inflammatory

The inflammatory intraperitoneal conditions originate as either acute inflammations of specific regions of the gastrointestinal tract (e.g. acute appendicitis, acute diverticulitis) or primary perforations of the gastrointestinal tract as a consequence of either benign disease (e.g. perforated duodenal ulcer) or malignant tumours (perforated gastric lymphoma, caecal carcinoma, etc.). Anastomotic leakage following resections with primary anastomosis of parts of the gastrointestinal tract is the most common cause of the postoperative acute abdomen. All the conditions in

Table 15.1 Acute abdomen: disease processes.

Inflammatory
Secondary bacterial peritonitis: localized, generalized
Primary bacterial peritonitis: generalized
Tertiary peritonitis: generalized, very poor prognosis

Traumatic
Injury to solid organs: acute intra-abdominal bleeding
Peritonitis secondary to intestinal injury

Obstructive
Acute intestinal obstruction (small bowel)
Chronic intestinal obstruction (colonic)

Vascular
Mesenteric infarction
Strangulated external/internal herniae
Volvulus (small or large intestine)

this category invariably lead to a localized or generalized bacterial peritonitis that is usually polymicrobial (caused by several bacteria). Some infections of the peritoneal cavity are primary *de novo*; in contrast these much rarer infections are caused by a single organism, usually *Streptococcus pneumoniae*.

Traumatic

Intra-abdominal injuries may be due to blunt or penetrating abdominal trauma (see Chapter 19). When solid organs such as the liver and spleen are involved, the clinical picture is dominated by acute hypovolaemia due to massive internal haemorrhage. In contrast, when the pancreas or gastrointestinal tract is traumatized, the symptoms and signs are those of peritonitis. Another group relates to injuries sustained inadvertently during the course of any operation, e.g. bile duct and bowel injuries during laparoscopic cholecystectomy. These are referred to as iatrogenic injuries. Not infrequently, they are missed at operation and the injury declares itself clinically with fever, sepsis, peritonitis and fistulae. These injuries usually proceed to litigation and emphasize the importance of good technique and impeccable perioperative care.

Obstructive

Obstructions of the gastrointestinal tract may involve the small intestine (acute) or the large bowel (chronic). The clinical picture of acute intestinal obstruction is dominated by vomiting, colicky abdominal pain and dehydration due to fluid and electrolyte losses, whereas chronic obstructions present with absolute constipation and marked abdominal distension. Unless the integrity of the wall of the obstructed bowel is compromised (as may happen in patients in whom the diagnosis is delayed or there is a primary adverse vascular event), there is no peritoneal contamination and therefore signs of peritonitis are absent.

Vascular

Acute intestinal ischaemia leading to infarction of segments of the gastrointestinal tract may be due to thrombotic or embolic occlusion of the mesenteric vessels, volvulus (twisting) of loops of small or large intestine, and external compression of the blood supply by bands or adhesions or the neck of external/internal herniae. Intestinal infarction is a serious condition that carries a high mortality. The clinical picture is dominated by severe pain, peritonitis, shock and, in some patients, rectal bleeding. Ruptured abdominal aortic aneurysm also comes in this category. Fortunately most aortic aneurysms do not sustain frank rupture but leak into the retroperitoneal tissues. Thus the bleeding is contained initially and this accounts for survival with emergency therapy in some of these patients (see Chapter 37).

Investigations

It is axiomatic that:
- clinical assessment, relief of pain and resuscitation come before imaging tests;
- only investigations essential to the emergency management of the patient are carried out;
- no patient with acute abdomen should be left unattended (medically) in a radiology department.

The basic investigations that are necessary in all patients with an acute abdomen are listed in Table 15.2. The essential blood investigations provide information on the following.
- Degree of hydration: osmolality, packed cell volume (PCV) and haemoglobin.
- Sepsis: white cell count (WCC), total and differential for leukocytosis; blood cultures (only in patients with rigors or shock without obvious blood loss).
- Urea and electrolyte imbalances.
- Chest X-ray is important, especially in the detection of free air under the diaphragm, which is always indicative of intestinal perforation or laceration (Fig. 15.1).
- Abdominal scout X-ray films for intestinal obstruction.

In addition, there are a number of special investigations that may be carried out in patients admitted with blunt abdominal trauma or acute undiagnosed abdominal pain. These include ultrasound examination, abdominal computed tomography (CT), peritoneal lavage and laparoscopy. These tests are only performed in trauma patients if the cardiovascular system is stable, i.e. the patient is not shocked.

03

Table 15.2 Investigations in patients with acute abdomen.

Essential
Haemoglobin, white cell count, packed cell volume
Urea, electrolytes and amylase
Chest X-ray and abdominal scout films (erect/supine)
Blood cultures for high fever and pyrexia

Special
Ultrasound and computed tomography
Peritoneal lavage
Mesenteric angiography
Laparoscopy

03

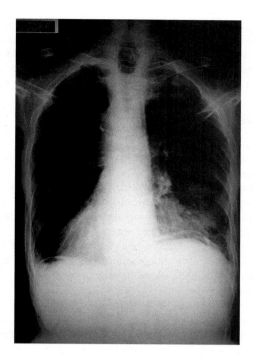

Figure 15.1 Perforated duodenal ulcer. Note presence of free air under the right diaphragm on the PA chest film.

Ultrasound examination and abdominal CT are both very useful in the detection of intraparenchymal haematomata, free fluid in the peritoneal cavity and localized inflammation, oedema and necrosis.

Peritoneal lavage is carried out after the insertion of a peritoneal dialysis catheter in the immediate subumbilical region. If blood or blood-stained fluid emerges immediately through the catheter, the test is positive. Otherwise, 1 L of Hartmann's solution is infused and then aspirated for examination. The test is considered positive if:

- red blood cells $> 100 \times 10^6$/L;
- white blood cells $> 500 \times 10^3$/L;
- amylase > 1100 U/L; or
- bile, bacteria or food particles are present.

Peritoneal lavage is most commonly used in the diagnosis of suspected blunt intra-abdominal trauma. Its one disadvantage is a 15–20% false-positive rate due to minor lesions, which stop bleeding and do not require laparotomy.

Emergency laparoscopy is extremely valuable in patients with acute lower abdominal pain, especially in females of childbearing age. It is carried out in the operating theatre under general anaesthesia and thus precedes the emergency operation if this is indicated on the basis of the laparoscopic findings. Emergency laparoscopy often resolves common diagnostic problems:

- Has the patient got acute appendicitis or acute pelvic adnexal disease (inflammatory, ruptured corpus luteum cyst or ectopic pregnancy)?
- Has the patient got mesenteric lymphadenitis (children)?
- Is there small bowel infarction?
- Has the patient sustained trauma to intra-abdominal organs (stab injuries of the abdomen)?

Peritonitis

Peritonitis is inflammation of the peritoneum. The peritonitis can be bacterial or chemical.

Bacterial peritonitis

Bacterial peritonitis is divided into four types.

1 *Secondary bacterial peritonitis*: the majority of the morbid processes lead to a breach in the integrity of the wall of the gastrointestinal tract, with transmigration of intestinal bacteria to the peritoneal cavity or actual perforation with escape of intestinal contents and substantial contamination of the peritoneal space. The consequence is an acute secondary bacterial peritonitis.

2 *Primary bacterial peritonitis*: primary bacterial peritonitis is a much rarer condition that occurs in otherwise healthy people in the absence of surgery or trauma and is the result of primary infection of the peritoneal lining by streptococcal organisms, usually in children and adult females.

3 *Spontaneous bacterial peritonitis*: develops in chronically ill patients, e.g. cirrhotic patients with ascites, renal failure patients on peritoneal dialysis, nephrotic syndrome.

4 *Tertiary peritonitis*: occurs in intensive care patients and is defined as the persistence or recurrence of intra-abdominal infection following apparently adequate therapy of secondary peritonitis. Patients who develop tertiary peritonitis have a significantly longer stay in the intensive care unit (ICU) and more advanced organ dysfunction reflected in higher ICU mortality than patients with uncomplicated secondary peritonitis. The most common infecting organisms in tertiary peritonitis are *Enterococcus, Candida, Staphylococcus epidermidis* and *Enterobacter.* These patients do not benefit from laparotomy, as the infection is diffuse and poorly localized. Tertiary peritonitis appears to be more a reflection than a cause of an adverse outcome.

Chemical peritonitis

In this instance the peritoneal inflammation is initially chemical in nature, e.g. early stages of perforated duodenal ulcer, extravasation of uninfected urine (bladder

injuries) or bile (after biliary operations). However, if treatment is delayed, secondary infection supervenes within a few hours. Thus chemical peritonitis represents the initial clinical phase of extravasation of visceral contents into the peritoneal cavity and almost invariably merges into acute secondary bacterial peritonitis.

Clinical manifestations

Irrespective of the exact aetiology, established peritonitis is usually accompanied by well-recognized systemic and local symptoms and signs.

Systemic manifestations

These emanate from the presence of a serious infection: the patient looks ill and is toxic with a high metabolic rate, pyrexia, tachycardia and leukocytosis. If bacteria have invaded the bloodstream (bacteraemia, septicaemia), attacks of rigors (shivering) are encountered; the patient feels cold even though his or her temperature is elevated above 38 °C. The combination of fluid and electrolyte losses (vomit, fluid inside the oedematous intestinal loops and peritoneal exudate that is sequestrated) and the enhanced insensible loss caused by the pyrexia lead to dehydration with dry mouth, loss of skin turgor and collapse of the peripheral veins.

Local symptoms

The pain of acute peritonitis is due to irritation of the somatic nerves supplying the parietal peritoneum. Its extent and exact location depend on whether the peritonitis is generalized or localized to a particular quadrant of the intra-abdominal cavity. It is always severe, constant and aggravated by movement (passive or active) and thus the patient lies still in the supine position and may at times draw up the knees to relax the abdominal musculature.

Local signs

The local or abdominal signs are elicited by a methodical sequence of inspection, palpation, percussion and auscultation of the abdomen and digital rectal examination.

Inspection
On inspection of the normal abdomen, the abdominal wall is seen to move with respiration; it bulges with inspiration as the diaphragm descends. This normal excursion is often absent in patients with peritonitis as the abdominal muscles over the area of peritoneal inflammation undergo reflex spasm.

Palpation
The same phenomenon accounts for the tight feel of the abdominal musculature noted during light palpation and often referred to as *guarding*. When marked, the abdominal muscles actually feel rigid (*rigidity*), although descriptions of board-like rigidity are exaggerated and have conveyed the wrong impression that deep palpation is necessary to elicit this sign. In fact, deep palpation is absolutely contraindicated in all patients with acute abdomen as it serves no purpose other than to inflict severe pain on the patient and thereby lose his or her confidence. Tenderness on light palpation elicited over the affected region is a most useful and reliable sign. *Rebound tenderness* is experienced by the patient when the pressure of the palpating hand is released. Considerable store has been laid on this physical sign in the past. More recent studies have cast some doubt on its value in clinical practice. Certainly it must be elicited with great gentleness.

Percussion
A more humane way to evoke rebound tenderness is to tap the affected area gently or better still ask the patient to cough, which, by moving the inflamed viscera against the inflamed parietal peritoneum, reproduces the localized pain.

Auscultation
Auscultation of the abdomen in patients with peritonitis reveals a silent abdomen (no identifiable borborygmi) due to absence of the normal peristaltic activity. At times, tinkling bowel sounds may be heard. These are due to passive movement of fluid within dilated loops of inflamed gut and signify the presence of a paralytic ileus.

Digital rectal examination
No examination of a patient with an acute abdomen is complete without a rectal examination. Although this is best carried out in the left lateral position, if the patient is in severe pain it may be conducted in the supine posture with flexion and abduction of the hip joints. The specific findings on digital rectal examination may include pelvic tenderness, boggy swelling in the rectovesical pouch and tenderness caused by movement of the cervix in the female.

Treatment of secondary bacterial peritonitis

Initial assessment and resuscitation

The diagnosis is established clinically and with certain key laboratory investigations (urea, electrolytes, osmolality, haemoglobin, WCC, serum amylase) and chest X-ray (air

03

Cause of peritonitis	Surgical treatment
Perforated acute appendicitis	Appendicectomy + peritoneal lavage
Gangrenous cholecystitis	Cholecystectomy + peritoneal lavage
Perforated duodenal ulcer	Suture closure + peritoneal lavage + postoperative eradication of *Helicobacter pylori*
Perforated gastric ulcer	Biopsy + closure of ulcer + peritoneal lavage
Perforated diverticulitis perforation	Drainage of localized pericolic abscess or colectomy for free + lavage
Perforated gastrointestinal neoplasm	Resection + lavage

Table 15.3 Causes of peritonitis and their surgical treatment.

under the diaphragm). Pain relief is a priority and should precede clinical examination. Analgesic medication (opioid) is administered intramuscularly (intravenously if patient is shocked). The view that analgesia should be withheld initially in these patients because it may mask physical signs is incorrect. Aside from being unkind, it reduces patient cooperation and confidence. Blood samples are taken for blood grouping if the patient is to undergo surgical treatment following resuscitation.

Intravenous fluid therapy and nasogastric suction

An intravenous line is set up for fluid and electrolyte replacement and all oral intake is stopped. A nasogastric tube is inserted and left draining continuously into a bag; the nursing staff check the patency of the tube by syringing and aspirating every hour.

Antibiotic therapy

Antibiotics are administered in all patients with evidence of intra-abdominal sepsis. If the infection is thought to arise from the upper gastrointestinal or hepatobiliary tract, a cephalosporin (active against Gram-negative aerobes) is sufficient. However, if the peritonitis is generalized or the disease is thought to originate from the colon, additional cover for Gram-negative anaerobes must be provided. This usually entails the administration of metronidazole in addition to the cephalosporin or aminoglycoside. The exact antibiotic regimen may be changed in the individual patient subsequent to clinical progress, bacterial culture and sensitivity tests.

Observations

If immediate surgery is not undertaken in any of these patients after they have been assessed by the more senior surgical staff, careful monitoring of their progress is carried out, with measurement of pulse, temperature, blood pressure and urine output and repeated physical examination of the abdomen. Provided the patient is improving, conservative management is continued; if deterioration is observed or the condition remains static, then further special tests or exploratory laparotomy is carried out.

Surgical treatment

Surgical treatment depends on the cause of the secondary bacterial peritonitis as established by laparotomy. The common acute intra-abdominal pathologies encountered and their treatment are shown in Table 15.3. The primary aim is to seal the perforation or remove the primary pathological source. This is followed by evacuation of pus with procurement of sample for culture, followed by abdominal lavage with several litres of warm isotonic saline. A perforated gastric ulcer must always be biopsied prior to closure because of the possibility of malignancy.

Primary bacterial peritonitis

By definition, this occurs in healthy individuals and the infecting organism is of the Gram-positive type, most commonly *Streptococcus pneumoniae* and group A streptococci. The disease is encountered in children, adolescents and adult females, in whom it may follow childbirth or chest and urinary tract infection. In most instances, the infection is haematogenous.

Infants and children usually present with acute abdominal pain, vomiting and fever, and abdominal signs indicative of peritoneal inflammation. Blood cultures may be positive. Treatment is with intravenous antibiotics in the first instance. Awareness of the condition is important as primary peritonitis is a rare condition, especially in children, and thus will be overlooked unless it is considered in the differential diagnosis of children presenting with an acute abdomen.

The disease in adults is confined to females. Although the infection is commonly pneumococcal, instances of gonococcal peritonitis have been reported. The typical patients are usually young adolescent girls. Some cases are reported in association with acute (non-perforated) appendicitis. The patients become pyrexial and develop abdominal pain, diarrhoea and clinical signs of peritonitis. In addition to antibiotic therapy, laparotomy is usually necessary to remove pus and for abdominal lavage. Culture of vaginal swabs is usually positive for pneumococcus in patients who develop the condition after childbirth. The prognosis of primary peritonitis with early diagnosis and treatment (antibiotics and abdominal lavage) is good, with recovery of the vast majority of patients. As the infection is most commonly due to *Streptococcus pneumoniae*, the initial antibiotic should be Augmentin (amoxicillin + clavulanic acid).

Spontaneous bacterial peritonitis

This carries a bad prognosis and has a definite mortality as a result of septic shock and multiorgan system failure. The groups of patients who are prone to develop spontaneous bacterial peritonitis (SBP) include:
- cirrhotic patients with ascites, Wilson's disease, chronic active hepatitis;
- renal failure patients on chronic peritoneal dialysis;
- patients with nephrotic syndrome.

These patients are all immunocompromised and exhibit reduced resistance to bacterial infection. The infecting organisms are often Gram-negative. About 30% of renal failure patients with SBP have no symptoms or signs directly referable to the abdomen. In other patients, the disease develops insidiously and localizing signs of peritonitis are minimal. The most common manifestations include abdominal pain, fever, tenderness and diminished or absent bowel sounds. The full-blown picture is accompanied by septic shock and is invariably fatal. Once suspected, a 100-mL specimen of ascitic fluid is taken for culture and Gram staining of the deposit after centrifugation and for measurement of polymorphonuclear cell count and pH. A polymorphonuclear cell count $> 250 \times 10^3/L$ and a pH < 7.37 are diagnostic and indicate the need for antibiotic therapy, even if the culture of the ascitic fluid is negative. A blood culture should also be taken.

In cirrhotic patients, the condition is a bacterial infection of ascitic fluid. The reported incidence of SBP in cirrhotics with ascites averages 20%. Most of the infections are aerobic and 50–60% of cases are caused by *Escherichia coli*. The aetiology is thought to involve:
- bacterial translocation from the gut to mesenteric lymph nodes;

- depressed activity of the reticuloendothelial phagocytic system;
- decreased antimicrobial capacity of ascitic fluid (low levels of C3, opsonins and fibronectin).

Diagnosis is based on clinical suspicion and analysis of ascitic fluid (WCC and culture in blood culture bottles). Treatment is with a third-generation cephalosporin. Despite documented cure of SBP, many patients (up to 30%) die during hospitalization from complications related to their end-stage liver disease. The long-term prognosis for patients with SBP is poor and they should be considered for liver transplantation.

As in cirrhotic patients, SBP in patients on chronic peritoneal dialysis can be culture positive or negative. The infection is caused by either Gram-positive cocci or Gram-negative bacilli. It can also arise as a consequence of catheter-related infections (subcutaneous tunnel or catheter exit site). The standard primary treatment of SBP in patients undergoing chronic peritoneal dialysis is intraperitoneal netilmicin combined with intermittent intraperitoneal vancomycin.

Haemoperitoneum

Haemoperitoneum is defined as free blood in the peritoneal cavity. It may arise from:
- intra-abdominal injuries, especially to solid organs;
- intra-abdominal operations;
- rupture of ectopic pregnancy;
- ruptured corpus luteum cyst;
- percutaneous interventions on the liver, e.g. core biopsy, transhepatic stenting;
- severe necrotizing pancreatitis;
- advanced peritoneal carcinomatosis;
- spontaneous rupture of primary liver tumour (rare);
- spontaneous rupture of an enlarged spleen (rare);
- spontaneous rupture of splenic aneurysm (rare).

Fortunately, intraperitoneal abdominal aortic aneurysms tend to leak into the retroperitoneal tissues, forming a haematoma rather than a haemoperitoneum in the first instance.

Clinical types

In the clinical context, haemoperitoneum is best considered as falling into two categories: progressive and stable.

Progressive haemoperitoneum

Progressive haemoperitoneum implies active continued intra-abdominal bleeding and is most commonly encountered with injuries to the solid organs (liver and spleen) or as an early complication after abdominal surgery. In

03

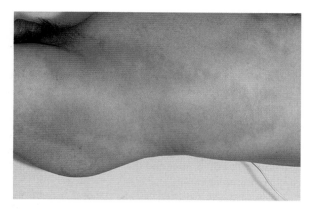

Figure 15.2 Grey Turner's sign in a patient with pancreatitis.

addition to obvious signs of hypovolaemic shock, there is progressive distension of the abdomen, which in severe injuries involving major vessels (e.g. hepatic veins) may become so tense as to obstruct venous return from the lower limbs. Postoperative bleeding is due either to slipping of a ligature on a blood vessel or reactionary bleeding or to oozing from raw surfaces (liver resections) or leaking arterial anastomosis. Reactionary bleeding occurs from cut small blood vessels that are missed at operation but which bleed subsequently as the blood pressure rises after recovery from surgery and anaesthesia. Bleeding from an arterial anastomosis may also be the result of infection. The signs and symptoms of progressive haemoperitoneum are dominated by the rapid loss of circulating blood volume, with the development of hypovolaemic shock. In this respect, the local abdominal signs, apart from increasing abdominal distension, are of minor importance. These patients only survive with prompt resuscitation and immediate surgical intervention.

Stable haemoperitoneum

A stable haemoperitoneum implies that the lesion which caused the haemoperitoneum in the first instance is no longer actively bleeding. Given time, the blood may track along tissue planes to appear in the flank (Grey Turner sign, found in patients with necrotizing pancreatitis; Fig. 15.2) or the periumbilical region (Cullen's sign, also found associated with necrotizing pancreatitis and rarely with missed ruptured ectopic pregnancy). The manifestations of patients with stable haemoperitoneum are not always clear-cut. The patient may appear clinically anaemic but this is best confirmed by haemoglobin estimation. Although free peritoneal blood acts as an irritant, the pain is not marked and tenderness is mild or absent. At

times the patient complains of shoulder-tip pain when lying supine. This is the result of diaphragmatic irritation. In equivocal cases raising the foot of the bed, thereby encouraging any free blood present to flow into the subdiaphragmatic spaces, enhances shoulder tip-pain. The abdomen may be distended and may have a doughy feel. Shifting dullness can sometimes be elicited.

Treatment

Progressive haemoperitoneum requires immediate surgical intervention with volume replacement (blood, colloids and crystalloids) during the surgery. Cross-matched blood should be available within 30 min in most hospitals nowadays and thus the need for transfusion of Group O Rh-negative non-cross-matched blood seldom if ever arises. The primary aim of the operation is to control the bleeding. Survival depends on this being achieved before substantial losses. In major liver injuries with massive bleeding that cannot be controlled at laparotomy, management is by packing of the entire supracolic compartment with gauze rolls and closure. The patient is re-explored 24 h later, when usually the condition has improved and control of bleeding by surgical means becomes feasible.

Patients with stable haemoperitoneum should be investigated without delay and some will require urgent surgical treatment when the diagnosis is confirmed.

Intestinal obstruction

Definitions and types

Intestinal obstruction may be complete (total blockage of the lumen) or incomplete (partial blockage). It may present acutely with dramatic symptoms when the obstruction is situated at any point between the second part of the duodenum and the caecum (acute intestinal obstruction). Alternatively, the presentation may be more insidious, over several weeks, when the obstruction is located in the colon (chronic intestinal obstruction). If the blood supply to the obstructed segment is not jeopardized, the obstruction is referred to as simple or mechanical, in order to distinguish it from those obstructions in which the blood supply is compromised at an early stage (strangulating intestinal obstruction).

Aetiology and pathophysiology

The various causes of mechanical intestinal obstructions can be grouped as extramural, intramural and intraluminal (Table 15.4).

Table 15.4 Causes of mechanical intestinal obstruction.

Extramural
Adhesions, bands
Herniae: external and internal
Compression by tumours (nodal tumour deposits)

Intramural
Inflammatory disease: Crohn's disease
Tumours: carcinomas, lymphomas, etc.
Strictures

Intraluminal
Faecal impaction
Swallowed foreign bodies
Bezoars
Gallstone

● *Extramural obstructions.* These are due to extrinsic compression of the walls of the gut by bands, adhesions or tumours (particularly secondary deposits in lymph nodes). Adhesive small-bowel obstruction secondary to previous peritonitis or surgical intervention is nowadays the most common cause of intestinal obstruction.
● *Intramural obstructions.* These are caused by lesions (neoplastic, inflammatory or cicatricial) arising from the wall of the intestine. The most common cause of this type of obstruction is carcinoma, usually of the colon.
● *Intraluminal obstructions.* Although intraluminal small-bowel obstructions are rare, chronic colonic intraluminal obstruction by impacted faeces in constipated elderly patients is quite common. The small-bowel lumen may be blocked by a swallowed object (children, mentally subnormal individuals) or a bolus composed of indigestible material (orange pith or hair bezoar, particularly in gastrectomized patients) or by a gallstone. The latter arises when a large gallstone in a chronically inflamed gallbladder that has become adherent to the duodenum erodes through the two organs by a process of pressure necrosis, thus entering the duodenum and becoming impacted lower down the small intestine, usually in the terminal ileum. The condition is known as gallstone ileus. By virtue of its origin it is always accompanied by a cholecystoduodenal fistula, which allows reflux of enteric contents and air into the biliary tract.

Specific types

Mechanical obstruction

Following the onset of obstruction, the distal bowel empties to a collapsed state whereas the proximal bowel becomes hyperactive, with vigorous peristaltic contractions, in an effort to overcome the obstruction. These cluster contractions are the cause of the severe colicky abdominal pain experienced by these patients. Additionally, the bowel proximal to the obstruction dilates due to the accumulation of swallowed air and increased intestinal secretions. The interface between air and fluid in the dilated loops accounts for the fluid levels seen in the erect abdominal film of these patients. The wall of the obstructed gut becomes oedematous. This is the result of increased transudation across the capillary membrane as the venous drainage of the affected segments is impaired by the distension. The fluid and electrolytes that accumulate in the lumen of the obstructed bowel and within its wall are effectively lost (sequestrated third-space losses) and contribute (together with vomiting) to the fluid and electrolyte deficit in these patients. Bacterial overgrowth occurs within the obstructed loops of intestine. Unless the distension is relieved, there is progressive occlusion (by stretching) of the intestinal intramural vessels such that, untreated, a mechanical intestinal obstruction leads to ischaemia and eventually necrosis with perforation of the bowel.

Strangulating obstruction

Here, in addition to the luminal obstruction, the viability of the gut is compromised because of impairment of its blood supply at an early stage. Common examples include strangulation caused by bands, adhesions and tight hernial sacs (strangulated herniae). There are special forms that merit separate attention, including intussusception, volvulus, closed-loop obstruction and mesenteric infarction.

Intussusception
This consists of telescoping of a loop of bowel inside itself (ileoileal, ileum inside ileum; ileocolic, ileum inside caecum or ascending colon; Fig. 15.3). It may or may not originate from a lead point, which is usually a swelling of the mucosa or submucosa (e.g. inflamed Peyer's patch, mucosal adenoma, submucosal lipoma). Intussusception occurs most commonly in infants and children usually 3–18 months of age, but may be encountered in adults. The blood supply of the involved bowel is compromised at an early stage and unless the intussusception is reduced early (e.g. by barium enema or surgery), infarction and peritonitis supervene.

Volvulus
Volvulus is a 360° twist of a loop or loops of intestine. The rotation causes early obstruction of the vascular

03

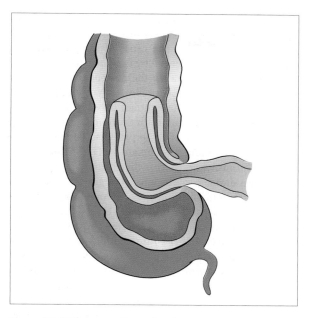

Figure 15.3 Diagram of ileocolic intussusception.

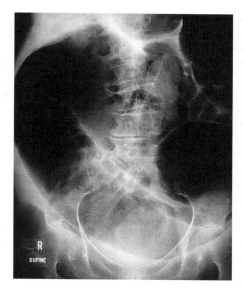

Figure 15.4 Plain abdominal X-ray showing a sigmoid volvulus.

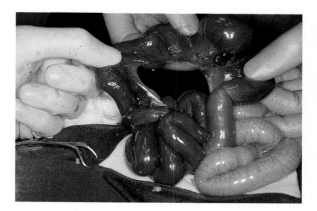

Figure 15.5 Infarcted midgut.

pedicle supplying the affected portion. Risk factors for small-bowel volvulus (which may affect the whole of the midgut) include adhesions or bands between the antimesenteric aspect of the bowel and the anterior abdominal wall and congenital malrotation of the gut. Volvulus of the sigmoid colon is encountered in the elderly, patients with chronic constipation and those with a redundant pelvic mesocolon (Fig. 15.4). Unless recognized early, volvulus leads to intestinal infarction, which often involves large segments of the gut.

Closed-loop obstruction
Although volvulus is an example of this type of obstruction, i.e. segment of the affected bowel closed at proximal and distal ends, the term 'closed-loop obstruction' is usually reserved for a complete obstruction of the left colon (usually by an annular carcinoma of the descending or sigmoid colon) in the presence of a competent ileocaecal valve. This prevents the proximal distended colon from decompressing into the small intestine. Meanwhile, small-bowel contents may continue to pass into the caecum through the one-way ileocaecal valve. The result is a rapid build-up of pressure in the colon, with the brunt being taken by the caecum, which becomes markedly distended to the point of ischaemia when it perforates, usually through a clear-cut hole (pistol-shot perforation).

Mesenteric infarction
In this serious condition, there is primary occlusion of the

blood supply to the intestine as a result of thrombotic or embolic disease of the mesenteric vessels. Most commonly, the superior mesenteric vessels are occluded, with infarction of the entire midgut from the level of the mid-duodenum to the junction of the proximal with the distal two-thirds of the transverse colon (long-loop infarction; Fig. 15.5). The condition, which affects patients who are elderly and suffer from cardiac and atheromatous vascular disease, is usually fatal. At times the extent of the infarction is less extensive, then resection may be followed by survival but the patient has insufficient small bowel for digestion and absorption and develops the short-gut syndrome. There is another type of small-bowel infarction encountered in patients with chronic hypoxia (chronic pulmonary disease, heart failure, etc.) and which is due

to hypoperfusion. The ischaemia is patchy and the mesenteric vessels appear patent, the block occurring in the small intramural vessels of the intestine (microcirculation). This variant is known as non-occlusive mesenteric infarction.

The same occlusive process may involve the vessels supplying the colon and lead to ischaemic colitis. This tends to affect predominantly the left colon and presents with a picture of acute inflammation not dissimilar from acute colonic diverticulitis. Fortunately the affected colon, although oedematous and inflamed, does not usually infarct and the process subsides with conservative management. However, a stricture of the left colon commonly situated just distal to the splenic flexure develops some weeks to months later.

Paralytic ileus

This term is used to describe a syndrome in which intestinal obstruction is due to absence of the normal peristaltic contractions. The common abbreviation 'ileus' is incorrect as this word, which is of Greek derivation, means 'to roll up'. Adynamic ileus is most commonly encountered after intra-abdominal surgery, when it is short-lived (few days) and often referred to as physiological ileus. The temporary cessation of intestinal motor activity is due to handling and exposure of the intestinal loops. On occasions, it is pathologically prolonged, when it is associated with postoperative intra-abdominal sepsis and fibrinous adhesion formation (postoperative ileus). In this setting the differentiation between mechanical and paralytic obstruction is difficult and often the clinical picture is mixed.

Paralytic ileus may also be caused by spinal injuries and by the accumulation of retroperitoneal blood or irritant exudates that disturb the functional activity of the coeliac plexus and splanchnic nerves (retroperitoneal haematoma from renal injuries, ruptured abdominal aneurysms, acute pancreatitis, etc.). Haemoperitoneum may also be accompanied by some loss of intestinal peristaltic activity. Infective paralytic ileus is the most serious and is secondary to peritonitis from any cause.

Clinical features

Symptoms

The cardinal symptoms of mechanical bowel obstruction are:
- vomiting;
- colicky abdominal pain;
- abdominal distension;
- absolute constipation.

Notwithstanding, the symptomatology may be varied and the clinical picture of acute small-bowel obstruction is quite different from that of chronic (colonic) obstruction.

Vomiting is a marked feature of high small-bowel obstruction but is rarely encountered in colonic obstruction. Initially, the vomit consists of food followed by bile-stained fluid, which later becomes faeculent. This is caused by bacterial overgrowth in the obstructed small intestine. Vomiting, together with the sequestration of fluid in the dilated loops, rapidly leads to dehydration with significant water and electrolyte deficits, particularly Na^+ and Cl^-. The dehydration leads to raised PCV and prerenal azotaemia, with elevation of blood urea and reduced urine output.

The *pain* in mechanical small-bowel obstruction is colicky in nature, situated in the centre of the abdomen around the umbilicus and accompanied by hyperperistaltic rushes that can easily be heard by the stethoscope. In colonic obstruction the pain is more of a discomfort and is situated in the suprapubic region. However, in the presence of closed-loop obstruction with marked caecal dilatation and impending perforation, localized pain is present in the right iliac fossa. Constant severe pain is ominous and indicates either infarction of the bowel or the onset of peritonitis. Paralytic ileus in itself is painless, except when secondary to peritonitis, when the pain is generalized and constant.

Abdominal distension becomes progressively more marked the lower the obstruction is situated and may reach extreme degrees in low colonic obstruction and paralytic ileus. It is caused by accumulation of gas and fluid within the obstructed bowel.

Following the onset of mechanical obstruction, the patient may have a bowel motion as the distal segment empties. Thereafter, there is *absolute constipation* (no passage of either flatus or faeces).

Physical signs

The physical signs of intestinal obstruction are usually clear-cut. Dehydration is accompanied by loss of skin turgor. Pyrexia is mild unless there is infarction and peritonitis. Fluid and electrolyte losses cause a reduction of circulating blood volume with some hypotension and persistent tachycardia. The distended abdomen is resonant to percussion on the anterior aspect but is dull towards the flanks. Auscultation confirms the presence of excessive peristaltic activity (borborygmi) that coincide with attacks of colic. In paralytic ileus bowel sounds are not heard; instead these are replaced by tinkling high-pitched sounds due to passive movement of fluid within the dilated loops.

Tenderness and rebound tenderness are indicative of ischaemic bowel or developing peritonitis (due to imminent or established perforation). They are usually accompanied by deterioration in the general condition of the patient and change in the character of the pain, which becomes severe and constant.

Rectal examination in small-bowel obstruction usually confirms an empty rectum. In colonic obstruction the findings may be:

● empty rectum;
● gross faecal loading (in obstruction due to faecal impaction);
● low neoplasm can be palpated by the examining finger.

Investigations

The essential investigations in patients with intestinal obstruction are haemoglobin, PCV, WCC, urea and electrolytes, chest X-ray, plain erect and supine abdominal films. Both the haemoglobin and PCV are elevated because of haemoconcentration. The raised blood urea is the result of an element of prerenal failure due to the hypovolaemia. The WCC is usually normal or slightly elevated unless there is bowel infarction and/or peritonitis. The serum Na^+ and Cl^- are low. Hyperkalaemia may be observed in patients with infarcted intestine.

The chest radiograph shows an elevated diaphragm, which is secondary to the abdominal distension. In addition there may be free air underneath the right diaphragm in patients with infective paralytic ileus (secondary to intestinal perforation). The erect abdominal film is taken to outline air–fluid levels. These are multiple and centrally placed in a ladder fashion in small-bowel obstruction (Fig. 15.6a). In large-bowel obstruction they are less numerous and located in the flanks and suprapubic regions (Fig. 15.6b). The supine film is used to assess distension of the intestine and helps to differentiate small from large intestine. Dilated jejunum often exhibits parallel soft-tissue shadows that extend the whole width of the involved segment (due to the folds of the small-bowel mucosa, so-called valvulae conniventes; Fig. 15.6a), whereas in the obstructed colon the haustra cause crescentic soft-tissue shadows that do not traverse the entire width of the bowel (Fig. 15.6b). Also, the obstructed colon has a sacculated outline. The obstructed ileum is relatively featureless. Other investigations that may be necessary are contrast examinations (water-soluble contrast swallow and meal, gentle barium enema) and sigmoidoscopy.

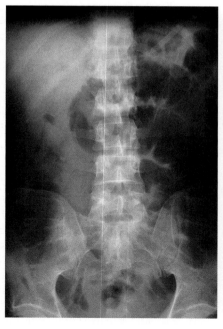
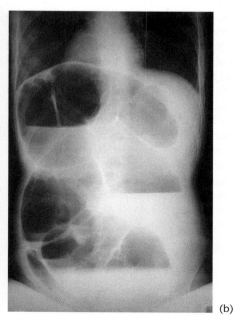

(a)   (b)

Figure 15.6 (a) Valvulae conniventes. Supine film showing a dilated jejunum in mechanical small-bowel obstruction. The soft-tissue markings extend the whole length of the dilated segment. The obstructed ileum is relatively featureless. (b) Haustral soft-tissue markings in colonic obstruction. They do not extend across the whole width of the affected segment. Note the presence of air–fluid levels.

Management

The management of intestinal obstruction is based on four principles:

- decompression of the obstructed gut;
- replacement of fluid and electrolyte losses;
- special conservative measures in certain situations;
- surgical intervention.

Decompression

Although various long tubes were used in the past, decompression is nowadays achieved by the insertion of a nasogastric sump suction tube (Salem). This is aspirated at least every hour and left draining into a bag in the intervening periods. The daily aspirate is measured and the amount used in calculating the daily fluid and electrolyte requirements (see Chapter 13). If the intestinal obstruction responds to conservative management, the daily amount of aspirate gradually reduces and its nature changes to clear, often bile-stained fluid.

Fluid and electrolyte therapy

Fluids and electrolytes are given through a peripheral venous line. As the major losses are water, sodium and chloride, the usual crystalloid solution consists of isotonic saline and 5% dextrose solution. Initially, large amounts are administered (1 L every 3–4 h) to replace the losses. Thereafter, maintenance intravenous fluid therapy is continued until return of normal bowel function. The usual daily requirements of potassium (40–120 mmol) are met by infusing 60–80 mmol of potassium chloride in divided doses over 24 h. If hypokalaemia is severe, up to 40 mmol may be infused over 1 h in 500 mL of fluid. It is important to remember that potassium must always be administered slowly and never given as a bolus injection because of the risk of cardiac arrhythmias and arrest.

Special conservative measures

For certain types of intestinal obstruction, additional specific measures may result in rapid relief of the obstruction, thereby avoiding surgical intervention. Examples include the passage of a rectal tube or flexible sigmoidoscope to deflate a sigmoid volvulus, barium contrast enema to reduce an early intussusception in an infant and manual removal of faeces and/or oil retention enema to deal with obstruction caused by faecal impaction.

Assessment of progress

It is important that the patient is assessed at frequent intervals to establish progress on conservative management. This is confirmed by relief of symptoms (vomiting and pain), improvement of the general condition and vital signs (pulse rate, temperature and blood pressure) and observations such as reduction in the amount of aspirate and abdominal girth and return of normal bowel sounds.

Surgical intervention

This is undertaken if the following apply.

- The underlying disease needs surgical treatment (obstructed hernia, obstructing carcinoma, etc.). In this respect, intestinal obstruction due to adhesions often settles with conservative management and therefore is not initially treated surgically unless there is clinical evidence of strangulation.
- The patient does not improve with conservative treatment.
- There are signs of strangulation or peritonitis.

Complications

The complications that may arise in patients with acute abdomen are outlined in Table 15.5. The acute complications develop early, usually during the same hospital admission. The most common is wound infection, which may be minor or major, i.e. requiring opening of the skin and subcutaneous tissue to drain the collection, necessary for healing by granulation (secondary intention). Some hospital-acquired infections (nosocomial) are more serious and can prove fatal, e.g. ventilator pneumonia. Hospital-acquired infections are often caused by resistant organisms, especially methicillin-resistant *Staphylococcus aureus* (MRSA). Aside from being difficult to treat, these

Table 15.5 Complications of acute abdomen.

Acute (early)
Nosocomial (hospital-acquired) infection: pneumonia, methicillin-resistant *Staphylococcus aureus* infection
Wound infection
Wound dehiscence
Abscess formation
Fistula formation
    External
    Internal

Chronic (late)
Incisional hernia
Wound sinus
Adhesions
    Recurrent small-bowel obstruction
    Bacterial overgrowth (blind loop)

03

infections may be spread to other patients unless special precautions are taken:

- all MRSA-infected patients must be isolated;
- all staff attending patients must wear disposable plastic aprons and gloves (discarded in a special disposable bin for incineration);
- hands are washed with antiseptic soap and then disinfected with alcohol.

Another serious early wound complication is total wound dehiscence, i.e. complete disruption of the abdominal wall. Often the skin edges remain approximated by the skin sutures but an obvious bulge is present in the subcutaneous layer with exudation of copious serosanguineous discharge. The treatment of wound dehiscence is immediate surgical intervention. The extravasated loops are washed and replaced in the peritoneal cavity and the abdominal wall closed in a single layer with large bites of non-absorbable sutures.

Intra-abdominal abscesses may be located in the various compartments of the subphrenic region (on the right or left side), in the pelvis or between loops of small intestine. The systemic manifestations of intraperitoneal abscesses include malaise, weight loss, intermittent pyrexia and persistent leukocytosis. There may or may not be any localizing signs. A subphrenic abscess may cause shoulder-tip pain. Intraloop abscesses (often multiple) induce prolonged ileus and a pelvic abscess (most commonly encountered after a perforated appendicitis) causes rectal tenderness and diarrhoea. These abscesses are easily located by either ultrasound or CT examination and many are drained percutaneously, avoiding the need for surgical intervention.

Intestinal fistulae may be external (enterocutaneous) or internal (between adjacent hollow viscera). Fistulae arise either from breakdown of an intestinal closure or anastomosis or because of delayed recognition or treatment of an intra-abdominal abscess, which then bursts, either between bowel and abdominal wall or between adjacent hollow viscera (e.g. colovesical fistula). An external high small-bowel fistula is a serious complication because most of the gastrointestinal secretions are lost through the fistulous opening (high-output fistula). As well as significant daily fluid and electrolyte losses, these fistulae lead to profound excoriation of the abdominal wall as this is digested by the activated pancreatic enzymes. These patients are managed by total parenteral nutrition and careful isolation of the fistulous discharge with the use of skin barriers and efficient sump suction drainage. Provided there is no distal obstruction or residual intra-abdominal abscess, the fistula usually heals with this conservative management. Colonic fistulae are much less serious and generally have a lower output. The same principles of management are adopted, except that nutrition is maintained enterally with low-residue or elemental diets.

Chronic complications include:

- incisional herniae, usually in patients who develop a postoperative wound infection;
- formation of intraperitoneal adhesions;
- persistent wound sinus.

Incisional hernias cause deformity and significant morbidity including strangulation. Thus if the patient is fit, repair is advocated. As the hernial defect is usually large, repair is carried out with a synthetic mesh as this carries the lowest incidence of recurrence. Intestinal adhesions cause considerable chronic disability because of recurrent attacks of small-bowel obstruction necessitating repeated hospital admissions and further surgical treatment. They are now the most common cause of intestinal obstruction. Currently several prophylactic treatments are being evaluated to reduce the formation of adhesions, e.g. intraperitoneal surfactant, Adept solution. Adhesions also cause chronic abdominal pain and may lead to the development of bacterial overgrowth (blind-loop syndrome) in the kinked small-bowel loops. The bacterial overgrowth results in malabsorption, anaemia and diarrhoea. A common chronic wound complication is the development of a persistent wound sinus. This is related to infection around a non-absorbable suture used in wound closure. Unless this is removed surgically, the sinus and the discharge persist, although one sinus may heal temporarily and then recur.

Intestinal pseudo-obstruction

This is sometimes referred to as Ogilvie's syndrome because he first described the condition in two patients with advanced cancer and involvement of the subdiaphragmatic autonomic plexus and postulated an imbalance between sympathetic and parasympathetic activity as the underlying cause. It is now thought to result from impairment of the reflex circuits within the enteric nervous system that ensure normal peristaltic progression. The syndrome is characterized by massive dilatation of the colon, suggesting distal organic colonic obstruction. This rare functional obstruction is usually encountered in elderly patients with severe extra-abdominal illness or injury (heart failure, sepsis, trauma, etc.). Other documented associations include chronic administration of hypnotics and sedatives, lead toxicity, hypothyroidism and various neurological disorders. The diagnosis is made by exclusion of organic disease. Air–fluid levels are often absent in this condition. Untreated the dilatation is progressive and when it exceeds 10 cm in the caecum, rupture with peritonitis may ensue. Treatment involves correction of the underlying cause, supportive management and decompression of the colon by passage of a rectal tube, sigmoidoscope or colonoscope.

The acute abdomen at a glance

Definitions

Acute abdomen: describes a group of life-threatening intra-abdominal conditions, characterized by peritonitis, that require emergency hospital admission ± surgery

Peritonitis: inflammation of the peritoneum (bacterial or chemical) that is always serious

Haemoperitoneum: the presence of free blood in the peritoneal cavity

Complete intestinal obstruction: total blockage of the intestinal lumen. Incomplete intestinal obstruction denotes only a partial blockage. Obstruction may be *acute* (hours) or *chronic* (weeks), *simple* (mechanical) or *strangulated* (blood supply compromised). A *closed-loop obstruction* is an obstruction of the colon in the presence of a competent ileocaecal valve

Causes
Inflammatory
- Acute inflammation of regions of the gastrointestinal tract
- Anastomotic leakage
- Secondary and primary peritonitis

Traumatic
- Blunt or penetrating trauma

Obstructive
- Small or large bowel

Vascular
- Thrombosis or embolus to mesenteric vessels
- Volvulus and strangulated herniae
- Adhesion or obstruction/infarction

Investigations
Essential
- Haemoglobin, WCC, PCV
- Urea, electrolytes, amylase
- Chest X-ray, supine and erect abdominal X-ray
- Blood cultures
- Group and save ± cross-match

Special
- Ultrasound and CT
- Peritoneal lavage
- Mesenteric angiography
- Laparoscopy/laparotomy

Peritonitis
Bacterial
- Secondary (from the gastrointestinal tract): common
- Primary (streptococcal): rare

- Spontaneous (seen in chronically ill): rare
- Tertiary (ICU patients): uncommon

Chemical
- HCl (early perforated duodenal ulcer)
- Extravasation of urine (ruptured bladder)
- Bile (leak post cholecystectomy)
- Amylase (pancreatitis)

Clinical features
Systemic features
Illness, toxicity, pyrexia, tachycardia, leukocytosis, rigors (bacteraemia/septicaemia), dehydration, loss of skin turgor, collapse of peripheral veins

Local symptoms
Pain (localized to one quadrant or generalized), severe, constant, aggravated by movement (active, e.g. coughing; passive, e.g. palpation)

Local signs
- Inspection: loss of normal abdominal movement on respiration
- Palpation: tenderness, guarding, rigidity, rebound tenderness (be gentle!)
- Percussion: tenderness
- Auscultation: silent abdomen
- Digital rectal examination: may elicit pelvic tenderness, boggy swelling, cervical tenderness in female

Management
Secondary bacterial peritonitis
- Resuscitate and investigate simultaneously
- Pain relief is a priority and should precede clinical examination
- Set up i.v. line and give crystalloids
- Place nasogastric tube if vomiting
- Give antibiotics:
   (a) If upper gastrointestinal pathology suspected, Gram-negative aerobe cover
   (b) If lower gastrointestinal pathology suspected, Gram-negative anaerobe cover
- Observe pulse, temperature, blood pressure, urinary output
- If unsure as to need for surgery, perform repeated physical examination ± special investigations
- Surgical treatment indicated for definite deteriorating peritonitis

Primary bacterial peritonitis
- Haematogenous spread of Gram-positive organisms (*Streptococcus pneumoniae*) to peritoneal cavity
- Occurs in children and adult females

- Treatment: antibiotics ± laparotomy to drain pus
- Prognosis is good

Spontaneous bacterial peritonitis
- Occurs in immunocompromised patients:
  (a) Cirrhosis + ascites, Wilson's disease, chronic active hepatitis
  (b) Chronic peritoneal dialysis
  (c) Nephrotic syndrome
- Usually Gram-negative organisms
- High risk of septic shock and multiorgan dysfunction syndrome
- Poor prognosis

Haemoperitoneum
Some common causes
- Intra-abdominal injuries (including iatrogenic)
- Intra-abdominal operations
- Ruptured ectopic pregnancy
- Ruptured corpus luteum cyst
- Retrograde menstrual flow
- Necrotizing pancreatitis

Progressive type
- Implies continued active intra-abdominal bleeding
- Clinical features of hypovolaemia + abdominal distension
- Requires prompt resuscitiation and surgery

Stable type
- Implies cessation of active bleeding
- Clinical features of peritoneal irritation
- (Abdominal ± shoulder-tip pain)
- May settle but some require surgery

Intestinal obstruction
Causes
- *Extramural*: adhesions, bands, volvulus, herniae (internal and external), compression by tumour (e.g. frozen pelvis)
- *Intramural*: inflammatory bowel disease (Crohn's disease), tumours (carcinoma, lymphoma), stricture, paralytic (adynamic) ileus
- *Intraluminal*: faecal impaction, foreign bodies, bezoars, gallstone ileus

Pathophysiology
- Bowel distal to obstruction collapses
- Bowel proximal to obstruction distends and becomes hyperactive. Distension is due to swallowed air and accumulating intestinal secretions
- Bowel wall becomes oedematous. Fluid and electrolytes accumulate in the wall and the lumen (third-space loss)
- Bacteria proliferate in the obstructed bowel
- As the bowel distends, the intramural vessels become stretched and the blood supply is compromised leading to ischaemia and necrosis

Clinical features
- Vomiting, colicky abdominal pain, abdominal distension, absolute constipation (i.e. neither faeces nor flatus)
- Dehydration and loss of skin turgor
- Hypotension and tachycardia
- Abdominal distension and increased bowel sounds
- Empty rectum on digital examination
- Tenderness or rebound tenderness indicates peritonitis

Investigations
- Haemoglobin, PCV: elevated due to dehydration
- WCC: normal or slightly elevated
- Urea and electrolytes: urea elevated, Na^+ and Cl^- low
- Chest X-ray: elevated diaphragm due to abdominal distension
- Abdominal X-rays: erect film demonstrates air–fluid levels; supine gives clue as to whether obstruction is in small bowel (central distension/valvulae conniventes shadows cross entire width of lumen) or large bowel (peripheral distension/haustral shadows do not cross entire width of bowel).
- Contrast studies, colonoscopy to show level of obstruction

Management
- Decompress the obstructed gut: pass a nasogastric tube
- Replace fluid and electrolyte losses: give Ringer's lactate or NaCl with K^+ supplementation
- Relieve the obstruction surgically if:
  (a) Underlying cause needs surgical treatment (e.g. hernia, colonic carcinoma)
  (b) Patient does not improve with conservative treatment, e.g. adhesion obstruction
  (c) There are signs of peritonitis or stangulation

Complications
Acute
- Nosocomial infections:
  (a) Pneumonia
  (b) MRSA
- Wound infection
- Wound dehiscence
- Abscess formation
- Fistula formation:
  (a) External
  (b) Internal

Chronic (late)
- Wound sinus
- Incisional hernia
- Adhesions:
  (a) Recurrent small-bowel obstruction
  (b) Bacterial overgrowth (blind loop)

Must know Must do

Must know
Pathophysiology of SIRS
Clinical features of MODS

Must do
Observe a patient with SIRS in an intensive care unit
**Look at a chest radiograph showing the features of
    ARDS**

Introduction

Over the last 30 years improvements in early resuscitation following major injury have meant that many very ill patients survive the initial traumatic insult (e.g. ruptured abdominal aortic aneurysm, road traffic accident) and are managed thereafter in intensive care units. Many of these patients subsequently develop a hypermetabolic state, similar to that seen with septic shock, that leads to sequential organ failure involving:

- lungs (acute respiratory distress syndrome, ARDS);
- kidneys (acute renal failure, ARF);
- gastrointestinal tract (liver failure, stress ulceration);
- central nervous system (confusion, encephalopathy);
- blood (disseminated intravascular coagulation, DIC);
- heart (cardiac depression).

The response to injury that occurs in the body and leads to this hypermetabolic state is called *systemic inflammatory response syndrome* (SIRS) and the sequence of failing end-organs is referred to as *multiple organ dysfunction syndrome* (MODS). Despite advances in organ support with volume ventilators, nutritional support and haemodialysis, MODS remains the leading non-cardiac cause of death in surgical patients, with a mortality of approximately 50%. This condition places enormous strains on healthcare resources, as intensive care medicine is extremely dependent on new technology and high personnel costs.

The cost to society, however, runs much higher because these patients are often young productive individuals. Added to this is the knowledge that those who survive the initial insult without developing multiple organ failure would expect, in most cases, near-perfect rehabilitation and a normal life expectancy.

Pathophysiology

The pathophysiology of SIRS/MODS is complex, although much research has focused on the role of the inflammatory response by cells of the immune system. It appears that one or more of many initiating factors (see below) causes a systemic hyperinflammatory response and it is the uncontrolled activity of this response that leads to organ failure (Fig. 16.1). A certain threshold level of injury is necessary for the development of SIRS, although this varies between individuals.

Initiating factors

No single initiating factor for the hyperinflammatory response has been isolated but a few suspects have been identified. It is likely that the clinical syndrome of SIRS results from the interaction of a number of proposed initiating mechanisms. Infection has long been known to cause a systemic inflammatory response (i.e. septic shock) but the realization that many patients in 'septic shock' had no focus of infection led to the idea that other initiating factors could precipitate a similar syndrome. It would seem that the presence of large areas of damaged or necrotic tissue can mimic an infectious focus. Thus it appears that a common factor in the host response to severe tissue injury from different causes is the initiation of an acute inflammatory response. Multiple organ failure may be due to an overvigorous manifestation of this normally protective defence mechanism.

Another view is that a shock toxin, thought to be a thrombogenic aminophospholipid that occurs only on the inner layer of all cell membranes, is liberated by cell

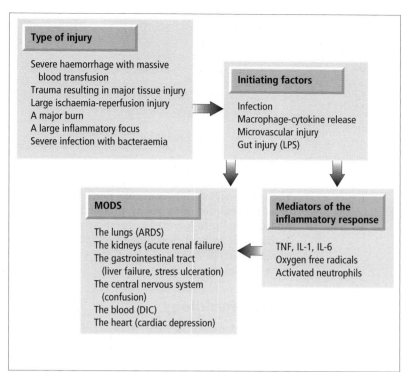

Figure 16.1 Pathophysiology of systemic inflammatory response syndrome.

03

destruction. It causes DIC, which may obstruct the micro-circulation of any and all organs producing MODS by microclots. These microclots may be lysed by plasminogen activator and circulation to the organs restored.

Infection

Uncontrolled infection accounts for 50% of cases of MODS. Sepsis has been defined as the presence of micro-organisms or their toxins (e.g. endotoxin) in the blood-stream together with the resultant host response. It has long been recognized that severe infection can lead to septic shock, with profound effects on haemodynamics and tissue perfusion. While most forms of circulatory shock induce cellular changes secondary to hypoxia, Gram-negative septic shock is associated with primary cellular dysfunction induced by bacterial endotoxins, which are composed of lipopolysaccharide (LPS) in the bacterial cell wall. LPS stimulates macrophages and endothelial cells to release cytokines that mediate the inflammatory response (Fig. 16.2). Gram-positive organisms (e.g. *Staphylococcus aureus*) release cytokines by adherence to macrophages, while their toxins act as superantigens that react directly with T cells, causing massive cytokine release (e.g. toxic shock syndrome).

Macrophage–cytokine release

Tumour necrosis factor (TNF)-α is detected in the serum of most patients with SIRS. TNF is a principal mediator of the inflammatory response and is released with inter-leukin (IL)-1 and IL-6 from macrophages. It is thought that persistent stimulation of the release of these cytokines leads to the inflammatory response and tissue injury.

Immune suppression and the compensatory anti-inflammatory response syndrome

Early observations in patients with SIRS documented major defects in T-cell function, with a central defect in IL-2 (T-cell growth factor) production. This apparent paradox of immune suppression coexisting with immune hyperstimulation (macrophages) may be explained by a two-phase response to injury. One possibility is that an exaggerated inflammatory response to injury may be counterbalanced by the release of potent anti-inflammatory cytokines, including IL-4, IL-10 and transforming growth factor (TGF)-β. This is known as the compensatory anti-inflammatory response syndrome (or CARS, a term used by Roger Bone who also coined the term SIRS). CARS may also be deleterious, resulting in opportunistic infection such as systemic candidiasis.

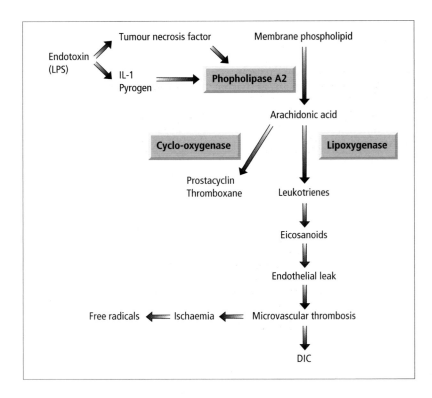

Figure 16.2 Role of endotoxin in promoting an inflammatory response.

Microcirculatory injury

Ischaemia–reperfusion may induce a systemic inflammatory response. Reperfusion of tissues after a period of ischaemia causes the release of toxic oxygen radicals (superoxide, O_2^-; hydrogen peroxide, H_2O_2; hydroxyl radical, OH^-) that cause tissue damage by lipid peroxidation. The resulting endothelial damage causes release of cytokines, initiating a systemic inflammatory response and end-organ failure.

Gut injury

The normal intestinal mucosa is an effective barrier against microorganisms and endotoxin. A number of adverse changes take place in the septic state that allow bacterial translocation (i.e. passage of bacteria from the gut to the systemic circulation) to occur.
● The nature of the microflora changes, especially in the presence of antibiotics, to a more pathogenic and more resistant pattern.
● Barrier function is lost through disappearance of tight junctions between epithelial cells, loss of mucus and increase in mucosal permeability.
● The Kupffer cells in the liver, which act as part of the reticuloendothelial system that provides the next line of defence, lose their filtering ability and allow bacteria and endotoxin to enter the portal and systemic circulations.
● Hepatocytes in the liver may also be damaged, with evidence of jaundice.
● *Candida* normally present in the gastrointestinal tract may migrate to the bloodstream and lungs, particularly when antibiotics are used.

The gut has been called the 'motor' of SIRS/MODS because it provides a reservoir of bacteria and endotoxin that sustains the inflammatory response. The inflammatory response in turn causes further intestinal injury. The absorptive power of the gut may also be lost because of damage to intestinal villi. Whenever possible, enteral feeding (to avoid further mucosal atrophy) should be the preferred mode of nutritional support in SIRS. However, if enteral feeding cannot be sustained, intravenous feeding (total parenteral nutrition, TPN) with its additional hazards is necessary.

Hyperinflammatory response

The interaction between initiating factors (endotoxin, ischaemia–reperfusion, etc.) and the host-mediated response results in changes in cellular metabolism, with

increased glucose and amino acid utilization. Mediators such as TNF (also called cachectin), IL-1 and IL-6 are released, resulting in a cascade of responses including:
- fever from endogenous pyrogen;
- priming of neutrophils to release reactive oxygen intermediates;
- promoting adherence of phagocytes to endothelium;
- activation of complement and release of prostaglandins and thromboxane A_2.

The mechanism by which the systemic inflammatory response causes end-organ failure is slowly being elucidated. The initial events occur at the microvascular endothelium. Thus, oxygen free radicals are released, neutrophil chemotactic factors are produced and surface adhesion molecules are expressed that enhance neutrophil adhesion and migration into the tissues. Further tissue damage is caused by release of destructive molecules from the trapped neutrophils (more oxygen radicals, elastase, collagenase and proteases). Tissue factor, which activates the extrinsic pathway of the coagulation system, is expressed on the cell surface of monocytes and endothelial cells. As a result, microthrombi are formed, interstitial oedema occurs and organ function deteriorates. Damage to cell membranes allows the free passage of calcium into the cell; this is toxic to mitochondrial function, with impairment of oxidative phosphorylation and ultimately cell death.

Clinical features

The patients at risk are those who have sustained a major biological insult, such as:
- severe haemorrhage requiring massive blood transfusion (e.g. liver trauma);
- trauma resulting in major tissue injury (e.g. crush injury);
- large ischaemia–reperfusion injury (e.g. reperfusion of a limb following embolectomy);
- major burn;
- large inflammatory focus (e.g. peritonitis, pancreatitis);
- severe infection with bacteraemia (e.g. ascending cholangitis).

Typically the patient seems to do well following resuscitation but after 2 or 3 days develops the characteristic hypermetabolic picture. In the early phase, blood pressure remains normal, peripheral vascular resistance is lowered and there is an increase in cardiac output. Later, with the development of shock the blood pressure falls, peripheral resistance decreases further and cardiac output remains high. There is a metabolic acidosis with a compensatory respiratory alkalosis. Typically there will be a leukocytosis (or leukopenia), thrombocytopenia and hyperglycaemia. Finally, cardiac output decreases with a profound fall in blood pressure and exacerbation of the metabolic acidosis; oxygen consumption falls, indicating inadequate oxygen perfusion.

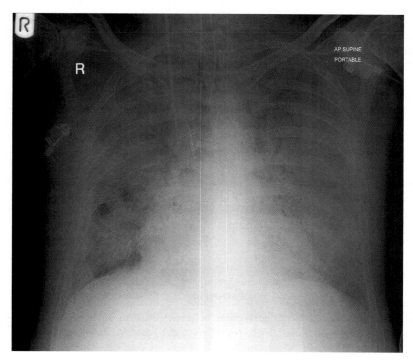

Figure 16.3 Chest radiograph of a patient with acute respiratory distress syndrome.

Table 16.1 Features of end-organ dysfunction.

System	Features
Respiratory (ARDS)	Increasing minute ventilation Decreased pulmonary compliance Arterial hypoxaemia and hypercapnia Diffuse fluffy pulmonary infiltrates on chest radiograph
Renal (ARF)	Oliguria Rising urea and creatinine
Liver	Jaundice Decreased protein synthesis (hypoalbuminaemia, prolonged PT)
Gastrointestinal	Gastric stress ulceration Adynamic ileus Acalculous cholecystitis Pancreatitis
Haematology	Leukopenia Disseminated intravascular coagulation
Central nervous system	Confusion Decreasing Glasgow Coma Score

ARDS, adult respiratory distress syndrome; ARF, acute renal failure; PT, prothrombin time.

03

The diagnosis of SIRS is made when two or more of the following are present:

- tachycardia;
- tachypnoea or hyperventilation; and
- fever and leukocytosis.

When two or more end-organs fail a diagnosis of MODS is made (Table 16.1).

Management

The best form of therapy is prevention and every effort should be made during resuscitation to avoid hypotension and gross sepsis (e.g. during bowel surgery) and to ensure adequate oxygenation and urinary output. The general aims of therapy are to:

- treat infection;
- ensure adequate tissue oxygenation;
- maintain nutritional support; and
- minimize systemic inflammation.

Management of the failure of the various end-organs must also be undertaken. This is largely supportive and is discussed in Chapters 11–15.

Treat infection

Eradication of the source of infection is a priority.

Removal of necrotic tissue or drainage of abscesses is essential. Nosocomial (hospital-acquired) infection must be prevented by aggressive physiotherapy, pulmonary toilet and care of central lines. Wounds must be kept clean and debrided, if necessary. Although no localized source of infection may be identifiable in SIRS, blood cultures are positive in one-third of patients. Antibiotic therapy is initiated on the basis of the most likely infecting organisms until the results of blood culture are available, when more specific antibiotic treatment can be initiated.

Adequate tissue oxygenation

Circulatory support with intravenous fluids is important, with constant monitoring of urine output and pulmonary artery pressure. Diuretics may be required to maintain urinary output but should only be used when adequate hydration has been achieved. Inotropic support with adrenaline or noradrenaline is indicated in situations where despite adequate filling pressures cardiac output and perfusion pressure (mean arterial pressure, MAP) are inadequate. Ventilatory support may be necessary, with supplementary oxygen or mechanical ventilation in severe cases. Oxygen delivery must be high as SIRS is associated with increased consumption of oxygen.

03

Nutrition

Adequate nutrition is essential in the management of patients with SIRS. Nutritional support restores the barrier function of the gut and should thereby reduce bacterial translocation. Whenever possible, enteral feeding is preferred because the enterocyte receives its energy substrates primarily from the gut lumen. However, if enteral feeding cannot be sustained, intravenous feeding (TPN) is necessary. Immune modulation via the addition of L-arginine has been shown to be moderately beneficial in SIRS but has not gained widespread acceptance as yet.

Minimize the systemic inflammatory response

- Corticosteroids have been used in the management of septic shock. However, their role is at best uncertain. A reduction in the damaging effects of the inflammatory response can be achieved with corticosteroids but only if given prior to the onset of sepsis so that the practical applications are limited.
- Generation of free oxygen radicals can be prevented by blocking the enzyme xanthine oxidase with allopurinol or by scavenging toxic radicals with superoxide dismutase. This has been shown to be beneficial in a number of experimental models and may be of future value in the clinical situation.
- Anti-TNF and anti-LPS monoclonal antibodies are among the newer approaches that show promise. They function by interrupting the inflammatory mediator cascade responsible for the persistent injurious response of the immune system to sepsis. However, results have been disappointing in the clinical setting.
- Other experimental treatments include IL-12 (restores helper T-cell balance), the opioid receptor antagonist naloxone (counteracts β-endorphin release) and non-steroidal anti-inflammatory agents (inhibit the arachidonic acid cascade).

The majority of clinical trials in the area of SIRS have been disappointing because of the difficulty in translating therapies found to be successful in tightly controlled animal models to critically ill patients, who represent a very heterogeneous population. The first breakthrough in terms of improved survival was recently achieved in trials of recombinant activated protein C (an anticoagulant protein) in patients with septic shock. It is likely that further progress will be made only with increased understanding of the very complex mechanisms involved. In addition, there is recent evidence that biological variation in the host immune response to trauma and sepsis may have a genetic basis. Identification of those individuals who are likely to have a poor outcome may lead to more focused clinical trials of immunomodulatory agents.

Prognosis

Overall, the prognosis for patients with SIRS remains poor. There are a number of factors that influence survival.
- Age: the very young and the very old have a poor outcome.
- Severity of the initial insult: the more severe the initial illness, the greater the chance of dying.
- Cardiac output: the ability to increase cardiac output during the hypermetabolic state is associated with better survival.
- Infection: identification of a septic source carries a better prognosis.
- End-organ failure: the more end-organs that fail, the worse the outlook. Patients with three or more end-organ failures rarely survive.

SIRS at a glance

Definitions

Systemic inflammatory response syndrome: a systemic inflammatory response characterized by the presence of two or more of the following:
- hyperthermia > 38 °C or hypothermia < 36 °C
- tachycardia > 90 beats/min.
- tachypnoea > 20/min or $Paco_2$ < 4.3 kPa
- neutrophilia > 12×10^9/L or neutropenia < 4×10^9/L

Sepsis syndrome: a state of SIRS with proven infection

Septic shock: sepsis with systemic shock not responsive to fluids

Multiple organ dysfunction syndrome: a state of derangement of physiology such that organ function cannot maintain homeostasis. Several organs may be involved:
- lungs (ARDS);
- kidneys (ARF);
- gastrointestinal tract (liver failure, stress ulceration);
- central nervous system (confusion);
- blood (DIC);
- heart (cardiac depression).

Compensatory anti-inflammatory response syndrome: an anti-inflammatory response that counteracts the systemic inflammation of SIRS. CARS is characterized by the release

of potent anti-inflammatory cytokines, including IL-4, IL-10 and TGF-β. It may also be deleterious, resulting in opportunistic infection such as systemic candidiasis.
- TNF-α is both released by and activates macrophages and neutrophils. It is cytotoxic to endothelial cells and parenchymal cells of end-organs. There is no clear evidence for the efficacy of anti-TNF therapies in SIRS.
- LPS released from Gram-negative bacterial cell walls activates macrophages via attachment of LPS-binding protein and activation of CD14 molecules on the cell surface. There is no proven value for anti-LPS antibody treatment.
- IL-6 and IL-1β cause endothelial cell activation and damage. They promote complement and chemokine release.
- High-dose intravenous steroids have little role in established SIRS (probably because of multiple pathways of activation). Steroids for early SIRS are unproven.
- Platelet-activating factor (PAF): implicated particularly in acute pancreatitis. No proven role for anti-PAF antibody treatment.
- Inducible nitric oxide synthase: synthesized by leukocytes, macrophages and Kupffer cells. It is active for up to 20 h and produces nitric oxide (NO) in nanomolar concentrations. NO is a potent vasodilator and a free radical scavenger. However, it can also form peroxynitrite (ONOO$^-$), a free radical that may cause cellular damage.

Common surgical causes
SIRS is more common in surgical patients than is diagnosed.

Pathophysiology

Common surgical causes of SIRS are:
- acute pancreatitis
- perforated viscus with peritonitis
- fulminant colitis
- multiple trauma
- massive blood transfusion
- aspiration pneumonia
- ischaemia–reperfusion injury

Management
Early treatment of SIRS may reduce the risk of MODS developing. The role of treatment is to eliminate any causative factor and support the cardiovascular and respiratory physiology until the patient can recover.
- Treat infection
- Ensure adequate tissue oxygenation
- Maintain nutritional support
- Minimize systemic inflammatory response
- May be role for recombinant activated protein C

Prognosis
Overall mortality is 7% for SIRS, 14% for sepsis syndrome, 40% for established septic shock, and 90% for three-system failure. Factors predicting poor outcome:
- very young and very old
- severe initial insult
- inability to increase cardiac output
- inability to find septic source
- multiple end-organ failure

03

Initiating factor $\longrightarrow$	Systemic hyperinflammatory $\longrightarrow$ response	Common end pathway $\longrightarrow$	Clinical picture
Infection:	Release of TNF-α, IL-1, IL-6	Endothelial cell activation	Tachycardia
Gram-negative bacteria:		Vasodilatation	Tachypnoea
endotoxin		Capillary leak	Fever
Gram-positive bacteria:		Intravascular coagulation	Leukocytosis
exotoxin			
Macrophage cytokine release			
Microcirculatory injury			
Gut barrier failure			

Evidence-based medicine

Hardaway, R.M. (1998) Traumatic and septic shock alias post-traumatic critical illness. *Br J Surg* **85**, 1473–1479. Review of evidence supporting shock toxin hypothesis.
http://www.ccforum.com/ Critical care forum of critical care and emergency medicine includes updates on clinical advances in the treatment of SIRS.
http://www.aast.org American Association for the Surgery of Trauma website.
http://www.emedicine.com/emerg/topic533.htm A comprehensive review of SIRS and sepsis with references.

Initial Management of the Severely Injured Patient

17

03

Must know Must do

Must know
Causes of death in injured patients
Immediate resuscitation measures in injured patients
Initial assessment of injured patients
Neurological assessment
Secondary survey of injured patients
Principles underlying definitive care of injured patients

Must do
Attend accident and emergency departments
Observe initial management of severely injured patients
Observe emergency operation for major orthopaedic, soft tissue and organ trauma
Talk to paramedics who bring in severely injured patients

Introduction

As a result of the chronic inability of humans to live at peace amongst themselves, their desire to go faster and further, and the increasing use of and illicit trade in mind-altering substances, there has emerged a modern epidemic — trauma. In the western world you are more likely to die as a result of trauma than any other cause in the first four decades of life.

There is no doubt it would be preferable to prevent 'accidents' rather than deal with their often disastrous consequences but it is, and will remain, the responsibility of those who treat trauma victims within the 'golden hour' to ensure they have a clear understanding of the basic principles of resuscitation and a system that will not fail them in the acute situation.

The golden hour

'The golden hour' should not be taken as a literal 60 minutes, although the concept of a limited time period following injury where lives may be saved or lost is a valuable one. It has been documented that 30% of trauma deaths occurring in hospital might be prevented, the majority by early (within an hour) correction of hypoxia, replacement of circulating blood volume and arrest of continuing haemorrhage.

Although the trimodal distribution of death (Fig. 17.1) is now thought to be more of a continuum, examination of its original form allows us to see where our efforts will be beneficial. The first peak of death is immediate (within minutes). These injuries affect vital structures (brainstem, upper spinal cord, great vessels including the heart) and death is probably inevitable. The second peak of deaths occurs in the first few hours: a substantial proportion of these are hypoxic and hypovolaemic deaths. The third peak occurs some weeks after the initial insult, probably in the intensive care unit (ICU), with death often due to multiorgan failure, which may have its origins in the hypoxic hypovolaemic phase. While we can have no effect on the first peak, our actions in the 'golden hour' may have a profound influence on subsequent mortality and morbidity.

Preparation

Every hospital that receives severely injured patients must be prepared for that purpose. Some units are large enough to provide prehospital medical teams to support ambulance technicians and paramedics, while smaller emergency units may depend on summoning inpatient specialists to provide the initial reception of the patient on arrival at hospital. Whatever system prevails it is clear that each individual involved must know their role and that lines of communication are clearly established and understood.

The resuscitation room should be appropriately equipped and the equipment should be checked at the beginning of every shift. Although there may be time for briefing of staff while waiting for the patient, individual roles should have been allocated at an earlier stage. Team members should have received appropriate training, understand what is expected of them and wear adequate

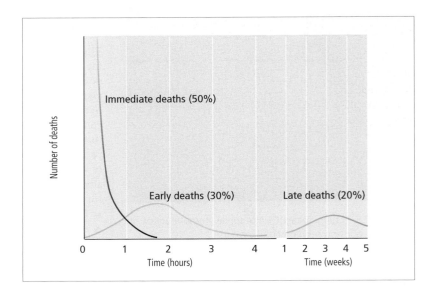

Figure 17.1 Trimodal distribution of death following trauma.

protective clothing. There should be a clear understanding of the dynamics of the team and the need to pass information to, and receive instruction from, the team leader.

Initial assessment

It is clear that a system requiring a detailed history and examination to be carried out before any treatment is instituted would be inappropriate for the severely injured patient. A different approach is required whereby vital functions are rapidly assessed and secured before treatment priorities are established. The process is known as initial assessment and can be divided into:
- primary survey and resuscitation;
- secondary survey;
- definitive care.

The importance of the primary survey cannot be overestimated. If life-threatening injuries are not identified and treated during this phase, then the quality of definitive care becomes irrelevant since the patient will not reach the operating theatre or the ICU.

Primary survey and resuscitation

The primary survey and resuscitation phases are grouped together because the two proceed simultaneously. If a life-threatening injury is uncovered, then it is dealt with immediately. It is essential that the correct sequence is followed, although given adequate personnel in the trauma team a number of assessments and activities can take place simultaneously. The elements of the primary survey are:

- airway and cervical spine control;
- breathing;
- circulation and haemorrhage control;
- disability/neurological impairment;
- exposure.

The first contact must include talking to the patient. If the patient responds verbally and sensibly, he or she has already conveyed reassuring information about the state of the airway, breathing and circulation.

Airway and cervical spine control

Patients who have been brought to hospital by ambulance and whose circumstances show the potential for cervical spine injury will almost certainly have had their spine immobilized. The initial approach to the patient should confirm that this is the case and that the equipment is correctly applied; this may have to be modified in the restless patient. Manual immobilization should be maintained until a semirigid collar, bolster splintage and tape or strapping is in place (Fig. 17.2). Airway management must proceed at the same time as the above, particularly if the patient has failed to provide a verbal response. Noisy respiration or evidence of trauma to the face or anterior neck should have raised awareness of a possible airway problem.

The initial measures to clear the airway involve anterior displacement of the mandible. This pulls the tongue musculature from the posterior pharyngeal wall. While either a chin lift or jaw thrust are acceptable, care must be taken that the neck remains unmoved. The opportunity should be taken to look inside the oral cavity and suction applied

03

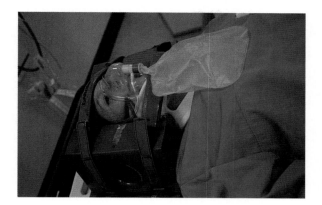

Figure 17.2 Trauma patient with spinal immobilization in place and receiving supplemental oxygen.

if there is evidence of blood or gastric contents. Dentures may also be removed. It is likely that if the airway requires manual methods to open it, then it will be jeopardized if manual support is withdrawn. There are a number of different options available at this stage, including oropharyngeal or nasopharyngeal airways. While these may be beneficial in the short term, they afford no protection for the lower airway. If there is doubt about the patient's ability to maintain a clear unsoiled airway or if there is an absent gag reflex, then a definitive airway should be secured. This is achieved by endotracheal intubation with or without the use of induction and neuromuscular blocking agents. This is a procedure that requires skill and practice and has an incidence of complications even in experienced hands. Unless an individual has the ability to intubate, then the airway should be maintained by other methods until skilled assistance arrives. Attempts by the inexperienced will almost certainly result in oesophageal intubation, which if unrecognized will prove fatal.

On rare occasions where there is severe disruption or swelling of the upper airway or it is not possible to intubate the trachea, a surgical airway is indicated. This is performed through the cricothyroid membrane. The area is relatively avascular and no significant structures are likely to be encountered during the procedure. A surgical cricothyroidotomy involves making an incision, forming an opening and then inserting a tube to maintain the opening. A needle cricothyroidotomy is performed by placing a cannula through the membrane, and attaching this to a high-flow oxygen source and a system for intermittently interrupting the gas flow.

Once the airway is secured, all injured patients should receive oxygen. If the patient is breathing spontaneously, oxygen should be given via a mask with a reservoir that will deliver approximately 80% oxygen (Fig. 17.2).

Breathing

The assessment of breathing should not commence until the airway has been secured. Attention should proceed downwards, with a check for tracheal deviation and inspection of neck veins before examination of all areas of the chest by inspection, palpation, percussion and auscultation. There are a number of traumatic conditions that present a threat to life in the immediate post-injury period and provided this logical and sequential approach to assessment of breathing and chest examination is adhered to, these will be uncovered as part of the primary survey. These conditions are:

- flail chest;
- open chest wound;
- massive haemothorax;
- tension pneumothorax;
- cardiac tamponade.

The first two conditions should be picked up on inspection; the others give rise to findings that will be elicited if the above assessment is carried out. As the examination progresses certain conditions will be excluded while the presence of others may be proven. Students should consider what examination findings will be present in each of these clinical presentations.

In tension pneumothorax, the intrathoracic pressure should be relieved by a needle thoracocentesis into the second intercostal space in the midclavicular line. A chest drain is required following the relief of pressure and this is positioned in the fifth intercostal space anterior to the midaxillary line. Massive haemothorax is treated with a chest drain inserted as above and cardiac tamponade may require a needle to be introduced into the pericardium from the xiphoid area. Open chest wounds can be covered with an occlusive dressing, which can function as a valve, but these patients must also have a chest drain inserted. Patients with flail chest require close observation and monitoring with supplemental oxygen and analgesia, although a proportion will require intubation and ventilation. The decision to carry this out at an early stage will be influenced by the severity of the underlying lung injury, the presence of other injuries and the premorbid state.

Other less immediately life-threatening chest injuries will be revealed following the secondary survey and chest X-ray. Provided the conditions above have been dealt with, the primary survey progresses to management of circulation.

Circulation and haemorrhage control

Provided the trauma team has adequate personnel, a number of tasks should occur simultaneously. An assessment of the patient's skin colour and 'feel' and the capillary

refill time should be carried out while monitoring is being attached to provide information on cardiac rate and rhythm, blood pressure and arterial oxygen saturation. If there is an identified source of bleeding, this should be controlled by direct pressure; with this in mind, staff should wear protective gloves and garments. While the classic signs of hypovolaemic shock (decreased systolic blood pressure and obvious tachycardia) are well known, these are late features that commonly only arise when at least one-third of the circulating blood volume is lost. The earlier, more subtle signs such as pallor, prolonged capillary refill and decreased pulse pressure must be sought so that early correction of blood loss can be guided.

Two large-bore cannulae should be inserted in large veins, the obvious site for these being the antecubital fossae. Also available is the femoral vein just below the inguinal ligament, with the artery as a palpable landmark just lateral. If direct peripheral percutaneous cannulation is difficult or not achieved, venous cut-down may be attempted. Insertion of a central line is also an option but requires skilled personnel. There is the potential for making a critical situation worse if further bleeding is caused or a pneumothorax created.

When vascular access is obtained, blood is drawn for routine haematological and biochemical analysis and cross-matching of blood. In the hypovolaemic patient, up to 2 L of warmed intravenous fluids (either colloids or crystalloids) are given while the patient is continually reassessed and monitored. The aim at this stage is to increase circulating volume so that the patient's remaining red cells receive a wider distribution. If the patient remains unstable, then more circulating red cells are required and blood should be administered; whether this is with type-specific or O-negative blood will be dictated by the patient's condition.

During the correction of hypovolaemia signs of adequate replacement of blood loss and stabilization are sought. If this takes some time or is not happening, the resuscitator must be aware that blood loss is large or likely to be continuing. If that blood loss is not external, then it must be internal in one of three areas: the thorax, the abdomen (intraperitoneal or extraperitoneal) or the pelvic girdle. If surgical colleagues have not already been involved, they must be summoned immediately. Even if relative stability has been achieved, blood loss may continue at a slower rate and the patient must be continually reassessed and closely monitored.

While hypovolaemia is the commonest type of 'shock' encountered in the trauma patient, it is not the only cause of a decrease in oxygen delivery to vital organs and tissues. Cardiogenic shock as a result of blunt or penetrating chest injury or myocardial infarction prior to an accident, neurogenic shock due to spinal cord injury, septic shock or even anaphylaxis may be present. These must be considered in all injured patients.

Disability

A basic assessment of neurological status is carried out as part of the primary survey. The AVPU scale, now widely used, describes the patient as:

● *A*lert
● Responding to *V*erbal stimuli
● Responding to *P*ainful stimuli
● *U*nresponsive.

As well as giving an indication of the patient's conscious level at any given moment, sequential assessment will indicate improvement or deterioration. In addition, the pupils are examined for size, reaction and any inequality. There is no purpose in carrying out even this basic neurological examination before hypoxia and hypovolaemia are corrected as any suboptimal response may be misinterpreted as a primary intracranial event rather than inadequate cerebral oxygenation.

A detailed examination with formal assessment using the Glasgow Coma Scale takes place after the primary survey is completed.

Exposure

Before the primary survey is complete, the patient must be fully exposed and viewed from both front and back. Once this inspection has been carried out the patient should be covered to prevent heat loss.

At this stage consideration is given to the insertion of a urinary catheter and gastric tube, provided there is no suspicion of urethral transection and rectal examination precedes passage of the catheter. Urinary output gives information on volume status and tissue perfusion, while a gastric tube allows decompression of the stomach and reduces the risk of aspiration. If there is the possibility of a base of skull fracture, the oral rather than the nasal route should be used. The presence of blood in urine or gastric aspirate indicates injury to the urinary or upper gastrointestinal tract and requires further investigation.

At the end of the primary survey, X-rays of chest, pelvis and lateral cervical spine should be obtained in patients who have sustained blunt trauma. Further X-rays are obtained in the secondary survey.

The primary survey is not complete until ABC has been secured and the patient is stable. This may not be achieved until the patient has undergone surgery to halt blood loss; if this is the case, the secondary survey should be carried out postoperatively. The importance of following the above system and repeating the primary survey in response to any deterioration in the patient's condition cannot be overstated.

03

Secondary survey

During this phase of initial assessment, a head-to-toe examination is carried out. Unless this is done in a methodical fashion, injuries will be missed. A full neurological examination is a necessity and the Glasgow Coma Score should be determined and sequentially recorded. Further investigations and involvement of other specialists is dictated by examination findings, and the gradual piecing together of clinical information will lead to a plan of action. In addition, information should be obtained about how the patient sustained their injuries and their past medical history.

If during the secondary survey there is any deterioration in the patient's clinical condition, the priority is to revert to the primary survey and reassess airway, breathing and circulation. The patient must be closely monitored throughout all activities and should not be moved or subjected to diagnostic procedures outside the resuscitation room until stabilized.

- Trauma is the leading cause of death up to the age of 40
- Major problems should be treated as they are identified
- Supplemental oxygen must be given to all trauma patients
- A cervical spine injury must be assumed in any patient with multiple injuries
- A lateral cervical spine X-ray must include the C7–T1 junction
- Most life-threatening chest injuries are treated by insertion of a tube or a needle and do not require surgery
- Hypotension and tachycardia may not be present until 30% of blood volume is lost
- The young and the elderly may have different physiological responses to injury
- The Glasgow Coma Scale has three parameters: eye opening, motor response and verbal response
- The severely injured patient must be constantly re-evaluated

Definitive care

Once the initial assessment has been carried out, a plan should be formulated for the patient's ongoing care. This may involve further investigation or transfer to the operating theatre for surgical intervention or to the ICU. There may be occasions when interhospital transfer is required. Before the patient leaves the resuscitation room a further re-evaluation should be carried out. Any equipment that might be required should be available in the form of a patient transfer kit. All patient records should be completed and the results of all investigations documented. X-rays and cross-matched blood should go with the patient. It is essential that there is clear communication between the referring and the receiving staff to ensure that all relevant information is passed on and that care is continuous. The mode of transport should be appropriate and the accompanying staff of the same competence as were involved in the resuscitation. It is useful to have a checklist in the resuscitation room to confirm that all the criteria for a successful transfer have been fulfilled.

Initial management of the severely injured patient at a glance

Definitions

Trauma: any injury caused by a mechanical or physical agent

The golden hour: a limited time period following injury when lives may be saved or lost depending on treatment given

The golden hour
30% of trauma deaths in hospital might be prevented by early (within an hour) treatment including:
- Correction of hypoxia
- Cessation of haemorrhage
- Restoration of circulating blood volume
  Death following injury is classically considered to have a trimodal distribution:
- Death immediately (50%): vital structures injured (brainstem, upper spinal cord, heart, great vessels)
- Death within a few hours (30%, reduced to 9% with good immediate care): mostly due to hypoxia and hypovolaemia; these are the preventable deaths
- Death weeks after injury (20%):
  (a) Multiorgan dysfunction syndrome secondary to systemic inflammatory response syndrome induced by injury (majority)
  (b) Raised intracranial pressure
  (c) Pulmonary embolism

Management
Preparation
- Good paramedical staff to recover patient, commence resuscitation and transport patient safely to hospital
- In hospital there should be a trained *team* with a recognized leader to deal with serious trauma. The team should comprise specialists in anaesthesia, orthopaedics, surgery and nursing

- Fully equipped resuscitation room; equipment must be checked daily
- Team members should wear protective clothing and roles and lines of communication should be clearly understood by all members

Assessment of the injured patient
Assessment and resuscitation are carried out simultaneously in a well-defined manner that has three elements:
- Primary survey and resuscitation
- Secondary survey
- Definitive care

Primary survey and resuscitation
The primary survey follows a logical sequence of assessments (ABCDE), and if a life-threatening problem is uncovered during this assessment it is dealt with immediately

A Airway and cervical spine control
- Ensure airway is clear and give O_2:
  (a) If patient talking freely, airway probably clear
  (b) Lift mandible anteriorly (make sure neck remains unmoved)
  (c) Suction oral cavity
  (d) Remove dentures
  (e) Place oropharyngeal or nasopharyngeal airway
  (f) Endotracheal intubation (no induction or muscle relaxant)
  (g) Cricothyroidotomy and minitracheostomy
- Ensure spine is immobilized:
  (a) Already immobilized by paramedics
  (b) Manual in-line immobilization
  (c) Semirigid collar, bolster splintage and strapping

B Breathing
Once airway is secure, check for tracheal deviation and neck veins and examine all areas of chest by inspection, palpation, percussion and auscultation. Look for and treat:
- Flail chest: intubation and positive-pressure ventilation
- Open chest wound: cover with occlusive dressing and insert chest drain
- Massive haemothorax: large-bore chest drain in fifth intercostal space, midaxillary line
- Tension pneumothorax: needle thoracocentesis in second intercostal space, midclavicular line, then chest drain
- Cardiac tamponade: needle aspiration via epigastric approach

C Circulation and haemorrhage control
- Assess skin colour and temperature while attaching pulse oximetry, blood pressure cuff and ECG leads
- Apply direct pressure to any identified bleeding source
- Insert two large-bore (size 14) cannulae in the antecubital fossae or the femoral vein
- Insert a central line (jugular or subclavian) if appropriately skilled personnel are available
- Draw and send blood for urgent cross-matching and baseline haematological and biochemical analysis
- If hypovolaemic give 2 L of warmed fluid (crystalloid or colloid)
- If still unstable after initial fluid give blood (type-specific or O-negative if patient's condition warrants)
- Look for internal bleeding: thorax, abdomen, pelvis
- Consider other causes of shock: cardiogenic, neurogenic, sepsis, anaphylaxis

D Disability
Basic assessment of neurological status:
A alert
V responding to verbal stimuli
P responding to painful stimuli
U unresponsive
Pupils are examined for size, reaction, inequality

E Exposure
- Patient must be fully exposed and viewed from the front and the back
At the end of the primary survey a urinary catheter and a nasogastric tube are placed and X-rays of chest, pelvis and lateral spine obtained. Once ABC has been secured and the patient is stable (which might be after an emergency laparotomy), a secondary survey can be carried out

Secondary survey
- Detailed head-to-toe examination of the patient
- Neurological examination and determination of Glasgow Coma Score
- 'Tubes and fingers in every orifice'
- Further investigation as warranted by findings
- Information regarding the injury
- Past medical history
- Continued monitoring of patient
- Revert to primary survey if patient becomes unstable

Definitive care
A clear plan should be formulated regarding patient's further care:
- Further investigation
- Transfer to operating theatre
- Transfer to ICU/HDU
- Interhospital transfer (e.g. to neurosurgical centre, burns unit)
  When transferring to another unit:
- Ensure that appropriate transport and equipment to transfer the patient safely is available
- Send all the documentation, X-rays and cross-matched blood with the patient
- Communicate with the receiving unit
- Remember the patient is the responsibility of the transferring unit until he or she physically reaches the receiving unit

03

Evidence-based medicine

American College of Surgeons Committee on Trauma (1997) *Advanced Trauma Life Support for Physicians.* American College of Surgeons, Chicago.

Driscoll, P., Gwinnutt, C., Le Duc Jimmerson, C. & Goodall, O. (1993) *Trauma Resuscitation: The Team Approach.* Macmillan, London.

Robertson, C. & Redmond, A. (1994) *The Management of Major Trauma.* Oxford University Press, Oxford.

Academic journals: *Journal of Trauma, Emergency Medicine Journal*

http://www.baem.org.uk   British Association of Accident and Emergency Medicine

http://www.amtrauma.org   American Trauma Society

Head Injury

18

Must know Must do

Must know

Differences between primary and secondary brain injury

Classification of head injuries

How to assess a patient with a head injury and to compute the Glasgow Coma Scale

Understand the pathophysiology of raised intracranial pressure and its management

Causes and treatment of intracranial haemorrhage

Classification of facial fractures

Must do

Follow a patient with a severe head injury, including stay in the intensive care unit

Follow a patient with a minor head injury

Examine computed tomographic scans showing the different types of intracranial haemorrhage

Talk to a professional involved in rehabilitation of a head injury patient

Introduction

More than 1 million patients present to UK emergency departments every year as a result of a head injury, which is thus one of the most common conditions seen in hospital. The causes of head injury are many and varied, although it is common to see 'head injury' as the only description of the incident in hospital notes. Every effort must be made to discover its underlying cause, paying particular attention to:

- the likely speed of impact;
- any events that may have led to the injury (e.g. epilepsy, subarachnoid haemorrhage, alcohol consumption);
- any events after its occurrence (e.g. vomiting, epilepsy, talking).

Pathology

The brain within the skull is liable to injury when deceleration occurs, i.e. when the neck flexes, extends or rotates. As the brain moves within the cranial cavity, it may strike sharp objects such as the sphenoid wing and the frontal and occipital poles. In addition, points where the brain is tethered, such as the foramen magnum and the cranial nerves, are also potential sites of injury. Shaking of the brain when the skull moves at high speed therefore results in haemorrhage in the subarachnoid space and at the frontal, temporal and occipital poles and in tearing of nerves and vessels. This damage can occur without the head being struck, for example in a high-speed car crash or in a fall from a height in which the body decelerates rapidly. It may also be associated with direct damage from a blow or a penetrating wound.

Primary damage

The impact from a direct blow to the head is absorbed by the scalp and the skull, which often fractures. The energy is then transmitted to the brain, damaging the tissue it strikes and causing brain movement within the skull. This damage occurring at the time of impact is called primary damage or concussion. Survival depends on the energy reaching the brain, which in turn depends on the velocity of impact (energy $= \frac{1}{2}m \times v^2$, where m is mass and v is velocity). Therefore hitting a brick wall at 70 mph (110 kph) will be fatal but a kick to the head playing rugby will probably not. Similarly, a shot from a high-velocity rifle will prove fatal but a shot from an air rifle will probably not. The mechanism is the same, the degree is different. Severe primary damage is characterized by coma from impact. The ability to talk, even a few simple words, after injury indicates that, whatever else may happen, the primary injury was not severe and the injury is theoretically survivable.

Secondary damage

Primary damage can be exacerbated by secondary damage (i.e. further insults to the damaged brain). These are important to understand as they can often be prevented and occasionally reversed, whereas nothing can be done about primary damage (except avoid the accident in the first place). The main secondary effects are respiratory complications, perfusion failure, intracranial haematoma, cerebral swelling, epilepsy, infection and hydrocephalus.

Respiratory complications

Hypoxia, hypercarbia or obstruction to breathing will have disastrous effects on a damaged brain and can worsen the clinical picture dramatically. Head-injured patients are especially prone to respiratory problems because of lack of central drive, airway obstruction, haemothorax or pneumothorax and/or aspiration pneumonia. It cannot be overemphasized that the most important aspect of care in the head-injured patient is care of the chest.

Perfusion failure

Perfusion failure will rapidly lead to cerebral ischaemia and a worsening of the clinical state. Head injury itself is rarely a cause of hypotension and other causes need to be investigated (e.g. ruptured spleen). Resuscitation must be rapid and patients with head injury accompanied by a systolic blood pressure of less than 60 mmHg for more than a few minutes rarely survive.

Intracranial haematomata

Intracerebral, subdural and extradural haematomata occur and can lead to deterioration following head injury.

Intracerebral and *acute subdural* haematomata are usually associated with severe primary injury and carry a bad prognosis. In contrast, *subacute subdural* and *extradural* haematomata are often associated with little or no primary injury and bleed slowly over a few hours or days; removal before intracranial pressure (ICP) is excessive can lead to complete recovery.

Cerebral swelling

If you sprain your ankle, it swells; if you injure your brain, it also swells. Because the brain is encased in a rigid box, cerebral swelling itself can cause damage by increasing ICP to levels at which cerebral perfusion fails. This leads to ischaemia, which in turn leads to more brain swelling and a further increase in ICP. This vicious circle tends to be worse in those with severe primary damage.

Epilepsy

Fits are common in head injury and cause ischaemia while they are occurring. They must be stopped rapidly using intravenous diazepam in small doses, followed by phenytoin or valproate to prevent recurrence.

Infection

The development of meningitis or an abscess after injury can reverse a good recovery and must be watched for and treated vigorously.

Hydrocephalus

An absorptive hydrocephalus can occur during recovery and may slow or reverse recovery; however, it is relieved by shunting.

Head injury at a glance

Definitions

Head injury: the process whereby direct or decelerating trauma to the head results in skull and brain damage

Primary brain injury: damage that occurs to the brain immediately as the result of the trauma

Secondary brain injury: damage that develops later as a result of complications

Epidemiology

Head injury is very common: 1 million patients each year present to accident and emergency departments in the UK with head injury and about 5000 patients die each year following head injuries

Pathophysiology
Direct blow
● May cause damage to the brain at the site of the blow (*coup injury*) or to the side opposite the blow when the brain moves within the skull and hits the opposite wall (*contrecoup injury*).

Rotation/deceleration
- Neck flexion, extension or rotation results in the brain striking bony points within the skull (e.g. the wing of the sphenoid bone)
- Severe rotation also causes shear injuries within the white matter of the brain and brainstem, causing axonal injury and intracerebral petechial haemorrhages

Crush
- Brain often remarkably spared direct injury unless severe (especially in children with elastic skulls)

Missiles
- Tend to cause loss of tissue with injury proportionate. Brain swelling less of a problem because the skull disruption automatically decompresses the brain
- Degree of primary brain injury is directly related to the amount of force applied to the head
- Secondary damage results from respiratory complications (*hypoxia, hypercarbia, airway obstruction*), hypovolaemic shock (head injury does not cause hypovolaemic shock: look for another cause), intracranial bleeding, cerebral oedema, epilepsy, infection, hydrocephalus

Clinical features
- History of direct trauma to head or deceleration
- Patient must be assessed fully for other injuries (full trauma survey)
- Level of consciousness determined by GCS: fully conscious, GCS = 15; deep coma, GCS = 3
- Pupillary inequalities or abnormal light reflex indicate intracranial haemorrhage
- Headache, nausea, vomiting, a falling pulse rate and rising blood pressure indicate cerebral oedema

Glasgow Coma Scale
Provides a simple method of monitoring global CNS function over a period rather than a precise index of brain injury at any one time

Investigations
- Skull X-ray: AP, lateral and Towne's views
- CT/MRI: show contusions, haematomata, hydrocephalus, cerebral oedema

Eye opening		Voice response		Best motor response	
Spontaneous	4	Alert and orientated	5	Obeys commands	6
To voice	3	Confused	4	Localizes pain	5
To pain	2	Inappropriate	3	Flexes to pain	4
No eye opening	1	Incomprehensible	2	Abnormal flexion to pain	3
		No voice response	1	Extends to pain	2
				No response to pain	1

Classification

There are four types of head injury.
- *Trivial*: little or no primary damage, no secondary effects.
- *Apparently trivial but potentially fatal*: little or no primary damage but underlying secondary effect (e.g. extradural haematoma).
- *Apparently hopeless but potentially salvageable*: moderate to severe but recoverable primary damage and avoidable or reversible secondary effects.
- *Hopeless*: overwhelming primary injury.

Management

The aims of management are to:
- recognize and treat those patients with apparently trivial but potentially fatal injuries at an early stage before brain damage occurs;
- recognize those with hopeless injuries and to withdraw treatment at an early stage;
- treat those with potentially salvageable severe injuries adequately and rapidly minimize secondary effects and allow complete or partial recovery.

Trivial head injury

If the patient is conscious, a history of the events leading up to the accident and subsequent to it is obtained. If the patient has sustained a period of unconsciousness, it is helpful to obtain corroboration of this from witnesses. Retrograde amnesia for events leading up to the accident is a significant factor in the history. The duration of unconsciousness and retrograde amnesia are indicative of the severity of the injury; if very transient and in the absence of other indications, they need not be a criterion for admission and further observation.

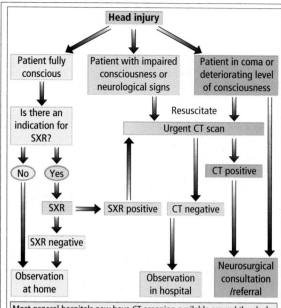

Most general hospitals now have CT scanning available around the clock. The ability to transfer images electronically from the general hospital to the neurosurgical unit means that a neurosurgical opinion on a patient can be obtained and a treatment plan decided on without having to transfer the patient to the neurosurgical unit. In many cases care can be given in the general hospital ICU with remote neurosurgical input. Only those patients that require burr holes, craniotomy or intracranial pressure monitoring need be transferred to the neurosurgical unit.

Table 18.1 Society of British Neurological Surgeons' guidelines for initial management of head injuries (1998).

Indications for skull radiography* after recent head injury
(A) Oriented patient
History of loss of consciousness or amnesia
Suspected penetrating injury
Cerebrospinal fluid or blood loss from the nose or ear
Scalp laceration (to bone or > 5 cm long), bruise or swelling
Violent mechanism of injury
Persistent headache or vomiting
In a child, fall from a significant height (which depends in part on the age of the child) and/or on to a hard surface; tense fontanelle, suspected non-accidental injury

(B) Patient with impaired consciousness or neurological signs
All patients, unless urgent CT is performed

Indications for admission to a general hospital
(A) Oriented patient
Skull fracture or suture diastasis
Persisting neurological symptoms or signs
Confusion or any other depression of the level of consciousness at the time of examination
Difficulty in assessing the patient (e.g. due to alcohol, young age, epilepsy, attempted suicide)
Inadequate social conditions or lack of responsible adult or relative
Coexistence of other medical conditions (e.g. coagulation disorders)

(B) All patients with impaired consciousness

Indications for urgent CT scanning and/or neurosurgical consultation
Coma, confusion or neurological signs persisting after resuscitation
Deteriorating consciousness or progressive neurological signs
Fractured skull in combination with:
    confusion or other impairment of consciousness
    epileptic seizure
    neurological symptoms or signs
Open injury with:
    depressed compound fracture of skull vault
    fractured base of skull
    penetrating injury
Unstable systemic state precluding transfer to neurosurgery
Diagnosis uncertain
Tense fontanelle or suture diastasis in a child

Indications for neurosurgical consultation after CT scanning
Abnormal CT scan
High- or mixed-density intracranial lesion
Midline shift
Obliteration of third ventricle
Relative dilatation of lateral ventricle(s)
Obliteration of basal cisterns
Intracranial air
Subarachnoid or intraventricular haemorrhage

CT scan normal but progress unsatisfactory

* Skull radiography is not necessary if CT is to be performed.

The questions to be asked include the following.
● Does this patient need a skull radiograph?
● Do I need to admit this patient to hospital?
● Do I need to refer this patient to a neurosurgeon?
These questions are easily answered by following guidelines laid down by a group of neurosurgeons under the auspices of the Kings Fund and first published by the Royal College of Surgeons in 1986. They have recently been updated and published in the *British Journal of Neurosurgery* (see Evidence-based medicine). The guidelines are shown in Table 18.1. The risk of a significant intracranial haematoma following head injury is 1 in 6000 among alert patients with no skull fracture, 1 in 120 among alert patients with a fracture and 1 in 4 among drowsy patients with a fracture.

An admitted patient needs regular neurological observation. Patients who suffered no loss of consciousness or who had no more than retrograde amnesia or brief loss of consciousness may be allowed home if they remain stable for 24 h. Simple fractures are not an indication for continued hospital stay. Compound fractures, i.e. associated with open scalp wounds or basal fractures with otorrhoea or rhinorrhoea, will need a more prolonged hospital stay.

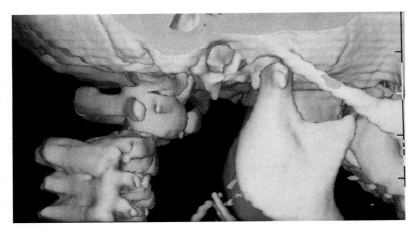

Figure 18.1 CT reconstruction of cervical spine C1/C2 fracture.

Traditionally prophylactic antibiotics have been given to these patients but are less commonly used nowadays. Persistent rhinorrhoea or otorrhoea requires surgical treatment to repair the skull base defect.

Following head injury, patients also need to be normally hydrated not fluid-restricted. An intravenous infusion should be used if the patient is too sleepy to drink or is vomiting.

The only other aspect of care is to deal carefully with any scalp wounds, remembering to:
- shave hair for at least 2 cm around the wound;
- remove foreign bodies;
- débride the skin edges;
- suture the scalp in a single layer, leaving stitches in for at least 7 days;
- use lidocaine with adrenaline to reduce bleeding.

Severe head injury

A person with a severe head injury will invariably arrive unconscious in the emergency department and the injury may be just one aspect of multiple trauma. It is important to stabilize the airway, breathing, circulation and exclude cervical fractures before concentrating on the head injury (Fig. 18.1). The management of head trauma is essentially the same whatever the cause and consists of intubation and ventilation, resuscitation, a thorough examination, imaging and decisions on treatment.

Intubation and ventilation

An unconscious patient with a head injury should be intubated to protect his or her airway. This usually involves sedation and paralysis and so ventilation will be required. There is no reason not to intubate. Traditional arguments against were that sedation prevented neurological monit-oring of any deterioration and that intubation put at risk an unstable cervical spine. Nowadays, patients with severe head injuries undergo computed tomography (CT) so the first reason is less applicable and, although the cervical spine is also commonly involved in fatal head injuries, it is rarely injured in a survivable head injury. Having intubated and ventilated the patient, ensure the chest is moving properly, that there is no haemothorax or pneumothorax, and check blood gases to ensure adequate oxygenation.

Resuscitation

Insert one or more large-bore cannulae, a central venous pressure line if necessary, and a urinary catheter. Make sure that the patient's blood pressure and pulse are normal and that he or she has a good urine output. If there is bleeding, find its source and stop it. Stop any fits with intravenous diazepam and phenytoin.

Assess the level of consciousness

Once the airway has been established and cardiovascular stability achieved, the next priority is to assess the level of consciousness. Response to verbal and painful stimuli provides a simple evaluation, although more objective analysis can be obtained by using the Glasgow Coma Scale (GCS) (Table 18.2). Any depression of consciousness is an indication for admission for observation. Confusion may arise if the patient has been taking alcohol or other drugs but this increases rather than diminishes the necessity for careful observation.

Thorough examination

A full neurological and general examination is conducted to establish the presence or absence of focal neurological

03

Table 18.2 Adult Glasgow Coma Scale.

	Score
Eye opening	
Spontaneous	4
To voice	3
To pain	2
No eye opening	1
Voice response	
Alert and orientated	5
Confused	4
Inappropriate	3
Incomprehensible	2
No voice response	1
Best motor response	
Obeys commands	6
Localizes pain	5
Flexes to pain	4
Abnormal flexion to pain	3
Extends to pain	2
No response to pain	1

03

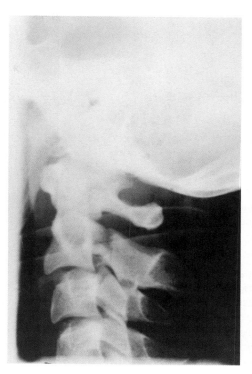

Figure 18.2 Radiograph of cervical spine showing fracture dislocation of the spine at C2/C3 level, so-called hangman's fracture.

signs. Pupillary inequalities or abnormal response to light are indicative of intracranial haemorrhage. A falling pulse rate and rising blood pressure are also indicative of increasing ICP. In the conscious patient, nausea and vomiting may suggest rising ICP due to bleeding. In the unconscious or semicomatose patient, vomiting may lead to aspiration into the air passage. Look at every part of the body. Pay particular attention to puncture wounds and the possibility of a spinal fracture.

Imaging

Accompanied by competent staff the patient should be imaged thoroughly. Skull (see Table 18.1), cervical spine (Fig. 18.2) and chest films are mandatory. If the patient has multiple injuries from a high-velocity injury, radiographs of the thoracic and lumbar spine, abdomen, pelvis and any suspected fractures should also be obtained. Nowadays, most multiple trauma patients will have CT of head, thorax and abdomen rather than radiography.

Treatment plan

There is no point in moving an unstable patient to another hospital for neurosurgery unless the instability is purely neurological. It is better to perform laparotomy or thoracotomy before transfer to stop bleeding and then to

move the patient afterwards. Even if the patient is being transferred, spend a few minutes closing wounds and splinting fractures. Even if these procedures are crudely performed, it is better than not doing them at all, and they can be tidied up later.

Frequently, patients who have suffered a serious head injury but do not have a neurosurgically remediable lesion (e.g. an extradural haematoma) are managed in the intensive care unit (ICU) of the admitting hospital. CT scanning is performed in the admitting hospital and the images are relayed electronically to the neurosurgical unit via an image link system. Based on the CT findings the neurosurgeons provide advice to the admitting hospital regarding treatment; these patients usually have some degree of cerebral oedema. Such a system reduces unnecessary transfers to the neurosurgical unit yet involves the neurosurgeons in the management of the patient's head injury. Modern minimally invasive ICP monitors (e.g. Codman, Micro-sensor, Cimino) are being increasingly used in district general hospitals without neurosurgical facilities by anaesthetists or other surgeons.

Transferring a neurosurgical patient

Some patients will have to be transferred to a neurosurgical unit for treatment. Indications for transfer include contusions, haematomata or hydrocephalus seen on CT scanning. Unconscious patients do not travel well and care must be taken to ensure the safest journey. The patient must be stable before the journey starts because treatment of a deteriorating patient in a moving ambulance or helicopter is very difficult. The most experienced doctor available, preferably an anaesthetist, and a nurse should travel with the patient. Lines and tubes must be well secured before setting out and adequate supplies of paralysing agents, sedatives and fluids must be taken.

Neurosurgical management

Neurosurgical management will depend on the CT findings. If a haematoma or hydrocephalus is evident, treatment with craniotomy or drainage is necessary. If no clots are shown, or after surgery, a decision must be made whether to ventilate the patient. Views differ about who should be ventilated; in the author's practice, patients with respiratory problems or those at risk of developing them are ventilated to prevent hypoxia.

Ventilation is also used along with sedation, diuretics and intermittent boluses of mannitol (an osmotic diuretic) to control ICP. Moderate hyperventilation works by reducing $P\text{co}_2$, which in turn reduces cerebral blood flow, although this mechanism tends to be effective for only 48–72 h. ICP monitoring is essential in these circumstances and is easily performed using a variety of methods. The most widely used technique is to insert a fine intraparenchymal wire sensor through a small twist-drill hole in the skull. The kits come prepacked with sensors and guarded drills and can be connected to the normal ICU monitoring systems (e.g. Codman, Micro-sensor, Cimino). Normal ICP is less than 10 mmHg. An ICP higher than 20 mmHg is worrying and needs to be treated; an ICP above 40 mmHg denotes severe problems and is rarely associated with a survivable injury. Note that these values apply to steady ICP levels. Coughing or chest physiotherapy may produce transient pressures of 60 mmHg or more but return to baseline when the stimulus stops.

The patient is ventilated with full nursing care (Table 18.3) for periods determined at the onset of ventilation (e.g. 48 or 72 h). After this period, if there are no problems and the ICP is low, sedation is stopped to allow the patient to waken. If the process runs smoothly, all well and good; however, if the patient becomes distressed or the ICP increases excessively, ventilation should be restarted for another set period. As the patient begins to wake, he or she

Table 18.3 Nursing the unconscious patient.

Elevate head 30°, turn patient frequently
Monitor arterial blood pressure, blood gases, ICP, serum sodium, glucose and osmolality
Endotracheal intubation, controlled ventilation
Control ICP: ventilation, intermittent boluses of mannitol
Enteral feeding, 2500 kcal/day (10 500 kJ/day)
Ulcer prophylaxis: proton pump inhibitors

ICP, intracranial pressure.

may be extubated as soon as the airway is secure. As soon as recovery begins, an active programme of physiotherapy, speech therapy and occupational therapy should be started to maximize rehabilitation.

Special problems

Children

Infants have a tendency to deteriorate dramatically after relatively minor injuries, becoming comatose and floppy and then recovering again rapidly (infant concussion syndrome). They also have a tendency to fit and may develop status epilepticus after minor trauma. Skull fracture and intracranial haematomata are less common in children than in adults. Non-accidental injury should always be borne in mind, especially when a child presents with acute subdural haematomata.

Depressed fracture

In a depressed fracture, bone is driven inwards and may penetrate the dura. CT scanning will show whether the dura is lacerated. Scalp lacerations over a depressed fracture must be closed urgently and the patient given antibiotics. He or she may then be transferred at leisure to a neurosurgical unit where a decision can be made regarding wound exploration. If there is a suspicion that the dura is lacerated, the fracture is always explored, although the indication for exploring a slightly depressed fracture is usually only cosmetic (Fig. 18.3).

Missile injuries

While high-velocity injuries are usually fatal, low-velocity injuries can be survivable. The patient should be resuscitated and transferred to neurosurgical care where the wound will invariably be explored to remove bone, skin and hair fragments. However, the missile itself can often be left undisturbed as the heat involved usually sterilizes it.

03

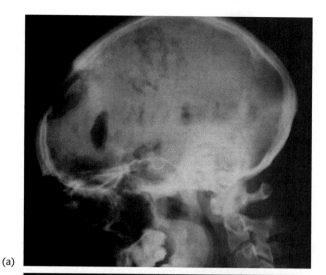

(a)

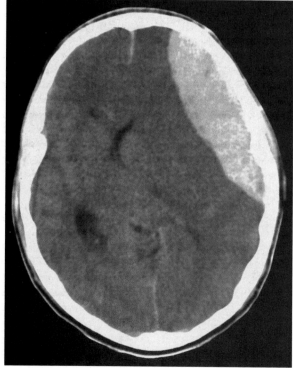

(b)

Figure 18.3 (a) Skull radiograph showing depressed fracture and air within the skull. (b) CT scan showing large extradural haematoma in the right frontal area with compression of the ventricles.

Basal fractures

Basal fractures may be accompanied by rhinorrhoea, periorbital haematoma and subconjunctival haemorrhage if the anterior cranial fossa is involved or otorrhoea if the middle cranial fossa is the site of injury. Subconjunctival haemorrhage, in which the blood tracks forwards from behind so that there is no posterior margin to the haematoma, is suggestive of anterior cranial fossa fracture. Direct injury to the eyeball produces a localized haematoma with visible margins. Periorbital bruising from direct injury is not confined by the orbicularis oculi, as is the case with intracranial (anterior fossa) injury.

Cerebrospinal fluid leak

Cerebrospinal fluid (CSF) leaks occur through the nose or ear, or silently down the back of the throat. Most clear up spontaneously within 2 weeks. Only a tiny percentage need surgical exploration to close the dural tear. Most neurosurgeons now advocate no treatment for CSF leaks, although traditionally broad-spectrum antibiotics (e.g. ampicillin and flucloxacillin) were given.

Cervical spine injury

Injury to the cervical spine may accompany a head injury and fractures and dislocations in this area are common after road traffic accidents and falls. If a patient complains of neck pain or weakness and/or numbness in the limbs or if there is loss of sphincter control, an injury to the cervical spine should be suspected. Precautions should be taken to prevent further damage. Extension and rotation of the neck should be prevented, preferably by halter traction. Skull callipers may be applied later. Sandbags may help prevent movement in the emergency situation. Collars should be maintained in position until radiography has been completed. Lateral radiographs of the cervical spine, including all seven cervical vertebrae, are done as soon as possible. Movement of the patient is especially hazardous: five individuals are needed to move the patient, keeping the head and neck immobile. Patients unconscious following a head injury should be assumed to have a cervical spine injury until proved otherwise by normal radiographs of the cervical spine (see Figs 18.1 & 18.2).

Other injuries

Even relatively minor head trauma can be complicated by injuries to the eyes, facial skeleton, ears and cranial nerves. The cooperation of ophthalmic, ear, nose and throat, plastic and faciomaxillary surgeons is therefore needed. More serious head injury may also be complicated by cervical

spine and carotid artery trauma, which may not be apparent at first.

Specific head injuries

Skull fractures

Skull vault

Skull vault fractures, if linear and closed, do not of themselves require treatment and are more an indication of the severity of the trauma: attention is concentrated on the associated brain injury. Penetrating injuries may cause compound fractures, with pieces of bone and foreign bodies penetrating the meninges or the brain itself. These obviously require careful exploration and wound toilet. Depressed skull fractures may lacerate meninges or brain and pressure from a depressed fracture may cause traumatic epilepsy.

Base of skull

Basal skull fractures have already been mentioned. They are usually anterior or middle cranial fossa fractures and may communicate with the exterior, with the risk of infection. Antibiotics should be given. In anterior cranial fossa fractures, persistent rhinorrhoea through the cribriform plate of the ethmoid may need formal repair.

Facial fractures

Nasal bone fracture

Nasal bone fractures are common and are accompanied by swelling, deformity and bleeding from the nose. Reduction is carried out to correct the deformity, although this is often delayed to allow resolution of swelling before reassessment for deformity. If there is dislocation of the septum, reduction is necessary to relieve the obstructed nasal passage.

Fracture of the zygoma

Direct injury, such as a blow on the neck, may produce a depressed fracture of the zygoma. There are three common fracture sites: the arch, the region of the infraorbital foramen and the frontomalar suture. On examination, circumorbital ecchymosis is evident, with the bruising confined to an area within the orbital rim. Subconjunctival haemorrhage is also present without a posterior border. The cheek appears flattened and a bony step can be felt in the infraorbital rim, with an area of paraesthesia below that in the distribution of the infraorbital nerve. Diplopia may occur and the patient may have unilateral epistaxis. Movement of the mandible may be restricted. Diplopia is usually temporary due to bruising of the inferior rectus and inferior oblique muscles. However, if there is entrapment of the muscles in the fracture, the diplopia may persist and an inability to elevate the affected eye can be demonstrated. Blowout fractures of the orbit are due to direct trauma to the eye, with collapse of the orbital floor into the antrum. Entrapment of the inferior extraocular muscles may cause persistent diplopia. Zygomatic arch fracture should be elevated via a temporal incision within 10 days of the injury. An orbital blowout fracture requires elevation through the antrum or may need prosthetic replacement.

Fractures of the maxilla

Le Fort has separated fractures of the maxilla into three categories (Fig. 18.4).

Le Fort I
This fracture traverses the lower nasal septum and maxillary antrum, separating the dentoalveolar portion of the

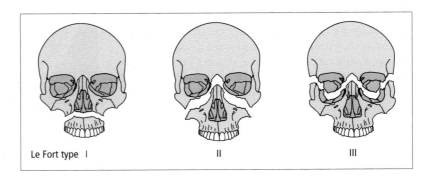

Figure 18.4 Le Fort classification of maxillary fractures.

Le Fort type   I   II   III

maxilla from the rest of the skull. The lower fragment is very mobile and dental occlusion is affected, giving an open bite.

Le Fort II

In this higher-level fracture, the line of the fracture extends through the nasal bones and medial portion of the orbit. Epistaxis and rhinorrhoea may occur. Periorbital bruising and subconjunctival haemorrhage are evident. Malocclusion is present with an anterior open bite.

Le Fort III

This is a very high fracture above the level of the zygomatic arch and including the whole maxilla, which is pushed downwards and backwards. There is extensive facial oedema and periorbital ecchymoses with subconjunctival haemorrhage. Involvement of the cribriform frontal sinuses in the line of the fracture gives rise to escape of CSF as rhinorrhoea.

Fractures of the mandible

These fractures often occur in two places, sometimes involving identical sites on both sides, sometimes involving quite different sites depending on the forces transmitted at the time of injury, e.g. a punch to the side of the jaw may cause a fracture through the premolar area on the side of the impact and a condylar fracture on the opposite side. The premolar area, angle of the jaw and the mandibular condyle are the common sites of fracture. The fracture is a compound fracture if it traverses a tooth socket, and the patient should accordingly be treated with antibiotics.

Clinically, a patient who sustains a mandibular fracture has a defective bite. Because of the upward pull of masseter and pterygoid muscles on the posterior fragment, posterior dental occlusion occurs prematurely and anterior dental occlusion cannot be achieved. The anterior fragment tends to be pulled downwards and backwards by the digastric muscles, thus further preventing occlusion. Damage to the inferior alveolar nerve may occur as it runs from mandibular to mental foramen, causing anaesthesia or paraesthesia in the area. A sublingual haematoma develops and a step may be felt in the line of the mandible.

Treatment is aimed at correcting the deranged dental occlusion and correcting the backward displacement of the horizontal ramus, which can obstruct the airway. As in any fracture, reduction with correct alignment of the fragments and immobilization achieves the desired result. Immobilization is achieved by fixing the upper and lower jaws together with cap splints or by direct wiring or plating of the fracture. Fixation for 4–6 weeks is usually required, except for unilateral condylar fractures where 10 days is deemed sufficient.

Intracranial haemorrhage

Extradural haemorrhage (Fig. 18.5 and Fig. 18.9)

An extradural haemorrhage is almost invariably caused by trauma, the only other cause being postoperative. Usually the patient has received a relatively minor blow that causes little primary brain damage but which fractures the skull. Beneath the fracture a dural vessel, most commonly the middle meningeal artery, is torn and the bleeding strips away the dura from the inner table of the skull. Bleeding is rapid and an enlarging haematoma collects between the skull and the dura mater and compresses the underlying brain. The signs of increased ICP quickly develop, with a rise in blood pressure, a fall in pulse rate, a dilated pupil and focal neurological signs, which include paresis or paralysis of the limbs on the opposite side and Jacksonian epilepsy. The patient gradually sinks into a coma and will die from raised ICP if no action is taken. Evacuation of the haematoma can only be carried out completely by craniotomy. Burr-holes placed over the clot to release some of it may be a life-saving procedure if there is not sufficient time for transfer to a neurosurgical unit, but if appropriate predictive care of a head injury has been carried out such heroics should not be neccessary. The possibility of an extradural haematoma should be considered in all those with a skull fracture (other than the fully alert patient) and a CT scan performed before further deterioration occurs.

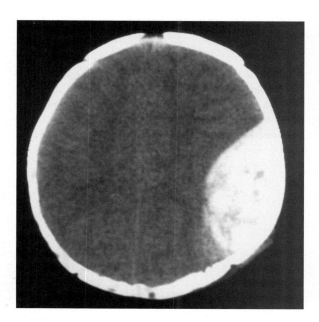

Figure 18.5 Extradural haematoma. CT scan showing large extradural haematoma in the left temporoparietal area with compression of the ventricles.

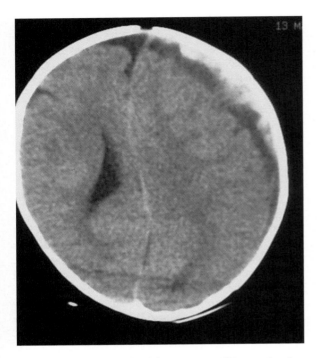

Figure 18.6 Acute subdural haematoma. CT scan showing large subdural haematoma in the left occipitoparietal area with compression of the left ventricles.

Acute subdural haematoma (Fig. 18.6 and Fig. 18.8)

Acute subdural haemorrhage carries a poor prognosis as it is usually associated with severe primary injury. This type of intracranial bleeding is more common than extradural haemorrhage and tends to occur in elderly patients who sustain a head injury because of the increased mobility of the brain within the skull cavity. It is accompanied by cerebral laceration or contusion and the patient tends to be in a confused or unconscious state from the time of the injury. The bleeding is the result of tearing of thin-walled veins traversing the space between the arachnoid and dura mater. The patient's neurological condition deteriorates progressively as the haematoma spreads. Even when the haematoma has been fully evacuated following craniotomy and incision of the dura mater, the patient may not fully recover because of the underlying brain injury or recovery may be slow.

Chronic subdural haematoma (Fig. 18.7)

Chronic subdural haemorrhage is seen in the elderly, alcoholics and infants. The most common cause in an infant is a non-accidental shaking injury and this possibility should always be considered. The condition develops over

03

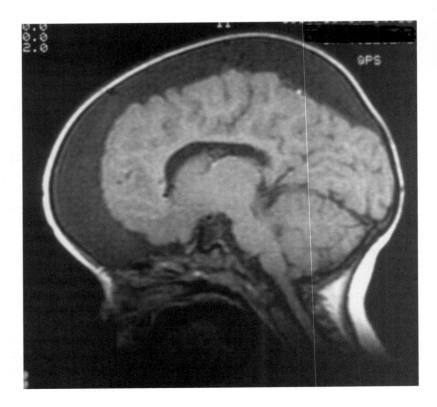

Figure 18.7 Chronic subdural haematoma. MRI scan showing large chronic subdural haematoma surrounding the cerebral cortex.

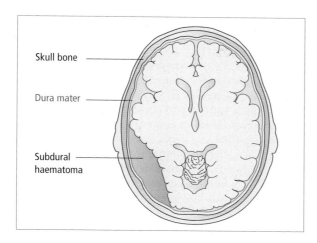

Figure 18.8 Subdural haematoma.

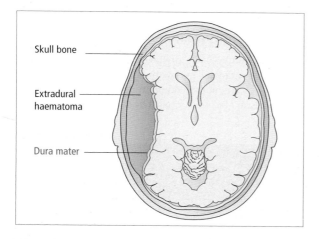

Figure 18.9 Extradural haematoma.

Table 18.4 Outcome from head injury related to Glasgow Coma Scale (GCS) on admission.

GCS on admission (maximum score 15)	Mortality (%)
15	1
8–12	5
< 8	40

Identification depends on a high index of suspicion if symptoms such as headache or mental confusion persist after a head injury, even a minor one. Clinical diagnosis can be confirmed by CT. Treatment is by evacuation of the clot at operation. Burr-holes are made and the dura, often stained greenish-blue by blood pigments from the underlying haematoma, is incised. The haematoma is usually watery and after release of fluid the subdural space is copiously irrigated.

Intracerebral haemorrhage

A patient with intracerebral haemorrhage following head injury is likely to be semicomatose or comatose on admission. The neurological deficit depends on the location and extent of the intracerebral bleeding. Much of the brain damage is irreversible, although further damage from surrounding cerebral oedema and ICP can be minimized by ensuring adequate oxygenation. The period of unconsciousness may be very prolonged, requiring attention to nutritional requirements and other problems such as decubitus calculi, bladder function and bed sores.

Outcome from head injury

Mortality

Survival after head injury depends largely on the level of consciousness on arrival in hospital, which reflects the severity of the primary injury. Those with a GCS score of 15/15 should have a mortality of no more than 1%; those scoring 8–12/15 have a mortality of 5%; those in actual coma on arrival with a score of 8 or less have a mortality of 40% (Table 18.4).

Morbidity

Only 30% of those in coma on arrival (GCS score < 8) will make a full recovery, while 20% will have some disability

a period of days or weeks so that the initial head injury, often minor, which precipitated the bleeding is forgotten. A small subdural bleed, often from a torn cortical vein, gradually enlarges over several days or weeks. The haematoma gradually enlarges, not as a result of continued bleeding but because of absorption by osmosis of CSF across the semipermeable membrane of the arachnoid into the clot. As the haematoma increases in size and the pressure rises, the patient exhibits drowsiness and confusion. Headache is not uncommon. Hemiplegia may develop. Pupillary changes develop late and are an indication of imminent cone formation. The symptoms may wax and wane depending on fluctuations in brain volume, which are dependent on changes in blood gases.

Table 18.5 Professionals involved in rehabilitation following head injury.

Nurses: help patients with all aspects of general healthcare

Doctors: coordinate medical care and prescribe medication as indicated

Physiotherapist: helps patients recover physical ability and competence

Occupational therapist: helps patients develop independence in carrying out everyday tasks

Clinical psychologist: assesses and provides help with patients' mental skills (memory, emotional problems)

Speech and language therapist: helps patients communicate more effectively using both the spoken and written word

Social worker: helps patient and families receive the practical help needed (e.g. benefits, accommodation, transport, housing)

but will be able to work and care for themselves; 10% will require full care, being severely disabled or in a persistent vegetative state.

Postconcussion syndrome

Those recovering from even minor trauma may take a long time to recuperate, suffering from the postconcussion syndrome. This is characterized by headaches, difficulty concentrating, dizziness and depression, and usually disappears after 3–6 months. Nothing can be offered except reassurance.

Other long-term effects

Survivors of more severe injuries often fail to return to their preinjury state as a result of personality change, memory impairment and depression, as well as any residual disability. Of those with a closed head injury, 5% develop epilepsy that may prevent return to work. Families are under great strain in these circumstances, and may benefit from contact with self-help groups such as Headway (http://www.headway.org.uk).

Rehabilitation after head injury

Rehabilitation aims to achieve the optimum levels of physical, cognitive and social competence for the patient followed by integration into the most suitable environment. A whole host of professionals are involved in rehabilitation of a patient following serious head injury but the patients who do best are those with very good family support (Table 18.5). Often patients will be admitted to a rehabilitation centre for a period of intensive assessment and therapy. The greatest visible progress occurs in the first 6 months, after which improvement is often more subtle and less obvious. It is important to bear in mind that progress does not stop after 2 years but may continue for 5, 10 or even more years after a head injury. Rehabilitation has two stages, the first being the formal intervention to improve the individual, and the second when the family and carers work to maintain that improvement.

Spinal injury

Spinal injury is about one-tenth as common as head injury but the basic pathology is the same. Such an injury may be complete (rendering the patient functionless below the level of the lesion) or incomplete (some function is preserved). Secondary effects, including hypoxia and perfusion failure, can also occur. However, compression of the cord is less common than compression of the brain following head injury. The causes of cord compression are bone fragments, haematomata and acute disc prolapses.

Management

Three fundamental questions must be answered when managing a spinal injury.
- At what level is the injury?
- Is the cord lesion complete or incomplete?
- Is the bony architecture stable or unstable?

Flaccid paraplegia with no preservation of sensation usually indicates a complete lesion. The sacral dermatomes are the most resistant to injury and sacral sparing is a cause for *slight* optimism. If the lesion is incomplete, every effort must be made to prevent deterioration. Thus the spine must be held in a stable position, hypoxia prevented and hypotension corrected. Early investigation with magnetic resonance imaging (MRI) will exclude cord compression.

If the bony architecture is displaced or thought to be unstable, it should be reduced and stabilized. When the cervical spine is injured this can be done with traction only, but if the thoracic and lumbar spines are involved open reduction may be required. It is now common to perform an early operative fixation with bone grafts and metal for both incomplete and complete lesions. This allows early mobilization, which in turn reduces the risk of chest complications and deep vein thrombosis. At the earliest opportunity the patient should be transferred to a spinal injuries unit.

03

Management of head injury at a glance

- Little can be done for primary brain injury apart from avoidance of head injury (seat-belts, helmets, don't drink and drive!)
- Prevention of secondary brain injury is the most important objective of head injury care

Trivial head injury
Patient is conscious, may be history of period of loss of consciousness. Retrograde amnesia for events prior to head injury is significant

Indications for skull X-ray
Oriented patient
- History of loss of consciousness or amnesia
- Suspected penetrating injury
- CSF or blood loss from the nose or ear
- Scalp laceration (to bone or > 5 cm long), bruise or swelling
- Violent mechanism of injury
- Persistent headache or vomiting
- In a child, fall from a significant height (depends in part on age of the child) and/or on to a hard surface; tense fontanelle, suspected non-accidental injury

Patient with impaired consciousness or neurological signs
- All patients, unless urgent CT is performed

Indications for admission
Oriented patient
- Skull fracture or suture diastasis
- Persisting neurological symptoms or signs
- Confusion or any other depression of the level of consciousness at the time of examination
- Difficulty in assessing the patient (e.g. due to alcohol, young age, epilepsy, attempted suicide)
- Inadequate social conditions or lack of responsible adult or relative
- Coexistence of other medical conditions (e.g. coagulation disorders)
All patients with impaired consciousness

Indications for urgent CT scanning ± neurosurgical consultation
- Coma, confusion or neurological signs persisting after resuscitation
- Deteriorating consciousness or progressive neurological signs
- Fractured skull in combination with:
  (a) Confusion or other impairment of consciousness
  (b) Epileptic seizure
  (c) Neurological symptoms or signs

- Open injury with:
  (a) Depressed compound fracture of skull vault
  (b) Fractured base of skull
  (c) Penetrating injury
- Unstable systemic state precluding transfer to neurosurgery
- Diagnosis uncertain
- Tense fontanelle or suture diastasis in a child

Indications for neurosurgical consultation after CT scanning
Abnormal CT scan
- High- or mixed-density intracranial lesion
- Midline shift
- Obliteration of third ventricle
- Relative dilatation of lateral ventricle(s)
- Obliteration of basal cisterns
- Intracranial air
- Subarachnoid or intraventricular haemorrhage
CT scan normal but progress unsatisfactory

Severe head injury
- Patient will arrive unconscious at hospital. Head injury may be part of a multiple trauma
- ABC: intubate and ventilate unconscious patients to protect airway and prevent secondary brain injury from hypoxia
- Resuscitate patient and look for other injuries, especially if the patient is in shock. Head injury may be accompanied by cervical spine injury and the neck must be protected by a cervical collar in these patients
- Treat life-threatening problems (e.g. ruptured spleen) and stabilize patient before transfer to neurosurgical unit. When transferring, ensure adequate medical supervision (anaesthetist + nurse) during transfer

Complications
Skull fractures
- Indicate severity of injury
- No specific treatment required unless compound, depressed or associated with chronic CSF loss (e.g. anterior cranial fossa basal skull fracture)

Raised ICP
- Trauma to the brain causes swelling but because the brain is encased in a rigid box (i.e. the skull) cerebral swelling results in raised ICP. If ICP rises above arterial blood pressure, cerebral perfusion fails. This leads to ischaemia, which in turn leads to more brain swelling and a further increase in ICP
- ICP tends to be worse in those with severe primary damage

• Ventilation is used with sedation, diuretics and intermittent boluses of mannitol (osmotic diuretic) to control ICP. Moderate hyperventilation reduces P_{CO_2}, which in turn reduces cerebral blood flow but this mechanism tends to be effective for only 48–72 h
• Monitoring is essential in patients with raised ICP:
    (a) Normal ICP < 10 mmHg
    (b) ICP > 20 mmHg is worrying and needs to be treated
    (c) ICP > 40 mmHg is severe and rarely associated with a survivable injury

Intracranial haemorrhage
• Extradural haemorrhage: tear in middle meningeal artery. Haematoma between skull and dura. Often a 'lucid interval' before signs of raised ICP ensue (falling pulse, rising blood pressure, ipsilateral pupillary dilatation, contralateral paresis or paralysis). Treatment is by evacuation of haematoma via burr-holes
• Acute subdural haemorrhage: tearing of veins between arachnoid and dura mater. Usually seen in elderly. Progressive neurological deterioration. Treatment is by evacuation via craniotomy but even then recovery may be incomplete
• Chronic subdural haematoma: tear in cortical vein. Haematoma enlarges slowly by absorption of CSF. Often the precipitating injury is trivial. Drowsiness and confusion, headache, hemiplegia. Treatment is by evacuation of the clot
• Intracerebral haemorrhage: haemorrhage into brain substance causes irreversible damage. Efforts are made to avoid secondary injury by ensuring adequate oxygenation and nutrition

Prognosis
Related to level of consciousness on arrival in hospital

GCS on admission	Mortality
15	1%
8–12	5%
< 8	40%

03

Evidence-based medicine

Dickinson, K., Bunn, F., Wentz, R., Edwards, P. & Roberts, I. (2000) Size and quality of randomised controlled trials in head injury: review of published studies. *Br Med J* **320**, 1308–11.
Society of British Neurological Surgeons (1998) Guidelines for the initial management of head injuries. *Br J Neurosurg* **12**, 349–52.

http://www.braintrauma.org/guideems.ns American Brain Trauma Foundation website with useful evidence-based guidelines for management of head injury.
http://www.crash.ucl.ac.uk/ CRASH investigators website describing update on corticosteroids in head injury trial.
http://www.rcsed.ac.uk/Journal/vol146–3/463000s.htm Modern management of head injuries.

Abdominal Trauma

19

Must know Must do

Must know

Causes, pathology, clinical features and principles of management of blunt and penetrating abdominal injuries

Core knowledge of liver, splenic and gastrointestinal injuries

Core knowledge of genitourinary injuries

Must do

Attend the accident and emergency department to witness initial management of patients with abdominal/genitourinary injuries

Observe peritoneal lavage

Observe a laparotomy for major intra-abdominal injury

Introduction

Injuries to the intra-abdominal organs may result from blunt, penetrating (stab, missile) or blast trauma. Blast injury is rare in civilian practice and is usually the result of explosions due to gas leaks or faulty household appliances. Penetrating trauma is not uncommon and results frequently from knife wounds and more rarely from bullet wounds. Blunt trauma remains one of the major public health problems, the vast majority of incidents being caused by road traffic accidents (RTAs). One-quarter of drivers involved in automobile accidents have a blood alcohol level exceeding 100 mg/L. Improved vehicle design, speed restrictions, road testing of old vehicles, breath analyser testing for alcohol and mandatory wearing of seat-belts have reduced the fatal injury rate. However, in the UK, 40 individuals still die every day from accidents, the vast majority being RTAs. In addition to the suffering, disfigurement and disability of the injured individual, trauma incurs a significant financial burden on the state.

Not only are valuable health service resources used to treat the patients initially but as most trauma victims are young active individuals at the height of their earning potential, there is a considerable loss of national revenue in lost years of productivity.

When plotted as a function of time after the accident/injury, the number of deaths caused by trauma forms three peaks (see Fig. 17.1, p. 189). The *first peak*, which accounts for 50% of all trauma-related deaths, consists of patients who die instantaneously or very soon after from irretrievable injuries. Few of these patients can be saved by healthcare systems, although the number of deaths is reduced by preventive measures such as legislation (alcohol testing, seat-belts, crash helmets for motorcycle and bike riders) and education.

The *second peak* occurs within hours of injury and accounts for 30% of trauma victims. These deaths, which are the result of severe blood loss, have been considerably reduced by the establishment of rapid transport from the scene of an accident to a hospital by a trauma system staffed by trained paramedics able to resuscitate the victim at the scene and during transport. The integration of pre-hospital care, rapid transport and immediate surgical treatment within a trauma system has been demonstrated to reduce preventable deaths due to trauma from 20–30% to around 9%.

The *third peak* of trauma deaths occurs days to weeks after injury and used to be caused by infection leading to multiple organ failure. Again, early resuscitation, rapid transport and aggressive hospital care has changed this late (infection) peak into three smaller peaks, the largest being due to uncontrollable intracranial hypertension following severe head injury. Sepsis now accounts for only 30% of late mortality (5% of all injury-related deaths), while the rest are caused by fatal pulmonary embolism.

Mechanism of injury

Traumatic injuries are due to the transfer of energy (mechanical, electrical, thermal, chemical) between the

environment and the patient. In civilian practice, the most common type of energy causing injury is kinetic energy, e.g. moving car, bullet, etc. Kinetic energy is expressed mathematically as half the mass of the object times its velocity squared ($KE = \frac{1}{2}m \times v^2$). Hence the speed of an object has a much greater impact on the energy product than its mass. This principle applies to all injuries, RTAs as well as high-velocity bullet injuries. The *impact force* is the total kinetic energy transferred to the victim at the point of impact. The impact force is also influenced by other factors, including the rate of onset of the energy, duration and direction of application. The resulting physical deformities (and hence injuries) of the victim's body produced by the impact force constitute the *strain*, which may be tensile (force acting along the longitudinal axis of victim) or shear (force acts perpendicular to the longitudinal axis of victim) or a combination of both. The tissues react to the impact force by a process of cavitation whereby layers or segments of tissue move rapidly away from the point of impact, creating an actual transitory cavity that collapses as the energy dissipates into the flesh. Temporary cavities are encountered in blunt trauma, where the effects of transitory cavitation is manifested as broken bones and soft-tissue disruption. A permanent cavity forms along the lines of an impact force that causes tearing or compression, leaving a permanent deformity in the affected tissues, e.g. penetrating trauma by knife or bullet.

Blunt trauma

Car occupant injuries

These are the most frequent type of injuries in most countries. The vast majority are caused by motor vehicle accidents (cars hitting each other, cars hitting an object, cars hitting pedestrians). When a car hits another object, there is rapid deceleration of both the car and its occupant. This translates into three rapid sequential collisions.
1 First collision: car hitting the object. Although the car stops, the occupant is still moving forward inside the car (at the same speed as the car was travelling).
2 Second collision: restraint devices or the interior of the car stops the occupant's forward movement.
3 Third collision: forward movement of the occupant's internal organs.

Factors that influence the severity of injury of the occupant include the following.
- Size of car: injury rate higher in occupants of smaller cars.
- Position of occupant within the car at the time of impact: related to risk of occupant hitting fixed structures within the car, e.g. steering wheel/column, windshield frame, etc.

- Occupant's body type: obese individuals have a lower incidence of facial and closed head injuries.
- Use and type of restraint device (seat-belts, airbags).
- Type of accident: rollover and ejection (worst), frontal (severe) and lateral (mild to severe).

Pedestrian injuries

The most common victims are children, the elderly and the inebriated. These severe multisystem injuries are caused by high kinetic energy transfer direct to the unprotected pedestrian from the moving car. There are three recognized impact sequences that contribute to these multisystem injuries. The first impact is caused by the bumper as it strikes the lower extremities of the victim (lower limb fractures). As the legs are displaced beneath the victim, the second impact occurs when the torso rolls up and hits the bonnet of the vehicle, causing abdominal, chest and spinal injuries. The momentum carries the victim forwards towards the windscreen of the car, with the potential for serious craniofacial, cervical spinal and cerebral injuries. The third impact occurs as the victim is thrown away from the car on to the ground. This distance can be considerable and depends on the speed of the car at initial contact. In general, the victim lands on one side of the body, causing additional injury to the extremities, head, spine, thorax and abdomen.

Children are usually struck anatomically higher than adults and thus sustain relatively fewer lower leg but more femur, pelvic, and torso injuries. As their mass is small, children may not be thrown clear of the vehicle and indeed are often dragged by the front of the vehicle or run over by the tyres.

Penetrating trauma

These injuries are caused by knives, firearms, impalement, etc. that separate and crush the tissues along the path of the penetrating object. Penetrating trauma is categorized by the energy level imparted by the source of injury:
- low-energy transfer (knife injuries, impalement following a fall);
- medium- to high-energy transfer (handguns, shotguns, rifles).

Because of the low energy transfer, knife injuries cause relatively little secondary damage. This is in sharp contrast to the significant secondary damage caused by bullet injuries. In the UK, knife injuries are often encountered at weekends, usually because of drunken brawls. Evaluation of knife wounds should always include a complete visual inspection of the victim in order to determine if there are additional stab wounds or associated injuries incurred from falling or attempts by the victim to defend/flee from

03

Table 19.1 Contents of the 'trauma' compartments of the abdomen.

Intrathoracic	True abdominal	Pelvic	Retroperitoneal
Diaphragm	Small and large intestine	Sigmoid colon	Kidney and ureters
Liver	Pregnant uterus	Rectum	Duodenum
Spleen	Distended urinary bladder	Small-bowel loops	Pancreas
Stomach		Bladder	Aorta
		Urethra	Inferior vena cava
		Ovaries and uterus	

the attacker. With prompt treatment, most victims survive knife wounds unless there is rapid exsanguination from a major artery or cardiac tamponade due to a stab wound of the heart. In general bullet injuries are much more serious and carry a high mortality. On inspection, there is always an entry wound but there may also be an exit wound. The trajectory of the bullet and the extent of cavitation (which depends on the velocity of the bullet) and fragmentation (shattering) determine the extent of the injury.

Surgical anatomy of abdominal injuries

In relation to trauma, the abdomen is divided into four components: intrathoracic, true abdominal, pelvic and retroperitoneal (Table 19.1).

• The intrathoracic abdomen is contained within the lower ribcage and includes the diaphragm, liver, spleen and stomach. All may be injured in blunt abdominal trauma but the spleen and liver are the most frequently affected organs and both present with evidence of internal haemorrhage.

• The true abdomen contains the small and large intestine, the urinary bladder (when distended) and the pregnant uterus. The clinical picture of these injuries is dominated by the development of peritonitis.

• The pelvic abdomen, which is surrounded by the bony pelvis, contains the rectosigmoid, urinary bladder, urethra, several loops of ileum and the female genital organs. Soft-tissue injuries often arise on a background of severe pelvic fractures, when the clinical picture is mixed with evidence of internal bleeding and the development of peritonitis.

• The retroperitoneal abdomen contains the kidneys and ureters, pancreas, the second and third parts of the duodenum and the great vessels (aorta and vena cava). Initially, physical findings may be minimal, although there is the ever-present risk of sudden vascular decompensation due to intra-abdominal rupture of a major retroperitoneal haematoma.

Management of trauma

History and examination

The initial management of all trauma patients is to ensure an adequate airway, arrest any bleeding and restore organ circulation. Assessment of injury depends on a detailed history of the trauma from the patient or witnesses and careful physical examination followed by haematological, urinary and radiological investigations. Investigation and management are carried out concurrently and the degree of initial investigation is determined by the stability of the patient.

The type and extent of trauma suffered by the patient determines the type of injuries he or she is likely to have sustained. The height of a fall and the manner of landing, the speed of the vehicle and the use of seatbelts, and type of penetrating injury are important facts to determine. The abdomen, pelvis and genitalia must be examined in detail. Generalized abdominal pain or tenderness may indicate a perforated viscus, free intraperitoneal blood or intraperitoneal urine. The presence of peritonism is an indication for peritoneal lavage and subsequent laparotomy if this is positive (see below). Contusions or subcutaneous haematomata may indicate deeper injuries to the pelvis or retroperitoneum. Rib fractures may be associated with splenic, hepatic or renal injuries, while pelvic fractures may be associated with bladder or urethral injuries. Perineal haematomata may be associated with urethral injuries. Blood at the external urinary meatus indicates a urethral injury unless proven otherwise. Gross or microscopic haematuria in a voided or catheter specimen suggests genitourinary tract injury and requires immediate assessment. The degree of haematuria does not correlate with the severity of the injury.

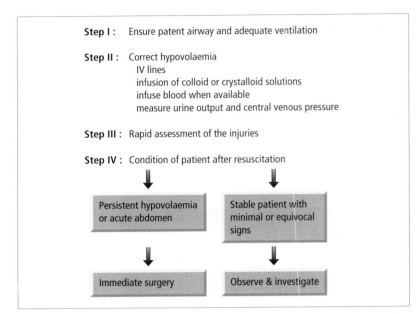

Step I :   Ensure patent airway and adequate ventilation

Step II :   Correct hypovolaemia
   IV lines
   infusion of colloid or crystalloid solutions
   infuse blood when available
   measure urine output and central venous pressure

Step III :   Rapid assessment of the injuries

Step IV :   Condition of patient after resuscitation

Persistent hypovolaemia or acute abdomen

Stable patient with minimal or equivocal signs

Immediate surgery

Observe & investigate

Figure 19.1 Management flow chart for unstable patients with abdominal injuries.

Resuscitation and urgent surgical intervention

The first priority in all injured patients is resuscitation, ensuring that there is an adequate airway, effective breathing and a circulation (see Chapters 11 and 12). The circulatory volume must be restored rapidly with crystalloid or colloid solutions while blood is being cross-matched and invasive monitoring should be established (urinary catheter and central venous line). Further management depends on the clinical picture, which is assessed as resuscitation proceeds.

The unstable patient

Immediate surgical intervention is essential if the patient is shocked and unstable and if positive signs indicative of an acute abdomen are present. The management flow chart of this clinical situation is outlined in Fig. 19.1.

Patients with massive intra-abdominal haemorrhage often reach the emergency room almost moribund, with profound hypotension, a grossly distended tense abdomen and blotchy lower limbs (due to compression of the iliac veins). They remain hypotensive (blood pressure < 80 mmHg, 10.6 kPa) despite rapid volume replacement. The cause is either a major vascular (vena cava, aorta, iliac artery) or organ (liver, spleen) injury, less commonly fracture of the pelvis. Laparotomy in these patients is usually fatal as the sudden decompression leads to the final fatal exsanguination. Some of these patients can be saved by prompt cross-clamping of the descending

thoracic aorta performed through a left anterolateral thoracotomy.

The stable patient

Frequent repeat clinical assessments are required in patients who are stable following resuscitation and in whom abdominal signs are equivocal. Either peritoneal lavage or laparoscopy is nowadays performed routinely in many centres, particularly when diagnosis is difficult. Computed tomography (CT) is preferred in the paediatric age group.

Peritoneal lavage

Peritoneal lavage is performed in patients with equivocal physical signs, depressed level of consciousness due to head injury or alcohol, spinal injury and penetrating trauma below the nipple line. It is performed by inserting a dialysis catheter under local anaesthetic into the peritoneal cavity through a small incision made in the midline below the umbilicus. A litre of saline or Ringer's lactate solution is infused over 5–10 min. The perfusate is then siphoned out by placing the empty perfusate bag below the level of the peritoneal cavity and the siphoned perfusate is examined. The criteria for a positive test are:

- red blood cells > 100×10^6/L;
- white blood cells > 500×10^3/L;
- amylase > 1100 U/L;
- the presence of bile, bacteria or food particles in the peritoneal effluent.

The overall diagnostic accuracy of percutaneous peritoneal lavage in the detection of intra-abdominal trauma

03

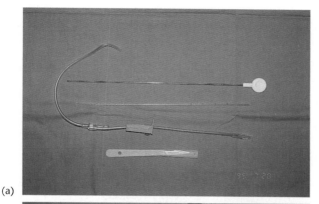

(a)

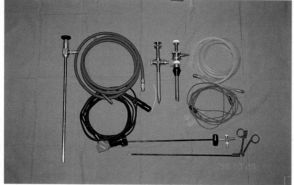

(b)

Figure 19.2 Equipment used for (a) peritoneal lavage and (b) diagnostic laparoscopy.

is 90%. One disadvantage of this test is the high false-positive rate (15–20%). This is due to minor lesions such as small lacerations that stop bleeding spontaneously by the time laparotomy is performed.

Laparoscopy

A small laparoscope (minilaparoscope) with an external diameter similar to that of the dialysis catheter can easily be inserted into the peritoneal cavity under intravenous sedation and local anaesthesia. Laparoscopy reliably excludes intra-abdominal injury and minor lacerations that do not require laparotomy (but which often yield a positive result with abdominal lavage). Laparoscopy is used in injured patients with stab wounds, a diminished level of consciousness and equivocal abdominal signs. The equipment used for peritoneal lavage and diagnostic laparoscopy is shown in Fig. 19.2.

Ultrasonography

Because haemoperitoneum and haematomata provide liquid–solid interfaces, high-resolution real-time ultrasonography is an extremely sensitive and accurate method of detecting intra-abdominal injury. Lesions of the liver and spleen give heterogeneous echo patterns. Haematomata appear as sonolucent (transparent) areas, while the presence of haemoperitoneum is identified by the crescent-moon sign.

Computed tomography

Contrast-enhanced CT scanning of the abdomen is used in the detection of abdominal injuries, provided the patient is haemodynamically stable (because the examination takes 45–60 min). It is particularly helpful in children where it is now the diagnostic procedure of choice. In children blunt abdominal injury, even with haemoperitoneum, is frequently treated non-operatively.

Angiography

The use of angiography in the diagnosis of solid organ damage has declined since the introduction of CT, although it is still valuable in confirming significant active bleeding and major disruption of the vascular pedicle of an organ. Isotope scintigraphy was used to detect injury to the solid organs but has been largely superseded by CT and ultrasound scanning of the abdomen.

Antibiotics in abdominal trauma

Systemic antibiotic therapy active against both aerobes and anaerobes is administered to patients with abdominal injuries. The risk factors for the development of infective complications are shock, missile/penetrating aetiology, colon injuries and old age. The most common causative aerobes are *Enterococcus*, *Escherichia coli* and *Klebsiella pneumoniae*, whereas the most commonly cultured anaerobes are *Bacteroides* species. The highest incidence of wound infection, abdominal abscess and mortality is encountered in colon injuries.

Specific intra-abdominal injuries

Hepatic injuries

Injuries to the liver include minor lacerations that do not require surgical treatment, moderately sized tears that need liver suture and severe injuries accompanied by extensive trauma to one or both lobes. The latter are life-threatening because of haemorrhage and other associated injuries. Stable patients with minor injuries are treated conservatively in the first instance. These patients are best followed up by serial CT scanning to monitor resorption of haemoperitoneum and the pattern of healing of intra-hepatic lesions. Surgical exploration is necessary if there is evidence of continued blood loss. Simple suture and resectional débridement are the two measures necessary

for the control of bleeding due to moderate injuries. In major injuries with bleeding from the vena cava or hepatic veins, the supracolic compartment of the abdomen is packed with gauze rolls. This usually controls the bleeding and allows resuscitation and transfer to a specialized hepatobiliary unit for definitive treatment.

Splenic injuries

Injuries to the spleen are usually sustained by blunt abdominal trauma: the spleen is the most commonly injured organ in RTAs. The injuries may consist of incomplete parenchymal tears, complete lacerations or severe fragmentation with avulsion of the hilar vessels. The clinical features of splenic injury include abdominal tenderness, hypotension and left lower rib fractures. Haematuria may be present. Left shoulder-tip pain, often stressed as a symptom of splenic injury, is in fact rare, being found in only 5% of patients. Associated chest injuries are very common. If in doubt, diagnosis can be confirmed by peritoneal lavage, minilaparoscopy or abdominal ultrasound scanning.

The surgical management of splenic injuries varies. The emphasis in recent years has been on splenic preservation whenever possible because of the risk of overwhelming postsplenectomy infection by encapsulated organisms, particularly *Streptococcus pneumoniae* (see box). In this respect, splenic preservation is particularly indicated in children, who are more at risk of this complication than adults. Indeed, some of these children are managed conservatively in the first instance, surgery being undertaken only if there is evidence of continued or renewed bleeding. In those patients who require surgery because of active bleeding, splenic preservation (by special suturing and haemostatic techniques) is attempted only if the condition of the patient is stable and there is no contamination of the peritoneal cavity. Otherwise splenectomy is performed, in which case autotransplantation of splenic slices in omental pouches may be undertaken in an attempt to preserve splenic immune function. All patients undergoing splenectomy should be vaccinated.

Diaphragmatic injuries

Injuries to the diaphragm are more commonly associated with abdominal than chest injuries. The majority follow RTAs but some are caused by crushing injuries and sharp localized blows such as a kick from a horse. The left diaphragm is more commonly injured than the right. Minor tears are usually unrecognized and may present several years later with incarcerated diaphragmatic hernia. More severe injuries are associated with multiple injuries and extensive herniation of the abdominal viscera — stomach,

Protection for patients following splenectomy

People who have had a splenectomy are at increased risk of severe infection. The risk is 12 times that expected in people with a normal spleen and children are the most vulnerable. The greatest period of risk is during the first 2 years after splenectomy but persists throughout life. The common pathogen is *Streptococcus pneumoniae*, although other bacteria with polysaccharide capsules (e.g. *Haemophilus influenzae*, *Neisseria meningitidis*) and malaria parasites also pose a significant risk. Patients who become infected may develop septicaemia with frightening speed and die within 24 h.

Prophylaxis against infection is achieved by vaccination and antibiotics. Three vaccines are now recommended: pneumococcal vaccine, *Haemophilus influenzae* type b (Hib) vaccine, and meningococcal groups A and C vaccine. These should be administered prior to or soon after splenectomy. Antibiotic prophylaxis should be given to children until the age of 16 and to everyone for 2 years following splenectomy (e.g. amoxicillin 500 mg daily for adults, 250 mg daily for children; patients allergic to penicillin should be given erythromycin). Some physicians recommend lifelong antibiotic prophylaxis. Asplenic patients travelling to endemic malarial areas should take antimalarial chemoprophylaxis as well as the usual physical precautions against mosquitoes, e.g. insect repellents, screens at night, etc.

colon, omentum, small bowel and spleen on the left side and liver on the right. Massive herniation leads to mediastinal shift, which causes respiratory distress and hypotension due to reduced cardiac output.

Pancreatoduodenal injuries

Injuries to the duodenum and head of the pancreas are more often due to penetrating than blunt abdominal trauma and usually give rise to peritonitis. Diagnosis is usually confirmed by peritoneal lavage, the effluent fluid from which will contain amylase. These are serious injuries and are accompanied by a high mortality and carry a substantial morbidity from the development of intra-abdominal sepsis and duodenal fistula. All these injuries require immediate surgical intervention. The vast majority of pancreatic fistulae that may complicate pancreatic injuries dry up within a short time following treatment with long-acting somatostatin, which has considerably simplified the management of this complication. Blunt injury to the upper abdomen may compress the pancreas against the vertebral column, leading to a traumatic pancreatitis and even transection.

03

Small intestinal injuries

Intestinal injury following blunt trauma may be due to:
- crushing of the intestinal loops between the vertebrae and anterior abdominal wall;
- a sudden increase in the intraluminal pressure of the bowel;
- tears at relatively fixed points along the attachment of the intestinal mesentery.

Preoperative diagnosis can be established by peritoneal lavage. The small bowel is more commonly injured than the colon. Associated intra-abdominal injury, most commonly spleen or liver, is present in 40% of patients. Early diagnosis and prompt surgical intervention are the most important determinants of a successful outcome. Surgical treatment consists of resection of devitalized segments of bowel and primary anastomosis. This is followed by thorough saline/antibiotic lavage of the peritoneal cavity before closure of the abdomen. The skin and subcutaneous tissues are left unsutured and packed with acriflavine gauze. Delayed primary suture is undertaken 5–7 days later.

Colonic injuries

Blunt injuries of the colon and rectum are rare and comprise 5% of all blunt injuries to the abdomen. As the force required to produce large-bowel injury needs to be considerable, associated injuries (e.g. liver, spleen, head, chest, pelvis and lower extremity) are common and adversely affect survival. The transverse colon is the most commonly affected segment, followed by the right colon, left colon and rectum. The lesions may consist of incomplete lacerations (seromuscular tears), haematoma or contusion with variable degrees of involvement of the adjacent mesentery or omentum, complete lacerations with faecal spillage and avulsion from the mesentery with full-thickness necrosis.

The operative management depends on the severity of the injury. Minor injuries are closed with primary suture with or without proximal defunctioning colostomy, depending on the extent of faecal contamination and colonic loading (Fig. 19.3a). Severe injuries are excised with exteriorization of the two ends as a proximal endcolostomy and distal mucous fistula (Fig. 19.3b). Restoration of continuity is performed a few months later. Following the definitive repair, a thorough peritoneal lavage with saline is necessary before closure. As with small-bowel injuries, the skin and subcutaneous tissues are left unsutured and packed; secondary suture is performed 5–7 days later.

Intra-abdominal genitourinary trauma

Approximately 10% of trauma patients seen in the accident and emergency department will have genitourinary trauma to a greater or lesser degree. Prior to catheter insertion the external urinary meatus must be examined for blood, which indicates the presence of urethral injury and the need for retrograde urethrography. When the catheter is passed, or if the patient voids spontaneously, the urine must be tested for blood immediately. Haematuria, gross or microscopic, is present in all patients with bladder or urethral injuries and in about 70% of patients with renal or ureteric injuries. In these patients retrograde cystography is performed prior to intravenous urography to rule out a bladder injury. Intravenous urography cannot reliably exclude a bladder injury.

Where a renal injury is suspected, intravenous contrast should be injected once the intravenous lines have been erected. A plain abdominal film at the time of injection and 5, 10 and 15 min after injection will establish the presence of two kidneys, their function and any injury present. Urinary extravasation on these films indicates the need for nephrotomograms. It is essential to establish the number of functioning kidneys prior to any surgical exploration. If a CT scan is readily available, a contrast study will more thoroughly delineate renal injury than an intravenous urogram. In the case of renal injury with urine extravasation that is being managed conservatively, ultrasonography is a useful means of follow-up.

Renal injuries

Injuries to the kidney are the most common injuries of the urinary system and account for approximately 50% of all genitourinary trauma. More than half these injuries involve patients under the age of 30 years and men are affected four times as frequently as women. Patients with renal abnormalities, such as hydronephrosis, are more prone to renal injury. Children are also at increased risk of renal injury because their kidneys are relatively larger than adults. Blunt trauma from RTAs and sporting mishaps account for 85% of renal injuries. Associated injury to other intra-abdominal organs occurs in approximately 40% of cases. Penetrating injury secondary to gunshot or stabbing occurs less frequently but associated organ injury occurs in approximately 80% of these patients. High-speed vehicle collisions may result in major renal vascular injury due to rapid deceleration.

Classification

Renal injuries are classified as minor, major and vascular.
- *Minor renal injury* (85% of all cases). These injuries consist of renal contusion (bruising), subcapsular

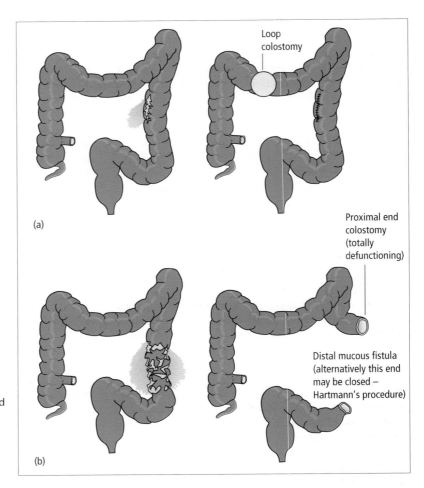

Figure 19.3 (a) Minor colonic injuries are closed with primary suture with or without proximal defunctioning colostomy depending on the extent of faecal soiling and colonic loading. (b) With major colonic injuries the injured colon is excised, the proximal end is exteriorized as an end-colostomy and the distal end exteriorized as a mucous fistula. Alternatively, the distal end may be closed and left intra-abdominally (Hartmann's procedure).

haematoma or superficial lacerations of the cortex not involving the collecting system. Most instances of blunt trauma result in minor renal injuries and approximately 40% of penetrating trauma produces similar injuries.

• *Major renal injury* (14% of all cases). These injuries consist of deep lacerations and are associated with retroperitoneal and perinephric haematomata. If the laceration extends into the collecting system, urine extravasation with a perirenal urine collection (urinoma) results. In their severest form, deep renal lacerations may cause complete disruption of the kidney.

• *Renal vascular injuries* (1% of all cases). These uncommon but very serious injuries are more frequent with penetrating trauma. They range from intimal tears with subsequent renal artery thrombosis to avulsion of segmental arteries or veins to partial or complete avulsion of the main renal pedicle.

Diagnosis

Any penetrating injury to the flank should be suspected of causing renal injury, whether or not haematuria is present. Blunt injury associated with flank or abdominal tenderness, fractured lower ribs or vertebral transverse bodies or producing haematuria should be suspected of causing renal injury. It is important to remember that haematuria, gross or microscopic, only occurs in 70% of renal injuries and that the degree of haematuria does not correlate with the severity of the injury. A rapid deceleration injury should be suspected as a potential cause of renal vascular injuries. Intravenous urography is the key to diagnosis and staging. If urine extravasation is noted, nephrotomograms are required to delineate the injury further. If the patient is stable, a contrast CT scan may be the investigation of choice because it gives a greater degree of detail with respect to the renal injury and may also be used to assess possible associated organ injuries. If there is non-visualization of a kidney, renal vascular injury must be suspected and urgent arteriography is indicated.

Treatment

Minor renal injuries are managed conservatively by strict bedrest, antibiotics and monitoring of vital signs, haematocrit and the injured kidney. Patients with major renal injuries pose difficult management questions. Most cases can be managed conservatively as described without significant problems. Indications for surgical intervention are:

- signs of continued blood loss, such as falling haematocrit;
- increasing size of retroperitoneal or perinephric haematoma; and
- marked urine extravasation or vascular injury.

The presence of associated organ injury may also call for surgical intervention. Smaller urinomas may be managed conservatively by frequent measurement using ultrasound examination to ensure decreasing size. Larger urinomas should be drained percutaneously and a urinoma that becomes infected (abscess) may require open surgical drainage. Where possible, exploration of renal injury due to blunt trauma should be avoided as the end-result is usually nephrectomy. In contrast, penetrating injuries almost always require surgical exploration.

Complications

- Bleeding at the time of injury and delayed bleeding within the first month of injury are important complications. In most cases bleeding ceases with conservative management but persistent bleeding or later heavy gross haematuria may require exploration.
- Urinomas and haematomas may result in fibrosis, leading to obstruction (hydronephrosis) that requires corrective surgery.
- Later complications include hypertension, arteriovenous fistula, hydronephrosis, stone formation, pyelonephritis and decreased function.

For these reasons, careful follow-up of patients following renal trauma is necessary. Thus patients should have an intravenous urogram 6 months after injury and blood pressure should be monitored regularly for a year after injury.

Ureteric injuries

Ureteric injuries are uncommon but their early recognition is critical as the nephrectomy rate may be as high as 30% when there is a delay in diagnosis. Most ureteric injuries are iatrogenic, with penetrating trauma the second most frequent cause. Blunt trauma to the ureter is rare and usually involves disruption of the ureteropelvic junction after rapid deceleration injuries; it occurs most frequently in children. The most common cause of iatrogenic injury is pelvic surgery, especially hysterectomy.

Surgery for carcinoma of the colon or rectum may be complicated by ureteric injury, especially where the tumour is extensive or ureteric abnormalities exist. Increasingly, endoscopic manipulation of stones with a basket or ureteroscope is being recognized as a potential cause of ureteral perforation or avulsion.

Injury to the ureter may be recognized at the time of surgery or may present in the postoperative period as pyrexia, flank or lower quadrant pain, paralytic ileus or fistula. Haematuria, gross or microscopic, is present in 90% of cases but diagnosis rests on intravenous urography. Delayed excretion with hydronephrosis is the most common finding, although extravasation may also be noted. A retrograde ureterogram will demonstrate the exact site of the obstruction or extravasation.

Early treatment is essential to preserve renal function. Stenting of ureteric repairs is an important determinant of a successful outcome. With prompt surgical intervention a satisfactory result can be anticipated in most cases.

Bladder injuries

Bladder injury complicates 10–15% of cases of fractured pelvis. About 90% of bladder injuries are associated with pelvic fractures. Other causes include direct trauma to the lower abdomen in a patient with a full bladder, iatrogenic injuries (endoscopy and pelvic surgery), penetrating injuries and, very rarely, spontaneous rupture of an overdistended bladder. When the pelvis is fractured, fragments may perforate the bladder, resulting in extravasation of urine into the retropubic space (extraperitoneal rupture). If the bladder is full and subjected to trauma, the perforation occurs at the weakest point, i.e. the dome, with extravasation of urine into the peritoneal cavity (intraperitoneal rupture).

Diagnosis

There is a history of blunt abdominal trauma. The patient may be unable to urinate or, if voiding occurs, gross or microscopic haematuria will be apparent. On examination the patient may be shocked due to blood loss from the pelvic fracture or associated organ injury. An acute abdomen, i.e. pain, tenderness and guarding progressing to rigidity, suggests a perforated viscus or free intraperitoneal blood or urine. Urine must be obtained for testing. If haematuria is present, a urethral or bladder injury is likely but associated renal injuries may also coexist. For this reason all patients with haematuria after trauma must have an intravenous urogram (see box below). If the patient has not voided spontaneously, a catheter is passed after inspecting the external urinary meatus for blood. If blood is present at the meatus, a retrograde urethrogram is necessary to rule out urethral injury before proceed-

Radiological investigations in the management of genitourinary trauma

Plain abdominal radiography

This will show fractures of the ribs or transverse processes of the vertebrae, indicating severe trauma and the possibility of associated renal injuries. Loss of renal outline, loss of psoas shadow, displacement of bowel gas suggesting a retroperitoneal haematoma or urinoma are other subtle manifestations of urinary tract injury. Pelvic fractures will also be seen and should raise the suspicion of bladder or urethral injuries.

Retrograde urethrogram

Prior to catheterization, the meatus should be inspected for blood. The presence of blood or difficulty in passing a catheter in the absence of blood at the meatus suggests a urethral injury and the need for a retrograde urethrogram. A size 12F Foley catheter is inserted to the fossa navicularis and the balloon inflated with 2–3 mL of water to hold the catheter in place; 20 mL of water-soluble contrast is gently injected through the catheter to outline the urethra.

Retrograde cystography

This is indicated in all patients with gross or microscopic haematuria on the voided or catheter specimen of urine. Contrast (300 mL) is infused through the catheter and a film of the distended bladder is taken. The bladder is allowed to drain by gravity and a second film is taken. This second picture is important in showing small amounts of extravasation.

Intravenous urography

After setting up the intravenous lines in a patient in whom renal injury is suspected, a bolus injection of contrast (2 mL/kg) is given. Films are taken at the time of injection and at 5-min intervals for 15–20 min. This investigation will establish the presence of two kidneys and their function. If urinary extravasation is present, nephrotomograms are necessary to delineate the degree of injury. If non-function is present, then absent perfusion due to a renal vascular injury must be considered and urgent arteriography is necessary.

Computed tomography

CT with intravenous contrast gives better definition of renal injuries than intravenous urography and may also assess the degree of associated intra-abdominal injuries. However, in the emergency situation intravenous urography suffices.

Ultrasonography

This investigation does not provide significant additional information in the immediate assessment of the trauma patient but it may be used to monitor patients with urinomas who are being managed conservatively.

ing. If this is normal, a cystogram is performed by infusing 300 mL of contrast medium and taking an X-ray. A further exposure is taken after gravity drainage of the contrast through the catheter as small perforations may be missed on the full film. A cystogram may reveal compression of the bladder by pelvic haematoma (teardrop bladder) on the first film, with extravasation on the drainage film in extraperitoneal rupture. In intraperitoneal rupture, contrast will outline the loops of bowel. In patients with intraperitoneal rupture, serum urea rises with a normal creatinine level due to reabsorption of urea across the peritoneum.

Recognition of bladder injury is important if mortality and morbidity are to be minimized. A fractured pelvis with haematuria indicates the need for urgent retrograde cystography.

Treatment

EXTRAPERITONEAL RUPTURE

Very minor ruptures in patients who do not have infected urine may be treated conservatively by catheter drainage alone. However, careful observation is necessary as the pelvic haematoma may become infected, resulting in a pelvic abscess. For the majority of cases, urgent surgical intervention is indicated. The bladder is repaired transvesically by suturing the tear with absorbable sutures, inserting suprapubic and urethral catheters and placing a drain in the retropubic space. A small hole may be made in the peritoneal cavity to inspect the intra-abdominal fluid. If this is blood-stained, full laparotomy is required. Drainage is maintained for 10 days to 2 weeks and a cystogram is performed prior to removal of the suprapubic catheter.

INTRAPERITONEAL RUPTURE

Intraperitoneal ruptures are approached transperitoneally. The bladder is drained by urethral and suprapubic catheters and the tear closed in layers with an absorbable suture. The peritoneal cavity is washed out to remove all urine and is also drained. Bladder integrity is checked by cystogram prior to removing the suprapubic catheter on the tenth postoperative day.

Penetrating abdominal trauma

Stab wounds

The vast majority of stab wounds are inflicted by knives and may be abdominal or thoracoabdominal. A high degree of suspicion of associated diaphragmatic laceration and pleuropulmonary injury is necessary in stab wounds of the upper abdomen as the direction of the knife thrust is often cephalad. Less commonly, stab wounds

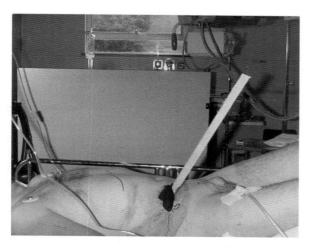

Figure 19.4 Impalement injury to the abdomen. Surprisingly, very little damage was caused by this injury. The caecum was perforated by the stake but the ureter and major vessels escaped injury. A right hemicolectomy was performed and the patient made an uneventful recovery.

occur from impalement injuries; these are usually serious and associated with major intra-abdominal trauma (Fig. 19.4).

The management of abdominal stab wounds has changed in recent years to selective surgical intervention, depending on the clinical state of the patient, the nature of the wound and the results of specific investigations, i.e. peritoneal lavage or laparoscopy. The indications for laparotomy following a stab wound include:

- hypovolaemic shock;
- peritonitis;
- evisceration of viscera or omentum through the wound;
- gastrointestinal bleeding;
- free air on abdominal films.

Wound exploration is useful in the management of the stable patient. In the absence of fascial penetration, wound toilet and primary suture are performed and the patient can usually be discharged from hospital after a short period of observation. Patients in whom wound exploration shows fascial penetration should have an abdominal lavage or laparoscopic examination followed by immediate laparotomy if indicated by the findings of either test.

Gunshot wounds

Gunshot wounds are considerably more serious than stab wounds and five times as lethal. Gunshot wounds to the abdomen are important because of their rising incidence worldwide and because they are accompanied by visceral injuries in the majority of cases. Some, especially those inflicted by high-velocity missiles, may not be initially accompanied by physical signs. For this reason all gunshot wounds of the abdomen should be explored, since physical examination and peritoneal lavage are unreliable in this situation. The propensity for visceral damage is directly related to the impact velocity and mass of the projectile. Thus, high-velocity missiles (usually from military weapons) impart a considerable amount of kinetic energy and produce extensive tissue damage, often remote from the site of injury. External contaminants are frequently introduced deep into the wounds caused by high-velocity missiles. Close-range use of the shotgun (favoured by bank robbers!) results in highly lethal injuries, with a reported mortality of 90% at a distance of less than 3 m.

Emergency laparotomy for abdominal injuries

This must not be delayed unduly, particularly if volume replacement proves difficult, suggesting significant active intra-abdominal bleeding. An adequate reserve of cross-matched blood must be available to cover the procedure. Adequate intravenous lines capable of rapid acceleration of inflow must be in place before the patient is anaesthetized. Muscle relaxation causes a further fall in blood pressure as the tamponade effect of the abdominal wall is diminished, and this effect is entirely lost as the surgeon opens the abdomen.

The operation is usually performed through a midline incision, as this can be readily extended from xiphoid to symphysis pubis and converted to a thoracoabdominal one when necessary. The first priority is control of haemorrhage. The next step concerns the operative treatment of hollow visceral injuries, especially those involving the colon, in order to minimize contamination. The abdominal exploration must be thorough, with a systematic inspection of all the quadrants and retroperitoneum (especially the second part of the duodenum) in order to avoid missed injuries. On completion, the peritoneal cavity is thoroughly lavaged with several litres of warm isotonic saline, especially in the presence of contamination from intestinal damage. Closure of the musculoaponeurotic layer of the abdominal wall is effected by absorbable monofilament material. The skin and subcutaneous tissues are left unsutured and the wound packed with acriflavine gauze if the peritoneal cavity has been contaminated by leakage of intestinal contents.

Pelvic genitourinary injuries

Urethral injuries

Urethral injuries are uncommon and usually occur in men in association with straddle injuries or pelvic fractures with disruption of the pelvic ring. Urethral injuries are rare in women.

Injuries to the bulbar urethra

These result from straddle injuries (e.g. falling astride a bicycle crossbar) or a direct kick to the perineum. Self-instrumentation or iatrogenic instrumentation may occasionally be responsible for injury to the bulbar urethra. These injuries vary from a simple contusion or bruise of the urethra to laceration. In addition to the history of direct trauma, bleeding from the urethra and perineal haematoma will be evident. No attempt should be made to pass a urethral catheter under any circumstances. A retrograde urethrogram is indicated to delineate the severity of the injury. If the urethra is intact (no extravasation), a urethral catheter may be passed. If extravasation is present on the retrograde urethrogram, a laceration of the bulbar urethra has occurred. A percutaneous suprapubic catheter may be inserted in those patients in whom bladder injury is not suspected. The catheter is left *in situ* for 3 weeks and a micturating cystourethrogram is performed prior to its removal to ensure resolution of the injury. A urethral stricture may develop subsequently at the site of injury.

If there is a possibility of associated bladder injury, then formal suprapubic cystostomy with inspection of the bladder and repair of any bladder laceration is necessary. Suprapubic drainage is maintained for 3 weeks and a voiding cystourethrogram performed prior to removal of the suprapubic catheter.

Injuries to the prostatomembranous urethra

Injuries to this portion of the urethra usually result from blunt trauma, which causes pelvic fractures with disruption of the pelvic ring. Because of the nature of the trauma, bladder injuries are often also present. Patients complain of lower abdominal pain and are unable to void. On examination urethral bleeding with a large, often palpable, pelvic haematoma will be noted. Rectal examination may reveal superior displacement of the prostate (gland impalpable) due to complete disruption of the membranous urethra. A urethral catheter should not be passed under any circumstances. A retrograde urethrogram is urgently indicated. Free extravasation of contrast into the perivesical space indicates complete disruption of the membranous urethra. Incomplete disruption, which is less common, manifests as minor extravasation with some contrast material passing into the bladder. A urinary catheter should not be passed in these cases as it may convert an incomplete disruption into a complete one.

The management of these injuries is somewhat controversial. However, most would agree that primary repair is a poor option because of the increased incidence of complications (stricture, impotence, incontinence) compared with delayed repair. Initial management consists of formal (i.e. operative) suprapubic cystostomy with inspection of the bladder for associated injuries. The suprapubic catheter is left *in situ* for 3 months, at which time a cystogram and urethrogram are performed to determine the extent of the resulting urethral stricture. The stricture is repaired by excision and anastomosis of the bulbar urethra to the apex of the prostate. This may be achieved through a perineal or transpubic approach. The suprapubic catheter is left *in situ* for a further month before repeating the radiological assessment of the urethra.

Using this management protocol, complications occur in a small percentage of patients. Stricture at the anastomosis site occurs in approximately 5% of patients and can be dealt with by urethrotomy. Impotence may occur in 10–15% of patients. Incontinence after repair is uncommon and usually resolves slowly. In contrast, primary repair is associated with strictures in about 50%, impotence in 50% and incontinence in 30% of patients.

Penile injuries

Most penile injuries result from accidents during sexual intercourse, resulting in a torn frenulum or fracture of the penile shaft. A torn frenulum presents as penile pain and bleeding after intercourse and is best dealt with by elongation of the frenulum (frenuloplasty). Penile fractures occur due to bending during sexual intercourse, resulting in a large and painful haematoma. Surgical correction of the tear in the tunica albuginea minimizes future penile deformity. Penetrating injuries and avulsion injuries occur much less frequently.

Scrotal and testicular injury

Blunt trauma to the scrotum may cause scrotal contusion alone or may also involve the testes. Abnormal testes, such as those with carcinoma, are more prone to trauma and this should be remembered when patients present with testicular injury after minimal trauma. In addition to the history of blunt trauma, examination will reveal a scrotal haematoma. Often the testis is impalpable and all such patients should have an urgent scrotal ultrasound. If ultrasonography confirms testicular injury, surgical exploration and repair are necessary. It is worthwhile noting that orchidectomy is a distinct possibility in these patients.

03

Abdominal trauma at a glance

Definitions

Kinetic energy (KE): the capacity of a body or system to do work that arises from its motion. It is expressed as $KE = \frac{1}{2}m \times v^2$, where m is mass and v is velocity. Hence the speed of an object has a greater impact on the energy produced than the mass

Impact force: the total kinetic energy transferred to the victim at the point of impact

Strain: the physical deformity of the victim's body produced by the impact force. There may be *direct deformity*, *tensile strain* (along longitudinal axis of victim) or *shear strain* (perpendicular to longitudinal axis of victim)

Cavitation: a process whereby a layer or segment of tissue moves rapidly away from the point of impact, creating an actual cavity that collapses quickly as the energy dissipates into the tissues

Motor vehicle injuries
- 40 people die every day in UK from accidents
- Majority are RTAs
- 25% have a blood alcohol level > 100 mg/L
- Most victims are young
- There is a huge financial cost in resuscitation, treatment, rehabilitation and lost years of productivity
- Pedestrian RTA victims are often children, the elderly, and the inebriated

Factors that influence severity of injury in RTAs
- Size of car: smaller is worse
- Position of victim in car
- Morphology of victim: more weight is better
- Use and type of restraint: three-point seat-belts, airbags
- Type of RTA:
  - (a) Lateral impact: least bad
  - (b) Frontal impact: bad
  - (c) Rollover and ejection: worst

Classification and surgical anatomy of abdominal injuries
Injuries may be:
- Blunt: most common injury in civilian life, mostly RTAs
- Penetrating:

(a) Low energy (knife): most survive with prompt treatment
(b) High energy (gun): mortality (generally high) depends on bullet velocity, fragmentation, and severity and site of injury

With respect to trauma, the abdomen is divided into four compartments:
- Intrathoracic abdomen: liver, spleen, diaphragm, stomach
- True abdomen: small and large intestine, pregnant uterus, distended bladder
- Pelvic abdomen: sigmoid colon, rectum, small bowel loops, bladder, urethra, ovaries and uterus
- Retroperitoneal space: kidneys and ureters, duodenum, pancreas, aorta, inferior vena cava

Management
1 Resuscitate patient and perform primary and secondary surveys as described in Chapter 17
2 Deal with abdominal injury:
  - (a) Unstable patient: surgery
  - (b) Stable patient: ultrasound, CT, peritoneal lavage, diagnostic laparoscopy, then surgery if indicated
3 Antibiotics: give aerobic and anaerobic cover

Peritoneal lavage
Indications
- Equivocal physical signs
- Depressed level of consciousness
- Spinal injury
- Penetrating trauma below nipple line

Technique
- Under local anaesthetic aseptically, insert dialysis catheter into peritoneal cavity in midline below umbilicus
- Infuse 1 L Ringer's lactate solution and siphon out after 5–10 min
- Positive if:
  - (a) red blood cells > 100×10^6/L;
  - (b) white blood cells > 500×10^3/L;
  - (c) amylase > 1100 U/L;
  - (d) presence of bile, bacteria or food particles in peritoneal effluent

Specific injuries

Site of injury (usual mechanism of injury)	Type of injury	Treatment
Liver (blunt)	Minor laceration Moderate-sized tears Severe injury	Observe, serial CT, surgery if evidence of continued bleeding Laparotomy, liver suture, resectional débridement Laparotomy, 'packing', refer to hepatobiliary unit
Spleen (blunt)	Incomplete parenchymal tears Lacerations Fragmentation	Conservative management, especially in children Splenic suturing and preservation if possible Splenectomy, vaccination against *S. pneumoniae* and *H. influenzae*
Diaphragm (blunt)	Traumatic rupture, usually left side	Early: laparotomy, reduce abdominal contents from chest and repair Late: presents as diaphragmatic hernia. Reduce and repair defect in diaphragm
Pancreas/duodenum (penetrating)	Blunt injury may fracture body of pancreas	Immediate surgery. May get duodenal or pancreatic fistula (treat with somatostatin). Very serious injuries with high mortality
Small intestine (blunt)	Crushing, tear from raised intraluminal pressure, tears at fixed points	Immediate surgery. Associated injury (spleen) in 40%. Resection of devitalized bowel with primary anastomosis. Stop mesenteric haemorrhage. Peritoneal lavage
Colon (rare, blunt and penetrating)	Minor injury Major injury	Immediate surgery. Primary closure ± proximal defunctioning colostomy/ileostomy. Peritoneal lavage Excision and exteriorization of two ends with reanastomosis at ~3 months
Kidney (blunt)	Minor injury (85%) Major injury (14%) Vascular (1%)	Conservative Conservative initially. Surgery only if continued blood loss, increasing haematoma, urine extravasation or vascular injury
Ureter (penetrating)	Usually iatrogenic (e.g. surgery for colorectal cancer)	If recognized immediately: repair with stenting (e.g. over 'Double-J' stent) If late diagnosis: attempt repair but high nephrectomy rate (30%)
Bladder (blunt) ± fractured pelvis	Extraperitoneal rupture Intraperitoneal rupture	Surgery and repair of bladder (absorbable sutures) + suprapubic and urinary catheters for ~14 days. Cystogram prior to catheter removal
Urethra (blunt)	Bulbar urethra ('saddle injury') Prostatomembranous urethra (fractured pelvic ring)	Bleeding from urethra/perineal haematoma. Immediate retrograde urethrogram: no extravasation, pass urinary catheter; extravasation, insert suprapubic catheter for 3 weeks. May develop urethral stricture ± Bladder injury. Per rectum examination reveals upward displacement of prostate. Retrograde urethrogram. Cystostomy + suprapubic catheter for 3 months
Scrotum and testis (blunt)	Abnormal testes more prone to injury	Scrotal ultrasound: if testicular injury, explore and repair Orchidectomy sometimes required
Penis (blunt, during sexual activity)	Torn frenulum Fractured shaft	Frenuloplasty Surgical repair of tear in tunica albuginea

03

Chest Trauma

Must know Must do

Must know

How to perform a primary survey of patients with chest injuries

How to interpret a chest X-ray performed for suspected trauma

Clinical features of major life-threatening chest injuries

How to detect respiratory distress, pneumothorax and haemopneumothorax

Indications for emergency thoracotomy for chest injuries

Must do

See patients with fractured ribs

Observe and follow a patient with severe chest injuries

Observe the insertion of an apical chest drain for pneumothorax

Observe the insertion of a basal chest drain for haemothorax

Introduction

Chest injuries are common in civilian life, although the overall mortality is usually less than 10%. Many of the patients who die following thoracic trauma do so after reaching hospital, in the so-called 'golden hour' described in the advanced trauma life support (ATLS) guidelines, indicating that the majority of chest problems are under the treatable umbrella of most doctors. Moreover, less than 15% of chest injuries end up requiring a thoracotomy, with most being managed in the emergency department and on the ward.

When considering trauma to the chest it is important to remember the anatomical structures present and how they could be damaged. Hence, viscera such as the lungs, heart and great vessels are at risk if the natural barrier of the ribcage is insufficient to prevent injury. In general, trauma to the chest can be considered to be either of the blunt type or the penetrating type. It is also important to remember that injuries to the chest can occur secondary to other traumatic processes and could significantly impair breathing. The best example of this is after severe burns to the chest, causing an encircling eschar that impairs the respiratory excursions of the thoracic cage. In both the blunt and penetrating types of chest trauma the forces causing the trauma can be either low velocity or high velocity. It is obvious therefore that the mechanism of injury is important because it determines the extent and type of damage sustained. It should also be recognized that the mechanisms that cause injury to the chest are identical to those that cause injuries to the abdomen, and frequently patients with thoracic injuries also have abdominal involvement. An important example of this is a rib fracture on the left side that leads to splenic laceration. It must also be remembered that if a patient has been stabbed in the upper abdomen with a knife, frequently the upstroke of the attacker leads to diaphragmatic and thoracic injury despite an abdominal entry.

The problems caused by thoracic trauma relate to the disruption of adequate gas exchange, leading to hypoxia, hypercarbia and acidosis. Other problems relate to shock secondary to disruption of major viscera in the chest.

Types of chest injury

As with all trauma, chest trauma should be managed according to the ATLS guidelines, which dictate that airway, breathing and circulation are examined sequentially, followed by disability and exposure of the patient. Following this primary survey and resuscitation of vital functions, a more detailed examination of the chest can occur followed by definitive care. It is therefore pertinent to divide the types of chest trauma into those encountered during the primary survey and those encountered during the secondary survey. The full spectrum of thoracic injuries is outlined in Table 20.1.

Primary survey chest injuries

Many of the problems that occur with trauma patients are secondary to thoracic cage trauma, the simplest example of which is fracture of a rib. The most common fractures are those of the lower ribs, usually the fifth to the ninth. Fractures of the lower ribs have significance because they

Table 20.1 Spectrum of thoracic trauma.

Chest wall trauma
Fractured ribs
Flail chest
Fractured sternum

Lungs and pleura
Simple pneumothorax
Tension pneumothorax
Haemothorax
Pulmonary contusion
Pulmonary laceration
Tracheobronchial disruption

Cardiovascular injuries
Cardiac trauma
Aortic disruption

Diaphragmatic injuries

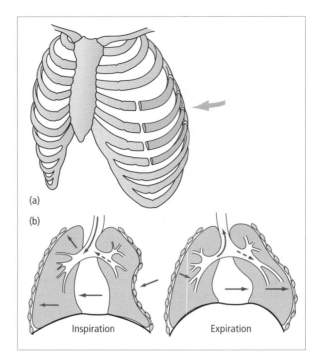

(a)

(b)

Inspiration   Expiration

Figure 20.1 (a) Rib fractures leading to the development of a flail segment with paradoxical movement. (b) Paradoxical respiration can lead to embarrassment of gaseous exchange.

03

can lacerate upper intra-abdominal viscera. It is also important to note that fractures of the upper four ribs, particularly the first rib, are indicative of extremely high-velocity trauma, as these ribs do not usually fracture because of their short, stout anatomy. Fractured ribs can also puncture the pleura and even the lung substance itself to cause a pneumothorax (see later). In more severe thoracic cage trauma, two or more consecutive ribs can be fractured in two or more places; this is the definition of a flail segment. A flail segment compromises a patient's breathing because the fractured segment undergoes paradoxical movement on inspiration (segment moves inwards rather than outwards) and hence impedes ventilation of the ipsilateral lung (Fig. 20.1a,b). Invariably, the degree of trauma causing a flail segment is likely to lead to underlying lung contusion and even laceration.

The consequences of rib fractures are treated individually. A simple rib fracture itself requires no specific treatment other than adequate analgesia. However, flail segments require specific therapy as well as adequate analgesia. This involves strapping of the segments and even positive pressure ventilation to compensate for poor oxygenation and to aid healing of the chest.

Finally, the anterior thoracic wall can also undergo severe trauma when the sternum is fractured. The mechanism of injury is usually a severe impact on a solid structure, the most common example being a collision where a driver of a motor vehicle is thrown onto the steering column. As one can imagine, a fracture of the sternum produces intense, deep pain. However, it is the risk of injury to the mediastinum that causes the greatest concern. Patients with sternal fractures should always be admitted and observed, and electrocardiography (ECG)

performed to look for electrical abnormalities. Cardiac enzymes should also be measured to ensure the myocardium has not sustained significant damage.

Pneumothorax

A pneumothorax is defined as air entering the pleural cavity secondary to trauma (Fig. 20.2). It is the most common pleural-related problem that any doctor is likely to encounter in practice. Many pneumothoraces are caused by trauma, although it should be remembered that they can occur in association with other diseases, e.g. bullous disease of the lung secondary to emphysema. The entrance of air into the pleural cavity leads to the collapse of the lung on that side. Pneumothoraces may be caused by fractures of the ribs secondary to blunt trauma or by a penetrating injury (e.g. a knife). In general, a pneumothorax can be either a tension pneumothorax or a simple pneumothorax.

A tension pneumothorax develops when a penetrating injury of the chest allows air from the external environment to enter the pleural cavity but not leave, the wound acting as a one-way valve. Eventually the accumulation of air in the pleural cavity displaces the mediastinum to the opposite side, thereby decreasing venous return and leading

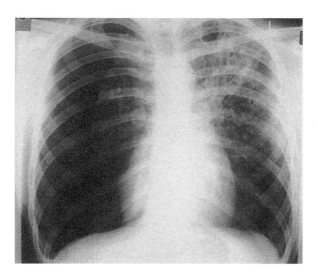

Figure 20.2 Chest X-ray showing a simple pneumothorax on the right and a lung contusion on the left.

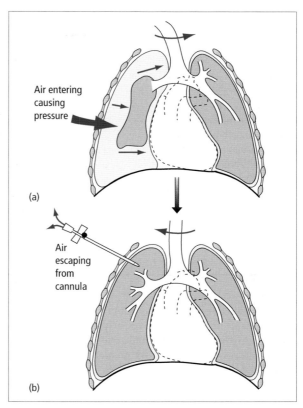

Air entering causing pressure

(a)

Air escaping from cannula

(b)

Figure 20.3 (a) The mediastinal shift that occurs due to a tension pneumothorax. (b) Release of tension pneumothorax after insertion of a cannula into the right second intercostal space.

to cardiac arrest that shows signs of electromechanical dissociation (Fig. 20.3a). A tension pneumothorax should be recognized at the time of the primary survey. The patient is typically short of breath and the trachea is displaced towards the side opposite the injury. The chest on the injured side also fails to expand and is hyperresonant to percussion. If, together with these findings, breath sounds are absent on the injured side, the patient should not proceed to chest X-ray. Immediate management is to relieve the build-up of air in the pleural cavity by decompression. A large-bore needle is inserted into the second intercostal space in the midaxillary line on the affected side. Successful decompression is heralded by a rush of air through the needle after insertion (Fig. 20.3b). This converts a tension pneumothorax into a simple pneumothorax.

Simple pneumothoraces are those where there is a defect in the chest wall that allows air to enter and leave the pleural cavity, causing the lung to collapse. However, because air does not accumulate in the pleural cavity there is no deviation of the mediastinum as seen in a tension pneumothorax. The initial management of an open pneumothorax is prompt closure of the defect with a sterile occlusive dressing large enough to overlap the edges of the wound and taped securely on three sides. This works as a flutter valve, preventing air from entering the pleural cavity when the patient inhales but allowing air to leave when the patient exhales.

Both types of pneumothoraces are definitively managed by the insertion of a chest tube to drain the air from the pleural cavity. The chest tube is traditionally inserted into the sixth intercostal space in the midaxillary line, the tube being aimed towards the apex of the lung. A tube of size 24F or greater is recommended. The tubing from the chest drain is attached to an underwater seal drainage system, where water in a bottle acts as an air lock. A negative pressure of approximately 5 mmHg may be attached to the system to aid adequate lung re-expansion (see Chapter 2).

The majority of simple pneumothoraces resolve in days when the re-expanded lung adheres to the chest wall due to the secretion of fibrin. A drain tube should only be removed if there is cessation of bubbling in the drainage bottle, even with suction. When the lung is fully expanded, this lack of bubbling needs to have been present for at least a day. It is important to tie a second pursestring suture to allow adequate closure of the drain site. After drain removal, a chest X-ray should be taken to confirm continued lung expansion.

03

Haemothorax

Trauma to the chest can also lead to the accumulation of blood in the pleural space. This is the definition of a haemothorax. Haemothoraces are most commonly associated with laceration or disruption of the lung parenchyma and are obviously more common in penetrating than blunt injuries. Haemothoraces can be defined as small or massive. A massive haemothorax is one where there is rapid accumulation of more than 1 L of blood in the chest cavity. This is most commonly caused by disruption of the hilar vessels of the lung, and hence the problems experienced by the patient would be not only those of hypoxia but also those of hypovolaemia. A massive haemothorax is recognized clinically by hypoxia, decreasing blood pressure, and a chest where there may be obvious signs of trauma and on the ipsilateral side decreased expansion, decreased percussion note and decreased breath sounds. Initial management involves the insertion of a large-bore chest tube into the sixth intercostal space in the midaxillary line. If a massive haemothorax is suspected, the blood from the chest can be used for autotransfusion. The subsequent management of the patient depends on the volume of blood loss. If over 1 L is immediately drained from the thoracic cavity, the patient requires an early thoracotomy. If less than 1 L is drained, the patient can be managed expectantly, with the decision for surgery based on the rate of continuing blood loss. If the rate of blood loss is 200 mL/h over the subsequent 2–4 h, the patient should be considered for surgery.

Cardiac tamponade

Cardiac tamponade is the accumulation of fluid in the pericardial sac, which restricts the filling and contraction of the heart and leads to shock. If this fluid is blood, it can come from disruption of the great vessels or the heart itself, most commonly as a result of penetrating injuries, although severe blunt trauma can also be a cause. As little as 20 mL of blood can cause symptoms. Cardiac tamponade is often missed until later in the assessment, although three classic diagnostic features occur, namely elevation of jugular venous pressure (JVP), decline in blood pressure and muffled heart sounds (known as Beck's triad). Additionally, the patient may demonstrate pulsus paradoxus and a rise in venous pressure with inspiration (also known as Kussmaul's sign). Transthoracic echocardiography can help in confirming the diagnosis. However, the diagnosis is often made only when pericardiocentesis is performed in a last-ditch effort to relieve the cardiogenic shock. In this procedure, a long spinal needle is

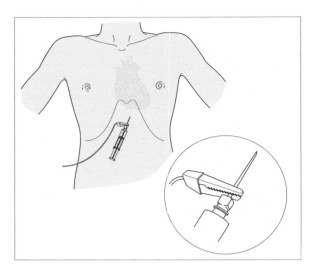

Figure 20.4 Site of insertion of a pericardiocentesis needle to decompress a cardiac tamponade.

inserted in the subxiphoid region and blood is evacuated. This procedure should always be performed under ECG monitoring. In very extreme situations, the thorax is opened and the pericardium evacuated (Fig. 20.4).

Secondary survey chest injuries

Haemothoraces and pneumothoraces can also cause death during the secondary survey period. However, the occurrence and discovery of visceral injuries that were not obvious initially tend to dominate the secondary survey.

Pulmonary contusion

One of the most common and often unrecognized problems associated with severe chest trauma is pulmonary contusion. This potentially lethal injury can often display subtle signs, where significant portions of the lung fail to function and cause the patient to become markedly hypoxic. The patient's injuries may often be sufficiently severe to require assisted ventilation and may also contribute to the development of adult respiratory distress syndrome (ARDS). More severe pulmonary injuries can lead to pulmonary laceration. However, this is most commonly observed with an associated fractured rib or secondary to penetrating trauma.

Aortic disruption

Traumatic disruption of the aorta is a common cause of death after trauma that involves very rapid deceleration

03

03

from great speeds, such as high-velocity road traffic accidents and falls from a great height. These patients are initially stable but continue to be hypotensive despite resuscitation, due to failure of the haematoma to contain the bleeding. There are usually few specific signs and symptoms. However, a high index of suspicion and a history of decelerating force will lead to inspection of the chest X-ray for specific signs of mediastinal widening. Also, if the patient is stable, angiography and even CT scanning will help confirm the diagnosis. Immediate referral to a cardiothoracic surgeon is imperative if the patient is to survive.

Diaphragmatic injury

Injuries to the diaphragm can occur as a result of huge compressional forces that cause the diaphragm to be torn from its attachments or secondary to penetrating trauma. This type of injury is usually associated with abdominal injury as well. Diaphragmatic trauma is yet another injury that is often missed or diagnosed late. Some patients may present years later with herniation through previous diaphragmatic defects caused by trauma. On chest X-ray these injuries may be recognized by an elevated diaphragm and can be confirmed by inserting contrast into the oesophagus and observing a high stomach.

Tracheobronchial disruption

Injury to the trachea or major bronchi is uncommon and fatal if overlooked. Patients who suffer severe tracheobronchial disruption usually die at the scene of the accident. However, those with a more minor degree of disruption are frequently recognized by the fact that they have a pneumothorax with associated subcutaneous emphysema, the pneumothorax persisting despite chest tube drainage. Frequently, definitive surgery is required to correct the abnormality.

Oesophageal disruption

The oesophagus is most commonly traumatized by penetrating trauma. However, the oesophagus can tear due to forceful expulsion of contents from the stomach during huge impacts. This causes gastric contents and air to leak into the mediastinum, resulting in mediastinitis and air in the subcutaneous tissues of the neck, recognized as surgical emphysema. Patients may also develop a pneumothorax, usually more common on the left than the right. The diagnosis is confirmed when particulate gastric matter is recovered from the chest tube. Prompt diagnosis and repair produce the best results in these patients.

Chest trauma at a glance

Definitions

Pneumothorax: the presence of air in the (normally potential) space between the visceral and parietal pleura in the chest cavity

Tension pneumothorax: a life-threatening condition that results from the continuing accumulation of air in the pleural cavity such that mediastinal structures (especially the great veins) are compressed and displaced laterally, inhibiting venous return and resulting in decreased cardiac output and ultimately cardiac arrest

Haemothorax: the presence of blood in the space between the visceral and parietal pleura in the chest cavity

Flail chest: a segment of chest wall that moves paradoxically on respiration (inward movement on inspiration and outward movement on expiration) secondary to multiple rib fractures such that there are more than two rib fractures in two or more consecutive ribs

Cardiac tamponade: abnormal compression of the heart as a result of the accumulation of fluid (e.g. blood) in the pericardial sac. A relatively small amount of fluid (~20 mL) can cause symptoms

Classification
- Type of injury: blunt or penetrating trauma
- Mechanism of injury: high- or low-velocity injury

Primary survey injuries
- Fractured ribs
- Flail chest
- Fractured sternum
- Pneumothorax
- Tension pneumothorax
- Haemothorax
- Cardiac tamponade

Secondary survey injuries
- Pulmonary contusion
- Aortic disruption
- Diaphragmatic injury
- Tracheobronchial disruption
- Oesophageal disruption

Clinical features and management

Anatomical region	Injury	Clinical features	Management
Chest wall	Fractured ribs	Usually 6th to 9th ribs. Fracture of 1st rib indicates high-velocity trauma	Adequate analgesia Breathing exercises
	Flail chest	Paradoxical chest wall movement on respiration	Adequate analgesia Strapping of flail segment Positive pressure ventilation
	Fractured sternum	Intense deep pain Look for cardiac injury	Adequate analgesia Cardiac monitor Check cardiac enzymes
Lungs and pleura	Simple pneumothorax	Dyspnoea Chest wall hyperresonant	Chest X-ray Chest drain if > 5–10% lung collapse (6th intercostal space midaxillary line)
	Tension pneumothorax	Dyspnoea Trachea deviated to opposite side Chest wall hyperresonant Cardiac arrest	Do *not* perform chest X-ray to confirm diagnosis Insert large-bore needle into the chest (2nd intercostal space, midclavicular line) Then chest X-ray and chest drain
	Open (sucking) pneumothorax	Open defect in chest wall	Cover defect with sterile occlusive dressing taped down on three sides
	Haemothorax	Penetrating injury Decreased expansion, dull percussion, reduced breath sounds	Insert large-bore chest drain If > 1 L blood discharges immediately, patient needs thoracotomy
	Massive (> 1 L) Small (< 1 L)	+ Hypoxia and shock + Dyspnoea	If < 1 L blood discharges immediately, observe If continuing blood loss of 200 mL/h, patient needs thoracotomy
	Pulmonary contusion or laceration	Hypoxia ARDS	May need ventilation
	Tracheobronchial disruption	Pneumothorax plus subcutaneous emphysema Persistent air leak from chest drain	Surgical repair
Cardiovascular	Cardiac tamponade (cardiac trauma)	Elevated JVP Decreased blood pressure Muffled heart sounds Pulsus paradoxus Rise in JVP on inspiration (Kussmaul's sign)	Pericardiocentesis Sternotomy and drainage of pericardium (Open repair of heart injury)
	Aortic disruption	History of rapid deceleration in high-velocity injury Hypotensive despite resuscitation	Chest X-ray shows widened mediastinum Diagnosis confirmed with contrast-enhanced CT Open surgical repair
	Venous injury	Rare History of penetrating injury Haemothorax	Surgical repair
Miscellaneous	Oesophagus	Mediastinitis Subcutaneous emphysema in neck Sometimes hydropneumothorax (L > R)	Urgent surgical repair Poor prognosis with mediastinitis
	Diaphragm (rupture or penetration)	History of compression force on abdomen History of penetrating trauma	Often present late with herniation of stomach into chest Reduction of stomach into abdomen and open repair of diaphragm

03

Musculoskeletal Trauma

21

03

Must know Must do

Must know

How to take a concise basic history from a patient who has had an accident or from relevant witnesses

Principles of assessment and resuscitation of the injured patient

General principles of fracture and soft-tissue management

Types of treatments available and the likely consequences for an individual patient such that you could answer sensible queries from the patient about what has happened or what may be about to happen

How to manage pain and shock

Common complications and consequences of injury or treatment

Must do

Attend the accident and emergency department to witness resuscitation/assessment of injured patients

Attend fracture clinic

Clerk patients in the orthopaedic wards recovering from major musculoskeletal trauma

Observe open reduction and fixation of major limb fractures

Attend rehabilitation sessions

Introduction

Fractures are a common medical problem: most people have broken a bone or know someone who has. Bones are familiarly regarded as inert things that are important for body structure. In reality, however, bones are dynamic living tissues with a very rich blood and nerve supply. The immediate consequences of fracture therefore are severe pain and blood loss, and the strategy of early management is to minimize pain with splints and analgesics and to anticipate the effects of blood loss, i.e. hypovolaemic shock. In the longer term, the rich blood supply must be re-established before bone will heal and so from the outset the state of the soft tissues becomes of central importance. Finally, it must be remembered that patients do not die from broken bones but from the results of associated injuries to the chest, head and abdomen and so fractures are not the first consideration when treating the injured patient.

History-taking after trauma

There are two principal reasons for taking a careful history after trauma: clinical and medicolegal.

Clinical history

Bones may be broken in many ways, including simple domestic accidents (the most common), high-velocity transport accidents and, more rarely, battle injuries. The following questions must be asked and answered (see box below).

● *What happened?* Once admitted to hospital, most fractures look the same whatever the mechanism of injury. However, there is a world of difference between a fracture caused by slipping off a step and a fracture caused by collision with a car; the first involves little energy transfer to the affected part of the body, while in the second a lot of energy is absorbed by the affected part. The amount of energy transferred to the body in an accident determines not only the bony injury but also the soft-tissue damage and the extent to which the blood supply is disrupted. Therefore, it is important to find out from the victim (*direct history*) and witnesses (*collateral history*) what exactly happened.

● *How did it happen?* How it happened can also help because injuries tend not to occur randomly but in some sort of pattern. For example, a pedestrian hit by a car tends to receive leg injuries from the bumper, pelvic and abdominal injuries from the bonnet and head injuries from the door pillar. Knowing something about these patterns permits the examiner to predict potential injuries.

● *Where and when did it happen?* It is also useful to know where and when it happened because a long delay between injury and treatment may limit therapeutic options.

● *What was the patient like before it happened?* Once the circumstances of the injury are appreciated, then the patient should have a full medical history taken. This is of course secondary to essential treatment required to protect the airway and control haemorrhage. It is important to establish as much as possible about the patient's previous general medical state. Often medical conditions may be associated with an injury. For example, the patient may have had a fit or collapsed with a hypoglycaemic attack. In the elderly, presentation with a fracture may represent a fall secondary to a myocardial infarction or a cerebrovascular accident. Many patients with fractures will need an anaesthetic and so the state of the cardiovascular and respiratory system must be established. The last time the patient ate or drank should be confirmed so that surgery can be delayed, if possible, until the stomach is empty, so reducing the risk of aspiration of vomit.

● *Who is the person?* Finally, the social history is extremely important. This may be obtained after the immediate treatment of the fracture has been carried out or may be obtained from a relative. The status of patients before injury must be established. Where do they live and with whom? Do they have stairs to climb into the house or flat or within the home? Can the older patient go to relatives after any hospital stay to rehabilitate?

Taking a history

● What happened? Was there a lot of violence involved or a simple fall?

● How did it happen? Can likely injuries be predicted from the patient's description of the incident?

● Where and when? Did it happen recently or has the patient come late?

● To whom did it happen? How does the patient live? Will they need some help at home later?

● What was the patient like before the accident? Has this patient other medical problems?

● Has an adequate history been taken and recorded? As a responsible professional you may have to account for youself in the future

---

Medicolegal aspects

Accidents have all sorts of consequences that affect the patient and the patient's family. They often result in insurance claims and litigation, not infrequently directed at the doctors and nurses who cared for the patient immediately after the accident. It is important therefore to keep meticulous notes at the time or as soon after the event as possible. This is particularly important when it is realized that it is often months or years before one may be called to give an account of an accident. For all concerned, legible and complete notes are essential.

Examination of the traumatized patient (see Chapter 17)

All patients need to have a full physical examination. Priorities should be established in the examination process as listed below.

1 Examine vital areas.
2 Examine injured areas.
3 Examine other areas at risk.
4 Do a general examination.

Vital areas

For patients with multiple injuries, airway protection and cardiorespiratory viability take precedence over everything else. Ask a simple question such as 'What is your name?' If you get a sensible answer, then the patient is conscious with a good airway. However, for most patients with a single or few injuries, the examination will concentrate on the injured part and the fitness of the patient for anaesthetic.

Injured area

Examination of the fracture site

The suspicion that a patient has sustained a fracture will have been raised from the history. The diagnosis should be confirmed by physical examination of the injured part and only rarely are radiographs needed to make the diagnosis. The signs of fracture are:

● deformity;
● tenderness;
● swelling;
● discoloration or bruising;
● loss of function; and
● crepitus.

Crepitus is perceived as a grating or grinding of the broken bone ends, although this sign should not be purposefully elicited as it will cause intense pain to the patient (Fig. 21.1).

Examination of the immediate vicinity of a fracture

● The skin may be partially damaged and present with or subsequently develop blisters. Such skin is only partially viable and may not tolerate being incised as part of an

03

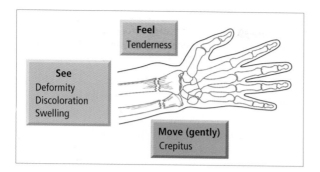

Figure 21.1 The cardinal features of a common fracture.

operation. If the skin has been breached, the fracture is described as an *open fracture* (see below).

● The subcutaneous fat will almost certainly be damaged and later necrosis may cause reddening of the skin with firmness and tenderness; this is easily mistaken for infection.

● The surrounding muscle will be damaged to some degree, contributing to limb swelling. If swelling is severe, the patient may develop a full-blown compartment syndrome (see later and Chapter 17).

● Damage to major vessels is surprisingly rare, except in extensive open injuries where there has been a lot of direct violence. Certain specific fractures (supracondylar elbow fractures and dislocated knee) are sometimes accompanied by arterial damage. Vessels are also at risk from compression (see section Compartment syndrome) and from damage to the intima that could cause thrombosis and occlusion. The features of vascular trauma are described in Chapter 37.

● Complete or incomplete division of nerves is rare except in penetrating wounds, in association with severe open fractures or with major trauma (e.g. brachial plexus injury). However, stretching (or neuropraxia) is not uncommon. The nerves are sometimes stretched around deformed fragments and this is sometimes exacerbated by swelling.

Other areas at risk

Certain types of injury are classically associated with other specific injuries and the discovery of one injury should alert the examiner to the possibility of the associated injury.

● *Head and spinal injuries.* The possibility that a patient with a head injury also has a spinal injury should constantly be borne in mind. If a blow is sufficient to render a patient unconscious, then the same violence could have broken the cervical spine, especially where it joins the head (at the atlas and axis) or where it joins the trunk (at the thoracocervical junction) (Fig. 21.2). If a patient is unconscious following a head injury, it is best to assume that he or she has a spinal injury until proven otherwise. Patients should be nursed with a collar and turned correctly (all in one piece and not twisted).

● *Rib fractures and pneumothorax.* The presence of fractured ribs should always raise the possibility of pneumothorax. The possibility of traumatic aortic dissection should be considered in a patient with a fractured left first rib following blunt trauma (see Chapter 20).

● *Femoral and pelvic injuries.* Pelvic injuries are sometimes seen in association with major long-bone injuries in the lower limb. Dislocation of a hip sometimes accompanies femoral fracture and ligamentous injuries to adjacent joints are always possible in any long-bone fracture.

● *Small injuries with big injuries.* It is wise to re-examine the patient on two or three occasions, including the next day, when small injuries are often discovered. It is often small injuries that lead to long-term problems: for example, it is extremely unfortunate if a patient with a well-treated long-bone fracture is still not at work because of an unrecognized and untreated fracture of some metatarsals.

Examination of the traumatized patient

● Is the patient conscious and responding sensibly? If not, resuscitation and airway protection take priority (ABC)

● If the injury is more localized, get the patient to show you where it hurts. Do not forget that some patients may be overwhelmed with pain in one area and forget a less sore injury elsewhere

● It is your job to examine the patient systematically to positively exclude injuries. It is easy to miss apparently minor injuries that become troublesome later

● Recognize associated injuries that commonly go together, e.g. ribs with pneumothorax, skull with neck, femur with pelvis

● Check the patient again on another occasion. You or the patient may have missed something

● When examining a limb always remind yourself about the areas at risk: skin, fat, muscle and tendon, bone, blood vessel, nerve, associated joints and ligaments

---

Investigation of fractures

Fracture architecture

Why is it important to describe the shape and degree of fragmentation of a fracture? In general, the shape of a

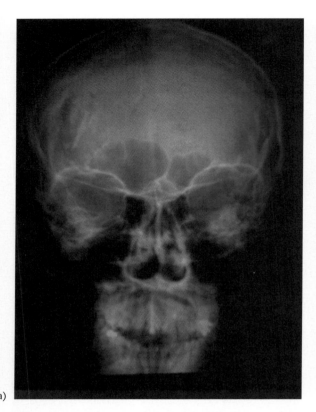

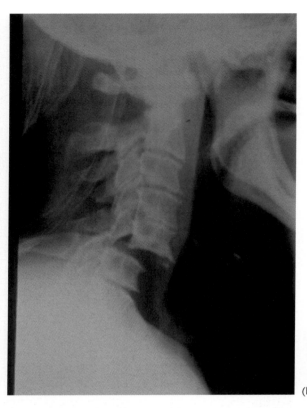

(a)

(b)

Figure 21.2 (a) This patient has an obvious fracture of the skull and is unconscious; (b) without careful examination and radiographic evaluation neck fractures such as these may be missed!

fracture reveals the amount of energy that has caused the damage and thus permits the correct treatment to be applied. In general, *spiral fractures* occur through twisting, which is a common low-energy mode of injury. Such injuries are usually associated with little soft-tissue damage and so the blood supply to the bone is preserved and therefore healing is unlikely to be a problem. In contrast, *oblique* and *transverse fractures* are caused by buckling or direct injury to the bone and involve a lot of energy, with soft-tissue stripping and damage to the blood supply. Such injuries require much consideration when the choice of treatment is being made. The types of fractures are summarized in Fig. 21.4.

Plain radiography of the injured area

The radiograph must show the part under investigation and it must be of diagnostic quality. The responsibility for achieving this rests solely with the clinician ordering the film. Dark films are dangerous because vital information

may be missed. Equally, it is important to make sure the whole of the site of injury is included in the investigation and so it is safest to include the joint above and the joint below the area in question.

Two films are usually taken at mutual right angles. Conventionally, an *anteroposterior* and a *lateral* view are taken. In this way, by always viewing conventional films the examiner recognizes deviations from normal patterns more easily. However, some injuries (e.g. of the hand) are best seen on *oblique* views. At least two views are needed to obtain a reasonably accurate impression of the extent of the fracture (Fig. 21.3).

The radiographic features of a fracture include:
- lucencies at the site of fractures;
- discontinuity in the cortex or surface of a bone or joint.

These features may be very obvious or quite subtle. The essence, however, is an index of suspicion and only rarely should the examiner be surprised by what is revealed by the radiograph (see box below).

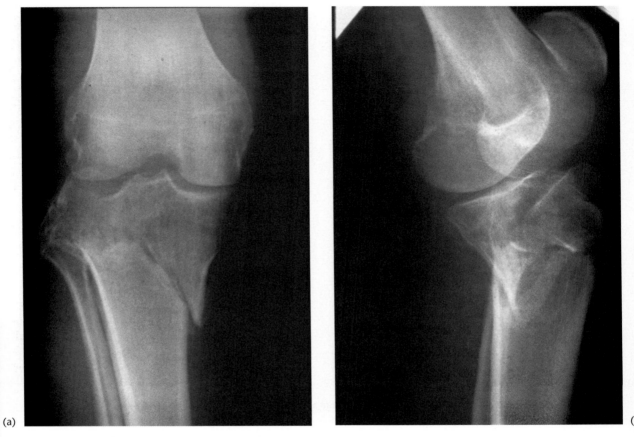

(a)   (b)

Figure 21.3 (a) A nasty tibial plateau fracture as seen on (b) to be even nastier on an oblique film.

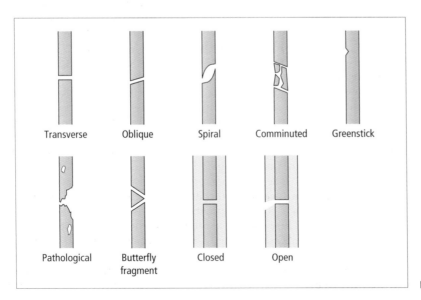

Figure 21.4 Fracture architecture.

How to describe a fracture

- Which bone is broken and on which side?
- Is the fracture open or closed?
- Where on the bone is it broken?
    - Intra-articular
    - Mid-shaft
    - Proximal or lower third
- What shape is the fracture?
    - Spiral
    - Oblique
    - Transverse
- How many fragments?
    - Simple
    - Butterfly
    - Comminuted
- Position of the distal fragment?
    - Displacement: anterior–posterior, medial–lateral
    - Angulation: anterior–posterior, varus–valgus
    - Rotation: internal–external

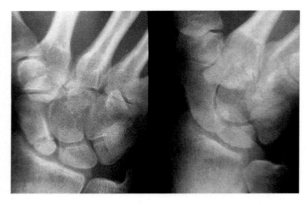

Figure 21.5 Special views are often required when a fracture is suspected. In this case an oblique view clearly shows that the scaphoid is fractured (left picture) but the fracture is not obvious on the conventional anteroposterior view (right picture).

Radiography of other areas

- Other films may be taken where injury to other areas is contemplated (see above). For example, if the skull is fractured, it is wise to X-ray the cervical spine; this is mandatory if the patient is unconscious.
- If the patient is to have an anaesthetic, a chest film will help exclude a small pneumothorax that may become lethally significant if the patient is intubated and given positive-pressure ventilation.
- In multiple lower limb injuries, it is wise to take a radiograph of the pelvis.
- On occasions it is useful to take radiographs of the opposite normal limb. This is particularly so in children, where epiphyseal centres of ossification can produce confusing pictures, with many apparently free-floating 'blobs' of bone. A comparison with analogous films of the other side may reveal a displaced fragment, often lying in the joint.
- It is also useful sometimes to X-ray the patient on two separate occasions. For example, scaphoid fractures are frequently invisible on an initial radiograph, only to be revealed on a film taken 2 weeks later. This radio-opacity is caused by the hyperaemia in the surrounding bone that occurs in the acute inflammatory phase following fracture. The improvement in fracture image with time is almost certainly due to resolution of the hyperaemia (Fig. 21.5).

Tomography

An alternative to waiting for radiolucency through areas of hyperaemia is to take tomograms. This is a radiographic technique where the X-ray beam and the film rotate around the limb so that only one point of the limb (the place that is potentially fractured) will be constantly in focus (see Chapter 3). In this way a detailed view of a small area of interest may reveal pathology. A good example is fracture of the odontoid peg, which is often lost among confusing shadows at the base of the skull.

Computed tomography

Computed tomography (CT) is essentially an extension of ordinary tomography but scans are repeated thousands of times and assembled into a single image by a computer. This represents a section of the body a few millimetres thick, usually taken in the transverse plane. CT scans are most useful in determining the extent of an injury but are less useful in primary diagnosis. In detail they are of value in planning an operation or determining the stability of a fracture, e.g. the spine.

Magnetic resonance imaging

Magnetic resonance imaging (MRI) works by aligning the body's hydrogen atoms (protons) in a magnetic field and bombarding them with radiofrequency (RF) waves. The RF waves cause the hydrogen atoms to spin as they acquire energy. Removal of the RF waves causes the protons to release the energy they have acquired. This energy release is picked up by detectors and converted into a grey-scale image. Each tissue produces a characteristic signal; compact bone gives off little or no signal, while soft tissue generally gives a good signal. MRI therefore has little place in the management of most fractures but is important for the assessment of spinal cord and spine trauma (see also Chapter 3).

03

Other investigations

In acute injuries few investigations apart from the plain radiograph are necessary.
● Ultrasound of a joint may help in elucidating an effusion.
● When there is doubt, radioisotope bone scanning can help determine whether a bone is fractured. This is most useful about 2 weeks after the injury. It is a highly sensitive test but does not provide any information about the fracture except that it is there. A useful example is the scaphoid fracture, which may be seen on a second X-ray at 2 weeks but there can still be doubt. A negative scan is very positive reassurance in such a situation and may help to allay lingering clinical doubt.

Investigating fractures

● Take a radiograph in two planes at right angles to each other to build up a mental three-dimensional image of the fracture
● If you cannot visualize the fracture adequately, take more films. Oblique films sometimes help
● If you still cannot see a fracture but suspect it clinically, do more tests. Your clinical judgement should always overrule negative investigations
● If you suspect associated injuries, use radiographs to exclude them: ribs–chest, skull–neck, femur–pelvis
● Sometimes it is necessary to take films on more than one occasion, e.g. scaphoid
● Use expensive tests specifically: CT for bones and joints, MRI and ultrasound for soft tissues, scintigraphy in specified circumstances

---

Management of fractures

How do fractures heal?

Bone has a natural tendency to heal and, unlike any other connective tissue, has a remarkable repair mechanism that ultimately results in bone regeneration and structural integrity; it is literally 'as good as new'. The pathology of fracture healing is summarized in Fig. 21.6.

This remarkable process and its mechanism remain poorly understood but there are a number of points worth noting.
● Bones heal in the presence of some movement. This is clear from the example of broken ribs, which unite efficiently (albeit painfully) with prodigious external callus formation. It appears that movement stimulates union but the movement must be small and must not be in certain directions. Essentially, bones are stimulated by micromovement directed along their axis and heal least efficiently if subject to shearing forces or large movements.
● The converse also holds true: although bones will heal if there is no movement, they do so very slowly and by an entirely different process that does not utilize natural external callus formation. This alternative method of fracture healing appears to be similar to the normal remodelling processes of bone, which are slow but sure.

Immediate management

Pain relief

● *Systemic pain relief* for fractures requires the use of opiates given in adequate doses in combination with an antiemetic to offset the adverse effects of opiates. In

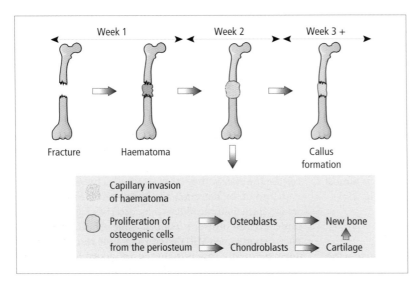

Figure 21.6 The pathology of fracture healing.

injured patients, intravenous rather than intramuscular opiates should be used. Clinicians, particularly when new, are often afraid to give adequate doses of opiates in the fear of affecting consciousness and clinical signs. In general, however, when serious head or visceral injury has been excluded, they may be used generously and early.

● *Local anaesthetic nerve blocks* are frequently effective. A femoral nerve block, for example, can remove the need for systemic drugs following femoral fracture, although the anxiolytic benefits of central nervous system agents should not be underestimated.

● *Splintage* can be applied to most fractures before arrival at hospital. This alone can relieve most intolerable pain. In general, a splint should encompass the joint above and below an injury. Simple expedients such as binding the arm to the chest, with or without a sling, or simply binding the legs together is often sufficient.

Blood loss

For most upper limb and peripheral lower limb fractures, blood loss is small and is tolerated even by the elderly. However, blood loss may be significant with major pelvic fractures (6+ units) and long-bone fractures, particularly the femur (2–3 units) and the tibia (1 unit). In general, all patients with long-bone injuries should be cross-matched for blood and a good-sized venous line established as soon as possible to ensure adequate resuscitation (see Chapter 6). For pelvic fractures two lines may be needed and a central venous line established to ensure transfusion is keeping up with loss.

Open fractures

Open (or, less meaningfully, *compound*) fractures are serious injuries (Fig. 21.7). Considerable violence is required

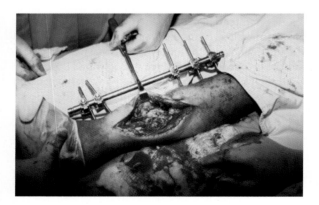

Figure 21.7 An open fracture undergoing surgery to clean the wound. An external fixator is in place.

to cause this type of injury and because there is a break in the skin, bacterial contamination of the bone occurs. The strategy of treatment is to clean the wounds as soon as possible and remove all dead tissue (débridement), thus preventing the development of infection. Open fractures are surgical emergencies and, provided the patient's general condition permits, formal surgical wound débridement should be performed as soon as possible and preferably within 6 h of injury. Wounds must be left open, and closed either as a secondary procedure after a few days or left to heal spontaneously. Such patients all need supplementary broad-spectrum antibiotics and some form of tetanus prophylaxis, i.e. tetanus toxoid booster to those with a previous immunization record or human antitetanus globulin for those with no previous active immunity.

Definitive management

The essential strategy of long-term fracture management must be to return patients to their preinjury level of function by the safest means. Functional requirements vary from individual to individual depending on many factors, including age, physical health and the patient's occupation. For example, a fractured wrist in a frail elderly patient with poor osteoporotic bone might be managed differently from that in a young fit, right-handed craftsman. In the former, a less than ideal reduction under local anaesthesia might be acceptable, allowing for early discharge and early mobilization of the wrist; the young patient may be prepared to spend many months ensuring a perfect result because this is required for his long-term health and employment security. The basic goals of management are reduction, immobilization and rehabilitation.

Reduction

In order to achieve acceptable function, a fracture should be reduced and held so that the anatomy of the bone is returned to as near normal as possible.

● If the fracture passes into a joint, then the anatomy should be restored accurately if acceptable function is to be achieved.

● If a fracture occurs through the shaft of a long bone, then it is desirable to return the anatomy to normal but the margin for error is much greater and something less than perfect is acceptable.

Closed reduction may be achieved by traction on the distal fragment and relocation of that distal part on to the proximal fragment by manipulation (e.g. Colles fractures). In order to achieve a reduction, adequate analgesia must be given; this is achieved by general or regional anaesthesia. The manipulative procedure usually involves

03

reversing the direction of the deforming force. If closed reduction is unsuccessful, then *open reduction* may be required, whereby the fracture site is opened surgically and the fragments are relocated directly under vision (e.g. unstable fracture of both forearm bones).

Holding

Once the fracture is adequately realigned, then it must be held in the normal position until the bone has become strong enough to support itself (*united*) and then protected until it is strong enough to bear some load (*consolidated*). Methods of immobilizing fractures are listed below. Over a longer period of time the bone architecture will return to normal or near normal depending on how much displacement occurred during treatment; this process is known as remodelling.

Casting

After the fracture has been manipulated, it may be held simply and effectively in a plaster of Paris cast until union occurs. The fracture must be held in a position that maintains it in three dimensions (tilt, twist and shift) and the cast must be the proper length. In order to ensure complete control of all dimensions of the fracture, it is necessary to control the joint above and below the fracture as otherwise joint movement may result in distortion in one or more dimensions. Plaster of Paris is relatively brittle, messy and very difficult to apply well. It is heavy and awkward, particularly in the elderly, and takes up to 3 days to dry fully. For these reasons, strong and light glass fibre and polyurethane resin materials have been developed. These are not as versatile as plaster of Paris and are better for secondary casts, which are applied after a week or two when the fracture swelling has settled (Fig. 21.8).

Functional bracing

Casts have a number of disadvantages: they are heavy, immobilize the joints and prevent access to the fracture site. The immobility imposed on a limb by a cast results in muscle wasting and joint stiffness. It is possible to overcome these disadvantages by the technique of functional bracing, i.e. freeing the joints while maintaining alignment at the fracture site. In order to maintain three-dimensional control of the fracture, it is necessary to support the cast at the joints by a combination of accurate moulding and the provision of hinges, which permit motion in one direction, usually flexion and extension. Functional bracing is highly dependent on a very accurate fit and can be used only after a few weeks when the pain and swelling have settled. In practice, functional bracing is used in the management of fractures of the tibia and fibula.

Internal fixation

Where accurate reduction and holding of fractures are required, internal fixation is performed. However, internal fixation is technically very demanding, has many complications and, most important of all, prevents natural healing. If fixation is to be used it can be achieved in a number of ways.

- *Apposition.* Once fractures are realigned, they may only need to be held in apposition for healing to proceed satisfactorily. This is particularly true in children. Apposition can be achieved simply by using semiflexible wires known as 'K' (for Kirschner) wires. They hold position without producing immobility and so healing occurs by natural callus formation. They can be left standing proud of the bone and can easily be pulled out once union is established and before consolidation.

- *Interfragmentary compression* is usually achieved by screws or occasionally by tension band wires. These achieve great accuracy and are particularly valuable in cancellous bone around joints. They are also useful in long bones, particularly in the upper limb, but in these situations extra support is required from an onlay device.

- *Onlay devices* are metal plates that are used to buttress weak structures around joints and to fix long bones in the upper limb. These very rigid systems inhibit natural bone union and, although they permit early movement, they ultimately delay healing and full load-bearing.

- *Intramedullary or inlay devices* are the most satisfactory method of fixation. They achieve alignment without unduly disturbing natural bone healing. They are a relatively inaccurate method of restoring anatomical position and so are not useful around joints. Their great strength makes them ideal devices for treating long-bone fractures, particularly in the lower limb.

External fixation

When fractures are open and associated with extensive soft-tissue damage and contamination, neither plaster casting nor internal fixation is appropriate. Plaster splints are unsuitable because the wounds become inaccessible for inspection and dressing, while internal fixation is hazardous because of the very high risk of wound infection.

A compromise solution is to apply an external fixation device, which consists of a strong metal rod (or series of rods) that runs parallel to the fractured bone and is attached to the bone by a series of pins. Such a device stabilizes the fracture and gives access to the soft tissues for dressings and secondary surgery such as skin grafting. A disadvantage of external fixators is the risk of infection at the pin sites.

Traction

Traction may be used to hold a fracture in a reduced

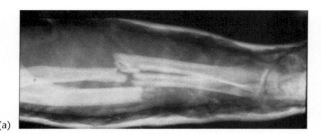

(a)

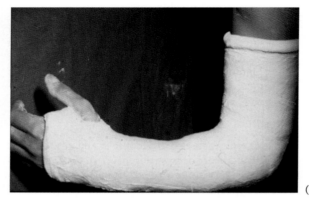

(b)

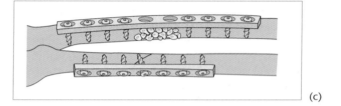

(c)

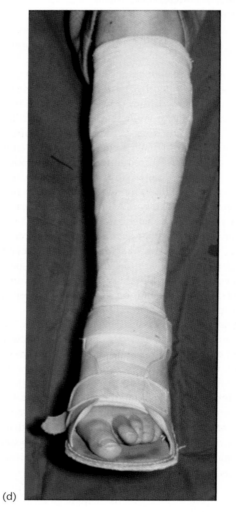

(d)

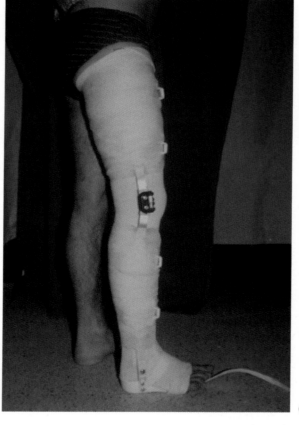

(e)

Figure 21.8 (a) A forearm midshaft fracture of radius and ulna; this may be treated in a plaster cast in children (b). (c) In adults it is usually plated following open reduction. (d) A tibia in a cast using modern resin materials. (e) Modern materials can be used to make sophisticated hinged casts that stabilise fractures but permit joint motion. A technique known as functional bracing.

03

position. Traction is achieved by the application of a relatively small weight (4.5–7 kg) to a limb. The weight exerts a pull along the axis of the broken bone, thus stimulating muscle contraction. The increased muscle tone acts like a splint, holding the broken bone in the position achieved at reduction.

Rehabilitation

Immobilization causes muscle atrophy and joint stiffness which, if not treated aggressively, may lead to contractures and post-traumatic syndromes (e.g. post-traumatic sympathetic dystrophy). Therefore, patients require intensive rehabilitation programmes to help them use their joints as soon as possible after the fracture, to exercise their muscles and begin to use and build up strength in the injured limb. Most of this work will be done under the supervision of physiotherapists and occupational therapists who work in close partnership with fracture surgeons (see also Chapter 10).

> ### Treatment of fractures at a glance
>
> - Treat the pain and exclude the risk of serious blood loss. Most low-energy fractures are not associated with blood loss, but pelvic and long-bone fractures are, so calculate the potential blood loss
> - Reduce the fracture: do this as simply and safely as possible. Restore function
> - Hold the fracture in a functional position. This may mean using:
>   (a) A cast
>   (b) Doing an operation and inserting fixation devices such as nails, plates or screws
>   (c) Applying external fixation where there is extensive soft-tissue damage
>   (d) Using weights to apply gentle traction
> - Rehabilitate the patient: work with the rest of the team of healthcare professionals including nurses, physiotherapists and occupational therapists

Complications of fractures

Early complications may occur either as a direct consequence of the injury or in association with the treatment. Late complications are generally related to the fracture but a few are unfortunately precipitated by treatment (or lack of it).

Infection

Bone infection (*osteomyelitis*) may occur after open frac-

tures or after internal fixation: it is notable that the most common cause of bone infection in the western world is surgery. Although infection may delay or prevent union, it is not inevitable that this will be so. Provided a fracture is held stable, it will unite despite infection. If there is movement and infection, then non-union is most likely. This phenomenon is poorly understood but if a fracture is infected, provided it is stable, it may be treated by drainage of pus and antibiotics until union has occurred.

Fat embolism

After fracture of a long bone, a small number of patients (usually men under the age of 20) suffer from fat embolism characterized by an increasing degree of respiratory distress, leading to adult respiratory distress syndrome (see Chapter 20). The cause of fat embolism remains unclear. It was originally thought to be due to fat from the marrow of the fractured long bone precipitating in the lungs. However, an alternative view is that there is a breakdown of tissue fats to free fatty acids, which precipitate a pneumonitis. The symptoms (initially tachypnoea and mild confusion) usually commence within 2–5 days of injury. The patient may have a petechial rash on the chest, neck and conjunctiva but this is not a universal finding. Fat globules may be found in the urine and sputum and are occasionally seen in the retinal vessels on fundoscopy. Early diagnosis depends on a high index of suspicion and appropriate investigation.

Blood gases will show a hypoxaemia (Pao_2 4.7–6.7 kPa) and respiratory alkalosis (from hyperventilation) and a chest radiograph diffuse opacities that increase to complete 'white-out' over the following few days. In severe cases the respiratory distress increases to the point where positive-pressure ventilation and positive end-expiratory pressure are required (see Chapter 11), but even with this level of support the condition carries a significant mortality. Unfortunately, younger men are more prone to the full-blown syndrome. Early diagnosis and treatment with oxygen and chest physiotherapy are helpful.

Renal failure

Patients with massive soft-tissue injury who are trapped for prolonged periods, particularly where they are shocked or the trapped limbs are relatively ischaemic, are prone to develop acute tubular necrosis. Again the key is to recognize the possibility and be prepared to support such patients with renal dialysis. The cause is purported to be the release of myoglobin and this is found in abundance in the renal tubules (see Chapter 14).

Compartment syndrome

Compartment syndromes may occur in the upper and lower limbs following a fracture with excessive localized soft-tissue swelling. Classically it occurs in the forearm, where it leads to Volkmann's ischaemic contracture, although any muscle compartment lined by a stout fascial sheath may be at risk (e.g. calf muscles). This condition is discussed more fully in Chapter 17.

Immobility

After injury the injured part needs a short period of rest followed by motion to aid rehabilitation. The whole person does not need to be immobilized and patients must begin to move and rehabilitate as soon after the injury as possible. Injury results in negative nitrogen balance and patients will lose lean body mass. The effects can be minimized by early mobilization, which will also discourage disuse osteoporosis and the migration of calcium into the blood (which can precipitate renal stone formation).

Delayed union and non-union

About 2% of all fractures fail to unite; this is known as non-union (Fig. 21.9). Delayed union is when fractures fail to unite within the expected time. If left to heal naturally, upper limb fractures heal in 6 weeks or so and lower limb fractures in 12 weeks. This rule of thumb is useful but must not be too strictly adhered to and will be modified depending on the degree of violence involved and how the fracture was treated. However, we may say that non-union is established at 20 weeks in the lower limb and 10 weeks in the upper. These are arbitrary but practical figures. Delayed union is even less specific and it is really a period between expected union and accepted non-union when the decision to intervene is contemplated. Non-union is most common in the tibia but may occur at any site. Why fractures demonstrate non-union is not fully understood but several factors have been implicated:

- excess movement;
- insufficient movement, e.g. rigid internal fixation;
- soft-tissue interposition;
- poor blood supply;
- infection;
- unstable fracture;
- excessive traction or separation of bone ends;
- intact fellow bone, e.g. fibula.

Treatment of non-union relies on removing any underlying cause and then stimulating union. Stabilizing the fracture sufficiently and then adding bone graft seems to stimulate union but how bone graft does this remains

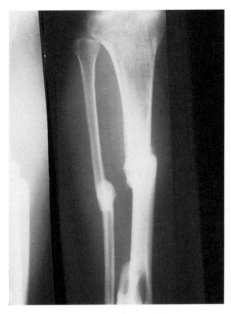

Figure 21.9 Non-union occurs most commonly in the tibia. If a tibial fracture has failed to heal at 20 weeks, a diagnosis of non-union is made. On X-ray, the fracture is still visible and the bone ends are sclerosed.

an enigma. Bone graft is usually autologous, being taken from the iliac crest and placed next to the fracture. The graft contains cells and minerals and humoral factors that probably mediate the repair by activating the hitherto deficient mechanism.

Malunion

Malunion implies that the fracture has been allowed to heal in a position that precludes normal function and usually implies failure of treatment or neglect. Regular review is the mainstay of fracture management and frequent radiological and clinical examination are essential to ensure that all is well.

Growth arrest

Children have a great capacity to remodel malunited fractures but are not able to remodel rotatory deformities. However, if a fracture breaches the germinal layer of the epiphyseal growth plate, distorted bone growth may occur. These are rare injuries and difficult to manage. All parents of children with epiphyseal injuries must be warned of this possibility if misunderstandings are to be avoided.

Complications

These can be early or late and a direct consequence of the injury or associated with the treatment applied

Early direct complications
Specific to the fracture
- Infection in open fractures
- Associated stretching or crushing of nerves
- Very rarely, damage to a blood vessel or its lining causes thrombosis
- Compartment syndrome caused by localized swelling

General
All these general complications should be anticipated and are very rare
- Fat embolism
- Renal failure
- Unrecognized hypovolaemic shock
- Muscle wasting due to immobility

Complications associated with treatment
- Infection of internally fixed fractures
- Surgical damage to vital structures such as nerves or blood vessels
- Compartment syndrome
- Pressure damage to skin or nerves from excessively tight bandages and splints

Late bone complications
- Malunion due to poor supervision of healing
- Non-union usually associated with:
  - (a) Excess movement
  - (b) Insufficient movement
  - (c) Poor local blood supply due to either anatomy (e.g. tibia) or a lot of trauma damage
- Growth arrest in children due to epiphyseal damage

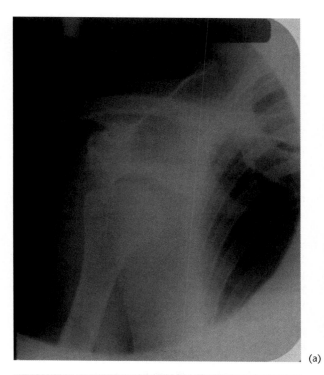

(a)

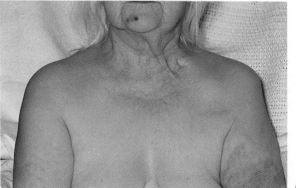

(b)

Figure 21.10 (a) A dislocated shoulder. (b) This is clinically detectable due to the loss of normal shoulder conture.

Post-traumatic (reflex) sympathetic dystrophy

This is a poorly understood syndrome characterized by persistent pain, swelling, hyperaesthesia, stiffness and disuse of a limb following an injury. If it persists, disuse osteoporosis may be seen on the radiograph. Treatment consists of physiotherapy with active and passive exercises and pain control. Chronic cases are extremely difficult to treat but pain clinics, vigorous rehabilitation and sympathectomy (in some patients) have been found to be helpful.

Dislocations

Dislocations of joints are serious problems and notoriously painful (Fig. 21.10). Before the days of anaesthesia

the reduction of a dislocated joint was exceptionally difficult because of the associated muscle spasm and the agony such a patient had to endure. Failure to reduce a joint was a serious consequence in terms of both pain and function. In modern times, reduction under anaesthesia ensures restoration of the joint surfaces. Nevertheless, dislocation is a potentially serious injury with long- and short-term consequences.

In the immediate term, apart from pain and loss of function, adjacent nerves and blood vessels may be compressed and thus urgent reduction is important. In the medium term, the ligaments of the joint will be disrupted to some degree. Although these usually repair naturally after closed reduction, in some circumstances the joint can become chronically unstable. This is seen most frequently in the shoulder and less commonly at the ankle. In the long term, a dislocated joint may lose the blood supply to the bone, which results in avascular necrosis. Even without this complication, dislocated joints seem more prone to late arthritis, seen most commonly at the hip.

The management of dislocation is first recognition and then assessment of the neurovascular status clinically, not least because it is essential to ensure that any nerve damage was present before treatment and not induced by manipulation. The joint is radiographed to ensure that there are no associated fractures that could be displaced further by the manipulation used to achieve reduction. Reduce the dislocation gently under sufficient anaesthesia to achieve muscle relaxation. Finally, hold the joint reduced in a position of function. Mobilise the joint gently as soon as pain permits but avoid full motion until ligaments have a chance to heal at 6–10 weeks.

Vascular problems need to be resolved immediately and continued features of ischaemia following reduction must be investigated to exclude vessel damage and thrombosis. Nerve lesions will not recover immediately, although most damage in association with dislocation is likely to be neuropraxia (see Chapter 22) and carries a good prognosis.

Common fractures and joint injuries

It would be inappropriate to list all fractures but some are commoner than others and some case knowledge for all doctors is prudent. The principles of reduction and holding have been discussed previously and some of the holding methods available and in common use have been described. Most injuries are of low velocity and the majority of broken bones are treated non-operatively in splints. There are a number of different reasons why fractures are held in different ways:

● it is important to be accurate in reduction and holding so that function is maintained;

● it is better for the general health of the patient, particularly when mobilization is paramount to good health;

● it is better to accept a less than perfect position and function in the interests of an individual's overall well-being;

● it is more cost-effective for the health service or an individual to have internal fixation;

● in multiple injuries, internal fixation can be life-saving.

Sometimes it is important to be accurate

When fractures are near joints and the congruity of the articular surface is severely disrupted, an operation may be necessary to achieve both reduction and fixation. In general, mid-shaft long-bone fractures will tolerate some degree of incomplete reduction in terms of angulation and length and will remodel. However, any rotatory deformity along the long axis of the bone will not be remodelled. Growing children also exhibit excellent potential for remodelling, but again not for rotation.

A good example of the need to be accurate is a fracture of both bones of the forearm. The radius articulates proximally and distally with the ulna and the two bones are further joined by a tough interosseous membrane. When the forearm is injured, both bones break or one bone breaks and either the proximal or distal joint dislocates. When both bones break, the angulation and shortening stop the ulna rotating as normal about the radius (Fig. 21.11). In adults, accuracy can only be assured by opening each fracture site and reducing the bones accurately under direct vision. Once reduced, holding with plates and screws protects the position until the soft tissues and then new bone consolidate the reduction. By holding the fracture firmly, the patient can immediately move the arm, thus restoring the important functional movements of pronation and supination as well as flexion and extension at the elbow and wrist.

The disadvantages of fixation are that a closed fracture is now open and thus at risk of infection. Also by opening the fracture an already damaged blood supply is inevitably damaged further and will therefore take longer to become re-established. It is important to remember that no fracture will heal until blood supply is restored locally. Thus, although accurate reduction is achieved, union is delayed and infection becomes a risk. Bones fixed in this way do not heal by callus formation as described earlier but by slow remodelling across the fracture site, a process sometimes referred to as primary bone healing. In a way, when fractures are repaired a race is set up: will the fracture heal and the bone become strong before the fixation device fails through fatigue? It requires exacting surgical skill to achieve reliable results and thus fixation, although very effective when it works, should be reserved for particular

03

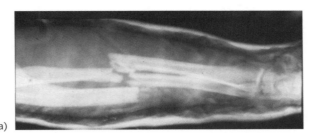

(a)

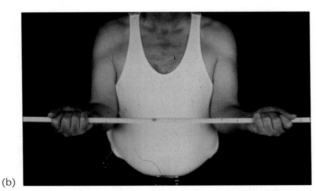

(b)

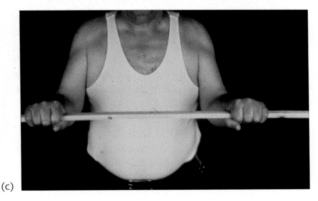

(c)

Figure 21.11 (a) This fracture has been treated with a cast and good alignment has not been achieved. (b,c) This denotes how pronation and supination requires accurate rotation of the forearm bones. This is only possible if such fractures are fixed following accurate reduction.

situations, such as the need to be accurate. Even though the evidence in the scientific literature shows that forearm fractures in adults treated by internal fixation do better than those manipulated and placed in plaster, in this case the risks outweigh the benefits for most adults. This risk–benefit question must be considered every time a surgeon decides to fix a fracture.

Sometimes an operation is better for the patient's general health

Older people who injure themselves are vulnerable if

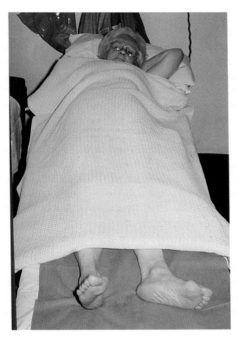

Figure 21.12 The diagnosis of extrascapular fracture of the neck of the femur can be made from the end of the bed. The patient's foot is externally rotated.

rested in bed too long. They may become disorientated in a new environment, are prone to chest and urinary infections and become rapidly susceptible to skin sores, muscle wasting and increasing osteoporosis. Older people are also more prone to falls for many reasons, such as poor eyesight and hearing, and have less adaptable cardiovascular and neurological function. Frequent falls, often but not always associated with osteoporosis, make older people particularly susceptible to fractures at the hip and wrist.

A broken hip means loss of mobility and immediate exposure to all the risks mentioned above. Early restoration of mobility is a priority, otherwise the factors that precipitated the fall are magnified and the risk to health and life becomes acute. For this reason, operating on hip fractures has been demonstrated to improve the chance of survival after such injuries. Even with appropriate treatment, one in four old people die within a year or so of their injury, not from the fracture but from the precipitating factors and their consequences post surgery. Clearly the balance between risk and benefit is a fine one but in this case the decision is in favour of surgery.

Any person admitted to hospital after a fall and who cannot walk should have hip fracture excluded clinically and if in any doubt radiologically (Fig. 21.12). There are two broad groups of hip fracture: those of the neck of the femur within the capsule of the joint (intracapsular) and

those through the line of the greater and lesser trochanters outside the hip capsule (extracapsular). If the fracture is intracapsular, it may not heal because of disruption of the blood supply. The older the patient and the more displaced the fracture, the less likely it is to heal. If the fracture is extracapsular, it will heal but not in a functional position (the leg will shorten). In either case, operation is essential if the patient is to avoid the risks of being confined to bed.

In younger intracapsular and all extracapsular fractures, reduction and internal fixation should be attempted as it is clearly better to have a healed normal hip than an artificial one if the state of the hip before fracture was otherwise normal. Any holding device needs to be strong enough to permit immediate mobilization of the patient. If the risk of failure of healing is high, then the head of the femur should be replaced with an artificial one. If the hip is otherwise healthy, it is quicker and safer to leave the natural acetabulum in place and perform a hemiarthroplasty. If the joint is arthritic, then a full replacement may be justified but this bigger operation carries more risk.

The complications of surgery are infection, device failure in soft bone, or dislocation of the artificial joint component(s). These compound the problems that may have been associated with the fall, such as stroke or myocardial infarction. In general it is better to treat the fracture within a few days and then treat any underlying medical conditions if the patient is fit enough for anaesthesia.

After surgery, early mobilization and rehabilitation is a vital step that requires a team approach involving physicians with a special interest in the elderly and the extensive network of healthcare professionals. The quality of the outcome is as much to do with good organization and teamwork as with good surgery.

Sometimes it is better to accept a less than perfect position

The objective of all fracture treatment is to return patients to as normal function as possible using the safest method, in a reasonable period of time and at effective cost. Perfect function is sometimes not achieved because the damage is not entirely retrievable and because accurate reduction and effective holding can sometimes only be accomplished by exposing people to unnecessary risk. A good example of this is a common fracture of the distal radius named after an Irish surgeon, i.e. Colles fracture.

Strictly speaking, a Colles fracture is a fracture of the distal 2 cm of the radius not involving the joint and results in dorsal angulation, posterior displacement and supination of the distal fragment; the fracture may include the tip of the ulna styloid but not the shaft of the ulna (Figs 21.13 & 21.14). It is commonly caused by a fall on to the out-

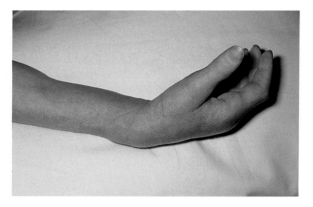

Figure 21.13 Typical 'dinner-fork' deformity seen in a patient with a Colles fracture.

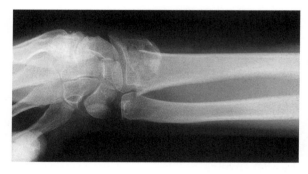

Figure 21.14 In a Colles fracture the radial fragment is shifted and tilted backwards and radially and impacted. There is usually also a fracture of the ulnar styloid.

03

stretched arm and may be produced by minimal force in older people with osteoporosis but requires more violence in young people with tougher bones.

The resulting 'dinner-fork' deformity is unsightly and results in collapse of the radius such that wrist joint function becomes difficult and positioning of the hand for routine tasks is sufficiently impaired to threaten independent living in often frail older people. Ideally, the fracture would be routinely reduced and held until union using a cast. However, the presence of osteoporotic bone frequently indicates that the fracture cannot be effectively held without it later collapsing to the same position as that seen immediately after injury. In practice, all Colles fractures tend to collapse to some degree. However, aggressive intervention is not always required as this may mean prolonged and difficult surgery and the risk of hospitalization in frailer people. These patients may be better served by accepting a less than perfect result, provided the wrist is not painful and displacement not gross. In such circumstances, some help with rehabilitation to achieve

acceptable activities of daily living may be a more pragmatic solution.

In younger people, Colles fracture is a serious injury and requires a major investment in time and resources by the surgeon and the patient in order to restore long-term function. It is vital to appreciate that this is by no means a second-class service for one particular group just because they are old. On the contrary, it is about ensuring that treatment is tailor-made for the patient: we treat people with fractures, not just broken bones.

Apart from malunion, the complications of Colles fracture include:

● acute compression of the median nerve, which may require operative intervention;

● late rupture of extensor tendons through attrition on displaced bone fragments;

● rare problems such as algodystrophy, which are seen more commonly at the wrist because wrist fractures are themselves very common.

Management after fracture consists of ensuring that a reasonable level of function is maintained over the 4–6 weeks of splintage. This may require physiotherapy and encouragement from clinicians and carers to ensure that patients maintain a good range of upper limb function.

Sometimes an operation is more effective for the patient and the health service

Fractures of major long bones such as the femur are potentially very serious injuries, especially if the fracture is open. Femoral fracture always implies that high energy transfer has occurred and soft-tissue damage will be extensive. However, the bone has a good blood supply and is surrounded by a large cuff of very vascular muscle. Provided bones can be held in alignment, the vast majority of even open femoral shaft fractures will heal with few complications. The issue is holding. Prior to the modern era of fracture fixation, patients with this injury were confined to bed on traction for many months. More recently, cast braces shortened the period of hospitalization but nonetheless was still 4–6 weeks followed by up to 6 months of rehabilitation. Effectively, if all went well, a patient with a fractured femoral shaft would lose almost a year of normal life, threatening employment and disrupting family relationships.

Intramedullary nailing, introduced during the Second World War and refined since the 1960s, has dramatically altered the pattern of post-fracture management and immeasurably improved quality of life for patients. Not least, hospital stays for isolated fractures may be as short as 5 days, with minimum outpatient supervision being required and huge cost savings for healthcare providers. Complications following nailing include malposition, especially in rotation, infection and associated damage to structures such as nerves. Non-union sometimes occurs but is relatively rare in the femur. In contrast, although other bones can be nailed in this way, the risk–benefit ratio will be different. For example, in tibial fractures the bone is not cocooned in well-vascularized muscle and so complications such as infection and non-union are higher than in femoral fracture; thus alternatives to nailing, especially in lower-energy tibial fractures, are seen as viable techniques. In the upper limb, the humerus may be nailed but the vast majority of these injuries heal perfectly well with satisfactory function if treated with a simple sling or cast brace; surgery to the humerus carries a very high complication rate in terms of radial nerve palsy. As with all decision-making, surgeons must be certain that any intervention they contemplate is weighted heavily in favour of improved quality of life for the patient, with acceptable risk and reasonable cost.

One other situation in this category is worth consideration. After pathological fracture following metastatic cancer, internal fixation is frequently deployed despite the severity of what is effectively a terminal illness. Fixation treats pain, permits nursing and medical management (mobilization, access to the fracture for adjuvant treatment such as radiotherapy) and improves the remaining quality of life for the individual.

Treating multiple injuries

After serious accidents, when the subject may have many fractures and damage to other systems such as the gut or chest and head, the indications for fixation assume a different perspective. The evidence from the literature overwhelmingly supports early and aggressive fixation of all major fractures, especially to the long bones and the pelvis. Such operations are very demanding but are often essential to save the patient's life. Multiple injuries treated conservatively lead to prolonged immobility, which is a major contributor to late death following injury. These major operations require massive resources in terms of intensive care, multidisciplinary teams, and highly skilled surgeons with regular experience of such operations. For these reasons, people involved in major injuries are best treated in regional centres supported by excellent mobile recovery services (paramedics and hospital-based retrieval teams).

Musculoskeletal trauma at a glance

Definitions

Fracture: a break in the continuity of a bone; fractures may be *transverse*, *oblique* or *spiral* in shape

Greenstick fracture: one in which only one side of the bone is fractured, the other simply bending (usually immature bones)

Comminuted fracture: one in which there are more than two fragments of bone

Complicated fracture: one in which some other structure is also damaged (e.g. a nerve or blood vessel)

Compound fracture: one in which there is a break in the overlying skin (or bowel wall) with potential contamination of the bone ends

Pathological fracture: fracture through a bone weakened by disease, e.g. metastasis

Common causes

Fractures occur when excessive force is applied to a normal bone or moderate force to a diseased bone, e.g. osteoporosis

Clinical features

- Pain
- Loss of function
- Deformity, tenderness and swelling.
- Discoloration or bruising
- Crepitus (not to be elicited!)

Investigations

- Radiographs in two planes (look for lucencies and discontinuity in the cortex of the bone)
- Tomography, CT, MRI (rarely)
- Ultrasonography and radioisotope bone scanning

Management

General
- Look for shock/haemorrhage and check ABC (see Chapter 17)

- Always consider multiple injury in patients presenting with fractures
- Look for injury in other areas at risk (head and spine, ribs and pneumothorax, femoral and pelvic injury)
- Compound fractures are a surgical emergency and require appropriate measures to prevent infection, including tetanus prevention
- Always image the joints above and below a long-bone fracture

The fracture

Immediate
- Relieve pain (i.v. opiates, nerve blocks, splints, traction)
- Establish good i.v. access and send blood for group and cross-match
- Open (compound) fractures require débridement, antibiotics and tetanus prophylaxis

Definitive
- Reduction (closed or open)
- Immobilization (casting, functional bracing, internal fixation, external fixation, traction)
- Rehabilitation (aim to restore patient to preinjury level of function with physiotherapy and occupational therapy)

Complications

Early
- Blood loss
- Infection
- Fat embolism
- Deep vein thrombosis and pulmonary embolism
- Renal failure
- Compartment syndrome

Late
- Non-union
- Delayed union
- Malunion
- Growth arrest
- Arthritis
- Post-traumatic sympathetic (reflex) dystrophy

03

Soft-tissue Trauma

22

Must know Must do

Must know

Soft-tissue injuries can be minimized with simple treatment

Principles of first aid for soft-tissue injuries

How to diagnose soft-tissue injuries by careful examination of the injured patient. Some basic anatomical knowledge is required to achieve this, particularly with nerve injuries

Not diagnosing apparently small and often remediable conditions can have serious social and economic consequences for patients

Importance of prophylaxis against infection and tetanus in soft-tissue injuries

Must do

Visit the accident and emergency department to observe treatment of soft-tissue injuries

Suture a minor laceration under vision

Administer a tetanus toxoid booster injection

Introduction

Although not usually life-threatening, soft-tissue injuries (i.e. injuries to ligaments, tendons, muscles and nerves) are important because they are common and result in morbidity for the patient and have important economic consequences through loss of work. Whenever the body receives a blow, the energy is transmitted through the soft-tissue layers and the bones to be dissipated as disruption, sound and heat. At low velocity such blows seldom break normal bones but will damage cells and tear soft tissues, causing bleeding followed by an acute inflammatory reaction. Acute inflammation is a physiological response to trauma and is associated with swelling, hyperaemia and pain. First aid consists of actions designed to reduce the effects of acute inflammation and to reduce pain. This may be achieved by applying:

- Rest,
- Ice,
- Compression and
- Elevation.

Ice should be wrapped in a cotton towel before being applied to the injured area as direct contact with the skin may lead to thermal injury. Compression of an injured limb should be supervised and not prolonged or performed without elevation; care should be taken to avoid hindering the circulation (see also compartment syndrome, Chapter 17). Elevation of the affected limb above the heart requires the patient to lie down and have the limb raised or sit with the whole arm elevated (Fig. 22.1). These simple measures can be applied to any injury and can reduce swelling effectively, thus facilitating definitive treatment.

Pain relief

The application of RICE, besides reducing swelling, will also help reduce pain. Simple oral analgesia often provides very effective pain relief and the anti-inflammatory properties of non-steroidal anti-inflammatory drugs (NSAIDs) make them particularly effective in soft-tissue injury. If used early and at relatively higher doses than normal, NSAIDs also help to reduce swelling and inflammation. Occasionally, opiates are required to provide pain relief. However, inordinate pain should alert the clinician to the possibility that some more serious condition such as a fracture or an impending compartment syndrome may have been missed.

Injuries to specific soft tissues

Fat and skin

Most superficial injuries to the fat and skin manifest themselves as bruising (*ecchymosis*) and blisters. The bruising may track along tissue planes but this is natural and simply an effect of gravity. Occasionally, fat necrosis causes an intense red reaction on the skin like an infection or cellulitis. If the patient is well and apyrexial, such reaction should not be treated with antibiotics. Haematomata in these layers may liquefy and cause fluid collections, which can be aspirated.

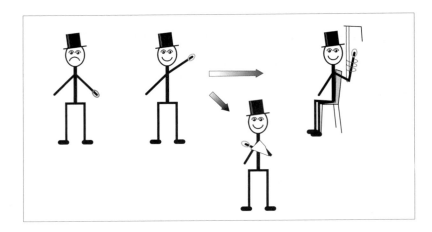

Figure 22.1 Immediate treatment of soft-tissue injury consists of RICE (rest, ice, compression and elevation).

Muscle

Dead muscle cells cannot regenerate. Healing following muscle injury is therefore by fibrosis, with compensatory hypertrophy of the surrounding muscle cells. However, deposition of fibrous tissue in muscle leads to stiffness. This process cannot be altered but early rehabilitation through movement will minimize stiffness and encourage muscle hypertrophy. Following muscle injury, physical therapy within the limits of pain should be instituted as soon as possible. Other techniques such as ultrasound may enhance recovery by dissipating the fibrous tissue.

Ligaments

Incomplete ligament injuries are referred to as *sprains*. Complete injuries are known as *ruptures* or *tears*.
● A sprain is caused by rupture of some, but not all, of the fibres of a ligament. A sprain generally does not cause the associated joint to become unstable but will cause dysfunction through pain. It should also be appreciated that the proprioceptive function of the ligament will be disrupted and this adds to the problems of recovery. Sprains do not require surgical intervention and, following the application of the first-aid measures described above (RICE), recovery is encouraged by exercise – initially non-weight-bearing exercises, rapidly progressing to gradual loading. Most sprains recover in a few weeks depending on the severity of injury and individual requirements, e.g. an athlete may require longer to achieve a high level of performance.
● Ruptures may render a joint unstable and also proprioceptively insensitive in certain planes of movement. Complete ruptures often present with less severe pain than sprains, presumably because of the associated nerve damage. Surprisingly, surgical intervention is seldom required

except in specific cases (e.g. cruciate ligament injuries). If joint motion is controlled by splintage early in treatment, then most ligaments will heal spontaneously.

Tendons

Tendon injuries generally arise from penetrating trauma, although they may be ruptured by excessive force. They occasionally rupture in middle and old age when subjected to normal forces. In these situations the tendon has undergone degenerative change due to either intrinsic collagen abnormalities or abnormal 'wear' against an osteophyte from an adjacent degenerative joint. Tendons usually require surgical repair, which can be technically challenging if function is to be restored. Postrepair physiotherapy to restore movement requires a balance between movement and a reduction in loading so that any repair is not damaged.

Common penetrating injuries to tendons occur in the hand. Extensor injuries are relatively benign and can be repaired fairly easily by direct suture with strong absorbable materials. The local blood supply enables predictable healing. Flexor injuries are more complex because the tendons pass through tight synovial-lined tunnels in the palm and the fingers. The blood supply is more tenuous than in extensor tendons. This leads to the double challenge of needing accurate repair with minimal damage to any remaining blood supply. Such injuries need the attention of specialist surgeons. Whenever a hand sustains a cut, then tendon (and nerve) injury must be specifically excluded.

Degenerative tendon injuries are commonly seen around the shoulder, affecting the tendon to the long head of biceps and the short tendinous sheath composed of the supraspinatus and infraspinatus muscles and the teres minor. Rotator cuff tears may occur through high-energy

03

trauma but more commonly occur in association with degenerative changes in the glenohumeral and acromio-clavicular joints. The patient may present with pain followed by loss of function (see painful arc syndrome, Chapter 21). Repair is technically difficult and sometimes all that may be done is to decompress the compromised tendon tissue by débriding degenerative osteophytes from around affected joints. This improves pain but unless the tear can be repaired there is no restoration of function.

Nerves

Stretching, crushing or cutting may injure nerves. Stretching or crushing may result in temporary loss of function. Such injuries may be associated with a fracture or a direct injury through pressure. Application of tight bandages or casts around a limb may cause nerve injury through pressure. It is important to document nerve injuries prior to treatment so that the relationship of the injury to the initial trauma is established and the clinician is not exposed to accusations that nerve injury has been caused by treatment.

Types of nerve injury

● *Neurotmesis* is complete anatomical division of a nerve with Wallerian degeneration. The nerve tissue distal to the division degenerates and only the support cells survive. New nerve tissue grows back as a series of processes from the damaged cells and so recovery can be prolonged and is usually never completed. Mixed sensory and motor nerves have a particularly poor prognosis, while simple sensory nerves such as those found in the fingers are most likely to recover well. *Tinel's sign* is used clinically to mark the level of nerve regeneration. The course of the nerve is percussed with a patella hammer from distally to proximally. A tingling sensation is felt when the level of regeneration is reached.

Complete division of a mixed peripheral nerve results in motor, sensory, vasomotor, sudomotor and trophic symptoms in the anatomical distribution of the nerve. Electromyography is useful in identifying the paralysed muscle groups. Cutaneous sensation is usually lost only over the area of skin *exclusively* supplied by the nerve. For most sensory nerves this area is quite small, as much of the nerve territory is overlapped by supply from adjacent nerves. Destruction of a mixed nerve leads to vasomotor and trophic disturbances related to damage to sympathetic fibres. The anaesthetic skin is dry, does not produce sweat and, when injured, heals slowly. Oedema and cold sensitivity are also recognized. After complete division, recovery is enhanced by surgical repair using fine sutures

Table 22.1 Factors that adversely affect nerve recovery following injury.

Older patients
More proximal levels of nerve injury
Injury caused by excessive trauma
Injuries to mixed nerves
Increasing distance between the nerve ends at the time of repair
Need to use nerve graft in repair

and magnification. However, even with most careful surgery, results are often disappointing.

● *Axonotmesis*: an injury in which the connective tissue survives but most of the axons of the nerve are damaged and Wallerian degeneration occurs. These injuries produce symptoms similar to neurotmesis but their prognosis is better.

● *Neuropraxia*: a minimal lesion producing paralysis without peripheral nerve degeneration. The most common cause is pressure. As the nerve remains in continuity and tissue damage is incomplete, recovery occurs fairly rapidly. It is important that the muscles and joints in the distribution of the nerve distal to injury are kept mobile so that rehabilitation, once recovery is established, is feasible.

The factors that influence recovery following nerve injury are summarized in Table 22.1.

Specific nerve injuries

Examination of all peripheral nerves can be considered under three headings: sensory loss, motor loss and trophic changes. An understanding of the anatomy of nerve supply is essential for understanding the lesions produced. The common upper limb nerve injuries are summarized in Table 22.2.

Footdrop

The common peroneal nerve may be compressed during medical management in situations where direct pressure may be applied to it. For example, a plaster cast may press on it or it may be subject to undue pressure while a patient is anaesthetized on the operating table. Of course because these potential hazards are recognized, then prevention by careful handling and padding to offer protection make these increasingly rare events. Occasionally the nerve may be stretched following major knee surgery or while treating fractures. In general, in all these cases, the nerve is likely to recover and the principle is to maintain passive motion and normal posture until the nerve recovers.

The effect of footdrop, i.e. loss of peroneal muscle ability to produce dorsiflexion, makes the gait clumsy

Table 22.2 Clinical features of some common upper limb peripheral nerve injuries.

	Cause	Motor	Sensory	Trophic
Brachial plexus injury				
Complete	Motor cycle accidents	Complete arm paralysis	Complete arm anaesthesia	Muscle wasting
Upper (C4–C6; Erb/Duchenne)	Motor cycle accident/ obstetric injury	Limb assumes 'waiter's tip' position	Decreased sensation over outer upper arm	Muscle wasting
Lower (C7, C8, T1; Klumpke)	Cervical rib/shoulder dislocation	Paralysis of the small muscles of the hand (may be a Horner's syndrome)	Sensory loss of inner side forearm and medial $3^1/2$ fingers	Wasting of muscles in hand
Radial nerve injury (Fig. 22.2)				
	Mid-shaft fracture of humerus 'Saturday night' palsy (falling asleep with arm draped over the back of a chair)	Wrist drop	Anaesthesia of a small area at base of thumb and index finger	Minimal wasting of long wrist extensors
Median nerve injury (Fig. 22.3)				
At the elbow	Fracture of lower end of humerus Elbow dislocation	'Pointing' index finger and 'simian hand' (loss of abduction and opposition of thumb)	Sensory loss over all palmar aspect and distal dorsal aspect of radial $3^1/2$ fingers	Thenar eminence wasting
At the wrist	Lacerations	Simian hand	Sensory loss over all palmar aspect and distal dorsal aspect of radial $3^1/2$ fingers	Thenar eminence wasting
Ulnar nerve injury (Fig. 22.4)				
At the elbow	Fracture of medial epicondyle of the humerus	Claw hand (*main en griffe*)	Palmar and dorsal medial $1^1/2$ fingers	Wasting of all small muscles of the hand apart from the thenar eminence
At the wrist	Lacerations	Marked claw hand	Palmar and dorsal medial $1^1/2$ fingers	Wasting of all small muscles of the hand apart from the thenar eminence

03

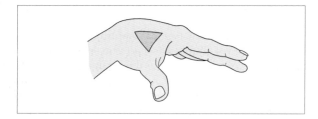

Figure 22.2 In radial nerve injury there is a characteristic wrist drop due to paralysis of the extensors of the wrist. There is only a very small area of anaesthesia at the base of the thumb and index finger as there is considerable sensory overlap from the median and ulnar nerves.

and inefficient. Classically, the patient has a high stepping knee gait to permit the floppy foot to come through during striding. Temporary splintage with a splint or orthosis will improve gait while the foot slowly recovers its functional power.

Wrist drop
The wrist is extended by the radial nerve, which is prone to damage when the humerus is fractured. Radial nerve palsy or wrist drop is even commoner following operations to repair the humerus by open reduction and internal fixation. Closed injuries as described carry a good prognosis and the principle is as usual to maintain function with

03

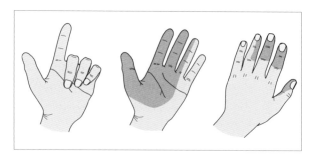

Figure 22.3 In high median nerve lesions the flexors of the wrist and fingers will be paralysed, except those supplied by the ulnar nerve, i.e. flexor carpi ulnaris and the medial half of flexor digitorum profundus. Thus when the patient attempts to flex the fingers, the index finger remains extended (pointing sign). With high and low lesions there will be failure to abduct and oppose the thumb, resulting in a simian or ape-like hand. Wasting of the muscles of the thenar eminence will be pronounced in all median nerve lesions. There will be sensory loss to the palmar surface of the lateral $3^1/2$ fingers and from the proximal interphalangeal joint distally on the dorsal surface of the same fingers.

splintage and therapy. In this case, a splint that maintains wrist extension and supports the metacarpophalangeal joints ensures the intrinsic muscles of the hand (supplied by ulnar and median nerves) continue to provide fine finger motion including finger extension. Physiotherapy is essential to provide the platform for recovery once nerve regeneration is established.

Sciatic nerve injuries

The sciatic nerve may be injured by penetrating trauma (e.g. an 'intramuscular' injection) or a posterior dislocation of the hip. There is paralysis of the hamstring muscles and all of the muscle groups below the knee. Only the muscles of the anterior compartment of the thigh are unaffected (as they are supplied by the femoral nerve). Sensory loss is also extensive, with complete anaesthesia below the knee except for a narrow strip along the medial side supplied by the long saphenous branch of the femoral nerve.

The common peroneal branch of the sciatic nerve is at risk of injury as it winds around the neck of the fibula. Unfortunately, this nerve often suffers iatrogenic injury because of an excessively tight plaster cast or inadequate protection from pressure while the patient is under anaes-

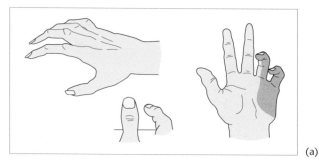

(a)

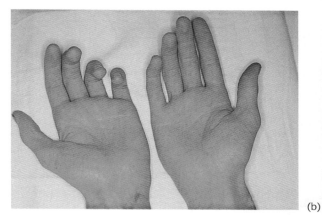

(b)

Figure 22.4 (a) Injury to the ulnar nerve produces a classical deformity known as claw hand or *main en griffe*. This occurs with both high and low lesions but the deformity is much more pronounced with low lesions. The clawed appearance results from the actions of the long extensors and flexors of the fingers. Wasting of all the small muscles of the hand (except the muscles of the thenar eminence) occurs and is seen most easily on the dorsum of the hand. (Weakness of the adductor pollicis accounts for *Froment's sign*: if the patient holds a piece of paper between the thumb and fingers, the terminal phalanx of the thumb of the affected hand flexes due to the unopposed action of flexor pollicis longus.) Sensory loss is to the medial $1^1/2$ fingers and affects both the dorsal and palmar surfaces. (b) A typical low ulnar nerve lesion: note the scar at the wrist.

thesia. Clinically, the patient has footdrop and anaesthesia on the dorsum of the foot. Most pressure-induced injuries are neuropraxias and as long as the paralysed part is managed carefully (by skin care, massage, passive joint movement and the use of spring-loaded 'lively' splints), a good outcome can be expected.

Soft tissue trauma at a glance

Definitions

RICE: a mnemonic for **R**est, **I**ce, **C**ompression and **E**levation, the mainstays of management of soft-tissue injuries

Neurotmesis: complete anatomical division of a nerve with Wallerian degeneration

Axonotmesis: a nerve injury that results in division of the axons but the connective tissues survive

Neuropraxia: a minimal nerve lesion producing paralysis without Wallerian degeneration

Causalgia: a pain syndrome characterized by severe burning pain with autonomic and trophic (denotes *nourishment, nutrition*) changes that may accompany a partial mixed-nerve injury. It is often helped by sympathectomy

Soft tissue injuries

Tissue	Type of injury	Treatment
Skin and fat	Ecchymosis (bruising)	RICE
	Fat necrosis	RICE
	Haematoma	RICE, aspirate if haematoma liquefies
Muscle	Tearing with healing by fibrosis	RICE with early movement ± ultrasound
Ligaments	Sprain (incomplete injury)	RICE + exercise when pain allows
	Rupture (complete injury	Splintage, RICE, occasionally surgery, e.g. anterior cruciate ligament
Tendons	Penetrating trauma (hand, wrist)	Surgical repair + physiotherapy
	Rupture (degenerative change)	
Nerves	Stretching, crushing or cutting	Neurotmesis: surgical repair
		Axonotmesis and neuropraxia: surgical repair not necessary. Maintain function while nerve recovers at rate of 1 mm/day. Recovery is usually excellent

03

Burns

23

03

Must know Must do

Must know

Pathophysiology of burns, including systemic response in major burns

How to assess severity and depth of burns

Indications for referral of patients to a major burns centre/department

Principles of general and local management of burns

Principles of intravenous fluid requirements in the severely burnt patient

Principles of rehabilitation of burn victims

Must do

See patients with minor burns

See at least one patient with a major burn, including any operative management, recovery and any subsequent plastic surgery

Observe skin grafting for burns

Introduction

Burn trauma represents one the most devastating conditions encountered in surgery. The correct treatment of these injuries is vital to ensure a favourable outcome and encompasses accurate assessment, careful resuscitation and precise surgical management. Much of the treatment of burns is controversial and the subject of debate. The aim of this chapter is to provide a framework for one method of managing a patient with major burns and to provide an overview of the complexities of dealing with these cases.

Epidemiology

Every year in the UK there are 13,000 hospital admissions for burns and around 300 burn-related deaths. Burns tend to affect specific groups of the population, particularly the vulnerable: the young, the old and the debilitated. Children between the ages of 1 and 5 are at high risk from scalding injuries. The elderly are at risk from scalds, contact and flame burns. Teenagers are often injured as a result of illicit activities involving accelerants or electrocution. The most common burns in adults are suffered by males aged between 17 and 30 years of age. These are mainly due to flame burns but also occur as a result of industrial accidents. Burn victims are often compromised by some other factor, such as alcoholism, epilepsy or psychiatric illness. All these problems need to be addressed when managing the patient.

Pathophysiology

Burn injuries result in a local and systemic response.

Local response

The three zones of a burn were described by Jackson in 1947 (Fig. 23.1). At the point of maximum damage there is a *zone of coagulation*. In this zone there is irreversible tissue loss due to coagulation of the constituent proteins. This is surrounded by a *zone of stasis*, characterized by decreased tissue perfusion. The tissue in this zone is potentially salvageable. The main aim of burns resuscitation is to increase tissue perfusion here and prevent any damage becoming irreversible. Additional insults, such as prolonged hypotension, infection or oedema, can convert this zone into an area of complete tissue loss. Finally, there is a *zone of hyperaemia*, where tissue perfusion is increased; this zone will invariably recover. In a burn wound, these zones are three-dimensional; loss of tissue in the zone of stasis will lead to the burn deepening.

Systemic response

The release of cytokines and other inflammatory mediators at the site of injury has a systemic effect once the burn reaches 30%. This systemic inflammatory response results in cardiovascular, respiratory, metabolic and immunological changes.

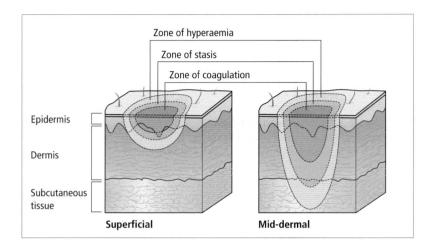

Figure 23.1 Jackson's burn zones.

Cardiovascular changes
- Increase in capillary permeability, leading to loss of proteins and fluids from the intravascular into the interstitial compartment.
- Peripheral and splanchnic vasoconstriction.
- Decreased myocardial contractility, possibly due to tumour necrosis factor α.

These changes, coupled with fluid loss from the burn wound, result in systemic hypotension and end-organ hypoperfusion.

Respiratory changes
- Bronchoconstriction secondary to inflammatory mediators.
- In severe burns, adult respiratory distress syndrome (ARDS) can occur.

Metabolic changes
- Up to threefold increase in the basal metabolic rate.
- Splanchnic hypoperfusion.

These two factors necessitate early and aggressive enteral feeding to decrease catabolism and maintain gut integrity.

Immunological: non-specific downregulation of the immune response, affecting both cell-mediated and humoral pathways.

Mechanisms of injury

Thermal injuries

Scalds

Of burns in children, 70% are caused by scalds. This type of burn also occurs frequently in the elderly. The common mechanisms are spillage of hot drinks/liquids or injuries caused by hot bathing water. Scalds tend to cause superficial to superficial dermal burns (see later for burn depth assessment).

Flame

Flame burns comprise 50% of adult burns. They are often associated with inhalational injury and other concomitant trauma. Flame burns tend to be deep dermal or full thickness.

Contact

In order to produce a burn by direct contact, the object touched must either have been very hot or the contact abnormally long. The latter is the more usual reason and these types of burns are commonly seen in epileptics, alcoholics and drug abusers. They are also seen in the elderly due to loss of consciousness; such a presentation requires a full investigation as to cause of the blackout. Contact burns tend to be deep dermal or full thickness.

Electrical injuries

Of all admissions to burn units, 3–4% are due to electrocution injuries. An electric current will travel through the body from one point to another, creating 'entry' and 'exit' points. The tissue between these two areas can be damaged by the current. The amount of heat generated and hence the amount of tissue damaged in an electrical injury is equal to $0.24V^2 \times R$ (where V is voltage and R is resistance). The voltage is therefore the main determinant of the degree of tissue damage, and it is logical to divide electrocution injuries into those caused by low-voltage domestic current and those caused by high-voltage currents. High-voltage injuries can be further divided into

03

'true' high-tension injuries caused by high-voltage current passing through the body and 'flash' injuries caused by tangential exposure to a high-voltage current arc, where no current actually flows through the body.

● Domestic electricity: low voltages tend to cause small, deep contact burns at the exit and entry sites. The alternating nature of domestic current can interfere with the cardiac cycle, giving rise to arrhythmias.

● 'True' high-tension injuries (when voltage is 1000 V or greater). There is extensive tissue damage and often limb loss. There is usually a large amount of soft and bony tissue necrosis. Muscle damage gives rise to rhabdomyolysis and there is a significant incidence of renal failure with these injuries. This injury pattern needs more aggressive resuscitation and débridement than other burns. Contact with voltage greater than 70,000 V is invariably fatal.

● 'Flash' injury: in this scenario, there has been an arc of current from a high-tension voltage source. The heat from this arc can cause superficial flash burns to exposed body parts, typically the face and hands. However, clothing can also be set alight, giving rise to deeper burns. No current actually passes through the patient's body.

A particular concern after an electrical injury is the need for cardiac monitoring. There is good evidence that if the admission electrocardiogram (ECG) is normal and there is no history of loss of consciousness, then cardiac monitoring is not required. If there are ECG abnormalities or a loss of consciousness, then 24-h monitoring is advised.

Chemical injuries

Chemical injuries are usually the result of industrial accidents but may occur with household chemical products. These burns tend to be deep because the corrosive agent continues to cause coagulative necrosis until completely removed. Alkalis tend to penetrate deeper and cause worse burns than acids. Cement is a common cause of alkali burns (Fig. 23.2).

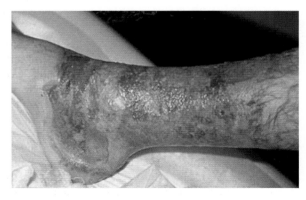

Figure 23.2 Cement chemical burn.

Certain industrial agents require specific treatments in addition to standard first aid. Hydrofluoric acid, widely used for glass etching and in the manufacture of circuit boards, is one of the more common culprits. It causes a continuing penetrating injury that is neutralized by calcium gluconate applied in a gel and/or injected into the affected tissues.

The initial management of all chemical burns is the same irrespective of the agent. All contaminated clothing must be removed and the area thoroughly irrigated. This is often best achieved by showering the patient, which has been shown to limit the depth of the burn. Litmus paper can be used to confirm removal of alkali or acid. Eye injuries should be irrigated copiously and referred to an ophthalmologist.

Initial management of major burns

The general approach to a major burn can be extrapolated to managing any burn. An accurate history and examination of the patient and the burn is vital. A systematic approach will ensure that key information is not missed.

History

The history in a burn injury can give valuable information about the nature and extent of the burn. The likelihood of inhalational injury, depth of the burn and suspicion of other injuries can all be ascertained from a comprehensive history. The exact mechanism of injury and any prehospital treatment must be established. The key points are as follows.

● Exact time and mechanism of the injury:
   (a) Type of burn, i.e scald, flame, electrical, chemical.
   (b) How was the person put out? How long were they alight for?
   (c) What first aid was carried out? If cooling was performed, what with and for how long?

● Likelihood of concomitant injuries (i.e. fall from height, road traffic accident, explosion).

● Likelihood of inhalational injury: did the burn occur in an enclosed space?

● Scalding injuries:
   (a) What was the liquid?
   (b) If tea/coffee, was there milk in it?
   (c) Was there a solute in the liquid? This will raise the boiling temperature and result in a worse injury.
   Boiling rice is a common cause in the UK.

● Electrocution injuries:
   (a) What voltage?
   (b) Was there a flash/arcing?
   (c) Contact time.

● Chemical injuries: what chemical?

● Any suspicion of non-accidental injury?

Burns at a glance

Definitions

Burn: the response of the skin and subcutaneous tissues to thermal injury

Partial-thickness burn: a burn that does not extend through all skin layers. Needle prick elicits bleeding and pain sensation

Full-thickness burn: extends through all skin layers into the subcutaneous tissues. It destroys all sources of skin epithelial regrowth. No bleeding or pain on needle prick

Deep dermal burn: extends through the epidermis and into, but not through, the deeper layers of the dermis. Needle prick elicits delayed bleeding and sensation of being touched but no pain

Escharotomy: an emergency surgical procedure where the burnt tissue (eschar) of a circumferential full-thickness or deep dermal burn on a limb or on the chest is divided

Epidemiology
- 13,000 burns and 300 burn deaths per annum in UK
- Children 1–5 years old: scalds
- Teenagers: flame, electrocution
- Adults (frequently males aged 17–30 years): flame burns, industrial accidents (flame, chemical, electrocution)
- Elderly: scalds, contact and flame burns

Pathophysiology
Local response
- Zone of coagulation: coagulation necrosis, irreversible tissue loss
- Zone of stasis: decreased tissue perfusion, potentially salvageable
- Zone of hyperaemia: increased tissue perfusion, invariably recovers

Systemic response
Mediated by cytokines and inflammatory mediators, present in burns of > 30%
- Cardiovascular: increased capillary permeability, vasoconstriction, decreased myocardial contractility
- Respiratory: bronchoconstriction, ARDS
- Metabolic: threefold increase in basal metabolic rate, splanchnic hypoperfusion
- Immunological: downregulation of both cell-mediated and humoral immune response

Mechanism of injury
- Thermal injury:
  (a) Scalds: superficial, superficial dermal
  (b) Flame: deep dermal or full thickness, inhalation injury
  (c) Contact: deep dermal or full thickness
- Electrical injury: heat generated = $0.24V^2 \times R$, thus voltage main determinant of degree of injury
  (a) Low voltage (< 1000 V): deep contact burns at entry and exit sites
  (b) True high voltage (> 1000 V): current goes through body. Extensive soft tissue and bone necrosis
  (c) Flash high voltage (> 1000 V): current does *not* pass through body. 'Flash' burn from heat generated by current arc from high-tension source. Exposed parts of body affected (face, hands)
- Chemical burns: deep necrotic burns

03

It is very important that the history be obtained at the point of admission. This may be the only time that a first-hand history is available because airway swelling may develop in the hours following injury and require intubation. A brief medical history should be taken (following the 'AMPLE' guidelines for ATLS).

Primary survey

The initial management of a severely burnt patient is similar to that of any trauma patient. A modified ATLS primary survey is performed, with particular emphasis being placed on assessment of the airway and breathing. It is important that the burn injury does not distract from this sequential assessment, otherwise serious associated injuries may be missed.

A: airway with cervical spine control

An assessment must be made as to whether the airway is compromised or is at risk of compromise. The cervical spine should be protected unless it is definitely not injured. Inhalation of hot gases will result in a burn above the vocal cords; this burn will become oedematous over the course of hours, especially after fluid resuscitation has begun. Consequently, an airway that is patent on arrival may occlude after admission.

Direct inspection of the oropharynx should be performed by a senior anaesthetist. If there is any concern about the patency of the airway, then intubation is the safest policy. However, unnecessary intubation and sedation could potentially worsen the patient's condition, so the decision to intubate should be made carefully (Fig. 23.3 & Table 23.1).

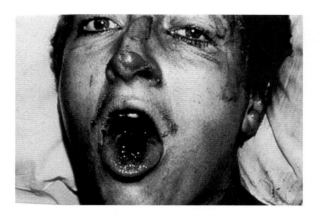

Figure 23.3 Patient at high risk of inhalational injury.

Table 23.1 Signs of inhalational injury and indications for intubation.

Signs of inhalational injury
History of flame burns/burns in an enclosed space
Full-thickness/deep dermal burns to the face, neck or upper
    torso
Singed nasal hair
Carbonaceous sputum/carbon particles in the oropharynx

Indications for intubation
Erythema/swelling of the oropharynx on direct visualization
Change in voice, with hoarseness/harsh cough
Stridor
Dyspnoea

B: breathing

All burn patients should receive 100% oxygen through a non-rebreathing mask on presentation. Breathing problems are considered as those that affect the respiratory system below the vocal cords. There are several mechanisms that can compromise respiration:
- mechanical restriction of ventilation;
- blast injury;
- smoke inhalation;
- carbon monoxide poisoning.

Mechanical restriction of breathing
Deep dermal or full-thickness circumferential burns of the chest can limit chest excursion and prevent aedequate ventilation. This requires immediate escaharotomy (see later).

Blast injury
If there has been a history of an explosion, blast lung can complicate ventilation. Penetrating injuries can cause

Table 23.2 Symptoms associated with different blood levels of carboxyhaemoglobin.

	Symptom
0–10%	Minimal symptoms (normal level in heavy smokers)
10–20%	Nausea, headache
20–30%	Drowsiness, lethargy
30–40%	Confusion, agitation
40–50%	Coma, respiratory depression
> 50%	Death

tension pneumothoraces and the blast itself can cause lung contusions and alveolar trauma and lead to ARDS.

Smoke inhalation
The products of combustion, though cooled by the time they reach the lungs, act as direct irritants to the lungs. This leads to bronchospasm, inflammation and bronchorrhoea. There is impaired function of type II pneumocytes and impaired ciliary action, both of which exacerbate the situation. The inflammatory exudate created is not cleared and atelectasis/pneumonia follows. The situation can be particularly severe in asthmatics. Non-invasive management can be attempted, with nebulizers and non-invasive positive-pressure ventilation with some positive end-expiratory pressure (PEEP). However, these patients may need a period of ventilation as this allows aedequate oxygenation and permits regular toiletting of the lungs.

CARBOXYHAEMOGLOBIN
Carbon monoxide binds haemoglobin with 40 times the affinity of oxygen. It also binds to other intracellular proteins, particularly the cytochrome oxygenase pathway. These two events lead to intracellular and extracellular hypoxia. The pulse oximeter will read spuriously high because it cannot differentiate between oxyhaemoglobin and carboxyhaemoglobin. However blood gases will reveal hypoxia, metabolic acidosis and raised carboxyhaemoglobin. The signs of carboxyhaemoglobinaemia are listed in Table 23.2. Treatment is with 100% oxygen as this displaces carbon monoxide from bound proteins six times faster than atmospheric oxygen. Patients with carboxyhaemoglobin levels greater than 25–30% should be ventilated. Hyperbaric therapy is rarely practical and has not been proven to be advantageous. It takes longer to shift the carbon monoxide from the cytochrome oxygenase pathway, so 100% oxygen should be continued until the metabolic acidosis has cleared.

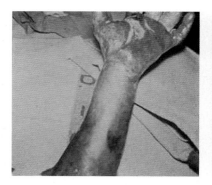
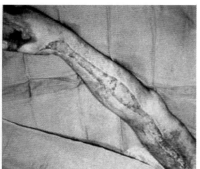

Figure 23.4 Escharotomies in upper limb.

C: circulation

Intravenous access should be established with large-bore cannulae placed preferably through unburnt tissue. The peripheral circulation must be checked. Any deep or full-thickness circumferential extremity burns can act as a tourniquet, especially once oedema secondary to fluid resuscitation has begun. If there is any suspicion of decreased perfusion due to circumferential burns, the tissue must be released with escharotomies (see later). Profound hypovolaemia is not the normal initial response in a burn. If a patient is hypotensive, it is due to a delayed presentation, cardiogenic dysfunction or an occult source of blood loss (chest, abdomen, pelvis).

D: neurological disability

The patient's score on the Glasgow Coma Scale should be assessed. Patients may be confused due to hypoxia or hypovolaemia.

E: exposure with environment control

The whole patient should be examined (including the back) to obtain an accurate estimate of the burn area. It is very easy for the burn patient, especially children, to become hypothermic. This leads to hypoperfusion and deepening of the burn wound. The patient should be covered and warmed as soon as possible.

F: fluids

The resuscitation regimen should be determined and begun. A urinary catheter should be placed.

Analgesia

Superficial burns can be very painful and therefore intravenous morphine should be used as this can be easily titrated against pain and respiratory depression.

Escharotomy

Any circumferential deep dermal or full-thickness burn on an extremity will not stretch as the underlying tissue swells due to burn wound oedema. This raises tissue pressure and can impair peripheral circulation but may only occur as fluid resuscitation causes oedema to develop. In addition, circumferential chest burns can limit chest excursion and impair ventilation. Both these situations require division of the burn eschar, a procedure known as escharotomy. Only the burnt tissue is divided, not any underlying fascia (differentiating this from a fasciotomy). Escharotomy is an emergency procedure that is performed at the bedside or in the trauma room. For extremities, incisions are made along the mid-lateral and/or medial aspects of the limbs, avoiding any underlying structures (Figs 23.4–23.6). For the chest, longitudinal incisions are made down each midclavicular line to the subcostal region. The lines are joined by a chevron incision running parallel to the subcostal margin. This creates a mobile breast-plate that moves with ventilation.

Escharotomies are best performed with a cutting diathermy as they tend to bleed. They are then packed with Kaltostat and dressed with the burn.

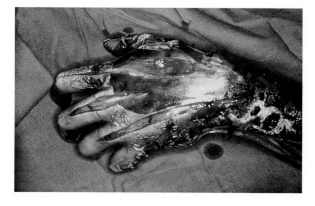

Figure 23.5 Escharotomies in lower limb.

03

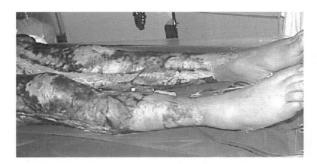

Figure 23.6 Escharotomies in hand.

Investigations

The number of investigations will vary with the type of burn but most patients require:
- full blood count, haematocrit, urea and electrolytes;
- group and save/cross-match;
- microbiology swabs of burn wounds.
  Electrical injuries also require:
- 12-lead ECG;
- cardiac enzymes (high-tension injury).
  Inhalational injuries require:
- chest X-ray;
- arterial blood gases (can be useful in any burn because base excess is predictive of amount of resuscitation required).

Any concomitant trauma requires its own investigations.

Assessment of burn area

The assessment of burn area tends to be done badly, even by those who are expert at it. There are three commonly employed methods of estimating burn area and each has a role in different scenarios. When calculating the burn wound area, erythema should not be included. Erythema may take a few hours to fade so it is inevitable that some overestimation will occur if the burn is estimated acutely.
- *Palmar surface*: the surface area of the patient's palm (i.e. *not* the fingers) is 0.8% (male) and 0.6% (female) of the total body surface area of the patient. Palmar surface area can be used to estimate relatively small burns (< 15%) or very large burns (> 85%, when unburnt skin is counted). For larger burns, it is inaccurate.
- *Wallace rule of nines*: this is a good quick way of estimating the area of medium to large burns in adults. The body is divided up into areas of 9% (Fig. 23.7) and the total burn area calculated. It is not accurate in children.
- *Lund and Browder chart*: if used correctly, this is the most accurate method. It is also the only chart that compensates for the variation in body shape with age

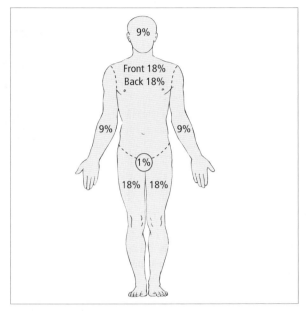

Figure 23.7 Wallace rule of nines.

(Fig. 23.8) and can therefore give an accurate assessment of burns area in children.

It is important that *all* of the burn is exposed and assessed. Pigmented skin can be difficult to assess and it may be necessary to remove all the loose epidermal layers in pigmented skin to get an idea of burn size.

Assessment of burn depth

Burns are best classified into two groups by the amount of skin loss.
- Partial thickness: the burn does not extend through all skin layers.
- Full thickness: the burn extends through all skin layers into the subcutaneous tissues (Fig. 23.9).

Partial-thickness burns can be further divided into superficial, superficial dermal and deep dermal.
- Superficial: the burn extends into the epidermis but not into the dermis (Fig. 23.10).
- Superficial dermal: the burn extends through the epidermis into the superficial layers of the dermis (Fig. 23.11).
- Deep dermal: the burn extends through the epidermis into the deeper layers of the dermis but not through the entire dermis (Fig. 23.12).

In reality, most burns will be a mixture of different depths. The assessment of depth is important for planning because the more superficial burns will tend to heal spontaneously but deeper burns will need surgical intervention.

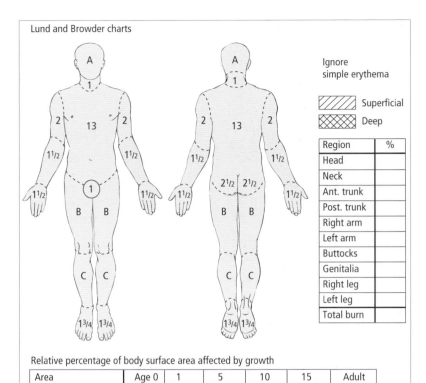

Figure 23.8 Lund and Browder chart.

Lund and Browder charts

Ignore simple erythema

⧄	Superficial
⧅	Deep

Region	%
Head	
Neck	
Ant. trunk	
Post. trunk	
Right arm	
Left arm	
Buttocks	
Genitalia	
Right leg	
Left leg	
Total burn	

Relative percentage of body surface area affected by growth

Area	Age 0	1	5	10	15	Adult
A = 1/2 of Head	9 1/2	8 1/2	6 1/2	5 1/2	4 1/2	3 1/2
B = 1/2 of one Thigh	2 3/4	3 1/4	4	4 1/2	4 1/2	4 3/4
C = 1/2 of one Leg	2 1/2	2 1/2	2 3/4	3	3 1/4	3 1/2

03

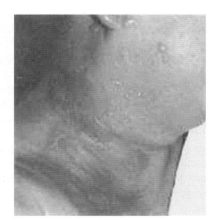

Figure 23.9 Full-thickness burn: flame.

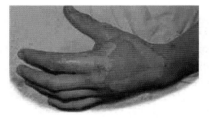

Figure 23.10 Superficial burn: scald.

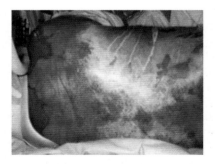

Figure 23.11 Superficial dermal burn: scald.

Burn depth estimation is not necessary for estimating resuscitation formulae.

The assessment of burn depth is very difficult. The history will give clues about the expected depth: a flash burn will probably be superficial and a flame burn that

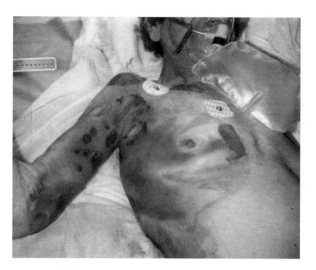

Figure 23.12 Deep dermal burn: flame.

03

was not rapidly extinguished will probably be deep. There are three elements that should be assessed: bleeding, sensation and appearance.

Bleeding. Test bleeding with a 21-gauge needle:
• brisk bleeding on a superficial prick means superficial/superficial dermal;
• delayed bleeding on a deeper prick means deep dermal;
• no bleeding means full thickness.

Sensation. Test sensation with a needle (as for bleeding):
• pain means a superficial/superficial dermal burn;
• pin can be felt but is not painful means deep dermal;
• no sensation means full thickness.

Appearance. Though obvious, it can be hard to judge burn depth by appearance as the burn is often covered in soot or dirt.
• A red glistening wound that obviously blanches is superficial.
• A paler, drier, but blanching wound is partial thickness.
• A dry, leathery, hard wound is full thickness.

It must be remembered that a burn is a dynamic wound and depth will change depending on the success of resuscitation. Initial estimates need to be reviewed later.

Once the burn's surface area and depth have been estimated, the wound should be washed and any loose skin removed. Any blisters should be deroofed for ease of dressing. The burn should then be dressed. For an acute burn that is to be referred to a burn centre, clingfilm is an ideal dressing as it will cover the wound but not alter the physical appearance of the burn. This allows accurate evaluation by the burn team later on. Flamazine should not be used on a burn that is to be referred as it makes assessment of depth by appearance difficult. Other burns are dressed according to depth (see later).

Prognosis

A rough estimate of prognosis can be given by adding the age of the patient to the percentage burn; this gives the percentage mortality. Inhalational injury increases mortality but it is arguable by how much. A decision should be made about whether resuscitation should be started or whether the patient should just be kept comfortable.

Resuscitation regimens

There is no ideal resuscitation regimen for burns and this is reflected by the continual change in the regimens in favour. It is vital to remember that all the fluid formulae are only *guidelines*. Their success relies on the adjustment of resuscitation against monitored physiological and investigative parameters. The main aim of these resuscitation formulae is to maintain tissue perfusion to the zone of stasis and prevent the burn deepening. This is not as easy as it sounds. Too little fluid will cause hypoperfusion; too much fluid will lead to oedema that will cause tissue hypoxia.

There are some important overall concepts about fluid resuscitation in burn patients. The greatest amount of fluid loss occurs in the first 24 h. For the first 8–12 h, there is a general shift of fluid from the intravascular to interstitial fluid compartment. This was thought mainly due to increased capillary permeability but other factors have also been shown to play a role. This means that any fluid given in this period will rapidly leave the intravascular compartment. Therefore colloids have no advantage over crystalloids in maintaining circulatory volume. Indeed, colloids could exacerbate the situation because they will leak out into the interstitial space, where they will increase the oncotic pressure and increase the flow of fluid from the circulation. Rapid fluid boluses are also of no benefit as a rapid rise in intravascular hydrostatic pressure only drives more fluid out of the circulation. However, much protein is lost through the burn wound so there is a need to replace this oncotic loss. Therefore some regimens use some colloid after 8 h, when the loss of fluid from the intravascular space is decreasing.

Burns greater than 15% in adults and 10% in children warrant formal resuscitation. Again, these are guidelines

and some discretion can be used by experienced staff. The most commonly used formula at present is actually a pure crystalloid resuscitation formula, the Parkland formula, devised by Charlie Baxter. It has the advantages that it is easy to calculate and that the titration is against urine output. The fluid for the first 24 h is calculated as follows:

4 mL × percentage total burn surface area × weight in kg = total fluid requirement in 24 h.

Half of the fluid is given in the first 8 h and half in the next 16 h. In children, maintenance fluid is required in addition, calculated by weight as:

4 mL/kg for 0–10 kg + 2 mL/kg for 10–20 kg + 1 mL/kg over 20 kg = rate in mL/h.

The start point for the timing is the time of injury not the time of admission. Any fluid already given should be deducted from the amount of fluid required. The formula ends at 24 h. For the next 24 h, colloid is begun at a rate of 0.5 mL × percentage total burn surface area × weight (kg) and maintenance crystalloid is continued at a rate of 1.5 mL × total burn surface area × weight (kg).

For example, a 25-year-old-man weighing 70 kg with a 30% flame burn is admitted at 16.00. His burn occurred at 15.00. He would need:

4 mL × 30% total burn surface area × 70 kg = 8400 mL in 24 h (4200 mL in first 8 h, 4200 mL over the next 16 h).

If he has already received 1000 mL from the emergency services, he needs a further 3200 mL in the first 8 h post burn, i.e. by 23.00. If it is now 16.00, he needs 3200 mL over the next 7 h, then 4200 mL over the next 16 h. Therefore, until 23.00 he needs 3200/7 = 457 mL/ h. After 23.00 for the next 16 h he needs 4200/16 = 262.5 mL/ h.

The maintenance fluid required for children is calculated as shown above. For example, a 24-kg child admitted with a resuscitation burn will need the following maintenance fluid:

4 mL/kg for first 10 kg (40 mL/h) + 2 mL/kg for next 10 kg (20 mL/h) + 1 mL/kg for next 4 kg (4 mL/h) = 64 mL/h.

The maintenance fluid given is usually dextrose-saline.

The end-point to aim for is a urine output of 0.5–1 mL/kg per h in adults and 1–1.5 mL/kg per h in children. High-tension electrical injuries will need significantly more fluid (up to 9 mL/kg per percentage burn surface area in the first 24 h) and a higher urine output (1.5–2 mL/kg per h). Inhalational injuries will also need more fluid.

The most commonly used crystalloid is sodium lactate solution (known as Hartmann's solution in the UK and Ringer-lactate in the USA). It comprises sodium chloride 0.6%, sodium lactate 0.25%, potassium chloride 0.04% and calcium chloride 0.027%. The colloid used is controversial. The Cochrane Report advised against the use of albumin but the review did not include many burn units and so may not be representative. Fresh frozen plasma is often used in children and albumin or a synthetic starch in adults.

It should be emphasized that the above regimen is a guideline only and that resuscitation should not be guided purely by urine output. Other physiological parameters (pulse, blood pressure, respiratory rate) and investigations (haematocrit, plasma sodium, base excess) are useful for giving an indication of the resuscitation status of the patient. The regimens should not be followed slavishly but adjusted according to response. Fluid rate should be changed gradually, between 20 and 30%.

Burn units will vary as to which resuscitation formula is used. It is best to contact the local burn unit and enquire how it wishes the patient to be resuscitated.

Referral to a burn unit

The National Burn Care Review has set guidelines about which patients warrant referral to a burn unit. Burns are divided into complex burns (i.e. those that require specialist intervention) and non-complex burns (i.e. those that do not require immediate admission to a specialist unit). Complex burns should be referred automatically.

A burn injury is more likely to be complex if associated with the following.

- Age: under 5 or over 60 years.
- Site: face, hands, perineum or feet (dermal/full-thickness loss) or any flexure (particularly the neck or axilla) or any circumferential dermal or full-thickness burn of the limbs, torso or neck.
- Inhalation injury: any significant injury, excluding pure carbon monoxide poisoning.
- Mechanism of injury:
    (a) chemical injury (> 5% total body surface area);
    (b) exposure to ionizing radiation;
    (c) high-pressure steam injury;
    (d) high-tension electrical injury;
    (e) hydrofluoric acid injury (> 1% total body surface area);
    (f) suspicion of non-accidental injury.
- Size (dermal/full-thickness loss):
    (a) paediatric (< 16 years old): > 5% total body surface area;
    (b) adult (16 years or over): > 10% total body surface area.

● Coexisting conditions: any serious medical conditions (cardiac dysfunction, immunosuppression, pregnancy) or any associated injuries (fractures, head injuries, crush injuries).

It is better to discuss all cases with the local burn unit as they will eventually be involved in the patient's care.

Subsequent management of burn injury

Superficial/superficial dermal burns

These heal spontaneously within 14 days unless there is secondary infection or the burn deepens. The aim is to provide a dressing that will keep the wound clean, create a suitable environment for healing and minimize pain. Various dressings are used.

Tulle gras (Jelonet, Bactigras)

The traditional method is to use tulle gras (Jelonet), either plain or containing an antiseptic solution such as chlorhexidine (Bactigras). This is adherent and can be difficult to remove once dried but provides a moist environment for healing. Gauze is placed over these wounds because they tend to exude fluid. The gauze may be changed as it soaks through but the tulle gras is usually left undisturbed for 5 days, unless there is concern about secondary infection.

Retention dressing (Hypafix)

A novel way of dressing burns is to use an adhesive dressing such as Hypafix. This sticks to the wound and prevents any shear forces from disrupting healing. The dressing can be kept clean by showering. Gauze will also be required to absorb the initial exudate. The adhesive in the dressing is oil-based so the application of any kind of oil (typically olive oil) dissolves the adhesive and permits removal of the dressing without disturbing the healing burn.

Interface dressings (Biobrane, Transcyte)

These bind to the raw epidermis and provide a semipermeable membrane that keeps the wound moist but prevents bacterial colonization. Transcyte has added growth factors that can accelerate wound healing. These dressings are only effective on superficial/superficial dermal burns and are expensive.

Topical antibacterial cream (Flamazine)

Topical bacterial creams are a popular way of dressing.

Silver sulfadiazine (Flamazine) has good Gram-negative cover and keeps the wound moist and clean. It can be used on its own or with a gauze layer on top. Unfortunately it tends to macerate the wound and can make burn depth assessment difficult. It also requires frequent dressing changes, which can be uncomfortable for the patient.

Deep dermal/full thickness

Deep dermal and full-thickness burns will need surgical intervention. There has been a major change in the way burns are managed in the last 30 years. Initially, there was a reluctance to remove the burn wound early, as this caused additional trauma to the patient and ran the risk of removing tissue that might have healed if left undisturbed. Therefore deep burns were left until 3 weeks when all unhealed areas were excised and skin grafted. However, it was subsequently shown that early removal of the burn wound limited the systemic inflammatory response and improved outcome. In addition, tangential excision allowed burnt tissue to be shaved off in layers, leaving healthy tissue behind. The modern approach to major burns is to remove the burn wound as soon as possible before the patient becomes unwell (< 48 h), resurface the burn and start rehabilitation. This allows faster healing, limits the stress from the burn wound and is associated with improved mortality.

The only innovation to this approach is the use of topical agents that bind to damaged proteins in the wound and inhibit the inflammatory response that the burn causes, e.g. cerium nitrate/silver sulfadiazine cream (Flammcerium). It is useful for large burns because it allows staged excision or for burns in the elderly who may need optimizing prior to surgery.

Surgery

Tangential excision involves shaving the burnt tissue off the healthy unburnt tissue below. This can be performed with a skin graft knife, Goulian hand-held blade for small areas or a mechanical dermatome. This approach is a team effort and requires skilled anaesthesia, as the patients cools down rapidly and blood loss can be large and dramatic. Infiltration of the burn and any skin donor sites with 1 in 1,000,000 adrenaline is effective at reducing blood loss, as is the use of tourniquets when excising burns on extremities. If the burn affects all the subcutaneous tissues, excision at the fascial layer can be performed (fascial excision). This leads to less blood loss but results in a poor cosmetic result with marked contour defects. Depending on the skill of the team and the stability of the patient, burns of up to 50% can be excised in one session.

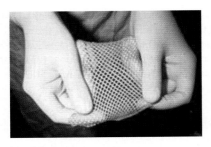

Figure 23.13 Meshed skin graft.

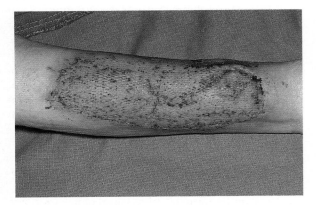

Figure 23.14 Healing meshed skin graft.

Resurfacing

Excising the burn wound is only part of the battle. The main challenge is to resurface the excised wound. There are various approaches to this.

Skin autografts

If the burn wound is less than 50% of total body surface area, then it can be covered with the patient's own skin (autograft). Split skin grafts are taken from unburnt areas and are usually meshed (i.e. have slit perforations placed in them) (Figs 23.13 & 23.14). This helps any exudate beneath the graft to ooze out and also allows the graft to be stretched to cover a larger area. The standard mesh ratio is 1 : 1.5. Wider meshing can cover a larger area but leaves bigger interstices to fill in. Meshed skin grafts heal with the mesh pattern visible so tend not to be used on the face. The grafts are secured with staples or tissue adhesive and then dressed. It is important to prevent shearing forces from disrupting the grafts so joints may be temporarily splinted.

In very large burns there may not be enough unburnt skin to provide autograft to cover the burn wound. Various alternatives to autografts are available.

Skin allografts

Cadaveric skin can be used as a temporary biological dressing. The storage solution decreases the antigenicity of the skin and the burn patient is relatively immuno-suppressed, so the graft is not rejected for a few weeks. This may allow autograft donor sites time to heal for regrafting.

Skin xenografts

Porcine skin can also be used as a temporary biological dressing.

Synthetic skin

There is much research being directed at creating artificial skin. Integra is the most commonly used variety and consists of an artificial neodermis and a silicone top layer. Once placed on the burn wound, the neodermis is vascularized over the course of a few weeks. The silicone layer is removed and a thin skin autograft placed on top. The use of Integra has allowed the rapid débridement and resurfacing of very large burns. Unfortunately it is prone to infection and can lead to hypertrophic scarring. Its overall usefulness in major burns is still being evaluated.

Cultured skin

An alternative approach is to grow the patient's own skin in culture. A small skin biopsy is taken on the day of admission and within 2–3 weeks sheets or suspensions of keratinocytes are available. Unfortunately, these keratinocytes are very delicate and are vulnerable to infection and shearing forces. The delay in culture is also a major drawback but this may be resolved in the future. However, cultured keratinocytes can be useful when used in conjunction with autografts, for filling in the interstices in a widely meshed skin graft.

Nutritional support

The systemic response to a burn injury leads to a three-fold increase in the basal metabolic rate. It is not possible for the patient to maintain an adequate calorie and protein intake by eating and hyperalimentation is required. Adequate nutrition is essential for ensuring wound healing and preventing gastrointestinal complications. Resuscitation burns should have a nasogastric or nasojejunal tube placed and enteral feeding commenced. There are various formulae for estimating the caloric requirements. The Curreri formula is commonly used (daily requirement = 25 kcal/kg + 40 kcal/percentage burn). Trace elements must also be measured and replaced. For the above reasons, it is obvious that a dietician is an important member of the burn team.

03

Microbiological support

Burn wound sepsis is a major problem. Infection can deepen a burn wound as well as worsening the general condition of the patient. Prophylactic antibiotics are of no benefit and may worsen the situation by selecting resistant bacterial strains. The best policy is strict wound care and repeated and regular wound cultures. Evidence of invasive infection should be treated with short courses of high-dose antibiotics to which the organism is sensitive. Topical agents can also be useful in decreasing the bacterial load. Organisms of particular concern include the β-haemolytic streptococci Lancefield group A, C and G. Skin grafts are particularly vulnerable to these organisms and grafting should not be performed on a wound colonized with them. Intravascular lines are associated with high infection rates in burn patients and so should be used sparingly.

Non-accidental injury

Of paediatric burns, 3–5% are due to non-accidental injury. As with other non-accidental injuries, the history and the pattern of injury may arouse suspicion.

History
- Delayed presentation.
- No explanation given for the burn.
- Implausible explanation for the burn.
- Inconsistency between age of the burn and age given by the history.

Injury pattern
- Obvious pattern from cigarettes, lighters, irons.
- No splash-marks in a scald injury: a child falling into a bath will splash; one that is placed into it may not.
- 'Tide-line' of scald: if the child is put into the fetal position, do the burns line up (i.e. what position was the child in when he/she was burned)?
- 'Doughnut sign': an area of spared skin surrounded by scald. If a child is forcibly held down in a bath of hot water, the part in contact with the bottom of the bath (e.g. the heels or buttocks) will not burn but the tissue around will.

Any suspicion of non-accidental injury should lead to immediate admission of the child to hospital, irrespective of how trivial the burn injury is, and the notification of social services. It should be remembered that the injury does not have to be deliberately caused for social services to intervene; inadequate supervision of children mandates their involvement.

Rehabilitation

There is no starting point for rehabilitation because it blends into the acute management phase. Physiotherapy is important initially for treating pulmonary problems and later for mobilizing the patient and regaining strength. Occupational therapists carry out much of the scar management for the patient. There is significant psychological trauma in a burn injury and a clinical psychologist has an important role in helping the patient come to terms with what has happened. Managing a burn patient is truly a team task and requires close cooperation between the various disciplines. Only if all members of the team work together will the patient have a good outcome.

Scar management

Hypertrophic scars are a major problem in children, pigmented skin and burns that take a long time to heal. There are several ways of preventing hypertrophy. Direct pressure on the scar can keep it flat. This can be achieved with adhesive tape, pressure garments or masks for facial burns. Silicone can also prevent hypertrophic scars and is applied as either a gel or a tape. Finally, direct steroid injections can cause a hypertrophic scar to involute, although these are painful and require general anaesthesia in children.

Secondary reconstruction

Secondary surgery addresses functional and cosmetic issues. The most common secondary procedure preformed is contracture release. This can be due to either the scar contracting or, in the case of children, the patient growing. Local flaps with or without tissue expansion or full-thickness skin grafts are often used. Minor cosmetic adjustments can have major psychological benefits for a patient and should be performed.

Assessment and management of burns at a glance

History
- Exact time, cause and mechanism
- Concomitant injuries
- Inhalational injury
- Non-accidental injury

Primary survey
A: airway (above vocal cords)
Evidence of inhalational injury
- Flame burns/enclosed space
- Burns to face, neck, upper torso
- Singed nasal hair
- Carbonaceous sputum

Intubate if:
- Erythema/oedema in oropharynx
- Voice change with hoarseness/harsh cough
- Stridor
- Dyspnoea

B: breathing (below vocal cords)
- Mechanical restriction: circumferential chest burns. Treatment: escharotomy
- Blast injury: lung contusion and alveolar trauma
- Smoke inhalation: bronchospasm, bronchorrhoea, inflammation, ciliary failure, atelectasis, pneumonia
- Carboxyhaemoglobin: CO binds haemoglobin and cytochrome oxygenase pathway proteins, extracellular and intracellular hypoxia, spurious readings on pulse oximetry, metabolic acidosis. Treatment: 100% O_2

C: circulation
- If profound hypovolaemia is present, look for cause other than burn
- Circumferential full-thicknes limb burns require escharotomy

D: neurological disability
- Score on Glasgow Coma Scale may be abnormal due to hypoxia/hypovolaemia

E: exposure
- Examine whole patient including back
- Cover patient to keep warm

F: fluids
- Determine and commence fluid regimen, place urinary catheter

- Monitor pulse, blood pressure, temperature, urinary output, give adequate analgesia i.v., consider nasogastric tube
- Give i.v. fluids according to Muir–Barclay formula: (%burn × weight in kg)/2 = one aliquot of fluid
- Give six aliquots of fluid over first 36 h in 4, 4, 4, 6, 6, 12 h sequence from time of burn
- Crystalloid (Ringer's lactate) and colloid (albumin or plasma) solutions are used

Pain relief
- Superficial burns are very painful so give i.v. morphine

Nutritional support
- Increased metabolic rate requires hyperalimentation with enteral feeding
- Daily caloric requirement is 25 kcal/kg + 40 kcal/%burn

Antibiotics
- Prophylactic antibiotics are not indicated
- Strict wound care and regular wound cultures required
- Invasive infection treated with short courses of high-dose antibiotic
- Give tetanus prophylaxis

Investigations
- Full blood count and haematocrit
- Urea and electrolytes
- Group and save/cross-match
- Swabs from burn for microbiology
- If inhalation suspected: chest X-ray; arterial blood gases, CO estimation
- ECG/cardiac enzymes with electrical burns

Burn assessment
- Generally poorly done
- Erythema is not included in calculation

Methods for assessing area of burn
- Palmar surface: area of patient's palm (no fingers!) = 0.8% (male) and 0.6% (female) of total body surface area. Useful for calculating small (< 15%) burns
- Wallace rule of nines: head 9%, torso front 18%, torso back 18%, right upper limb 9%, left upper limb 9%, right lower limb 18%, left lower limb 18%, perineum 1%
- Lund and Browder chart: widely available and very accurate

03

Methods for assessing depth of burn

| Burn depth | Response to needle prick | | Appearance |
	Bleeding	Sensation	
Superficial	Brisk	Pain	Red, glistening, blanches
Deep dermal	Delayed	Touch but no pain	Pale, not moist, blanches
Full thickness	None	None	Dry, leathery, hard

Referral to burn unit

- Age < 5 or > 60 years
- Site: face, hands, feet, perineum, flexure (neck/axilla/groin), circumferential
- Inhalational injury
- Mechanism: chemical (> 5% total body surface area), ionizing radiation, high-pressure steam, high-tension electrical, hydrofluoric acid (> 1% total body surface area), non-accidental injury
- Size: paediatric (age < 16 years), > 5% total body surface area; adult > 10% total body surface area
- Coexisting medical conditions or associated injuries

Management

Superficial
- Heals spontaneously in 14 days
- Needs dressing (tulle gras, retention dressing, interface dressing, topical antibacterial cream) to keep wound clean

Deep dermal/full thickness
- Excise burn wound as soon as possible after resuscitation (usually < 48 h after burn)
- Resurface wound with:
  (a) Skin autograft (patient's own skin, possible if burn < 50% total body surface area)
  (b) Skin allograft (cadaver skin as temporary biological dressing)
  (c) Skin xenograft (porcine skin as temporary biological dressing)
  (d) Synthetic skin (artificial neodermis and silicone top layer)
  (e) Cultured skin (culture patient's own skin)

Rehabilitation
- Physiotherapy (pulmonary problems and mobilization)
- Occupational therapy (contractures)
- Clinical psychology (psychological trauma)

Complications

Immediate
- Compartment syndrome from circumferential burns: limb burns leading to limb ischaemia, thoracic burns leading to hypoxia from restrictive respiratory failure
- Prevent by urgent escharotomy

Early
- Hyperkalaemia (from cytolysis in large burns): treat with insulin and dextrose
- Acute renal failure (combination of hypovolaemia, sepsis, tissue toxins): prevent by aggressive early resuscitation, ensuring high GFR with fluid loading and diuretics, treat sepsis
- Infection (beware *Streptococcus*): treat established infection (10^6 organisms in wound biopsy) with systemic antibiotics
- Stress ulceration (Curling's ulcer): prevent with antacid or histamine H_2-blocker

Late
- Contractures

Prognosis

- Age of patient + %burn = %mortality (e.g. 60 year old + 40% burn = 100% mortality)
- Mortality increased with inhalational burn

Must know Must do

Must know

Surface anatomy of common external abdominal herniae

Clinical symptoms and signs of common external abdominal herniae and their complications

Complications of external abdominal herniae

Principles of operative management of common external abdominal herniae

Must do

Examine patients with inguinal, femoral, paraumbilical and incisional herniae

Observe elective repair operations for external abdominal herniae

Follow the management of patient(s) admitted as emergency with obstructed/incarcerated external abdominal hernia

Introduction

Disorders of the abdominal wall are commonplace in surgical practice. The majority of problems encountered are in the form of herniation, with inguinal herniae forming a significant bulk of outpatient referrals and theatre operating time.

Swellings in the wall

Haematoma of rectus sheath

A haematoma of the rectus sheath presents as a swelling in the anterior abdominal wall, usually below the umbilicus, and is associated with sudden abdominal wall strain such as sneezing or coughing. This causes a tear in a branch of the inferior epigastric artery and the rapid formation of a haematoma. Clinically, the patient experiences severe abdominal pain with nausea and vomiting accompanied by pyrexia and leukocytosis. The abdominal wall swelling is tender and takes several weeks to resolve. No interven-

tion is needed if the diagnosis is certain. If not, the haematoma should be evacuated and the artery ligated.

Desmoid tumour

These slow-growing non-metastasizing tumours arise from the rectus abdominis muscles and may attain a very large size. The histology of the tumour is variable and may resemble a low-grade fibrosarcoma. It is easily palpated and is rendered more prominent by contraction of the abdominal muscles. It may be associated with Gardner's syndrome and may be related to childbirth injuries.

Common abdominal herniae

A hernia is defined as the protrusion of a viscus or part of a viscus through an abnormal opening. Herniae may occur in the brain (e.g. after head injury), in muscle through its fascial covering, internally in the abdomen (internal hernia) or externally through a weak normal opening (inguinal and femoral herniae) or an abnormal opening (e.g. incisional hernia) in the abdominal wall. The common external abdominal herniae are presented here (Table 24.1; Figs 24.1 & 24.2).

Inguinal hernia

Inguinal hernia is a common complaint, occurring mostly in men. It is twice as frequent as femoral hernia and in males more than 90% of herniae are inguinal.

Inguinal herniae may occur at any age. In children they are generally associated with developmental disorders such as persistent processus vaginalis or testicular maldescent. Inguinal hernia is also common in young adult males and this is also related to a congenital defect such as a persistent processus, which may be precipitated from potential to actual existence by physical effort (Fig. 24.3).

Anatomy
Inguinal canal
The anterior wall of the inguinal canal is formed by the aponeurosis of the external oblique and in its lateral half

	Site of defect	Treatment
Umbilical	Umbilicus	Observe
Paraumbilical	Just above umbilicus	Surgical repair (Mayo)
Epigastric	Midline between umbilicus and xiphisternum	Surgical repair
Inguinal		
Indirect	Deep inguinal ring	Infant: herniotomy only
		Adult: herniotomy/herniorrhaphy (Sholdice, Darn; occasionally truss)
Direct	Posterior wall	Herniorrhaphy
Femoral	Femoral canal	Surgical repair (femoral, Lotheissen, McEvedy)
Incisional	Previous abdominal wound	Surgical repair (occasionally Marlex mesh)

Table 24.1 Common abdominal herniae and their management.

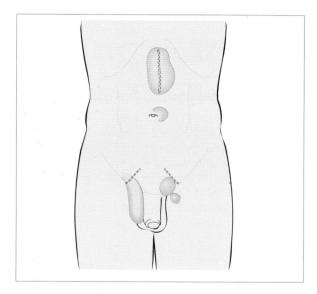

Figure 24.1 Diagram of common herniae: incisional, periumbilical, indirect inguinoscrotal (right), direct inguinal and femoral (left).

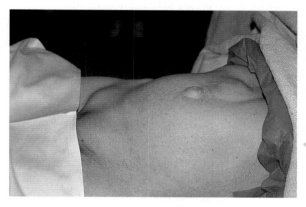

Figure 24.2 Femoral (right), inguinal (left) paraumbilical and incisional herniae in one patient. Courtesy of Mr K. Mealy.

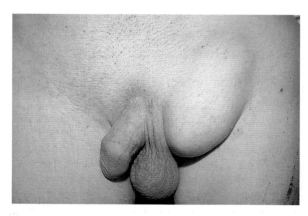

Figure 24.3 Inguinal hernia.

by the internal oblique and transversus abdominis muscles. The floor of the canal is formed by the inguinal ligament and the roof of the canal by the conjoint tendon, which consists of the fused inferior borders of internal oblique and transversalis abdominis. The posterior wall of the canal consists of the transversalis fascia, with a portion of the medial end formed by the insertion of the conjoint tendon (Fig. 24.4a).

At its lateral end the transversalis fascia is penetrated at the deep inguinal ring by the spermatic cord, with the

04

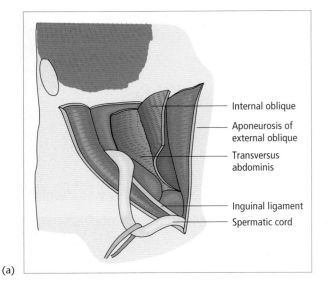

(a)

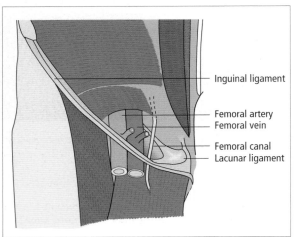

(b)

Figure 24.4 Anatomy of (a) the inguinal and (b) the femoral canal.

inferior epigastric artery passing upwards and medial to it. Thus an indirect inguinal hernia as it emerges through the deep ring within the spermatic cord has the conjoint tendon laterally and above it, the inferior epigastric artery medially and the inguinal ligament inferiorly.

Femoral canal

The femoral canal is bounded anteriorly by the inguinal ligament, posteriorly by the fascia over the pectineus muscle, medially by the lacunar ligament and laterally by the femoral vein. The canal often contains a named lymph gland (of Cloquet; Fig. 24.4b).

Clinical features

An indirect inguinal hernia occurs when a sac develops by emerging through the deep inguinal ring and passing through the inguinal canal in the spermatic cord adjacent to the vas deferens and surrounded by the coverings of the cord. The sac, if sufficiently large, may emerge through the external inguinal ring or descend into the scrotum. It may contain omentum or small bowel and has the potential to become irreducible and strangulated. On examination an indirect inguinal hernia is detectable above and medial to the pubic tubercle. The latter may be detected by palpating laterally along the pubic ramus or by invaginating the scrotum in the male, when it can be felt underneath and just lateral to the spermatic cord. Unless incarcerated, an inguinal hernia has an impulse on coughing and, if reducible, can be controlled by pressure over the internal inguinal ring, which is situated at the mid-inguinal point 1 cm above the pulsation of the femoral artery.

A direct inguinal hernia occurs as a result of a weakness in the transversalis fascia and is common in the elderly because of aetiological factors such as chronic cough, chronic strain during micturition due to prostatic hypertrophy, or chronic constipation. A direct hernia usually appears as a diffuse bulge that cannot be controlled by pressure over the internal ring. It is above and lateral to the pubic tubercle and does not enter the scrotum. A direct inguinal hernia has a wide neck, in contrast to the narrow neck of an indirect hernia. In consequence, a direct hernia is much less likely to strangulate.

Strangulation

Strangulation of an inguinal hernia develops when constriction occurs at the neck of the sac, cutting off the blood supply of the contents. Initially the venous blood supply is obstructed. This causes swelling of the contents (omentum or bowel) and eventually a combination of oedema and constriction interrupts the arterial blood supply and gangrene supervenes in the strangulated loop (Fig. 24.5).

These changes are accompanied by severe local pain, with irreducibility of the hernia and tenderness. The symptoms of small-bowel obstruction are also evident, with colicky abdominal pain, nausea and vomiting.

When the hernia first becomes obstructed it is possible to reduce it by manipulation. It is important, however, to ensure that the hernia is not reduced en masse into the abdominal cavity with the contents still strangulated by the constricting neck of the sac. An irreducible hernia *per se* does not indicate strangulation and may be incarcerated with an adequate blood supply but completely irreducible.

04

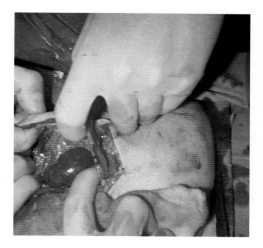

Figure 24.5 Strangulated inguinal hernia (operative photograph).

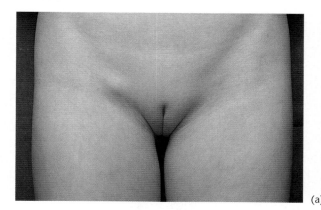

(a)

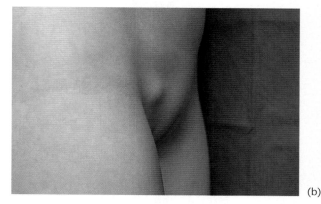

(b)

Figure 24.6 Femoral hernia: (a) anterior and (b) lateral views.

Management

Ideally, all inguinal herniae should be repaired by elective surgical operation. Surgery is usually performed under general anaesthesia but local or regional anaesthesia is also used. Surgical repair classically consists of two elements: excision of the hernial sac (herniotomy) and repair or buttressing of the weakness in the posterior inguinal canal (herniorrhaphy). In infants (always indirect herniae), the internal and external rings are superimposed and only a herniotomy is required for effective treatment. Laparoscopic repair of adult inguinal herniae is also performed by some surgeons.

Complications of hernia repair include the following.
- Haematoma: may be in the wound or scrotum.
- Acute urinary retention: this frequently follows bilateral repair.
- Wound infection: this should be rare as hernia repair is a clean operation, but in practice infection occurs in 5–8%.
- Chronic pain: trapping of the ilioinguinal nerve.
- Testicular pain and swelling followed by atrophy usually means that the repair is too tight and the testicular artery is compromised. Testicular atrophy will occur when the swelling subsides.
- Recurrence of hernia occurs in about 5% of patients but the rate is higher when surgical technique is poor.

Occasionally a truss may be used to control an inguinal hernia if the patient is unfit for or refuses surgery. However, trusses are unsatisfactory, do not treat the hernia and the patient is still at risk of incarceration and strangulation.

Femoral hernia

A femoral hernia emerges through the femoral canal and may be felt as a soft swelling below and lateral to the pubic tubercle (Fig. 24.6). It is a protrusion of peritoneum through the femoral canal, below which it emerges subcutaneously. It is usually a small sac and may contain omentum or small bowel. Because of its position below the inguinal ligament it must be distinguished from a saphena varix, which disappears on pressure or on lying down and has a cough impulse. It must also be distinguished from femoral artery aneurysm, enlarged lymph nodes or, on very rare occasions, a psoas abscess.

Strangulation

Femoral herniae often strangulate. Because of their small size, femoral herniae do not provide local signs and symptoms comparable to inguinal hernia and the swelling of a strangulated femoral hernia may be impalpable. However, there is evidence of small-bowel obstruction and this should stimulate a careful search for a hernia.

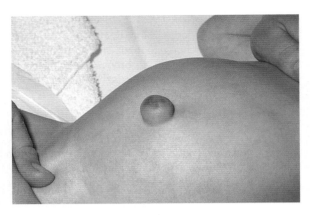

Figure 24.7 Congenital umbilical hernia.

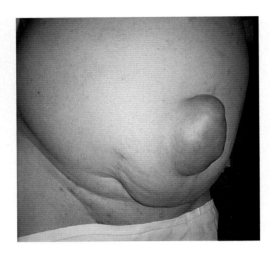

Figure 24.8 Paraumbilical hernia.

Management

Because femoral herniae are more likely to lead to strangulation than inguinal herniae, they should always be repaired without delay. A truss should not be used. Surgically, the hernia may be approached from below (femoral approach) or from above via the inguinal canal (Lotheissen approach) or via the rectus abdominis muscle (McEvedy approach). The contents of the sac are emptied, the sac is excised and the femoral canal is obliterated with three interrupted non-absorbable sutures.

Umbilical hernia

True umbilical hernia is common in infants (especially in Africans) and is due to a persistent defect in the abdominal wall at the umbilicus. The majority close spontaneously and surgical closure is rarely necessary. Intervention is required in the unlikely event of strangulation or incarceration (Fig. 24.7).

Paraumbilical hernia

These herniae occur in obese adult women and are prone to strangulate. The defect occurs through the midline just above the umbilicus (Fig. 24.8). The sac may contain omentum or small intestine or both and, because of the narrow neck, strangulation is relatively common. With long-standing herniae, adhesions occur between the contents and the wall of the sac so that the hernia becomes irreducible.

Strangulated herniae are repaired as an emergency. Long-standing herniae should be repaired electively. The Mayo repair is commonly used. With this technique the contents of the sac are freed from its walls and reduced. The sac is excised and the fascial defect is repaired trans-versely with the upper flap overlapping the lower, thereby doubling the strength of the repair.

Epigastric hernia

These usually small but often quite painful swellings occur in the midline between xiphisternum and umbilicus. The swelling most frequently consists of herniation of extraperitoneal fat through a small defect in the linea alba. Sometimes it carries a peritoneal sac with it that may contain omentum but this is rare. Pain is localized to the site with tenderness on pressure, but it may also simulate the symptoms of peptic ulcer. Clinical examination reveals a tender swelling in the midline. Sometimes incarcerated fat becomes devascularized and necrotic.

Treatment is surgical and may be carried out under local anaesthesia, enlarging the defect, excising the fat and suturing the defect with non-absorbable sutures.

Incisional hernia

This is a hernia that protrudes through a defect in an old abdominal wound. Wound infection predisposes to incisional hernia. The margins of the defect in the abdominal wall under the old incision can often be felt and the hernia is easily demonstrated by asking the supine patient to raise his or her head off the pillow (thus tensing the abdominal muscles; Fig. 24.9). An incisional hernia often contains bowel that is adherent to the peritoneal sac. Surgical repair requires excision of the sac and identification and apposition of the margins of the hernia. Occasionally, with a very large incisional hernia, it is not possible to bring the muscle edges together and a polypropylene mesh (Marlex) has to be inserted to close the abdominal wall defect.

04

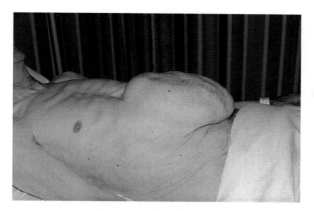

Figure 24.9 Large incisional hernia.

Unusual herniae

Inguinal variations

- *Sliding hernia (hernia en glissade)*. Some inguinal herniae are sliding herniae, i.e. retroperitoneal structures such as large bowel herniate into the inguinal canal and scrotum, dragging their overlying peritoneum with them. Thus the peritoneal sac itself is empty and the contents of the hernia lie behind the sac. These can often be quite difficult to repair.
- *Littré's hernia*. This is an unusual hernia in which the sac of an inguinal hernia contains a Meckel's diverticulum.

- *Maydl's hernia (hernia-en-W)*. In this rare form of inguinal hernia, two loops of intestine are incarcerated in the sac. The intervening loop of small intestine that remains in the abdominal cavity becomes strangulated by compression of its mesenteric vessels at the neck of the sac.

Richter's hernia

This is a variant of strangulated hernia. When a Richter's hernia is present, only part of the circumference of the small bowel is strangulated. As a consequence, while the patient is still able to pass flatus, he or she experiences colicky abdominal pain and vomiting and radiological evidence of small-bowel obstruction is present.

Spigelian hernia

This is an interstitial hernia of the abdominal wall. The defect occurs at the lateral border of the rectus abdominis, emerging through a defect in the transversus and internal oblique fascia halfway between the umbilicus and the pubic symphysis. The swelling is diffuse and difficult to palpate as it is covered by the external oblique. It may be identified by its position above and medial to the location of an inguinal hernia.

Obturator, gluteal and lumbar herniae

These are excessively rare herniae that occur with herniation through the obturator foramen and the gluteal and lumbar regions. It is likely that most doctors will never see any of them.

04

Abdominal herniae at a glance

Definition

Hernia: the protrusion of a viscus or part of a viscus through an abnormal opening in its coverings

Types
Common
- Umbilical/paraumbilical
- Inguinal (direct and indirect)
- Femoral
- Incisional

Uncommon
- Epigastric
- Gluteal, lumbar, obturator

Pathophysiology
- Defect in the abdominal wall may be congenital (e.g. umbilical hernia, femoral canal) or acquired (e.g. an incision) and is lined with peritoneum (the sac)
- Raised intra-abdominal pressure further weakens the defect, allowing some of the intra-abdominal contents (e.g. omentum, small-bowel loop) to migrate through the opening
- Entrapment of the contents in the sac leads to incarceration (unable to reduce contents) and possibly strangulation (blood supply to incarcerated contents is compromised)

Clinical features
Patient presents with a lump over the site of the hernia

Femoral herniae
- Femoral herniae are below and lateral to the pubic tubercle, usually flatten the groin crease and are 10 times more common in women than men
- Half present as a surgical emergency due to obstructed contents, and 50% of these will require small-bowel resection

Inguinal herniae
- Inguinal herniae start off above and medial to the pubic tubercle but may descend broadly when larger; they usually accentuate the groin crease
- Most are benign and have a low risk of complications
- Indirect inguinal herniae can be controlled by digital pressure over the internal inguinal ring, may be narrow-necked and are common in younger men (3% per annum present with complications)
- Direct inguinal herniae are poorly controlled by digital pressure, are often broad-necked and are commoner in older men (0.3% per annum strangulate)

Incisional herniae
- Incisional herniae bulge and are usually broad-necked, poorly controlled by pressure and accentuated by tensing the recti
- Large chronic incisional herniae may contain much of the small bowel and may be irreducible/unrepairable due to the 'loss of the right of abode in the abdomen' of the contents

True umbilical herniae
- Present from birth and are symmetrical defects in the umbilicus due to failure to close

Paraumbilical herniae
- Develop due to an acquired defect in the periumbilical fascia

Management
- Assess the hernia for:
  - (a) Severity of symptoms
  - (b) Risk of complications (type, size of neck)
  - (c) Ease of repair (size, location)
  - (d) Likelihood of success (size, 'loss of right of abode')
- Assess the patient for fitness for surgery, impact of hernia on lifestyle (job, hobbies)
- Surgical repair is usually offered in suitable patients for:
  - (a) Herniae at risk of complications whatever the symptoms
  - (b) Herniae with previous symptoms of obstruction
  - (c) Herniae at low risk of complications but symptoms interfering with lifestyle, etc.
- Principles of surgery:
  - (a) Herniotomy: excision of the hernial sac
  - (b) Herniorrhaphy: repair of the defect

Complications of surgery
- Haematoma (wound or scrotal)
- Acute urinary retention
- Wound infection
- Chronic pain
- Testicular pain and swelling leading to testicular atrophy
- Hernia recurrence (about 5%)

04

Disorders of the Oesophagus

25

Must know Must do

Must know

Symptoms and investigation of patients with
  oesophageal disease

Principles of oesophageal function tests

Medical, interventional and operative management of
  reflux disease and common oesophageal motility
  disorders

Principles of management of oesophageal cancer

Must do

Clerk a patient with dysphagia due to benign disease

Follow the management of a patient with oesophageal
  cancer from time of diagnosis

Attend sessions in the flexible endoscopy suite to
  observe upper gastrointestinal endoscopy for
  diagnosis of oesophageal disease and for stenting of
  inoperable oesophageal cancer

Learn how to interpret a barium swallow

Anatomy and physiology

The oesophagus is a muscular tube that transports food from the pharynx to the stomach. It is divided into three parts.

- Upper: extends from the cricopharyngeus to the level of the carina.
- Middle: extends from the level of the carina to halfway between the carina and the oesophagogastric junction.
- Lower: the remaining segment that joins the stomach. Clinically, the term 'cardia' is used to describe the junction between the oesophagus and stomach. It contains the squamocolumnar junction, which forms the serrated Z-line that marks an abrupt change from the tough pale squamous epithelium of the oesophagus to the columnar epithelium of the stomach. A zone of junctional epithe-

lium is interposed between the squamous lining of the oesophagus and the gastric mucosa.

The lower oesophagus is the most important site of communication between the portal and systemic venous systems in view of the development of varices in patients with portal hypertension. The lymphatics form extensive plexuses such that lymph flows long distances in the large submucosal plexus before passing through the muscular coat to the draining lymph nodes. These are grouped into three main tiers: the first lies alongside the oesophagus (para-oesophageal), the second is composed of mediastinal lymph nodes, and the third comprises the deep cervical, supraclavicular, tracheobronchial and coeliac nodes (from above downwards). In general, lymph drainage from the upper two-thirds of the oesophagus proceeds in a proximal direction, whereas the lower third drains distally to the subdiaphragmatic region and coeliac lymph nodes.

Two nerve plexuses in the oesophageal wall (Meissner's plexus in the submucosa, Auerbach's plexus in the muscularis) form networks of ganglion cells, which receive axons from the vagus. Swallowing is coordinated by the swallowing centre in the medulla oblongata. This receives and coordinates sensory inputs from peripheral mechanoreceptors in the pharynx and oesophagus and sends motor impulses to the pharynx and upper oesophagus that initiate the swallowing reflex. The parasympathetic fibres to the oesophagus are predominantly motor and travel in the glossopharyngeal, vagus and recurrent laryngeal nerves to the myenteric plexus. The sympathetic nerve supply consists of preganglionic fibres derived from spinal cord segments T5 and T6. The postganglionic sympathetic fibres then reach the oesophagus as a periarterial plexus.

The swallowing mechanism has three stages.

1 The first is *voluntary* and initiates the process. The food bolus is rolled posteriorly into the pharynx upwards and backwards against the palate by the tongue.

2 The *pharyngeal stage* is reflex. As food enters the pharynx it stimulates mechanoreceptors that trigger a series of

automatic pharyngeal muscular contractions such that the soft palate is pulled upwards, preventing entry of food into the nasal cavities. The vocal cords adduct and the larynx is pulled upwards against the epiglottis, preventing passage of food into the trachea. The upward movement of the larynx enlarges the opening of the oesophagus and stimulates relaxation of the tonically active upper oesophageal sphincter (cricopharyngeus). The muscular wall of the pharynx then contracts from above downwards, propelling the food bolus into the oesophagus.

3 The *oesophageal stage* is also involuntary and propels food from the pharynx to the stomach by peristaltic waves. Primary oesophageal peristalsis is a continuation of the pharyngeal peristaltic wave and travels all the way from the pharynx to the stomach in approximately 8 s. If the primary peristaltic wave fails to move all the food into the stomach, secondary peristaltic waves result from distension of the oesophagus by the retained food and these continue until all the food empties into the stomach. Tertiary oesophageal contractions occur spontaneously and are non-propulsive. They are encountered in various oesophageal motility disorders but also occur in healthy individuals.

Symptoms of oesophageal disease

The specific symptoms of oesophageal disease are dysphagia, regurgitation, odynophagia, chest pain and water brash.

Dysphagia

Dysphagia is difficulty in swallowing or a sensation of food bolus arrest or delay. The patient feels the food sticking and often points to a particular site on the sternum. Dysphagia for solids implies significant disease, whereas dysphagia for liquids only is more likely to be of functional origin (oesophageal motility disorder), in which case it may be intermittent. Persistent and progressive dysphagia indicates mechanical narrowing of the oesophageal lumen and is usually associated with regurgitation. Eventually, the patient is unable to swallow saliva and exhibits constant drooling. Obstructive dysphagia is first experienced when 20–30% of the oesophageal lumen is lost; most patients usually present when 50% of the oesophageal lumen is compromised.

Sensation of a substernal lump (globus)

When this occurs during fasting it is termed 'globus hystericus'. It is a neurotic symptom in patients with emotional instability but requires thorough examination to exclude organic disease.

Regurgitation

Regurgitation of gastric or oesophageal fluid into the throat accompanied by a sour taste is often postural and occurs predominantly in the supine position especially at night, with the regurgitated material staining the pillow. Postural regurgitation is a very common symptom of reflux disease. It is precipitated by meals and activities that raise intra-abdominal pressure, i.e. bending and straining. Regurgitation may also occur as an overflow of accumulated food in the oesophagus proximal to a stenosing lesion. This spillback into the pharynx and mouth at night may lead to aspiration pneumonitis.

Odynophagia

This complaint consists of localized pain, usually in the lower sternal region, which occurs immediately on swallowing certain foods or liquids. It indicates oesophagitis. Hot drinks, acid citrus beverages, coffee and heavily spiced foods are among the most frequent dietary items that induce this symptom. It can be severe enough to condition patients not to eat or drink the offending item, or food in general. Odynophagia signifies mucosal damage by reflux, radiation, viral or fungal infections.

Heartburn

This is the most common symptom of oesophageal disease and occurs in up to 50% of the population. It is due to reflux of gastric juice. Some patients complain of severe heartburn, yet on endoscopy there is little or no evidence of inflammation. These individuals may still have reflux in association with an abnormally sensitive oesophageal mucosa. Heartburn is often worsened by recumbency and increase in intra-abdominal pressure, and may follow fatty meals or alcoholic beverages. Heartburn is temporarily relieved by antacids.

Chest pain

Oesophageal anterior chest pain consists of a tightening or gripping pain that closely simulates angina pectoris. Thus it may radiate to the back, jaw, arm and ear and may even be relieved by sublingual nitrates. This type of pain is commonly found in patients with reflux oesophagitis or oesophageal motility disorders.

Water brash

This symptom is uncommon and is restricted to patients with reflux disease. It is due to excessive salivation, the mouth becoming full of fluid that has a salty taste and is clear and frothy.

04

Table 25.1 Investigations for oesophageal disease.

	Test	Indications

Radiology	Chest radiograph
	Contrast swallow
	CT
		Aspiration pneumonitis; oesophageal perforation,
		  dysphagia, motility disorders; reflux disease, staging of
		  malignant disease

Ultrasound	External Endoscopic	Diaphragmatic screening Staging of malignant disease
Radioisotope studies	Labelled liquid or solid bolus studies	Oesophageal transit, reflux disease
Endoscopy	Fibreoptic with biopsy, cytology	All patients with oesophageal symptoms, especially dysphagia
Physiological	Stationary and ambulatory manometry 24-h pH monitoring Bilitec	Pre-pH monitoring: reflux disease Oesophageal motility disorders: non-cardiac chest pain Alkaline reflux disease

Investigations

These are outlined in Table 25.1.

Radiography

A chest radiograph is necessary in all patients admitted acutely with oesophageal symptoms in order to detect the following.
● Aspiration pneumonitis.
● Mediastinal widening from nodal involvement in patients with oesophageal tumours.
● Outline any soft-tissue shadows and fluid gas levels: intrathoracic stomach, achalasia.
● Mediastinal emphysema and/or pleural effusion: patients with oesophageal perforations or suture line dehiscence after an oesophagectomy.

The standard contrast investigation is the barium swallow, which is particularly useful in the following.
● Patients with dysphagia from any cause.
● Patients with gastro-oesophageal reflux should have this investigation to determine the presence or absence of a hiatus hernia and to exclude oesophageal shortening.
● Patients with previous surgery to the oesophagus or oesophagogastric junction.
● Patients with known benign or malignant strictures about to undergo surgery or endoscopic therapeutic manoeuvres.

Barium swallow is inaccurate for the detection of gastro-oesophageal reflux. Its main value lies in the demonstration of an associated hiatus hernia and in detecting stricture formation (Fig. 25.1). A contrast swallow is an essential investigation in patients suspected of oesophageal perforation or leaking oesophageal anastomosis.

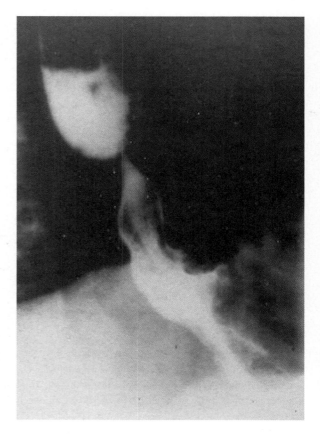

Figure 25.1 Barium swallow showing irregular annular stricture in the middle third of the oesophagus that proved to be an annular carcinoma on endoscopy and biopsy.

04

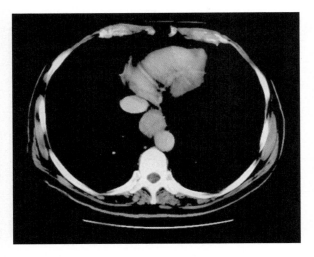

Figure 25.2 CT cross-section showing oesophageal cancer abutting but not involving the descending thoracic aorta.

Computed tomography

Computed tomography (CT) is very useful for the preoperative assessment of oesophageal malignancy (Fig. 25.2). It reliably assesses the extent of mural invasion and the size of the lesion. Aortic invasion can be predicted with accuracy if there is more than 90° contact. It is also used for the detection of distant metastases including pulmonary metastases but not small peritoneal deposits.

Ultrasound

Endoscopic ultrasonography provides accurate staging of a tumour in terms of intramural involvement and enlargement of adjacent lymph nodes. Ultrasonically, five oesophageal layers can be distinguished. The first two layers correspond to the superficial and deep mucosa, the third layer to the submucosa, the fourth layer to the muscularis propria and the fifth layer to the adventitia (Fig. 25.3). Endoscopic ultrasound provides sufficient information on lymph nodes such that rounded, sharply demarcated, homogeneous, hypoechoic lymph nodes are most likely malignant.

Radioisotope studies

These are used to evaluate oesophageal transit of liquid and solid boluses in individuals with motility disorders. Standardized solid bolus tests are more reliable and the study is carried out with the patient in the erect position. The normal transit time for this test is 10 s. Special software can generate time vs. radioactivity curves and special techniques generate a condensed image that outlines the spatial transit of the labelled bolus. Prolonged transit times are encountered in oesophageal motility disorders. The condensed image shows a striking sinuous outline resulting from oscillations of the bolus in patients with achalasia and diffuse oesophageal spasm (Fig. 25.4).

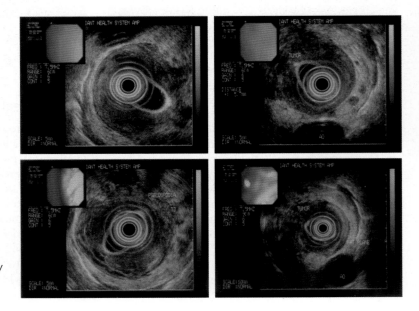

Figure 25.3 Endoscopic ultrasound showing sequences of an oesophageal cancer extending by 'pseudopodia' into the adventitia/fat plane. Enlarged probably involved para-oesophageal lymph nodes are seen in top-right sequence.

04

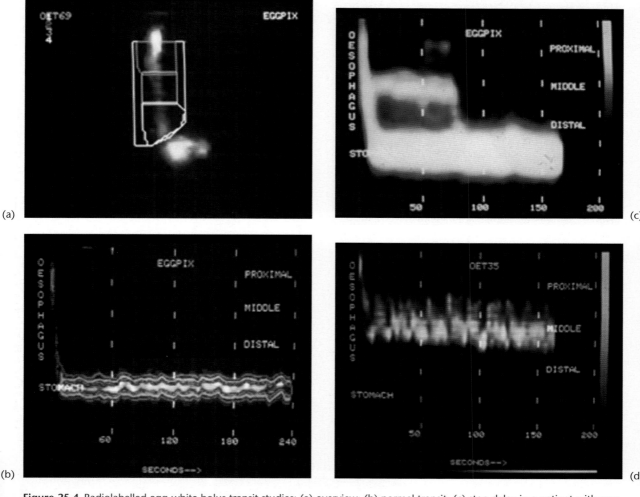

Figure 25.4 Radiolabelled egg-white bolus transit studies: (a) overview; (b) normal transit; (c) step delay in a patient with non-specific motility disorder; (d) oscillatory pattern in diffuse oesophageal spasm.

Endoscopy

Flexible endoscopy is essential in all patients with dysphagia. It provides direct visual information on the presence or absence of pathology. Both biopsy and brush cytology are used to confirm oesophageal malignancy. Endoscopic biopsies are also necessary in the diagnosis and histological grading of reflux oesophagitis and in the detection of Barrett's epithelium and its surveillance in patients with long-standing reflux disease (Fig. 25.5).

Physiological tests

These include manometry, pH monitoring and tests to assess bile reflux.

Oesophageal manometry

This is used to measure the activity of the oesophageal musculature and oesophageal sphincters by recording intraluminal pressure profiles caused by contractions. Intraluminal pressure recording is carried out by a system of water-perfused catheters (Fig. 25.6) or by solid-state strain-gauge transducers built into catheters. The information obtained is analysed according to established criteria in order to diagnose oesophageal motility disorders. Prolonged ambulatory manometric studies are particularly useful for patients with non-cardiac chest pain who may have transient motility disturbances in the oesophagus.

04

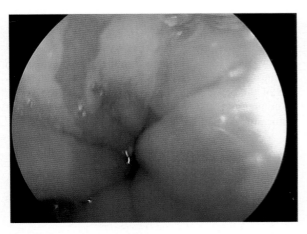

Figure 25.5 Upper gastrointestinal endoscopy: pinkish red Barrett's columnar mucosal change in a patient with gastro-oesophageal reflux.

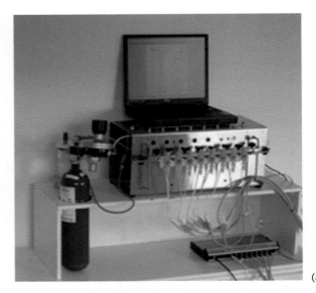

(a)

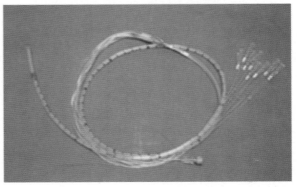

(b)

Figure 25.6 Perfusion manometry: (a) Arndorfer system; (b) multilumen catheter.

04

24-Hour pH monitoring

This technique involves the transnasal placement of a pH measuring electrode in the lower oesophagus. The pH electrode monitors the changes in intra-oesophageal pH over 24 h, with the information stored in a portable logger (Fig. 25.7). A 24-h pH profile is thus obtained that provides information on frequency, duration and pattern of reflux episodes together with temporal correlation with symptoms. A reflux episode is defined as a pH drop to below pH 4. Specially designed software analyses the data in two ways.

● Reflux event analysis. All individual reflux episodes are identified and characterized: number, mean duration, number of long reflux events > 5 min, duration of the longest reflux episode.

● Cumulative oesophageal exposure analysis: depicts the frequency distribution of the oesophageal pH data for the erect and supine parts of the study as well as for the whole period of study.

The indications for 24-h ambulatory pH monitoring are as follows.

● Definitive diagnosis of gastro-oesophageal reflux in patients who are sufficiently symptomatic to have warranted endoscopy but in whom endoscopy is normal.

● Investigation of patients suspected of having gastro-oesophageal reflux as a cause of atypical symptoms, such as non-cardiac chest pain, respiratory and laryngeal symptoms, in whom the relevant investigations have been normal and to correlate such symptoms with reflux episodes.

● When established gastro-oesophageal reflux responds poorly to medical therapy and particularly when surgical treatment is contemplated.

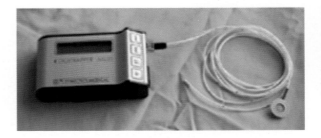

Figure 25.7 Ambulatory 24-h pH logger.

24-Hour oesophageal bile monitoring (by spectrophotometry)

This test uses an optical fibre sensor capable of detecting bilirubin in the oesophagus as a marker of

enterogastro-oesophageal reflux. The ambulatory spectrophotometer transfers the signals to a data logger and a 24-h profile can be recorded. The data are then downloaded to a computer. It is important to use a standard diet that avoids coloured food substances and beverages during the test. The test is indicated in:
- patients with symptomatic gastro-oesophageal reflux with poor response to an adequate dose of proton pump inhibitor;
- patients with complications of gastro-oesophageal reflux disease such as Barrett's metaplasia, strictures and ulcers;
- patients with reflux symptoms after gastrectomy.

Bernstein's acid perfusion test

This detects oesophageal mucosal sensitivity to acid and is very useful in the determination of the oesophageal origin of chest pain. A nasogastric tube is positioned in the middle of the oesophagus. Infusion is initially started with isotonic saline and then switched to 0.1 M HCl without informing the patient.

Gastro-oesophageal reflux disease

Gastro-oesophageal reflux disease (GORD) is the most common upper gastrointestinal disorder in western

---

Oesophageal symptoms at a glance

Definitions

Dysphagia: difficulty with swallowing, which may be associated with ingestion of liquids, solids or both. Most causes of dysphagia are oesophageal in origin

Heartburn: an aching, burning sensation felt behind the lower part of the sternum, caused by reflux of acid from the stomach into the oesophagus

Regurgitation: when fluid from the stomach flows back into the mouth producing a sour taste. It is frequently postural and indicates gastric reflux

Water brash: sudden secretion of a quantity of saliva into the mouth as a reflex response to reflux

Odynophagia: painful swallowing and usually indicates oesophagitis

Causes of dysphagia
Mural
- Carcinoma of the oesophagus: progressive, weight loss and anorexia, anaemia
- Reflux oesophagitis: preceded by heartburn, anaemia, nocturnal regurgitation
- Achalasia: liquids > solids, frequent regurgitation, recurrent chest infections due to aspiration, long history, younger patients or old age
- Tracheo-oesophageal fistula: recurrent chest infections, childhood (congenital), late adulthood (post trauma, deep X-ray therapy, malignancy)
- Caustic stricture: history of corrosive ingestion, chronic dysphagia
- Scleroderma: slow onset, skin and hair changes apparent
- Chagas' disease: *Trypanosoma cruzi*, South America, arrhythmias, colonic dysmotility

Intramural
- Foreign body: acute distress, marked retrosternal discomfort, difficulty in swallowing saliva

Extramural
- Pulsion diverticulum: intermittent symptoms, unexpected regurgitation
- External compression: mediastinal lymph nodes, left atrial hypertrophy, bronchial malignancy

Investigation of dysphagia
Any new symptom of progressive dysphagia should be assumed to be a carcinoma until proven otherwise

All patients
- Full blood count: anaemia more common with tumours than reflux
- Liver function tests: exclude hepatic disease

Oesophagogastroduodenoscopy (OGD)
- Moderate risk
- Differentiates between tumour, reflux, stricture and achalasia
- Allows biopsy and possible treatment (e.g. placement of endoprosthesis)

Barium swallow
- Low risk
- Good for detecting fistula, reflux, high tumour, diverticulum
- ? Dysmotility:
  (a) Achalasia: video barium swallow
  (b) Neurogenic cause: oesophageal manometry
- ? Extrinsic compression: chest X-ray (AP and lateral)

CT
- Chest and mediastinum

countries. Minor gastro-oesophageal episodes occur in most people but they are short-lived and exposure of the lower oesophageal mucosa to acid pH < 4 does not exceed 5% in 24 h. Reflux in excess of this is considered pathological. In many patients the symptoms are mild and intermittent with no significant mucosal damage. In 10% of patients, the acid-induced mucosal injury causes oesophagitis, which may lead to further major complications such as:

- ulceration (bleeding);
- stricture/webs;
- columnar metaplasia (Barrett's columnar epithelium);
- oesophageal shortening.

Approximately 10% of patients with columnar metaplasia develop dysplasia in the metaplastic segment of the oesophagus.

Pathophysiology

The disease develops as a result of failure of the normal antireflux mechanisms, with chemical injury to the squamous lining of the oesophagus. The antireflux mechanisms include:

- competence of the lower oesophageal sphincter (LOS) 'complex';
- oesophageal clearance of refluxed material;
- mucosal resistance to the damaging effects of the refluxate.

The LOS is the single most important factor accounting for the competence of the gastro-oesophageal junction. Several drugs, hormones and food substances are known to influence the contractile activity of the LOS (Table 25.2). The normal resting pressure of the LOS is 10–25 mmHg. Temporary inhibition of the LOS occurs just prior to the arrival of a primary peristaltic wave induced by swallowing in order to allow entry of food into the stomach. The sphincter relaxes and contracts immediately the food bolus passes through. The length of the intra-abdominal segment of the oesophagus is another important factor in the competence of the LOS. The diaphragmatic crural mechanism exerts its antireflux effect mainly during deep inspiration or sudden increases in intra-abdominal pressure, e.g. coughing or sneezing. The acute angle of His is also thought to be important by providing an abrupt insertion of the oesophagus into the stomach. The mucosal rosette at the lower oesophagus provides substance for the valve and thus closure of the lumen when the LOS is contracted. Between 25 and 50% of patients with GORD have impaired peristaltic function.

Table 25.2 Effect on lower oesophageal sphincter pressure (high-pressure zone) by hormones, drugs and foodstuffs.		Decrease pressure	Increase pressure
	Hormones/peptides	Glucagon Secretin Cholecystokinin Vasoactive intestinal peptide Gastric inhibitory polypeptide Progesterone Oestrogens Serotonin (N receptors) Histamine (H$_2$ receptors) Enkephalins	Gastrin Motilin Bombesin Histamine (H$_1$ receptors) Serotonin (M receptors)
	Prostaglandins	E$_1$, E$_2$, A$_2$	F$_2$
	Drugs	Atropine Antihistamines Calcium blockers Ganglion blockers Tricyclic antidepressants	Metoclopramide Domperidone Cisapride Cholinergic drugs Anticholinesterases
	Foodstuffs	Caffeine Fats Chocolate Alcohol	Protein meal
	Other	Smoking	

04

Aetiology

The factors that promote reflux and damage include the following.

- Primary weakness of the smooth muscle of the LOS.
- Short length of the intra-abdominal segment of oesophagus.
- Defective hormonal and neural control of the sphincter: most commonly dietary induced and transient.
- Abnormally high number of transient LOS relaxations.
- Presence of a hiatus hernia. This results in a change of the pressure environment, shortening of the LOS and changes in the anatomy and reflexes of the gastric cardia. Approximately 50% of patients with reflux symptoms and 90% of patients with reflux oesophagitis have a hiatus hernia. However, many patients with a hiatus hernia are asymptomatic and 40–50% have no oesophagitis.
- Delayed gastric emptying: present in up to 40% of patients with GORD.

The principal components of the refluxate (gastric juice) are HCl and pepsins. Bile salts also produce severe mucosal damage. Clinically, pure acid and pepsin reflux occurs in 40% of patients and mixed reflux of gastric and duodenal juices occurs in 60% of patients. Pure alkaline reflux is uncommon and occurs after gastric resections.

Pathology

The histological changes of early damage include widening of the basal layer and extension of the dermal papillae to more than two-thirds of the epithelium. With more severe damage there is an accumulation of inflammatory cells and the epithelial thickness is reduced. The papillae become widened and extend to the surface, when superficial necrosis and ulceration supervene. These acute superficial ulcers heal without fibrosis. However, if the ulceration and inflammation reach the submucous layer or beyond, fibrosis ensues and the mucosa may undergo metaplasia to columnar epithelium (Barrett's columnar epithelium).

Infection with *Helicobacter pylori* protects against the development of GORD and its complications. This protective effect depends on the extent of *Helicobacter*-induced gastritis with reduction of acid secretion. Thus reflux oesophagitis may develop after therapy to eradicate *H. pylori* as gastric acid secretion returns to normal.

Clinical features

The typical symptoms of GORD are heartburn, regurgitation and dysphagia. Symptoms are aggravated by posture and can be especially severe at night and after large meals and activities that increase intra-abdominal pressure, e.g. bending, stooping. Other symptoms include pain on swallowing hot or spicy foods (odynophagia) and water brash. Dysphagia may be due to spasm or oedema of the inflamed lower oesophagus, in which case it remits with improvement of the oesophagitis consequent on treatment. In some patients dysphagia may be secondary to a motility disorder or stricture formation. A scoring system introduced by DeMeester is useful for assessing the extent of symptomatic severity (Table 25.3). The severity of the disease is assessed by endoscopy (Table 25.4).

Table 25.3 DeMeester's scoring system for symptoms of gastro-oesophageal reflux.

Symptoms	Grade	Description
Heartburn		
None	0	No heartburn
Minimal	1	Occasional episodes
Moderate	2	Reason for medical visit
Severe	3	Interference with daily activities
Regurgitation		
None	0	No regurgitation
Minimal	1	Occasional episodes
Moderate	2	Predictable on position or straining
Severe	3	Episodes of pulmonary aspiration with chronic nocturnal cough or recurrent pneumonitis
Dysphagia		
None	0	No dysphagia
Minimal	1	Occasional episodes
Moderate	2	Requires fluids to clear
Severe	3	Episode of meat impaction requiring medical treatment

Table 25.4 Los Angeles classification of oesophagitis.

Grade	Description
Grade A	One (or more) mucosal break no longer than 5 mm that does not extend between the tops of two mucosal folds
Grade B	One (or more) mucosal break more than 5 mm long that does not extend between the tops of two mucosal folds
Grade C	One (or more) mucosal break that is continuous between the tops of two or more mucosal folds but which involves less than 75% of the circumference
Grade D	One (or more) mucosal break that involves at least 75% of the oesophageal circumference

Table 25.5 Drug therapy in gastro-oesophageal reflux disease.

Drug class	Drug(s)	Mode of action
Antacids with silicone	Dimethylpolysiloxane	Defoaming agents
Antacids with alginate	Antireflux floating alginate	Antacid platform on top of gastric juice
Prokinetic drugs	Bethanechol, metoclopramide, domperidone	Motility enhancing (improve clearance)
Antisecretory drugs	Cimetidine, ranitidine, famotidine	Histamine H_2-receptor blockers
	Omeprazole, lansoprazole, rabeprazole	Proton pump inhibitors
Mucosal protectors	Carbenoxolone with alginate, sucralfate, misoprostol	Various actions

Atypical presentation with chest pain can mimic ischaemic heart disease. In other patients, especially children, presentation may be with pulmonary symptoms including asthma. Some patients present with laryngeal symptoms, manifest as a persistent dry cough or changes in voice or choking episodes. The clinically useful tests for establishing the diagnosis are flexible endoscopy with biopsy followed by pH monitoring. Oesophageal manometry is of limited value except in patients with dysphagia without stricture, where manometry is used to assess the motility of the oesophageal body. Barium swallow is necessary prior to surgical treatment to demonstrate the presence, type and size of any hiatus hernia.

Treatment

Management is conservative in the first instance and is designed to reduce chemical damage and improve oesophageal clearance. Dietary advice includes the avoidance of large meals, especially within 3 h of retiring to bed. Postural advice includes sleeping propped up by raising the head of the bed. Medical treatment is good at controlling heartburn but less effective at reducing regurgitation. The various drugs used alone or in combination in the medical treatment of GORD are shown in Table 25.5. Although antacids provide some symptomatic relief in mild cases, this is short-lived and these agents do not heal oesophagitis. Histamine H_2-receptor antagonists can achieve symptomatic control and endoscopic healing

of oesophagitis after 3 months, followed by maintenance therapy indefinitely. If symptoms persist despite H_2-receptor antagonists, the treatment is changed to proton pump inhibitors (e.g. omeprazole, lansoprazole). Therapy with high-dose proton pump inhibitors for 8 weeks results in healing of endoscopic oesophagitis in 90%. Again, recurrence of oesophagitis is universal unless maintenance therapy is administered indefinitely. The additional use of prokinetic agents is used to reduce oesophageal exposure time. The γ-aminobutyric acid B-receptor ($GABA_B$) agonist baclofen is useful for control of transient LOS relaxations. The conservative management of neutral/alkaline reflux after gastric surgery is difficult and seldom effective.

Surgical treatment

The majority of patients with GORD will have limited periods plagued with episodes of reflux controlled by lifestyle adjustments and pharmacological agents with or without maintenance therapy. Approximately 10–15% of patients will be referred for antireflux surgery. The indications for surgical treatment are as follows.
● Failure of medical therapy: includes failure to control symptoms despite high-dose proton pump inhibitor therapy for 6 months.
● Development of complications in young or fit patients and patients with high-grade oesophagitis from the outset.

04

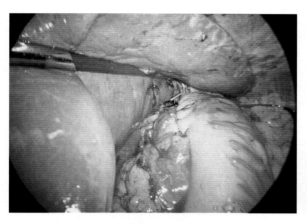

Figure 25.8 Operative photograph of laparoscopic total fundoplication.

- Persistence of reflux in children beyond 2 years.
- Reflux after previous upper abdominal surgery.
- Atypical symptoms: respiratory, pharyngeal and dental problems.
- Patient preference, especially in young patients.
  The most commonly performed operations are:
- loose (floppy) total fundoplication;
- partial anterior fundoplication;
- partial posterior fundoplication.

All these antireflux surgical procedures can be performed by laparoscopy (Fig. 25.8) and this approach has largely replaced the traditional open method (Fig. 25.9). Loose total fundoplication consists of a circumferential 2–3 cm loose wrap of gastric fundus around the mobilized abdominal oesophagus, with preservation of the vagal trunks. In anterior partial fundoplication, the mobilized fundus is brought in front of the oesophagus and sutured to it and to the adjacent oesophagogastric junction and to the right crus, in effect achieving a 180° wrap around the front of the oesophagus. In posterior crurally fixed partial fundoplication, the fundus is brought behind the mobilized oesophagus, sutured to the right and left crura and then to either side of the oesophagus (Fig. 25.10).

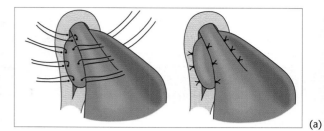

(a)

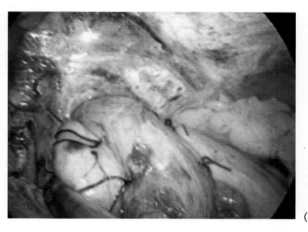

(b)

Figure 25.10 Toupet crurally fixed posterior partial fundoplication: (a) schematic drawing; (b) completed laparoscopic posterior partial fundoplication.

Benign oesophageal strictures

These arise most commonly secondary to long-standing reflux disease and less commonly by oesophageal/gastric resections or ingestion of corrosive agents. These patients present with dysphagia and their management entails the following.

- Establishing an accurate diagnosis of the nature of the stricture and its cause.
- Dilatation of the stricture to obviate dysphagia.
- To establish a long-term treatment strategy for the individual patient. This may be medical (proton pump

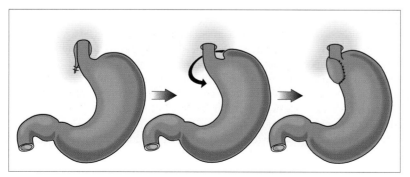

Figure 25.9 Open total fundoplication.

Gastro-oesophageal reflux disease at a glance

Definitions

Gastro-oesophageal reflux disease: a condition caused by the retrograde passage of gastric contents into the oesophagus resulting in inflammation (*oesophagitis*), which manifests as dyspepsia. The majority of GORD is benign and uncomplicated

Barrett's oesophagus: metaplastic change of the squamous epithelium of the lower oesophagus to specialized gastric epithelium as a consequence of long-standing reflux

Hiatus hernia: an abnormal protrusion of the proximal stomach through the oesophageal opening in the diaphragm resulting in a more proximal position of the oesophagogastric junction and predisposition to gastro-oesophageal reflux. *Sliding* (common) and *rolling* or *para-oesophageal* (rare) types are recognized

Pathophysiology
- Failure of normal mechanisms of gastro-oesophageal continence (LOS pressure, length of intra-abdominal LOS, angle of His, sling fibres around the cardia, crural fibres of the diaphragm, mucosal rosette, presence of hiatus hernia, delayed gastric emptying)
- LOS pressure reduced by smoking, alcohol and coffee

Clinical features
- Retrosternal burning pain radiating to epigastrium, jaw and arms (oesophageal pain is often confused with cardiac pain)
- Regurgitation of acid contents into the mouth (water brash)
- Back pain (a penetrating ulcer in Barrett's oesophagus)
- Dysphagia from a benign stricture

Investigations
- Patients over the age of 45 or with suspicious symptoms should have malignancy excluded as a cause when first presenting with symptoms of GORD
- Barium swallow and meal: sliding hiatus hernia, oesophageal ulcer, stricture
- Oesophagoscopy: assess oesophagitis, biopsy for histology, dilate stricture if present
- 24-h pH monitoring: assess degree of reflux

Management
General
- Lose weight and avoid smoking, coffee, alcohol and chocolate
- Avoid tight garments and stooping

Medical
- Exclude carcinoma by OGD in patients over 45 years and with symptoms suspicious of malignancy
- Control acid secretion with H_2-receptor antagonists (e.g. ranitidine) or proton pump inhibitors (e.g. omeprazole)
- Minimize effects of reflux (give alginates to protect oesophagus)
- Prokinetic agents (e.g. metoclopramide, cisapride) improve LOS tone and promote gastric emptying

Surgical
- Surgery for GORD should be reserved for complications or patients resistant to medical therapy
- Antireflux surgery (e.g. Nissen fundoplication) may be performed by laparotomy or laparoscopy. Indicated for:
  (a) Complications of reflux
  (b) Failed medical control of symptoms
  (c) ? Long-term dependence on medical treatment
  (d) ? 'Large-volume' reflux

Complications
- Benign stricture of the oesophagus
- Barrett's oesophagus (see below)
- Bleeding

Barrett's oesophagus
Definition and aetiology
- Columnar epithelium lining the lower anatomical oesophagus
- May be related to eradication of *H. pylori* and increasing incidence of GORD
- LSBO (> 3.0 cm) is more likely to develop dysplasia and neoplastic progression than SSBO (< 3.0 cm)

Diagnosis
- Can only be confidently made by biopsy but appearance of 'reddish' mucosa in the lower oesophagus is typical on OGD

Complications
Risk of adenocarcinoma:
- 2%: no dysplasia present
- 20%: low-grade dysplasia present
- 50%: high-grade dysplasia present

Treatment
- Follow-up OGD (close surveillance if low-grade dysplasia), H_2-receptor blockers and proton pump inhibitors
- Oesophagectomy if high-grade dysplasia because of risk of carcinoma

04

presents acutely with respiratory distress in the neonatal period. In adults most are asymptomatic but a few present with digestive symptoms due to herniation of the colon, stomach or small bowel.

Parasternal hernia (through foramen of Morgagni or Magendie)

This rare hernia is more common on the right and occurs through a triangular anterior defect lateral to the sternum. It is usually asymptomatic in the first years of life but may cause episodes of pain and tenderness in the right subcostal region and intermittent obstructive symptoms. Surgical treatment is recommended because of the risk of intestinal obstruction and strangulation.

Traumatic diaphragmatic hernia

Traumatic rupture of the diaphragm results from penetrating or blunt trauma to the abdomen and chest. The tendinous portion, especially on the left side, is the site of rupture in the majority. The rupture may present acutely following the injury or escape detection until several months to years later. The symptoms are related to the size of the herniated contents and to the onset of mechanical complications such as intestinal obstruction, strangulation, haemorrhage or progressive cardiorespiratory insufficiency. The diagnosis is usually established on chest films in which a space occupying lesion or bowel gas shadow is seen. Herniated spleen may be ruptured and accompanied by severe haemorrhage resulting in total opacification of the left chest and hypovolaemic shock. Otherwise, air fluid levels may be observed (colon, small bowel). Contrast studies may be needed to confirm the diagnosis. In acute rupture any associated injuries take precedence over the diaphragmatic injury. However repair of the acute tear is performed at the same emergency operation. Late presenting cases are operated upon electively.

Hiatus hernia

Three types of hiatus hernia are recognized:
- type 1, axial or sliding;
- type 2, para-oesophageal;
- type 3, mixed para-oesophageal and sliding.

Axial (sliding) hernia accounts for the majority. The gastro-oesophageal junction and a variable portion of the adjacent stomach slide upwards into the mediastinum carrying with them a peritoneal sac (Fig. 25.12a). This results in incompetence of the cardio-oesophageal junction. The symptoms and complications of this type of hernia are those of GORD. In *para-oesophageal hernia*, the fundus of the stomach rotates in front of the oesophagus and herniates through the hiatus into the mediastinum

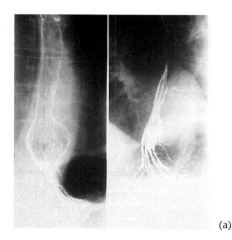

(a)

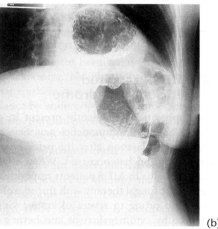

(b)

Figure 25.12 Contrast studies: (a) sliding hiatus hernia; (b) rolling hiatus hernia.

(Fig. 25.12b). As the cardio-oesophageal junction remains *in situ* within the abdomen, GORD is not a clinical feature and symptoms when present are caused by pressure on the heart (palpitations) or lungs (dyspnoea). Para-oesophageal hernia is found predominantly in the elderly. In large herniae the entire stomach and pylorus may be found within the chest inside a large hernial sac, which may also contain the spleen and transverse the colon. These large herniae can strangulate, with infarction and perforation of contents. *Mixed hernia* resembles a large para-oesophageal hernia but the gastro-oesophageal junction is also herniated above the diaphragm. It is a late stage of the para-oesophageal variety and has both pressure and reflux symptoms. Approximately 20% of patients with large para-oesophageal/mixed herniae may present acutely with severe upper gastrointestinal haemorrhage or strangulation/infarction/perforation of the intrathoracic stomach.

04

Treatment

If clinical assessment and appropriate investigations establish that the symptoms are due to the hiatal hernia, surgical correction is advisable if the patient is fit. The principles of treatment (by open or laparoscopic approach) are:

- excision of sac;
- reduction of hernia;
- antireflux repair (usually total fundoplication).

Oesophageal motility disorders

Oesophageal motility disorders are classified as follows.

- Primary: the oesophagus is the major site of involvement.
- Secondary: the oesophageal abnormalities are due to generalized neural, muscular or systemic diseases, or metabolic, inflammatory or neoplastic disorders.

The recognized primary oesophageal motility disorders are shown in Table 25.7. The differentiation of the main primary varieties is based largely on the symptoms, manometric profile and radiological appearances.

Achalasia

Achalasia is the most common primary oesophageal motility disorder and is caused by inflammation of the myenteric plexus, leading to fibrosis with decrease or loss of myenteric ganglion cells and selective destruction of non-cholinergic, non-adrenergic inhibitory neurones. The manometric profile includes absence of peristaltic contractions and incomplete relaxation of the LOS in response to swallowing. In addition, LOS pressure is usually elevated (> 25 mmHg). Loss of propulsive peristaltic contractions and defective sphincter relaxations lead to stasis of food in the oesophagus, which progressively dilates and lengthens, thereby assuming a sigmoid shape in advanced cases. The mucosa of the oesophagus often shows oesophagitis, with mucosal ulceration secondary to bacterial proliferation. Leucoplakia is commonly encountered in long-standing cases. The main symptoms are dysphagia, regurgitation and chest pain. The dysphagia is mainly for solid food, with variable degrees of liquid dysphagia. Initially it is intermittent, of variable severity and may be aggravated by emotional stress and cold liquids. Often patients find that swallowing is improved by drinking liquids or by repeated swallowing. When oesophageal dilatation is minimal, odynophagia as well as spontaneous episodes of chest pain may simulate angina pectoris. Respiratory symptoms when present are due to pulmonary complications. The classic radiological features include dilatation of the oesophageal body, a beak-like tapering of the oesophagus at the gastro-oesophageal junction (Fig. 25.13).

Achalasia may be treated by:

- botulinum toxin injection (temporary relief only);
- pneumatic dilatation;
- surgical myotomy.

Botulinum toxin binds to presynaptic receptors and

Table 25.7 Manometric criteria for oesophageal motility disorders.

Motility disorder	Manometric criteria
Achalasia	Simultaneous contractions (aperistalsis) High LOS pressure Incomplete LOS relaxation
Diffuse oesophageal spasm	Simultaneous contractions (> 10% of swallows) Intermittent normal peristalsis
Nutcracker oesophagus	High amplitude (> 140 mmHg) peristaltic contractions
Hypertensive LOS	High resting LOS pressure (> 45 mmHg) Normal LOS relaxation Normal peristalsis
Non-specific motility disorders	Non-propagated contractions Retrograde contractions Low amplitude (< 30 mmHg) contractions Prolonged duration (> 6 s) contractions Multipeaked and disordered contractions Aperistalsis in oesophageal body with normal LOS Abnormal LOS function

LOS, lower oesophageal sphincter.

04

04

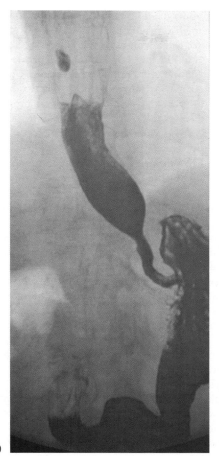

(a)

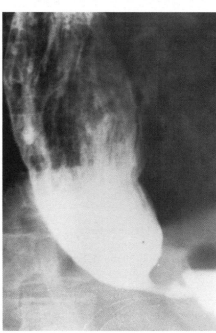

(b)

Figure 25.13 Barium swallow: (a) early achalasia; (b) late achalasia.

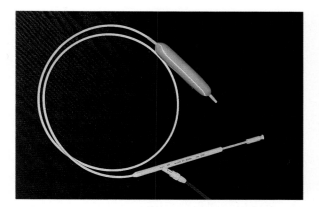

Figure 25.14 Oldbert oesophageal balloon for dilatation of achalasia.

irreversibly inhibits axonal acetylcholine release. When injected into the LOS, the toxin reduces sphincter pressure. Symptomatic improvement is obtained in 50% but the effect is not lasting. Pneumatic dilatation using low-compliance balloon dilators (Fig. 25.14) is effective in 70% but many patients have recurrence of their symptoms within 5 years. These can be treated by repeat dilatation or surgical myotomy. The indications for surgical treatment of achalasia (Heller's cardiomyotomy) are as follows:

- children and young adults;
- after failure of pneumatic dilatation or botulinum toxin injection therapy;
- patients with coexistent pathology requiring surgical intervention;
- patient's preference.

The modern anterior cardiomyotomy is performed via a laparoscopic approach (Fig. 25.15).

Chagas' disease

This is the result of infestation with *Trypanosoma cruzi* (endemic in rural parts of Latin America). The parasite invades the reticuloendothelial system, muscles and nerves. Destruction of the myenteric plexus leads to a condition that simulates achalasia radiologically, manometrically and clinically. Laparoscopic cardiomyotomy is the treatment of choice.

Diffuse oesophageal spasm

Diffuse oesophageal spasm is characterized by multiple spontaneous contractions and by simultaneous swallowing-induced repetitive contractions of large amplitude and long duration that alternate with periods of normal

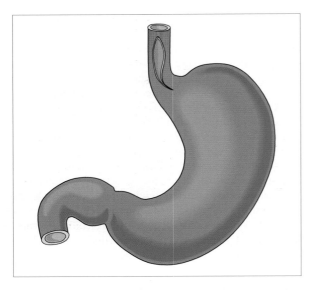

Figure 25.15 Diagram of Heller's cardiomyotomy.

peristalsis. LOS resting pressure is normal, with normal relaxation in response to swallowing. Patients may progress from diffuse oesophageal spasm to achalasia. The major clinical symptoms are substernal midline chest pain, odynophagia and dysphagia. Pain is most commonly constricting and is often misdiagnosed as ischaemic heart disease because it radiates to the back, neck and jaws. Dysphagia is also common but of variable severity. However, weight loss is not a significant feature. The barium swallow may demonstrate the typical corkscrew oesophagus (Fig. 25.16). The oesophageal radionuclide transit test shows an oscillatory or non-clearance pattern. Treatment with long-acting nitrates can provide temporary relief of symptoms. Benzodiazepines and psychotropic drugs may be effective in some patients and pneumatic dilatation may help. Surgical intervention is considered only after the above measures have failed and consists of a long oesophageal myotomy (Fig. 25.17).

Nutcracker oesophagus

This condition is characterized by high amplitude (> 140 mmHg) peristaltic contractions and hypertrophy of the muscle walls of the oesophagus. These strong contractions may be limited to the distal oesophagus or are present throughout the whole oesophagus. Nutcracker oesophagus is more often associated with non-cardiac chest pain than with dysphagia. The pathophysiology of nutcracker oesophagus is unclear but some patients have GORD and antireflux surgery may alleviate the symptoms. Medical therapy with antispasmodics is usually unsuccessful.

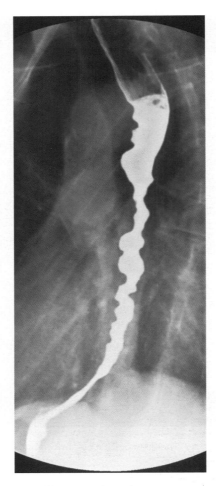

Figure 25.16 Diffuse oesophageal spasm: contrast swallow demonstrating corkscrew oesophagus.

04

Non-specific oesophageal motility disorders

Non-specific oesophageal motility disorders produce a variety of symptoms, e.g. dysphagia, non-cardiac chest pain, regurgitation, heartburn and globus sensation. Patients have manometric features that do not fit any recognized specific pattern, although often they exhibit delayed oesophageal transit. Some patients with gastro-oesophageal reflux exhibit these manometric findings, suggesting a possible association between the two disorders. Non-specific motility disorders are difficult to treat, although some are helped by antisecretory agents, sedatives and psychotropic agents.

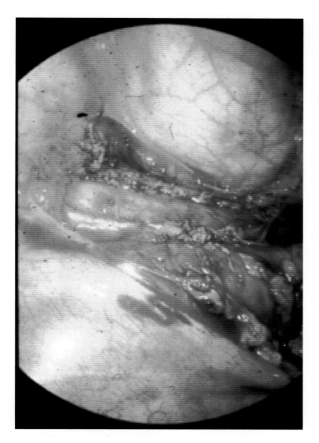

Figure 25.17 Thoracoscopic long myotomy for diffuse oesophageal spasm.

Motility disorders secondary to systemic disorders

The systemic disorders that may cause abnormal oesophageal motility include:

- progressive systemic sclerosis (most common cause);
- dermatomyositis;
- lupus erythematosus;
- rheumatoid arthritis;
- diabetes mellitus.

The oesophageal motor disorder in patients with systemic sclerosis is characterized by severe incompetence of the LOS and weakness leading to complete loss of peristaltic activity of the distal two-thirds of the oesophagus. The myopathy is confined to the smooth muscle portion of the oesophagus, the upper striated segment remaining normal. There is no specific medical therapy, although prokinetic agents are often used with variable results. GORD is treated with proton pump inhibitors.

Oesophageal diverticulae

Oesophageal diverticulae may be congenital or acquired. Congenital diverticulae are very rare and are due to incomplete duplication of the oesophagus. Acquired diverticulae are classified into pulsion and traction varieties. Pulsion diverticulae arise as a consequence of pathological elevation of the intraluminal oesophageal pressure, causing herniation of the mucosa through a weak area in the muscular wall. Traction diverticulae are the consequence of inflammatory adhesions between the oesophagus and mediastinal structures, particularly lymph nodes. The subsequent fibrous contracture pulls the oesophageal wall (mucosa and muscle) to form a pouch.

The types of oesophageal diverticulae include pharyngo-oesophageal (Zenker's) diverticulum, mid-thoracic diverticulae and epiphrenic diverticulae.

Pharyngo-oesophageal (Zenker's) diverticulum

This diverticulum is secondary to cricopharyngeal dysfunction and less commonly to an oesophageal motility disorder. It develops as a midline mucosal outpouching on the posterior aspect of the pharyngo-oesophageal junction between the fibres of the inferior pharyngeal constrictor and the transverse fibres of the cricopharyngeus and usually manifests on the left side. With enlargement, it comes to lie to the side (usually left) behind the oesophagus. The diverticulum consists mainly of mucosa and submucosa. Symptoms include high dysphagia, coughing and spluttering with meals with risk of aspiration. Pharyngo-oesophageal diverticulum is three times more common in males and usually occurs in late middle age and in the elderly. As the condition progresses, the patient complains of regurgitation, constant throat irritation, gurgling noises during swallowing, chronic cough and recurrent chest infections due to aspiration. With compression of the oesophagus, dysphagia becomes more severe and attacks of coughing and spluttering are experienced with each meal. The diagnosis is confirmed by a barium swallow.

The management is operative, the surgical options being as follows.

- Diverticulectomy.
- Endoscopic division of the septum in elderly poor-risk patients with large dependent diverticulae: stapled division of the septum formed by the opposed walls of the diverticulum and the oesophagus.

Mid-thoracic diverticulae

These may be congenital, traction or pulsion. The congen-

ital and traction varieties have a similar radiological appearance (tented triangular shape with a wide neck) and possess a muscular coat. The congenital ones are thought to represent foregut duplications and the traction types are secondary to fibrous adhesions to healed tuberculous lymph nodes.

Epiphrenic diverticulae

The majority of epiphrenic diverticulae are acquired and of the pulsion variety. The symptoms are largely due to the underlying disorder. If the pouch is small, it usually resolves after successful therapy of the motility disorder or reflux disease. Excision of the diverticulum is indicated if the pouch is dependent and has a narrow neck.

Sideropenic dysphagia (Paterson–Kelly or Plummer–Vinson syndrome)

This syndrome is associated with iron-deficiency anaemia and affects predominantly postmenopausal females. Symptoms include dysphagia, microcytic hypochromic anaemia, glossitis, atrophic inflammation of the mucosa of the pharynx and upper oesophagus with areas of hyperkeratosis, ulceration and the formation of high, usually anteriorly placed, oesophageal webs. The dysphagia is thought to result more from oesophageal spasm associated with the inflamed atrophic mucosa than partial obstruction by the oesophageal webs. Patients with this condition require long-term follow-up because of the risk of upper oesophageal cancer.

Oesophageal perforations

Perforation of the oesophagus constitutes a serious life-threatening condition and is accompanied by a high morbidity, prolonged hospital stay and an appreciable mortality. Survival depends on prompt recognition and early surgical intervention for the majority of cases, although there is a place for non-operative management in selected patients. The categories are outlined in Table 25.8. The most common cause is endoscopy, especially when associated with dilatation and/or intubation of strictures.

From the clinical standpoint, oesophageal perforations are classified into two groups.
● Early (acute): recognized immediately or within a few hours; carries a good prognosis with a low mortality.
● Late (chronic): missed injuries, diagnosed beyond 24 h of onset. Transmural oedema of the oesophagus precludes safe primary suture closure, high mortality from sepsis.

The early manifestations of an oesophageal perforation are pain, tachycardia and fever. Patients with cervical injuries often develop a nasal voice. Hematemesis may be

Table 25.8 Categories of oesophageal perforation.

Iatrogenic
  Instrumental
  Postoperative
Swallowed foreign bodies
External trauma: usually penetrating
Corrosive ingestion
Spontaneous
  Neonatal
  Intramural haematoma (incomplete perforation)
  Mallory–Weiss syndrome
Progressive disease
  Peptic ulceration
  Hiatus hernia
  Tumours

a feature of incomplete injuries of the thoracoabdominal segment. Supraclavicular swelling and crepitus (subcutaneous emphysema) are observed in 60% of cervical and 30% of midoesophageal injuries. In thoracic injuries, respiratory distress is common and is accompanied by dullness on percussion and diminished air entry and breath sounds on the affected side (effusion). Upper abdominal tenderness with rebound and infrequent or absent bowel sounds indicates perforation of the abdominal segment of the oesophagus. However, these abdominal signs may be absent with small perforations. The first intimation of perforation may be the development of a subphrenic abscess.

In late perforations, clinical evidence of established sepsis is present with fever, cardiovascular instability or fully developed septic shock. The diagnosis is confirmed by plain and contrast radiology. Endoscopy is not required for complete injuries; its main indication is in diagnosis of incomplete (intramural) perforation and Mallory–Weiss syndrome (mucosal tears).

Spontaneous oesophageal injuries

Three conditions are included in this category:
● intramural haematoma (incomplete perforation);
● mucosal laceration (Mallory–Weiss syndrome);
● complete spontaneous perforation (Boerhaave syndrome).

Intramural haematoma

This is an extremely rare lesion that arises as an oesophageal mucosal tear associated with submucosal bleeding with dissection of this plane by the expanding intramural haematoma A contrast radiological swallow demonstrates a double-barrel oesophagogram (Fig. 25.18).

04

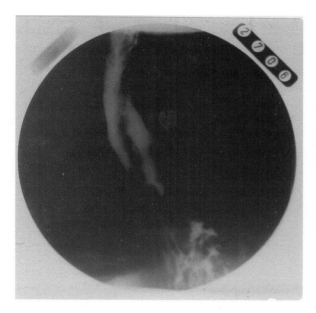

Figure 25.18 Incomplete perforation of the oesophagus showing 'double-barrel' oesophagogram.

The condition is self-limiting and seldom progresses to complete perforation.

Mallory–Weiss syndrome

This syndrome consists of painless haematemesis after vomiting, retching and straining usually induced by excess alcohol intake. There is a high incidence of GORD. The lesion consists of a longitudinal mucosal tear involving the mucosa alone or the mucosa and submucosa on the gastric side of the oesophagogastric junction. The tear, which may be single or multiple, is located on the lesser curve in the majority. The condition is commoner in males and a history of alcoholism is frequently present. Hypovolaemia requiring blood transfusion is present in one-third of patients. Treatment is by endoscopic photocoagulation or electrocoagulation.

Boerhaave syndrome

This is a rare syndrome of acute gastric distress, forceful vomiting, severe chest pain and collapse due to a complete tear of the lower thoracic oesophagus, just above the cardia. The condition occurs usually between the ages of 40 and 60 years, with a male to female ratio of 2 : 1. There is frequently a long history of indigestion and chronic gastrointestinal disease such as duodenal ulcer, reflux oesophagitis and hiatal hernia. The manifestations consist of sudden severe epigastric pain radiating to the left chest and shoulder and upper abdomen, which develops after a violent retching episode or straining. Dyspnoea and shock rapidly supervene. Physical findings include surgical emphysema in the neck, dullness and diminished air entry over the base of the left lung, tenderness and guarding in the upper abdomen and absent or infrequent bowel sounds. The condition may simulate very closely myocardial infraction, perforated peptic ulcer, pulmonary embolism, dissecting aortic aneurysm and severe acute pancreatitis. The chest radiograph shows a left-sided pleural effusion and contrast swallow establishes the diagnosis.

Management of oesophageal perforations

The management of oesophageal perforations consists of resuscitation, antibiotic therapy with broad-spectrum antibiotics and surgical intervention. However, there are certain specific indications for adopting non-operative management.
- Incomplete injuries: traumatic perforation in the neonate, intramural haematoma and Mallory–Weiss syndrome.
- Complete injuries: these include minor guidewire-induced subdiaphragmatic perforation and certain thoracic perforations. The accepted criteria for a conservative approach in thoracic injuries are a localized perforation contained within the mediastinum, minimal symptoms or clinical sepsis.

Conservative management consists of oral intake, antibiotic therapy, nasogastric aspiration, parenteral nutrition and underwater seal pleural drainage if the radiograph shows a pleural effusion. The condition of the patient is monitored closely and surgical intervention is undertaken if there is lack of progress or deterioration. All other injuries require surgical treatment. Several options are available and treatment is tailored to the individual patient. Factors such as delay in presentation, underlying oesophageal disease, location of the perforation and cause of the perforation all influence the results of therapy. Overall, the aims of treatment are to seal the leak while maintaining gastrointestinal continuity, drain the infected area and the oesophageal contents, and treat sepsis aggressively.

Tumour of the oesophagus

The only important benign tumour of the oesophagus is leiomyoma, which has a predilection for the lower oesophagus. The majority are small and asymptomatic but larger ones can project into the lumen of the oesophagus and cause dysphagia. Treatment is by localized resection or enucleation.

Malignant oesophageal neoplasms are mostly carcinomas and carry a poor prognosis, with an overall 5-year survival of 5%. In the West, cancer of the oesophagus is predominantly a disease of elderly men. Carcinoma of the oesophagus is some 20–30 times more common in China, Iran and the Transkei region of South Africa than in the West. The aetiology of squamous cell cancer and adenocarcinoma of the oesophagus is different.

There is a good correlation between excess alcohol intake and smoking and incidence of oesophageal cancer. Vitamins (A, B_{12}, C, E, folic acid and riboflavin) and trace elements (iron, zinc, selenium and molybdenum) are thought to be protective. Certain disorders predispose to the development of squamous cancer of the oesophagus, e.g. achalasia, Plummer–Vinson syndrome, strictures associated with lye ingestion and human papilloma virus infection. Adenocarcinoma of the oesophagus is closely linked to Barrett's columnar epithelium. There is a clear racial, gender and site predilection for oesophageal adenocarcinoma. Thus 95% of patients are white, men outnumber women 5 : 1, and approximately 80% of patients have tumours in the distal third of the oesophagus or in the gastro-oesophageal junction.

Pathology

The predominant histological type throughout the world is squamous cell carcinoma but adenocarcinoma, especially of the lower oesophagus and gastro-oesophageal junction, is commoner in the West where the peak incidence of the disease is found over the age of 60 years.

Macroscopically, the disease assumes one of three forms:
- stenosing (Fig. 25.19a);
- polypoid (fungating, protruded) (Fig. 25.19b);
- ulcerative (excavated).

Growth of oesophageal cancer (squamous cell carcinoma or adenocarcinoma) occurs by intra-oesophageal spread, direct extension and lymphatic or haematogenous metastases. Squamous cell carcinoma more typically invades adjacent structures compared with adenocarcinoma. Distant metastases are present in 25–30% of patients at the time of diagnosis. The liver, lungs and bones are the most frequent sites. Early cancer of the oesophagus (confined to mucosa/submucosa) is only detected by screening. Both types spread to regional lymph nodes once the muscle coat is involved.

Diagnosis

The majority of patients in the West present with advanced disease. Dysphagia may not be experienced until two-thirds of the oesophageal lumen is obliterated

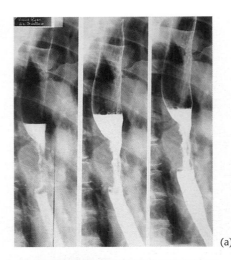
(a)

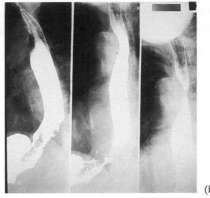
(b)

Figure 25.19 (a) Squamous carcinoma of the middle third of the oesophagus; (b) adenocarcinoma of lower third of the oesophagus.

04

(Fig. 25.20). Oesophageal obstruction results in malnutrition, weight loss, regurgitation and occasionally aspiration. Some patients may have palpable cervical lymph nodes and hepatic or cutaneous metastases at presentation. The key investigations for establishing the diagnosis are barium swallow and endoscopy with biopsy and cytology. Once a diagnosis is made, the tumour is staged as this influences management in the individual case. The most common clinical staging system is the TNM classification (Table 25.9), which correlates well with prognosis. CT and endoscopic ultrasonography are used to assess depth of invasion of the oesophageal wall and infiltration of adjacent structures by the tumour. Bronchoscopy is performed in proximal oesophageal tumours to exclude bronchial involvement. This, together with vocal cord and phrenic nerve paralysis, involvement of mediastinal structures (especially aorta) and distant metastases, indicate inoperability.

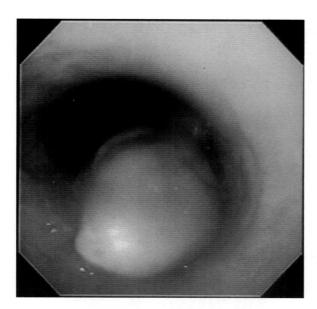

Figure 25.20 Flexible endoscopy showing a polypoid carcinoma of the lower oesophagus encroaching on about one-third of the oesophageal lumen. The lesion was confirmed as adenocarcinoma on biopsy/histology.

Treatment

The treatment of patients with oesophageal cancer depends on the stage of the disease and the condition of the patient. Some patients with resectable lesions are unfit for surgery by virtue of significant comorbid disease. The nutritional state of the patient must also be considered and assessed. In malnourished patients, a period of enteral nutrition is undertaken for a few weeks before surgery. Surgery constitues the primary treatment for resectable disease in fit patients. The aim of surgery is an R0 resection (complete macroscopic and microscopic removal of tumour) for cure, although palliation of dysphagia is an important secondary objective.

Treatment of patients who are unfit or have locally advanced disease is by chemoradiation. This is followed by restaging. Surgery is considered in fit patients whose disease is downstaged by the treatment.

Non-operative treatment

Radiotherapy

Treatment by supervoltage external beam radiotherapy may be curative (radical) or palliative to relieve dysphagia and metastatic bone pain. It can also be given as an adjunct to surgical treatment, either in the form of multimodality treatment or after oesophagectomy to improve locore-gional control. There are certain contraindications to radical radiotherapy. These include large tumours (> 9.0 cm) and the presence of a tracheal broncho-oesophageal fistula. The main disadvantages of radical radiotherapy are the development of a fibrous stricture in half the patients treated. Brachytherapy (intracavity irradiation) with caesium or iridium pellets loaded into an applicator and placed in the lumen of the oesophagus is another technique used for palliation of dysphagia.

Chemotherapy

Several agents are used in combination treatment regimens for oesophageal cancer. These include 5-fluorouracil (5-FU), cisplatin, vindesine, mitomycin C, paclitaxel and etoposide. Paclitaxel achieves a high response rate in metastatic oesophageal cancer and also acts as a radiation sensitizer. Most combination regimens have 5-FU with or without leucovorin. The second mst common agent used in combination regimens is cisplatin.

Table 25.9 TNM staging system for oesophageal cancer.

Primar tumour (T)

TX	Primary tumour cannot be assessed
T0	No evidence of primary tumour
Tis	Carcinoma *in situ*
T1a	Tumour invades lamina propria
T1b	Tumour invades submucosa
T2	Tumour invades muscularis propria
T3	Tumour invades adventitia
T4	Tumour invades adjacent structures

Regional lymph nodes (N)

NX	Regional lymph nodes cannot be assessed
N0	No regional lymph node metastasis
N1	Regional lymph node metastasis

Distant metastasis (M)

MX	Presence of distant metastasis cannot be assessed
M0	No distant metastasis
M1	Distant metastasis

Stage grouping

Stage 0	Tis	N0	M0
Stage I	T1	N0	M0
Stage IIA	T2	N0	M0
	T3	N0	M0
Stage IIB	T1	N1	M0
	T2	N1	M0
Stage III	T3	N1	M0
	T4	Any N	M0
Stage IV	Any T	Any N	M1

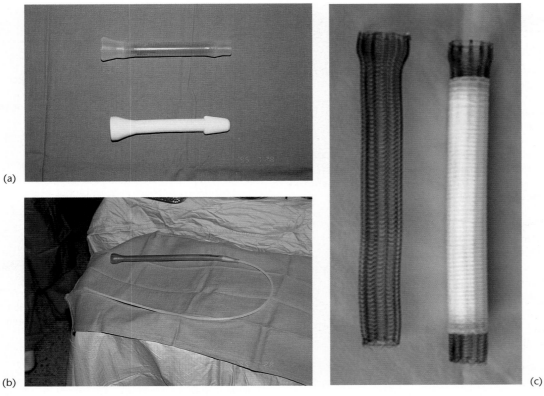

Figure 25.21 Oesophageal stents: (a) plastic introduced endoscopically after dilatation; (b) Celestin introduced by railroading during surgery for inoperable lesions; (c) Ultraflex self-expanding stents (covered and uncovered) introduced endoscopically or under radiological control.

The combination of cisplatin and 5-FU produces complete response rates averaging 10%.

Multimodality treatment

The combined use of chemotherapy and radiation therapy for the primary treatment of oesophageal cancer produces better response rates with improved survival than either modality alone. Preoperative chemotherapy (neoadjuvant) followed by surgery is used to downstage advanced tumours and thus increase the resectability rate and improve survival. The addition of radiotherapy to chemotherapy preoperatively offers possible survival advantages.

Palliation of advanced oesophageal cancer

Palliation is most commonly directed to relief of dysphagia. There are several methods to achieve this and they fall into two categories: recanalization or intubation. Surgical bypass is seldom used nowadays. The recanalization treatments include the following.

- Photocoagulation using Nd:YAG laser together with dilatation.
- Photodynamic ablation using haematoporphyrin derivative followed by irradiation with red light (wavelength 630 nm): this combination causes necrosis of tumour by highly reactive species such as singlet oxygen.
- Endoscopic-guided fulguration of advanced oesophageal neoplasm with the BICAP probe.
- Intratumour injection of absolute alcohol under endoscopic control: used as an adjunct to stenting to deal with tumour overgrowth/ingrowth.

Intubation is still the most widely used method for palliation of dysphagia in inoperable oesophageal cancer. The main advantage of intubation is that the treatment is performed in a single session, with dramatic restoration of swallowing. Plastic tubes have been replaced by self-expanding metallic stents as these provide excellent palliation and are relatively easy to insert. Several types are available (Fig. 25.21). Some patients develop a malignant tracheo-oesophageal fistula (spontaneously or after radiotherapy) that can be sealed with covered self-expanding metallic stents.

04

Oesophageal carcinoma at a glance

Definition

Oesophageal carcinoma: malignant lesion of the epithelial lining of the oesophagus

Epidemiology
- Male/female ratio 5 : 1
- Age 50–70 years
- High incidence in areas of China, Iran, Russia, Scandinavia and among the Bantu in South Africa
- Adenocarcinoma has the fastest increasing incidence of any carcinoma in the UK

Aetiology
- Alcohol consumption and cigarette smoking
- Chronic oesophagitis and Barrett's oesophagus
- Stricture from corrosive (lye) oesophagitis or human papilloma virus infection
- Achalasia
- Plummer–Vinson syndrome (oesophageal web, mucosal lesions of mouth and pharynx, iron-deficiency anaemia)
- Nitrosamines

Pathology
- Histological type: 90% squamous carcinoma (upper two-thirds of oesophagus); 10% adenocarcinoma (lower third of oesophagus)
- Macroscopically may be stenosing, polypoid or ulcerative
- Spread: lymphatics, direct extension, vascular invasion

Clinical features
- Majority of patients in West present with advanced disease
- Dysphagia progressing from solids to liquids
- Weight loss and weakness
- Aspiration pneumonia
- Evidence of distant disease (cervical nodes, hepatic or cutaneous metastases)

Investigations
To make the diagnosis
- Barium swallow: narrowed lumen with 'shouldering'
- Oesophagoscopy and biopsy: malignant structure

To assess whether tumour is operable
- Transluminal ultrasound may help assess local invasion
- Bronchoscopy: assess bronchial invasion with upper third lesions
- CT (helical): assess degree of spread if surgery is being contemplated
- Laparoscopy to assess liver and peritoneal involvement prior to surgery

Management
Only a minority of tumours are successfully cured

Palliation
Recanalization
- Photocoagulation by Nd:YAG laser plus dilatation
- Photodynamic ablation using haematoporphyrin plus red light irradiation
- Endoscopic-guided fulguration with BICAP probe
- Endoscopic intratumour injection of absolute alcohol
- Brachytherapy: intraluminal irradiation with caesium or iridium wires

Intubation
- Most widely used method of palliation
- Intubation with expanding endoprosthesis (has replaced Atkinson or Celestin tubes)

Curative treatment
- Surgical resection is curative only if lymph nodes are not involved
- Reconstruction is by gastric 'pull-up' or colon interposition

Other treatment
- Combination therapy with preoperative external beam irradiation and chemotherapy followed by surgery may offer survival advantage

Prognosis
- Following resection, 5-year survival rate is about 15%
- Overall 5-year survival (palliation and resection) is only about 4%

Evidence-based medicine

Delattre, J.-F., Avisse, C., Marcus, C. & Flament, J.-B. (2000) Functional anatomy of the gastroesophageal junction. *Surg Clin North Am* **80**, 241–60.

Katzka, D.A. & Castell, D.O. (1998) Esophageal manometry and modern medicine. *Dig Dis Sci* **16**, 189–91.

Lew, J.I., Gooding, W.E., Ribeiro, U. Jr *et al.* (2001) Long-term survival following induction chemoradiotherapy and esophagectomy for esophageal carcinoma. *Arch Surg* **136**, 737–42.

Rice, T.W. (2000) Clinical staging of esophageal carcinoma. CT, EUS, and PET. *Chest Surg Clin N Am* **10**, 471–85.

04

Disorders of the Stomach and Duodenum

26

Must know Must do

Must know

Types of dyspepsia

Alarm symptoms of serious upper gastrointestinal disease

Investigation of patients with dyspeptic symptoms

Acute complications of upper gastrointestinal disorders

Tests for *Helicobacter pylori*

Spectrum of disease caused by *Helicobacter* organisms

Clinical features and management of patients with gastric tumours

Must do

Follow the course of a patient admitted with haematemesis

Follow the course of a patient admitted with perforated duodenal ulcer

Attend the endoscopy suite to observe upper gastrointestinal endoscopies

Perform a faecal occult blood test

Insert a nasogastric tube in a patient under supervision

Attend an operation for resection of gastric cancer

Learn how to interpret barium swallow/meal for the detection of organic disease

Learn how to detect free gas under the diaphragm on the PA chest film

Introduction

The stomach is divisible into three parts: fundus, body and pyloric region (antrum and pyloric canal). Its most important physiological function is to act as a receptacle for ingested food, which is partially digested and hydrolysed by acid and pepsin into semifluid chyme and then delivered into the small intestine. The stomach possesses the property of adaptive relaxation, i.e. increase in capacity without a significant rise in intraluminal pressure.

Adaptive relaxation is mediated by stretch reflexes and vagal afferents and is therefore greatly impaired after gastric surgery. The mucosa lining the proximal stomach contains the parietal and chief cells, whereas the mucosa lining the more muscular antropyloric segment secretes an alkaline mucus but contains specialized endocrine (G) cells that release gastrin under the influence of gastrin-releasing peptide. The parietal cells secrete acid and intrinsic factor, whereas the chief cells are responsible for the production and secretion of pepsinogens that are then converted to active pepsins by HCl.

Dyspepsia

Gastroduodenal disease produces varied symptoms described by the term 'dyspepsia'. Dyspeptic symptoms are extremely common in the general population. An agreed international definition is 'episodic or persistent abdominal symptoms, often related to the intake of food, which patients or physicians believe to be due to disorders of the proximal portion of the digestive tract'. The symptoms included in this generic definition of dyspepsia are:

- pain or discomfort in the upper abdomen;
- nausea and vomiting;
- early satiety;
- epigastric fullness and regurgitation.

There are two categories of dyspepsia: organic and non-organic (no demonstrable focal lesion). The prevalence of organic dyspepsia increases above the age of 40–45 years. There are four subgroups of dyspeptic patients based on the predominant symptoms:

- ulcer-like;
- reflux-like;
- dysmotility-like;
- non-specific.

Symptoms alone do not differentiate between organic and non-organic disease. Hence history does not always predict the underlying cause of dyspepsia and for this reason investigation by endoscopy is necessary for certain groups:

04

- age > 45 years;
- patients who are *H. pylori* positive;
- patients with a history of using non-steroidal anti-inflammatory drugs (NSAIDs);
- patients with alarm/sinister symptoms (loss of appetite, weight loss, bleeding).

Alarm symptoms

Loss of appetite, weight loss, recent-onset dyspepsia, constant upper abdominal pain and evidence of bleeding are regarded as alarm or sinister symptoms and thus require urgent endoscopy, particularly if the patient is over 40 years of age. Weight loss and loss of appetite associated with early satiety/abdominal discomfort are suspicious of a gastric neoplasm.

Investigations

Endoscopy and radiology

Upper gastrointestinal endoscopy is necessary for the following groups of patients.
- Individuals > 45 years old testing positive for *H. pylori*, with persistent symptoms despite eradication treatment.
- Individuals > 45 years old, never investigated, *H. pylori*-negative and no intake of NSAIDs, with persistent symptoms despite acid-lowering treatment.
- Individuals > 45 years old with a previous history of gastric ulcer, no *H. pylori* testing or *H. pylori* test negative, with persistent symptoms despite acid-lowering drugs.
- Gastrointestinal bleeding: acute and chronic.

Contrast swallow and meal examination is seldom used in the investigation of patients with dyspepsia because endoscopy has a higher diagnostic yield and permits biopsy with histological diagnosis. However, contrast radiology is needed in:
- patients with gastric cancer undergoing surgery (precise location of lesion);
- patients with hiatus hernia undergoing surgery (type and size of hernia);
- suspected perforation/anastomotic leak (water-soluble contrast must be used).

Barium studies are unreliable in the assessment of a patient with acute upper gastrointestinal bleeding. Endoscopy is the preferred investigation in this situation.

Endoscopic ultrasonography

Flexible endoscopic ultrasonography enables identification of the layers of the oesophagus and stomach and provides the most accurate staging of oesophageal and gastric

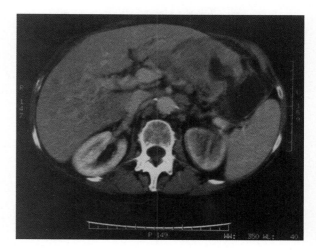

Figure 26.1 Hydro-helical CT showing gastric carcinoma.

tumours. In the stomach endoscopic ultrasonography is used for:
- pretreatment staging of early gastric cancer (detection of submucosal involvement);
- staging and follow-up of lymphomas of gastric mucosa-associated lymphoid tissue (MALT);
- diagnosis of stromal (mesenchymal) tumours.

Deep involvement of the submucosa in early gastric cancer is associated with a significantly increased risk of lymph node spread. Endoscopic ultrasonography is also capable of identifying advanced gastric cancer and infiltration of adjacent organs but is unreliable in detecting lymph node involvement.

Helical computed tomography

Computed tomography (CT) is useful in the staging and assessment of operability of patients with gastric cancer. The technique involves ingestion of water (hydro-CT) or dilute contrast by the patient followed by helical CT scanning with the patient in the prone position (Fig. 26.1). This technique allows documentation of extent of mural involvement, extragastric extension and involvement of retrogastric organs such as the pancreas. Helical CT also enables detection of lymph node enlargement, especially of the coeliac/para-aortic lymph nodes.

Gastric emptying

Measurement of gastric emptying is indicated in patients with symptomatology indicative of abnormal emptying (delayed or rapid). Delayed gastric emptying is encountered in diabetic patients and those with dysmotility disorders. A variety of radionuclide 'meals' are used. The

patient drinks or ingests the meal and the radioactivity in the stomach is then monitored with an external gamma camera, thus obtaining radioactivity–time curves. The most useful index is the half-emptying time ($T_{1/2}$), i.e. the time taken for half of the ingested meal to leave the stomach. Assessment of both liquid and gastric emptying is necessary to document the pattern of abnormal gastric emptying.

Plasma gastrin

This is indicated if clinical or gastric secretory features suggest the possibility of Zollinger–Ellison syndrome. The reported levels of plasma gastrin vary between laboratories but values greater than 200 pg/mL are regarded as abnormally high. Values in excess of 1000 pg/mL are virtually diagnostic of a gastrinoma, provided that the patient is secreting acid. The reason for this proviso is that in an achlorhydric patient, e.g. one with pernicious anaemia, there is no fall in antral pH to inhibit gastrin secretion.

Gastroduodenal disease: *Helicobacter pylori* infection

Helicobacter pylori infection (Fig. 26.2) is acquired by oral ingestion. In the stomach, the bacteria localize on the epithelial surface beneath the viscid mucous layer where they exert pathological effects via the elaboration of various enzymes/toxins. One of the toxins induces cellular vacuolization. This vacuolizing cytotoxin is much more commonly encountered in patients with duodenal ulceration than those with gastritis without ulceration. Not all patients with *H. pylori* infection develop gastroduodenal disease. Factors that determine development of gastroduodenal disease include:

- host factors;
- virulence and genetic type of the organism;
- age of the host;
- environmental factors (smoking, diet especially the protective effect of fruit and vegetables).

Virulence is associated with the 'cag pathogenicity island' (segment of DNA) that contains 40 genes. One of these is the cytotoxin-associated gene A (*cagA*) that codes for the protein CagA, which is detected by antibody tests. The pathogenicity island is associated with the vacuolating toxin and hence mucosal damage and inflammation. Long-standing inflammation then leads to atrophy and intestinal metaplasia. The *H. pylori* antigens also induce the appearance of MALT follicles in the gastric submucosa. Hence the entire spectrum of gastroduodenal disease caused by *H. pylori* includes:

- gastroduodenitis;
- duodenal and gastric ulcers;
- atrophic gastritis;
- carcinoma of the body and antrum of the stomach;
- MALT-associated gastric lymphoma.

Tests for *H. pylori* infection

The most commonly performed are the rapid urease tests, which are carried out on endoscopic biopsies. These tests use kits such as the *Campylobacter*-like organism (CLO) (Fig. 26.3), Hpfast and Pyloritec and provide a result within 3 h of endoscopy. Other tests include culture in a microaerobic environment, polymerase chain reaction, histology of the antrum and corpus (Giemsa or Warthin–Starry silver stain), ^{13}C urea breath test, and serology for detection of *H. pylori*-specific antibodies (Table 26.1).

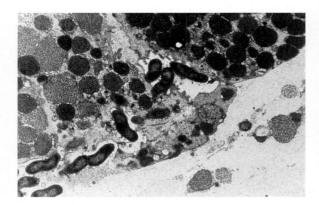

Figure 26.2 *Helicobacter pylori.*

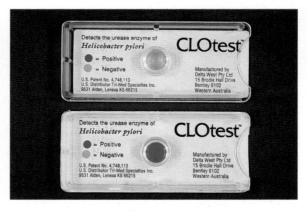

Figure 26.3 *Campylobacter*-like organism (CLO) test for *Helicobacter pylori.*

Test	Sensitivity (%)	Specificity (%)
Rapid urease tests	90	100
Culture	98	100
Polymerase chain reaction	97	100
Histology of antrum and corpus	98	99
^{13}C breath test	100	100
Serology	98	88

Table 26.1 Comparative sensitivity and specificity of the various tests used for diagnosis of *Helicobacter pylori* infections.

Dyspepsia at a glance

Definition

Dyspepsia: a feeling of discomfort or pain in the upper abdomen or lower chest. There may also be symptoms of nausea ± vomiting, early satiety and epigastric fullness. *Indigestion* may be used by the patient to mean dyspepsia, regurgitation or flatulence. Dyspepsia may be organic or non-organic (i.e. no demonstrable focal lesion)

Causes

Oesophagus
- Reflux oesophagitis: retrosternal dyspepsia, worse after large meal or lying down, associated symptoms of regurgitation, pain on swallowing
- Oesophageal carcinoma: new-onset dyspepsia in older patient, weight loss/dysphagia/haematemesis, failure to respond to acid-suppression treatment

Stomach
- Gastritis: recurrent episodes of epigastric pain, transient or short-lived symptoms, may be associated with diet, responds well to antacids or acid suppression
- Gastric ulcer: typically chronic epigastric pain, worse with food, 'food fear' may cause weight losss, exacerbated by smoking/alcohol, occasionally relieved by vomiting
- Carcinoma of the stomach: progressive symptoms, weight loss/anorexia, iron-deficiency anaemia, early satiety, epigastric mass

Duodenum
- Duodenal ulcer: epigastric and back pain, chronic exacerbations lasting several weeks, relieved by food especially milky drinks, relieved by bedrest, commoner in young men, associated with *H. pylori* infection
- Duodenitis: often transient, mild symptoms only, associated with alcohol and smoking

Gallstones
- Dyspepsia is rarely the only symptom. Often associated with right upper quadrant pain
- Should only be considered as cause of dyspepsia after normal oesophagogastroduodenoscopy (OGD) and ultrasound demonstrating gallstones

Alarm symptoms
- Loss of appetite
- Recent-onset dyspepsia
- Constant upper abdominal pain
- Weight loss
- Evidence of bleeding

Helicobacter pylori
- Bacterium acquired by oral ingestion, found in the stomach and duodenum of a high percentage of patients with gastroduodenal disease
- Not all patients with *H. pylori* get disease and not all patients with disease have *H. pylori*
- Bacteria are found on the epithelial surface of the stomach and duodenum below the mucus layer
- Cause disease by the action of toxins, especially vacuolizing cytotoxin which causes cellular vacuolization

Factors that predispose to gastroduodenal disease
- *H. pylori* virulence and genetic type
- Host factors: age
- Environmental factors: smoking, diet

Gastroduodenal disease caused by H. pylori
- Gastroduodenitis
- Gastric and duodenal ulcers
- Atrophic gastritis
- Carcinoma of the stomach (body and antrum)
- MALT-associated lymphoma

Tests for H. pylori
- Rapid urease test on gastric biopsies
- Culture of gastric biopsies
- Polymerase chain reaction
- Histology of antrum/corpus

- ^{13}C-urea breath test
- Serology

Eradication
- Dual therapy: antibiotic + PPI (e.g. omeprazole)
- Triple therapy (used most often): acid inhibition (e.g. one

of omeprazole, lansoprazole, pantoprazole, ranitidine bismuth citrate) + antibacterial treatment (e.g. two of clarithromycin, amoxicillin, metronidazole) for 1 week is highly effective in eradicating *H. pylori*
- Quadruple therapy: PPI, bismuth, metronidazole and tetracycline.

Algorithm for investigation of dyspepsia

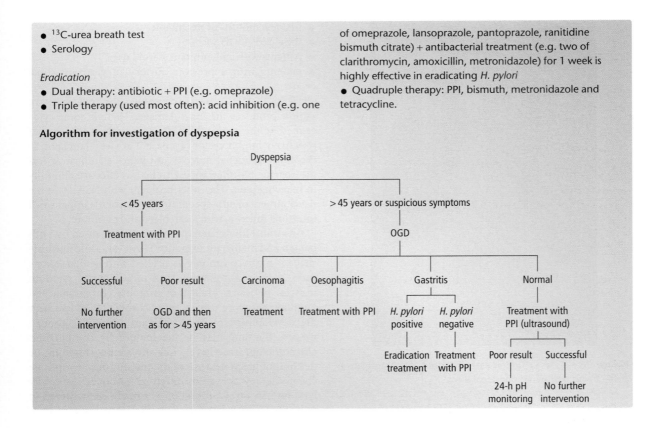

Acute gastroduodenal disorders

These include perforated ulcers, upper gastrointestinal bleeding and pyloric stenosis.

Perforation

Perforation can occur in both acute and chronic peptic ulcers. NSAIDs are prone to cause peptic ulceration, with an increased risk of both perforation and bleeding. Acute perforations may also accompany stress, such as burns, multiple injuries, sepsis, etc. Some perforated gastric ulcers are malignant.

The moment of perforation is often identified by the patient as sudden excruciating epigastric pain, which becomes generalized quickly. The physical signs include tenderness with guarding, which is initially localized to the upper abdomen but soon becomes generalized. Abdominal distension is a late feature and is due to paralytic ileus. A variable degree of peripheral circulatory failure may be present, with tachycardia, hypotension, a cold periphery and decreased urinary output. Respiration will often be shallow. The diagnosis is confirmed by the presence of free air underneath the right diaphragm on the

chest radiograph (Fig. 26.4). If a pneumoperitoneum is not seen radiologically, the diagnostic problem is to differentiate a sealed perforation from acute pancreatitis/ cholecystitis. Contrast radiology with a water-soluble contrast medium may be required for this purpose.

Initial treatment is directed towards correction of hypovolaemia and any electrolyte imbalance. Either colloids or crystalloids can be used for resuscitation. Pain relief should be given as soon as the physical signs have been assessed. Antibiotics are not recommended routinely since the initial peritonitis is chemical. However, if surgery is delayed beyond 8 h from perforation or if the patient has chronic respiratory problems, the use of a broad-spectrum antibiotic is necessary.

Patients with perforated ulcers can be managed successfully with a non-operative approach using nasogastric suction, intravenous fluids, antibiotics and analgesics, and intravenous proton pump inhibitors (PPIs). This approach is reserved for poor-risk elderly patients and carries a high incidence of abscess formation in the subphrenic region that will subsequently require drainage. Operative closure of the perforation and peritoneal lavage is the correct treatment in patients who are fit for surgery and anaesthesia. Insertion of drains is not generally

04

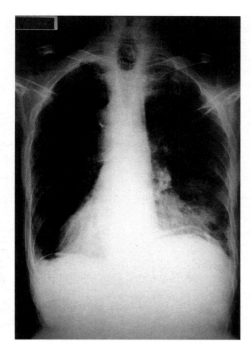

Figure 26.4 Free air underneath the right diaphragm in a patient with perforated duodenal ulcer.

recommended. In patients undergoing emergency surgery for perforated gastric ulcer, biopsy is essential as 10% of perforated gastric ulcers are due to malignant disease.

Upper gastrointestinal bleeding

Bleeding from the gastrointestinal tract may be caused by lesions located in the foregut (oesophagus, stomach and duodenum), midgut (small bowel up to mid transverse colon) and hindgut (distal colon and rectum). The bleeding may be acute when the patient presents with hypovolaemia, or chronic when the clinical picture is that of symptomatic anaemia.

The common causes of acute upper gastrointestinal haemorrhage are:

- chronic peptic ulceration;
- NSAID-induced bleeding;
- oesophagogastric varices.

Irrespective of the cause, the vomited blood (haematemesis) may be fresh (in severe active bleeding as from ruptured oesophageal varices) or chemically altered (because acid digestion simulates 'coffee grounds'). Extensive gastrointestinal bleeding also gives rise to the passage of black foul-smelling liquid faeces known as melaena.

Patients taking NSAIDs have a threefold risk of gastrointestinal haemorrhage, surgery and death compared with non-users. The risk from bleeding is greatest in:

- first few months of treatment;
- the elderly (> 65 years);
- patients with concomitant steroid use;
- patients with a previous history of gastrointestinal events.

Of all the NSAIDs known to cause bleeding or perforation, aspirin produces the most damage. There is some evidence that the newer NSAIDs (e.g. nabumetone) that selectively inhibit cyclooxygenase-2 are less damaging to the gastroduodenal mucosa and hence significantly less ulcerogenic but they appear to be less effective clinically in relieving pain. The other problem with NSAIDs is the development of non-specific ulceration of the upper small intestinal mucosa, which can bleed and perforate.

Gastrointestinal haemorrhage may be caused by both benign and malignant tumours. However, acute haemorrhage is more commonly associated with benign lesions such as neurofibromatosis and mesenchymal (smooth muscle) tumours. Malignant tumours (carcinoma and lymphomas) more usually cause chronic blood loss with the development of iron-deficiency anaemia, although massive bleeding may be precipitated by combination chemotherapy (see later). Life-threatening bleeding or perforation from necrosis of the tumour may complicate chemotherapy for gastrointestinal tumours, especially lymphomas. Stress ulceration is usually encountered in critically ill patients nursed in the intensive care unit, although its incidence has declined.

Other causes of acute upper gastrointestinal bleeding include Dieulafoy's lesion, portal hypertensive gastropathy and watermelon stomach.

- *Dieulafoy's lesion (exulceration simplex)* consists of a nodule containing a visible vessel covered with normal mucosa. Treatment is by endoscopic electrocoagulation or sclerotherapy.
- *Portal hypertensive gastropathy* develops in some patients with cirrhosis and portal hypertension with progressive liver damage and affects predominantly the fundus but may be generalized.
- *Diffuse vascular ectasia (watermelon stomach)* consists of ectatic mucosal sacculated vessels in the lamina propria traversing the antrum and sometimes the duodenum. The endoscopic appearance bears some resemblance to the stripes of a watermelon. The bleeding is often recurrent requiring multiple transfusions. Portal hypertensive gastropathy and diffuse gastric vascular ectasia are probably related.

The treatment of acute upper gastrointestinal haemorrhage is based on the following principles.

- Resuscitation: volume replacement with crystalloids, colloids and blood.
- Early endoscopy: for diagnosis and endoscopic control of bleeding.

● Combined management by gastroenterologists and surgeons with early recourse to surgery if bleeding continues or recurs.

Sometimes there is clear evidence of upper gastrointestinal bleeding without apparent cause. In these patients, mesenteric angiography and small-bowel enteroscopy often locate the source of the bleeding.

Chronic gastrointestinal bleeding is unnoticed by the patient and for this reason is referred to as *occult*. The constant drain results in depletion of iron stores and thus the development of iron-deficiency (hypochromic microcytic) anaemia. When discovered this must always be investigated as follows:

● faecal occult blood;
● upper gastrointestinal endoscopy;
● flexible sigmoidoscopy and barium enema or colonoscopy if upper gastrointestinal endoscopy is negative.

Carcinoma of the caecum and ascending colon most commonly presents as iron-deficiency anaemia as does carcinoma of the stomach.

Pyloric stenosis (gastric outlet obstruction)

Pyloric stenosis is rarely due to stenosis at the pylorus. More commonly, the obstruction is on one side of the pylorus, either in the first part of the duodenum due to chronic scarring from a duodenal ulcer or in the antrum due to a carcinoma (Fig. 26.5). True pyloric stenosis can arise from a pyloric channel ulcer or very rarely from a

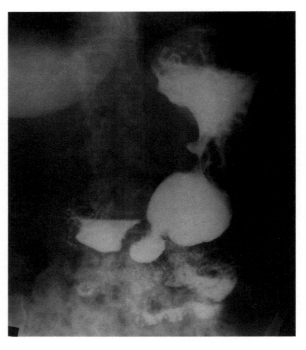

Figure 26.6 Barium meal showing hour-glass deformity caused by a lesser curve ulcer in the middle third of the stomach. The deformity resolved with medical treatment. However, some of these deformities are fibrotic in nature (contractures) when obstructive symptoms persist depite ulcer healing. These require dilatation or surgical treatment.

congenital web or adult hypertrophic pyloric stenosis. Some instances of gastric stenosis are caused by inflammatory oedema surrounding an active ulcer and these often resolve with conservative treatment (Fig. 26.6). The common causes of gastric outlet obstruction are:

● chronic duodenal ulceration/fibrosis;
● antral gastric carcinoma;
● carcinoma of the head of the pancreas.

Rare causes include a variety of benign tumours, lymphomas, Crohn's disease, duodenal haematoma, adult pyloric hypertrophy, annular pancreas and mucosal diaphragm.

Benign pyloric stenosis usually occurs in a patient with long-standing symptoms of ulceration. Vomiting and anorexia supervene. The typical vomiting of pyloric stenosis is projectile and the vomitus is characterized by an absence of bile and the presence of partially digested food eaten hours or even days previously. With repeated vomiting and failure to eat, the patient often becomes constipated, although in some cases diarrhoea may develop. Examination usually shows an underweight patient, dehydration and often a degree of iron-deficiency

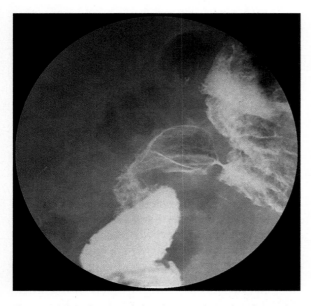

Figure 26.5 Barium meal showing gastric outlet obstruction caused by fibrosis following healing of chronic duodenal ulcer.

04

anaemia. A succussion splash may be present and visible contractions passing across the upper abdomen from left to right may be observed on inspection.

Prolonged vomiting of gastric contents results in characteristic electrolyte disturbances. Initially, the major loss is fluid rich in hydrogen and chloride ions so that dehydration is accompanied by hypochloraemic alkalosis. At this stage the serum sodium is usually normal and hypokalaemia may not be obvious. More marked metabolic changes supervene as a result of continued losses and secondary changes in renal function. Initially, the urine is characterized by a low chloride content and is appropriately alkaline because of enhanced bicarbonate excretion compensating for the metabolic alkalosis but at the expense of sodium. If gastric losses continue, the patient becomes progressively hypovolaemic and hyponatraemic. In an attempt to conserve circulating volume, sodium is retained by the kidneys and exchanged for hydrogen ions and potassium. At this late stage, the patient has a metabolic alkalosis and, paradoxically, an acid urine. As a secondary effect of the alkalosis, the concentration of plasma ionized calcium may fall so that disturbances of consciousness and tetany may be apparent.

The priority in management of the advanced case of pyloric stenosis is correction of the fluid and electrolyte

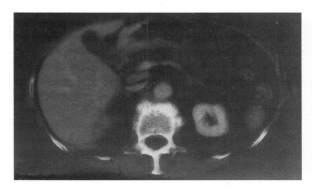

Figure 26.7 CT showing pyloric obstruction by an antral carcinoma.

disturbances. Rehydration is achieved by saline infusions with potassium supplements as indicated by electrolyte determinations. Gastric lavage is performed with a wide-bore tube using isotonic saline daily until the returning fluid becomes clear. The surgical treatment of pyloric stenosis caused by duodenal ulceration/fibrosis is truncal vagotomy and posterior gastroenterostomy. In western countries the majority of cases of gastric outlet obstruction are caused by distal gastric cancer (Fig. 26.7).

Haematemesis at a glance

Definitions

Gastrointestinal bleeding: any blood loss from the gastrointestinal tract (from mouth to anus), which may present with haematemesis, melaena, rectal bleeding or anaemia

Haematemesis: vomiting of blood, usually caused by upper gastrointestinal disease

Melaena: the passage per rectum of black treacle- or tar-like stool that contains altered blood, usually the result of proximal bowel bleeding

Causes
Oesophagus
- Reflux oesophagitis: small volumes, bright red, associated with regurgitation
- Bleeding varices: sudden painless vomiting of copious volumes of dark-red blood. History of alcohol abuse and evidence of portal hypertension
- Trauma during vomiting (Mallory–Weiss syndrome): bright red bloody vomit usually preceded by forceful vomiting without blood
- Oesophageal carcinoma (rare): scanty, blood-stained debris, associated weight loss, dysphagia and anergia

Stomach
- Erosive gastritis: small volumes, bright red, may follow alcohol or NSAID ingestion. May be history of dyspepsia
- Gastric ulcer: often large bleed, painless, 'coffee grounds', history of peptic ulcer
- Carcinoma of the stomach: usually anaemia, associated weight loss, anorexia, dyspepsia. Rarely large bleed
- Gastric leiomyoma (rare): spontaneous moderate-sized bleed
- Dieulafoy's disease (rare): younger patients, spontaneous large bleed. Very difficult to diagnose

Duodenum
- Duodenal ulcer: past history of ulcer, usually haematemesis and melaena, back pain, hunger pain, NSAID use
- Aortoduodenal fistula (rare): usually infected graft after repair of abdominal aortic aneurysm. Sentinel bleeds followed by massive haematemesis and per rectum bleed. Usually fatal

Investigations
- Full blood count: carcinomas, reflux oesophagitis
- Liver function tests: liver disease (varices)

- Clotting screen: liver disease, bleeding diatheses
- OGD (key investigation): high diagnostic accuracy, allows therapeutic manoeuvres
- Barium studies: useful in demonstrating reflux, in

patient who may be unfit for OGD (rare), and to demonstrate small-bowel lesions
- Angiography: sometimes helpful in eliciting cause of occult gastrointestinal bleed

Algorithm for investigation and management of haematemesis

Haematemesis
|
Baseline bloods, group and cross-match, resuscitate

Minor bleed — Major bleed
|
Continued resuscitation, urgent OGD

Minor bleed:
- Observation
  Monitor haemoglobin
  and fluid balance
  Scheduled OGD

Major bleed:
- Peptic ulcer → Endoscopic therapy
- Varices → Endoscopic therapy / Sengstaken tube / Surgery
- Gastritis → i.v. treatment with PPI / Early feeding

No further bleeding → i.v. treatment with PPI

Rebleed or high risk → Surgery (usually just oversew bleeding point + PPI)

Peptic ulcer disease

Worldwide, duodenal ulcers are more common than gastric ulcers and there is a significantly higher incidence of duodenal ulceration in males of all age groups. Dietary factors, drug ingestion (NSAIDs) and smoking are important in the aetiology. The most common causes are environmental ulcerogens (chemical or infective) acting in consort with factors that impair gastric mucosal resistance to injury and healing of mucosal lesions thereby leading to chronicity. The most important infective agent responsible for peptic ulceration (duodenal and gastric) is *H. pylori*. Not all patients who are infected with this organism develop ulcers. The risk of peptic ulceration is determined by the severity of the *H. pylori*-associated gastritis. The organism impairs the mucus–bicarbonate protective layer and is responsible for the chronicity and the tendency to relapse, as evidenced by the permanent healing when infection is eradicated by appropriate antibiotic therapy. Strains of *H. pylori* with vacA signal-sequence type S1A are associated with severe gastritis and duodenal ulcers, whereas vacA S2 strains cause mild gastric mucosal inflammation without ulceration.

The most important group of chemical ulcerogens is constituted by aspirin and other NSAIDs. These are the most common cause of peptic ulceration in *H. pylori*-negative individuals. However, these drugs are not specific gastroduodenal ulcerogens as they also induce damage and ulceration of the small and large intestine. There are a number of differences between ulcers caused by *H. pylori* and those caused by NSAIDs.

- NSAID-associated ulcers are more likely to cause gastrointestinal haemorrhage. Thus, overall 75% of patients with upper gastrointestinal bleeding from peptic ulcers are on NSAID medication.
- Gastric ulcers caused by *H. pylori* are rarely encountered on the greater curve (5%), being most commonly situated on the lesser curve (85%). In contrast, NSAID-associated ulcers (in the absence of *H. pylori* infection) occur along the lesser and greater curvatures in 35 and 45% respectively.

Infection with *H. pylori* and use of NSAIDs is encountered in 20% of patients. Eradication of the infection does not influence the healing and recurrence of gastric and duodenal ulcers associated with chronic NSAID medication.

04

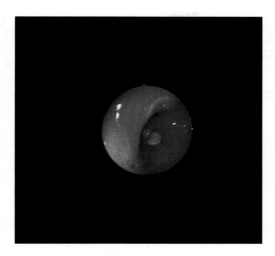

Figure 26.8 Upper gastrointestinal endoscopy showing duodenal ulcer.

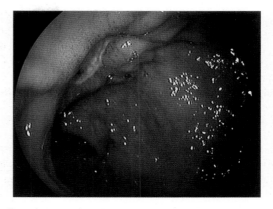

Figure 26.9 Upper gastrointestinal endoscopy showing gastric ulcer.

Although some 30–40% of duodenal ulcer patients exhibit acid hypersecretion, the overlap between the acid secretory status of these patients and controls is considerable. Gastric acid is an important factor in the chronicity of the disease and suppression of acid secretion by medical or surgical treatment undoubtedly permits healing in the majority of patients. The secretory characteristics of the usual duodenal ulcer patient include increased acid secretory capacity, increased gastrin response to food and insulin, increased sensitivity to gastrin and defective inhibition of acid secretion. There is an increased concentration of pepsins in the gastric juice of patients with duodenal ulceration, especially pepsin I (the most mucolytic). The disruption of the mucus–bicarbonate layer by pepsin I exposes the underlying mucosa to injury by ulcerogens and impairs healing by removal of the protective mucus cap (blister effect). Stress induces gastric hypersecretion and can lead to acute (stress) ulceration in seriously ill patients.

Clinical features

Chronic duodenal ulcer (Fig. 26.8) occurs in all age groups but the peak incidence is between 25 and 50 years of age. There is a significantly higher incidence of duodenal ulceration in males, with a sex ratio of 2–4 : 1. Duodenal ulceration is a remitting disease characterized by periods of activity and quiescence. Exacerbations are associated with periods of stress, dietary or alcoholic indiscretions and smoking. Early in the history of the disease, remissions may be associated with complete healing of the ulcer, but as the disease progresses there is a tendency towards fibrous scarring. Typically, epigastric pain is

experienced during fasting (hunger pain) when the stomach is empty and there is nothing to buffer the acid secretions. Relief usually follows eating, ingestion of milk or alkalis. Failure to produce relief, particularly if the pain radiates to the back, is suggestive of posterior ulcer penetration into the pancreas. The postprandial pain relief lasts for varying periods but usually averages several hours before pain recurs; it often occurs at night, awakening the patient. Vomiting is not usually a feature of uncomplicated disease but may develop in severe exacerbation of an inflamed ulcer with surrounding gross oedema of the duodenal bulb or result from fibrosis causing organic outlet obstruction (pyloric/duodenal stenosis). As patients are constantly nibbling food to ward off painful indigestion, they are usually overweight. Other than this, physical signs may amount to no more than diffuse epigastric tenderness, although this is sometimes well localized. Occult bleeding may produce marked iron-deficiency anaemia. The presence of a succussion splash indicates delayed gastric emptying.

Chronic gastric ulcer (Fig. 26.9) is less common, the ratio of gastric to duodenal ulcers varying from 1 : 4 to 1 : 20. There are two types of gastric ulcer.
● Type I: occurs in the body of the stomach along the lesser curve.
● Type II: pyloric channel ulcer and includes prepyloric ulcers.
The natural history, acid secretory profile and therapeutic response of type II ulcers are similar to those of duodenal ulcer. Type I chronic gastric ulcer may arise in a normal mucosa or on a mucosal background of atrophic gastritis. The disease is not associated with hyperacidity and indeed hypoacidity is frequently encountered, particularly in patients with atrophic gastritis. There is a male preponderance but this is not as marked as in duodenal ulceration and the peak incidence is encountered after middle

age. The main clinical feature is pain, or a feeling of acute discomfort and fullness in the epigastrium. Unlike duodenal ulcer, the pain of gastric ulceration is not experienced during fasting when the stomach is empty. Indeed, the converse is true, as eating produces or exacerbates the pain. For this reason, patients are afraid of eating and because of the reduced dietary intake they are usually underweight. It is important to stress that this symptom complex of indigestion immediately after meals and weight loss is indistinguishable from that produced by gastric cancer and clinically it is impossible to differentiate between the two disorders. Nausea and vomiting are more common symptoms than in duodenal ulcer, even in the absence of outlet obstruction. Although periodicity with remission and relapse of symptoms is encountered, this is not as obvious as in duodenal ulceration. Aside from weight loss, physical examination is not usually rewarding, with epigastric tenderness being the only fairly consistent finding. Gastric ulcers may obstruct, perforate or bleed.

Medical treatment

Before the pathogenic role of *H. pylori* was recognized, medical therapy was based on acid suppression. The main problem with both histamine H_2-receptor antagonists and PPIs is recurrence, which is universal unless maintenance therapy is continued indefinitely. In patients who are *H. pylori* positive, eradication therapy constitutes first-line treatment. There are several eradication regimens administered over a 1–2 week period:
- dual therapy (antibiotic + omeprazole);
- bismuth-based triple therapy;
- triple therapy with PPI and two antibiotics (clarithromycin + amoxicillin or metronidazole);
- quadruple therapy (PPI, bismuth, metronidazole and tetracycline);
- ranitidine bismuth citrate and two antibiotics.

However, eradication therapy has some limitations.
- Incidence of *H. pylori* ulcers is declining rapidly in many countries, and in some *H. pylori* infection prevalence rates are now 10%.
- Eradication therapy fails in 10–19% of patients due to non-compliance or bacterial resistance.
- Treatment-related issues: eradication regimen used and its duration.
- Reinfection.

Indications for surgical treatment

The need for elective surgery for duodenal ulcer disease has declined substantially and is now largely restricted to the treatment of complicated disease. However, the situation may change as the prevalence of *H. pylori* infection declines. Even in *H. pylori*-positive patients, gastroenterologists now acknowledge the real problem with failures of eradication therapy since long-term acid suppression therapy is costly and attended by poor compliance. The operations used for peptic ulcer disease are:
- closure of perforation;
- under-running of bleeding ulcer;
- truncal vagotomy and drainage;
- highly selective vagotomy;
- truncal vagotomy and antrectomy;
- partial gastrectomy.

The alternative to truncal vagotomy and drainage is highly selective vagotomy, which is the most physiological procedure since it denervates the parietal cell mass but leaves the antropyloric segment innervated and therefore obviates the need for a drainage procedure. Avoidance of drainage leads to a virtual abolition of the alimentary adverse effects, although diarrhoea can still occur. The drawback of highly selective vagotomy is the higher incidence of recurrent ulceration documented by some long-term reports.

The objectives of surgery for gastric ulcer are the removal of the ulcer, thus dealing with the problem of possible malignancy, and prevention of further ulcer recurrence. Ideally, the ulcer should be removed as part of a gastrectomy procedure but on occasion local excision of the ulcer is combined with vagotomy.

Complications of gastric surgery

A useful classification of the sequelae of gastric surgery is shown in Table 26.2.

Table 26.2 Sequelae of gastric surgery.

Recurrence of the disease: recurrent ulcer, recurrence of gastric carcinoma
Nutritional consequences: weight loss, iron-deficiency anaemia, B_{12} deficiency
Milk intolerance
Bone disease
Dumping symptoms
Reactive hypoglycaemia
Bile vomiting
Diarrhoea
Small stomach syndrome
Mechanical complications: afferent/efferent loop obstruction, jejunogastric intussusception, gastro-oesophageal reflux
Others: bezoar formation, gastric carcinoma

04

Peptic ulcer at a glance

Definition

Peptic ulcer: a break in the epithelial surface of the oesophagus, stomach or duodenum (rarely Meckel's diverticulum) caused by the action of gastric secretions (acid and pepsin) and, in the case of duodenal ulceration, infection with *H. pylori*. Worldwide, duodenal ulcers are commoner than gastric ulcers and occur more frequently in males

Common causes

- Infection with *H. pylori*
- NSAIDs and the usual suspects (alcohol, cigarettes, 'stress')
- Imbalance between acid/pepsin secretion and mucosal defence
- Defects in mucosal defence (e.g. mucus secretion)
- Acid hypersecretion occurs because of increased numbers of parietal cells (or rarely in response to gastrin hypersecretion in Zollinger–Ellison syndrome)

Clinical features

Duodenal ulcer and type II gastric ulcer (i.e. prepyloric and antral)
- Male/female ratio 4 : 1, 25–50 years
- Epigastric pain during fasting (hunger pain), relieved by food/antacids, typically exhibits periodicity
- Boring back pain if ulcer is penetrating posteriorly
- Haematemesis from ulcer penetrating gastroduodenal artery posteriorly
- Peritonitis if perforation occurs with anterior duodenal ulcer
- Vomiting if gastric outlet obstruction (pyloric stenosis) occurs (note succussion splash and watch for hypokalaemic hypochloraemic alkalosis)

Type I gastric ulcer (i.e. body of stomach)
- Male/female ratio 3 : 1, 50+ years
- Epigastric pain induced by eating
- Weight loss
- Nausea and vomiting
- Anaemia from chronic blood loss

Investigations

- Full blood count: to check for anaemia
- Urea and electrolytes: rarely indicate Zollinger–Ellison syndrome
- Faecal occult blood
- OGD: necessary to exclude malignant gastric ulcer in:
  (a) Patients > 45 years at first presentation
  (b) Concomitant anaemia
  (c) Short history of symptoms
  (d) Other symptoms suggestive of malignancy
- Barium meal: best for patients unable to tolerate OGD or evaluation of duodenum in cases of pyloric stenosis
- Urease breath test: non-invasive method of assessing presence of *H. pylori* infection. Used to direct therapy or confirm eradication

Management
Medical
Majority of chronic duodenal ulcers are related to *H. pylori* infection and respond to eradication therapy

General management
- Avoid smoking and foods that cause pain
- Antacids for symptomatic relief
- H_2 blockers (ranitidine, cimetidine)

Specific management: eradication of H. pylori *infection*
- Dual therapy: antibiotic + PPI (e.g. omeprazole)
- Triple therapy (used most often): acid inhibition (one of omeprazole, lansoprazole, pantoprazole, ranitidine bismuth citrate) + antibacterial treatment (two of clarithromycin, amoxicillin, metronidazole) for 1 week is highly effective in eradicating *H. pylori*
- Quadruple therapy: PPI, bismuth, metronidazole and tetracycline
- Re-endoscope patients with gastric ulcer after 6 weeks because of risk of malignancy

Surgical
- Only indicated for failure of medical treatment and complications
- Elective for duodenal ulcer (rare now): highly selective vagotomy
- Elective for gastric ulcer: Billroth I gastrectomy
- Perforated duodenal/gastric ulcer: simple closure of perforation and biopsy
- Haemorrhage: endoscopic control by sclerotherapy, undersewing bleeding vessel ± vagotomy
- Pyloric stenosis: gastroenterostomy ± truncal vagotomy

Nutritional consequences

Loss of weight is very common after gastric surgery and tends to be more marked after gastrectomy. Significant weight loss is usually encountered in patients who experience a poor result and who have severe postcibal symptoms. Microcytic hypochromic anaemia is very common after vagotomy and drainage and gastric resections,

especially in females. Prophylactic treatment with oral iron (300 mg q.d.s.) is nowadays recommended in all patients after gastrectomy and truncal vagotomy and drainage. Macrocytic anaemia is the result of vitamin B_{12} deficiency, caused by malabsorption of this vitamin after total gastrectomy due to the loss of intrinsic factor. The megaloblastic anaemia takes several years to develop due to the large body stores of vitamin B_{12}. Bone disease develops several years after gastric resection with duodenal exclusion as the duodenum is the major site of calcium absorption. The majority of patients are females, who develop osteomalacia 10–20 years after gastrectomy. However, cases with features of both osteomalacia (bone demineralization) and osteoporosis (loss of bone substance) are well documented. The biochemical features (raised alkaline phosphatase and serum calcium) and radiological changes (rarefaction) usually predate the clinical symptoms by several months to years. The clinical features of postgastrectomy bone disease include generalized bone pains, weakness due to associated myopathy and the development of stress fractures. Treatment is with oral calcium and vitamin D supplements or with bisphosphonates.

Dumping

This is one of the most common complaints and consists of postprandial vasomotor (systemic) and gastrointestinal symptoms (Table 26.3). Dumping syndrome is associated with rapid gastric emptying. The vasomotor symptoms (palpitation, vasodilatation, hypotension and fainting/

Table 26.3 Manifestations of dumping syndrome.

Vasomotor (systemic)
Weakness
Tiredness
Dizziness
Headache
Fainting/wanting to lie down
Warmth
Palpitations
Dyspnoea
Sweating

Gastrointestinal
Fullness
Epigastric discomfort/heaviness
Nausea
Vomiting
Distension
Excessive borborygmi/distension
Diarrhoea

having to lie down, etc.) occur within minutes of eating and are due to hypovolaemia accompanied by diminished peripheral resistance. The attacks are typically precipitated by high-carbohydrate meals. The hypovolaemia is secondary to a massive outpouring of fluid from the vascular compartment into the bowel lumen as a consequence of the hyperosmolar nature of the intestinal contents resulting from rapid gastric emptying. Patients with mild to moderate dumping symptoms are managed satisfactorily with dietary manipulations. They are advised to eat small dry meals rich in protein and fat but low in carbohydrate. Additives that slow gastric emptying, such as methoxypectin or bran, are beneficial. However, remedial gastric surgery is required for patients with severe symptoms.

Reactive hypoglycaemia

This is relatively uncommon but often coexists with other symptoms, including vasomotor dumping and diarrhoea. The symptoms of reactive hypoglycaemia occur 2–3 h after a meal and include sweating, tremor, difficulty in concentration and, rarely, fainting. The diagnosis is confirmed by an extended oral glucose tolerance test, which documents initial hyperglycaemia followed by exaggerated insulin and enteroglucagon release and hypoglycaemia. Reactive hypoglycaemia usually responds to dietary measures, including low-carbohydrate, high-protein meals.

Bile vomiting

Vomiting of bile or bile-stained fluid before or after meals is a common complaint after gastric surgery. It may be a manifestation of:
- recurrent ulceration;
- enterogastric reflux;
- intermittent obstruction of the afferent or efferent loop of a gastroenterostomy;
- cardio-oesophageal incompetence.

Extrinsic loop obstruction

This rare complication occurs after truncal vagotomy and gastroenterostomy and usually affects the afferent loop. Obstruction of afferent or efferent loops is usually chronic and intermittent but may be acute. The symptoms of chronic afferent loop obstruction include fullness, cramp-like pain and nausea within 1 h of eating. The attack culminates in vomiting of copious amounts of bile-stained fluid that relieves the symptoms. The presentation of acute afferent loop obstruction is with severe colicky abdominal pain, nausea and vomiting characteristically

04

free of bile. Abdominal tenderness is present. The condition may be complicated by the development of acute pancreatitis, jaundice and necrosis with perforation. Acute jejunogastric intussusception is a serious condition characterized by severe epigastric pain, vomiting, haematemesis, a palpable abdominal mass and high small-bowel obstruction. Urgent surgical intervention is required because of the risk of strangulation and gangrene.

Gastro-oesophageal reflux/oesophagitis

Vagotomy itself does not affect the oesophageal high-pressure zone but damage to the oesophageal attachments, particularly the phreno-oesophageal membrane, during surgery may cause cardio-oesophageal incompetence. If this is associated with enterogastric reflux, a severe form of oesophagitis due to reflux of bile and pancreatic juice (neutral or alkaline) may ensue and lead to stricture of the lower oesophagus.

Diarrhoea

Severe explosive diarrhoea is a rare disability, being encountered in 2% of patients after truncal vagotomy. It is often accompanied by dumping symptoms and is precipitated by food. Severe intractable diarrhoea is characterized by extreme urgency and often causes incontinence during an acute attack. The exact mechanism of intractable explosive diarrhoea is unknown. Malabsorption of bile salts and/or fatty acids consequent on intestinal denervation has been implicated. Small-bowel transit is markedly accelerated. Medical management is with a low animal fat diet, intestinal sedatives (codeine phosphate, Lomotil) and bile-salt binding agents such as cholestyramine. Although temporary improvement can be obtained in this way, long-term benefit is rarely achieved with conservative management.

Small-stomach syndrome

This term is reserved for the inability to eat experienced by some unfortunate patients, usually females, after extensive gastrectomy. The patient usually complains of a multiplicity of symptoms that preclude an adequate oral intake. The condition leads to gross malnutrition and is refractory to conservative management. Some patients can be managed by elemental diets administered via a Clinifeed tube and an IVAC pump or via a feeding jejunostomy. Although many can be trained to use this in their homes and maintain an adequate nutritional state in this way, quality of life is poor. Thus, if the patient's age and general condition are satisfactory, surgical intervention designed to reconstruct a gastric reservoir and restore duodenal continuity is indicated.

Other complications

These include the formation of bezoars and the development of gastric carcinoma. The factors implicated in the formation of bezoars include hypoacidity, impaired proteolytic activity, inadequate mastication and loss of the antral pump. The majority of bezoars that develop after gastric surgery consist of undigested vegetables/fruit (notably orange pith). Bezoars can cause chronic symptoms such as nausea, vomiting, abdominal discomfort, halitosis and early satiety. Treatment is initially conservative by enzymic (cellulase) digestion or endoscopic fragmentation/removal. Surgical intervention is undertaken if medical/endoscopic therapy fails or because of the development of a complication.

Gastric surgery (partial gastrectomy, gastroenterostomy) predisposes to the development of gastric carcinoma in the stomach remnant.

Gastritis

The classification of gastritis (Table 26.4) recognizes two categories (atrophic and non-atrophic) and has five histological components that are each graded as mild, moderate or severe:
1 chronic inflammation (mononuclear infiltrates);
2 activity (acute polymorphonuclear infiltrates);
3 atrophy (loss of normal glands);
4 intestinal metaplasia;
5 extent of colonization of biopsies by *H. pylori* in non-metaplastic epithelium.

Extensive lymphoid follicle formation is indicative of *H. pylori* infection and may lead to the development of

Table 26.4 Classification of gastritis.

Common
Non-atrophic gastritis (*H. pylori*)
Atrophic gastritis
   Type A (autoimmune)
   Type B (associated with *H. pylori* infection)
Reflux gastritis (enterogastric reflux)
Stress gastritis (seriously ill patients)
Erosive gastritis (drugs and alcohol)

Rare
Lymphocytic gastritis
Granulomatous gastritis (tuberculosis, Crohn's disease)
AIDS gastritis (cryptosporidiosis)
Eosinophilic gastritis

MALT lymphomas. From a clinical standpoint, it is useful to consider gastritis as either acute, when the condition is likely to be associated with acute pain and bleeding, or chronic, when vague non-specific symptoms predominate and the risk to the patient lies in progression of the condition to peptic ulceration or to dysplasia and development of gastric cancer.

Lymphocytic gastritis

This is a rare form of gastritis but is commonly encountered among patients with coeliac disease, in whom it is present in 15–45%. It results from an abnormal immunological reaction to unidentified luminal antigens. Histologically, it is characterized by infiltration of the gastric epithelium with T lymphocytes. Although some patients do not exhibit any specific endoscopic features, in the majority a distinctive appearance consisting of nodularity, erosions and enlarged mucosal folds (referred to as varioliform gastritis) is observed.

Reactive/erosive gastritis

This is the result of gastric mucosal damage by exogenous and endogenous irritants. Histologically, there is foveolar hyperplasia, severe congestion, oedema and fibrosis of the lamina propria with a paucity of inflammatory cells. Reactive gastritis is commonly caused by drugs (e.g. the condition is present in 25–45% of NSAID users) and alcohol. The usual locations of drug-induced damage are the antral and prepyloric regions. The lesions are produced by blockade of the cyclooxygenase pathway, with reduction of the cytoprotective gastric prostaglandins. Thus prostaglandin-sparing NSAIDs (non-acetylated salicylates such as carprofen and nabumetone) and low-dose steroids are less likely to cause erosive gastritis. Alcohol-induced mucosal damage affects in addition the mucosal microvessels, which undergo necrosis with resulting haemorrhage and thrombus formation. Other causes of haemorrhagic erosions include cor pulmonale, severe infections such as pneumonia, cirrhosis and blood disorders. Reflux gastritis due to enterogastric reflux of bile is a form of reactive gastritis with a distinctive pathological change that consists of subnuclear vacuolization of the foveolar epithelium.

Gastritis in acquired immunodeficiency syndrome

In patients with AIDS, vomiting due to gastric outlet obstruction from gross inflammatory oedema of the pyloric ring is caused by infection with *Cryptosporidium*, when cryptosporidial oocysts can be recovered from the stool. An interesting observation is the low prevalence of *H. pylori* infection in human immunodeficiency virus (HIV)-positive patients with low CD4 counts (< 200/dL) compared with HIV-negative patients. This low prevalence is also accompanied by a reduced incidence of peptic ulcers. Gastric toxoplasmosis due to infection with *Toxoplasma gondii* is rare in AIDS patients but when it occurs it causes abdominal pain.

Eosinophilic gastritis

This occurs as part of eosinophilic gastroenteropathy in infants and children and has an allergic basis. The pyloric region and adjacent duodenum become diffusely thickened due to oedema of the submucosal and muscle layers, which are also infiltrated with eosinophils. The antrum is the area of the stomach most severely affected. There is elevation of serum IgE and this correlates with the severity of the disease. In the majority of patients there is a peripheral eosinophilia. Some cases arise as a complication of polyarteritis nodosa, when they tend to be severe and life-threatening. The clinical features of eosinophilic gastritis include symptoms of delayed gastric emptying, e.g. early satiety, nausea and vomiting, and gastrointestinal bleeding. Treatment is with sodium cromoglicate and/or prednisolone.

Granulomatous and Crohn's gastritis

Granulomatous gastritis is very rare. The largest subgroup of cases (50%) is due to Crohn's disease. The reported estimates of Crohn's gastritis in patients with established intestinal Crohn's disease vary from 6 to 24% of cases. Crohn's gastritis may occasionally be the presenting form of the disease. The microscopic features are similar to those of intestinal Crohn's disease and non-caseating granulomas are present in one-third of cases. In addition, there is focal chronic active ulceration with erosions of the epithelium in the absence of *H. pylori* infection. Involvement of the duodenum is common. Granulomatous gastritis also includes tuberculous gastritis. Tuberculous infection of the stomach is almost always secondary to active pulmonary disease. It produces multiple ragged ulcers and discrete tubercles may be visualized at endoscopy. Serosal inflammation is common and there is marked locoregional lymphadenopathy. Treatment is with antituberculous chemotherapy.

Gastric tumours

Gastric tumours may be benign or malignant. The benign group includes non-neoplastic gastric polyps. Carcinoma is the predominant malignant gastric tumour; lymphoma

04

is much less common and may occur as a primary lesion or as secondary involvement from lymphomas arising elsewhere. The most common, stromal (mesenchymal) neoplasms are the smooth muscle tumours. Although most of these are benign (leiomyoma), some are malignant (leiomyosarcoma).

Non-neoplastic gastric polyps

The usual site of non-neoplastic polyps of the stomach is the antropyloric region. Various types are recognized, the most common being the *regenerative (hyperplastic)* variety. These have an inflammatory origin and occur in association with gastritis and peptic ulceration. The *inflammatory fibroid polyp* is a rare lesion most commonly found in the gastric antrum and can be sessile or pedunculated. It is usually associated with hypochlorhydria. *Myoepithelial hamartoma* is composed of glands surrounded by smooth muscle and arises from the submucosal layer of the antrum and pylorus, forming smooth sessile masses. The *hamartomatous polyps* of Peutz–Jeghers syndrome may occur in the stomach but very rarely become malignant. Heterotopic pancreatic tissue is again most commonly found in the antropyloric region.

Neoplastic polyps

These are adenomas. They occur predominantly in the antrum and may be either sessile or pedunculated. They are analogous to colonic adenomas and histologically consist of atypical glands with pseudostratified epithelium showing nuclear abnormalities and high mitotic figures. Like the colonic counterparts they are categorized as *adenomatous (tubular adenoma)*, *tubovillous* and *villous*. All have malignant potential, which is however low and size dependent. Endoscopic removal and surveillance are recommended.

Polyposis syndromes

Multiple gastric polyps of varying types can be found in:
- familial colonic polyposis and the related Gardner's syndrome (gastric polyps occur in 50% of patients);
- Peutz–Jeghers syndrome (occur in 20% of patients);
- generalized juvenile polyposis and related Cronkhite–Canada syndrome;
- Cowden's syndrome (multiple hamartoma syndrome).

Giant gastric folds and Ménétrier's disease (hypertrophic gastropathy)

Giant gastric folds (or large gastric folds) are found in

both benign and malignant diseases, and their differentiation may be difficult. Sometimes, even endoscopic biopsy cannot establish a definitive diagnosis. The causes of giant gastric folds are:
- gastric varices;
- gastric lymphangiectasis;
- gastritis;
- gastric carcinoma (scirrhous type);
- gastric lymphomas;
- Ménétrier's disease.

Ménétrier's disease (hypertrophic gastropathy) can occur in both children and adults and consists of giant hypertrophy of the mucosal folds of the stomach associated with marked protein-losing enteropathy. The giant folds are usually centred along the greater curvature, with sharp demarcation between the abnormal and normal gastric mucosa. Histology shows marked foveolar hyperplasia with inflamed and oedematous stroma. There is gastric hypersecretion in terms of volume but the acid content is low. Often polyps form in this condition. The patient may develop acute or, more commonly, chronic blood loss leading to anaemia. The protein-losing enteropathy can result in severe hypoproteinaemia correctable only by gastrectomy. The condition predisposes to gastric malignancy. There is an association between hypertrophic gastropathy and cytomegalovirus infection. A similar morphological change with prominent gastric folds may be encountered in Zollinger–Ellison syndrome.

Carcinoma of the stomach

This disease continues to carry a poor prognosis, especially in western countries where the overall 5-year survival averages 10%. A better outcome is obtained in Japan, where the improved survival is due to an active screening programme resulting in earlier diagnosis and an aggressive surgical approach. There has been a decline in the incidence of gastric cancer during the past 30 years throughout the world. The exact reason for this is unknown but increased consumption of fresh vegetables and fruit may be responsible. The protective vegetables include dark-green, cruciferous and allium vegetables (onions, garlic and leeks). Increased dietary carotene, vitamin C and calcium are also protective.

The male preponderance (2 : 1) is encountered worldwide. The disease is rarely seen before 40 years of age and the incidence rises sharply with age to reach a maximum between 70 and 80 years. In contrast to the overall decline in the incidence of gastric cancer, tumours of the upper third of the stomach including the oesophagogastric junction have increased and now account for approximately 40% of gastric cancers.

04

Aetiology

Gastric carcinogenesis is a multistep process: *chronic gastritis* leads to *atrophy* and *intestinal metaplasia*, which then changes to *dysplasia* (preinvasive neoplasia). The underlying mechanism for this stepwise carcinogenesis consists of a series of genetic changes that ultimately result in a clone of neoplastic cells that escapes the normal growth control checks and is thus able to proliferate and disseminate. Different gene mutations and growth factors are involved in this cascade. Although the results of several epidemiological studies have failed to demonstrate specific causative factors, the following have been implicated:

- *H. pylori* gastritis;
- highly spiced salted or pickled foods;
- polycyclic hydrocarbons, especially those generated by high-temperature pyrolysis of animal fat and aromatic amino acids in grilled and barbecued meats;
- inorganic dusts (miners and potters);
- high consumption of animal fat;
- high salt consumption (osmotic damage to gastric mucosa);
- protein malnutrition (may lead to achlorhydria);
- viral infections (which may damage the gastric mucosa and cause temporary achlorhydria);
- excess alcohol consumption;
- tobacco smoking;
- dietary nitrates (drinking water and vegetables);
- refluxed bile acids (as tumour promoters).

The recognized risk factors in the development of gastric carcinoma are:

- persistent infection with *H. pylori*;
- atrophic gastritis and pernicious anaemia;
- previous partial gastrectomy;
- adenomatous and regenerative (hyperplastic) gastric polyps;
- familial polyposis;
- hypogammaglobulinaemia;
- blood group A;
- type III intestinal metaplasia.

The most researched risk factor has been atrophic gastritis in view of the high incidence of carcinoma (threefold to sixfold increase). The incidence of gastric atrophy increase with age and is frequently encountered in patients above the age of 60 years. In addition to *H. pylori*, other factors can cause primary damage of the gastric mucosa with the development of atrophic gastritis. There is now evidence for the progression of gastric atrophy to intestinal metaplasia, dysplasia and carcinoma *in situ*.

The most important histological marker of gastric cancer is dysplasia. Dysplasia is graded histologically (either by subjective or morphometric quantitative methods) into mild, moderate and severe based on architectural parameters. Severe dysplasia is now regarded as *in situ* gastric cancer. Thus while mild to moderate dysplasia merit endoscopic surveillance only, when severe dysplasia is diagnosed a second biopsy is mandatory within a few weeks. If severe dysplasia is confirmed, gastrectomy should be performed.

Pathology

The most useful classification is the Lauren (or DIO) classification. This recognizes two main groups. The first is known as *intestinal gastric cancer* (I) because the gastric carcinoma cells exhibit a striated (brush) border and generally resemble intestinal cells. They tend to form localized expanding or ulcerated lesions and are frequently surrounded by intestinal metaplasia. The second group is known as *diffuse gastric cancer* (D) because the lesion infiltrates the gastric wall without forming large discrete masses. Diffuse cancer carries a worse prognosis than the intestinal variety and often arises from apparently normal gastric mucosa. Intestinal and diffuse cancers account for 90% of all gastric carcinomas. The remainder have a mixed morphology and are referred to as other (O), hence the alternative name, DIO classification. However, the majority of the tumours in the 'other' category behave like intestinal gastric cancers. Within each category (intestinal or diffuse), the tumours are graded pathologically into well differentiated, poorly differentiated and undifferentiated.

Diffuse gastric carcinomas are made of neoplastic cells that lack cohesion and therefore tend to invade the stomach wall with no tendency to form tubular or glandular structures. They are highly invasive tumours. The well-known linitis plastica (leather-bottle stomach) is a classic example of the diffuse type of gastric cancer. Various antibodies are used for the detection of shed surface tumour-associated antigens in the peripheral blood of patients with gastric carcinoma (CEA, CA19-9, CASO, CA125, CA72-4). These tumour markers are used to detect recurrence after surgical treatment and progression of the disease. The only reliable marker in patients with gastric cancer is CA72-4.

Early gastric cancer

This is cancer limited to the mucosa and submucosa. It is becoming increasingly relevant in western countries as with early-access endoscopy, early gastric cancer is diagnosed more frequently. The macroscopic type of early gastric cancer seen endoscopically and the extent of submucosal invasion (superficial or deep) determined by endosonography appear to determine the incidence of spread to the level 1 regional lymph nodes. Overall

04

some 15% of early gastric cancers have lymph node deposits. Early gastric cancer assumes different endoscopic appearances:

- protruding;
- superficial (elevated, flat or depressed);
- excavated.

The prognosis with adequate resection is excellent, with 5-year survival rates exceeding 80%.

Advanced gastric carcinoma

This is defined as a tumour that involves the muscularis propria of the stomach wall and accounts for 90% of gastric carcinomas diagnosed in the UK (Fig. 26.10). In the vast majority of cases, spread to the regional lymph nodes is present alone or in association with peritoneal and hepatic deposits. Advanced gastric carcinoma is further classified into macroscopic types first described by Borrmann.

Staging and spread of gastric cancer

The TNM system is used for staging (Fig. 26.11). The important prognostic factors are depth of invasion of the stomach wall by the tumour and lymph node spread. The diffuse type of gastric cancer spreads rapidly through the submucosal and subserosal lymphatic plexuses and penetrates the gastric wall at an early stage. The intestinal variety remains localized for a while and has less tendency to disseminate. With both cancers, spread to the lymph nodes along the greater and lesser curvatures tends to occur once the muscular coat of the stomach is invaded by the neoplasm (level 1 nodes). Thereafter, spread occurs to the nodes along the coeliac axis and its trifurcation, to the nodes in the splenic hilum, the root of the mesentery, the retropancreatic nodes and the hepatoduodenal nodes (level 2 nodes). Involvement of the para-aortic nodes above and below the transverse colon then ensues (level 3 nodes). Metastatic spread is usually to the peritoneal cavity and the liver. The most common organs involved by direct extension are the omentum, transverse colon and mesocolon, pancreas and the left lobe of the liver.

Clinical features

Early gastric cancer is often asymptomatic. When present, early symptoms are vague and include indigestion, malaise, early satiety, postprandial fullness and loss of appetite. Weight loss is a significant feature of the disease but usually signifies an advanced lesion. Lesions of the cardia may present with dysphagia, and circumferential growths of the middle third and the pyloric antrum cause obstructive symptoms with vomiting after meals.

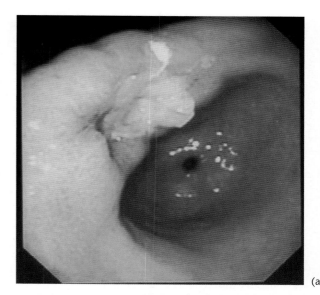

(a)

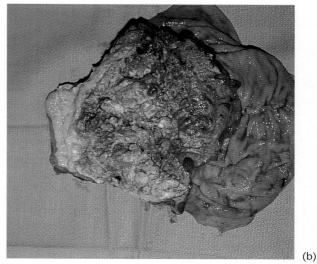

(b)

Figure 26.10 (a) Early gastric cancer of the excavating type: on histology the lesion involved the mucosa and submucosa only with no nodal involvement (T_1N_0); (b) Gastrectomy specimen for advanced gastric cancer: the lesion reached the serosa and had involved regional nodes close to stomach margins (T_3N_1).

The most common presentation is that of recent dyspepsia in a patient above the age of 45 years. There are no specific features to the cancer dyspepsia. All patients who present with indigestion require full investigation including endoscopy to establish the diagnosis before treatment is started. The most frequent reason for delay in the diagnosis of cancer of the stomach is a period of symptomatic

Staging of gastric cancer

Surgical Stage grouping is based on T, N, P, H and M with each of these components being defined as follows:

T - Primary tumour

T_1 Tumour limited to the mucosa and submucosa
T_2 Tumour involves the muscularis propria or subserosa
T_3 Tumour penetrates the serosa
T_4 Tumour involves contiguous structures

N - Regional lymph nodes

N_0 No metastases to the regional lymph nodes
N_1 Involvement of the perigastric lymph nodes within 3 cm of the primary tumour
N_2 Involvement of the regional lymph nodes more than 3 cm from the primary including those located along the left gastric, common hepatic, splenic and coeliac arteries

P - Peritoneal metastases

P_0 No peritoneal metastases
P_1 Peritoneal metastases to adjacent but not distal peritoneum
P_2 A few metastases to the distant peritoneum
P_3 Numerous metastases to distant pneumoperitoneum

H - Hepatic deposits

H_0 No hepatic deposits
H_1 Metastases limited to one lobe
H_2 A few metastases in both lobes
H_3 Numerous metastases to both lobes

M - Distant metastases

M_0 No evidence of diatant metastases
M_1 Evidence of distant metastases

N.B. Involvement of lymph nodes beyond level N_2, i.e. N_3, N_4 is regarded as distant metastases according to the new classification.

On the basis of the above, the surgical grouping is:

		P_0, H_0, M_0				P_0 H_1 $N_{0,1,2}$
		N_0	N_1	N_2	N_3	
P_0 H_0 M_0	T_1	Ia	Ib	II	IIIa	
	T_2	Ib	II	IIIa	IIIb	IVa
	T_3	II	IIIa	IIIb	IVa	
	T_4	IIIa	IIIb	IVa		
P_1 H_0 $T_{1,2,3}$		IVa				

Figure 26.11 TNM system for staging of gastric cancer.

therapy before referral for endoscopy is undertaken. Anaemia, which is often present at the time of diagnosis, is usually of the iron-deficiency type. Evidence of weight loss is present on examination and hypoalbuminaemia is frequent. Although often stressed, enlarged left supraclavicular lymph nodes are a rare physical finding. A palpable epigastric mass usually signifies incurable, though not necessarily a non-resectable, tumour. Jaundice, hepatomegaly or ascites indicate advanced incurable disease and limited survival.

The key investigations are upper gastrointestinal endoscopy with multiple biopsy and brush cytology and bar-ium meal. Other tests are used to detect extragastric disease and stage the tumour. These include chest radiography, liver function tests, hydro-helical CT with the patient in the prone position and gastric endosonography.

Treatment

In advanced gastric cancer, adequate surgical resection remains the only effective treatment that offers a chance of long-term survival. Furthermore, palliative resection when-ever feasible is more effective in relieving symptoms than bypass or intubation procedures. The

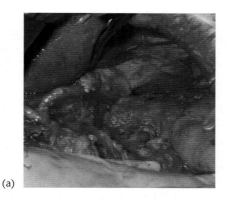

(a)

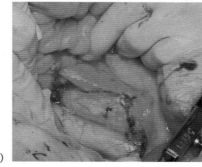

(b)

Figure 26.12 D$_2$ total gastrectomy with level 2 nodal clearance for gastric cancer: (a) nodal clearance of supracolic compartment showing the bared common hepatic and splenic artery; (b) nodal clearance of infracolic compartment exposing aorta and vena cava.

04

principles underlying a potentially curative resection of gastric carcinoma are:

- appropriate resection with adequate tumour-free margins;
- regional lymph node clearance corresponding to the location of the primary tumour in the stomach;
- safe and well-functioning reconstruction.

Adequate gastrectomy with removal of level 1 and 2 lymph nodes is the standard treatment for patients with tumours invading the muscularis propria (advanced) (Fig. 26.12). When the tumour is confined to mucosa and submucosa (early), alternative methods can be employed and provided adequate selection of cases is undertaken, survival is not compromised. There are four alternatives:

- interventional flexible endoscopic treatment (submucosal resection, photodynamic ablation);
- laparo-endoluminal resection;
- transgastrostomal endoscopic surgery;
- laparoscopic gastric resections (totally laparoscopic, laparoscopically assisted and hand-assisted).

Chemotherapy

The most widely used effective regimen, in view of its efficacy and acceptable toxicity, is that developed at the Royal Marsden Hospital. This consists of epirubicin (50 mg/m^2 i.v. in 3-weekly boluses), cisplatin (60 mg/m^2 in 3-weekly infusions) and 5-fluorouracil (200 mg/m^2) administered daily by continuous infusion through a central Hickman line for 3 weeks. The full treatment consists of six cycles. In advanced or recurrent disease, the Marsden regimen exhibits a higher response rate than other regimens, averaging 40% overall with 15–20 complete response rates.

Mesenchymal tumours

These include smooth muscle tumours, neurogenic tumours (schwannomas) and neoplasms of uncommitted mesenchymal cells, often considered as a less-differentiated variant of leiomyomas and classified as gastrointestinal stromal tumours.

The term 'gastrointestinal sarcoma' covers smooth muscle tumours, gastrointestinal stromal tumours and neurogenic tumours with malignant potential. These sarcomas are rare. The most common site is the stomach (50%), followed by small bowel and duodenum (Fig. 26.13). The usual clinical presentation, irrespective of site, is with pain or bleeding (acute or chronic). Some are asymptomatic and may be found accidentally during operation, while others present acutely with tumour perforation. Large tumours may cause massive intraperitoneal bleeding.

Although often classified into benign (leiomyoma) and malignant (leiomyosarcoma), the histological differentiation between the two may be difficult. However, the majority of gastric smooth muscle tumours are benign. They are encountered in the upper and middle thirds and rarely in the antrum. Malignant tumours tend to be larger, show necrotic and haemorrhagic change and have a mitotic rate. Local resection with a surrounding cuff of normal tissue is safer than enucleation as this has a high recurrence rate. For lesions larger than 5.0 cm a formal gastrectomy with lymphadenectomy is necessary.

Gastric lymphomas

Primary Hodgkin's disease is extremely rare in the gastrointestinal tract and in practice all gastrointestinal lymphomas are of the non-Hodgkin's type, arising from either B or T cells. The stomach is the major organ involved. A significant proportion of gastric lymphomas show low-grade histology and arise from MALT. Such MALT lymphomas may be associated with *H. pylori* infec-

Histologically, PGL consists of follicle centres (non-neoplastic component) that are surrounded and invaded by a malignant cellular infiltrate consisting of centrocyte-like cells and a variable proportion of plasma cells (some reactive, some neoplastic). This malignant infiltrate extends into the surrounding mucosa, where it forms characteristic lymphoepithelial lesions, and to the submucosa where it induces dense sclerosis. Lymph node spread from B-cell MALT lymphoma is usually limited to the gastric regional lymph nodes. The lymphoma that arises in patients with coeliac disease is a T-cell lymphoma.

MALT lymphomas arise from sites normally devoid of lymphoid tissue and are preceded by chronic inflammatory, usually immune, disorders that induce the accumulation of lymphoid tissue in the first instance. The stomach is the most common site of MALT lymphoma. In the vast majority, gastric lymphoma arises on a background of *H. pylori* infection/gastritis and much less commonly *H. heilmannii*.

Clinical features

PGL is the most common extranodal lymphoid tumour in the West and accounts for 60% of gastrointestinal lymphomas. The clinical course varies with the grade of the lesion, being slow and indolent in low-grade MALT tumours. PGL has only a marginal male predominance. The age distribution is wide, with a mean around 55–60 years. The early symptoms are indistinguishable from those of gastric carcinoma and always include upper abdominal discomfort and dyspepsia, although nausea, vomiting and weight loss are less common. Some patients develop diarrhoea. Ulceration of the tumour may lead to bleeding and perforation; indeed some patients with high-grade aggressive tumours present as an emergency with acute bleeding or perforation. The risk of both complications is enhanced by chemotherapy. The prognosis is influenced by the grade (low, low-intermediate, high-intermediate) irrespective of age. Within each grade the adverse prognostic factors in patients with non-Hodgkin's lymphoma are:

- age > 60 years;
- elevated lactate dehydrogenase (×1 normal);
- performance status;
- stage of the disease.

A palpable mass is present in at least 20% of patients but its detection does not signify inoperability. Occult blood is found on testing in 50% of patients. The erythrocyte sedimentation rate is grossly elevated. The diagnosis is confirmed by endoscopy with multiple biopsy. The criteria for establishing PGL include absence of superficial lymphadenopathy and splenomegaly, normal chest X-ray, no hepatic involvement and appropriate histology.

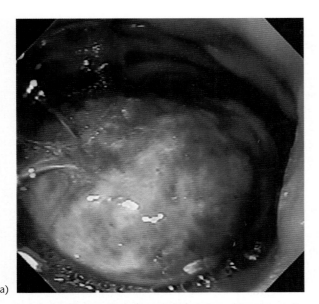

(a)

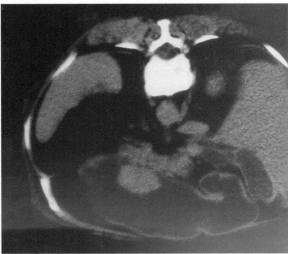

(b)

Figure 26.13 (a) Endoscopic appearance of malignant smooth muscle tumour (gastrointestinal sarcoma): the patient presented with upper gastrointestinal bleeding. (b) CT scan of the tumour.

tion and may undergo complete regression following eradication of *H. pylori*.

Pathology

Primary gastric lymphoma (PGL) tends to infiltrate the wall of the stomach in a diffuse fashion, causing mucosal thickening with a tendency to ulceration and indeed perforation. The antrum is the most common site.

04

Stage I

Involvement of a single lymph node region (I) or single extralymphatic organ or site (IE)

Stage II

Involvement of two or more lymph node regions on the same side of the diaphragm (II) or localized involvement of an extralymphatic organ or site (IIE)

Stage III

Involvement of lymph node regions on both sides of the diaphragm (III) or localized involvement of an extralymphatic organ or site (IIIE), the spleen (IIIS) or both (IIISE)

Stage IV

Diffuse or disseminated involvement of one or more extralymphatic organs with or without associated lymph node involvement

Table 26.5 Ann Arbor staging of lymphomas.

Asymptomatic patients are designated as distinct from those with symptoms (B), which include fever, sweats, or weight loss < 10% body weight.

Treatment

Treatment depends on the stage of the disease (Table 26.5). The majority of patients with stage I disease are positive for *H. pylori*/*H. heilmannii*. Eradication of the infection is followed by complete regression of MALT lymphoma in 50% of cases. The recommended eradication regimens used vary considerably. The most common first-line treatment (except in patients with known allergy or intolerance) is a full-dose PPI, clarithromycin 500 mg and amoxicillin 1000 mg, all given twice daily for 10 days. Eradication must be confirmed preferably by culture. Although complete remissions of low-grade gastric MALT lymphomas after cure of *H. pylori* infection appear to be stable, there are insufficient results to conclude that these patients are permanently cured. Eradication is not indicated in patients with high-grade tumours and in patients who are *H. pylori* negative. In *H. pylori*-negative stage I tumours, first-line treatment rests between radiotherapy and chemotherapy. Surgery is reserved for treatment failures or complications.

The management in patients with stage II disease entails surgery (total/partial gastrectomy) followed by chemotherapy initially with m-VEPA (vincristine, cyclophosphamide, prednisolone and doxorubicin). This is followed by consolidation chemotherapy with VEMP. Using this management, the reported postoperative overall and disease-free survival rates at 10 years are 82 and 92.0% respectively. The prognosis of patients with stage III/IV disease is poor. Initially treatment is with chemotherapy or chemo-irradiation. Surgical resection is carried out for patients who respond to chemotherapy but have residual disease.

Carcinoid and other endocrine tumours

Gastric carcinoids are rare. There is an established association between the atrophic gastritis and chronic hypergastrinaemia of pernicious anaemia. Initially these patients develop hyperplasia of the gastrin-producing G cells of the antral mucosa and of the argyrophil endocrine cells (enterochromaffin) of the fundic mucosa. This is followed in time by the development of a spectrum of neoplastic change, varying from diffuse hyperplasia of the argyrophil cells to discrete often multiple carcinoid tumours. The prevalence of gastric carcinoids in patients with pernicious anaemia averages 5%. Fundal enterochromaffin tumours also occur in some patients with Zollinger–Ellison syndrome after prolonged therapy with omeprazole.

Gastric carcinoids, though generally slow growing and indolent, can metastasize especially if they exhibit atypical histology and are larger than 2.0 cm. They are rarely symptomatic and the majority are discovered during endoscopy or contrast examination of the stomach. They do not have a distinctive macroscopic appearance and can form smooth elevations covered by intact mucosa, polypoid projections or ulcerative lesions, which can cause chronic blood loss and microcytic hypochromic anaemia. However, overt haematemesis is rare. Gastric carcinoids are best treated by local resection, although some advocate and practise endoscopic resection (especially for small tumours) followed by endoscopic surveillance. The use of antrectomy (to abolish the source of gastrin) in patients with diffuse hyperplasia and microcarcinoidosis is being evaluated in some centres. The prognosis following resection is good even in the presence of regional node deposits and hepatic metastases.

Gastric tumours at a glance

Definition

Gastric tumour: benign or malignant lesion of the stomach

Benign gastric tumours
Non-neoplastic gastric polyps
- Regenerative (hyperplastic)
- Inflammatory fibroid polyp
- Myoepithelial hamartomas
- Peutz–Jeghers syndrome (hamartomatous polyps)

Polyposis syndromes
- Familial colonic polyposis and related Gardner's syndrome: gastric polyps in 50% of patients
- Peutz–Jeghers syndrome: gastric polyps in 20%
- Generalized juvenile polyposis and related Cronkhite–Canada syndrome
- Cowden's syndrome (multiple hamartomas syndrome)

Causes of giant gastric folds
- Gastric varices
- Gastric lymphangiectasis
- Gastritis
- Gastric carcinoma (scirrhous)
- Gastric lymphomas
- Ménétrier's disease

Carcinoma
Key points
- Majority of tumours are unresectable at presentation
- Tumours considered candidates for resection should be staged with CT and laparoscopy to reduce the risk of an 'open and shut' laparotomy
- Most tumours are poorly responsive to chemotherapy

Epidemiology
- Male/female ratio 2 : 1
- Age 50+ years
- Incidence has decreased in western world over last 50 years; still common in Japan, Chile and Scandinavia

Aetiology
- *H. pylori* gastritis
- Diet (smoked fish, pickled vegetables, benzpyrene, nitrosamines)
- Atrophic gastritis
- Pernicious anaemia
- Previous partial gastrectomy
- Familial hypogammaglobulinaemia
- Gastric adenomatous polyps
- Blood group A

Pathology
- Multistep process: chronic gastritis → atrophy → intestinal metaplasia → dysplasia → carcinoma
- Histology: adenocarcinoma
- Advanced gastric cancer (penetrates muscularis propria): polypoid, ulcerating or infiltrating (i.e. linitus plastica)
- Early gastric cancer: confined to mucosa or submucosa
- Spread: lymphatic (e.g. Virchow's node); haematogenous to liver, lung, brain; transcoelomic to ovary (Krukenberg tumour)

Clinical features
- Often asymptomatic
- History of recent dyspepsia (epigastric discomfort, postprandial fullness, loss of appetite)
- Anaemia
- Dysphagia
- Vomiting
- Weight loss
- Presence of physical signs usually indicates advanced (incurable) disease

Investigations
- Full blood count
- Urea and electrolytes
- Liver function tests
- OGD: see the lesion and obtain biopsy to distinguish from benign gastric ulcer
- Barium meal: space-occupying lesion/ulcer with rolled edge. Best for patients unable to tolerate OGD
- Helical CT: stages disease locally and systemically
- Laparoscopy: excludes undiagnosed peritoneal or liver secondaries prior to consideration of resection

Management
Early gastric cancer (10%)
- Cancer is limited to mucosa and submucosa
- Aggressive treatment with resection. Curative treatment (resectable primary and local nodes) involves surgical excision with clear margins and locoregional lymph node clearance (D2 gastrectomy)
- With adequate resection, prognosis is good (80% 5-year survival)

Advanced gastric cancer (90%)
- Cancer involves muscularis propria of the stomach wall
- Majority of tumours are unresectable at presentation
- Palliation (metastatic disease or gross distal nodal disease at presentation):
  (a) Gastrectomy: local symptoms, e.g. bleeding
  (b) Gastroenterostomy: malignant pyloric obstruction
  (c) Intubation: obstructing lesions at the cardia

04

- Other treatment: combination chemotherapy with etoposide, Adriamycin and cisplatin may induce regression. Most tumours are poorly responsive to chemotherapy
- Prognosis: overall 5-year survival (palliation and resection) is only about 5%

Gastrointestinal sarcomas

- Smooth muscle tumours
- Gastrointestinal stromal tumours
- Neurogenic tumours (schwannomas)
- Leiomyoma
- Leiomyosarcoma

Gastric lymphomas

- Gastrointestinal lymphomas are almost always non-Hodgkin's type, arising from B or T cells
- PGL arise from MALT and are low grade histologically. Often background of *H. pylori* infection
- Common in antrum
- Diffuse infiltration of wall of stomach with tendency to ulcerate
- Histology: follicle centres surrounded by malignant cellular infiltrate, dense sclerosis

Clinical features
- Marginal male preponderance
- Age 55–60 years
- Dyspepsia (nausea, vomiting, weight loss)
- Bleeding or perforation
- Palpable mass in 20%

Criteria for establishing PGL
- Appropriate histology
- Absence of superficial lymphadenopathy
- Absence of splenomegaly
- Normal chest X-ray
- No hepatic involvement

Staging of lymphoma (modified Ann Arbor staging)
- Stage I: disease confined to a single extralymphatic organ
- Stage II: localized involvement of one organ/site + one or more lymph node groups on one side of the diaphragm:
    (a) II_1: regional adjacent lymph node involved
    (b) II_2: regional non-confluent lymph node involved
- Stage III: localized involvement of one organ/site + lymph node groups on both sides of the diaphragm
- Stage IV: diffuse disseminated disease of more than one organ + lymph node involvement

Treatment
Stage I disease
- Eradication of *H. pylori* infection causes complete regression of stage I MALT lymphoma in 50% of patients
- *H. pylori*-negative stage I disease: radiotherapy or chemotherapy

Stage II disease
- Surgery (gastrectomy) + chemotherapy
- Prognosis is good (85% 10-year disease-free survival)

Stage III and IV disease
- Chemotherapy or chemoirradiation
- Surgery for responders with residual disease
- Poor prognosis

04

Evidence-based medicine

Gabriel, S.E., Jaakkimainen, L. & Bombardier, C. (1991) Risk of serious gastrointestinal complications related to use of non-steroidal anti-inflammatory drugs. A meta-analysis. *Ann Intern Med* **115**, 787–96.

Isaacson, P.G. (1999) Gastrointestinal lymphomas of T- and B-cell types. *Mod Pathol* **12**, 151–8.

(1998) Japanese classification of gastric carcinoma. *Gastric Cancer* **1**, 10–24.

Talley, N.J., Evans, J.M., Fleming, K.C. *et al.* (1995) Non-steroidal anti-inflammatory drugs and dyspepsia in the elderly. *Dig Dis Sci* **40**, 1345–50.

Disorders of the Liver

27

Must know Must do

Must know

Clinical manifestations and investigation of patients with liver disease

Diagnosis and management of patients with chronic liver disease

Clinical features and management of acute and chronic liver failure

Clinical features, types and principles of management of patients with portal hypertension

Diagnosis and principles of management of primary and secondary hepatic tumours

Clinical features and principles of management of liver cysts and abscesses

Must do

Clerk and follow patients with jaundice/chronic liver disease

Learn how to interpret liver function tests

Learn how to detect hepatomegaly, splenomegaly, ascites, spider naevi

Observe a liver biopsy

Examine CT and ultrasound images of liver cysts, liver abscesses and liver tumours

Visit the emergency endoscopy suite to observe variceal banding/sclerotherapy

Anatomy of the liver

The liver is the largest organ in the body and is shaped like a wedge tapering to the left with three surfaces. The anterosuperior surface is marked by the umbilical fissure, in the depths of which is inserted the round ligament (obliterated umbilical vein). The falciform ligament divides the anterosuperior surface into right and left lobes. The posterior surface is formed of the bare area of the right lobe. The gallbladder is attached to the inferior surface anteriorly and the area between the gallbladder and the umbilical fissure forms the quadrate lobe. Behind this is the transverse hilar fissure that contains the main divisions of the portal vein, hepatic artery and common hepatic duct. The hepatic parenchyma separating the hilar fissure lobe from the vena cava forms the caudate lobe. The anterosuperior surface of the liver touches the diaphragm and its upper margin reaches the level of the fourth interspace on the right side. Inferiorly the right liver reaches the costal margin. The lesser sac lies below the liver and behind the lesser omentum and communicates with the rest of the peritoneal cavity through the foramen of Winslow. The inferior vena cava lies in a gutter on the posterior surface and receives the hepatic and phrenic veins.

The surgical segmental anatomy differs from the classical anatomical description of right and left lobes. The liver is a paired organ (right and left livers) fused along a line extending from the middle of the gallbladder fossa anteriorly to the left edge of the suprahepatic inferior vena cava posteriorly. The right liver receives the right portal vein, hepatic artery and bile duct and the left liver the corresponding left portal vein, hepatic artery and bile duct. Each liver is formed of anatomically distinct segments. The right liver has four segments (5, 6, 7, 8) and the left liver three (2, 3, 4). The caudate lobe, which has a separate venous drainage to the inferior vena cava, constitutes segment 1 (Fig. 27.1). Each segment contributes hepatic veins that coalesce to form the three main veins: the right hepatic drains segments 5–8; the middle hepatic drains from both livers (segments 4 and 5); and the left hepatic drains segments 2–4.

The portal vein, formed behind the head of the pancreas by the junction of splenic and superior mesenteric veins, passes along the edge of the lesser omentum. It receives the left coronary (left gastric) draining the cardio-oesophageal region and divides at the hilum of the liver into right and left branches. There are major anastomotic sites between the portal and systemic systems that open in the presence of obstruction to portal blood flow.

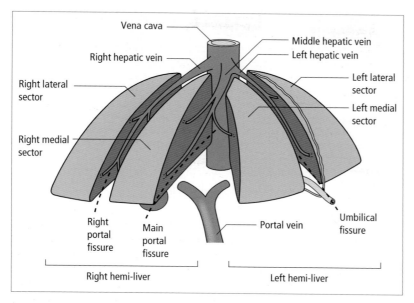

Figure 27.1 Surgical segmental anatomy of the liver.

- Cardio-oesophageal junction: left gastric (coronary) vein to the azygos system.
- Communications with retroperitoneal veins of Sappey.
- Umbilicus: recanalized left umbilical vein to abdominal parietal veins (caput medusae).
- Communications with the inferior rectal plexus.

The common hepatic duct, formed by the union of the right and left hepatic ducts, passes in front of and to the right of the portal vein and receives the cystic duct at a variable point in its course to form the common bile duct. The common hepatic artery runs to the left of the common bile duct, giving off the main cystic artery and branches to the common bile duct prior to division into right and left branches.

Investigations

Hepatic functional reserve

This is the residual functional capacity of the liver following chronic disease and can be difficult to assess. Scoring systems used for this purpose are based on standard liver function tests, nutritional state, muscle wasting, water and salt retention with ascites. The most commonly used is the Child–Pugh score/grading and the Paul Brousse Hospital classification (Tables 27.1 & 27.2). The prothrombin time after administration of vitamin K is a very good test of the synthetic function of the liver. An elevated prothrombin time that does not normalize with vitamin K analogue therapy is indicative of severe functional decompensation.

Table 27.1 Child–Pugh classification of disease severity in cirrhotic patients.

	A	B	C
Albumin (g/L)	> 35	30–35	< 30
Bilirubin (μmol/L)*	< 25	25–40	> 40
Prothrombin (s > normal)†	< 4	4–6	> 6
Prothrombin (%)	> 64	40–65	< 40
Ascites	None	Controlled	Refractory
Encephalopathy	None	Minimal	Advanced

* The bilirubin value has to be adjusted for patients with primary biliary cirrhosis: A = 5–7; B = 8–10; C = 11 or more.
† In the original Child–Turcotte classification, nutrition was used but this has been substituted with prothrombin activity.

Table 27.2 Paul Brousse Hospital classification system.

Parameter	Number of criteria
Albuminaemia < 30 g/L	1
Hyperbilirubinaemia > 30 μmol/L	1
Encephalopathy	1
Clinical ascites	1
Coagulation factors II and V 40–60%	1
Coagulation factors II and V < 40%	2

Category A, none of the criteria
Category B, one to two criteria
Category C, three or more criteria

Imaging

A plain abdominal film may give helpful information about liver size and the position of the diaphragm. Rarely, a small gas–fluid level may be seen within an abscess. Ultrasonography is the investigation of choice in patients with suspected biliary tract disease. In patients with cholestasis, dilated intrahepatic bile ducts signify the presence of large duct obstruction. The demonstration of gallbladder disease is good and gallstones are diagnosed with an accuracy of 95%. The patency of the portal vein and other major vascular channels including surgical shunts is readily established with duplex ultrasound scanning. Ultrasound is used in the screening of liver parenchyma for focal lesions (e.g. liver cysts, abscesses) and solid primary and secondary liver tumours. Ultrasonography is also used during liver surgery and by the interventional radiologist for guidance of needles and catheters into intrahepatic collections.

Helical computed tomography (CT) is invaluable in the diagnosis of focal disease: tumours, cysts or abscesses and liver injuries. Often intravenous contrast is administered during the investigation. Intra-arterial contrast-enhanced helical hepatic CT can also be used to obtain CT angiography (CT-A, CT-AP). Magnetic resonance imaging (MRI) provides the best detailed images of the liver parenchyma.

Needle biopsy

This is indicated in patients with undiagnosed liver disease and selectively in some with focal abnormalities of the liver. The procedure is only performed once the prothrombin time is shown to be normal or not grossly deranged and the platelet count greater than 60×10^6/L. A special needle, the Tru-cut needle, is used to obtain a core of liver substance. For diffuse liver disease (e.g. cirrhosis), the procedure may be carried out by the blind percutaneous technique. Most centres now undertake liver biopsy with ultrasound guidance and this reduces the risk of iatrogenic damage.

The important indications for liver biopsy are:
- chronic liver disease;
- cholestatic jaundice without dilatation of the biliary tract on ultrasonography;
- unexplained hepatomegaly;
- drug-induced liver disease.

Suspect malignant lesions of the liver that are considered operable should not be biopsied as this may cause spillage and peritoneal implantation. In contrast if the lesion is judged to be inoperable, biopsy for histological confirmation is mandatory.

The complications of liver needle biopsy include:
- pleural effusion;
- haemorrhage from the liver and thoracic wall;
- intrahepatic haematoma;
- hepatic arteriovenous fistulae;
- haemobilia;
- accidental puncture of the gallbladder and large bile ducts leading to bile peritonitis;
- tumour cell implantation.

Laparoscopy with contact ultrasonography

This is useful in the investigation of patients with jaundice, chronic liver disease, ascites of unknown origin, and in the diagnosis and staging of both primary and secondary hepatic tumours. Laparoscopic contact ultrasonography has added considerably to the diagnostic yield of laparoscopy for the detection and staging of hepatic tumours. Laparoscopy detects small hepatic secondary deposits in the liver and peritoneal seedlings that are too small to be detected by CT and MRI.

Clinical features of liver disease

Many of the symptoms of liver disorders are non-specific. Fatigue, malaise, headache, myalgia and fever are commonly found with hepatitis. Confusion, forgetfulness, poor concentration and personality change are central nervous symptoms of advanced end-stage disease. Anorexia and nausea are common in all forms of hepatic and biliary disease, as is pain in the right hypochondrium. Jaundice is the most obvious symptom of chronic liver disease and is often accompanied by dark urine, pale stools and pruritus. Chronic liver disease may show stigmata, including:
- hepatosplenomegaly;
- palmar erythema;
- finger clubbing;
- leuconychia;
- spider naevi in the territory of the superior vena cava (Fig. 27.2);
- skin changes including bruising;
- muscle wasting;
- water and salt retention leading to oedema and ascites (Fig. 27.3);
- gynaecomastia and testicular atrophy.

On palpation, the hepatomegaly may be smooth or nodular. The hepatomegaly regresses as the liver becomes shrunken with progression to end-stage chronic liver disease. Splenomegaly indicates presence of portal hypertension. Liver tenderness is present in acute hepatitis.

04

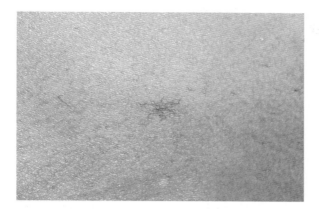

Figure 27.2 Spider naevus in a patient with alcoholic cirrhosis.

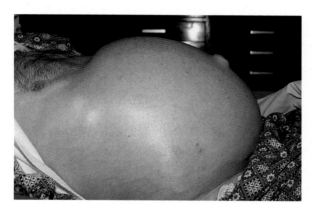

Figure 27.3 Gross ascites and muscle wasting in a patient with advanced chronic liver disease.

04

Cirrhosis

Cirrhosis is the end-result of hepatocyte death. Confluent necrosis leads to fibrotic bridges and the regeneration of surviving hepatocytes causes distortion of hepatic architecture. Not uncommonly, early cirrhosis is discovered during routine investigation or is found incidentally at laparotomy. It may also be encountered as progression of known chronic liver disease. In some cases presentation is late with advanced disease associated with muscle wasting and ascites, gastrointestinal haemorrhage, jaundice or hepatic encephalopathy. The prognosis varies with the underlying disease, some of which can be reversed with appropriate therapy, e.g. haemochromatosis.

Renal disease is very common in patients with chronic liver disease and may, for a while, be subclinical. The hepatorenal syndrome is encountered in patients with end-stage liver disease but may also complicate the post-operative period after surgery for variceal bleeding. The urine output may not be significantly reduced but, despite this, sodium, potassium and water retention are pronounced and blood urea and creatinine rise sharply. Renal failure may also complicate infection of the ascitic fluid (primary bacterial peritonitis). Hepatorenal failure does not usually recover with renal dialysis and the best chance of reversal is improvement of liver function.

Congenital hepatic fibrosis (fibropolycystic disease)

This is a rare congenital disorder that is inherited as an autosomal recessive trait. It leads to development of portal hypertension with variceal bleeding. Because of the association with other disorders characterized by dilated bile ducts or cysts (Caroli's syndrome), the disease is better known as fibropolycystic disease. There is enlargement of the portal spaces by pronounced fibrosis and bile ductule proliferation. The ductules are dilated to varying degrees but still communicate with the main intrahepatic biliary tree. Some of the bile ductules may become so dilated as to form microcysts. The portal fibrosis results in obstruction of the sinusoidal circulation within the liver and hence the development of portal hypertension. Usually the condition presents with severe gastrointestinal bleeding from oesophageal varices. Despite the portal hypertension and repeated episodes of variceal haemorrhage, liver function remains good. The best treatment is by selective decompression by Warren shunt after the acute episode has been controlled by endoscopic banding. Sclerotherapy is avoided in these patients because of the risk of portal vein thrombosis.

Hepatic encephalopathy

Hepatic encephalopathy covers a spectrum of neuropsychiatric disorders encountered in patients suffering from chronic liver disease. Hepatic coma is present in acute liver failure (*acute fulminant encephalopathy*). In chronic liver disease, the hallmarks of hepatic encephalopathy are intellectual impairment, reduced level of consciousness and abnormalities on psychometric testing. The encephalopathy in chronic liver disease may be subclinical (mild) or overt, either as recurrent reversible episodes (often precipitated by bleeding) or as a persistent condition.

The encephalopathy of acute liver failure is different from that encountered in chronic liver disease and portosystemic shunting. Cerebral oedema is frequently present in acute liver failure and rarely encountered in chronic liver disease. However, the exact mechanisms involved in the production of encephalopathy in both instances remain uncertain. Five hypotheses have been advanced:
- ammonia toxicity;
- multiple synergistic neurotoxins;

- false neurotransmitters secondary to abnormal plasma amino acid profile;
- overactivity of γ-aminobutyric acid (GABA) neurotransmission;
- depressant cerebral effects of benzodiazepine-like substances.

The most common precipitating cause of acute encephalopathy in patients with chronic liver disease is gastrointestinal haemorrhage, usually due to ruptured varices. When severe, the patient becomes deeply comatose. Other precipitating factors include hypokalaemic alkalosis, diuretic therapy, sedation, sepsis and portosystemic surgical shunting.

The principles of management of patients with hepatic precoma or coma include the correction of any precipitating cause (e.g. withdrawal of sedatives and administration of suitable antagonists), correction of fluid and electrolyte disturbances, arrest of haemorrhage and treatment of sepsis (including primary peritonitis in ascitic patients). In the presence of a gastrointestinal bleed, purgation with oral magnesium sulphate and the use of enemas is needed to reduce the intestinal protein load (and thus the production of ammonia by intestinal organisms). This is accomplished by the administration of neomycin or metronidazole and lactulose.

Fulminant liver failure

Acute fulminant liver failure is defined as severe encephalopathy occurring within 6–8 weeks of the onset of the illness. It is the consequence of acute massive hepatocellular damage in a previously normal liver caused by:
- poisoning/overdose, e.g. paracetamol and ecstasy (3,4-methylenedioxymethamphetamine);
- viral infections (hepatitis A, B or C virus);
- halothane anaesthesia;
- mushroom poisoning (*Amanita phalloides*);
- drugs.

The disease still carries a high mortality despite newer methods of treatment. Patients with hepatotoxicity caused by paracetamol or infected with hepatitis A or B virus are more likely to recover than patients with other drug-induced liver failure or non-A non-B hepatitis. Biochemical evidence of massive liver cell necrosis in these patients includes marked elevations of transaminases and deepening jaundice. The coma is accompanied by gross cerebral oedema with raised intracranial pressure (ICP). There is multisystem involvement, with clotting failure, renal impairment, fall in peripheral resistance, pulmonary insufficiency and increased susceptibility to serious infections.

The treatment of fulminant liver failure is supportive and carried out in the intensive care unit. The useful therapeutic measures that have contributed to improved survival are:
- early ventilatory support for encephalopathy;
- prophylactic antibiotics and antifungal agents;
- inotropic support;
- renal support with haemofiltration/dialysis;
- extraction of poisons;
- ICP monitoring and reduction of cerebral oedema by 20% mannitol infused intravenously;
- *N*-acetylcysteine infusion.

The infusion of *N*-acetylcysteine is well established in the treatment of liver failure caused by paracetamol and survival in these patients has improved from 40 to 83%. Liver transplantation is used for patients who do not respond to supportive therapy. Newer forms of artificial hepatic support may bide time until a donor becomes available. These include the extracorporeal liver assist (using a pig's liver) and the bioartificial liver device based on isolated hepatocytes.

Hepatic abscess

Abscesses of the liver are of two types: pyogenic and amoebic. Pyogenic hepatic abscess is caused by the following.
- Bile duct infection with ascending cholangitis: *Escherichia coli* and anaerobic Gram-negative organisms.
- Ascending pylephlebitis from any inflammatory process within the abdomen: complicated diverticulitis.
- Staphylococcal/streptococcal bacteraemia: haematogenous.
- Direct extension from intra-abdominal suppuration, e.g. gangrenous cholecystitis, penetrating peptic ulcer disease and subphrenic collections.
- Trauma to the liver with subsequent infection.
- Cryptogenic: a significant group of patients in the geriatric population with no obvious cause. These have an insidious onset and non-specific symptoms such that at the time of diagnosis, the abscess is usually very large. The infecting organisms are commonly *Peptostreptococcus* and *Streptococcus milleri* but other microbes including *Bacteroides fragilis* may be involved.

Irrespective of aetiology, liver abscesses are found much more commonly in the right lobe. Untreated pyogenic liver abscess carries a high mortality, especially when multiple and in the presence of hyperbilirubinaemia and comorbid disease. Common manifestations include high fever, rigors, profuse sweating, anorexia and vomiting. Pain is a relatively late symptom. These features are less striking in hepatic amoebiasis where the fever is usually low grade. However, pain is a more common feature with amoebic abscess and is aggravated by movement and coughing. About half the patients with amoebic abscesses have diarrhoea. Hepatomegaly is common, particularly

04

with amoebiasis. An abscess in the left lobe may present as a painful epigastric swelling. Anaemia and leukocytosis are usually present and the erythrocyte sedimentation rate is markedly elevated. Disturbances of liver function tests are not diagnostic and may be absent in amoebiasis.

Blood cultures are usually positive in patients with pyogenic abscesses. Clinical suspicion of hepatic abscess is confirmed by ultrasonography or CT. Diagnostic aspiration is safe and provides material for culture of organisms responsible and hence the appropriate antibiotic therapy. Chest radiography is necessary to outline basal lung changes (consolidation and effusion) in complicated cases. An elevated immobile diaphragm is often encountered in large abscesses. A plain film of the abdomen may demonstrate gas in the abscess cavity. Extension through the diaphragm may lead to thoracic empyema or rupture into the bronchus with expectoration of large volumes of pus ('anchovy paste' in amoebic abscesses).

Initial management of a hepatic abscess is usually non-surgical with administration of antibiotics. Closed percutaneous drainage under ultrasound or CT control is then performed. Deterioration in the general condition of the patient and failure of the abscess to decrease in size are indications for open surgical drainage. Amoebic abscesses are treated with metronidazole with or without chloroquine. Aspiration of the amoebic abscess is not required routinely and is usually reserved for patients when there is no response within 2 days. Rupture of an amoebic abscess into the lung and bronchus can usually be treated successfully by antibiotics and postural drainage.

Subphrenic extrahepatic abscess

Abscesses around the liver occur in six defined spaces. Superiorly, the falciform ligament divides the left and right subphrenic spaces, the latter being divided into anterior and posterior spaces by the triangular ligament. The infrahepatic region has three spaces: two on the left side including the lesser sac and the space immediately below the lateral lobe of the left hepatic lobe. Subphrenic collections may contain a mixture of pus and gastrointestinal secretions and are often large. While any intra-abdominal sepsis may cause any of these abscesses, most follow gastrointestinal operations complicated by postoperative leaks, spontaneous perforation of hollow organs or accidental abdominal trauma. Primary causes include pancreatitis, cholecystitis, perforated peptic ulcer, perforated diverticular disease and perforated acute appendicitis.

Clinically, suspicion of a perihepatic collection is aroused by fever with rigors, leukocytosis and pain. Nonspecific abdominal symptoms and general ill health are common, though in some patients attention is drawn to respiratory symptoms resulting from inflammatory pulmonary changes secondary to a subdiaphragmatic collection. When an abscess is subhepatic, tenderness is elicited and a mass may be palpated. Diagnosis and location of subphrenic abscesses is by CT scanning. Once diagnosed, drainage of the abscess is mandatory. Many collections can be aspirated and a catheter left in place under radiological guidance. Open surgical drainage may be necessary for multilocular collections and for the presence of thick pus with necrotic slough. Culture of the infected fluid is taken at the time of drainage.

Non-parasitic hepatic cysts

Some are traumatic and have no epithelial lining; others are clearly similar to dermoid cysts. The majority of hepatic cysts are lined by cuboidal or columnar epithelium, contain serous fluid and do not communicate with the biliary tract. These are known as simple cysts and are multiple in 50% of cases. They can grow to a large size and in so doing cause pressure atrophy of the surrounding hepatic parenchyma. They are generally regarded as developmental abnormalities from aberrant bile ducts. Symptomatic cysts are commoner in females and huge cysts are almost exclusively found in women above the age of 50 years. Most simple hepatic cysts are asymptomatic. Symptoms are caused by pressure effects as cysts increase in size, e.g. vomiting, upper abdominal pain. Clinical examination reveals a non-tender smooth mass in the liver. Jaundice is very unusual and liver function tests are usually normal. The diagnosis is confirmed by ultrasonography. Complications are uncommon but include intracystic bleeding that causes sudden severe pain and increase in size, fistulation with the intrahepatic biliary tract or duodenum, bacterial infection, compression of the bile duct with obstructive jaundice, and compression of the vena cava or portal vein. Differentiation is from parasitic cysts and from adult polycystic disease of the kidney, where multiple serous hepatic cysts are often present. Only symptomatic cysts require treatment. This consists of fenestration (deroofing), nowadays carried out laparoscopically. Caroli's syndrome is characterized by congenital multifocal dilatations of the segmental bile ducts. In 50% of cases Caroli's syndrome is associated with congenital hepatic fibrosis.

Hepatic cystadenoma is rare and affects predominantly females, forming a large multiloculated cyst filled with mucinous fluid and lined by cuboidal epithelium. In places the lining epithelium forms polypoid projections. Although benign, the lesion is liable to complications, notably cholestasis due to compression of the bile duct, intracystic bleeding, infection, rupture and malignant degeneration. Hepatic cystadenoma must be excised completely even when asymptomatic.

04

Hydatid cysts

This infestation is endemic in certain countries, e.g. South America, Australasia, New Zealand, France and certain areas of the USA and the UK. Humans are a secondary host and become infected by ingesting vegetables and water fouled by dogs or more directly by handling parasite-infested dogs. After ingestion, the embryos hatch within the duodenum and then migrate through the gut wall into the mesenteric circulation to lodge within the liver. The embryo becomes a small vesicle with an inner germinal epithelium that produces secondary or daughter brood cysts containing scolices and hooklets. Hydatid cysts caused by *Echinococcus granulosus* are unilocular, as distinct from the multilocular alveolar type due to *Echinococcus multilocularis*. This forms a spongy collection of cysts and carries a poor prognosis.

Many years elapse before the cyst reaches significant size. In most patients general health remains good. Anteriorly located cysts present as smooth rounded tense masses. Secondary infection results in tender hepatomegaly, rigors and pyrexia associated with a deep-seated continuous pain. Intrabiliary rupture may give biliary colic and usually causes jaundice and fever. Intraperitoneal rupture produces severe pain and shock classically associated with pruritus and urticaria. Some of the implanted brood cysts induce a profound fibrous reaction that sterilizes the infection but other cysts reappear in various parts of the peritoneal cavity years later. Intrathoracic rupture may be preceded by symptoms of diaphragmatic irritation, and rupture into bronchus leads to blood-stained sputum that frequently becomes bile-stained. An unruptured cyst may show on plain radiograph as a calcified reticulated shadow. Following intrabiliary rupture, gas may enter the cyst leading to partial collapse of the cyst wall (Camellotte sign). Ultrasonography reveals an echogenic cyst. Eosinophilia is present in 25% of patients. The complement fixation test is positive in 93% of patients.

The treatment of hydatid cysts of the liver is surgical or radiological. Medical treatment with mebendazole and albendazole is started before surgery. Surgical treatment involves removing the cyst without contaminating the peritoneal cavity. Marsupialization of large cysts is indicated for secondary infection. Cysts with extensive calcification are usually sterile and best left alone. There have been good reported results of percutaneous ultrasound-guided treatment of hepatic hydatid cysts. This involves *p*uncture, *a*spiration, *i*njection (of scolicidal agents) and *r*easpiration (PAIR). In patients with cysts larger than 6 cm in diameter, PAIR is followed by percutaneous drainage (PAIR-PD).

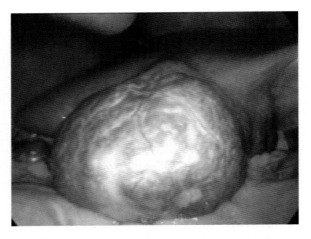

Figure 27.4 Laparoscopic view of hepatic haemangioma.

Liver tumours

Benign tumours of the liver are commonly asymptomatic and discovered accidentally during investigation, usually by ultrasound, and during laparotomy for other conditions. More rarely, they reach sufficient size as to cause symptoms or complications. Benign tumours include:

- haemangioma;
- hamartoma;
- focal nodular hyperplasia;
- adenoma.

Haemangiomas

Haemangiomas (Fig. 27.4) are the most common benign tumours of the liver, usually found in adults between the ages of 30 and 70 years, but only rarely produce symptoms. They are frequently situated just beneath the liver capsule and are normally of the cavernous type. Histologically, the lesion is composed of blood-filled endothelial-lined spaces separated by a variable degree of fibrous tissue and inflammatory changes, both of which result from episodes of spontaneous thrombosis.

Adenomas

Adenomas are rare. There is an established increased incidence related to use of the contraceptive pill, particularly in women over 30 years of age on high-oestrogen pills. There is also an increased incidence in patients with type I glycogen storage disease and galactosaemia. Up to 30% of adenomas are multiple. The differentiation between liver cell adenoma and well-differentiated hepatocellular (lamellar) carcinoma may be difficult and the two may coexist. Hepatic adenoma carries a risk of spontaneous

04

rupture with severe haemorrhage. If the diagnosis is certain and the lesion asymptomatic, it is monitored by ultrasound and α-fetoprotein (AFP) every 6–12 months for at least 10 years. Oral contraception is stopped. Adenomas that do not regress on follow-up should be excised.

Focal nodular hyperplasia

Focal nodular hyperplasia is a separate entity from liver cell adenoma and is regarded as a response to parenchymal injury or to an anomalous arterial supply to a local area of liver tissue. The lesion is usually small and may be multiple (20%), although large lesions presenting as an abdominal mass may occur especially in pregnant females and children of both sexes. There is no aetiological association with oral contraception. Macroscopically, focal nodular hyperplasia consists of a firm mass, the cut surface of which reveals a central scar with radiating fibrous septa. The microscopic findings are akin to cirrhosis, with regenerating nodules and fibrosis. Focal nodular hyperplasia is not premalignant and the natural history is such that it may be observed without serious risk.

Adenomatous hyperplasia

This ill-defined pathological entity refers to sizeable nodules that develop in chronic liver disease. In cirrhosis, adenomatous hyperplasia forms part of the spectrum of morbid pathological change that includes small benign regenerative nodules, large-size regenerative nodules (adenomatous hyperplasia), atypical adenomatous hyperplasia (dysplastic borderline lesions considered as low-grade hepatocellular carcinomas by some pathologists) and frank hepatocellular carcinoma. There is some debate as to the malignant potential of adenomatous hyperplasia: some reports have indicated that cancer can develop from the intervening hepatic parenchyma, whereas others consider the transition from regenerative nodules to adenomatous hyperplasia, dysplasia and carcinoma to be the norm.

Primary hepatocellular carcinoma

Primary hepatocellular carcinoma (HCC) is the most common malignant tumour worldwide and its geographical distribution closely parallels the incidence of hepatitis B virus (HBV) and hepatitis C virus (HCV) infection. Although the highest prevalence is encountered in the Far East and sub-Saharan Africa, it is also common in selected populations within the USA and Europe. The disease usually develops on a background of cirrhosis (cirrhomimetic) but can originate in normal or non-cirrhotic hepatic parenchyma (non-cirrhomimetic) (Fig. 27.5).

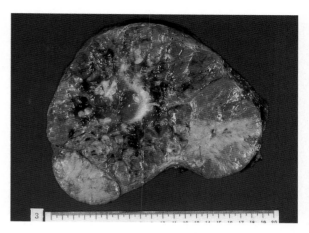

Figure 27.5 Laparoscopic view of hepatocellular carcinoma arising in a cirrhotic liver.

The disease is more common in males and, although slow-growing, is associated with a poor prognosis and frequently fatal outcome, with a median survival of 4 months in patients with symptomatic disease.

There is a strong association between the development of HCC and the presence of chronic (necro-inflammatory) liver disease with or without a background of HBV/HCV disease. The risk is increased 94-fold in HBsAg-positive males. There is also a high incidence in areas of endemic HCV infection and antibodies to HCV are often found in patients with HCC. Alcoholic liver disease is also common in patients who develop the disease. Aflatoxin B, a mycotoxin that contaminates grain and nuts particularly in West Africa, is involved in some cases that arise in this region.

Fibrolamellar HCC is a distinct variant with specific histological, histochemical and clinical features that occurs in young adults. This tumour has a better prognosis, with cure rates of 50% after resection. The histology shows large polygonal cells in a dense fibrous stroma that forms bands or lamellar structures.

Clinical features

In the early stages, HCC is asymptomatic and is only discovered by screening (ultrasound and AFP) in individuals at risk of the disease. The predominant symptom is an abdominal mass that produces a dragging sensation. Other symptoms include anorexia, weight loss, abdominal or chest pain, vomiting, fever and weakness. Jaundice and peripheral stigma of chronic liver disease may be present in patients with HCC in a cirrhotic liver. Also, jaundice may supervene from the growth of HCC into the bile ducts (icteric hepatoma). Some liver tumours at all ages

04

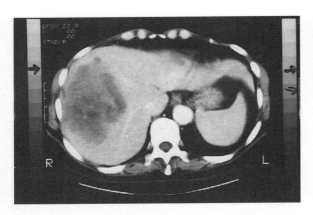

Figure 27.6 CT angiography showing primary hepatocellular carcinoma. The patient had a rising α-fetoprotein level.

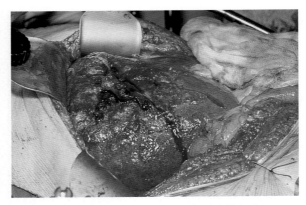

Figure 27.7 Large hepatocellular carcinoma arising in a non-cirrhotic liver treated by right hepatectomy.

present acutely with rupture and massive intraperitoneal bleeding.

Physical findings include hepatomegaly or hepatic mass. A bruit is heard in about 10% of patients. Ascites is common and is sometimes blood-stained. Laboratory studies frequently show abnormalities of liver function tests but these may reflect underlying chronic liver disease. Haematological abnormalities may include anaemia due to intratumoral haemorrhage or polycythaemia due to anomalous erythropoietin release. Serum AFP levels are elevated in about one-third and are a useful cancer marker after resection. Serum AFP is more likely to be elevated in undifferentiated cancers and is a valuable marker for screening the cirrhotic population for HCC development. A rising level of AFP or a level greater than 500 ng/mL in patients with chronic liver disease or cirrhosis requires ultrasonographic examination of the liver and CT to exclude HCC (Fig. 27.6).

Treatment

Surgical resection remains the first-line treatment of HCC even in patients with cirrhosis, provided their hepatic reserve is good (Fig. 27.7). The best results are obtained in patients with small, encapsulated, well-differentiated tumours. The 5-year survival rate after resection averages 35–38%. Recurrence after resection is common and reaches 55% at 5 years. Hepatic transplantation is indicated in cirrhotic patients with small tumours and patients with large fibrolamellar carcinoma. Chemotherapy is used in some patients with unresectable lesions, although the results are generally poor. Some response to interferon alfa can occur in patients with HCC arising on a background of cirrhosis due to HBV or HCV. Transarterial chemoembolization with gelatin sponge and/or ethiod-

ized oil (with or without added chemotherapeutic agents such as cisplatin or doxorubicin) may impart an objective response in some patients with unresectable disease. Targeted interstitial radiotherapy with ^{131}I-labelled antibodies to ferritin and AFP with the aim of targeting the radiation dose to the tumour achieves a 50% partial response rate.

Metastatic disease of the liver

The liver is the most common site of metastatic disease from gastrointestinal, bronchial and breast cancers (Fig. 27.8). Although many patients appear physically well when liver metastases are first detectable, as the disease progresses malnutrition, jaundice, ascites and cachexia are inevitable. By the time liver metastases become symptomatic, there is usually massive involvement. Detection of early asymptomatic disease in patients with colorectal cancer is important as some of these may be cured or prolonged survival obtained following resection. Macroscopically, secondary tumour deposits in the liver are classified as:
● discretely nodular (single or multiple, unilateral or bilateral);
● miliary (widespread small seedling deposits);
● diffusely confluent disease (involving multiple segments or lobes).

Only the discretely nodular disease is potentially treatable, and cure is rarely obtained if involvement is greater than 30% of the hepatic substance. The most common systemic chemotherapy regimen for treating colorectal hepatic deposits is high-dose infusion of 5-fluorouracil through a Hickman line with folinic acid. Significant response is obtained in 30% but the duration of response is measured in months. Newer agents (e.g. Raltitrexed) are marginally more effective. Transarterial chemoembolization

04

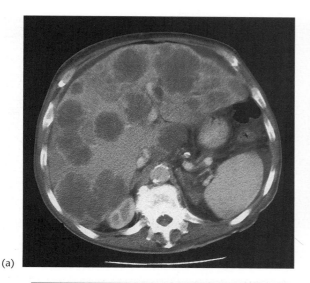

(a)

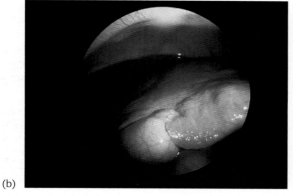

(b)

Figure 27.8 (a) CT showing multiple deposits from primary colorectal cancer. (b) Laparoscopic view of secondary deposits.

is beneficial in secondary ocular melanoma, advanced carcinoid syndrome and deposits from islet cell tumours. Secondary deposits can also be treated by *in situ* ablation, i.e. local destruction of the tumour. This can be achieved by the following:

- rapid freezing (cryotherapy; Fig. 27.9);
- radiofrequency heating probes (Fig. 27.10);
- microwave heating;
- interstitial laser hyperthermia;
- heating by high-intensity focused ultrasound;
- chemical ablation by alcohol, hot saline, acetic acid injection.

Currently, *in situ* ablation of liver tumours is used:

- when the disease is inoperable, either because of multiple deposits in both lobes or in the case of HCC because the functional reserve of the liver precludes safe resection (Child–Pugh categories B and C);
- in conjunction with resection for bilateral disease.

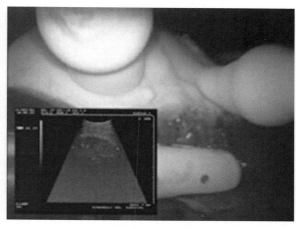

Figure 27.9 Laparoscopic cryotherapy for secondary tumour deposits from primary colorectal cancer.

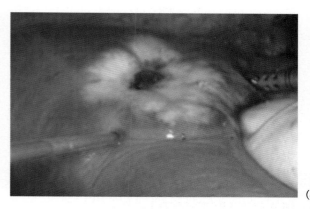

(a)

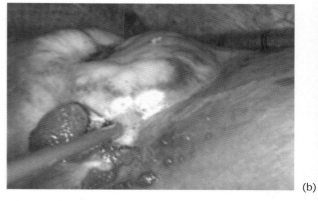

(b)

Figure 27.10 Laparoscopic radiofrequency thermal ablation of secondary deposit.

In situ ablation can be carried out at open surgery, percutaneously or via the laparoscopic approach. The major advantage of the percutaneous and laparoscopic routes is that the procedure can be repeated several times.

04

Portal hypertension

Portal hypertension is present when portal vein pressure exceeds 20 cm of saline. The most common cause is obstruction to portal blood flow. This may result from extrahepatic compression or thrombosis of the portal vein, from compression of portal venous radicles within the liver from a wide variety of liver diseases or from obstruction to the outflow from the liver. Rarely, anomalous arterioportal fistulae result in a rise in portal venous flow and pressure (Table 27.3).

Portal hypertension in patients with cirrhosis is the result of a combination of increased portal venous resistance (postsinusoidal) and increased splanchnic blood flow. Posthepatic outflow block may result from occlusion of the hepatic veins (Budd–Chiari syndrome). The thrombosis may be caused by protein C deficiency, the contraceptive pill or ingested toxins that include senecio or bush tea poisoning (veno-occlusive disease). Other patients have congenital diaphragm in the suprahepatic vena cava. Patients with posthepatic block may present with bleeding varices but more commonly the presenting features are intractable ascites, painful hepatomegaly with rapidly deteriorating liver function. Portal hypertension may also follow thrombosis of the splenic vein from pan-

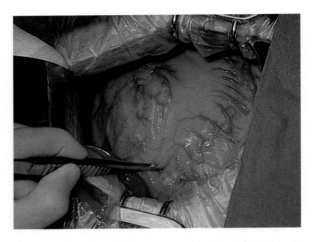

Figure 27.11 Sectorial portal hypertension due to thrombosis of splenic vein in patient with chronic pancreatitis. Operative photograph during splenectomy showing prominent left gastroepiploic veins.

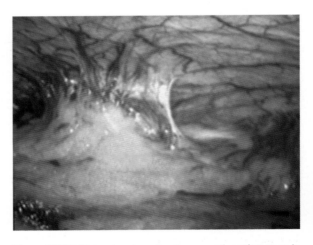

Figure 27.12 Natural portosystemic connections that open in portal hypertension. From the clinical standpoint, the most important is the connection between the azygos system and the left gastric (coronary) vein.

Table 27.3 Pathogenesis of portal hypertension.

Increased blood flow into portal venous system (no obstruction)
Hepatic and splenic arterioportal fistulae (rare)

Extrahepatic outflow obstruction
Hepatic vein thrombosis
Budd–Chiari syndrome
Veno-occlusive disease
Tricuspid incompetence
Right heart failure

Extrahepatic inflow obstruction
Congenital malformation of portal vein
Portal vein thrombosis
Splenic vein thrombosis (sectorial portal hypertension)
Portal vein compression, e.g. nodes

Intrahepatic obstruction
Presinusoidal
  Periportal fibrosis
  Schistosomiasis
Postsinusoidal
  Cirrhosis (alcoholic, nutritional, postnecrotic, biliary)
  Veno-occlusive diseases
  Haemochromatosis
  Wilson's disease
  Congenital hepatic fibrosis

creatitis or tumour. In this instance, portal hypertension is left-sided (sectorial) and the varices affect the short gastric and gastroepiploic veins (Fig. 27.11).

Obstruction to portal venous flow is followed by enlargement of natural portosystemic communications (Fig. 27.12). Rarely, portal venous blood is shunted away from the liver by an enlargement of the umbilical vein that connects with a collection of engorged veins at the umbilicus (caput medusae). This only becomes prominent if the patient develops a paraumbilical hernia containing an omental plug. The major risk of haemorrhage is from the

04

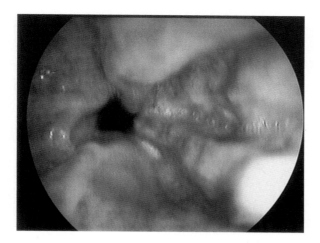

Figure 27.13 Endoscopic view of large oesophageal varices.

oesophagus and stomach. In the oesophagus the varices are large, tortuous and thin-walled with a tendency to rupture. Three columns tend to develop and run upwards to communicate with the azygos system. Blood flow from the spleen courses through the short gastric vessels to the gastric fundus (fundal varices) that link with enlarged collaterals at the cardia. In the stomach there is also venous engorgement of the gastric mucosa, with a tendency to erosive gastritis and a widespread diffuse haemorrhage (portal hypertensive gastropathy).

Patients with portal hypertension may develop:
● hypersplenism;
● ascites;
● gastrointestinal bleeding from gastro-oesophageal varices.

Splenomegaly is frequently associated with portal hypertension and may lead to anaemia, leukopenia and thrombocytopenia. The hypersplenism may improve after portal vein decompression. The development of fluid retention and ascites is extremely common in chronic liver disease and portal hypertension and its incidence correlates with the degree of advancement of the disease. A varying proportion of patients with chronic liver disease develop portal hypertension and only about half of these patients bleed from their varices. Approximately 30% of patients sustain their first variceal haemorrhage within 2 years of diagnosis. Large varices (Fig. 27.13) are more likely to bleed than small ones and varices that are observed to increase in size over a period of 1 year will almost certainly bleed at some point. Aside from size (grades II, III), the risk factors that predispose to variceal haemorrhage are:
● portal pressure;
● cherry-red spots;

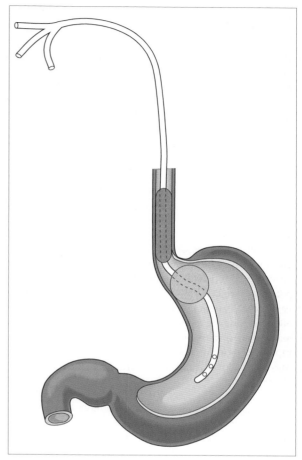

Figure 27.14 Balloon tamponade trilumen tube may be used to control major bleeding from oesophageal varices.

● overlying varices;
● red whale markings; and
● blue varices (as opposed to white).

There is commonly a minor warning bleed of a mouthful of bright red blood followed some hours later by a major haemorrhage of fresh blood produced without retching. Unless bleeding is massive and continuing, every attempt is made to localize the source of bleeding by fibreoptic endoscopy. This is performed as soon as the patient has been resuscitated and is haemodynamically stable. In addition to blood volume replacement and correction of electrolyte and acid–base imbalance, methods to prevent the development of encephalopathy or minimize its severity are instituted.

The mainstays of modern management are balloon tamponade (Fig. 27.14) followed by sclerotherapy or banding of the varices, or primary control with sclerother-

apy/banding. The major standby in the immediate control of variceal haemorrhage remains balloon tamponade. Problems arise with this technique when it is used as the only means of control over a long period. The major disadvantage of balloon tamponade is the accumulation of pharyngeal and oesophageal secretions with aspiration into the bronchial tree. Once control of bleeding is obtained, time is spent for full resuscitation with blood transfusion. Balloon tamponade is discontinued after 12–24 h but the tube is retained initially so that gastric and oesophageal aspiration may continue. By this time, the management follows a well-established pathway.

Endoscopic sclerotherapy

Many clinicians now proceed to variceal injection at the time of diagnostic endoscopy without resorting to balloon tamponade. Sclerotherapy is very effective in the arrest of bleeding from variceal haemorrhage and in reducing the incidence of subsequent bleeding episodes. Sclerotherapy is repeated until all the varices are obliterated. Sclerotherapy has a number of complications:
- oesophageal ulceration, perforation or stricture;
- adult respiratory distress syndrome;
- mediastinitis;
- bacteraemia (10%) with endocarditis (especially in patients with prosthetic valves);
- anaphylactic reactions (ethanolamine oleate);
- pneumatosis intestinalis;
- pneumoperitoneum;
- portal/mesenteric vein thrombosis.

Thus sclerotherapy should be used cautiously, especially in low-risk patients (Child–Pugh category A) who may later require a shunt operation. Sclerotherapy also aggravates portal gastropathy, is difficult to apply and is less effective in the control of gastric varices.

Endoscopic band ligation of varices

Endoscopic ligation of varices is achieved by rubber O bands mounted on a tubular attachment at the end of the flexible endoscope that are dislodged around the base of the varix after this is sucked inside the ring. Compared with endoscopic sclerotherapy, endoscopic ligation of varices is as effective or more effective in controlling active variceal bleeding and eradicating varices; furthermore, it is accompanied by a significantly lower morbidity (bacteraemia and infective complications, treatment-induced ulcers and stricture formation).

Gastric varices are difficult to control by endoscopic sclerotherapy and endoscopic ligation and are generally considered indications for trans-internal jugular portosystemic shunt (TIPSS) or surgical shunting.

Drug therapy

Drug therapy may be used in both the initial control of bleeding and the prophylaxis against further bleeding. The efficacy of continuous intravenous infusion of vasopressin (or its analogue terlipressin) in the control of variceal haemorrhage remains unconfirmed. Arrest of bleeding can be obtained by the synthetic long-acting analogue of somatostatin (octreotide). Pharmacological lowering of portal venous pressure by β-blockers (propranolol and nadolol) has been employed to prevent bleeding after initial control by sclerotherapy; various reports suggest a reduction of subsequent bleeds by 30%. However, propranolol therapy results in an elevation of blood ammonia and this increases the incidence of encephalopathic episodes.

Surgical treatment

Some 85% of patients with bleeding varices can be controlled by non-surgical measures. Only 15% continue to bleed or bleeding recurs soon after standard nonoperative management. The majority of these patients are high-risk candidates whose liver function is poor from end-stage liver disease. Portosystemic shunting is contraindicated in this group and continued bleeding is managed by oesophageal transection.

Two groups of patients are considered for shunting. The first consists of patients in whom bleeding has been arrested and who have good liver function (Child–Pugh categories A/good B). Since the expected survival of these patients is good, elective surgical therapy by portosystemic shunting is appropriate. The other group concerns patients with end-stage liver disease (Child–Pugh category C) who have been controlled by sclerotherapy. These patients can be considered for hepatic transplantation. For this reason, surgery is avoided and percutaneous TIPSS is employed to achieve portal decompression and thus avoid further bleeding episodes prior to hepatic transplantation (Fig. 27.15). TIPSS has been used in low-risk patients but follow-up has demonstrated an unacceptably high thrombosis rate beyond 6 months.

Direct surgical obliteration

This is undertaken in patients in Child–Pugh category C who continue to bleed and are not considered candidates for transplantation. It consists of transabdominal lower oesophageal transection using a circular stapling gun introduced via a gastrotomy. The device is used to transect and remove the segment of oesophagus immediately adjacent to the cardia. For bleeding gastric varices, a gastrotomy with double, separate, straight, non-cutting linear stapling

04

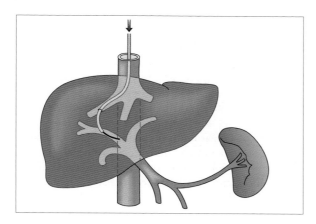

Figure 27.15 Schematic representation of trans-internal jugular portosystemic shunt: a metal stent is placed percutaneously via the internal jugular vein to establish communication between the portal vein and the hepatic venous system.

across the anterior and posterior walls is performed. The procedure may be extended by adding a splenectomy if significant hypersplenism is present.

Surgical portosystemic shunt

Surgical shunting by decompression of the portal venous system reduces the incidence of variceal bleeding. Total shunts include portacaval (between portal vein and inferior vena cava), lienorenal (between spleen and left renal vein) or mesentericocaval (between superior mesenteric vein and inferior vena cava) (Fig. 27.16). These shunts decompress the portal venous system very effectively but at the same time direct portal blood, with its hepatotrophic factors, away from the diseased liver. Their main disadvantage is encephalopathy, although this is less of a problem with lienorenal and mesentericocaval shunts.

Selective decompression of the oesophagogastric junction is achieved by the Warren distal splenorenal shunt (Fig. 27.17). In this operation, diversion of blood from the cardia is via the short gastric veins into the splenic, which is anastomosed to the left renal vein. The objective is to preserve portal venous flow to the liver and hence reduce the incidence and severity of encephalopathy.

Prophylactic therapy

This applies to patients who have never bled from their varices. Prophylactic surgical shunting is contraindicated because it does not impart any benefit but merely substitutes the risks of haemorrhage with deterioration of liver function and encephalopathy. Prophylactic pharmacological therapy with β-blockers may be used to prevent

bleeding episodes. However, this medical therapy can result in significant deterioration of liver function. For this reason case selection seems sensible and it seems appropriate to limit this prophylactic treatment to patients with low risk factors for bleeding and good liver function.

Extrahepatic portal block

Infants and children with this condition will generally stop bleeding and require only blood transfusion. Recurrent haemorrhage in the early years is the rule but becomes less frequent in teenage and young adult life. Ideally, these patients may be managed with banding. Adult patients are amenable to stapling procedures and it is important that the site of bleeding between staples is accurately localized. Careful follow-up with endoscopy and sclerotherapy for residual varices is appropriate.

Budd–Chiari syndrome

This is a syndrome of abdominal pain with intractable ascites associated with obstruction to the hepatic venous system. Strictly speaking, the term 'Budd–Chiari syndrome' should be restricted to those patients with occlusion (usually thrombosis) in the major hepatic veins and/or adjacent suprahepatic vena cava, and the term 'veno-occlusive disease' to obliteration (usually by sclerosis) of the smaller intrahepatic veins following ingestion of certain alkaloids, after chemotherapy, bone marrow transplantation and irradiation of the liver. Budd–Chiari syndrome is more common in women and some cases are caused by oestrogen/progesterone oral contraceptives. Others are the result of haematological disorders, such as polycythaemia, paroxysmal nocturnal haemoglobinaemia, antithrombin III deficiency and haemolytic anaemias. Collagen disorders such as lupus erythematosus, sarcoidosis and rheumatoid arthritis also predispose to the disorder. About one-third of cases are associated with obstruction of the superior vena cava (fibrosis from trauma; primary or secondary tumours of the liver, adrenal, kidney or vena cava itself; congenital webs).

The condition may present acutely with severe abdominal pain and vomiting and a large tender liver with ascites. It may progress rapidly over a few weeks to hepatic failure, coma and death. The more chronic form presents in similar fashion but at a reduced tempo and with less evidence of hepatic failure. There is usually peripheral oedema, which extends to the thighs if the vena cava becomes obstructed. Ultrasound examination indicates absence of the hepatic veins and a hepatic scintiscan may be grossly abnormal, with poor general uptake except the caudate lobe which may show normal or greater than normal

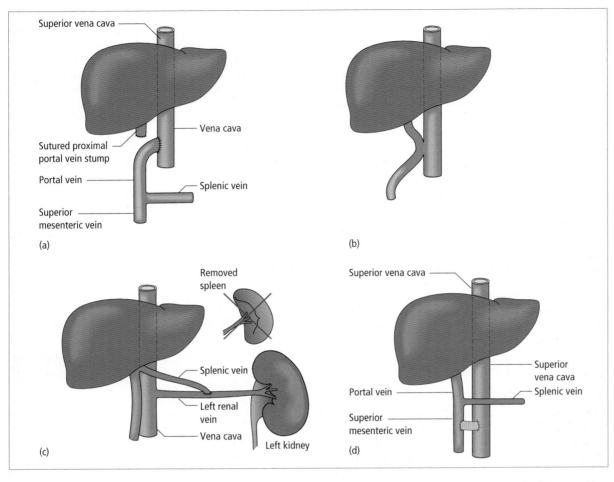

Figure 27.16 Types of total shunts: (a) end-to-side portacaval; (b) side-to-side portacaval; (c) distal splenorenal; (d) interposition mesocaval between vena cava and superior mesenteric vein.

04

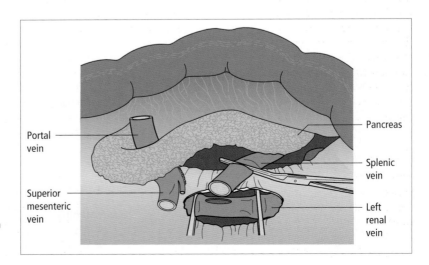

Figure 27.17 Warren selective splenorenal shunt that decompresses portal hypertension and varices through the short gastric and hence the splenic vein.

uptake. Diagnosis is established by hepatic venography/inferior vena cavography.

Mild cases can be managed with a low-sodium diet and diuretics and spontaneous improvement appears to occur in some patients, presumably as the veins recanalize. The ascites has to be managed by portal and hepatic decompression. A side-to-side portacaval shunt can accomplish this provided the inferior vena cava is not obstructed. A prosthetic mesoatrial shunt between the superior mesenteric vein and the right atrium is used in the presence of caval occlusion. Inferior vena caval webs or diaphragms can be dealt with by balloon angioplasty or surgical 'membranotomy' through the right atrial appendage. Hepatic transplantation is indicated in patients with chronic Budd–Chiari syndrome and deteriorating hepatic function or after failed shunt surgery.

Hepatic artery aneurysm

Hepatic artery aneurysms account for 20% of all splanchnic artery aneurysms. The most common cause is atheroma but some are infective while others are caused by trauma. The risk of rupture is high and may occur into the peritoneal cavity (usually fatal), bile duct (causing haemobilia), portal vein (with the development of an arteriovenous fistula) and duodenum (with massive upper gastrointestinal haemorrhage). Most are encountered in middle age and are commoner in males. Patients may present with non-specific pain in the right upper quadrant, when the aneurysm is discovered by ultrasound examination and the lesion confirmed by CT angiography. Sometimes the pain resembles biliary colic with jaundice and evidence of upper gastrointestinal haemorrhage. Acute presentation with sudden collapse and peritoneal signs indicates free rupture into the peritoneal cavity.

Even asymptomatic hepatic aneurysms should be treated because of the risk of rupture. Intrahepatic aneurysms are managed by percutaneous embolization. Extrahepatic aneurysms require surgical treatment, although transcatheter embolization may also be used.

Disorders of the liver at a glance

Functions of the liver
Metabolic
Glucose homeostasis
- Converts glucose to glycogen
- Releases glucose from glycogen
- Gluconeogenesis from amino acids

Lipid metabolism
- Converts free fatty acids to triglycerides
- Secretes lipoproteins

Synthetic
Synthesizes serum proteins (except immunoglobulins):
- Albumin
- Clotting factors
- Complement and other acute-phase proteins
- Specific binding proteins, e.g. copper, iron, vitamin A

Storage
- Glycogen
- Triglycerides
- Iron and copper
- Lipid-soluble vitamins (A, D, E, K)

Catabolic
Endogenous substances
- Hormones, e.g. oestrogen
- Serum proteins

Exogenous substances (detoxification)
- Drugs
- Industrial chemicals
- Products of bacterial metabolism in gut (endotoxin)

Excretory
- Bile salts
- Cholesterol
- Lecithin
- Bile pigment

Investigations
Blood
- Liver function tests
- Coagulation screen

Imaging
- Plain abdominal radiograph
- Ultrasonography
- Contrast-enhanced CT

Biopsy
- Needle
- Laparoscopy ± biopsy

Clinical signs of liver disease
- Hepatosplenomegaly
- Palmar erythema

- Finger clubbing
- Leuconychia
- Spider naevi in territory of superior vena cava
- Muscle wasting
- Oedema/ascites (water and NaCl retention, decreased protein synthesis)
- Gynaecomastia

Diseases of the liver
Infection/infestation
Hepatitis
- Acute: caused mostly by viral infection (HAV, HBV, HCV)
- Chronic: aetiology uncertain (persistent acute hepatitis, drugs, autoimmune)

Liver abscess
- Pyogenic:
   (a) Ascending cholangitis (*E. coli*)
   (b) Ascending pylephlebitis
   (c) Haematogenous (staphylococci/streptococci)
   (d) Extension of intra-abdominal abscess
   (e) Post trauma
   (f) Cryptogenic
- Amoebic

Hydatid disease
- *Echinococcus granulosus* or *E. multilocularis* causing large cysts in the liver

Cirrhosis
- Alcohol causes a spectrum of disease from fatty liver to hepatitis to cirrhosis
- Biliary:
   (a) Primary: chronic autoimmune destructive disease of intrahepatic bile ducts
   (b) Secondary: destruction of liver from long-standing obstruction of extrahepatic biliary tree
- Haemochromatosis
- Wilsons's disease
- α_1-Antitrypsin deficiency
- Glycogen storage disease

Toxic injury
Causes a spectrum of disease from clinically trivial to cholestasis to fulminant necrosis
- Viral infections
- Drugs: tetracycline, halothane, carbamazepine, paracetamol, ecstasy
- Chemicals: carbon tetrachloride, aflatoxin

Neoplasia
- Benign:
   (a) Haemangioma
   (b) Hamartoma
   (c) Focal nodular hyperplasia
   (d) Adenoma
- Secondary: gastrointestinal tract, breast, lung, pancreas, melanoma
- Primary:
   (a) Hepatocellular carcinoma
   (b) Cholangiocarcinoma
   (c) Hepatoblastoma (children)
   (d) Sarcoma (usually haemangiosarcoma)

Hepatic failure
Severe encephalopathy occurring within 6–8 weeks of the onset of illness

Causes (see Toxic injury above)
- Encephalopathy may be precipitated by gastrointestinal bleed in patient with cirrhosis

Clinical
- Jaundice
- Encephalopathy:
   (a) Intellectual impairment
   (b) Reduced level of consciousness
   (c) Abnormal psychometric tests
- Coma, cerebral oedema and raised ICP
- Systemic inflammatory response syndrome/multiple organ dysfunction syndrome

Treatment
- Remove the poison if possible
- Ventilation and ICP monitoring for coma
- Prophylactic antibiotics + antifungal agents
- Ionotropes as indicated
- Renal support + haemofiltration/dialysis
- *N*-Acetylcysteine infusion for paracetamol poisoning
- Liver transplantation

Portal hypertension
Present when portal vein pressure > 20 cm saline

Causes
Obstruction to portal blood flow
- Prehepatic: portal vein thrombosis or compression
- Hepatic: compression of portal venous radicles in liver, e.g. from cirrhosis (also increased splanchnic blood flow in cirrhotics)
- Posthepatic: occlusion of hepatic veins draining liver, e.g. Budd–Chiari syndrome

Increased blood flow
- Arterioportal fistulae cause rise in portal venous flow and pressure

04

Consequences
- Splenomegaly and hypersplenism
- Ascites
- Gastrointestinal haemorrhage from varices

Management of gastrointestinal bleeding (see also Chapter 12)
- Endoscopic sclerotherapy

- Endoscopic band ligation of varices
- Drugs: vasopressin, somatostatin, β-blockade
- TIPSS
- Surgery:
  (a) Direct surgical ablation: lower oesophageal transection
  (b) Surgical portosystemic shunts

Child–Pugh classification of hepatic reserve

	A (good)	B (moderate)	C (poor)
Serum albumin (μmol/L)	> 35	30–35	< 30
Serum bilirubin (g/L)	< 25	25–40	> 40
Prothrombin time prolongation (s)	< 4	4–6	> 6
Ascites	None	Controlled	Refractory
Encephalopathy	None	Minimal	Advanced

Evidence-based medicine

Freeny, P.C. (1997) Helical computed tomography of the liver: techniques, applications and pitfalls. *Endoscopy* **29**, 515–23.

Jalan, R. & Hayes, P.C. for British Society of Gastro-enterology (2000) UK guidelines on the management of variceal haemorrhage in cirrhotic patients. *Gut* **46** (Suppl.), 1–15.

Mahfouz, A.-E., Hamm, B. & Taupiz, M. (1997) Hepatic magnetic resonance imaging: new techniques and contrast agents. *Endoscopy* **29**, 504–14.

Must know Must do

Must know

How to investigate patients with jaundice

Principles of management of patients with jaundice due to large bile duct obstruction

Symptoms, management and treatment of patients with gallstones

Complications of gallstone disease

Clinical features and management of patients with ductal calculi and cholangitis

Pathology and principles of management of bile duct injuries/strictures

Clinical features and principles of management of patients with bile duct tumours

Must do

Clerk patients with large bile duct obstruction

Clerk patients with acute cholecystitis

Examine the urine for bilirubin and urobilin in patients with jaundice

Examine ultrasound scans showing gallstones, acute cholecystitis and dilated intrahepatic ducts

Observe diagnostic and interventional endoscopic retrograde cholangiopancreatography (ERCP) being performed on patients

Observe magnetic resonance cholangiopancreatography (MRCP) in a patient with large bile duct obstruction

Observe a laparoscopic cholecystectomy

Anatomy

The union of the right and left hepatic ducts in the porta hepatis forms the common hepatic duct and this receives the cystic duct to form the common bile duct. The gallbladder is a pear-shaped sac situated on the inferior surface of the right liver. It is divided into fundus, body and neck, which leads to the cystic duct. The neck often has an abnormal sacculation (Hartmann's pouch). The arterial supply of the gallbladder is by means of the cystic artery. The lower end of the common bile duct deviates to the right before entering the duodenum. In 90% of cases, the main pancreatic duct (of Wirsung) joins the postero-medial wall of the transduodenal segment of the bile duct to form a common channel. A localized dilatation of the common channel to form the ampulla of Vater is uncommon and separate opening of the two ducts into the duodenum is rarer still. An important variation of the anatomy of the Vaterian segment is the condition of pancreas divisum, which results from failure of fusion of the ventral and dorsal pancreas during embryological development. The duct of the ventral pancreas, which normally forms the main pancreatic duct, remains rudimentary and drains the lower portion of the pancreatic head and the uncinate process. The rest of the pancreas is drained through the duct of the dorsal anlage (duct of Santorini), which opens through the small accessory papilla.

Investigation of biliary tract disorders

Ultrasonography is the first-line investigation for biliary tract and pancreatic disease. It provides information on:
- presence of gallstones (90% accuracy);
- presence of gallbladder disease;
- dilatation of biliary tract and hepatic parenchymal disease, e.g. tumour deposits;
- lesions in the pancreas.

Ultrasound examination of the gallbladder is used as the initial diagnostic procedure for acute cholecystitis since it detects tenderness over the gallbladder, pericholecystic fluid collections and gallbladder wall oedema/thickening (ultrasonographic signs of cholecystitis), in addition to sludge and stones. The ultrasonographic documentation of a dilated biliary tract is the first step in the investigation of patients with cholestatic jaundice. In icteric patients, its accuracy in the diagnosis of extrahepatic bile duct

04

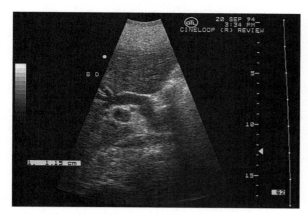

Figure 28.1 Ultrasound showing dilated (and hence obstructed) intrahepatic biliary tract.

obstruction exceeds 90% (Fig. 28.1). As ultrasound examination does not give accurate information on the exact site and extent of the lesion causing the extrahepatic obstruction, further investigation with computed tomography (CT) or MRCP/ERCP is required. Ultrasound examination is unsatisfactory for technical reasons in the following:

- obesity;
- following previous surgery;
- ascites;
- gaseous distension of upper abdominal viscera.

MRCP provides detailed imaging the entire biliary tree (intrahepatic and extrahepatic) and pancreatic ductal system without the administration of contrast (Fig. 28.2). It detects stones as small as 2 mm in the bile duct even when this is not dilated. MRCP is displacing diagnostic ERCP. Percutaneous transhepatic cholangiography, although highly accurate in detecting the level and cause of biliary obstruction, is kept in reserve because of its morbidity due to the following:

- bacteraemia;
- bile leakage;
- haemorrhage (free bleeding into the peritoneal cavity and haemobilia);
- bile embolization;
- intrahepatic arterioportal fistula;
- pneumothorax;
- contrast reactions.

Certain lesions can be treated or palliated by ERCP, e.g. endoscopic stone removal, endoscopic nasobiliary drainage, and stent insertion for inoperable malignant large bile duct obstruction (therapeutic ERCP). Diagnostic ERCP has a very low morbidity (largely due to pancreatitis) but the morbidity of interventional (therapeutic) ERCP is much higher (6–10%).

The radionuclides used for biliary scintiscanning are ^{99m}Tc-labelled compounds of IDA (iminodiacetic acid) and EHIDA (diethylacetanilido-iminodiacetic acid). These agents (γ-ray emitters) are administered intravenously, whereupon they are selectively taken up by hepatocytes and secreted into the bile. EHIDA cholescintiscanning is the most accurate test of acute cholecystitis. EHIDA scintigraphy is also very useful for the functional evaluation of surgically constructed bilioenteric anastomoses.

Jaundice

Jaundice (hyperbilirubinaemia) is a syndrome of varied aetiology that is recognized clinically when serum bilirubin exceeds 40 μmol/L. The excess bilirubin may be either conjugated or unconjugated and may result from:

- excess bilirubin production;
- impaired uptake by the hepatocyte;
- failure of conjugation;

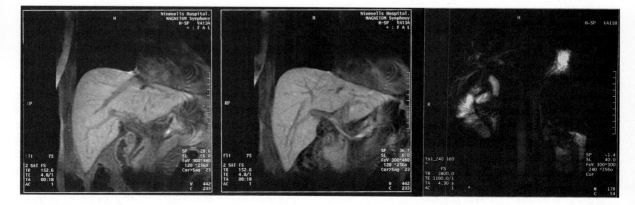

Figure 28.2 Magnetic resonance imaging of the liver and biliary tract. The biliary tract is shown by special T_2 weighted sequences.

- impaired secretion of conjugated bilirubin into the bile canaliculi;
- impairment of bile flow subsequent to secretion by hepatocytes (*cholestatic* or *obstructive jaundice*).

The cholestatic defect may be congenital but much more commonly is acquired as a result of:
- haemolysis;
- liver disease (acute or chronic);
- adverse drug reaction;
- biliary tract obstruction (intrahepatic or extrahepatic).

In clinical practice, hepatocellular and cholestatic jaundice comprise the majority of cases. *Hepatocellular jaundice* is due to parenchymatous liver disease, which may be acute (viral hepatitis, liver cell necrosis, acute alcoholic hepatitis, etc.) or chronic (various types of cirrhosis – primary biliary, etc.). The principal defect is the failure of secretion of conjugated bilirubin into the bile canaliculi. Serum transaminases are grossly elevated, especially in acute disease. In patients with alcohol-related liver disease, γ-glutamyltransferase (γ-GT) is elevated. Acute hepatitis due to viral infection or drugs may also cause a cholestatic picture, in which case alkaline phosphatase and 5′-nucleotidase are elevated. The hyperbilirubinaemia is predominantly of the conjugated variety, with the presence of bilirubin in the urine.

Cholestatic jaundice is the result of impaired bile flow to the duodenum subsequent to the secretion of conjugated bilirubin into the bile canaliculi. The block may be intrahepatic (drugs, hepatitis, obstruction of the intrahepatic biliary tree) or extrahepatic. The latter is known as *large bile duct obstruction* and constitutes the most important surgical subgroup of cholestatic jaundice as it is always the result of organic disease, e.g. ductal calculi, pancreaticobiliary cancer.

The biochemical features of cholestasis include the following.
- Conjugated hyperbilirubinaemia.
- Elevation of alkaline phosphatase, 5′-nucleotidase and γ-GT. The enzyme 5′-nucleotidase is the most reliable since its level is not influenced by bone disease and the enzyme is not induced by alcohol.
- Minimal or no elevation of serum transaminases.
- Presence of bilirubin in the urine: conjugated bilirubin is water soluble and is therefore filtered in the glomerulus.
- Elevation of serum cholesterol and bile acid, although these are not routinely measured in patients with cholestatic jaundice.

These biochemical markers of cholestasis do not distinguish between intrahepatic and extrahepatic obstruction.

In *haemolytic jaundice*, the unconjugated hyperbilirubinaemia results from haemolysis. Bilirubin is not present in the urine because the unconjugated pigment is insoluble in water and is carried in the plasma bound to albumin. The excess bilirubin production is accompanied by increased secretion of the conjugated pigment in the bile and therefore increased production of urobilinogen by bacterial decomposition in the distal small intestine. The urine therefore contains an excess amount of urobilinogen and urobilin.

Jaundice at a glance

Definition

Jaundice (*icterus*): yellowing of the skin and sclera from accumulation of the pigment bilirubin in the blood and tissues. The bilirubin level has to exceed 35–40 µmol/L before jaundice is clinically apparent

Classification

Prehepatic (haemolytic) jaundice
Haemolytic/congenital hyperbilirubinaemias
- Excess production of unconjugated bilirubin (from red blood cells) exhausts the capacity of the liver to conjugate the extra load, e.g. haemolytic anaemias (hereditary spherocytosis, sickle cell disease, hypersplenism, thalassaemia)

Hepatic (hepatocellular) jaundice
Hepatic unconjugated hyperbilirubinaemia
- Failure of transport of unconjugated bilirubin into the cell, e.g. Gilbert's syndrome

- Failure of bilirubin-glucuronide glucuronosyltransferase activity, e.g. Crigler–Najjar syndrome

Hepatic conjugated hyperbilirubinaemia
- Hepatocellular injury results in failure of excretion of bilirubin into the biliary system. Causes include:
  (a) Infections: viral hepatitis
  (b) Poisons: carbon tetrachloride, aflatoxin
  (c) Drugs: paracetamol, halothane

Posthepatic (obstructive) jaundice
Posthepatic conjugated hyperbilirubinaemia
- Anything that blocks the release of conjugated bilirubin from the hepatocyte or prevents its delivery to the duodenum. These are the most common causes of jaundice that present to a surgical service, e.g. gallstones blocking common bile duct, periampullary carcinomas, portal lymphadenopathy, sclerosing cholangitis

04

| Type of jaundice | Haemolytic | Hepatocellular | | Obstructive |
		Early	Late	
Serum bilirubin				
Unconjugated	Elevated	Normal/elevated	Normal/elevated	Normal
Conjugated	Normal	Normal	Elevated	Very elevated
Urinary bilirubin	Normal/elevated	Elevated	Elevated	Very elevated
Urinary urobilinogen	Normal/elevated	Normal	Decreased	Very decreased
Liver function tests				
Alkaline phosphatase	Normal	Normal	Elevated	Very elevated
γ-GT	Normal	Elevated	Elevated	Very elevated
Transaminases	Normal	Elevated	Very elevated	Normal/elevated
Lactate dehydrogenase	Normal	Elevated	Very elevated	Normal/elevated
Reticulocytes	> 2%	Normal	Normal	Normal

Courvoisier's law

'A palpable gallbladder in the presence of jaundice is unlikely to be due to gallstones'

- Usually caused by a neoplastic stricture obstructing the distal common bile duct
- Causes include periampullary tumours (pancreas, ampulla, duodenum, distal common bile duct), pancreatic stricture (chronic pancreatitis) or portal lymphadenopathy

Sclerosing cholangitis

- Obscure uncommon disorder of uncertain aetiology
- Results in fibrous obliteration of the biliary tract leading to jaundice, cirrhosis and portal hypertension
- Associated with inflammatory bowel disease especially ulcerative colitis
- Only effective treatment is hepatic transplantation

Management

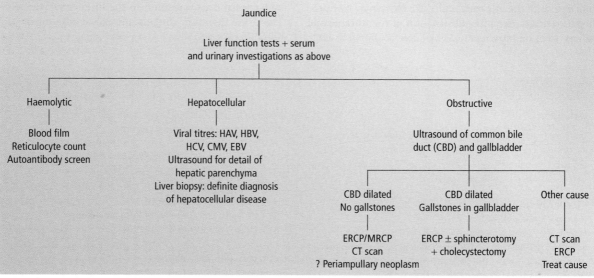

Management of large bile duct obstruction

A well-conducted history and physical examination will allow a correct diagnosis of the cause of the jaundice in 80% of patients. Surgical obstructive jaundice (large bile duct obstruction) is always accompanied by dilatation of the biliary tract. In essence, the management entails:

- establishing the cause of the jaundice;
- assessment of the general condition of the patient;

- staging in patients with tumours;
- appropriate treatment (which may be surgical, endoscopic or radiological).

Malignant large bile duct obstruction may be inoperable either because the lesion is not resectable or because the patient's grade on the American Society of Anesthesiologists (ASA) scale precludes major surgical intervention. In this situation management is directed towards palliation by non-surgical means.

Preoperative management of obstructive jaundice

Adequate preparation of the patient for surgery is essential in obstructive jaundice. Preparation entails the correction of metabolic abnormalities, improvement of the general condition, and institution of specific measures designed to minimize the incidence of complications associated with prolonged or severe cholestasis such as:

- infections (cholangitis, septicaemia, wound infections);
- disorders of the clotting mechanism;
- renal failure;
- liver failure;
- fluid and electrolyte abnormalities.

The conjugation and metabolism of drugs and anaesthetic agents is impaired because of hepatocyte malfunction. Hypokalaemia is frequently present and should be corrected. A viral screen is necessary and when the serology is positive, special precautions must be taken in both the ward and the operating theatre to avoid spread of the infection. Postoperative sepsis after biliary tract surgery is generally due to bacteria in the bile and the use of short-term prophylactic antibiotics significantly lowers the incidence of sepsis only in patients who have bacteria in the bile at the time of surgery. Prophylactic antibiotics are therefore administered to:

- all jaundiced patients;
- patients with rigors and pyrexia;
- patients undergoing emergency biliary procedures/operations;
- elderly patients;
- patients with common duct stones even if not jaundiced;
- patients undergoing secondary biliary intervention.

The most common disorder of coagulation encountered in large bile duct obstruction is a prolonged prothrombin time resulting from deficiency of vitamin K-dependent factors consequent on the malabsorption of this vitamin. The intramuscular injection of phytomenadione (10–20 mg) will reverse the clotting deficiency within 1–3 days. There is an association between severe conjugated hyperbilirubinaemia and postoperative renal failure but the underlying mechanism for this impairment is not known, although reduced glomerular filtration is

present. Adequate hydration and preoperative induction of a natriuresis/diuresis reduces the incidence of postoperative renal failure in jaundiced patients. It is currently routine practice to administer intravenous fluids (5% dextrose saline) for 12–24 h before surgery followed by an osmotic diuretic (mannitol) or a loop diuretic (furosemide) administered intravenously at the time of induction. All patients undergoing surgery should be catheterized and the urine output measured hourly.

Liver failure is usually encountered in patients with prolonged complete large bile duct obstruction or those patients with pre-existing chronic hepatocellular disease (e.g. cirrhosis, chronic active hepatitis). If the jaundice is severe (> 150 µmol/L) or the patient shows signs of impending liver failure, a period of decompression is indicated before surgery. This is achieved by insertion of a plastic endoprosthesis or by endoscopic sphincterotomy in patients with periampullary cancer. Other prophylactic measures against encephalopathy include correction of hypokalaemia, the restricted use of sedatives, hypnotics and potent analgesics, and the prompt treatment of infection.

Cystic disease of the biliary tract

Cystic disease of the biliary tract is rare in western countries. Most instances are thought to represent congenital weakness of the common bile duct with distal obstruction caused by an anomalous acute or 90° angle at the junction between the pancreatic duct and the common bile duct, resulting in an abnormally long common channel. Several types are recognized.

- Type I: diffuse choledochal cystic dilatation, the most common.
- Type II: localized dilatation of the supraduodenal bile duct.
- Type III: supraduodenal diverticulum.
- Type IV: intraduodenal diverticulum or choledochocele.
- Type V: solitary intrahepatic cyst.
- Type VI: multiple intrahepatic cysts (Caroli's syndrome).
- Type VII: multiple intrahepatic and extrahepatic cysts.

There is a high incidence of cystic disease in the Japanese and a strong female predominance worldwide (70% of reported cases in the West). About 25% of cases are diagnosed during the first year of life; one-third become clinically manifest over the next 10 years. The symptoms include cholestatic jaundice, abdominal mass and pain. Complications of the disease are recurrent cholangitis and pancreatitis, hepatic abscess, calculous disease, rupture of the cyst with biliary peritonitis (rare) and portal vein thrombosis. There is also an increased risk of cholangiocarcinoma. The treatment of choledochous cysts is surgical excision. The treatment of patients with intrahepatic

04

cystic disease is difficult; when localized, partial liver resection is possible.

Gallstones

The current mean prevalence in Europe is 18.5%. Based on chemical composition, gallstones are classified into cholesterol, black pigment and brown pigment stones.

Cholesterol stones. These are preceded by the formation of biliary sludge and account for the vast majority of gallstones encountered in western countries. They have a protein matrix but are composed predominantly of cholesterol, with varying amounts of bile pigments and calcium salts deposited on the periphery. Cholesterol gallstones do not commonly harbour bacteria and are not usually associated with infected bile. They are often radio-lucent but cast strong acoustic shadows on ultrasono-graphy (Fig. 28.3). Cholesterol stones are often multiple and medium-sized, but when solitary attain a large size and have a radiating crystalline cross-sectional appearance.

Black pigment stones. Black pigment stones account for 25% of gallstones in the West, although their prevalence is higher in the Far East. They are composed of bilirubin polymers without calcium palmitate, small amounts of cholesterol and a matrix of organic material. Associated infection is present in less than 20% of patients. Black pigment stones are usually multiple, small, irregular and dark-green to black in colour. Although haemolytic states predispose to the formation of black pigment stones, most occur in patients without detectable chronic haemolysis.

Brown pigment stones. In contradistinction to the above types, brown pigment stones form in the bile ducts (primary ductal calculi) and are associated with infection of the biliary tract. Scanning electron microscopy of fresh specimens demonstrates bacteria inside crevices and pits of these amorphous soft stones in 98% of cases. Brown pigment stones contain calcium bilirubinate, calcium palmitate and only small amounts of cholesterol bound in a matrix of organic material.

Pathogenesis

There is an increased prevalence of gallstones in females and the frequency of gallstones increases with age in both sexes. The importance of genetic and ethnic factors is exemplified by the unusually high prevalence of gallstones in Native Americans, particularly the Pima tribe. Certain risk factors are known to increase the prevalence of gallstones, while others induce symptomatic disease in patients with silent gallstones without necessarily enhancing the overall frequency (Table 28.1). The modern 'mini' contraceptive pill does not appear to enhance the overall risk of gallstone formation, although it may be associated with an increased risk of symptomatic disease in young women.

The formation of cholesterol stones involves seven processes:
- supersaturation of bile with cholesterol;
- incomplete transfer of cholesterol from biliary vesicles to bile salt micelles;

Table 28.1 Risk factors for gallstone prevalence and symptomatic gallstone disease.

Increased prevalence
Female sex*
Obesity*
Age*
Genetic and ethnic factors*
Diet depleted in fibre and high in animal fats*
Diabetes mellitus*
Ileal disease and resection
Haemolytic states†
Infections of the biliary tract†
Parasitic infestations†
Cirrhosis†
Cystic fibrosis

Precipitation of symptomatic disease
Pregnancy
Clofibrate
Thiazide diuretics
?Oral contraception

* Increased prevalence of cholesterol stones.
† Increased prevalence of pigment stones.

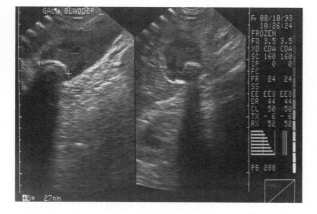

Figure 28.3 Gallstones detected by ultrasonography.

- formation of abnormal high-cholesterol-containing biliary vesicles;
- aggregation and fusion of unstable vesicles;
- cholesterol crystallization (nucleating and antinucleating factors);
- biliary sludge formation;
- stone growth.

The outstanding biochemical abnormality associated with the formation of cholesterol gallstones is the secretion of bile supersaturated with cholesterol. Under normal physiological conditions, cholesterol is secreted by hepatocytes into the hepatic bile as cholesterol–phospholipid vesicles. Within the bile, a phase change occurs due to the relative high concentrations of bile acids, and micelles form. These are essentially molecular aggregates in which the cholesterol and phospholipid molecules form a central core surrounded by bile salt molecules. This mechanism is invoked to maintain cholesterol (which is water insoluble) in solution. The lithogenic index is the ratio of the actual amount of cholesterol that can be dissolved in the bile sample. The source of the supersaturated bile is the liver. Excess cholesterol secretion in the bile is well documented in obese patients and is thought to result from increased activity of the enzyme β-hydroxy-β-methylglutaryl-CoA reductase. Most non-obese patients with cholesterol gallstones have reduced absorption as the cause of the diminished bile salt pool. Although gallstones develop only in individuals with supersaturated bile, many patients with this abnormality never develop gallstones. Thus other factors are involved. These include the persistence of cholesterol–phospholipid biliary vesicles, kinetic balance between nucleating and antinucleating factors, and biliary sludge. The latter is composed of mucin, calcium, monoconjugated bilirubin and cholesterol and is now thought to be the direct precursor of gallstones.

That the gallbladder plays an important role in gallstone formation (both cholesterol and black pigment) is evidenced by the fact that 85–90% of stones are encountered in this organ rather than in the bile ducts. The gallbladder may alter the physicochemical composition of bile, favouring nucleation and crystal growth by abnormal absorption/secretion, defective surface pH, stasis caused by impaired gallbladder emptying and stratification of bile or by providing essential nucleating factors.

The pathophysiology of black pigment stones is largely unknown. They are common in cirrhotic patients who have an elevated concentration of monoconjugated bilirubin and a lower bile salt concentration than normal. Mucins may be involved in the development of pigment stones, especially those forming in the intrahepatic ducts.

Brown pigment stones are caused by infection with Gram-negative bacteria (*Escherichia coli* and *Bacteroides fragilis*), which elaborate and release β-glucuronidase. This is implicated in the hydrolysis of conjugated bilirubin, with consequent precipitation of insoluble calcium bilirubinate. Brown pigment stones are encountered in biliary tract conditions associated with stasis and infection, such as chronic obstructive disease, indwelling biliary endoprostheses and around non-absorbable suture material or metal clips used in biliary tract surgery.

Clinical features

Often non-specific, the symptoms may be acute, chronic or absent when gallstones are diagnosed as an incidental finding during the investigation of patients for unrelated disorders. In patients with chronic symptoms, it is important to exclude other disorders that might be responsible. The common coexisting diseases are:

- colonic motility disorders and diverticular disease;
- gastritis and peptic ulceration;
- reflux oesophagitis and hiatal hernia;
- pancreatitis;
- colonic cancer;
- ischaemic heart disease.

Silent gallstones heavily outnumber symptomatic ones and there is no indication for cholecystectomy in patients with asymptomatic gallstones. The clinical presentation varies and may be acute or chronic (Table 28.2). The stones induce chronic inflammation of the gallbladder. These patients complain of recurrent attacks of epigastric or right hypochondrial pain, often radiating to the right side of the back and, less commonly, to the shoulder blade. The pain is more often persistent than intermittent. Episodes of biliary colic, with severe intermittent peaks of pain lasting a few minutes to several hours, may subside spontaneously or progress to cystic duct obstruction and acute cholecystitis. Nausea and vomiting may accompany the episodes of chronic pain and the severe attacks of biliary colic. Jaundice and dark urine may follow an attack of biliary colic and indicate common bile duct obstruction

Table 28.2 Spectrum of symptomatic gallstone disease.

Chronic cholecystitis
Acute biliary colic/acute cholecystitis
Jaundice due to large bile duct obstruction
Cholangitis/septicaemia
Acute gallstone pancreatitis
Biliary fistulous disease
Gallstone ileus

04

by a calculus. Jaundice often subsides after a few days but may persist as a major presenting symptom. The only reliable sign, which is found infrequently, is tenderness in the right upper quadrant. More often than not, the clinical features of chronic cholecystitis are non-specific and confirmation by ultrasound examination is necessary.

Acute biliary colic and acute cholecystitis

Acute biliary colic consists of severe colicky abdominal pain usually accompanied by nausea and vomiting. The duration of severe pain, which makes the patient restless, varies from 30 min to several hours. Biliary colic may merge into acute obstructive cholecystitis. However, resolution of the severe colicky pain without the development of acute cholecystitis is common and many patients give a history of recurrent episodes of biliary colic. Acute cholecystitis is usually obstructive in nature from impaction of a stone in Hartmann's pouch/cystic duct. Much less commonly, acute cholecystitis is acalculous (not associated with gallstones). Acute cholecystitis in the elderly may result from cystic duct obstruction due to carcinoma of the gallbladder. In acute obstructive cholecystitis, the initial inflammation is chemically induced, although infection supervenes in established disease. Cultures of gallbladder bile taken during open cholecystectomy are positive in only 15–30%, with the predominant microorganisms being *E. coli*, *Klebsiella* spp. and *Streptococcus* spp. The inflammation resolves in the majority of patients with conservative management as the rising tension in the gallbladder lumen from the outpouring of inflammatory exudate lifts the walls of Hartmann's pouch off the impacting stone. When this drops into the gallbladder lumen, cystic duct drainage leads to resolution. This fortuitous sequence is not encountered in 20% of patients, in whom patchy gangrene and/or perforation with a large inflammatory phlegmon or peritonitis supervene. The sequence of events following the acute inflammatory process may vary as follows.

● Resolution (most common) with scarring, abnormal function or non-function of the gallbladder.
● Persistence of the infection: the gallbladder becomes distended with pus (empyema of the gallbladder).
● Resolution of the inflammatory process within the gallbladder with persistence of cystic duct obstruction: mucocele (hydrops) of the gallbladder.
● Gangrene and acute perforation leading to localized (pericholecystic) abscess or frank biliary peritonitis.
● Chronic perforation with the development of bilioenteric and biliobilial fistulae.

Known pre-existing gallbladder disease may be present or chronic symptoms over several months to years may precede the acute presentation. Alternatively, acute obstructive cholecystitis may be the first intimation of gallstone disease. In mild cases, the patient complains of right upper quadrant pain. Pyrexia, severe pain and tenderness in the right hypochondrium with rebound reflect more severe inflammation. In these instances, Murphy's sign (inspiratory arrest due to pain on inspiration during gentle palpation of the right subcostal region) is usually present. Nausea, vomiting, ileus, mild abdominal distension and toxicity are also encountered in severe disease. Jaundice is present in 25% of patients with acute obstructive cholecystitis but common duct stones are found in only half these patients. A tender palpable mass in the right subcostal region is found in 25% of cases and signifies one of the following:
● empyema of the gallbladder;
● omental phlegmon;
● abscess due to localized perforation;
● carcinoma of the gallbladder, if the patient is elderly.

Laboratory tests are frequently non-specific, their value being to rule out other conditions particularly acute pancreatitis. Most patients have a neutrophil leukocytosis ($> 10 \times 10^9$/L) together with some abnormality of the liver function profile. The levels of serum bilirubin and alkaline phosphatase do not invariably correlate with the presence of ductal calculi but are suggestive and clinical jaundice warrants investigation with endoscopic retrograde cholangiography. Other laboratory findings include minor elevations of serum amylase, below the diagnostic threshold for acute pancreatitis. Other conditions that need exclusion are perforated peptic ulcer, acute pancreatitis or retrocaecal appendicitis, viral hepatitis, right-sided pyelonephritis, pneumonia and myocardial infarction.

Acute acalculous cholecystitis

This usually occurs in critically ill patients in whom acute inflammation of the gallbladder arises in the absence of gallstones, although biliary sludge is often present. This condition now accounts for up to 8% of patients. Acute acalculous cholecystitis does not always arise on a background of a critical illness. It also occurs in elderly patients, usually men with atheromatous vascular disease and/or diabetes. The exact pathology is not known but the inflammation develops as a consequence of prolonged distension of the gallbladder, bile stasis and inspissation (biliary sludge) that cause mucosal injury and thrombosis of vessels of the seromuscular layer of the gallbladder. Culture of the aspirated gallbladder bile is positive in only 38% of cases. The diagnosis of acute

acalculous cholecystitis is often difficult. The early manifestations include fever, leukocytosis and tenderness in the right hypochondrium. The diagnostic methods used are CT, ultrasonography and isotope scintiscanning. In the absence of significant gangrene, cholecystostomy (performed percutaneously) is performed particularly in critically ill patients.

Complications of acute cholecystitis

The important complications of all forms of acute cholecystitis are empyema, perforation and gangrene. All require urgent surgical intervention. Empyema of the gallbladder is uncommon and presents as a tender mass in the right hypochondrium in elderly patients in whom systemic signs, including pyrexia and leukocytosis, may be minimal. Cultures of the gallbladder contents are positive in 80%. Patchy gangrene of the fundus of the gallbladder is encountered in 10% of patients with obstructive cholecystitis. It is more common in elderly patients, diabetics and patients with empyema of the gallbladder and acute acalculous cholecystitis. Perforation may be localized (with the formation of a pericholecystic abscess) or free, resulting in a generalized infective biliary peritonitis that carries a high mortality (30%). A localized perforation may involve the duodenum, with the development of a cholecystoduodenal fistula and resolution of the inflammatory episode. However, the bilioenteric fistula persists and passage of a large stone through this may eventually cause gallstone ileus.

Treatment of acute cholecystitis

Initial management consists of intravenous fluid and electrolyte replacement, nasogastric suction and parenteral analgesia. Systemic antibiotics (third-generation cephalosporin) are administered to prevent septic complications. Anaerobes are associated with more severe mixed infections, particularly in the elderly, and require combination

therapy using metronidazole with an aminoglycoside and/or penicillin.

The timing of surgery (cholecystectomy) is dictated by the severity of the attack. Table 28.3 summarizes the indications for emergency/urgent surgical intervention. At times, the precarious condition of the patient precludes a lengthy operation or the anatomy may be so obscured by the inflammatory mass as to render the cholecystectomy hazardous. In these situations, a cholecystostomy should be performed. In seriously ill unfit patients, the only viable option may be percutaneous ultrasound-guided cholecystostomy.

In patients with established non-progressive disease, there are two management options:
- delayed (interval, subsequent admission) cholecystectomy;
- early (same admission) cholecystectomy.

The interval approach entails conservative management of the acute episode with discharge of the patient after complete resolution. Subsequently, the patient is admitted some 2–3 months later for an elective cholecystectomy. Early cholecystectomy must be distinguished from emergency cholecystectomy. Following initial conservative management, the patient is operated electively on the next available operating list. The results of several prospective clinical trials comparing early vs. interval cholecystectomy have shown a clear benefit from early cholecystectomy performed during the same hospital admission in fit patients. Cholecystectomy (interval or early) is nowadays performed by the laparoscopic approach (Fig. 28.4).

Table 28.3 Indications for emergency surgical intervention in patients with acute cholecystitis.

Progression of the disease despite conservative treatment
Failure to improve within 24 h especially in patients > 60 years old
Presence of an inflammatory mass in the right hypochondrium
Detection of gas in the gallbladder/biliary tract
Established generalized peritonitis
Development of intestinal obstruction

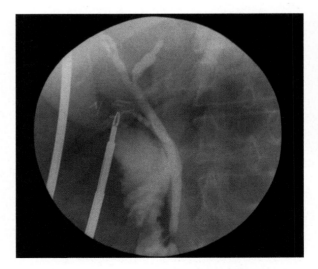

Figure 28.4 Laparoscopic cholecystectomy: intraoperative cholangiogram is performed during the cholecystectomy.

Gallstone disease at a glance

Definition

Gallstones: round, oval or faceted concretions found in the biliary tract containing cholesterol, calcium carbonate, calcium bilirubinate or a mixture of these elements

Epidemiology
- Male/female ratio 1 : 2
- Age > 40 years
- High incidence of mixed stones in the West; pigment stones commoner in the East

Pathogenesis
- Cholesterol stones: imbalance in bile between cholesterol, bile salts and phospholipids producing lithogenic bile. Associated with inflammatory bowel disease
- Bilirubinate stones: chronic haemolysis, infection with β-glucuronidase-producing bacteria
- Mixed stones: associated with anatomical abnormalities, stasis, previous surgery, previous infections

Pathology
- Gallstones passing through biliary system may cause biliary colic or pancreatitis
- Stone obstruction at the gallbladder neck with superimposed infection leads to cholecystitis
- Obstruction of common bile duct with superimposed infection leads to septic cholangitis
- Migration of a large stone into the gut may cause intestinal obstruction (gallstone ileus)

Clinical features
90% of gallstones are (probably) asymptomatic

Biliary colic
- Severe colicky upper abdominal pain radiating around the right costal margin ± vomiting
- Periodicity of hours, often onset at night; spontaneously resolves after several hours
- Differential diagnosis: myocardial infarction, peptic ulcer exacerbation, gastro-oesophageal reflux disease

'Chronic cholecystitis'
- Uncertain diagnosis suggested by vague intermittent right upper abdominal pain, distension, flatulence, fatty food intolerance
- May indicate recurrent mild episodes of cholecystitis
- Differential diagnosis: chronic peptic ulcer disease, gastro-oesophageal reflux disease

Acute obstructive cholecystitis
- Constant right hypochondrial pain, pyrexia, nausea ± jaundice

- Tender in right upper quadrant with positive Murphy's sign
- Leukocytosis
- Unresolved may lead to empyema of the gallbladder
- Differential diagnosis: myocardial infarction, basal pneumonia, pancreatitis, appendicitis, perforated peptic ulcer, pulmonary embolus

Cholangitis
- Abdominal pain, high fever/rigors, obstructive jaundice (Charcot's triad), severe right upper quadrant tenderness
- Differential diagnosis: myocardial infarction, basal pneumonia, pancreatitis, acute hepatitis

Obstructive jaundice
- Upper abdominal pain, pale/clay-like stools, dark-brown urine, pruritus
- May progress to cholangitis if common bile duct remains obstructed

Pancreatitis (see Chapter 29)
- Central/epigastric pain, back pain, fever, tachycardia, epigastric tenderness

Investigations
- Full blood count: acute inflammatory complications, picture of underlying haemolytic anaemias
- Urea and electrolytes
- Liver function tests: pattern of obstructive jaundice
- Plain X-ray of the abdomen shows only 10% of gallstones
- Ultrasound: detects 90% of gallstones. Assesses size of, and possible presence of stones in, common bile duct
- Other investigations rarely required (when ultrasound impossible, e.g. obesity): oral cholecystography, intravenous cholangiography, HIDA scanning
- ERCP: suspected or proven common bile duct stones. Allows stone removal or stent to be placed to bypass any risk of obstruction
- Oesophagogastroduodenoscopy: to exclude peptic ulcer disease as a cause for uncomplicated disease symptoms

Management
Asymptomatic
- No treatment required unless diabetic or undergoing major immunosuppression (risk factors for cholecystitis)

Prophylactic
- An attack of acute pancreatitis, cholangitis or obstructive jaundice is usually an indication for prophylactic cholecystectomy

Biliary colic
- Elective cholecystectomy, now usually performed laparoscopically, for classic symptoms with ultrasound-proven gallstones

Chronic cholecystitis
- Elective laparoscopic cholecystectomy only if no evidence of peptic ulcer disease or other cause for symptoms

Acute cholecystitis
- Intravenous fluids, antibiotics, early or interval cholecystectomy

Empyema
- Percutaneous (ultrasound- or CT-guided) drainage of gallbladder and interval cholecystectomy

Ascending cholangitis
- Prompt and energetic treatment mandatory if septicaemia/systemic inflammatory response syndrome is to be avoided
- Intravenous fluids, antibiotics, ductal drainage (now usually by ERCP, sphincterotomy and extraction of stones)
- Mortality 15–20% among patients requiring urgent decompression for severe cholangitis

Complications of cholecystectomy
- Leakage of bile from cystic duct or gallbladder bed
- Jaundice due to retained ductal stones. Retained stones can be treated by ERCP or if a T-tube is in place by extraction with a Dormia basket down the T-tube track (Burhenne manoeuvre)
- Injury to the common bile duct

Acalculous chronic gallbladder disease

Chronic inflammation of the gallbladder in the absence of gallstones is due to adenomyomatosis or cholesterolosis of the gallbladder and these may be grouped as acalculous chronic gallbladder disease. Both can give rise to vague symptoms not dissimilar to those of chronic cholecystitis. Thickening and 'polypoid' lesions/diverticulae may be documented by high-resolution ultrasound. In many instances, the diagnosis is made on pathological examination of the excised gallbladder.

Ductal calculi

The majority of ductal calculi are found in the common bile duct. In the West only an estimated 5% of ductal calculi are located in the intrahepatic ducts, although multiple intrahepatic calculi are common in eastern countries. Ductal calculi may be:
- secondary calculi from migration of gallstones;
- primary calculi arising *de novo* within the bile ducts.

Primary ductal calculi are brown pigment stones (infected) and are encountered in:
- stasis of the biliary tract;
- parasitic infestations;
- recurrent pyogenic cholangitis (Far East);
- indwelling endoprostheses.

Clinical features

The majority of ductal calculi (Fig. 28.5) are symptomatic and by and large incur a significant morbidity. Ductal calculi may present with:

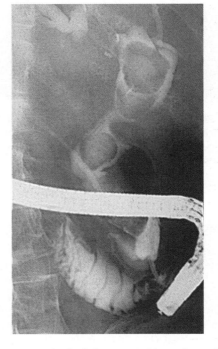

Figure 28.5 Ductal calculi documented by endoscopic retrograde cholangiopancreatography.

- recurrent bouts of biliary colic accompanied by intermittent jaundice;
- episodic upper abdominal pain and dyspepsia;
- stone impaction with progressive jaundice;
- cholangitis;
- gallstone pancreatitis;
- secondary biliary cirrhosis and portal hypertension.

04

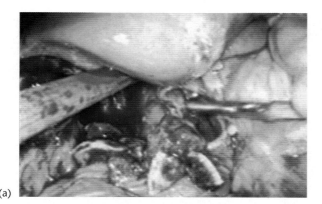
(a)

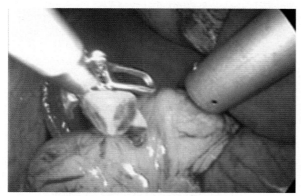
(b)

Figure 28.6 Laparoscopic surgery for ductal calculi: (a) direct extraction of multiple calculi via a choledochotomy; (b) extraction with a wire (Dormia) basket via the cystic duct suitable for small stones.

04

Management

The current treatment for ductal calculi is endoscopic sphincterotomy and stone extraction. In patients requiring cholecystectomy for symptomatic gallstone disease, endoscopic stone extraction is performed before the operation. However, single-stage treatment with ductal stone clearance at the time of laparoscopic cholecystectomy is also practised (Fig. 28.6). In fit patients single-stage laparoscopic surgical treatment is gaining favour among laparoscopic surgeons. However, endoscopic stone extraction is mandatory for:

- poor-risk patients;
- patients with cholangitis;
- patients with severe pancreatitis;
- in some patients with failed laparoscopic stone extraction as an alternative to conversion;
- retained or recurrent stones after cholecystectomy.

Ductal calculi discovered soon after cholecystectomy

Retained ductal calculi following biliary tract surgery are either diagnosed in the immediate postoperative period or present with recurrent symptoms, usually within 2 years of cholecystectomy without exploration of the common bile duct. Ductal stones presenting beyond this interval are generally considered to be of the primary variety.

The various methods available for the non-surgical management of retained stones are:

- flushing;
- dissolution;
- percutaneous stone extraction via the T-tube tract;
- endoscopic sphincterotomy and stone extraction.

The first three options are applicable only to patients with an indwelling T-tube, whereas endoscopic stone extraction can be used in all patients. All the above methods are performed under antibiotic cover because of the risk of cholangitis and septicaemia. Endoscopic sphincterotomy with stone extraction is the most effective method of dealing with the problem of retained stones.

Cholangitis

Acute bacterial cholangitis is a serious life-threatening emergency caused by infection of an obstructed biliary tract. The systemic manifestations result from bacteraemia. The most common obstructing agent is an occluding stone in the common bile duct, followed by bile duct strictures (including sclerosing cholangitis) and, less commonly, tumours of the bile ducts, pancreatic head and periampullary lesions. Cholangitis may also complicate bilioenteric anastomoses, spontaneous bilioenteric fistulae, cystic disease of the biliary tract and duodenal diverticulae. Cholangitis may also occur following instrumentation of the biliary tract, e.g. after ERCP. In the Far East, recurrent pyogenic cholangitis is common.

The infection is most commonly caused by Gram-negative organisms. The classic triad of symptoms consists of pain in the right hypochondrium, intermittent fever and jaundice (Charcot's biliary fever). Aside from toxicity, the high intermittent pyrexia is accompanied by severe rigors. The pain varies in intensity and may be severe. There is usually tenderness in the right hypochondrium that, if marked, suggests the presence of abscess formation. Nausea and vomiting are frequent accompaniments. Hypotension is found in patients with severe cholangitis, when renal failure is usually present.

Prompt and energetic treatment is mandatory. Resuscitative measures include intravenous fluids. A blood culture is taken and systemic antibiotics commenced

(cephalosporin with metronidazole or piperacillin, or imipenem). The majority respond to this treatment but some do not and these require emergency biliary decompression. For most patients endoscopic decompression by sphincterotomy and extraction of calculi is generally favoured, especially if the patient is elderly. If the calculi cannot be extracted, a temporary pigtail stent is inserted endoscopically to drain the proximal biliary tree into the duodenum. The alternative is surgical exploration with ductal clearance and insertion of a T-tube. The overall reported mortality of patients requiring urgent decompression for severe cholangitis is 15–20%.

Sclerosing cholangitis

This is an obscure disorder of uncertain aetiology that results in progressive fibrous obliteration of the biliary tract. Often, sclerosing cholangitis occurs as a secondary complication of inflammatory bowel disease, usually ulcerative colitis. The disease progresses invariably to cirrhosis and the development of portal hypertension. Sclerosing cholangitis occurs more commonly in males and usually presents in the fifth decade. The symptoms include vague ill health, asthenia, pain in the right hypochondrium, jaundice and itching, pyrexia and attacks of rigors. The liver is often palpable and tender. Liver function tests demonstrate a cholestatic picture and bilirubin is detected in the urine. Serum transaminases are mildly elevated. The majority of patients are HBsAg-negative. Contrast radiological visualization shows pruning of the biliary tree (scanty ducts) and stricture formation, which may be localized or diffuse. Differentiation from hilar and diffuse cholangiocarcinoma may be difficult on radiological grounds and even after histological examination of biopsy specimens. There is no effective medical or surgical therapy for the condition and these patients are treated by hepatic transplantation.

Biliary disorders in acquired immunodeficiency syndrome

Patients suffering from AIDS are prone to develop acute acalculous cholecystitis, papillary stenosis and a cholangiopathy that closely simulates sclerosing cholangitis. Both papillary stenosis and cholangiopathy with intrahepatic and extrahepatic strictures are frequent and are thought to be caused by infection with cytomegalovirus and *Cryptosporidium*, although in some patients these pathogens are absent. In these cases, the biliary tract changes may be caused by direct invasion of the bile duct mucosa by human immunodeficiency virus. The diagnosis is confirmed by ERCP. Patients with papillary stenosis obtain biochemical improvement and relief of pain by endoscopic sphincterotomy.

Haemobilia

Major (profuse) haemobilia is rare but when it occurs spontaneously is caused by rupture of an intrahepatic aneurysm. Nowadays, significant haemobilia is most commonly encountered as a complication of percutaneous radiological interventions on the liver and following hepatic trauma. The vascular injury within the hepatic parenchyma caused by transhepatic radiological interventions results in an arteriovenous fistula or pseudoaneurysm or direct vascular–biliary connection. If the bleeding is marked, blood clots with biliary colic complicate the clinical picture. Treatment is by percutaneous embolization of the bleeding site. The second most common cause is blunt or penetrating hepatic trauma. Traumatic haemobilia may be treated by direct ligation of the vessels inside the liver haematoma or by percutaneous selective arterial embolization. Minor haemobilia may also be caused by stones, primary hepatic tumours including angiomas, gallbladder and bile duct polyps, parasitic infestations and extracorporeal shock-wave lithotripsy for ductal calculi.

Bilioenteric fistulae

The vast majority of external biliary fistulae occur in the postoperative period and may result from the following:
- leakage of bile from a slipped cystic duct ligature or cut accessory bile duct;
- trauma to the extrahepatic biliary tree during cholecystectomy, gastric surgery or pancreatectomy;
- dislodged T-tube after common bile duct exploration;
- leakage from bilioenteric anastomosis;
- hepatic resections.

Postoperative external biliary fistulae occurring in association with jaundice indicate bile duct trauma or a missed obstructive lesion of the biliary tract. These patients require urgent investigation with ultrasonography/CT and ERCP.

Internal fistulae are usually spontaneous and arise from chronic or acute perforation of the gallbladder into an adjacent organ. Others are due to malignant infiltration arising from or involving the gallbladder, e.g. carcinoma of the hepatic flexure, duodenum or gallbladder. The symptoms of non-malignant internal fistulae involving the gallbladder are similar to those of chronic cholecystitis but jaundice and cholangitis are more common and radiology of the abdomen shows gas or barium in the biliary tree. The most frequent of the internal fistulae is the

04

liver may be enlarged or the gallbladder may be palpable. Ascites is encountered in advanced disease. Anaemia is present in 50% of patients and is due to chronic hae-mobilia. Even in the presence of a normal serum bili-rubin, the majority of patients have an elevated alkaline phosphatase. Few patients with stage I or II disease are diagnosed preoperatively. Although ultrasound examina-tion of the gallbladder identifies advanced disease, it misses the early potentially curable lesions. Useful diagnostic information is obtained by CT angiography or magnetic resonance imaging (MRI). The highest diagnostic yield is obtained by laparoscopy with contact ultrasonography and this is nowadays regarded as the gold standard for diagnosis and staging of this tumour.

Treatment of cancer of the gallbladder is surgical, although opinions vary as to the exact operative proced-ure that should be performed. For stages I–III, the best results are reported with extended cholecystectomy. Initially, the gallbladder is removed and the diagnosis confirmed by frozen section. If positive and the tumour is stage I–III, a 3-cm resection of surrounding hepatic parenchyma is performed together with lymph node clearance. If the tumour is advanced, some advocate an aggressive approach with right lobectomy and regional node clearance. Long-term survival is only very rarely encountered after aggressive major resections. Thus even if resectable, patients with stage II–IV disease are generally regarded as incurable in view of the uniformly poor prog-nosis. In inoperable patients with jaundice and itching, palliation can be achieved by endoscopic/radiological stenting with a metal expanding endoprosthesis or sur-gically by round ligament segment III bypass. The response of gallbladder cancer to radiotherapy and chemotherapy is poor.

A frequently encountered problem relates to patients in whom unsuspected gallbladder cancer is found after laparoscopic cholecystectomy on pathological examina-tion of the resected specimen. In these cases, the port wound through which the gallbladder was extracted should be excised full thickness. Thereafter, if the cancer is pT_1 (confined to mucosa/submucosa) no further action is needed except for careful follow-up. If the tumour involves the muscularis, then hepatic resection (segments 4, 5) and lymph node clearance is wise provided the patient's general condition is good.

Tumours of the bile ducts

A variety of benign tumours of the bile duct, including adenoma and papilloma, have been reported but they are rare and far less common than cholangiocarcinomas. Benign bile duct tumours have a tendency to recur after excision and some have been reported to undergo malig-

Table 28.4 High-risk groups for development of cholangio-carcinoma.

Parasitic infestation of the biliary tract
Cystic disease of the biliary tract
Chronic typhoid carriers
Ulcerative colitis
Sclerosing cholangitis

nant change. Benign bile duct tumours present with jaun-dice and occult chronic gastrointestinal haemorrhage (haemobilia).

The prevalence of carcinomas of the biliary tract and gallbladder in England and Wales is 2.8 per 100,000 in females and 2 per 100,000 in males. Contrary to gallbladder cancer, there is a slight preponderance of males. The age at presentation varies but the peak incidence is in the sixth decade. Bile duct carcinoma is very common in Far East countries where parasitic infestation is endemic. The median age at presentation of cholangiocarcinomas in areas of endemic infestation with *Opisthorchis viverrini* is 52 years. The aetiology of bile duct cancer is unknown. The association with gallstones is much less marked than it is with carcinoma of the gallbladder, although ductal calculi are found in 20–50% of patients who develop cholangiocarcinoma. Bacterial-induced endogenous car-cinogens derived from bile salts have been implicated and their role is supported by the findings of some epidemi-ological studies and the higher incidence in typhoid carriers. Cholangiocarcinoma is seen with increasing fre-quency in certain clinical groups (Table 28.4).

The tumours are best classified into anatomical site of origin.
- Intrahepatic: from the minor hepatic ducts (intrahep-atic cholangiocarcinomas).
- Proximal: from the right and left hepatic ducts, hilar confluence and proximal common hepatic duct (Klatskin tumours).
- Middle: from the distal common hepatic duct, cystic duct and its confluence with the common bile duct.
- Distal: from the distal common bile duct, ampullary and periampullary regions.
The gross appearance of extrahepatic cholangiocarcino-mas assumes one of three forms: stricture (scirrhous vari-ety), nodular or papillary. The scirrhous variety can be very difficult to distinguish from sclerosing cholangitis even on histological grounds. These tumours are generally confined to the proximal ducts (hilar) and form grey annular thickenings with clearly defined edges. The nodular tumours form extraductal nodules in addition to intraluminal projections. The papillary variety is most commonly found in the distal bile duct and periampullary

04

region. These lesions are friable and may fill the duct lumen with vascular neoplastic tissue and tend to bleed in the ductal lumen causing haemobilia. The majority of tumours are adenocarcinomas of varying differentiation. All cholangiocarcinomas are slow-growing, locally infiltrative but have a special predilection for perineural spread and do not metastasize beyond the liver. The best prognosis is encountered after resection, especially of distal ampullary and periampullary lesions.

In patients with intrahepatic cholangiocarcinomas, mild abdominal pain is the most frequent presenting clinical symptom. Presentation with jaundice is uncommon. If a mass lesion is detected by imaging (CT, MRI, etc.), preoperative biopsy is ill-advised since it may result in local implantation. The main presentation in patients with extrahepatic cholangiocarcinomas is obstructive jaundice, which is progressive and accompanied by itching and anorexia. Weight loss is not evident until the disease is advanced. Dull upper abdominal pain is a frequent symptom. Some patients present acutely with cholangitis or acute cholecystitis. The duration of symptoms is usually short. In the West, distal bile duct stones and proximal extrahepatic malignant biliary obstructions may coexist. These stones probably predate the development of the malignant obstruction and are found in 12–18% of patients with proximal tumours. Physical examination reveals hepatomegaly. Microcytic hypochromic anaemia is present in patients with papillary tumours at the lower end of the bile duct and in the periampullary region. The faeces of these patients have a characteristic silvery appearance due to a combination of steatorrhoea and altered blood. A palpable gallbladder is present in patients with distal tumours. CT does not permit sufficiently precise anatomical localization to predict the exact site and resectability of the tumours. The definitive investigation is MRCP. ERCP is indicated for ampullary and periampullary lesions.

Resection (for both intrahepatic and extrahepatic lesions) is the best method of treatment and is indicated for all operable tumours in fit individuals. The percutaneous insertion of iridium-192 wire has been used to provide local irradiation (brachytherapy) with good results. Survival benefit has been reported from postoperative radiotherapy after resection of hilar (Klatskin) tumours. Cholangiocarcinomas of the bile ducts are generally regarded to be unresponsive to chemotherapy, although response rates have been documented with mitomycin C, doxorubicin and FUDR.

Non-surgical palliation

In patients who are considered inoperable on preoperative assessment and those who are too old and frail or have serious cardiorespiratory disease, palliation of jaundice is best achieved by percutaneous transhepatic or endoscopic stenting. The endoprosthesis has to be large (8–10F) and may require replacement if it becomes blocked with calcium bilirubinate encrustation. Self-expanding wire biliary endoprostheses are now used frequently for these malignant strictures. Their big advantage over plastic stents is that they can be introduced through a small-calibre sheath and on expansion have a much larger lumen. These self-expanding metal stents are contraindicated in patients with polypoid tumours as the fronds of the neoplasm project through the wire framework into the lumen. Approximately 15% of patients develop stent occlusion at a mean interval of 4 months after insertion of metal stents. In 80% occlusion is due to tumour overgrowth and in 20% to debris. Occlusion by tumour ingrowth is treated by internal plastic stents. Occlusion by debris is effectively cleared by sweeping the stent with a balloon catheter.

Distal tumours

These include:
- distal bile duct tumours;
- ampullary tumours;
- periampullary carcinoma;
- primary duodenal carcinoma.

Ampullary tumours can be either adenomas or adenocarcinomas. Some arise in association with familial polyposis coli. Ampullary carcinomas have a higher resectability rate and better prognosis than periampullary carcinomas, although the prognosis is poor when the disease is advanced. Several studies have now shown that preoperative staging is best achieved by endoscopic ultrasound, which has a high accuracy of tumour (T) staging although it is less reliable in detecting lymph node involvement. The options for treatment of ampullary tumours include local excision, pancreaticoduodenectomy and endoscopic management (endoscopic papillectomy and debulking, endoscopic stenting).

Periampullary tumours are generally more advanced than ampullary lesions and include ampullary carcinomas that have spread to involve the adjacent mucosa, although they are considered to be distinct from primary duodenal carcinoma. By definition this includes tumours located within 1 cm of the papilla. When operable and in fit patients, the treatment is pancreaticoduodenectomy. Local excision (transduodenal papilloduodenectomy) is indicated in frail patients. The resection includes the papilla, distal bile duct and pancreatic duct with surrounding pancreatic tissue. Following excision, the pancreatic and common bile duct are sutured together and then to the defect in the medial wall of the duodenum.

04

Tumours of the biliary tract at a glance

Definition

Tumours of the biliary tract: benign or malignant lesions of the gallbladder or the bile ducts

Benign tumours

- Benign gallbladder tumours are usually found incidentally and are adenomas or papillomas
- A gallbladder polyp > 10 mm on ultrasound should be treated by cholecystectomy
- Papillomas and adenomas of the bile ducts are very rare

Carcinoma of the gallbladder

- Most common malignancy of the biliary tree
- Aetiology: unknown but increased incidence with calcified gallbladder and gallstones (typhoid carriers, South American Indians, obesity)
- Majority are adenocarcinomas (very rarely carcinoid, melanoma or ACTH apudoma)
- Staging
  I: confined to mucosa/submucosa
  II: muscle layer involved
  III: serosa involved
  IV: spread to cystic node
  V: invasion of liver and local organs
- Usually found accidentally during cholecystectomy or at histological examination

- May present as mass in right upper quadrant. Anorexia, weight loss, anaemia, haemobilia, jaundice
- Most are advanced (stage IV–V) at time of diagnosis
- Wide surgical excison for early-stage (I–III) disease recommended
- Palliation only (e.g. stenting for relief of jaundice) for advanced disease
- Prognosis is poor in majority of patients, who have advanced disease

Cholangiocarcinoma

- Uncommon tumours, 2–3 per 100,000
- Age of onset: sixth decade
- Common in Far East where parasitic infestation (*Opisthorchis viverrini*) is endemic
- Classification
- Majority are adenocarcinomas and are slow-growing
- Patients present with jaundice
- Definitive investigation is MRCP
- Resection is indicated for operable tumours
- Brachytherapy (local irridation via percutaneous iridium-192 wire) gives good results
- In inoperable patients, palliation is achieved by percutaneous transhepatic or endoscopic stenting

	Duct of origin	Type
Intrahepatic	Minor hepatic ducts	Scirrhous
Klatskin tumour	Right and left hepatic ducts and hilar confluence	Scirrhous
Middle	Distal common hepatic duct, cystic duct	Nodular
Distal	Common bile duct and (peri)ampullary	Papillary

Evidence-based medicine

Coakely, F.V. & Schwartz, L.H. (1999) Magnetic resonance cholangiopancreatography. *J Magn Reson Imaging* 9, 157–62.

Cuschieri, A., Croce, E., Faggioni, A., *et al.* (1999) EAES multicentre prospective randomized trial comparing two-stage vs. single-stage management of patients with gallstone disease and ductal calculi. *Surg Endosc* 13, 952–7.

Kiviluoto, T., Siren, J., Luukkonen, P. & Kivilaakso, E. (1998) Randomised trial of laparoscopic vs. open cholecystectomy for acute and gangrenous cholecystitis. *Lancet* 351, 321–5.

Kubo, H., Chijiiwa, Y., Akahoshi, K., Hamada, S., Matsui, N. & Nawata, H. (1999) Pre-operative staging of ampullary tumours by endoscopic ultrasound. *Br J Radiol* 72, 443–7.

Strasberg, S.M., Hertl, M. & Soper, N.J. (1995) An analysis of the problem of biliary injury during laparoscopic cholecystectomy. *J Am Coll Surg* 180, 101–25.

Disorders of the Pancreas

Must know Must do

Must know

Clinical features, diagnosis and management of acute pancreatitis

Clinical features and principles of management of chronic pancreatitis

Clinical features and principles of management of tumours of the exocrine pancreas

Core knowledge of endocrine pancreatic tumours and their presentation

Must do

Clerk patients with alcoholic- and gallstone-associated acute pancreatitis

Clerk and follow the management of patients with carcinoma of the pancreas

Examine CT angiography scans of necrotizing acute pancreatitis

Examine CT scans of pancreatic pseudocysts

Examine CT scans of cancer of the pancreas

Anatomy and physiology

The pancreas is a large central retroperitoneal gland overlying the vertebral column in the supracolic compartment of the abdomen. It has a complex vascular supply and venous/lymphatic drainage and is surrounded by the duodenum and upper jejunum. It has two components:

● exocrine, concerned with secretion of enzymes necessary for digestion of foodstuffs

● endocrine, which elaborates important hormones essential for metabolism.

The exocrine pancreas consists of lobules composed of acinar glands that drain via the main pancreatic duct into the duodenum. The exocrine secretion contains water and bicarbonate ions and digestive enzymes secreted as inactive precursors (zymogens) into the duodenum in response to neural and hormonal influences. Enzyme activation begins after the zymogens enter the duodenum, where mucosal enterokinase cleaves trypsinogen into trypsin, which activates the other enzymes.

The endocrine pancreas consists of the islets of Langerhans, which comprise four recognized cell types.

● A cells (α cells): synthesize, store and secrete glucagon.

● B cells (β cells): synthesize, store and release insulin; also form islet amyloid-associated polypeptide and pancreastatin.

● D cells: secrete somatostatin and probably gastrin.

● F cells: secrete pancreatic polypeptide (HPP).

The main stimulus for insulin secretion is an increase in blood glucose levels (hyperglycaemia). Insulin causes the blood glucose concentration to decrease but further insulin secretion is inhibited by glucose concentration via a negative feedback mechanism. Other stimuli for insulin release include amino acids (arginine and lysin) and other hormones (glucagon, growth hormone, cortisol, placental lactogen, oestrogens). Insulin release is also enhanced by free fatty acids in order to prevent ketoacidosis which would otherwise occur during fasting in normal individuals.

Glucagon secretion is stimulated by low blood glucose levels (hypoglycaemia). It has catabolic actions and initiates glycogenolysis, increasing glucose formation from non-glucose precursors and enhancing the breakdown of fat into free fatty acids and glycerol. Glucagon also stimulates gluconeogenesis from plasma amino acids and inhibits protein synthesis.

Somatostatin is an inhibitory hormone. It inhibits growth hormone, insulin and glucagon secretion, gastric acid and pepsin secretion, the release of pancreatic enzymes and intestinal motility. It reduces splanchnic blood flow. The physiological function of HPP remains unknown.

Investigations

These may be categorized as follows.

● Imaging: radiology, ultrasonography, computed tomography (CT), magnetic resonance imaging (MRI), endoscopic retrograde cholangiopancreatography (ERCP).

● Test of pancreatic exocrine function: faecal fat excretion, secretory tests.

● Tests of endocrine function:

  (a) fasting blood glucose;

04

361

(b) hormone assays (insulin, C-peptide, glucagon, gastrin, somatostatin, etc.);

(c) provocation tests: calcium infusion test (insulinoma and gastrinoma), glucagon test (insulinoma), secretin test (gastrinoma).

- Estimation of serum markers: enzymes (amylase), tumour-associated antigens (pancreatic oncofetal antigen, CA19-9).
- Pancreatic biopsy and cytology.

Plain radiography is useful for detection of pancreatic calcification, which is present in:

- some types of chronic pancreatitis;
- hereditary pancreatitis;
- cystic neoplasms of the pancreas;
- pancreatic lymphangiomas/haemangiomas.

Ultrasonography is a very useful investigation for the detection of pancreatic disease. CT is carried out to confirm localized or diffuse enlargement of the gland detected by ultrasound examination. ERCP is used to visualize the duodenum, ampulla of Vater and to cannulate the pancreatic duct and in patients with suspected pancreatic cancer and chronic pancreatitis, although magnetic resonance cholangiopancreatography (MRCP) is replacing diagnostic ERCP for this purpose. Likewise, endoscopic ultrasonography (EUS) is very useful in the evaluation of the jaundiced patient where it detects lesions in the head of the pancreas that can be sampled by EUS-guided fine-needle aspiration cytology.

Congenital anomalies

Ectopic pancreas

The most common site for ectopic pancreatic tissue is the wall of the stomach, duodenum or jejunum. The majority of cases remain asymptomatic. However, some give rise to abdominal pain, abnormal gastric emptying (by lesions situated in the pyloric region), peptic ulceration, gastrointestinal haemorrhage or intussusception.

Annular pancreas

This consists of a ring of pancreatic tissue, continuous with the head of the pancreas, surrounding the second part of the duodenum proximal to the ampulla of Vater. It may cause duodenal obstruction with half of the cases presenting during the first year of life. There are often associated intrinsic abnormalities, e.g. atresia or stenosis of the duodenum, Down's syndrome, malrotation of the mesentery, imperforate anus, oesophageal atresia and congenital heart disease. Vomiting is the main symptom and jaundice may be present. The diagnosis is comfirmed by contrast radiological studies. Other patients with annular

pancreas present for the first time between the ages of 21 and 70 years and these cases often have co-existing duodenal ulcer disease. The treatment is either duodenoduodenostomy or duodenojejunostomy.

Pancreas divisum

Pancreas divisum is discussed in Chapter 28.

Pancreatitis

Clinically, pancreatitis (inflammation of the pancreas) may be acute or chronic but acute disease may lead to the chronic condition. Thus a patient who survives severe acute (necrotizing) pancreatitis may sustain irreparable damage to the pancreas that precludes normal restitution and the disease then progresses to chronic pancreatitis. Likewise, recurrent attacks of acute pancreatitis from any cause may lead to the chronic disease.

Acute pancreatitis

The exact mechanism that initiates pancreatic inflammation and autodigestion and the factors that determine the severity of the disease (mild to moderate self-limiting or a necrotizing severe often fatal disease) remain unclear. There is an established association with specific disorders:

- alcoholism;
- biliary tract stone disease (gallstone-associated pancreatitis);
- viral infections (mumps and coxsackie B viruses), *Mycoplasma pneumoniae* (usually mild);
- metabolic disorders (hypercalcaemia);
- drug therapy (diuretics and steroids);
- ERCP;
- trauma including surgery and pancreatic biopsy;
- postoperative (splenectomy, gastrectomy, bile duct exploration);
- fulminant liver failure.

The first two account for 95% of cases. Gallstone pancreatitis most commonly occurs in patients older than 60 years, may be severe and accompanied by serious complications but recurrences are prevented by cholecystectomy. In contrast, alcoholic pancreatitis is a recurring disease often of young males unless the patient abstains from alcohol. The first attacks are usually severe, although subsequent ones tend to be mild. The recurring episodes of inflammation cause progressive destruction of the gland, leading to chronic pancreatitis or chronic relapsing pancreatitis.

Clinical features

Acute pancreatitis is classified as (i) mild (oedematous) acute pancreatitis or (ii) severe (necrotizing) acute pancreatitis. Distinction between the two is difficult at the *onset* of the disease. The clinical manifestations of acute pancreatitis can be misleading and the disease can coexist with acute cholecystitis or bacterial cholangitis. Acute pancreatitis is rare in children and young adults, in whom it is usually associated with infections, trauma and drugs or is hereditary.

The onset of symptoms is usually sudden, pain being the major initial symptom in the vast majority. The severity of the pain is variable though always constant. The location of the pain is diffuse epigastric with radiation to the flanks and back. Some patients may adopt certain postures to alleviate the pain. Bending forwards, or much more commonly, the patient draws up the knees to ease the abdominal discomfort. Other common symptoms include nausea, vomiting, retching and hiccups. In severe disease, tachypnoea and dyspnoea may be marked. The physical findings vary with the severity of the disease but fever, tachycardia, epigastric tenderness and muscle guarding are frequent. Hypotension usually indicates severe disease. Mild jaundice is frequently present as is abdominal distension caused by paralytic ileus.

In severe disease, there is renal failure or progressive ventilatory difficulty leading to acute respiratory distress syndrome (ARDS). The abdominal tenderness and ileus become more marked. A palpable epigastric mass may be felt several days after the onset of the disease (indicating the development of a pseudocyst or marked peripancreatic fat necrosis). Rarely in severe haemorrhagic disease, a bluish discoloration of the skin around the umbilicus (Cullen's sign) or in the loins (Grey Turner's sign, Fig. 29.1) may be encountered.

The diagnosis is confirmed by marked elevation of serum amylase to a value exceeding five times normal for the laboratory. Although hyperamylasaemia can be encountered in other acute disorders, e.g. infarcted small bowel, the levels are much lower. However, amylase levels in the blood decline within a few days of onset and thus may be normal if the determination is carried out late in the course of the disease. Persistence of hyperamylasaemia indicates the development of local complications such as pseudocyst formation or pancreatic abscess. As amylase clearance is increased threefold for 1–2 weeks in patients with acute pancreatitis with normal renal function, increased urinary output of amylase persists longer than hyperamylasaemia and may thus be helpful in the diagnosis of late cases. Other biochemical abnormalities that may be present in severe disease include hyperglycaemia and hypocalcaemia.

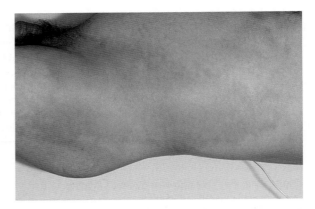

Figure 29.1 Grey Turner sign in a patient with severe necrotizing pancreatitis.

A plain radiograph of the abdomen and chest may show intestinal distension in the region of the pancreas (sentinel jejunal loop, colon cut-off, duodenal ileus) or a generalized paralytic ileus. Haziness in the supine plate of the abdomen is caused by retroperitoneal fluid accumulation and may be associated with obliteration of the psoas shadow. The chest x-ray may show basal atelectasis, sub-diaphragmatic fluid collection, or pleural effusions.

The common acute disorders that require exclusion are:
- acute cholecystitis and acute cholangitis (both may coexist with acute pancreatitis);
- perforated peptic ulcer;
- acute appendicitis;
- acute upper small-bowel obstruction.

The early identification of severe disease (day 1 or 2 of admission) is important as timely administration of broad-spectrum antibiotics decreases the incidence of pancreatic and peripancreatic infection. Thus imipenem (Meropenim) when administered within 48 h of onset and maintained for 10 days in patients with severe (necrotizing) pancreatitis reduces the incidence of pancreatic/peripancreatic infection from 40% to 20%.

The differentiation of mild from severe acute pancreatitis is not possible on clinical features alone and disease-severity scores are needed to confirm severe disease. Ranson developed 11 objective criteria and confirmed that the risk of death and/or major complications can be determined objectively by five parameters on admission to hospital and six parameters within the initial 48 h of admission (Table 29.1). In patients with less than three of these 11 prognostic factors, the mortality rate is low (1%); with three to four factors, 18%; with five to six factors, 50%; and with more than six factors, 90%. A similar system based on parameters obtained within 48 h was

04

On admission	Within 48 h
Age > 55 years	Haematocrit fall > 10%
White cell count > 16×10^9/L	Blood urea nitrogen rise > 5 mg/dL
Blood glucose > 10 mmol/L	Serum calcium < 2.0 mmol/L
Aspartate aminotransferase > 250 U/dL	Pa_{O_2} < 8 kPa
Lactate dehydrogenase > 350 U/L	Base deficit > 4 mEq/L
	Estimated fluid sequestration > 6 L

Table 29.1 Ranson's prognostic grading system for acute pancreatitis (three or more positive criteria signifies severe acute pancreatitis).

Table 29.2 Imrie (Glasgow) prognostic grading system for acute pancreatitis (all within 48 h).

Age > 55 years
White cell count > 15×10^9/L
Blood glucose > 10 mmol/L and patient not diabetic
Serum albumin < 32 g/L
Blood urea > 16 mmol/L with no response to i.v. fluids
Lactate dehydrogenase > 600 U/L
Aspartate aminotransferase/alanine aminotransferase
    > 100 U/L
Serum calcium < 2.0 mmol/L

proposed by Imrie and is sometimes known as the Glasgow grading (Table 29.2). Both systems have been replaced by the APACHE II scoring system, which gives better differentiation and has the added advantage that it can be used *at any time* in the course of the disease. The APACHE II system allocates three sets of points: A, B and C.
- A: assessment of clinical parameters, e.g. vital signs, electrolytes, arterial blood gases, etc.
- B: points allocated in accordance with age.
- C: points added for comorbid disease or chronic health of patient.

The APACHE II score is the sum of A, B and C; if this exceeds 9, the patient has severe acute pancreatitis. Mortality is very high if the score increases after admission.

Urinary trypsin activated peptide (TAP), serum trypsinogen-2 and C-reactive protein (CRP) are also useful in the differentiation of mild from severe disease. In this respect CRP is only reliable as an index of severity after the second or third day of the disease. CRP levels in excess of 100 mg/dL usually indicates necrotizing pancreatitis.

Treatment

Once diagnosis is established, initial treatment is conservative with:

- correction of hypovolaemia by replacement of fluid, electrolytes, blood or plasma;
- serial clinical, haematological, respiratory and biochemical assessment;
- ultrasound examination of gallbladder and biliary tract;
- CT scanning of the pancreas;
- analgesia;
- nasogastric suction except in very mild attacks;
- enteral feeding or parenteral hyperalimentation, depending on severity;
- antibiotics for severe disease (Meropenim and Cilastin);
- ERCP in selected cases of severe disease (for ampullary obstruction, associated bacterial cholangitis).

Careful monitoring of vital signs, hourly urine output and central venous pressure measurements is important. Arterial blood gases *must* be measured during the first few days in view of the risk of respiratory failure. Severe cases are managed in the HDU or ICU if they need respiratory support. Medical treatment is continued for patients with severe disease unless they develop complications or the pancreatic necrosis becomes infected. Patients with mild (not severe) gallstone-associated pancreatitis are best treated with laparoscopic cholecystectomy (with operative cholangiography) on the next available operating list (early cholecystectomy). Thus the indications for surgical treatment are as follows:

- when the diagnosis is in doubt;
- for patients with mild gallstone-associated acute pancreatitis (early cholecystectomy);
- for patients with severe pancreatitis who do not improve with medical treatment and are found to have infected pancreatic necrosis by CT-guided aspiration of peripancreatic fluid;
- for the treatment of complications (pseudocyst, pancreatic abscess).

Acute pseudocysts (Fig. 29.2), usually discovered by ultrasound scanning, are managed expectantly for up to 6 weeks as spontaneous resolution is common. Surgical treatment is undertaken if the cyst has not resolved, by which time it has a thick (mature) wall. Most commonly

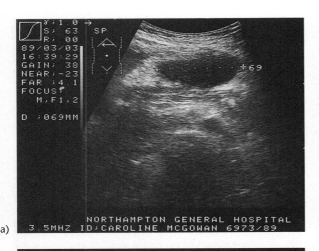

(a)

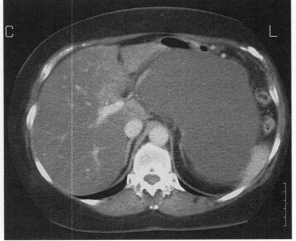

(b)

Figure 29.2 (a) Ultrasound scan and (b) a CT of acute pancreatic pseudocyst.

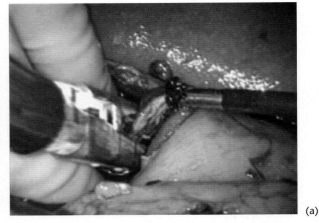

(a)

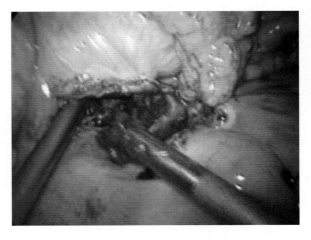

(b)

Figure 29.3 Hand-assisted laparoscopic cystogastrostomy for mature pancreatic pseudocyst: (a) stapling of walls of the stomach and cyst wall together; (b) completed anastomosis.

the treatment consists of surgical internal drainage of the cyst into the stomach (cystogastrostomy) and can be performed laparoscopically (Fig. 29.3). Alternatively, some retrogastric pseudocysts can be treated by the endoscopic insertion of a stent between the cyst cavity and the stomach. Patients with infected pancreatic necrosis are very ill and their only chance of survival is necrosectomy (removal of necrotic pancreatic/peripancreatic tissue) followed by irrigation of the lesser sac with hypertonic crystalloid solution for several days (Fig. 29.4).

Recurrent acute pancreatitis is caused by:
- alcohol abuse;
- missed biliary tract disease including biliary sludge;
- papillary stenosis/papillitis (rare);
- pancreas divisum;
- familial.

Figure 29.4 Laparoscopic necrosectomy for infected pancreatic necrosis.

04

The most common congenital abnormality leading to recurrent pancreatitis is pancreas divisum (see Chapter 28).

Surgical treatment of chronic pancreatitis

Patients with chronic pancreatitis present a management problem. Where the disease is caused by alcohol abuse, abstinence is essential and is as important as the surgical procedure in determining the outcome. The indications for surgical treatment in patients with chronic pancreatitis are:

- Intractable pain requiring opioid medication
- The development of complications (lower bile duct obstruction, duodenal obstruction, bleeding from microaneurysms or splenic vein thrombosis, pancreatic cysts, pseudocysts and suspicious mass lesion).

The most common cause necessitating surgical intervention is intractable chronic pain. If the main pancreatic duct is not dilated (narrow-duct pancreatitis, Fig. 29.5a), the treatment is bilateral thoracoscopic splanchnicectomy (section of all splanchnic nerve roots that carry sensory fibres from the pancreas). Substantial and lasting pain relief is obtained in 70% of cases. Resection is reserved for patients who do not respond or have an inflammatory 'pseudotumour' (usually in the head of the pancreas). If the ductal system is dilated, pain can be relieved by pancreaticojejunostomy (Peustow's operation), which consists essentially of a long anastomosis between the dilated duct and a Roux-loop of jejunum (Fig. 29.5b).

Some patients develop frank obstructive jaundice. In these patients, it is often impossible to exclude an underlying cancer preoperatively and even at laparotomy. For these patients, a total pancreatoduodenectomy may be performed. If cancer can be excluded, a biliary bypass by choledochojejunostomy is performed.

Tumours of the exocrine pancreas

Benign neoplasms of the non-endocrine pancreas are exceedingly rare and of no clinical significance. Thus for clinical purposes, all tumours of the exocrine pancreas are regarded as malignant.

Pancreatic cancer

This is pancreatic ductal adenocarcinoma and originates in the head of the pancreas (in about 70% of cases). It has to be differentiated from cancer arising from the periampullary region (ampulla, duodenum or lower bile duct), which has a much better prognosis. The incidence of pancreatic adenocarcinoma has tripled over the past 40 years throughout the western world. It continues to carry a dismal prognosis, with 5-year survival rates of 1–2%. Cancer

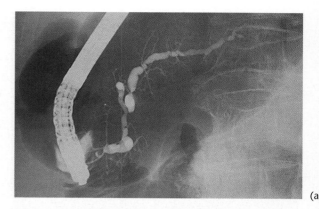

(a)

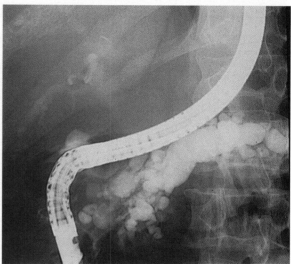

(b)

Figure 29.5 Endoscopic retrograde cholangiopancreatography in chronic pancreatitis: (a) narrow-duct disease; (b) dilated-duct disease suitable for pancreaticojejunostomy (Peustow's operation).

of the pancreas is more common in older people and is relatively uncommon below the age of 50 years.

The exact causative factors are unknown but there is an association with cigarette smoking and diabetes mellitus. Patients with hereditary chronic pancreatitis have a higher risk of developing pancreatic cancer than the general population.

Clinical features

Irrespective of site, the disease is asymptomatic in the early stages and, when located distally (in the body and tail), pancreatic ductal adenocarcinoma is usually inoperable when the diagnosis is made.

Pancreatitis at a glance

Definition

Pancreatitis: an inflammatory condition of the exocrine pancreas that results from injury to the acinar cells. It may be acute or chronic

Aetiology
- Gallstones and alcohol abuse account for 95% of cases of acute pancreatitis
- Other causes include idiopathic, congenital structural abnormalities, drugs, viral infections, hypercalcaemia, hypothermia, hyperlipidaemia and trauma (ERCP)

Pathology
Acute
Mild injury
- Acinar (exocrine) cell damage with enzymatic spillage, inflammatory cascade activation and localized oedema
- Local exudate may also lead to increased serum levels of pancreatic enzymes (amylase, lipase, colipase)

Moderate injury
- Increasing local inflammation leads to intrapancreatic bleeding, fluid collections and spreading local oedema involving the mesentery and retroperitoneum
- Activation of the systemic inflammatory response leads to progressive involvement of other organs

Severe injury
- Progressive pancreatic destruction leads to necrosis, profound localized bleeding and fluid collections around the pancreas
- Spread to local structures and the peritoneal cavity may result in mesenteric infarction, peritonitis and intra-abdominal fat 'saponification'
- Persisting accumulation of inflammatory fluid in the lesser sac is a pseudocyst, i.e. does not have an epithelial lining

Chronic
- Recurrent episodes of acute inflammation lead to progressive destruction of acinar cells with healing by fibrosis
- Incidental islet cell damage may lead to endocrine gland failure

Clinical features
- Mild/moderate pancreatitis: constant upper abdominal pain radiating to back, nausea, vomiting, pyrexia, tachycardia ± jaundice
- Severe/necrotizing pancreatitis: severe upper abdominal pain, signs of hypovolaemic shock, respiratory and renal impairment, silent abdomen, retroperitoneal bleeding with flank and umbilical bruising (Grey Turner and Cullen's signs)

Management
- Most pancreatitis is mild and resolves spontaneously
- All patients should have a cause sought by imaging and the severity assessed by recognized criteria
- Attempt to confirm diagnosis: serum amylase > 1000 U diagnostic (may be clinical diagnosis)
- Normal or mildly elevated serum amylase does *not* exclude pancreatitis
- Assess disease severity (Imrie/Ranson criteria or APACHE II system)
- Resuscitate the patient:
  - (a) Mild/moderate disease: i.v. fluids, analgesia, monitor progress with pulse, blood pressure, temperature
  - (b) Severe pancreatitis: full resuscitation in ICU with invasive monitoring
- Establish the cause: ultrasound to look for gallstones

Further management
- No proven use for routine nasogastric tube or antibiotics
- Consider vitamin supplements and sedatives if alcoholic cause
- Proven common bile duct gallstones may require urgent ERCP
- Failure to respond to treatment or uncertain diagnosis warrants abdominal CT scan
- Suspected/proven infection of necrotic pancreas: antibiotics ± surgical débridement

Complications of acute pancreatitis
Acute
- Pancreatic abscess: usually necrotic pancreas present
- Intra-abdominal sepsis
- Necrosis of the transverse colon
- Respiratory failure (ARDS) or renal failure (acute tubular necrosis)
- Pancreatic haemorrhage

Subacute/chronic
- Pseudocyst formation: may need to be drained internally or externally
- Chronic pancreatitis

Chronic pancreatitis
- Usually caused by chronic alcohol abuse
- Presents with intractable abdominal pain and evidence of exocrine pancreatic failure (steatorrhoea) and eventually diabetes as well
- Medical treatment is with analgesia and exocrine pancreatic enzyme replacement
- Surgical treatment is by drainage of dilated pancreatic ducts or excision of the pancreas in some cases. Splanchnicectomy is performed sometimes for intractable pain

04

Progressive cholestatic jaundice, with dark urine and pale stools, occurs in the majority of patients with carcinoma of the head of the pancreas, the incidence of jaundice as a presenting feature decreasing with more distal location. Weight loss and anorexia are also common symptoms even in the early stages. Nausea, epigastric bloating, change in bowel habit and vomiting are occasionally present. Pain can also be experienced. In advanced disease, haematemesis and melaena may result from direct invasion of the duodenal mucosa by tumour and duodenal obstruction may supervene. Fever and rigors may accompany the jaundice (bacterial cholangitis) and tend to occur in long-standing biliary obstruction. A palpable gallbladder (Courvoisier's sign) is present in one-quarter of patients with resectable tumours. The liver is often enlarged on palpation.

In distal cancer (body and tail), pain and weight loss are the two main consistent symptoms. The pain is dull and localized to the epigastrium or the back and radiates to either upper quadrant. Severe pain indicates advanced disease with involvement of the retroperitoneal nerves. At presentation, weight loss is usually substantial. Haematemesis may be due to bleeding gastric varices from occlusion of the splenic vein with sectorial portal hypertension. Migratory thrombophlebitis (Trousseau's sign) can be present but indicates advanced disease and is not specific to pancreatic cancer. On rectal examination a rectal shelf may be evident in the rectovesical or rectovaginal pouch (Blumer's shelf). There may be evidence of ascites, and distant metastases may be present in the supraclavicular fossa (Troisier's sign).

Thin-section CT (pancreatic protocol) or MRI provides the best diagnostic yield in suspect cases, supplying information on pancreatic mass, its relationship to the superior mesenteric artery and vein and to the coeliac axis, patency of the portal vein, and liver metastases. Until recently, ERCP combined with cytology has been used to differentiate choledocholithiasis from malignant obstruction of the distal common bile duct when a mass was not seen on CT. MRCP and EUS have replaced ERCP for this purpose because of their high diagnostic rate and avoidance of pancreatitis (Fig. 29.6). Staging laparoscopy is used to detect inoperable disease (especially peritoneal deposits) and thus avoid unnecessary laparotomy.

Surgical treatment

For resectable cancer of the head of the pancreas (judged by preoperative staging), the surgical treatment is resection by pancreaticoduodenectomy (Whipple's operation) in which the following are removed en bloc: head and neck of the pancreas, duodenum, distal half of the stomach, lower common bile duct and gallbladder and upper

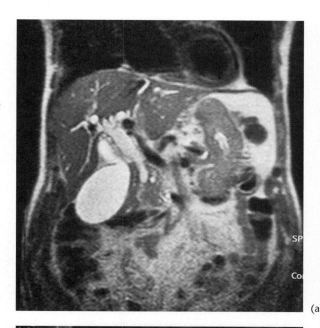
(a)

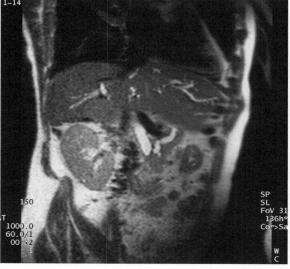
(b)

Figure 29.6 (a) Magnetic resonance cholangiopancreatography showing a large inoperable pancreatic adenocarcinoma with dilated gallbladder and dilated and obstructed common bile duct; (b) another view from the same patient showing dilated and obstructed bile and pancreatic ducts, giving the 'double duct' sign.

jejunum with the regional lymph nodes (Fig. 29.7). An alternative is the modification known as the pylorus-preserving pancreaticoduodenectomy in which the stomach and duodenum are preserved to eliminate post-gastrectomy symptoms. Cancers of the body of the pancreas are rarely operable but when they are, resection

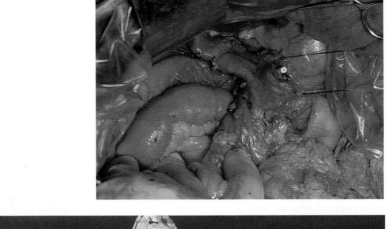

(a)

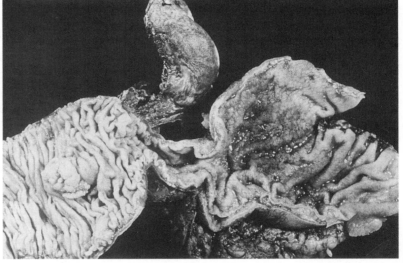

(b)

04

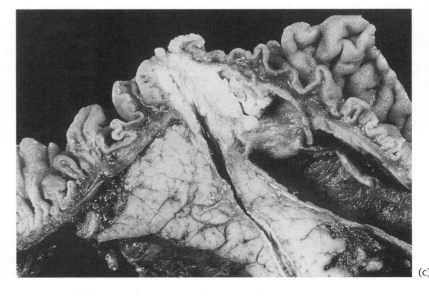

(c)

Figure 29.7 Pancreaticoduodenectomy (Whipple's procedure). (a) Photograph during surgery before reconstruction showing the exposed portal vein after resection of the specimen. The transected pancreas is held up with two stay sutures to the right of the portal vein. (b) Whole specimen consisting of gallbladder, head of pancreas, duodenum (opened showing the periampullary tumour) and antrum of stomach. (c) Close-up of the periampullary carcinoma. This patient is still alive 10 years after the operation.

consists of total pancreatoduodenectomy. Operable cancers of the tail are treated by distal pancreatosplenectomy. Survival after resection is improved by chemotherapy with irradiation using infusional 5-fluorouracil and external beam supervoltage radiotherapy. Newer agents such as gemcitabine are currently being studied in combination with radiation as an alternative to 5-fluorouracil. Even so 5-year survival is rare after resection of pancreatic cancer. In contrast, excellent 5-year survival (50% or more) is obtained after Whipple's operation for periampullary cancers.

Palliation of inoperable disease

This is aimed at relief of:
- jaundice and pruritus;
- vomiting due to duodenal obstruction;
- pain.

Relief of jaundice and pruritus is achieved by endoscopic or transhepatic (radiological) stenting using self-expanding metallic stents, which have largely replaced plastic stents for this purpose. Endoscopic/radiological stenting has replaced surgical biliary bypass, cholecystojejunostomy (Fig. 29.8) or choledochojejunostomy unless duodenal obstruction is also present when a double bypass (biliary bypass and gastrojejunostomy) is needed. Severe pain is often present and requires palliation with any of the following:
- percutaneous coeliac plexus block with 50 mL of 50% alcohol or 20 mL of 6% phenol;
- bilateral thoracoscopic splanchnicectomy;
- opioid analgesia.

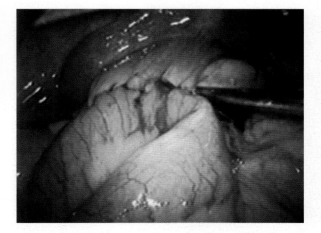

Figure 29.8 Laparoscopic cholecystojejunostomy for relief of jaundice in a patient with inoperable pancreatic cancer.

Tumours of the endocrine pancreas

Pancreatic endocrine tumours may be benign or malignant. Compared with pancreatic adenocarcinoma, endocrine tumours, even when malignant, are slow-growing and many metastasize only to regional lymph nodes. Hence curative surgical excision is possible in a significant proportion of patients. Normal islet cells also synthesize the protein chromogranin along with specific peptide hormones. Elevated plasma levels of chromogranin or neurone-specific enolase are thus useful markers for pancreatic endocrine tumours. The important clinical syndromes associated with overproduction of hormones by pancreatic islet cell tumours are:
- insulinoma — hyperinsulinism (autonomous hypoglycaemia);
- overproduction of gastrin with intractable ulceration — gastrinoma (Zollinger Ellison syndrome).

Hyperinsulinism

This may be caused by:
- B-cell neoplasia (insulinoma), most common endocrine tumour;
- B-cell hyperplasia/microadenomatosis, rare, occurs in infants.

The excess circulating insulin manifests as symptomatic hypoglycaemia. Insulinoma is the most common endocrine tumour in adults. The majority are benign solitary tumours occurring with an even distribution in the head, body and tail (Fig. 29.9). Multiple tumours are associated with multiple endocrine neoplasia type 1 (MEN1) syndrome (see later). Malignant insulinoma (B-cell carcinoma) is rare and tends to be larger than 2 cm at presentation. It invades local tissues and spreads to regional lymph nodes and liver (Fig. 29.10). Primary hyperinsulinism is rare in infants and children and is then usually caused by B-cell hyperplasia/microadenomatosis.

Most of the symptoms are the result of adrenergic hyperactivity consequent on episodes of hypoglycaemia, e.g. weakness, sweating, hunger, palpitations and tremor. In addition, the hypoglycaemia has direct cerebral effects leading to headaches, visual disturbance, dizziness, confusion, aggressive behaviour, seizures and coma. The diagnosis is initially suspected by documenting the relationship of the symptoms to fasting or physical exercise with relief of symptoms on eating. Thus the diagnosis of insulinoma is based on:
- recognition of the symptom complex and relation to fasting and exercise;
- documentation of fasting hypoglycaemia;
- demonstration that the plasma insulin concentration is inappropriately high for the plasma glucose level.

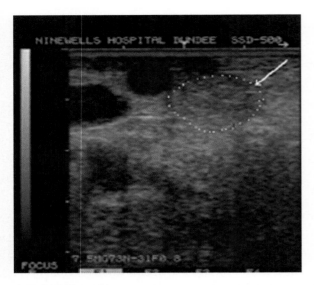

Figure 29.9 Benign insulinoma localized by laparoscopic contact ultrasonography. The insulinoma, which was above the splenic vein on the posterior surface of the pancreas, appears as a hypoechoic oval lesion.

The hypoglycaemia must be differentiated from reactive postprandial (reactive hypoglycaemia) hyperinsulinism. In these patients, the low plasma glucose occurs only in response to meals. Patients with reactive hypoglycaemia never have symptoms when fasted. In contrast, fasting hypoglycaemia in an otherwise healthy individual usually indicates an insulinoma in the adult or islet cell hyperplasia in the neonate or infant and all insulinoma

patients will develop symptomatic hypoglycaemia during a 72-h fast.

Most insulinomas are small benign adenomas (< 1.5 cm) and may be wholly embedded in the pancreas. Thus, preoperative localization may be difficult but should be attempted in all patients using angiography, MRI, angio helical CT, somatostatin scan and EUS (for tumour in head). Preoperative localization proves unsuccessful in 30% of patients with biochemically-confirmed insulinoma (occult insulinomas). Hence the importance of thorough exploration of the pancreas by manual palpation and contact ultrasound examination during surgery. Intraoperative contact ultrasound of the pancreas (Fig. 29.9) has proved invaluable for the identification of occult insulinomas during open and laparoscopic surgery. Preoperative measurement of immunoreactive insulin in blood sampled from selective catheterization of small pancreatic veins via the percutaneous transhepatic route is performed when preoperative imaging tests fail to localize the tumour. This may help to indicated the probable site and thus guide the intraoperative exploration.

Surgical management

If the diagnosis is confirmed biochemically but the insulinoma is occult, the surgeon carries out a thorough exploratory laparotomy. The entire pancreas and peripancreatic area are examined visually, by palpation and by contact ultrasound examination during the operation. Full mobilization of the gland is required for this purpose. Insulinomas are slightly firmer than normal pancreas to palpation. All enlarged lymph nodes in the peripancreatic region and any liver lesions found are submitted for

04

Figure 29.10 Malignant insulinoma diagnosed by magnetic resonance cholangiopancreatography (white arrow) before surgery, which consisted of radical distal hemipancreaticosplenectomy with lymph node clearance.

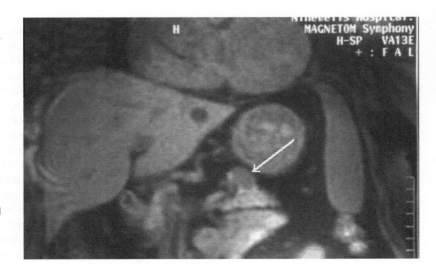

frozen section histological evaluation to exclude metastatic disease. Solitary insulinomas are enucleated through the cleavage plane between the capsule and the pancreatic parenchyma. Distal pancreatectomy or, very occasionally, pancreaticoduodenectomy with pyloric preservation are indicated only for deeply situated tumours that cannot be enucleated safely. Subtotal pancreatectomy is undertaken for multiple tumours throughout the gland, as seen in MEN1 patients. Malignant insulinoma is treated by total pancreatectomy with regional lymphadenectomy. Even if the tumour is inoperable, as much tumour mass is removed as is safely possible since debulking provides good palliation with resolution of hypoglycaemic symptoms and increases the likelihood of successful chemotherapy.

The results of surgical treatment of insulinoma suggest that about 75% of patients are cured, with some 10% developing diabetes following extensive pancreatic resection. About 10–15% of patients have persistent or recurrent hypoglycaemia requiring reoperation at some time. The major operative complications include pancreatitis, abscess, fistula and pseudocyst formation.

Neonatal and infantile hyperinsulinism

Autonomous hyperinsulinism accounts for 20–30% of all cases of unremitting hypoglycaemia in neonates and infants. Such hypoglycaemia can lead to irreversible central nervous system damage and thus requires early recognition, thorough investigation and expeditious treatment. These patients require a high intravenous and/or oral glucose intake to prevent brain damage in addition to specific treatment with diazoxide, somatostatin or a variety of other agents (epinephrine, diphenylhydantoin, glucocorticoids, glucagon, growth hormone). Urgent surgical intervention is required when medical management fails to control the hypoglycaemia caused by the hyperinsulinaemia. The underlying pathology in the vast majority of neonates and infants with hyperinsulinism consists of nesidioblastosis, B-cell adenomatosis or islet cell hyperplasia. Hence imaging techniques used to localize islet cell tumours in adults are inappropriate and have no place in the management of these children. Likewise, palpation of the pancreas at operation and biopsies for frozen section histological examination are noncontributory. The correct surgical treatment consists of 80–90% extended distal pancreatectomy with splenic preservation. If postoperative monitoring of glucose levels indicates that the resection has been inadequate, medical therapy is reinstated and consideration given to reoperation in all neonates with persistent unremitting hypoglycaemic episodes after surgery. The reoperation consists of near total (95%) pancreatectomy with preservation of the distal bile duct and duodenum. Permanent exocrine or endocrine insufficiency is unusual in infants less than 3 months of age because of the considerable regenerative capacity of the infantile pancreas.

Medical treatment

Therapy with diazoxide to reduce excess insulin secretion is indicated for persistent hypoglycaemia in the preoperative phase and when operation is unsuccessful or contraindicated because of the poor condition of the patient. Diazoxide is a benzothiadiazine that inhibits the release of secretory granules from normal islet B cells and insulinoma cells. The dose has to be individualized because of variable individual efficacy. Close monitoring of patients is essential as there are serious side-effects such as oedema, bone marrow depression, hyperuricaemia, cardiomyopathy and hirsutism in females. Long-acting analogues of somatostatin (octreotide) are also effective in the treatment of hyperinsulinism in inoperable patients with insulinoma. Octreotide both inhibits secretion of peptide by the hyperfunctioning islet tumour cells and reduces target organ receptivity. Two-thirds of patients have obtained good symptomatic relief with this treatment. However, there are little or no antitumour effects in malignant insulinoma. Streptozotocin selectively destroys pancreatic islet cells by inhibiting DNA synthesis, is the chemotherapeutic agent of choice for metastatic insulinoma. Objective tumour regression occurs in about 60% of patients and survival is doubled in those who respond to the drug. Combinations of octreotide, streptozotocin and diazoxide are often useful in treating functioning malignant insulinoma.

Gastrinoma (Zollinger–Ellison syndrome)

The syndrome was first described by Zollinger and Ellison in 1955 in two patients with fulminant intractable peptic ulcer disease, marked gastric acid hypersecretion in conjunction with a non-beta islet cell tumour of the pancreas. Zollinger and Ellison were the first to suggest that the excessive gastric acid secretion responsible for the peptic ulceration was caused by a hormone secreted by the tumour. They indicated erroneously that glucagon was the responsible factor. Subsequently, Gregory Tracey and Grossman extracted the peptide hormone gastrin from the stomach and the tumours which were characterized as non-beta, non-alpha. A radioimmunoassay was developed for gastrin and the hormone was found to be markedly elevated in the plasma of patients with Zollinger–Ellison syndrome.

Clinical features and diagnosis

The incidence of Zollinger–Ellison syndrome is approximately 1 in 100,000. The disease is more common in men than women, the male/female ratio being 3 : 2. Zollinger–Ellison syndrome has been reported in patients ranging in age from 7 to 90 years but the majority of patients are between the third and fifth decades. It should be stressed that the syndrome is very rare, and only 1 in 750 patients with peptic ulcer disease will have an underlying gastrinoma.

About one-quarter of patients with Zollinger–Ellison syndrome have a gastrinoma as part of MEN1 syndrome. Gastrinomas in patients with MEN1 are less likely to be malignant but are almost always multifocal. This is in contrast to patients with sporadic gastrinoma in whom the disease is more often malignant but somewhat less often multifocal. Overall, gastrinoma is malignant in about half of patients and arises in the pancreas in 75%. The most common extrapancreatic primary tumour site is the duodenum. Tumours in this location are solitary in about half of cases. Much less commonly, primary gastrinomas are found in the greater omentum, lymph nodes, liver and gastric antrum. Malignant gastrinomas metastasize to regional lymph nodes and liver.

Peptic ulcer disease is present in over 90% of gastrinoma patients. All patients with ulcers have severe dyspeptic pain, which does not respond well to medical treatment (including eradication therapy). Coexisting diarrhoea is a common complaint and is the presenting symptom in a few patients (5%) with gastrinoma. As a result of large fluid and potassium losses in the colon, these patients develop dehydration, wasting and weakness from hypokalaemia. The diarrhoea results primarily from the incessant severe gastric acid hypersecretion and the accompanying rapid gastric emptying. Thus a continous large acid load is delivered to the duodenum and upper jejunum with lowering of the intestinal pH to a level that inactivates pancreatic lipase and other digestive enzymes. In addition the severe acid load induces a direct intestinal mucosal injury with ulceration further aggravating the malabsorption and steatorrhoea. Hypergastrinaemia also increases intestinal motility and inhibits water and salt absorption from the jejunum.

The majority of patients with Zollinger–Ellison syndrome are diagnosed late, usually after several years of symptoms and repeated gastric operations in the past for intractable ulcer disease. However, with increasing awareness of the disease during the past decade, the interval between onset of symptoms and diagnosis of the disease has been considerably reduced. Nowadays, the vast majority of patients are diagnosed prior to being subjected to any elective gastric surgery. All of the known complications of peptic ulcer disease are encountered in patients with the Zollinger–Ellison syndrome. Acute upper GI haemorrhage and duodenal perforation are very common (20% each), whereas vomiting and other symptoms of gastric outlet obstruction are less than ordinary peptic ulcer disease. Dr Wilfred Sircus of Edinburgh referred to patients with the Zollinger–Ellison syndrome as 'recurrent ulcerators, persistent perforators, and bleeders unto death.' Severe, refractory reflux oesophagitis is common. When present, physical signs include weight loss, epigastric tenderness and intestinal hypermotility. Intra-abdominal tumour masses are rarely palpable but hepatic enlargement secondary to massive metastatic deposits is occasionally seen at initial presentation. The diagnosis of Zollinger–Ellison syndrome should be considered in any patient with:

- severe peptic ulcer disease refractory to medical therapy, including eradication of *Helicobacter pylori*;
- multiple peptic ulcers or ulcers in unusual locations such as the distal duodenum or jejunum;
- recurrent peptic ulcer disease following an acid-reducing operation;
- peptic ulcer disease in association with a strong family history of ulcer disease or MEN1; or
- peptic ulcer disease in association with any other component of MEN1 (e.g. hypercalcaemia).

The upper GI endoscopy usually shows large gastric mucosal folds and diffuse inflammation or frank ulceration distal to the duodenal bulb and barium contrast radiology may demonstrate ulcers in the distal duodenum and upper gastrointestinal tract. The diagnosis is confirmed by radioimmunoassay of fasting plasma. A basal gastrin level greater than 100 pg/mL strongly supports the diagnosis of gastrinoma. The majority of patients have fasting gastrin levels exceeding 200 pg/mL. Hypergastrinaemia can occur in association with gastric hypochlorhydria or achlorhydria, e.g., pernicious anaemia, chronic atrophic gastritis, gastric cancer, prior vagotomy or histamine H_2-receptor antagonist or omeprazole therapy, but the levels are well below 200 ph/mL. However for added confirmation it is important to measure gastric basal acid output in all patients suspected of the disease.

The principal circulating form of gastrin in patients with the Zollinger–Ellison syndrome is G-34 or 'big gastrin'. This is a precursor of the active gastrin, a situation that is analogous to insulinomas where elevated levels of precursor forms of insulin are found. There is little or no correlation between the level of the fasting plasma gastrin and the tumour mass. Gastric outlet obstruction secondary to ordinary duodenal ulcer disease, antral G-cell hyperfunction or hyperplasia, and retained gastric

04

antrum after Billroth II gastrectomy are other conditions associated with peptic ulcer in which elevated basal plasma gastrin levels may be found. These can be differentiated from gastrinoma by a number of provocative tests. The best of these is the secretin stimulation test. Following intravenous injection of secretin (2 µg/kg), the plasma gastrin level rises within 5–10 min to a level 200 pg/mL greater than the basal level in patients with gastrinoma, but not in those with other conditions. The meal provocation test may be used to differentiate gastrinoma from antral G-cell hyperfunction. In this test, a standard meal is ingested by the patient and causes a marked rise in plasma gastrin levels in patients with G-cell hyperfunction but no rise or only a minimal one in gastrinoma patients.

A basal level acid output greater than 15 mmol/h strongly supports the diagnosis as does a value greater than 5 mmol/h in the patient who has had previous acid-reducing gastric surgery for peptic ulcer disease. Upper gastrointestinal endoscopy and a standard barium meal and follow-through should be performed in all patients suspected of the disease. In addition to the mucosal abnormalities often found with these studies, on rare occasion a duodenal or antral polypoid lesion has proved to be a gastrinoma on biopsy. All patients diagnosed as having Zollinger–Ellison syndrome should be further investigated to exclude the presence of MEN1 syndrome (see later).

Tumour localization

Preoperative techniques to localize gastrinomas are not often successful. External abdominal ultrasonography is rarely helpful as gastrinomas are usually small and deeply in the pancreas. Approximately two-thirds of gastrinomas can be identified with thin section current-generation CT scanners. However, tumours smaller than 7 mm are virtually never identified preoperatively by this technique. MRI is useful because islet cell tumours produce an unusually intense signal. Since most gastrinomas are hypovascular, visceral angiography is of little benefit in preoperative localization. Both EUS and octreoscan are useful in detection of gastrinomas and other neuroendocrine tumours. The combination of both increases the sensitivity. The sensitivity of EUS depends on the endoscopist and ranges from 70 to 95%. Octreoscan detection rate depends on the level of density of somatostatin receptors in the tumour.

Thus the current preoperative imaging tests are no more capable of localizing the tumour any more reliably than careful intraoperative exploration by the experienced surgeon. Intraoperative contact ultrasonography may prove valuable in the localization of small tumours within the pancreatic gland. Experience with this technique remains limited at present but early reports suggest that half of non-palpable tumours can be localized by this method. Intraoperative upper GI endoscopy with transillumination of the duodenal wall is also useful for the intraoperative localization of duodenal gastrinomas.

Medical treatment

Proton pump inhibitors (PPIs) that inhibit the potassium-hydrogen ATPase of the parietal cell are the most powerful and specific inhibitor of gastric acid secretion and constitute the mainstay of the medical treatment of patients with Zollinger–Ellison syndrome. They control acid hypersecretion in approximately 98% of gastrinoma patients although the dose required in the individual patient is highly variable. An increase in dose appears necessary over time in one-quarter of patients. PPIs are now the only antisecretory drugs for all gastrinoma patients.

Surgical treatment

Prior to the advent of PPIs, total gastrectomy was required in virtually all gastrinoma patients to prevent mortality from the acute complications of peptic ulceration. With PPIs the situation has changed and gastrectomy is rarely indicated nowadays in view of the satisfactory control of acid secretion by these agents in the majority of patients. The role of surgery has thus changed to control of the tumour itself. In 30% of patients the tumour(s) can be removed by local excision or enucleation with a 30% 5-year disease-free survival.

Patients with liver metastases and/or MEN1 syndrome are treated medically and total gastrectomy only performed when medical therapy has failed. All young and middle-aged patients without metastatic liver disease on preoperative imaging are treated by elective laparotomy with a view to complete tumour excision. Even patients with involvement of regional lymph nodes can be cured by adequate regional lymphadenectomy. The pancreatic tumour itself is removed by enucleation or distal pancreatectomy only and major resections avoided. Successful removal of all gastrin-secreting tumours is confirmed by serial negative plasma gastrin responses to secretin stimulation. However, long-term follow up is necessary because of tumour recurrence and these are detected by a rise in the fasting serum gastrin level.

Results with chemotherapy for advanced hepatic metastases are poor. Streptozotocin and 5-fluorouracil are the only drugs with some therapeutic efficacy. Octreotide can be effective in controlling the symptoms and hypergastrinaemia in patients with inoperable disease. Gastrinoma patients with MEN1

syndrome and hyperparathyroidism should have parathyroid surgery performed before surgical removal of the gastrinoma(s).

Often the parathyroidectomy provides marked amelioration of ulcer symptoms and marked reduction of gastric acid secretion and plasma gastrin levels. As these effects are transient, resection of the gastrinoma should not be delayed.

Vipoma (Werner–Morrison syndrome, pancreatic cholera)

The syndrome of watery diarrhoea, hypokalaemia and achlorhydria in association with an islet cell tumour of the pancreas was initially described by Werner and Morrison in 1958. A number of hormones have been identified in these tumours but vasoactive intestinal polypeptide (VIP) is now known to be the causative agent in the majority of cases. VIP stimulates pancreatic, intestinal and gallbladder water and electrolyte secretions as well as pancreatic enzyme secretion and secretion of potassium by the colonic mucosa. VIP inhibits absorption of water and electrolytes in the small intestine and colon and also inhibits acid and pepsin secretion in the stomach.

Patients with this condition develop profuse secretory diarrhoea causing severe dehydration and hypokalaemia. Acidosis usually accompanies the hypokalaemia and patients suffer from lethargy and weakness as a result of the dehydration and electrolyte abnormalities. Virtually all patients sustain significant weight loss; a majority have abdominal colic and a few experience cutaneous flushing. Slightly less than half of the tumours are malignant and metastases to the liver are often found at the time of diagnosis. The primary tumour is located in the body and tail of the pancreas in approximately 75% of cases, and is almost always solitary. Forty per cent are malignant and usually larger than 3 cm before causing symptoms. Extrapancreatic vipomas include ganglioneuromas and neuroblastomas and are capable of causing the identical clinical syndrome.

The diagnosis is confirmed by assay of plasma levels of VIP, which exceed 190 pg/mL. The tumour is easily localized because of its usual large size by external and endoscopic ultrasonography, CT and angiography. Tumours less than 1 cm are difficult to detect by CT.

Medical treatment consists of fluid and electrolyte replacement and maintenance therapy. Usually large volumes (5 L or more) of intravenous crystalloids are required per day. Glucocorticoids or octreotide are helpful in controlling the diarrhoea. Octreotide is effective in 90% of patients with marked amelioration of the diarrhoea, dehydration and electrolyte losses.

The definitive treatment of vipoma is surgical excision of the tumour whenever possible. Debulking of metastatic disease often provides effective palliation. Since the majority of non-metastatic cases are caused by large solitary pancreatic tumours, enucleation or distal pancreatectomy are often curative. Patients who are inoperable or who develop recurrent disease may obtain symptomatic benefit from therapy with long-acting somatostatin analogues. Streptozotocin is also reasonably effective in palliation but immediately following administration, diarrhoea and electrolyte losses may be exacerbated for several days. The prognosis is poor with advanced disease, and thromboembolic complications due to excessive dehydration are often responsible for major morbidity and mortality. The occasional patient with pancreatic cholera secondary to prostaglandin E_2 hypersecretion may obtain dramatic relief with indomethacin.

Glucagonoma

Glucagonoma is a very rare tumour arising from the A-cell of the pancreatic islet. It gives rise to a characteristic syndrome consisting of severe skin rash, weight loss, diabetes mellitus, deep venous thrombosis, anaemia and hypoaminoacidaemia. Glucagonoma is considerably more common in females and is a disease of middle age. The majority of tumours (60–70%) have already metastasized at the time of diagnosis, predominantly to the liver. The typical skin rash consists of necrolytic migratory erythema with symmetrical erythematosus lesions that have crusted erosions and involve the perineum, groin, thighs, buttocks and lower limbs. The systemic manifestations include weight loss, weakness, lethargy and hyperglycaemia due to the metabolic and catabolic effects of high plasma glucagon levels. Most patients are diabetic but ketonaemia rarely develops because the circulating insulin level is not increased. Panhypoaminoacidaemia is always present and is responsible for the skin rash and any neurological deficits that may develop. The anaemia is normocytic and normochromic and does not respond to iron and vitamin therapy.

The diagnosis is confirmed by finding elevated plasma glucagons concentration. Normal values range between 50 and 150 pg/mL. Values of glucagon greater than 1000 pg/mL are often encountered. In most patients glucagon release from the tumour can be induced by the administration of arginine or tolbutamide. Pancreatic polypeptide levels are elevated in half of patients. The tumour is localized by CT, EUS, MRI and octreotide scintigraphy.

The definitive treatment is surgical. Operative exploration is indicated even for advanced metastatic disease as debulking procedures may significantly alleviate the debilitating catabolic effects of the excess glucagon. When

04

surgical resection is not an option, selective arterial embolization and chemotherapy are indicated. Streptozotocin combined with 5-fluorouracil can produce reduction in both tumour size and glucagon levels. Dimethyltrizenoimidazole carboxamide is effective in providing symptomatic relief and healing or improvement of skin lesions. Octreotide is highly efficacious in both the preoperative management and as palliative therapy. It reduces circulating glucagon levels, improves the skin rash, attenuates the severity of the systemic manifestations and helps to restore positive nitrogen balance with parenteral nutrition. Use of the somatostatin analogue is indicated in all cases regardless of the stage of disease or surgical plan. Treatment with interferon alfa can prolong survival and control the symptoms of the disease. Combination treatment with interferon alfa and octreotide or chemotherapy gives the best results.

Somatostatinoma

This is a very rare somatostatin-secreting tumour which occurs mostly in middle-aged predominantly female patients in the pancreas or the duodenum. Over 80% of the tumours have metastasized to the liver at the time of diagnosis. Most tumours produce other hormones such as VIP, pancreatic polypeptide, gastrin, calcitonin or cortisol. The clinical syndrome is often non-specific. Abdominal pain is the most common presenting symptom and this may relate to the high prevalence of gallstones. Other symptoms and signs include diarrhoea, diabetes mellitus (25%), weight loss, anorexia, hypochlorhydria, steatorrhoea and anaemia. Symptoms not related to excessive somatostatin levels are present in some patients, e.g., tachycardia, flushing, hypertension, hypokalaemia and hypoglycaemia.

Ideally, treatment is by surgical excision of the pancreatic or duodenal lesion. Debulking of advanced tumours may be efficacious and some patients benefit from adjunctive therapy with streptozotocin and 5-fluorouracil. The 5-year survival is poor (15%).

Human pancreatic polypeptide tumour

HPPomas are rare and arise from pancreatic polypeptide-secreting cells (also known as D2-cells or F cells). They do not give rise to a specific clinical syndrome although a few are associated with diarrhoea and a pruritic rash. The identification of the disease is difficult because elevated levels of pancreatic polypeptide in the plasma are found in many patients with various islet cell tumours of the pancreas (gastrinoma, glucagonoma) and carcinoid tumours. Most HPPomas grow to a large size and as they are usually located in the head of the pancreas, resection involves pancreaticoduodenectomy. Chemotherapy with streptozotocin may benefit patients with unresectable and/or metastatic disease.

Non-functioning endocrine pancreatic tumours

Some 10–15% of islet cell tumours have been diagnosed without any accompanying symptoms or signs other than those relating to a mass lesion. These tumours usually present late, often with hepatic metastatic disease although most are slow growing. The best treatment for non-functioning islet cell tumours is surgical resection. Chemotherapy is effective in some of these tumours.

Further therapeutic possibilities for the treatment of advanced islet cell malignancies

Many islet cell tumours have a high concentration of somatostatin receptors; pick-up radiolabelled octreotide, and can be localized by scintigraphy. The radiotherapeutic value of radiolabelled octreotide is under investigation. There are reports of successful outcome of metastatic glucagonoma treated with peptide receptor radiotherapy demonstrating decrease in tumour burden and in circulating glucagon levels. If all extrahepatic tumours can be eradicated, there are successful instances of orthotopic liver transplantation for multiple liver metastases. Cryotherapy of liver metastases and percutaneous injection of the lesions with ethanol under ultrasound guidance are being investigated in limited numbers of patients.

Multiple endocrine neoplasia type 1 syndrome (MEN1; MEA1 Wermer's syndrome)

MEN1 syndrome is inherited as an autosomal dominant disorder but exhibits considerable phenotypic variability. The pancreas, parathyroid glands and pituitary are involved in all patients. The pancreas is inevitably involved, with diffuse islet cell disease consisting of micronodular and macronodular hyperplasia and often with multiple tumours secreting multiple peptide hormones. Hyperparathyroidism is present in 85% of cases, with hyperplasia of all four glands, in sharp contrast with the very low incidence of parathyroid hyperplasia in isolated primary hyperparathyroidism. Pancreatic abnormalities occur in the vast majority of MEN1 patients, with non-B-cell tumours (especially gastrinoma) being most common.

Chromophobe adenomas and particularly prolactinomas are the most frequent pituitary lesions. When small, these tumours may be asymptomatic but in male patients are associated with antiandrogenic manifestations due to excess prolactin. Tumours producing growth hormone cause acromegaly. Adrenocortical non-functioning adenomas and rarely glucocorticoid-secreting adrenal lesions, have been documented. Other occasional associations of MEN1 include thyroid nodules, bronchial and intestinal carcinoids and lipomas.

All patients with endocrine pancreatic tumours should be investigated for additional manifestations of MEN1 syndrome. Screening of all available family members is also indicated.

Multiple endocrine neoplasia type 2 syndrome (MEN2; MEA2; Sipple's syndrome)

This is inherited as an autosomal dominant and is not associated with pancreatic disease. It consists of hyperparathyroidism, medullary carcinoma of the thyroid gland and phaeochromocytoma. MEN2b is a variant, also inherited as an autosomal dominant but unlike MEN2, has a very low incidence of parathyroid disease. It is characterized by multiple mucosal neuromas, intestinal ganglioneuromatosis leading to megacolon and constipation, a Marfanoid habitus and characteristic facies (thickened lips and alae nasi), in association with the medullary carcinoma of the thyroid and phaeochromocytoma.

Pancreatic tumours at a glance

Definitions

Pancreatic adenocarcinoma: malignant lesion of the head, body or tail of the pancreas

Periampullary carcinomas: arise around the ampulla of Vater and include tumours of the pancreas, duodenum, distal bile duct and the ampulla itself

Endocrine pancreatic tumours: cause a variety of syndromes secondary to the secretion of active peptides

Tumours of exocrine pancreas
Epidemiology
- Male/female ratio 2 : 1
- Age 50–70 years
- Incidence of pancreatic carcinoma is increasing in the western world

Aetiology
- Predisposing factors: smoking, diabetes, chronic pancreatitis

Pathology
- Site: 55% involve head of pancreas, 25% body, 15% tail, 5% periampullary region
- Macroscopic: growth is hard and infiltrating
- Histology: 90% ductal, 7% acinar cell, 2% cystic, 1% connective tissue origins
- Spread: lymphatics to peritoneum and regional nodes, via bloodstream to liver and lung. Metastases often present at time of diagnosis

Clinical features
Head of pancreas or periampullary
- Painless progressive jaundice with a palpable gallbladder (Courvoisier's law: a palpable gallbladder in the presence of jaundice is unlikely to be due to gallstones)
- Occasionally, duodenal obstruction causing vomiting

Body of pancreas
- Back pain, anorexia, weight loss, steatorrhoea
- New aching back pain and vague symptoms may be only presenting features

Tail of pancreas
- Often presents with metastases, malignant ascites or unexplained anaemia

Investigations
- Ultrasound: may see mass in head of pancreas and distended biliary tree, facilitates needle biopsy
- CT: demonstrates tumour mass, facilitates biopsy, assesses involvement of surrounding structures and local lymph node spread
- ERCP: very accurate in making diagnosis; obtain specimen or shed cells for cytology and stent may be placed to relieve jaundice
- Barium meal: widening of the duodenal loop with medial filling defect, the reversed '3' sign

04

Management
Palliation
- Pancreatic adenocarcinoma is usually incurable at time of diagnosis
- Jaundice can be relieved by placing a stent through the tumour either transhepatically or via ERCP
- Duodenal obstruction may be relieved by gastrojejunostomy
- Pain may be helped with a coeliac axis block

Curative treatment
- Rarely, surgical (Whipple's) resection of small tumours of the head of the pancreas is curative if lymph nodes are not involved

Prognosis
- 90% of patients with pancreatic adenocarcinoma are dead within 12 months of diagnosis
- Important to obtain histology from tumours around the head of the pancreas as the prognosis of non-pancreatic periampullary cancers (distal common bile duct tumours, ampullary tumours, duodenal tumours) is considerably better (50% 5-year survival) following resection

Tumours of endocrine pancreas
May be benign or malignant but usually slow-growing. All are rare

Islet cell tumour	Syndrome
Insulinoma	Hyperinsulinism
Gastrinoma (part of MEN1 syndrome)	Zollinger–Ellison syndrome
Vipoma	Werner–Morrison syndrome
Glucagonoma	Glucagonoma syndrome
Somatostatinoma	None
Non-functioning islet cell tumours	None

Evidence-based medicine

Cuschieri, A., Shimi, S.M., Crosthwaite, G., *et al.* (1992) Bilateral endoscopic splanchnicectomy. In: G.P. Burns & S. Bank (eds) *Disorders of the Pancreas.* McGraw-Hill, New York.

Knaus, W.A., Draper, E.A., Wagner, D.P., *et al.* (1985) APACHE II: a severity disease classification system. *Crit Care Med* **13**, 818–29.

Wiersema, M.J., Hawes, R.H., Lehman, G.A., *et al.* (1993) Prospective evaluation of endoscopic ultrasonography and endoscopic retrograde cholangiopancreatography in patients with chronic abdominal pain of suspected pancreatic origin. *Endoscopy* **25**, 555–64.

Must know Must do

Must know

Causes and clinical manifestations of hypersplenism

Causes and management of patients with
    splenomegaly

Adverse effects of splenectomy

Must do

Clerk and follow the management of a patient with
    idiopathic thrombocytopenic purpura

Learn to detect an enlarged spleen by palpation

Observe a patient undergoing laparoscopic
    splenectomy

Examine a blood film from a splenectomized patient

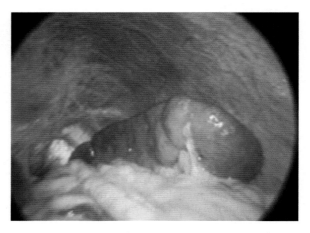

Figure 30.1 Appearance of normal spleen during laparo-scopic antireflux surgery: the organ is well inside the lower ribcage.

Anatomy and physiology

The spleen is situated in the left upper quadrant tucked under and against the left dome of the diaphragm and overlain by the lower left 9th to 11th ribs (Fig. 30.1). It has to enlarge two to three times before becoming palpable. Accessory spleens (splenunculi) are present in 10% of adults and are most commonly situated near the hilum but may occur in other sites They are important in relation to splenectomy for haematological disorders, because if left behind they may hypertrophy and cause recurrence of the disease.

The spleen removes damaged or senescent red cells from the circulation (culling) and remodels the surface of maturing erythrocytes to achieve the ideal ratio between membrane surface area and cell volume. Hence target cells, which have excess membrane, appear in the peripheral blood after splenectomy. Intraerythrocytic inclusions are removed by the spleen, e.g. Howell–Jolly bodies (nuclear remnants), siderotic granules (haemosiderin aggregates) and Heinz bodies (aggregates of denatured haemoglobin). These appear in the peripheral blood after splenectomy. The spleen is very efficient in clearing par-ticulate matter from the circulation. Following splenectomy, the primary antibody response is decreased and the secondary response is abnormal in that there is impaired switching from IgM to IgG antibody subtypes. The spleen also produces non-specific effectors of the immune response, e.g. tuftsin, which opsonizes particulate matter thereby facilitating phagocytosis. The spleen opsonizes pneumococci and is involved in the alternative pathway of complement activation. Loss of these immune functions accounts for the increased susceptibility to sepsis after splenectomy, especially in infants and children.

Hypersplenism

This is a syndrome of splenomegaly combined with destruction of formed blood elements leading to one or more of the following:

- anaemia;
- leukopenia < 4–5×10^9/L;
- thrombocytopenia $< 100 \times 10^9$/L.

Primary hypersplenism is when the destruction of normal

04

blood elements is caused by a primary lymphoreticular disorder, as distinct from *secondary hypersplenism* where the hyperactivity is associated with splenomegaly from other causes, e.g. liver disease. In both states, the bone marrow is unable to maintain normal numbers of circulating cells or platelets. Splenectomy is potentially curative of the cytopenias that occur in hypersplenism but there are other alternatives.

Hyposplenism

Hyposplenism is confirmed by the appearance of defective red cells in the peripheral circulation. The common causes of hyposplenism are summarized in Table 30.1. The most frequent cause is surgical splenectomy. Splenic hypoplasia forms part of the syndrome of Fanconi's anaemia (congenital hypoplastic anaemia). Acquired hyposplenism occurs in patients with coeliac disease and other gastrointestinal disorders, e.g. Crohn's disease, ulcerative colitis. Circulating autoantibodies and immune complexes in clinical autoimmune disorders, e.g. systemic lupus erythematosus (SLE), can cause a functional hypoplastic state secondary to Fc-receptor blockade. The hyposplenism of sickle cell anaemia is related to the extent of splenic infarction. Hyposplenism is also a feature of patients with full-blown human immunodeficiency virus (HIV) infection. These patients usually present with *Mycobacterium avium*

Table 30.1 Causes of asplenism/hyposplenism.

Splenectomy
Splenic agenesis
Atrophy
    Coeliac disease
    Inflammatory bowel disease and collagenous colitis
    Systemic amyloidosis
    Old age
    Dermatitis herpetiformis
    Sickle cell anaemia
    Systemic lupus erythematosus

complex infection, which often complicates HIV-related immune thrombocytopenic purpura (ITP).

Postsplenectomy sepsis

The risk of overwhelming sepsis is increased after splenectomy, with the greatest risk in infants and children up to 5 years old. Apart from age, the risk is also influenced by the nature of the disease necessitating splenectomy, with trauma having the lowest risk and thalassaemia the highest (Table 30.2). Some of the estimates of risk have been questioned because the majority of reported data are based on single case reports of pneumococcal infections with bacteraemia. Community-acquired pneumococcal pneumonia with bacteraemia is common in patients with normal splenic function and is seldom reported because of its established occurrence in susceptible groups.

Streptococcus pneumoniae is responsible for 60% of septic episodes in asplenic patients, although infections by other encapsulated bacteria (e.g. *Haemophilus influenzae*, *Haemophilus pertussis*, *Neisseria meningitidis*) are also common, as are infections by Gram-negative bacteria. The syndrome of overwhelming postsplenectomy infection (OPSI) begins insidiously with a non-specific viral-like illness with rapid progression to a fulminant infection with high fever, rigors, vomiting, dehydration, hypotension and coma, unless halted by effective resuscitation and aggressive antibiotic therapy. The mortality rate of OPSI exceeds 50%. Treatment is with intravenous broad-spectrum antibiotics effective against encapsulated cocci in the first instance until blood culture results become available. Intravenous colloids are used to correct the hypovolaemia using central venous pressure as a guide to therapy.

The prevention of OPSI is based on vaccination, administration of oral penicillin and patient education. Prophylactic antibiotic therapy is recommended (together with vaccination) in children and some would extend it indefinitely to adults. Vaccination is carried out at least 10–14 days prior to splenectomy for maximum effective immunization and includes polyvalent pneumococcal vaccine and *Haemophilus* vaccines. Immunization after

Indication	Incidence of sepsis (%)
Trauma	1.4
Immune (idiopathic) thrombocytopenia	2.0
Incidental (iatrogenic injury)	2.1
Congenital spherocytosis	3.5
Acquired haemolytic anaemia	7.5
Portal hypertension	8.2
Reticulosis/lymphomas	11.5
Thalassaemia	24.8

Table 30.2 Risk of postsplenectomy sepsis with indication for splenectomy. Modified from Singer, D.B. (1973) Postsplenectomy sepsis. *Perspect Pediatr Pathol* **1**, 285–311.

splenectomy (trauma cases) is much less effective but is advisable. All patients should carry a 'splenectomy card'.

Splenic infarction

Infarction of the spleen has a variable clinical presentation, ranging from patients with acute life-threatening complications (splenic rupture, splenic abscess) to others where symptoms are minor or absent. There is a high risk of infarction in patients with sickle cell disease and those with splenomegaly due to chronic myeloid leukaemia and myelosclerosis. Splenic infarction may also be due to thromboembolic disorders (atrial fibrillation), diabetic microvascular disease and acute torsion of an *ectopic (wandering) spleen*. A variety of other disorders may be complicated by the development of splenic infarction, e.g. falciparum malaria, acquired immunodeficiency syndrome (AIDS), severe necrotizing pancreatitis. The splenic infarction in patients with AIDS is due to arterial thrombosis of the coeliac trunk and is associated with thrombocytopenia and a coagulopathy.

The age range of splenic infarction varies widely. The most common symptoms are acute upper left quadrant abdominal pain, fever, chills and malaise. However one-third of patients are asymptomatic. Physical examination reveals tenderness and guarding maximal in the left upper abdomen. Splenic infarction results in a capsular inflammatory reaction causing irritation of the left diaphragm, with left basal pleurisy/effusion and left shoulder pain (Kerr's sign). The diagnosis is confirmed by abdominal computed tomography (CT). Initially, management is conservative with analgesia and antibiotics. Surgery is indicated if the diagnosis is in doubt or for complications (splenic abscess, bleeding from splenic rupture) when splenectomy is indicated.

Splenomegaly

There are several causes of splenomegaly (Table 30.3) and the relative incidence varies in different parts of the world. In the West the distribution is as follows:
- hepatic diseases, most commonly cirrhosis;
- haematological disease;
- infectious diseases (16%, increasingly AIDS);
- inflammatory non-infectious disease;
- primary splenic disease;
- others (3%, e.g. congestive heart failure, endocarditis).

The spleen may enlarge transiently in a variety of acute bacterial and viral infections, chronic infections and in subacute bacterial endocarditis. Parasitic infections such as malaria cause massive congestive splenomegaly and these very large spleens can rupture. AIDS now accounts for 60% of splenomegaly caused by infectious disease. Portal hypertension causes mild to moderate spleno-

megaly unless it is part of Budd–Chiari syndrome or follows splenic vein thrombosis. Splenomegaly accompanies both hereditary and acquired red cell defects. The increasing splenic size predisposes these patients to increased destruction of the abnormal red cells. Splenomegaly regularly accompanies myeloproliferative disorders, e.g. myelosclerosis, leukaemia or lymphoma.

Clinical features

When palpable, the spleen is at least two to three times normal size. Pressure symptoms of splenomegaly are present when the spleen becomes massively enlarged and include chronic dragging abdominal pain or pain when lying on the side, abdominal discomfort and early satiety. In addition patients may complain of attacks of colicky left upper quadrant pain. Physical examination shows a left upper quadrant mass that disappears beneath the costal margin such that it is impossible to reach its superior limit. The enlarged spleen lies against the abdominal wall and is dull to percussion. Capsular inflammation of the spleen may produce a rub heard with the stethoscope. Physical examination must include a careful search for lymphadenopathy and stigmata of chronic liver disease. The cause of splenic enlargement is identified by history, physical examination and a few key tests. Haematological causes are fully characterized by a peripheral blood smear and a bone marrow biopsy. Serological testing identifies most infectious cases, e.g. AIDS, mononucleosis (positive Paul–Bunnell test, rising anti-Epstein–Barr virus titre). Patients with a history of travel or those living in endemic areas should have blood smears examined for malaria or a marrow biopsy examined for Leishman–Donovan bodies.

The size, shape and consistency of the spleen is accurately visualized by either CT or ultrasonography. The splenic blood vessels can be imaged using either duplex ultrasound or high-dose contrast helical CT. Splenic ultrasound is used for:
- detection of accessory spleens;
- confirmation of splenomegaly but not its cause;
- differentiation of solid from cystic intrasplenic focal masses;
- detection of calcification, wall thickening, internal debris, and gas within cystic-type lesions;
- detection of splenic cavernous haemangiomas;
- diagnosis of splenic infarction;
- diagnosis of splenic trauma and monitoring of patients with splenic injuries managed conservatively.

An accurate assessment of the spleen's function can be obtained by injection of labelled platelets, cells (red, white) or carrier molecules and radiotracer studies. The splenic uptake rate of ^{99m}Tc-labelled sulphur colloid or Tc-labelled tin colloid provides a sensitive and quantitative assessment of splenic function.

04

Table 30.3 Disorders producing splenomegaly.

Infections
Acute
Hepatitis
Mononucleosis
Salmonellosis
Toxoplasmosis
Cytomegalovirus
Abscess

Subacute
AIDS
Bacterial endocarditis
Tuberculosis
Brucellosis
Malaria

Chronic
Fungal disease
Syphilis
Bacterial endocarditis

Congestive
Intrahepatic portal hypertension
Cirrhosis
Wilson's disease
Haemochromatosis
Congenital hepatic fibrosis

Prehepatic portal hypertension
Portal vein thrombosis

Posthepatic portal hypertension
Budd–Chiari syndrome
Congestive cardiac failure

Segmental (left-sided portal hypertension)
Splenic vein occlusion

Haematological
Haemolytic disorders
Hereditary cell membrane defects
Autoimmune haemolytic states (warm antibodies)
Thalassaemia
Sickle cell disease
Haemoglobin C disease

Myeloproliferative disorders
Myeloid metaplasia
Polycythaemia vera
Essential thrombocythaemia

Miscellaneous
Primary splenic hyperplasia

Megaloblastic anaemia
Iron deficiency

Malignant
Haematological malignancies
Acute or chronic leukaemias
Leukaemic reticuloendotheliosis
Malignant lymphomas
Malignant histiocytosis
Myelomatosis

Primary intrinsic malignancies
Lymphosarcoma
Plasmacytoma
Fibrosarcoma
Angiosarcoma

Intrinsic secondary malignancies
Carcinoma
Melanoma

Benign
Haemangioma
Lymphangioma

Inflammatory or granulomatous
Felty's syndrome
Systemic lupus erythematosus
Rheumatic fever
Serum sickness
Sarcoidosis

Storage disease
Gaucher's disease
Wilson's disease
Niemann–Pick syndrome
Histiocytosis X
Hurler's syndrome
Tangier disease

Miscellaneous
Cysts
Parasitic
Pseudocysts
Congenital
Traumatic

Others
Hyperthyroidism
Osler–Weber–Rendu syndrome
Splenic mastocytosis
Albers–Schönberg disease

Table 30.4 Indications for splenectomy.

Definite
Non-salvageable spleen injury
En-bloc resection of adjacent neoplasms (usually proximal
    gastric cancer)
Neoplasms of the spleen (usually lymphomas)
Splenic abscess
Echinococcal cysts
Bleeding gastric varices due to sinistral portal hypertension
    (splenic vein thrombosis)

Desirable (selective)
Hereditary spherocytosis
Immune (idiopathic) thrombocytopenic purpura
AIDS-related thrombocytopenic purpura
Autoimmune haemolytic anaemia
Sickling syndromes (sickle cell disease and sickle β-
    thalassaemia)

Debatable
Non-parasitic splenic cysts
Thalassaemia syndromes
Lymphoma with specific cytopenia or pancytopenia
Thrombotic thrombocytopenic purpura
Myeloproliferative disorders

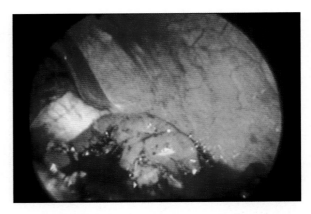

Figure 30.2 Laparoscopic splenectomy: detached spleen prior to removal.

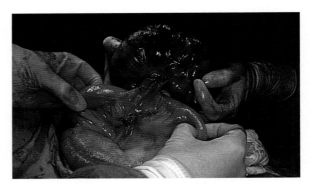

Figure 30.3 Emergency splenectomy for necrotic wandering spleen following torsion of the splenic vessels. Courtesy of Professor R.J.C. Steele, University of Dundee.

The indications for splenectomy are shown in Table 30.4. All patients undergoing elective splenectomy should be immunized against *Streptoccoccus pneumoniae* and *Haemophilus* spp. and this should be carried out 2 weeks before surgery. If the platelet count is low, platelet transfusion to a level greater than 60×10^9/L is indicated both prior to and for the first few days following operation. If the thrombocytopenia is caused by immune disease (e.g. ITP), then preoperative platelet transfusions are less useful, whereas human IgG increases the platelet count. Because of its advantages (fewer perioperative complications, reduced morbidity, shorter hospital stay), laparoscopic splenectomy is now preferable to open operation for some but not all disorders requiring splenectomy. It is the procedure of choice for benign disease especially when the spleen is not very enlarged, e.g. ITP, AIDS-related thrombocytopenic purpura and acquired haemolytic anaemia (Fig. 30.2).

Ectopic (wandering) spleen

Ectopic (wandering) spleen is rare and occurs more commonly in women (7 : 1). It is due to lax attachments of the spleen to the retroperitoneum and long splenic vessels, such that the spleen 'wanders' the quadrants of the abdomen (Fig. 30.3). It may present acutely with abdominal pain due to torsion that may progress to infarction,

with hypersplenism (due to congestion), or simply with an abdominal mass with or without associated pain. The diagnosis is confirmed by CT or duplex ultrasonography. Treatment of ectopic spleen is by splenopexy (viable spleen) or splenectomy when the spleen is infarcted.

Splenic cysts

Splenic cysts are primary or secondary. Secondary cysts are more common and develop after splenic injuries, hence the name 'traumatic splenic pseudocysts' (no lining epithelium). Splenic traumatic pseudocysts may be totally asymptomatic but have a tendency to enlarge (Fig. 30.4). The time interval between initial injury and presentation or diagnosis is extremely variable. Some traumatic pseudocysts remain asymptomatic and are discovered accidentally during investigation by ultrasound. Others develop abdominal pain and a palpable mass. Acute presentation with rupture is well documented. Surgical

04

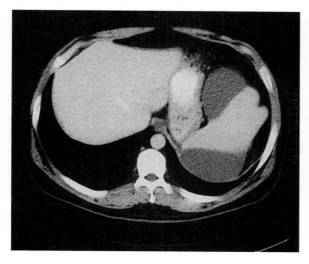

Figure 30.4 Computed tomography showing traumatic cysts at the poles of the spleen following blunt traumatic injury. The lesions were treated laparoscopically with splenic preservation.

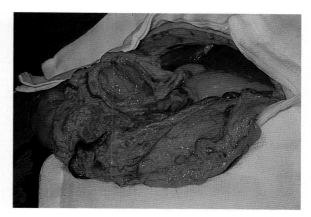

Figure 30.5 Sectorial (sinistral, left-sided) portal hypertension following splenic vein thrombosis in a patient with chronic pancreatitis. Note engorged and prominent left gastroepiploic veins. The patient presented with bleeding gastric varices.

treatment is only necessary for large symptomatic cysts after confirmation of the diagnosis by ultrasound or CT. Spleen-preserving excision is possible unless the cyst is very large or presents acutely with rupture and bleeding.

Primary splenic cysts have an epithelial lining and can be:

- epithelial;
- dermoid;
- lymphangiomatous;
- mucinous cystic lesions;
- parasitic (hydatid).

Splenic tumours

Apart from lymphomas, primary and secondary tumours of the spleen are both rare. Vascular tumours include primary angiosarcoma, haemangioma and haemangioendotheliomas. Secondary tumour deposits are very rare, with a reported frequency of 2–5%. Cutaneous melanoma can metastasize to the spleen, and direct involvement from pancreatic and retroperitoneal sarcomas can occur.

Splenic vein thrombosis

Most commonly, this occurs as a complication of acute or chronic pancreatitis. It can also be caused by pancreatic cancer. Isolated splenic vein thrombosis results in splenomegaly and sectorial or left-sided portal venous hypertension. The condition is characterized by varices involving the short gastric and gastroepiploic veins. The most common presentation is with bleeding gastric varices in patients with normal or good liver function (Fig. 30.5). Treatment is by splenectomy.

Disorders of the spleen at a glance

Functions of the spleen
- Removes damaged and senescent red blood cells from circulation
- Remodels the surface of maturing red blood cells
- Removes intraerythrocytic inclusions:
    (a) Howell–Jolly bodies (nuclear remnants)
    (b) Siderotic granules (haemosiderin aggregates)
    (c) Heinz bodies (denatured haemoglobin)
- Removes particulate matter from the circulation

- Produces non-specific effectors of immune response, e.g. tuftsin
- Opsonizes pneumococci
- Involves an alternative pathway of complement activation

Hypersplenism
- Syndrome of splenomegaly and destruction of formed elements of blood resulting in:

(a) Anaemia
(b) Leukopenia
(c) Thrombocytopenia
- Primary hypersplenism: caused by primary lymphoreticular disorder
- Secondary hypersplenism: results from hyperactivity associated with splenomegaly due to some other cause, e.g. liver disease

Hyposplenism
- Caused by failure or absence of the spleen
- Characterized by appearance of defective red blood cells and increase in platelets in the circulation

Causes
- Splenectomy
- Splenic agenesis
- Atrophy caused by:
  (a) Coeliac disease
  (b) Inflammatory bowel disease
  (c) Systemic amyloidosis
  (d) Old age
  (e) Dermatitis herpetiformis
  (f) Sickle cell anaemia
  (g) SLE

Overwhelming postsplenectomy infection
- After splenectomy there is an increased risk of overwhelming sepsis
- Greatest risk in infants and children up to 5 years of age
- Risk depends on reason for splenectomy:
  (a) Least after trauma and ITP
  (b) Greatest after lymphomas and thalassaemia
- Usually caused by encapsulated bacteria: *Streptococcus pneumoniae* (60%), *Haemophilus influenzae*, *Neisseria meningitidis*
- Mortality rate for OPSI > 50%
- Prevention by vaccination (preferably 10–14 days before splenectomy), oral penicillin (probably indefinitely) and patient education (carry splenectomy card)

Splenic infarction
Causes
- Sickle cell disease
- Splenomegaly secondary to chronic myeloid leukaemia and myelosclerosis
- Thromboembolism
- Diabetic microvascular disease
- Acute torsion of ectopic spleen

- Complication of falciparum malaria, AIDS, necrotizing pancreatitis

Clinical features and diagnosis
- Asymptomatic in 30%
- Acute left upper quadrant abdominal pain, fever, chills and malaise
- Tenderness and guarding in left upper abdomen
- Left basal effusion and left shoulder pain
- Diagnosis: CT

Management
- Conservative: analgesia and antibiotics
- Splenectomy for complications only: abscess, rupture

Splenomegaly
- Spleen has to be enlarged two to three times to be clinically palpable

Disease groups that result in splenomegaly
- Hepatic disease: portal hypertension
- Haematological disease: haemolytic disorders, myeloproliferative disease
- Infectious disease: hepatitis, mononucleosis, AIDS, malaria, bacterial endocarditis
- Malignant disease: leukaemias, lymphomas, myelomatosis, lymphosarcoma
- Granulomatous disease: SLE, sarcoidosis, rheumatic fever, Felty's syndrome

Ectopic (wandering) spleen
- Rare phenomenon due to long attachments of the spleen to the retroperitoneum
- Torsion may occur leading to splenic infarction

Splenic cysts
Primary
Primary splenic cysts are rare and classified as:
- Epithelial
- Dermoid
- Lymphangiomatous
- Mucunious cystic lesions
- Hydatid

Secondary
- Secondary (pseudocysts) are seen more often than primary but are not common
- Develop after splenic injury

04

Evidence-based medicine

Allen, K.B., Gay, B.B. Jr & Skandalakis, J.E. (1992) Wandering spleen: anatomic and radiologic considerations. *South Med J* **85**, 976–84.

Brigden, M.L. & Pattullo, A.L. (1999) Prevention and management of overwhelming postsplenectomy infection: an update. *Crit Care Med* **27**, 836–42.

Grotto, H.Z. & Costa, F.F. (1991) Hyposplenism in AIDS. *AIDS* **5**, 1538–40.

Must know Must do

Must know

Symptoms and investigations of patients with suspected small-bowel disease

Clinical features, pathology and management of patients with Crohn's disease

Pathology, clinical features and principles of management of small-bowel tumours

Acute appendicitis and appendiceal tumours

Short-gut syndrome and its management

Must do

See/clerk patients with Crohn's disease and follow their management

Examine enema films of small-bowel Crohn's disease and small-bowel tumours

Observe an operation for Crohn's disease

Physiology

The small intestine is divided into two anatomical portions: the jejunum, which constitutes the proximal two-fifths; and the thinner ileum, which occupies the right iliac fossa and pelvis. The lining mucosa is folded into villi to increase the absorptive surface area and these are covered by tall columnar absorptive cells (enterocytes) that have microvilli at their luminal surfaces (brush border). Goblet cells, found interspersed among the enterocytes, synthesize the mucinous glycoprotein essential for maintaining the surface glycocalyx. At their bases, the villi are surrounded by intestinal crypts that contain stem cells from which the surface epithelium is constantly replaced by a process of cell division and migration. The primary function of the small intestine is the absorption of nutrients but it is also involved in digestion by brush-border enzymes that are essential for the final hydrolysis of peptides and carbohydrates.

Normally, the digestion and absorption of fluid, elec-trolytes, iron, folate, carbohydrate, fat and protein is completed in the jejunum. However, absorption of bile salts and vitamin B_{12} only occurs in the terminal ileum, which contains specific transport sites. The critical length of small bowel required for maintenance of oral nutrition is 100 cm. Below this length some form of parenteral nutritional support is needed. Another function of the small intestine is the synthesis of peptide and amine intestinal hormones. These are located within the enteroendocrine cells and in the neurones of the myenteric plexus. They influence intestinal secretion and transport, growth and differentiation, splanchnic haemodynamics and the release of insulin.

Intestinal microflora

The small-bowel microflora plays an important role in intraluminal metabolism of various substances. Obstruction and stasis increase the bacterial population substantially. Even in the absence of obstruction, this bacterial overgrowth may produce adverse consequences including malabsorption. The normal intestinal mucosa is able to resist invasion by pathogenic bacteria but this antimicrobial barrier can break down under certain pathological states, with translocation of pathogens to the blood and lymph. This bacterial translocation underlies one of the mechanisms held responsible for systemic inflammatory response syndrome.

Small-bowel investigations

Radiology

This includes plain radiography, barium studies, fistulography, computed tomography (CT) and mesenteric angiography.

Plain radiography

This is a useful investigation in the management of

patients with acute abdominal disorders. Intestinal obstruction is confirmed by dilated gas/fluid-filled loops of small bowel that can be distinguished from large bowel by the more central distribution and the ladder-like valvulae conniventes. Thickening of the small bowel is inferred when there is a significant gap between the gaseous luminal outline of adjacent loops of small bowel. Plain chest radiographs identify free air in the peritoneal cavity and hence perforation of hollow viscera.

Barium studies

Most common disorders of the small intestine are investigated by barium small-bowel follow-through as part of a barium meal study. However, small-bowel enema (enteroclysis), in which contrast medium is instilled via a Bilbao–Dotter tube directly into the upper jejunum, carries a higher diagnostic yield especially for small-bowel tumours. Injection of contrast into the fistula (contrast fistulography) is of value especially in Crohn's disease. Fistulography also enables the diagnosis of associated abscess cavities and strictures and provides anatomical information essential for the appropriate surgical intervention.

Mesenteric angiography

Selective mesenteric angiography is used to detect angiodysplastic lesions and vascular tumours in the small bowel, which can be the cause of occult or frank gastrointestinal bleeding. If a bleeding point is identified during mesenteric angiography, the radiologist can place a superselective catheter into the appropriate branch of the superior mesenteric artery to lie as close as possible to the lesion. The catheter is then left *in situ*. At operation the surgeon then injects dye (methylene blue) through it to identify the segment of small bowel in which the bleeding lesion is present.

Isotope studies

External isotope scintigraphy following the intravenous administration of radiolabelled compounds or isotope-labelled autologous cells can be useful in the investigation of patients with occult intestinal bleeding. Radionuclide studies are also helpful in detecting inflamed intestine and in estimating intestinal transit time.

Intestinal bleeding

Some lesions that bleed into the small intestine (e.g. Meckel's diverticulum, polyps, tumours, vascular malformations) may not be detectable by barium studies or angiography. Radionuclide studies may help to identify these lesions. Two isotope methods are used.

- Intravenous injection of labelled technetium pertechnetate ($^{99m}TcO_4$), which is taken up by the ectopic gastric mucosa: method of choice for the detection of bleeding Meckel's diverticulum with an accuracy rate of 90%.
- Intravenous injection of Tc-labelled autologous red cells: these are cleared slowly from the vascular compartment and allow repeated examination by external scintiscanning over 24 h.

Estimation of small-bowel transit time

Small-bowel transit studies can be performed by external scintigraphy after administration of liquid and solid meals incorporating ^{99m}Tc-labelled sulphocolloid or diethylenetriaminepentaacetic acid (DTPA). These estimate gastric emptying and small-bowel transit time at the same time. The detection of caecal radioactivity is used as the end-point for the estimation of small-bowel transit time.

Detection of small-bowel inflammatory disease

When injected intravenously, In-labelled autologous leukocytes home to areas of inflammation and abscess formation. Sucralfate (aluminium salt of polysulphated sucrose) binds selectively to areas of mucosal ulceration. Radiolabelled sucralfate is thus a useful technique for detection of inflammatory bowel disease of both large and small intestine. The labelled suspension of sucralfate is administered by mouth and serial isotope scans of the abdomen are carried out at 2, 6, 20 and 24 h. It gives a lower radiation dose than barium studies and is used as a screening test and for serial assessment of disease activity.

Investigations for malabsorption

Malabsorption is defined as the inability to absorb sufficient nutrient to sustain normal health and may be caused by gastric, small-bowel or pancreatic disorders. The most common clinical feature is steatorrhoea (malabsorption of fat), which produces foul-smelling, floating and difficult-to-flush stools. Symptoms attributable to malabsorption of carbohydrate and protein are less common and consist of abdominal discomfort and bloating. Unabsorbed carbohydrate is fermented to lactic acid in the large bowel and induces diarrhoea. Tests of malabsorption include:
- faecal fat estimation;
- mucosal biospy;
- Schilling test;
- radionuclide tests of bacterial overgrowth;

04

- tests of carbohydrate malabsorption;
- hydrogen breath tests.

Estimation of faecal fat

This is the most sensitive test for disorders of digestion and absorption. The daily faecal fat output is estimated by collecting faecal samples over 3–5 days while the subject consumes a standard diet containing 80–100 g of fat; the normal value is less than 6 g/day (80 mmol triglyceride). Other tests, such as the ^{14}C triolein breath test and oxalate loading test, are less reliable.

Small-bowel mucosal biopsy

Mucosal biopsy from the distal duodenum obtained by upper gastrointestinal endoscopy is used to search for abnormalities of villous architecture, e.g. subtotal villous atrophy in coeliac disease.

Schilling test

The absorption of vitamin B_{12} in the terminal ileum requires the presence of intrinsic factor and the R protein in gastric juice. In the Schilling test, radiolabelled vitamin B_{12} (1 μg) is administered orally immediately after an intravenous injection of the unlabelled vitamin (1000 μg), which ensures saturation of body stores. Normal subjects will excrete 10% or more of the radiolabelled vitamin in their urine. If abnormally low excretion is documented, the test is repeated but labelled vitamin B_{12} is given together with intrinsic factor. Abnormally low excretion of labelled vitamin in the urine not altered by intrinsic factor indicates the presence of ileal disease. In contrast, after total gastrectomy or in patients with pernicious anaemia, the administration of intrinsic factor normalizes urinary excretion of the labelled vitamin. Both stages of the test are invalidated by dehydration and renal disease. Bacterial overgrowth may cause malabsorption of the vitamin and an abnormal Schilling test but this will revert to normal after a course of antibiotic therapy.

^{14}C-Glycocholate and ^{14}C-D-xylose breath tests

The ^{14}C-glycocholate breath test detects bacterial overgrowth in the small intestine. The labelled glycocholate is administered orally so that it mixes with the endogenous bile salts in the intestine. Normally, bile salts are largely reabsorbed intact in the terminal ileum and enter the enterohepatic circulation, only a small amount reaching the colon. Here the bile salts are deconjugated by colonic bacteria and the glycine metabolized to yield CO_2, which is absorbed and eliminated in expired air. In bacterial overgrowth, most of the ingested labelled salt is deconjugated by small-bowel bacteria and excess $^{14}CO_2$ is produced and eliminated in expired air. False-positive results are obtained in the presence of ileal disease. The ^{14}C-D-xylose test is more reliable in this respect.

Breath tests for carbohydrate malabsorption

Analysis of breath $^{14}CO_2$ following the ingestion of ^{14}C-lactose is a convenient test for lactose intolerance resulting from lactase deficiency. This test is as accurate as the lactose tolerance test. In lactose malabsorption, excess sugar reaches the colon and the resulting fermentation produces hydrogen. A proportion of this gas is absorbed and eliminated in expired air. Mass spectrometry is used to detect the hydrogen in end-expiratory air. Both $^{14}CO_2$ and the breath hydrogen test give false-positive results in patients with bacterial overgrowth.

Hydrogen breath test for measurement of small-bowel transit time and bacterial overgrowth

The hydrogen breath test is a reliable method for determining small-bowel transit time. Repeated measurements of hydrogen in end-expiratory air are taken every few minutes after the ingestion of mashed potatoes and baked beans (non-absorbable oligosaccharides). When the meal reaches the caecum, the resulting bacterial fermentation induces a sustained rise in breath hydrogen concentration. Thus the test measures oral–caecal transit time. However, if the meal is radiolabelled with technetium, both gastric emptying and small-bowel transit times can be calculated.

Small-bowel enteroscopy

Endoscopy of the small bowel can be performed by using a long balloon-tipped small-bowel enteroscope or a 'push' enteroscope. With the former, the balloon is inflated after the endoscope has entered the duodenum and this enables gut peristalsis to carry the tip of the enteroscope to the caecum (established by radiological screening). Inspection of the bowel is performed as the instrument is withdrawn. Small-bowel enteroscopy is used to investigate recurrent obscure bleeding. The limitations of this type of enteroscopy include the time required to perform the procedure and the inability to obtain biopsy. On the other hand, the push enteroscope enables procurement of biopsies, but only the first 60 cm or so of the small bowel beyond the duodenojejunal flexure can be visualized by this technique.

Small-bowel tumours

Small-bowel tumours are rare. A number of gastrointestinal disorders are associated with an increased risk, including:
- Crohn's disease (adenocarcinoma);
- coeliac disease (lymphoma);
- dermatitis herpetiformis;
- Peutz–Jeghers syndrome (carcinoma);
- radiation enteritis (lymphoma).

Benign tumours

The majority of small-bowel tumours are benign. They include epithelial tumours (tubulous and villous adenomas), lipomas, haemangiomas and neurogenic tumours. Small-bowel adenomas may occur in association with familial adenomatous polyposis (FAP). Many benign small-bowel tumours are asymptomatic. The most common presentation is with intestinal obstruction due to intussusception. Chronic blood loss from a benign small-bowel tumour may cause iron-deficiency anaemia.

The diagnosis is made by small-bowel follow-through or small-bowel enema. In the majority, however, the disease is diagnosed at emergency laparotomy for small-bowel obstruction. Treatment is by resection.

Malignant tumours

Malignant small-bowel tumours present late, usually when the tumour has spread beyond the confines of the bowel wall (T3/4). The important malignant small-bowel tumours include:
- adenocarcinoma (40%);
- carcinoid tumours (30%);
- lymphoma (25%);
- mesenchymal tumours (5%).

The usual presentation is with acute small-bowel obstruction often preceded by recurrent attacks of central abdominal colic. Thus in the majority the diagnosis is made at emergency laparotomy. If clinical suspicion is raised before the onset of acute intestinal obstruction, the tumour may be identified by small-bowel enema, small-bowel enteroscopy, mesenteric angiography and CT.

Adenocarcinoma

These adenocarcinomas are mucus-secreting tumours. They occur most commonly in the duodenum (periampullary region and third part/duodenojejunal junction) and jejunum. These sites account for 80% of cases, while 20% of small-bowel adenocarcinomas originate in the ileum. Intestinal adenocarcinomas spread primarily to the regional lymph nodes, liver and peritoneal cavity.

The aetiology is not known but there is an increased incidence of small-bowel adenocarcinomas in patients with hereditary polypoid syndromes (FAP, Peutz–Jeghers syndrome). There is also an increased risk in Crohn's disease and coeliac disease.

The median age at diagnosis is 60 years and the sex distribution is equal. The symptoms include abdominal discomfort, which is usually postprandial and colicky in nature, nausea and vomiting, particularly in patients with duodenal carcinomas and weight loss. Gastrointestinal bleeding may be occult, leading to iron-deficiency anaemia, but may also be overt with melaena or frank rectal bleeding. Intestinal obstruction indicates advanced disease, although a relatively small polypoid tumour may lead to intussusception. Patients with duodenal carcinomas often present with obstructive jaundice. The carcinoma that develops in Crohn's disease occurs in a younger age group (40–50 years) predominantly in males and involves the ileum in 75%.

Surgical resection is the only effective treatment. Pancreaticoduodenectomy is performed for periampullary tumours, although segmental resection may be possible for tumours of the third and fourth parts. Jejunal and ileal tumours are resected with a minimum of 5 cm of healthy margin on either side of the lesion together with the associated mesentery and regional lymph nodes. Carcinomas of the terminal ileum usually require formal right hemicolectomy. The 5-year survival rate for adenocarcinoma of the small intestine averages 15%. Carcinomas arising in patients with Crohn's disease carry a dismal prognosis.

Carcinoid tumours

Carcinoid tumours arise from specialized enterochromaffin cells (stain with potassium chromate) of the crypts of Leiberkühn. Carcinoid tumours occur predominantly in the gastrointestinal tract and can be classified into three groups.
- *Foregut tumours*: arise in the stomach, biliary tract and bronchus, consist of regularly shaped cells with trabecular arrangement and round granules, exhibit an argyrophilic reaction, i.e. the cells can only be stained with metallic silver in the presence of a reducing agent.
- *Midgut tumours*: arise in the jejunum, ileum and right colon, cells are pleomorphic and arranged in nests separated by connective tissue, exhibit both argentaffin (can be stained directly with metallic silver without reducing agent) and argyrophilic staining properties.
- *Hindgut tumours*: arise in the left colon and rectum, cells are arranged in a trabecular pattern containing round granules but do not stain with silver.

Foregut tumours produce 5-hydroxytryptophan (5-HTP), 5-hydroxytryptamine (5-HT, or serotonin),

histamine and substance P. Midgut tumours produce 5-HT, kallikrein and possibly prostaglandins. Tumours of the hindgut do not usually secrete active peptides. In addition, midgut and foregut tumours may contain and secrete a variety of hormones, including insulin, somatostatin, adrenocorticotrophic hormone (ACTH), gastrin, antidiuretic hormone (ADH), parathormone, glucagon, vasoactive intestinal polypepetide (VIP), calcitonin, β-melanocyte stimulating hormone (β-MSH), cholecystokinin and growth hormone. The histology does not differentiate between benign and malignant carcinoid tumours. In general, tumours smaller than 1 cm are rarely malignant. Tumours between 1 and 1.9 cm may be malignant and tumours larger than 2 cm are usually invasive and exhibit metastatic spread. These more aggressive lesions invade the bowel wall mesentery, parietal peritoneum and adjacent organs. Metastatic spread involves the regional lymph nodes and liver in particular but other sites such as the lung and the bones may be involved. The most common sites of gut carcinoids are the appendix, small intestine and rectum in that order. The majority of carcinoid tumours of the small intestine are malignant, 40% are multiple and in 30% there is an associated malignant neoplasm, usually an adenocarcinoma. The age at presentation of intestinal carcinoids varies between 45 and 55 years. Duodenal carcinoids may present with vomiting due to obstruction or as an endocrine syndrome. Carcinoids of the jejunum or ileum present with diarrhoea, intestinal obstruction, palpable abdominal mass and, much less commonly, massive gastrointestinal haemorrhage or intestinal infarction. Resection of the tumour (with wide margins of healthy tissue), regional lymph nodes and associated mesentery is the standard treatment. Radiotherapy has been used for inoperable tumours but the results are disappointing.

Carcinoid syndrome

The carcinoid syndrome is very rare and produced by less than 10% of all carcinoid tumours. In the majority of cases the primary tumour originates in the small intestine. The syndrome is invariably associated with the presence of hepatic involvement by tumour and the clinical manifestations are the result of inappropriate secretion of 5-HT, 5-HTP, kallikrein, histamine, prostaglandin and ACTH. The clinical features include the following.

● Several types of flushing syndromes, intestinal colic and diarrhoea, bronchospasm, hypoproteinaemia and oedema. The cutaneous flushing episodes affect the upper part of the body and are accompanied by sweating, itching, oedema, palpitations and hypotension.
● Cardiac lesions (tricuspid insufficiency or pulmonary stenosis).
● Pellagra-like skin lesions (photosensitive dermatitis).
● Neurological signs.
● Peptic ulceration and neuralgia.

Biochemical confirmation of the diagnosis is achieved by determination of 5-hydroxyindoleacetic acid (5-HIAA), the urinary metabolite of 5-HT and 5-HTP.

Hepatic deposits should be resected when possible, otherwise hepatic arterial embolization or *in-situ* ablation is performed. Both are covered with antiserotonin therapy. Chemotherapy is also used for palliation. Drugs that are effective include cyclophosphamide, Adriamycin, 5-fluorouracil, 5-fluorodesoxyuridine and streptozotocin, used singly or in combination. The best results are obtained by prolonged infusion chemotherapy either through the hepatic artery or a tributary of the portal vein. Pretreatment with antiserotonin therapy is necessary to prevent a carcinoid crisis during chemotherapy. Antiserotonin therapy can be undertaken with agents that either reduce the production of 5-HT or antagonize its effects (Table 31.1).

Lymphoma

Primary intestinal lymphoma is much rarer than intestinal involvement by primary extraintestinal lymphomatous disease. Thus the vast majority of primary gut lymphomas are non-Hodgkin's and are classified as B-cell or T-cell lymphomas, each further subdivided into low grade and high grade. Most are B-cell lymphomas arising from cells of the mucosa-associated lymphoid tissue (MALT) and referred to as MALT lymphomas. The most common types of intestinal lymphoma are:
● MALT lymphoma;
● Centrocytic lymphoma;
● Mediterranean lymphoma;
● Burkitt-type lymphoma;
● Polymorphic T-cell lymphoma.

MALT lymphoma

MALT lymphomas are mostly low-grade tumours that have a tendency to remain localized for long periods and to metastasize late to other MALT sites. Some are high-grade tumours and carry a less favourable prognosis. Microscopically, low-grade tumours form well-defined growths with deep invasion of the bowel wall, whereas high-grade tumours involve extensive segments of the bowel and form large strictured lesions with a tendency to ulceration.

Centrocytic lymphoma

This is less common and forms superficial diffuse lesions that do not invade deeply into the bowel wall. The affected mucosa develops a convoluted heaped-up appearance,

Table 31.1 Antiserotonin drugs and their effects.

Drug	Effect
Parachlorophenylalanine	Relieves diarrhoea
Phenoxybenzamine	Administered to achieve α-adrenergic blockade. It may relieve attacks precipitated by emotion, diet, exercise and alcohol
Chlorpromazine	Has antikinin effects and may control flushing
Methysergide maleate	Most potent serotonin antagonist. May relieve flushing, diarrhoea and bronchospasm
Cyproheptadine	Less potent antiserotonin agent. May relieve diarrhoea and less frequently reduce intensity of flushing
Prednisolone	May relieve facial oedema, diarrhoea and the flushing symptoms of bronchial carcinoids but not when the symptoms are caused by gastrointestinal tumours
Long-acting somatostatin analogue (octreotide)	Abolishes flushes due to gastrointestinal carcinoids and diarrhoea
Ketanserin	May reduce diarrhoea
Calcitonin	Same effects as somatostatin

hence the alternative name of malignant lymphomatous polyposis. Many patients develop a centrocytic leukaemia and peripheral lymphadenopathy.

Mediterranean lymphoma

This is related to immunoproliferative small intestinal disease (IPSID), which occurs mainly in the Middle East or the Mediterranean basin and in South Africa. The diseased mucosa shows a heavy plasma-cell and B-lymphocyte infiltration. The abnormal plasma cells secrete a fragment of IgA (α or heavy chain) that can be detected in the plasma and duodenal juice. A malignant B-cell lymphoma develops in some patients suffering from IPSID.

The macroscopic features of Mediterranean lymphoma are highly variable and range from diffuse thickening of the upper small intestine with enlargement of the associated mesenteric lymph nodes to localized, often multiple tumours.

Burkitt-type lymphoma

This primary high-grade B-cell lymphoma affects the ileocaecal region, particularly in children, although other sites of origin may occur. It is an aggressive tumour that invades and permeates through the bowel wall at an early stage and is usually advanced at the time of presentation. It has a tendency to recur after surgical resection and for this reason resection should always be followed by adjuvant chemotherapy.

Polymorphic T-cell lymphoma

This often develops in patients suffering from coeliac disease but can arise in the absence of this condition. The tumour may occur in any part of the small bowel, but the jejunum is the most common site. The lesion is often mul-

tifocal and can form ulcers, strictures, plaques, nodules or diffuse thickening. In general the prognosis is poor and the disease tends to become disseminated at an early stage.

Clinical features and management of small-bowel lymphoma

Small-bowel lymphoma may occur at any age but the peak incidence is in the sixth decade. It is commoner in males. The presentation may be acute or insidious. Acute presentation is with intestinal obstruction or perforation leading to peritonitis. The chronic symptoms include malaise, abdominal pain, weight loss, diarrhoea and anaemia. The erythrocyte sedimentation rate (ESR) is elevated and hypoproteinaemia is frequently present. In patients with coeliac disease the lymphoma causes a return of symptoms previously controlled by diet, with abdominal pain, diarrhoea and rapid weight loss. In the Middle East, IPSID affects children and is associated with growth retardation, malabsorption, bacterial overgrowth, hypoproteinaemia with oedema and ascites, and parasitic infestations particularly giardiasis. It can also present with intestinal obstruction, perforation and massive haemorrhage.

In all cases the most common physical finding is a mobile abdominal mass. The diagnosis is often established by means of small-bowel contrast enema, CT and laparoscopy. In IPSID, the abnormal α-chain is detected by immunocytochemistry of tumour sections and by immunoelectrophoresis with monospecific IgA antibody of serum and duodenal juice. The staging of small-bowel lymphoma is shown in Table 31.2.

Patients presenting with acute abdominal disease are treated by emergency resection. Adjuvant treatment is administered soon after recovery from the operation and usually consists of combination chemotherapy (CHOP,

04

Table 31.2 Modified Ann Arbor clinical staging of lymphoma.

Stage I
Disease confined to a single extralymphatic organ

Stage II
Localized involvement of one organ or site plus involvement of one or more lymph node groups on one side of the diaphragm
  II_1: regional adjacent lymph node involvement
  II_2: regional non-confluent node involvement

Stage III
Localized involvement of organ or site plus involvement of lymph node groups on both sides of the diaphragm

Stage IV
Diffuse disseminated disease with involvement of more than one organ plus lymph node enlargement

CMOPP, etc.) or radiotherapy. In uncomplicated lymphoma, elective surgery is followed by chemotherapy or radiotherapy in patients with stage I and stage II disease. Chemotherapy alone is indicated for more advanced disease but the prognosis in these cases is poor. Complete remissions can occur in patients with IPSID after treatment with tetracycline but patients with established lymphoma are generally treated as outlined above.

Mesenchymal tumours (gastrointestinal stromal tumours)

These include smooth muscle tumours, neurogenic tumours and neoplasms of uncommitted mesenchymal cells, often considered a less-differentiated variant of leiomyomas. With all mesenchymal tumours the distinction between the benign and malignant forms is often difficult even on histological grounds. In general, malignant tumours are larger, more often ulcerated and exhibit marked cellularity and necrosis, although an individual tumour can be confirmed benign if the patient is disease-free for at least 3 years after surgical excision. Smooth muscle tumours may occur anywhere in the small intestine but are more commonly found in the jejunum and ileum. The term 'gastrointestinal sarcoma' covers all mesenchymal tumours with malignant potential as judged histologically. These sarcomas are rare.

The majority of gastrointestinal stromal tumours present in middle age with a long history. The symptoms and signs include recurrent episodes of gastrointestinal bleeding (most commonly melaena), abdominal pain, weakness and rarely weight loss. Acute presentation with intestinal obstruction or perforation can also occur. A palpable abdominal mass is present in about one-third of patients and this is usually mobile. Some are asymptomatic and may be found accidentally during operation. A significant percentage of gastrointestinal sarcomas present acutely with tumour perforation or massive intraperitoneal bleeding.

Proximal lesions may be diagnosed by flexible endoscopy or push enteroscopy. Selective mesenteric angiography carries the highest diagnostic yield in patients with gastrointestinal bleeding. A small enema may also demonstrate the tumour.

Gastrointestinal stromal tumours do not respond to radiotherapy or chemotherapy. The treatment is therefore surgical excision with a wide healthy margin and removal of the regional lymph nodes and associated mesentery.

Small-bowel tumours at a glance

Definition

Small-bowel tumours: benign or malignant lesions of the duodenum, jejunum or ileum; they are rare and most are benign

Predisposing factors
- Crohn's disease: adenocarcinoma
- Coeliac disease: lymphoma
- Dermatitis herpetiformis
- Peutz–Jeghers syndrome: adenocarcinoma
- Radiation enteritis: lymphoma

Benign tumours
Types
- Epithelial tumours (tubulous and villous adenomas)
- Lipomas
- Haemangiomas
- Neurogenic tumours

Presentation and management
- Often asymptomatic
- May present with obstruction or anaemia
- Diagnosis: small-bowel enema
- Treatment: resection

Malignant tumours
Adenocarcinoma (40%)
- 80% in duodenum
- Predisposing conditions:
  (a) FAP
  (b) Peutz–Jeghers syndrome
  (c) Crohn's disease
  (d) Coeliac disease
- Male/female ratio 1 : 1, age 60 years
- Abdominal discomfort, nausea and vomiting, weight loss
- Anaemia

- Obstructive jaundice if tumour in ampulla
- Surgical resection
- 5-year survival: 15%

Carcinoid tumours (30%)
- Enterochromaffin cells of the crypts of Leiberkühn
- Sites: appendix, small bowel, rectum
- Size:
  (a) < 1 cm never malignant
  (b) 1–1.9 cm may be malignant
  (c) > 2 cm usually malignant
- Usually malignant, multiple (40%) and associated with a malignant neoplasm (30%)
- Age at presentation: 45–55 years
- Clinical features: diarrhoea, intestinal obstruction, abdominal mass
- Treatment: resection
- Prognosis: generally good.

Embryological site	Anatomical sites involved	Peptides that may be secreted	Hormones that may be secreted
Foregut	Stomach, biliary tree, bronchus	5-HTP, 5-HT, histamine, substance P	ACTH, ADH, calcitonin, cholecystokinin, gastrin, glucagons, growth hormone, insulin, β-MSH, parathormone, somatostatin, VIP
Midgut	Jejunum, ileum, right colon	5-HT, kallikrein, ?prostaglandins	
Hindgut	Left colon and rectum	No active peptides secreted	No hormones secreted

Carcinoid syndrome
- Rare syndrome found in < 10% of patients with carcinoid tumours, always associated with hepatic carcinoid involvement
- Caused by inappropriate secretion of peptides (5-HT, 5-HTP, kallikrein, histamine, ACTH)

Clinical features
- Cutaneous flushing syndromes affecting the upper part of the body
- Intestinal colic, diarrhoea, bronchospasm
- Cardiac lesions: tricuspid incompetence, pulmonary stenosis
- Photosensitive dermatitis
- Neurological signs, peptic ulceration and neuralgia
- Biochemical diagnosis: urinary 5-HIAA, the metabolite of 5-HT and 5-HTP

Treatment
- Remove hepatic deposits: surgery or embolization if surgery not possible
- Antiserotonin therapy: several agents (see Table 31.1)
- Chemotherapy for palliation: via hepatic artery or portal vein tributary

Lymphoma (25%)
- Non-Hodgkins lymphoma
- B-cell or T-cell lymphoma
- Low grade or high grade

Types
- MALT lymphoma
- Centrocytic lymphoma
- Mediterranean lymphoma
- Burkitt-type lymphoma
- Polymorphic T-cell lymphoma

Clinical features
- Age 60+ years, male > female
- Acute presentation: intestinal obstruction or perforation
- Insidious presentation:
  (a) Malaise, abdominal pain, weight loss, diarrhoea, anaemia
  (b) Rasied ESR, hypoproteinaemia
- Diagnosis: small-bowel contrast enema, CT, laparoscopy

Management
- Emergency resection for acute presentation
- Chemotherapy/radiotherapy for stage I or II disease (see Table 31.2)

04

Mesenchymal tumours (5%)
● 'Gastrointestinal sarcoma' is term used to describe all mesenchymal tumours with malignant potential on histology

Types
● Smooth muscle tumours
● Neurogenic tumour
● Uncommitted mesenchymal cells

Clinical features
● Present in middle age

● Long history, gastrointestinal bleeding, abdominal pain, weakness, weight loss
● Intestinal obstruction/tumour perforation
● Intraperitoneal bleeding
● Palpable abdominal mass
● Diagnosis: endoscopy for proximal lesions, contrast small-bowel enema, angiography

Treatment
● Surgery (do not respond to chemotherapy or radiotherapy)

Crohn's disease

This is an idiopathic chronic inflammatory condition that can affect any part of the gastrointestinal tract and may be associated with systemic manifestations. The disease is localized to:
● ileocolic region in 60% of patients;
● small bowel alone in 20%;
● colon alone in 20%.
Perianal disease may accompany more proximal disease. Other sites (e.g. mouth, oesophagus, stomach) are extremely rare. Crohn's disease is common in North America and northern Europe.

Pathology

Crohn's disease is segmental, with areas of involvement sharply demarcated from the contiguous normal bowel, at least macroscopically. There may be several diseased segments with normal intervening bowel (skip lesions). The disease starts as mucosal inflammation with small aphthoid ulcers but progresses to involve all layers, so that in advanced disease the serosal surface is inflamed with a tendency for it to be encroached by swollen, oedematous and foreshortened mesentery. The transmural inflammation is associated with narrowing of the bowel lumen. Mucosal oedema accounts for the characteristic cobblestone appearance of the mucosa and is followed by sloughing and linear ulceration of the mucosa. Pseudo-polyps and mucosal bridges may form and the ulcers, which are typically deep and fissuring, penetrate into the muscle layers and may lead to perforation and fistula formation. Regional lymphadenopathy is invariably present and usually the result of reactive hyperplasia.

The histological features of Crohn's disease are characterized by transmural inflammation consisting of chronic inflammatory cell infiltrates including eosinophils, crypt abscess formation, oedema, non-caseating epithelioid cell granulomas containing giant cells (Langhans' cells), dilatation and sclerosis of the intestinal lymphatics, and lymphoid aggregates with or without germinal centres. These granulomas are found in the bowel wall in 50–60% of cases and to a lesser extent in the regional lymph nodes. They constitute the most important feature for histological diagnosis.

The aetiology of Crohn's disease remains obscure. The hypotheses include genetic factors, infective agents (attenuated L-bacterial forms), immunological mechanisms and vasculitis. A susceptibility locus for Crohn's disease has been mapped to chromosome 16.

Clinical features

The peak incidence is in the third decade with equal sex distribution. However, Crohn's disease may also affect children and the elderly. The clinical manifestations are extremely varied and depend on the location and extent of disease. Often the disease presents with other clinical syndromes:
● pseudo-appendicitis syndrome;
● small-bowel obstruction;
● abscess and fistula formation;
● diarrhoea;
● growth retardation.
Some patients, especially children, present with acute abdominal pain in the right iliac fossa simulating acute appendicitis. At operation it may be difficult to differentiate acute Crohn's ileitis from acute terminal ileitis due to *Yersinia* infection and for this reason resection is avoided. Another presentation is with acute or subacute small-bowel obstruction (Fig. 31.1). Patients with intermittent subacute obstructive episodes develop bacterial overgrowth with malabsorption, hypoproteinaemia and malnutrition. Other patients present with abscess formation from bowel perforation or with an inflammatory phlegmon consisting of a mass of inflamed regional lymph nodes without

04

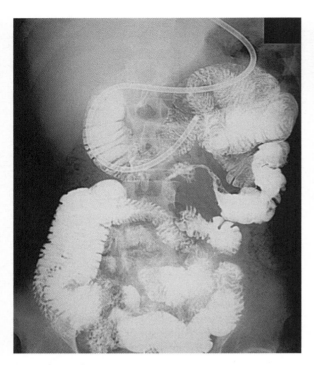

Figure 31.1 Small-bowel enema (enteroclysis) demonstrating ileal Crohn's disease.

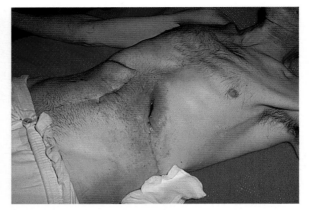

Figure 31.2 Jejunal fistula with excoriation of the abdominal wall in a patient with severe and extensive small-bowel Crohn's disease.

Diagnosis

The diagnosis of Crohn's disease is based on clinical signs and endoscopic, radiological and histological findings. Certain laboratory tests are important: full blood count, ESR, serum electrolytes, serum proteins and, in particular, serum albumin. The indices of disease activity are:

- ESR;
- serum, α_1-glycoprotein;
- C-reactive protein;
- OKT9 lymphocyte positivity.

Small-bowel disease is usually detected by small-bowel enema or follow-through. Narrowing of the lumen, nodularity of the mucosal pattern, thickening of the ileocaecal valve, mucosal irregularity and deep ulcerations (rose-thorn ulceration) and fistula formation are all characteristic features of Crohn's disease. Long narrow strictures result and produce the string sign of Kantor (Fig. 31.3). Skip lesions are characteristic, with normal bowel between the diseased areas. External fistulae and sinuses are evaluated by direct injection of contrast media or by magnetic resonance imaging.

Complications

In addition to the local complications, Crohn's disease may give rise to:

- sclerosing cholangitis;
- skin problems (e.g. pyoderma gangrenosum and erythema nodosum);
- arthritis;
- uveitis;
- obstructive uropathy;
- renal calculi.

perforation of the bowel. In addition to pain and tenderness, abscess formation causes malaise, weight loss, fever and anorexia. The most common site of abscess formation is in the right iliac fossa. Free perforation of Crohn's disease into the peritoneal cavity with widespread peritonitis is rare. Presentation with a perianal fistula in association with perianal abscess is very common. These perianal complications are a significant feature of Crohn's disease and may be present months or years before intestinal symptoms are noticed. Other fistulae (enterocutaneous) usually become evident following drainage of abdominal abscesses (Fig. 31.2). Enterovesical fistulae present with urinary symptoms (cystitis and pneumaturia).

Diarrhoea is a predominant symptom in patients with Crohn's disease, especially in patients with terminal ileal/ileocolic involvement. Diarrhoea associated with colonic disease is accompanied by the passage of mucus and blood from the rectum and is very similar to the symptomatology of ulcerative colitis. Growth retardation is common in children. Following an appropriate bowel resection, growth resumes the normal pattern but compensatory growth does not occur. It is therefore essential to treat these children while their bones are still capable of growth.

04

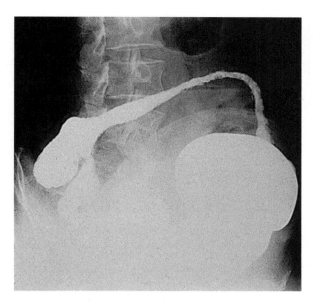

Figure 31.3 Extensive Crohn's disease of the colon exhibiting the string sign of Kantor.

Treatment

Medical

In patients with extensive disease, correction of nutritional deficiencies is necessary and oral feeding with elemental diet reduces the foreign protein load presented to the inflamed mucosa. Parenteral nutrition is indicated in:

- intestinal failure with gross nutritional deficiencies and severe hypoalbuminaemia;
- malnourished patients prior to surgery;
- in obtaining remission in patients with severe active disease;
- in patients with enterocutaneous fistulae.

Long-term home parenteral nutrition is reserved for patients with extensive small-bowel disease or resection and intestinal failure. Patients are taught to self-administer the parenteral feeds and to care for their central lines, and it offers a reasonable quality of life. Some patients require only intermittent supplemental intravenous feeding and manage reasonably well with oral modified or elemental diets in the intervening periods. Home parenteral nutrition is supervised by the medical and nursing staff of specialized nutrition units.

Glutamine added to either parenteral or enteral diets improves intestinal healing and nitrogen utilization. Supplemental folate therapy (0.2 mg/day) is indicated during acute exacerbations and particularly during parenteral nutrition. Reduced serum concentrations of trace elements are also found in patients with severe active inflammatory bowel disease and require correction as they are essential components of metalloenzymes and metalloproteins.

5-Aminosalicylic acid (5-ASA) is the initial treatment of choice in mild to moderate Crohn's disease and for the maintaining remission. Sulfasalazine, a combination of 5-ASA and sulfapyridine, is not recommended for small-bowel disease because of adverse effects (headaches, nausea, oligospermia). Preparations containing 5-ASA alone are now used and are formulated to allow targeting of the drug at sites of active disease, e.g. slow-release mesalazine (Pentasa) or pH-dependent-release mesalazine (Asacol). Cortiscosteroids are used in severe disease and in cases not responding to 5-ASA therapy. Budesonide, a highly potent semisynthetic steroid, in a dose of 5 mg/day is as effective as 40 mg of prednisolone daily. It reduces steroid-associated adverse effects and may become the drug of choice in the management of patients with active Crohn's disease.

For particularly severe disease that relapses or is dependent on steroids, a number of modulators of the cellular immune response can provide benefit, such as azathioprine and 6-mercaptopurine. Therapy with a monoclonal antibody against tumour necrosis factor (TNF)-α (Infliximab) is efficacious in fistulating disease and has a relatively low incidence of adverse effects. Antibiotics have their place, particularly in the treatment of perianal Crohn's disease, and some (ciprofloxacin and metronidazole) can induce symptomatic remission in active Crohn's disease.

Surgical

Surgical intervention is only indicated for complications of the disease and for active disease that does not respond to medical therapy. Other factors that influence the decision to operate and the type of operative procedure include the anatomical site of disease and whether the operation is being performed as an emergency or an elective procedure. The extra-gastrointestinal manifestations of Crohn's disease are not an indication for operative intervention. The emphasis of surgical treatment is on maximal preservation of intestine, with resections being strictly limited to the diseased segment. Bypass is only carried out when there is no other alternative. Conservative (non-resectional) surgery is indicated in patients with multiple previous resections and 'burnt-out' strictures for which stricturoplasty is used.

Operations for Crohn's disease are followed by a high incidence of postoperative complications, such as anastomotic leakage, fistula formation, intra-abdominal abscess and haemorrhage. One of the unresolved problems is the high incidence of recurrence following resection, up to

Crohn's disease at a glance

Definition

Crohn's disease: idiopathic chronic transmural inflammatory disorder of the alimentary tract

Epidemiology
- Male/female ratio 1 : 1.6
- Young adults
- High incidence among Europeans and Jews

Aetiology
- Unknown
- Impaired cell-mediated immunity
- Genetic link probable but candidate genes unknown
- No proven link to mycobacterial infection or measles virus hypersensitivity
- Smoking associated with recurrence

Pathology
Macroscopic
- May affect any part of the alimentary tract. Ileocolic region in 60% of patients, small bowel only in 20% and colon only in 20%
- Skip lesions in bowel (affected bowel wall and mesentery are thickened and oedematous, frequent fistulae)
- Affected bowel characteristically 'fat wrapped' but mesenteric fat
- Perianal disease characterized by perianal induration and sepsis with fissure, sinus and fistula formation

Histology
- Transmural inflammation in the form of lymphoid aggregates
- Non-caseating epithelioid cell granulomas with Langhans' giant cells. Regional nodes may also be involved

Clinical features
Acute presentation (uncommon)
- Right iliac fossa peritonitis (like appendicitis picture)
- Generalized peritonitis (due to free perforation)

Subacute presentation (common)
- Right iliac fossa inflammatory mass: usually associated with fistulae or abscess formation
- Widespread ileal inflammation: general ill health, malnutrition, anaemia, abdominal pain

Chronic presentation
- Strictures: intermittent colicky abdominal pains associated with eating

- Diarrhoea: prominent in patients with ileal or ileocolic disease
- Malabsorption: due to widespread disease often with previous resections
- Growth retardation in children: due to chronic malnutrition and chronic inflammatory response suppressing growth

Extraintestinal features
- Eye: episcleritis, uveitis
- Joints: arthritis
- Skin: erythema nodosum, pyoderma gangrenosum
- Liver: sclerosing cholangitis, cirrhosis
- Urinary: obstructive uropathy, renal colic

Perianal disease
- Is common and may be the presenting feature
- Fissure in ano, fistula in ano, perianal sepsis

Investigations
- Full blood count: macrocytic anaemia
- Small-bowel enema: narrowed terminal ileum, string sign of Kantor, stricture formation, fistulae
- Abdominal ultrasound: right iliac fossa mass, abscess formation
- CT: right iliac fossa mass, abscess formation
- In-labelled white-cell scan: areas of inflammation

Indices of disease severity
- ESR
- Serum α_1-glycoprotein
- C-reactive protein
- OKT9 lymphocyte positivity

Management
Medical
- Nutritional support: enteral and parenteral feeding
- Indications for total parenteral nutrition:
  (a) Intestinal failure with severe nutritional deficiency
  (b) Malnutrition prior to surgery
  (c) To achieve remission in severe active disease
  (d) Enterocutaneous fistulae
- Anti-inflammatory drugs: 5-ASA, mesalazine, steroids. Sulfasalazine (5-ASA + sulfapyridine) is not recommended for small-bowel Crohn's disease because of adverse effects
- Antibiotics: only for specific complicating bacterial infections
- Immunosuppressive agents: azathioprine, 6-mercaptopurine, cyclosporin, anti-TNFα (for fistulating disease)

04

Surgical
● Surgery is common but never curative and should be used sparingly when necessary for:
    (a) Complications (peritonitis, obstruction, abscess, fistula)
    (b) Failure of medical treatment and symptomatic
    (c) Growth retardation in children
● Principles: resect minimum necessary

Prognosis
● Crohn's disease is a chronic problem and recurrent episodes of active disease are common
● 75% of patients will require surgery at some time
● 60% of patients will require more than one operation
● Life expectancy of Crohn's disease patients is little different from the 'normal' population

Intestinal obstruction at a glance

Definitions

Complete intestinal obstruction: total blockage of the intestinal lumen, whereas *incomplete obstruction* denotes only a partial blockage. Obstruction may be *acute* (hours) or *chronic* (weeks), *simple* (*mechanical*), i.e. blood supply is not compromised, or *strangulated*, i.e. blood supply is compromised

Closed loop obstruction: both the inlet and outlet of a bowel loop is closed off

Common causes
● Extramural: adhesions, bands, volvulus, herniae (internal and external), compression by tumour (e.g. frozen pelvis)
● Intramural: inflammatory bowel disease (Crohn's disease), tumours, carcinomas, lymphomas, strictures, paralytic (adynamic) ileus, intussusception
● Intraluminal: faecal impaction, foreign bodies, bezoars, gallstone ileus
● Small-bowel obstruction is often rapid in onset and commonly due to adhesions or hernia
● Large-bowel obstruction may be gradual or intermittent in onset, is often due to carcinoma or strictures and *never* due to adhesions

Pathophysiology
● Bowel distal to obstruction collapses
● Bowel proximal to obstruction distends and becomes hyperactive. Distension is due to swallowed air and accumulating intestinal secretions
● Bowel wall becomes oedematous. Fluid and electrolytes accumulate in the wall and lumen (third-space loss)
● Bacteria proliferate in the obstructed bowel
● As the bowel distends, intramural vessels become stretched and the blood supply is compromised leading to ischaemia and necrosis

Clinical features
● Vomiting, colicky abdominal pain, abdominal distension, absolute constipation (i.e. neither faeces nor flatus)
● Dehydration and loss of skin turgor

● Hypotension, tachycardia
● Abdominal distension and increased bowel sounds
● Empty rectum on digital examination
● Tenderness or rebound indicates peritonitis

Investigations
● Cause should be sought and confirmed wherever possible prior to operation
● Haemoglobin, packed cell volume: elevated due to dehydration
● White cell count (WCC): normal or slightly elevated
● Urea and electrolytes: urea elevated, Na^+ and Cl^- low
● Chest X-ray: elevated diaphragm due to abdominal distension
● Abdominal supine X-ray:
    (a) Small-bowel obstruction: central loops, valvulae conniventes shadows cross entire width of lumen
    (b) Large-bowel obstruction: peripheral distribution/ haustral shadows do not cross entire width of bowel
    (c) Look for cause (gallstone, characteristic patterns of volvulus, herniae)
● Single-contrast large-bowel enema: ?large-bowel obstruction (site and cause)
● CT: ?small-bowel obstruction (site and cause)
● Sigmoidoscopy: to show site of obstruction

Management
● Decompress the obstructed gut: pass nasogastric tube
● Replace fluid and electrolyte losses: give Ringer's lactate or saline with K^+ supplementation
● Monitor the patient: fluid balance, urinary catheter, temperature, pulse, respiration, blood tests
● Request investigations appropriate to likely cause
● Relieve obstruction surgically if:
    (a) Underlying cause needs surgical treatment (e.g. hernia, colonic carcinoma)
    (b) Patient does not improve with conservative treatment (e.g. adhesion obstruction)
    (c) Signs of strangulation or peritonitis are present
● Tachycardia, pyrexia and abdominal tenderness indicate the need to operate whatever the cause

60% at 15 years. Young patients and those with ileocolic disease have the highest and earliest recurrence and the worst ultimate prognosis. Maintenance medical therapy does not influence recurrence rate. The majority of recurrences occur at or near the anastomosis and in patients with ileorectal anastomosis the recurrent disease often involves the ileum.

Many patients with Crohn's disease undergo multiple resections and a significant percentage of these develop short-gut syndrome. At present the majority of these patients are managed by home parenteral nutrition.

Radiation enteropathy

The immediate effect of radiation on the gastrointestinal tract is arrest of cell division in the intestinal crypts. Radiation exposure also causes oedema and ulceration of the mucosa. Eventually the mucosa becomes thinner with stunted villi, leading to malabsorption of varying degrees. In addition the damaged bowel becomes fibrotic, with the appearance of atypical fibroblasts in the submucosa and ischaemia due to the development of proliferative endarteritis and vasculitis. Obliteration of the intestinal lymphatics with lymphatic ectasia complicates the pathological picture. The oedema is most marked in the submucosal layer. The serosa becomes thickened, opaque and greyish white and dense adhesions develop between adjacent intestinal loops.

Radiation-induced bowel disease is common especially when the pelvis is irradiated, usually for rectal or gynaecological cancer. The most common symptoms referable to chronic bowel damage are vague abdominal discomfort, diarrhoea, mild rectal bleeding and the passage of mucus. The interval between the time of radiation and onset of symptoms varies considerably from 2 months to 2 years. Intestinal obstruction may be acute or subacute and recurrent. Occasionally, acute presentation with infarction may occur and this carries a high risk of perforation and mortality. Diagnosis is established by contrast radiology of the small and large intestine.

Management is conservative in the first instance, with correction of nutritional deficiencies and the use of intestinal sedatives (codeine phosphate, Lomotil and diphenoxylate hydrochloride). Prednisolone enemas provide symptomatic benefit in patients with radiation proctitis. Some patients with extensive small-bowel disease and severe malabsorption require parenteral nutrition. Emergency surgery is indicated for infarction with perforation or acute intestinal obstruction that fails to settle with conservative treatment. The radionecrotic bowel is ideally excised, with primary anastomosis or exteriorization of the bowel ends in the presence of ischaemia and sepsis. Elective surgery is undertaken for chronic severe symptoms due to stricture or internal fistula formation.

Intestinal tuberculosis

Intestinal tuberculosis can be classified into four macroscopic forms: hypertrophic, ulcerative, fibrotic and ulcerofibrotic, with the first two accounting for the majority of cases.
- *Hypertrophic type*: affects predominantly the ileocaecal region and is characterized by marked thickening of the submucosal and subserosal layers. It is generally regarded as a low-virulence infection in a patient with a high degree of immunological resistance.
- *Ulcerative type*: involves largely the terminal ileum where multiple deep transverse ulcers develop and extend to the serosa and may give rise to perforation. The serosal surface is thickened and studded with tubercles. Healing may result in multiple strictures with intervening and dilated segments of ileum.
- *Fibrotic type*: affects the terminal ileum, caecum and ascending colon. It leads to shortening and considerable narrowing of long segments of the bowel and may be accompanied by generalized peritoneal tuberculosis.

Patients with the hypertrophic type of intestinal tuberculosis are not usually very ill, although they exhibit the systemic manifestations of tuberculosis. The intestinal infection itself causes recurrent episodes of subacute intestinal obstruction, with colicky abdominal pain and vomiting or a mass in the right iliac fossa. The ulcerative type presents acutely with perforation or with subacute intestinal obstruction. The fibrotic variety also presents with acute or subacute intestinal obstruction. The diagnosis of abdominal tuberculosis can be difficult. Attempts to culture mycobacteria from gastric washings, faeces, peritoneal fluid and tissue biopsies may be negative. Barium studies show features of altered motility and stenotic radiological changes that may be indistinguishable from Crohn's disease. In many instances, the diagnosis is only made at laparotomy.

In the absence of intestinal obstruction or perforation the treatment is conservative, with rest, adequate nutritional intake and antituberculous chemotherapy using combinations of rifampicin, isoniazid and ethambutol for 12 months. Surgical treatment is indicated for intestinal obstruction or perforation. Ileocaecal resection and right hemicolectomy are the standard operations for ileocaecal disease and the results are good.

Human immunodeficiency virus enteropathy

Gastrointestinal problems are very common in patients

with acquired immunodeficiency syndrome (AIDS). In the majority these are caused by opportunistic infection with protozoal organisms, various bacterial species, viruses and fungi; however, in one-third of patients no identifiable pathogens can be isolated from the stool but DNA probe studies identify human immunodeficiency virus (HIV)-1 in the enterochromaffin cells, base of the crypts and lamina propria. The gastrointestinal symptoms common in AIDS are diarrhoea, weight loss and abdominal pain. Other clinical features include fever, sore throat, lymphadenopathy and arthralgia. All AIDS patients with gastrointestinal symptoms require endoscopy and stool culture. If a specific infection is established, treatment is directed to eradicating the organism responsible. Symptomatic relief can be obtained using non-specific anti-diarrhoeal therapy.

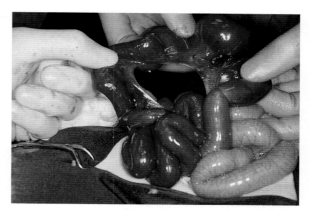

Figure 31.4 Small-bowel infarction caused by volvulus.

Short-gut syndrome (intestinal failure)

The intestinal decompensation that follows massive resection of the small intestine (< 100 cm residual small bowel) is due to sudden reduction of the absorptive area and a greatly reduced transit time, which further aggravates malabsorption and in extreme cases limits the extent of digestion. Malabsorption of fats and proteins is invariable. Carbohydrate absorption is less severely affected and is the first to recover. Spill-over of primary bile salt conjugates into the colon, where bacterial action converts them to deconjugated and dehydroxylated derivatives, contributes to the diarrhoea characteristic of short-gut syndrome. This severe diarrhoea can amount to several litres in the first few weeks after resection. Lactose intolerance may occur in some patients after extensive small-bowel resection.

Multiple/major resections leading to short-gut syndrome are necessitated by:

- Crohn's disease;
- mesenteric infarction (Fig. 31.4);
- radiation enteritis;
- midgut volvulus;
- multiple fistulae;
- small-bowel tumours.

Crohn's disease is the most common cause as it often necessitates repeated resections over a number of years. Patients with a residual small-bowel length of less than 2 m have a diminished work capacity and those with less than 100 cm require home parenteral nutrition on an indefinite basis. Infants and neonates seem to tolerate extensive small-bowel resections better than adults and a minimum of 30 cm of small intestine can support both nutrition and growth.

The critical length of residual small bowel necessary to avoid intestinal failure is influenced by the site of resection and the retention or otherwise of the ileocaecal valve. Thus ileal resections are less well tolerated than jejunal resections because the active transport sites for bile salts and vitamin B_{12} are localized in the ileum. An intact ileocaecal valve slows transit time and limits the degree of bacterial colonization of the residual intestine.

The main clinical features are weight loss and incessant watery diarrhoea. Perianal excoriation is frequent because of the diarrhoea and the low pH of the stool. With time, structural and functional changes occur in the residual bowel as part of the process of adaptation and are characterized by dilation of the remaining intestine and enlargement of the villi. These changes are accompanied by gradual improvement in the absorption of water, electrolytes, carbohydrate and protein. The enhanced absorption results from an increased cell population in the intestinal villi. Both luminal and humoral factors are involved in this adaptive hyperplasia. Luminal factors include alimentary secretions and ingested nutrients. The maintenance of adequate intraluminal nutrition by oral ingestion is essential for the adaptive response. Enteroglucagon is the most important hormone involved in the adaptive response. The stimulus for its release is exposure of the residual bowel to luminal nutrition. Other factors that may contribute to compensation by the residual intestine include changes in the motility pattern leading to a gradual slowing of the transit time and increased absorption of water-soluble substances by the colon.

The complications associated with short-gut syndrome include:

- gastric hypersecretion;
- cholesterol gallstones;

Table 31.3 Sequential management of patients after massive resection of the small bowel.

Stage of decompensation
Total parenteral nutrition
Oral sips of water/hypotonic solutions

Transition to enteral feeding
Parenteral nutrition plus gradually increasing supplement of enteral feeds
Full enteral feeding

Final stage
Normal low-fat (medium-chain triglyceride) diet plus supplements in patients with > 1 m of residual small bowel
Enteral feeding plus intermittent parenteral feeding in patients with about 1 m of residual small bowel
Home parenteral nutrition in patients with no effective residual small bowel

- hepatic disease;
- impaired renal function and stone formation;
- metabolic bone disease;
- growth failure in children.

Treatment

The treatment of short-gut syndrome is centred around supporting the patient during the initial stage of decompensation and through the critical stage of adaptation, which may last up to 3 months. At the end of this time the stage of equilibrium is reached and the patient with residual small intestine enters the final stage of rehabilitation. In patients with massive small-bowel resection, indefinite total parenteral nutrition via a permanent tunnelled silicon feeding line is the only option for survival. It is essential that these patients receive a programme of training in the management of intravenous feeds and care of feeding lines so that they can eventually carry out parenteral nutrition themselves in their own homes, usually at night.

In the immediate postoperative period, total parenteral nutrition is essential. Accurate fluid balance must be maintained by daily charting of input and output volumes, which should include all measured losses. Histamine H_2-receptor antagonists or proton pump inhibitors are administered to suppress gastric secretion. Initially only small amounts of weak hypotonic fluids or water are given to avoid a dry mouth. When the patient's condition becomes stable, transition to an oral diet is started in those patients with an adequate length of small intestine. Feeding is started gradually, initially with isotonic carbohydrate and electrolyte solutions. Thereafter, elemental diets are infused at a rate of 25 mL/h via a nasogastric feeding tube. The rate and concentration are gradually increased until the patient is receiving 100–120 mL/h of full-strength diet, with care to avoid gastric dilatation and pulmonary aspiration. Diarrhoea is often accentuated at the start of enteral feeding but is controlled by intestinal sedatives (loperamide hydrochloride, diphenoxylate hydrochloride, codeine phosphate). Somatostatin infusion may be necessary in some patients with severe diarrhoea.

In patients in whom the ileum has been resected, vitamin B_{12} is administered parenterally at 3-monthly intervals on an indefinite basis. The sequential medical management of patients after massive resection of the small intestine is summarized in Table 31.3. Currently, home total parenteral nutrition is the only option for the majority of patients with intestinal failure.

Vascular abnormalities

Vascular abnormalities of the small bowel include angiodysplasia, phlebectasia, telangiectasia (hereditary haemorrhagic telangiectasia or Osler–Weber–Rendu disease) and haemangiomas.

- *Angiodysplasias.* These are the most common and form in the mucosa/submucosa of the gastrointestinal tract. They consist of a cluster of arteriolar, venular and capillary vessels and are less common in the small bowel than the right colon. The aetiology is uncertain but they are thought to arise on a background of chronic mucosal ischaemia secondary to arterial venous shunting, decreased perfusion pressure and lowered oxygen tension in the terminal branches of the superior mesenteric arteries.
- *Phlebectasia.* These lesions consist of a meshwork of dilated veins having a normal endothelial lining and situated in the submucosal layer of the intestine.
- *Hereditary haemorrhagic telangiectasia.* This rare inherited disorder is characterized by multiple telangiectasias of the lips, mouth, nasopharynx and gut. The lesion consists of arteriolar dilations due to a congenital weakness of

04

the arterial muscle and absence of elastin in the medial coat.

● *Haemangiomas*. These are rare, congenital, non-hereditary malformations of blood vessels (vascular hamartomas). They may occur in the small or large intestine.

The clinical presentation of angiodysplasias and cavernous haemangiomas is with rectal bleeding, which can be massive and incur a mortality. In hereditary haemorrhagic telangiectasia gastrointestinal bleeding is rarely severe and patients may present with anaemia or intermittent melaena. Likewise, in phlebectasia the bleeding is usually mild although severe bleeding can occur.

The diagnosis of small-bowel vascular lesions is confirmed by angiography performed during a bleeding episode. Treatment consists of resection of the affected segment of small bowel.

Peutz–Jeghers syndrome. This is an inherited autosomal dominant disorder characterized by jejunal or ileal polyps and mucocutaneous pigmentation. The polyps are hamartomatous in nature and consist of a fibromuscular stroma covered with well-differentiated epithelium. Rarely, the polyps may be localized in the stomach, duodenum or large bowel. The patients have pigmentation on the lips and buccal mucosa. This abnormal pigmentation usually appears in infancy but symptoms from polyps do not usually occur until the second decade. These consist of attacks of intestinal colic that predate acute intestinal obstruction from intussusception or intraluminal obstruction by a large polyp. Bleeding from the polyps is common but is usually chronic and occult, leading to iron-deficiency anaemia. There is a small risk of malignant transformation. Surgical treatment is also indicated for intestinal obstruction and haemorrhage.

Vermiform appendix and Meckel's diverticulum

The vermiform appendix is narrow, of variable length (5–15 cm) with its base attached to the posteromedial surface of the caecum close to the junction of the ileum and caecum. However, the position of the appendix is very variable: below or behind the caecum (retrocaecal); preileal; or lesser pelvis, when it may lie close to the ovary, fallopian tube and ureter. The submucosal layer of the appendix has lymph follicles. When these enlarge in response to infection, the swollen submucosal layer can block the lumen of the appendix.

Acute appendicitis

Development of appendicitis is related to swelling of the lymphoid tissue in the submucosa in response to viral or bacterial infection. This may then proceed to inflammation. The presence of gangrene or perforation is associated with the presence of faecoliths. Approximately 50% of cases of gangrenous or perforated appendicitis are associated with a faecolith in contrast with uncomplicated appendicitis. Overall, about 20% of all patients with acute appendicitis have perforation at the time of operation. This is much higher at the extremes of age (below 5 and above 60 years).

The aetiology of acute appendicitis remains unclear. Diet may be involved (reduced fibre content) as the disease is very common in the West but rare in Africa. Acute appendicitis is commoner in urban populations compared with rural districts, an observation attributed to the high incidence of enteric infections in densely populated areas. There has been a steady decline in the incidence of the disease during the last 50 years and this has been linked to improved domestic and food hygiene. Consumption of green vegetables and tomatoes may be protective. In elderly patients there is some evidence that chronic intake of non-steroidal anti-inflammatory drugs may increase the risk.

Clinical features

In the majority of patients with acute appendicitis, pain starts in the umbilical region and consists of a dull ache or colic (presumably from obstruction of the appendiceal lumen). After a variable period, the pain shifts to the right lower quadrant of the abdomen as the inflamed appendix irritates the parietal peritoneum. However not all patients experience this shift of pain and the presentation may start with discomfort in the right lower quadrant. Patients usually report that movement and coughing induce sharp exacerbation of the pain. Nausea and vomiting are common and anorexia is almost inevitable. About 20% of patients have diarrhoea and this may lead to a mistaken diagnosis of gastroenteritis.

In children it is important to ask about a sore throat or flu-like symptoms as these often accompany mesenteric adenitis. Female patients in particular should be asked about dysuria, frequency and cloudy/strong-smelling urine because urinary tract infection can often cause lower abdominal pain. Likewise, a menstrual history is essential. A missed period may point to an ectopic pregnancy. Pain at mid-cycle may indicate that the pain is due to ovulation (mittelschmerz) and vaginal discharge may indicate pelvic inflammatory disease.

Patients with acute appendicitis usually have a sustained tachycardia, mild pyrexia and abdominal tenderness. A very high temperature (> 39°C) indicates probable abscess formation or some other diagnosis such as a viral illness. It is then useful to ask the patient to cough

while watching the facial expression. If coughing produces obvious pain, the patient should be asked to indicate the site of maximum pain. In acute appendicitis the patient points to the right iliac fossa. The tongue is usually furred. The tonsils should also be inspected particularly in children, as pharyngitis may be associated with mesenteric adenitis. The site of maximal tenderness on palpation is close to McBurney's point (junction between the upper two-thirds and lower one-third of a straight line joining the umbilicus and the anterior superior iliac spine). However, in patients with an inflamed retrocaecal appendix the pain may be considerably higher and more lateral than this, and in pelvic appendicitis the pain may be lower and almost in the midline. Indeed, with a low pelvic appendix, tenderness may only be detectable by rectal examination. Right lower quadrant guarding is found in about 90% of patients with acute appendicitis; if the appendix has perforated causing generalized peritonitis, the area of guarding extends beyond the right lower quadrant. Rebound tenderness may be elicited by pressing gently into the right lower quadrant of the abdomen and then suddenly releasing the hand, watching the patient's face for signs of discomfort. Another approach is to percuss the area; this elicits the same response and is kinder. When the amount of tenderness permits, careful palpation of the right iliac fossa for a mass should be carried out. This may indicate the presence of an appendiceal abscess or an appendix mass (phlegmon) created by omentum wrapped around the inflamed appendix. It may also indicate some other pathology such as a perforated caecal carcinoma or Crohn's disease. Rectal examination should always be done and elicits tenderness on the right.

The diagnosis of acute appendicitis is made largely on clinical grounds but there are some investigations that may be of value:
- WCC;
- plain abdominal X-ray;
- urinalysis;
- ultrasound (especially in females to exclude acute gynaecological pathology);
- laparoscopy (especially in female patients in the reproductive age);
- aspiration cytology;
- CT (selective use for right iliac fossa mass).

The majority of patients have a polymorphonuclear leukocytosis ($> 12 \times 10^9$/L). In a patient with clear-cut symptoms and signs of acute appendicitis, a plain abdominal X-ray is of little or no diagnostic value. However, it is indicated if there is some clinical suspicion of intestinal obstruction or ureteric colic. Ultrasound examination of the pelvis is particularly useful in female patients (exclusion of gynaecological pathology), in distinguishing between an appendix mass and an abscess, and in making

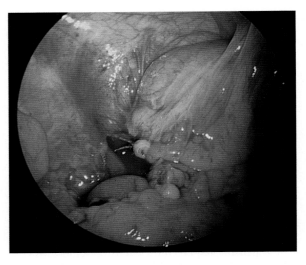

Figure 31.5 Laparoscopic appendicectomy.

a specific diagnosis of appendicitis, although this is not as yet routine practice. CT may occasionally be useful in establishing the diagnosis where a right lower quadrant mass is present. Some practise the aspiration cytology test: peritoneal fluid is aspirated using a fine catheter introduced immediately below the umbilicus; the test is positive if more than 50% of the cells are neutrophils. This indicates the presence of infection.

Laparoscopy has an established role in the diagnosis of acute appendicitis. It is valuable in women of childbearing age where there are a number of different causes of right lower quadrant pain and tenderness. Use of laparoscopy in males and in children is less well established but whenever there is a diagnostic problem and the surgeon is unhappy about prolonged observation, then laparoscopy is appropriate in any patient who has not had previous extensive abdominal surgery. In expert hands, laparoscopy can also be used to carry out appendicectomy (Fig. 31.5).

A urinalysis should always be carried out to exclude the possibility of urinary tract infection.

Complications

Complications of acute appendicitis are secondary to gangrenous or perforated appendicitis and can therefore be avoided by early diagnosis and treatment. The important complications are:
- appendix abscess;
- appendix mass;
- generalized peritonitis, particularly in the very young or elderly;

04

- intraperitoneal abscess formation, either subphrenic or multiple small intraloop abscesses;
- faecal fistula usually following drainage of an abscess;
- recurrent intestinal obstruction due to the formation of adhesions;
- portal pyaemia;
- wound infection;
- overwhelming sepsis and death.

Treatment

The treatment is appendicectomy. Prophylactic antibiotics should be used in all patients. Metronidazole alone, administered as a suppository, is appropriate. In patients with perforated appendicitis, appendicectomy is followed by peritoneal lavage with saline containing an antibiotic. These patients require intravenous antibiotics (metronidazole and cefuroxime) for 5 days postoperatively.

The treatment of patients presenting with an appendiceal mass is conservative in the first instance. A high intermittent fever and a high WCC together with a tender mass indicate formation of an appendiceal abscess. This can be confirmed by ultrasound or CT scanning and insertion of a percutaneous drain is the current treatment of choice. This may be followed by the development of a faecal fistula but this normally heals spontaneously. If no abscess develops, conservative treatment is maintained until resolution.

Neoplasms of the appendix

These are rare and include carcinoids, adenocarcinoma, mucinous neoplasms and lymphoma. The vast majority of tumours of the appendix present as acute appendicitis and the diagnosis is made on histology after appendicectomy.

Carcinoids

The appendix is the most common site for carcinoid tumour formation and carcinoid tumour of the appendix is the most common appendiceal neoplasm. The vast majority are found incidentally at the time of appendicectomy, usually at the tip of the appendix. Rarely they arise at the base of the appendix and may then obstruct the lumen causing acute appendicitis. The vast majority of appendiceal carcinoids are less than 1 cm in diameter and these do not metastasize. Carcinoid tumours greater than 1.5 cm in diameter can and do metastasize. Thus while appendicectomy is curative for a carcinoid less than 1 cm in diameter, tumours greater than 1.5 cm require a right hemicolectomy with radical removal of the ileocaecal lymph nodes.

Adenocarcinoma

This is a rare tumour and accounts for approximately 15% of all malignant tumours of the appendix. It may arise from the base of the appendix. Treatment is right hemicolectomy irrespective of exact location.

Mucinous neoplasms

Simple mucocele of the appendix is rare. It arises as a sequel to obstruction of the appendix without the onset of infection. The appendix becomes distended by mucoid secretion and the normal mucosa becomes replaced by a single layer of mucus-secreting cells. Eventually the lesion may calcify. Malignant mucocele on the other hand is a papilliferous cystadenoma or cystadenocarcinoma consisting of mucus-secreting cells. It often leads to pseudomyxoma peritonei following rupture and spillage of the mucus-secreting cells.

Meckel's diverticulum

Meckel's diverticulum is a remnant of the vitello-intestinal duct and is present in about 2% of the population. It arises from the antimesenteric side of the ileum. It has the same microscopic structure as the adjacent small bowel and its own blood supply from the adjacent small-bowel mesentery. Although the majority are situated 60 cm from the ileocaecal valve, as many as 25% occur more proximally. The length and shape of the diverticulum is also variable and although 85% are blind-ended, the rest have an attachment to the anterior abdominal wall that is related to its embryological origin.

The diverticulum frequently contains ectopic tissue, most commonly gastric mucosa but also pancreatic, duodenal or colonic tissue. The presence of ectopic gastric mucosa can influence the clinical presentation as it is associated with peptic ulceration secondary to acid and pepsin secretion. The majority of Meckel's diverticula do not cause problems and remain asymptomatic. However the following complications may arise:

- inflammation of the diverticulum;
- peptic ulceration of the small bowel;
- bleeding;
- intestinal obstruction.

Meckel's diverticulum can become inflamed in the same way as the vermiform appendix and gangrene and perforation of the diverticulum may ensue. Ectopic gastric mucosa may ulcerate and bleed. Intestinal obstruction may result from intussusception, with the diverticulum acting as a lead point. It can also occur because of persistence of the band between the apex of the diverticulum and the anterior abdominal wall (remnant of the vitello-

intestinal duct) inducing a small-bowel volvulus. In addition, entrapment of small bowel can occur through a defect caused by a mesodiverticular band.

Clinical features

The clinical features of symptomatic Meckel's diverticulum are those of its complications. Otherwise the diverticulum is discovered accidentally during investigations or surgery for other conditions. Acute Meckel's diverticulitis produces a symptom complex very similar to appendicitis but normally the pain persists in the central abdominal area without a shift to the right lower quadrant. This usually occurs in children and frequently a diagnosis of acute appendicitis is made.

Peptic ulceration of the neck of a Meckel's diverticulum or the ileum can lead to bleeding that presents either as melaena or fresh rectal bleeding. Again this nearly always occurs in children. Intestinal obstruction may present with the typical clinical features of small-bowel obstruction. However, infarction of the bowel is likely with volvulus or entrapment of the small bowel by the band. In such cases the patient becomes rapidly ill with peritonitis. The diagnosis of Meckel's diverticulum is usually made at operation but in the child suffering repeated episodes of brisk rectal bleeding or melaena, a technetium scan may be of value.

Treatment

The treatment of a Meckel's diverticulum is excision of the diverticulum together with a wedge of adjacent ileum.

Acute appendicitis at a glance

Definition

Acute appendicitis: inflammation of the vermiform appendix

Epidemiology
- Most common surgical emergency in the western world
- Rare under 2 years of age, common in second and third decades, but can occur at any age

Pathology
- 'Obstructive': infection superimposed on luminal obstruction from any cause
- 'Phlegmonous': viral infection, lymphoid hyperplasia, ulceration, bacterial invasion without obvious cause

Clinical features
- Periumbilical abdominal pain, nausea, vomiting
- Localization of pain to right iliac fossa
- Mild pyrexia
- Patient is flushed, tachycardia, furred tongue, halitosis
- Tender (usually with rebound) over McBurney's point
- Right-sided pelvic tenderness on rectal examination
- Peritonitis if appendix perforated
- Appendix mass if patient presents late

Investigations
- Diagnosis is clinical, but WCC (almost always leukocytosis) and C-reactive protein (usually raised) are helpful
- Ultrasound: for appendix mass and if in doubt to rule out other pelvic pathology (e.g. ovarian cyst)
- Laparoscopy: commonly used to exclude ovarian pathology prior to appendicectomy in young women
- Helical CT: in elderly patients or where other causes are considered possible. CT should be used whenever there is real concern about the differential diagnosis to prevent inappropriate surgical exploration

Differential diagnosis
- In children under 10 years old, 7 of 10 cases of right iliac fossa pain are non-specific and self-limiting
- Mesenteric lymphadenitis in children
- Most common differential diagnosis in young adults is ovarian pathology in females (e.g. pelvic inflammatory disease, urinary tract infection, ectopic pregnancy, ruptured corpus luteum cyst)
- More rarely: Crohn's disease, cholecystitis, perforated duodenal ulcer, right basal pneumonia, torsion of the right testis, diabetes mellitus in younger and middle-aged patients
- Right iliac fossa peritonism over the age of 55 years should raise the suspicion of other causes
- Occasionally: perforated caecal carcinoma, sigmoid diverticulitis, caecal diverticulitis in elderly patients

Management
- Acute appendicitis: appendicectomy
- Appendix mass: i.v. fluids, antibiotics, close observation. Then:
  (a) If symptoms resolve, interval appendicectomy after a few months
  (b) If symptoms progress, urgent appendicectomy ± drainage

Complications
- Appendix mass/abscess
- Generalized peritonitis (elderly/very young)
- Wound infection
- Intra-abdominal abscess (pelvic, right iliac fossa, subphrenic)

04

- Adhesions
- Faecal fistula
- Abdominal actinomycosis (rare!)
- Portal pyaemia

Meckel's diverticulum

Definition

Meckel's diverticulum: remnant of the vitello-intestinal duct forming a blind-ending pouch on the antimesenteric border of the terminal ileum, present in 2% of the population

Clinical features

- Most are asymptomatic
- May present with rectal bleeding, mimic appendicitis (Meckel's diverticulitis), be a lead point for intussusception or cause a volvulus
- Ectopic gastric mucosa in a Meckel's diverticulum is responsible for gastrointestinal bleeding and may be detected by technetium pertechnetate scan in 70% of cases

Management

- Surgical excision, even if found incidentally

Disorders of the Colon and Rectum

32

Must know Must do

Must know

Pathology, manifestations, diagnosis and clinical management of diverticular disease and inflammatory bowel disease

Aetiology, pathology, clinical features and management of colorectal cancer

Colonic obstruction

Common benign anorectal conditions and their management

Must do

Clerk and follow the management of patients with diverticular disease, ulcerative colitis and Crohn's disease, and cancer of the colon and rectum

Observe flexible sigmoidoscopy and colonoscopy

Observe banding, injection or surgical treatment of haemorrhoids

Learn to recognize fistula *in ano*, fissure *in ano* and pilonidal sinus

Observe operations for resection of colon and rectal cancer

Diverticular disease

A diverticulum is an outpouching of part or all of a viscus (the term 'diverticulum' is derived from the Latin for 'place of ill repute'). Diverticula can be acquired or congenital.

Congenital diverticula

Congenital diverticula are distinguished from the acquired type by being composed of all the layers of their containing viscus. The most famous example of a congenital diverticulum is Meckel's diverticulum. This is a remnant of the vitello-intestinal duct and is typically found approximately 60 cm from the ileocaecal junction. The majority of cases of Meckel's diverticulum are asymptomatic, although some present with acute inflammation and rectal bleeding if the diverticulum contains gastric-type mucosa.

Congenital diverticula may also be found in the caecum and may bleed, leading to anaemia and melaena. Inflammation of a solitary caecal diverticulum will present like acute appendicitis or as an inflammatory mass resembling an appendix phlegmon or an appendicular abscess. It may also present in a less acute fashion, giving rise to suspicion of caecal carcinoma.

Acquired diverticulosis

Acquired diverticula are usually composed of mucosa and are pulsion in nature, implying that the mucosal lining of the viscus has been forced out through a defect. Usually, the diagnosis of diverticular disease implies acquired diverticula of the colon and hence the terminology used needs to be accurate and unambiguous.

- Diverticulum: one outpouching.
- Diverticula: multiple outpouchings.
- Diverticular disease/diverticulosis: the condition of having diverticula.
- Diverticulitis: acute inflammation of a diverticulum/diverticula.

Aetiology

Diverticular disease is a common condition of the colon in most countries where the diet is deficient in fibre. In the UK the disease can affect approximately 35% of the population over 60 years of age. As a result of poor diet the normal segmental contractions of the colon are more vigorous and prolonged, raising intraluminal pressure. This eventually leads to herniation of the mucosa through the circular muscle of the colonic wall where the anterior and posterior branches of the marginal artery enter. This

04

gives rise to two rows of diverticula adjacent to the append-ices epiploicae. The disease is slightly more common in females and there is an increasing incidence from the fourth or fifth decade onwards.

Pathology

Diverticula are mainly found in the sigmoid colon, although they may also be seen more proximally. They emerge between the taenia coli and may contain faeco-liths. The circular muscle of the colon is thickened and the taenia are thickened also, causing shortening of the colon.

Clinical presentation

In the majority of patients, diverticular disease is asymp-tomatic. However a number of patients present with one or more of the following complications:
- painful diverticulosis;
- acute diverticulitis;
- perforation of a diverticulum;
- obstruction due to fibrosis (following multiple attacks of inflammation);
- fistula (usually colovesical or colovaginal);
- pericolic abscess;
- haemorrhage.

Painful diverticulosis
A number of patients present with intermittent attacks of pain, principally located in the left iliac fossa and accom-panied by either constipation or alternating constipation and diarrhoea with mucus. The pain may be transient or persist for some days and is relieved temporarily by pass-ing flatus. An increase in dietary fibre will usually produce relief in a week or so, although it may initially cause exac-erbation of the symptoms.

Acute diverticulitis
This complication of colonic diverticulosis produces a more generalized picture of malaise, anorexia and fever, with local signs of tenderness, rigidity and a palpable mass in the left iliac fossa. Abdominal distension may occur and a sentinel loop of small bowel may sometimes be seen in plain films of the abdomen. Frequency and haematuria are the result of adherence of the inflamed loop of colon to the bladder. Treatment includes bedrest, intravenous fluids, analgesia and antibiotics. In almost all patients the acute attack will subside with this regimen.

Perforation
In some patients acute inflammation may progress to per-foration. Such a perforation may become walled off as a pericolic abscess or may perforate freely into the peritoneal cavity, causing generalized faecal peritonitis. If signs of generalized peritonitis are absent, the patient may be treated conservatively but any exacerbation of symptoms is an indication for laparotomy.

Formerly, drainage of local collections of pus, repair of the perforation with an omental patch and a proximal defunctioning colostomy was the recommended treat-ment. Such treatment was associated with a high postop-erative mortality. Nowadays, resection of the inflamed and perforated segment is recommended, with proximal colostomy and closure of the distal colon. This is known eponymously as Hartmann's procedure. Restoration of colonic continuity is undertaken 6 months later.

Obstruction
An episode of acute inflammation may be complicated by acute large-bowel obstruction due to occlusion of the bowel lumen, although this is likely to subside with reso-lution of the inflammation. Repeated attacks of inflam-mation, with thickening of the bowel wall and fibrous stricture formation, may precipitate recurring attacks of subacute obstruction. Small-bowel obstruction due to adherence of a loop of small intestine to a sigmoid inflammatory mass may also occur (see later). Distinction from colonic cancer may be difficult and the two may coexist.

Fistula
Adherence of the inflamed colon to adjacent organs may cause fistula into the small bowel, vagina or bladder. A fistula involving the small intestine may cause diarrhoea or subacute obstruction. Communication with the vagina or uterus will be evident from discharge of faecal material through the vagina. Colovesical fistula presents as intrac-table cystitis and, if the fistula is large enough, with pneu-maturia. Resection of the inflamed loop of colon and repair of the fistula is the appropriate treatment.

Haemorrhage
Severe acute haemorrhage may occur in elderly patients with diverticular disease due to erosion of the vessels adjacent to the diverticulum. The haemorrhage usually occurs without warning and is not usually associated with complications of the diverticulosis such as inflammation. The acute bleed is treated conservatively in most cases, although resection of the affected sigmoid loop may be necessary to avoid repeated attacks. The bleeding must be distinguished from that caused by angiodysplasia. The location of the bleeding can sometimes be identified at sigmoidoscopy. Angiography is required to demonstrate angiodysplasia.

Diverticular disease at a glance

Definition

Diverticular disease (or diverticulosis): a condition in which many sac-like mucosal projections (diverticula) develop in the large bowel especially the sigmoid colon. Acute inflammation of a diverticulum causes diverticulitis

Epidemiology
- Male/female 1 : 1.5
- Age: forties and fifties onwards
- High incidence in the western world, where it is found in 50% of people over 60 years

Aetiology
- Low fibre in the diet causes an increase in intraluminal colonic pressure, resulting in herniation of the mucosa through the muscle coats of the colonic wall
- Weak areas in wall of colon where nutrient arteries penetrate to submucosa and mucosa

Pathology
Macroscopic
- Diverticula mostly found in (thickened) sigmoid colon
- Emerge between the taenia coli and may contain faecoliths

Histology
- Projections are *acquired* diverticula as they contain only mucosa, submucosa and serosa and not all layers of intestinal wall

Clinical features
- Mostly asymptomatic
- Painful diverticulosis: left iliac fossa pain, constipation, diarrhoea
- Acute diverticulitis: malaise, fever, left iliac fossa pain and tenderness ± palpable mass and abdominal distension
- Perforation: peritonitis + features of diverticulitis
- Large-bowel obstruction: absolute constipation, distension, colicky abdominal pain and vomiting
- Fistula:
  (a) To bladder (cystitis, pneumaturia, recurrent urinary tract infections)
  (b) To vagina (faecal discharge from vagina)
  (c) To small intestine (diarrhoea)
- Lower gastrointestinal bleed: painless, spontaneous (distinguish from angiodysplasia)

Investigations
- Diverticulosis: barium enema (colonoscopy)
- Diverticulitis: full blood count, white cell count, urea and electrolytes, chest X-ray, CT

- Diverticular mass/paracolic abscess: CT
- Perforation: plain film of abdomen, CT
- Obstruction: Gastrografin or dilute barium enema, colonoscopy to exclude underlying malignancy
- Fistula:
  (a) Colovesical: midstream urine, cystoscopy, barium enema
  (b) Colovaginal: colposcopy, flexible sigmoidoscopy
- Haemorrhage: colonoscopy, selective angiography
- 'Diverticular' strictures should be biopsied in case of underlying colon carcinoma

Management
Medical
Painful or asymptomatic
- High-fibre diet (fruit, vegetables, wholemeal bread, bran)

Acute diverticulitis
- Majority of acute attacks are resolved by non-surgical treatment
- Antibiotics and bowel rest
- Radiologically guided drainage for localized abscess

Surgical
Elective (uncommon)
- Elective surgery should be reserved for recurrent proven symptoms and complications (e.g. stricture) or rarely failed medical treatment
- Elective left colon surgery without peritonitis: resect diseased colon and rejoin the ends (primary anastomosis)

Emergency (common)
- Emergency surgery for complications has a high morbidity and mortality and often involves an intestinal stoma
- Emergency left colon surgery with diffuse peritonitis: resect diseased segment, oversew distal bowel (i.e. upper rectum) and bring out proximal bowel as end-colostomy (Hartmann's procedure)
- Emergency left colon surgery with limited or no peritonitis: resection of diseased segment and rejoining the ends (primary anastomosis) may be safe
- Complicated left colon surgery (e.g. colovesical fistula): resection, primary anastomosis (may have defunctioning proximal stoma)

Prognosis
- Diverticular disease is a 'benign' condition but there is significant mortality and morbidity from the complications

04

Vascular lesions of the colon

Angiodysplasia

Angiodysplastic lesions of the colon occur in the elderly and give rise to recurrent episodes of severe bleeding or chronic anaemia due to persistent slow blood loss. These anomalous vessels are mostly confined to the caecum and right side of the colon and can only be identified at angiography. Intra-arterial infusion of vasopressin or embolization with injection of Gelfoam into the appropriate vessels may be employed to stop bleeding. Right hemicolectomy may be a more certain means of providing a cure.

Ischaemic colitis

Ischaemic colitis occurs in elderly patients who have arteriosclerosis, blood disorders with increased viscosity or who have had surgical interference with the colonic blood supply (e.g. resection of an aortic aneurysm). If sufficiently acute and severe, the interference with the blood supply may cause gangrene. If less severe or more chronic, the condition may be transient or the end-result may be stricture.

The patient presents with severe, crampy, left-sided abdominal pain followed by bloody diarrhoea. The degree of pain and tenderness reflects the severity of the condition. If severe symptoms persist, gangrene should be suspected and laparotomy and resection undertaken. Conservative measures with intravenous fluids and antibiotics are appropriate for less severe forms of ischaemia. When the acute symptoms have subsided, barium studies may show lateral indentations in the column of barium ('thumb-printing'), indicating mucosal oedema. If later stricture formation occurs, the lesion may resemble a stenosing colonic carcinoma on barium studies. Resection may be required for subacute obstruction.

Volvulus of the colon

Caecal volvulus

Poor fixation of the caecum in the right iliac fossa may result in volvulus. The torsion is clockwise and may cause acute closed-loop obstruction with rapidly supervening gangrene and generalized peritonitis. The condition may resolve spontaneously but more frequently requires surgical intervention. Early intervention allows resection of the gangrenous caecum in the right iliac fossa.

Sigmoid volvulus

Volvulus of the sigmoid colon tends to occur in elderly,

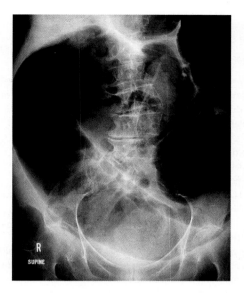

Figure 32.1 Plain abdominal radiograph showing a sigmoid volvulus.

constipated, institutionalized patients who are mentally defective. In addition to the above interrelated factors, there is a redundant sigmoid loop on a narrow mesentery. Torsion occurs around the mesenteric axis. A varying degree of obstruction occurs, from chronic to subacute to acute obstruction and strangulation. The patient presents with abdominal distension and tenderness and plain radiographs of the abdomen demonstrate a grossly dilated loop of large bowel (Fig. 32.1). Decompression of the loop with a flatus tube or sigmoidoscope may be possible in subacute obstruction. More often, laparotomy is required. Fixation of the untwisted loop to the left iliac fossa may be sufficient if the bowel is viable. If not, resection should be carried out. It is probably wisest to defer reconstruction of the colon to a later date and limit the emergency operation to a Hartmann's procedure. Resection of the sigmoid loop and end-to-end anastomosis are indicated for recurrent obstruction.

Chronic inflammatory bowel disease

By convention, the term 'inflammatory bowel disease' is confined to two conditions: ulcerative colitis and Crohn's disease of the colon. Although easily distinguished from one another in their classical presentations, in some patients there is sufficient overlap in symptomatology, radiological findings and histological features to make either diagnosis a possibility (i.e. indeterminate colitis). However, an accurate diagnosis is important as this has implications for prognosis and treatment.

Ulcerative colitis

In ulcerative colitis the proximal extent of the inflammation is variable but the rectum is almost always involved. The small intestine is not affected except for the backwash ileitis that may occur in patients with proximal colonic disease and an incompetent ileocaecal valve.

Extracolonic manifestations of ulcerative colitis include:
● eye disorders (iritis, interstitial keratitis, retrobulbar neuritis);
● arthritis (sacroiliitis, ankylosing spondylitis);
● skin disorders (pyoderma gangrenosum, erythema nodosum);
● renal calculi and pyelonephritis;
● blood disorders (hypochromic anaemia, deep vein thrombosis and haemolytic anaemia);
● hepatic disease and cholangitis.

Aetiology

A genetic origin for the disease is suggested by its ethnic and familial associations and its association with human leukocyte antigen (HLA)-B27 phenotypes. Ulcerative colitis may also have an autoimmune basis. It is no longer seriously regarded as a psychosomatic illness, although psychological stresses may be involved in its onset.

Clinical features

Ulcerative colitis presents in the third and fourth decades and is more common in females. Colonic symptoms are diarrhoea, with passage of mucus and pus, and rectal bleeding. Abdominal pain is often present. Systemic symptoms include anorexia and weight loss. A low-grade pyrexia usually accompanies the symptoms. The disease may pursue a mild and chronic course and the disease in these patients is usually confined to the distal colon and rectum.

A more severe and progressive form of the disease may run a rapid course and produce complications such as toxic megacolon, perforation and severe bleeding. Fulminant ulcerative colitis may develop *de novo* or occur as an exacerbation of chronic disease. The patient develops profuse diarrhoea and bleeding and rapidly becomes hypovolaemic and shocked and the abdomen distended and painful. Toxic megacolon and perforation may ensue. These patients are desperately ill and in this situation require rapid resuscitation and urgent colectomy.

Investigations

● Plain films of the abdomen are useful in the severely ill patient (Fig. 32.2a). They can demonstrate air under the diaphragm if a perforation has occurred and will show the progressive colonic dilatation in patients with toxic megacolon.
● In chronic ulcerative colitis, a barium enema will demonstrate loss of haustrations and the rigidity and shortening aptly described as 'lead-pipe' appearance (Fig. 32.2b). Diffuse narrowing can also be noted, as well as a fuzzy appearance at the margins of the barium outline due to mucosal ulceration.
● Sigmoidoscopy will demonstrate an inflamed friable mucosa that bleeds easily on contact. Mucosal ulceration is unusual but may be present in severe cases.

Pseudopolyps may also be seen (Fig. 32.2c). Biopsy confirms the diagnosis, with an inflammatory infiltrate of lymphocytes, plasma cells, eosinophils and mast cells in the mucosa and submucosa. The crypts of Lieberkühn are inflamed and crypt abscesses develop that coalesce and cause ulceration.

Treatment
Medical
● Sulfasalazine (Salazopyrin), a combination of sulfapyridine and 5-aminosalicylic acid, may induce remission in acute attacks and is effective in the prevention of relapse. It is less effective than steroids and is used only in mild cases or as maintenance therapy. Adverse effects that may inhibit its use include nausea, vomiting, headache, skin rashes and blood dyscrasias.
● Occasionally, azathioprine is used in combination with sulfasalazine to reduce relapse frequency in resistant cases.
● Steroids, used topically (Predsol enemas) or orally (30–40 mg prednisolone), are probably the treatment of choice in mild ulcerative colitis. For moderately severe cases a higher oral dose is appropriate, but with severe acute disease intravenous hydrocortisone is required with transfer to high oral dosage of prednisolone when improvement takes places.
● High-fibre diet and bulk-forming agents such as methylcellulose may be useful; occasionally antidiarrhoeal drugs such as codeine phosphate are required.

Surgical
Surgery is indicated if medical treatment fails to control an acute episode or if relapses are too frequent. Surgery may also be necessary because of complications such as perforation or toxic megacolon and because of the risk of cancer in ulcerative colitis of more than 10 years' duration (see below).

Classically, surgery for ulcerative colitis consists of removing the colon, rectum and anus (panproctocolectomy) and creating a permanent ileostomy. Because ulcerative colitis is confined to the large bowel, this

04

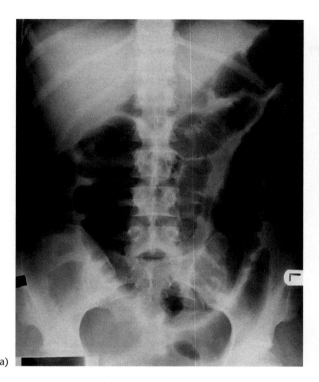

(a)

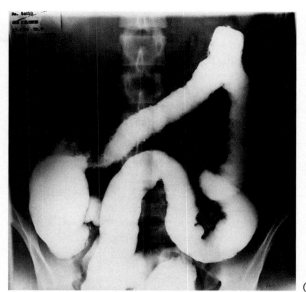

(b)

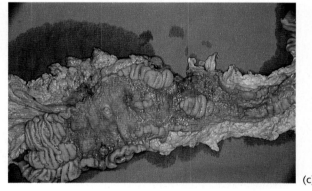

(c)

Figure 32.2 Appearances of ulcerative colitis. (a) Plain abdominal film: note the dilated colon, mucosal oedema, 'thumb-printing', thickened haustra, absence of faeces and small-bowel obstruction. (b) Barium enema: note the shortened narrow colon, loss of haustrations and the 'lead-pipe' colon. (c) Pathology specimen: note the presence of superficial ulceration and pseudopolyposis (regenerative tissue from surviving islands of mucosa).

04

procedure is curative but leaves the patient with one of the following ileostomies.

● A well-functioning spout ileostomy (*Brooke ileostomy*; Fig. 32.3) gives very satisfactory results, with abolition of all intestinal symptoms and greatly improved general health. Problems such as retraction, prolapse or obstruction of the ileostomy may occur, and refashioning of the ileostomy may be necessary.

● The *Koch ileostomy* provides a continent stoma; this involves the construction of a reservoir and a continent valve with the stoma in the right iliac fossa. Evacuation is carried out by catheter. Disruption of the valve mechanism with incontinence and occasional fistula formation are complications. This procedure is rarely performed now.

More recently, surgeons have attempted to preserve the anal sphincters by performing a colectomy but retaining a short rectal stump that is then stripped of its mucosa. To maintain continence a reservoir (ileal pouch) is created

from the distal ileum and anastomosed to the anus. The construction of an ileal pouch (usually J-shaped) and pouch–anal anastomosis enables the removal of all diseased mucosa with preservation of sphincter function and anal continence. Stool frequency is high (six to eight motions per day) and continence of flatus not assured. There may also be some soiling at night.

Complications

Perforation. Perforation may occur during an acute attack or in association with toxic megacolon. The patient develops generalized peritonitis and septic shock but the clinical features may be masked if the patient is on steroid therapy. The mortality is around 30%.

Toxic megacolon. In toxic megacolon the inflammatory process involves the full thickness of the bowel wall, with coalescence of crypt abscesses, destruction of the muscle

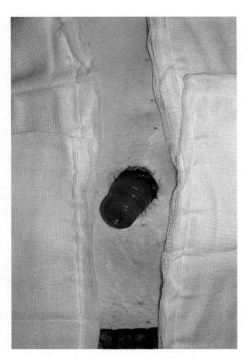

Figure 32.3 Brooke ileostomy: unlike a colostomy, an ileostomy has a long spout.

layer and the myenteric plexus and severe dilation of a very friable colon. Signs and symptoms include pyrexia, tachycardia, anaemia, hypovolaemia and electrolyte disturbance. The abdomen is distended, bowel sounds are absent and blood pressure is low. Perforation is imminent and if intense medical treatment does not elicit an immediate response, emergency colectomy is needed. The mortality is 20–30%.

Carcinoma. Patients with extensive ulcerative colitis involving the entire colon in whom the disease has been present for more than 10 years have a significantly higher risk of developing cancer than the general population. Because of the confusion between the symptoms of ulcerative colitis and those of a tumour, diagnosis is often late and the prognosis is poor. Hence, the need for surveillance in patients at risk.

Crohn's disease

Although originally called regional ileitis because of its classical presentation, Crohn's disease can occur anywhere in the gastrointestinal tract (see earlier), including the colon and frequently perianally. Its symptomatology is very varied, ranging from chronic diarrhoea, abdominal

---

Ulcerative colitis at a glance

Definition

Ulcerative colitis: a chronic inflammatory disorder of the colonic mucosa, usually beginning in the rectum and extending proximally to a variable extent

Epidemiology
- Male/female 1 : 1.6
- Age 30–50 years
- High incidence among relatives of patients (up to 40%) and among Europeans and Jews

Aetiology
- Genetic origin: increased prevalence (10%) in relatives, associated with HLA-B27 phenotype
- May have autoimmune basis
- Smoking protects against relapse

Pathology
Macroscopic
- Disease confined to colon; rectum always involved; may be 'backwash' ileitis
- Only the mucosa is involved, with superficial ulceration, exudation and pseudopolyposis

Histology
- Crypt abscess, inflammatory polyps and highly vascular granulation tissue
- Epithelial dysplasia with long-standing disease

Clinical features
Proctitis
- Mucus, pus and blood per rectum
- Diarrhoea with urgency and frequency

Left-sided colitis and total colitis
- Symptoms of proctitis plus increasing features of systemic upset, abdominal pain, anorexia, weight loss and anaemia with more extensive disease

Extraintestinal features
- Joints: arthritis (25%)
- Eye: uveitis (10%)
- Skin: erythema nodosum, pyoderma gangrenosum (10%)
- Liver: pericholangitis, fatty liver (3%)
- Blood: thromboembolic disease

Severe/fulminant disease
- 6–20 bloody bowel motions per day

04

- Fever, anaemia, dehydration, electrolyte imbalance
- Colonic dilatation/perforation (toxic megacolon)

Investigations
- Full blood count: iron-deficiency anaemia
- Stool culture: exclude infective colitis before treatment
- Plain abdominal radiograph: colonic dilatation or air under diaphragm indicates perforation in fulminant colitis
- Barium enema: loss of haustrations, shortened 'lead-pipe' colon
- Sigmoidoscopy: inflamed friable mucosa, bleeds to touch
- Colonoscopy: extent of disease at presentation, evaluation of response to treatment after exacerbations, screening of long-standing disease for dysplasia
- Biopsy: typical histological features

Management
General principles
- Majority controlled by medical management; surgery is usually only required for poor control of symptoms or complications
- Acute attacks require close scrutiny to avoid major complications
- Long-term colitis carries a risk of colonic malignancy

Medical
- Basic: high-fibre diet, antidiarrhoeal agents (codeine phosphate, loperamide)
- First-line therapy: anti-inflammatory drugs (sulfasalazine, 5-aminosalicylic acid, corticosteroids)

- Second-line therapy:
  (a) Other immunosuppressive agents (azathioprine, cyclosporin)
  (b) Enemas if disease confined to rectum
  (c) Oral preparations for more extensive disease
  (d) Intravenous immunosuppressives for acute exacerbations

Surgery
Indications
- Failure of medical treatment to control chronic symptoms
- Complications: profuse haemorrhage, perforation/toxic megacolon, risk of cancer (greater with longer disease, more aggressive onset and more extensive disease)
- Dysplasia or development of carcinoma

Operations
- For acute attacks/complications: total colectomy, end-ileostomy and preserved rectal stump
- Electively: proctocolectomy with end (Brooke) ileostomy *or* proctocolectomy with preservation of anal sphincter and creation of ileoanal pouch (e.g. J-shaped pouch)
- Ileoanal pouch reconstruction offers good function in the majority of cases where surgery is required

Prognosis
- Ulcerative colitis is a chronic problem that requires constant surveillance unless surgery, which is drastic but curative, is performed

pain and weight loss to the clinical features of acute appendicitis, pyrexia, vomiting and right iliac fossa pain. It may also present as an abdominal mass, as acute intestinal obstruction and with multiple perianal fissures and abscesses. The extraintestinal manifestations of Crohn's disease include arthritis and skin conditions such as erythema nodosum and pyoderma gangrenosum. Crohn's disease gives rise to chronic ill health and children fail to thrive, have retarded growth and are generally malnourished. The aetiology of Crohn's disease is unknown but heredity and autoimmune reactions may play a part.

Pathology

In contrast to ulcerative colitis, the inflammation of Crohn's disease involves the full thickness of the bowel wall. Crypt abscesses are rare but non-caseating granulomas are present (Fig. 32.4). The bowel serosa is involved, as are the mesentery and regional lymph nodes. Macroscopically the bowel wall is reddened and thickened. The mucosa has a cobblestone appearance with deep fissured ulcers surrounded by oedematous mucosa. The mesen-

tery is shortened and thickened and lymph nodes are enlarged and show a hyperplastic reaction. Fistulae may occur to the skin, to adjacent loops of bowel or to the bladder or vagina.

Investigations

Barium enema may show the extent of the lesions (Fig. 32.5a). Sigmoidoscopy and colonoscopy allow visualization of Crohn's lesions located in the colon or rectum (Fig. 32.5b). The disease is patchy in distribution and the rectum is often uninvolved. The histological features obtained on biopsy are chronic inflammatory infiltrate with lymphocytes and non-caseating granulomas. The fissured ulcers are narrow and deep.

Treatment

Differentiation between ulcerative colitis and Crohn's disease is important as treatment strategies are different in the two conditions, with surgery playing a minor role in the management of Crohn's disease (Table 32.1).

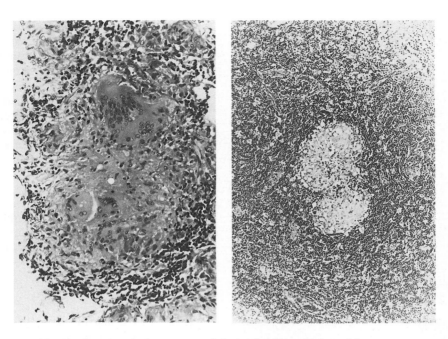

Figure 32.4 Non-caseating granulomas: note the presence of giant cells with multiple nuclei.

Table 32.1 Comparison of the features of ulcerative colitis and Crohn's disease.

	Ulcerative colitis	**Crohn's disease**
Aetiology	HLA-B27 phenotype	Unknown
Pathology		
Macroscopic	Rectum (always), colon, terminal ileum (backwash ileitis)	Any part of gastrointestinal tract, skip lesions
	Mucosa only, superficial ulceration, pseudopolyps	Full-thickness (hosepipe), fissures, mesentery involved
Microscopic	Crypt abscesses	Non-caseating granulomas
Clinical		
Bowel features	Rectal bleeding, diarrhoea	Abdominal pain and mass, malaise, diarrhoea, perianal disease
Extraintestinal features	Iritis, arthritis, blood, skin and renal disorders (see text)	Erythema nodosum
		Pyoderma gangrenosum
Complications	Haemorrhage, perforation, toxic megacolon, carcinoma	Stricture, fistulae
Radiology	Barium enema: shortened narrowed colon, loss of haustrations, 'lead-pipe' colon	Barium meal and follow-through, barium enema: altered mucosal pattern, 'string sign', deep penetrating ulcers
Management		
Medical	Sulfasalazine	Dietary manipulation
	Steroid enema	Sulfasalazine, metronidazole
	Systemic steroids	Systemic steroids, azathioprine
	Azathioprine	
Surgery	Panproctocolectomy and ileostomy	Only for complications and limited to localized
	Ileal pouch	resections and stricturoplasties

HLA, human leukocyte antigen.

04

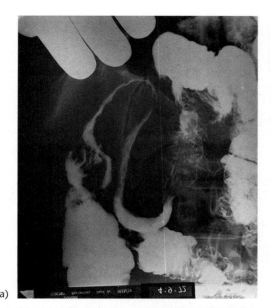

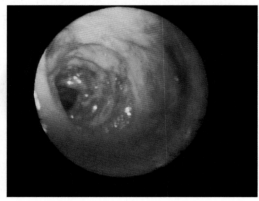

(a)

(b)

Figure 32.5 Crohn's colitis: (a) barium enema; (b) endoscopic view.

tion. Acute regional ileitis should be treated conservatively as it is often due to *Yersinia* infection and will resolve completely. Crohn's disease involving the colon may require resection with ileorectal anastomosis or, if the rectum is involved, panproctocolectomy with ileostomy. Sphincter-saving operations or reservoirs are not suitable in Crohn's disease. The treatment of Crohn's perianal disease is essentially the treatment of abscess by drainage and the laying open of fissures and fistulae. Metronidazole may be beneficial.

Colonic polyps

Polyps may occur anywhere in the gastrointestinal tract. Polyps occurring in the colon or rectum include hamartomatous lesions of juvenile polyposis, adenomatous polyps and villous papillomas.

Juvenile polyps

Juvenile polyps occur in infants and young children. They may be single or multiple, are pedunculated and found mainly in the rectum and distal colon. There is a familial tendency and they are more common in male children. The polyps are vascular and secrete mucus. They have little malignant potential. When identified they should be removed endoscopically.

Adenomatous polyps

Adenomatous polyps are pedunculated, vary in size from a few millimetres to several centimetres and occur mainly in the rectum and sigmoid colon (Fig. 32.6). They are often asymptomatic but may produce anaemia from chronic occult bleeding. Rarely they may initiate an

Supplementary diet to correct malnutrition is important in the management of Crohn's disease. Elemental diets may help and supplements of oral iron are needed. In severe malnourished states total parenteral nutrition is required. This may also be useful in accelerating remission of an acute exacerbation. Sulfasalazine may be used for acute episodes and maintenance therapy. Metronidazole may benefit patients with perianal disease. Prednisolone may be necessary to induce remission in severe acute attacks of inflammation. Azathioprine may sometimes be of benefit.

The surgical treatment of Crohn's disease is largely the treatment of its complications. Strictures may require dilation, adhesions may need to be divided in obstruction and localized segments of small bowel may require resec-

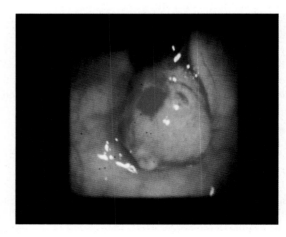

Figure 32.6 Endoscopic view of a colonic polyp of rectum.

intussusception. They may also give rise to crampy abdominal pain. If a lot of mucus is secreted, spurious diarrhoea may occur, although this is more common with villous papillomas. Adenomatous polyps have malignant potential and should be removed when diagnosed.

Villous papillomas

Villous papillomas are sessile lesions that spread around the circumference of the bowel and secrete copious amounts of mucus. The mucus discharge produces spurious diarrhoea. Significant losses of potassium may occur, giving rise to a metabolic acidosis with lethargy, muscle weakness and mental confusion. There is a significant risk of malignant change. Some are small enough to be amenable to endoscopic removal with a snare or diathermy coagulation, but larger masses may need wide excision after infiltration of the submucosa with dilute adrenaline solution. The cut edges of normal mucosa are then approximated. Where malignant change has occurred in a polypoid lesion, a formal resection of colon or rectum should be carried out.

Familial polyposis

Familial polyposis coli is an inherited autosomal dominant condition in which hundreds of adenomas develop throughout the colon and rectum early in the second decade of life. The patient may be relatively asymptomatic but bleeding, abdominal pain and diarrhoea are all likely symptoms. The risk of developing carcinoma is virtually 100% within 15 years. The most appropriate treatment is panproctocolectomy with ileal pouch–anal anastomosis.

Gardner's syndrome

In this condition the patient develops multiple colorectal adenomas in association with sebaceous and dermoid cysts, osteomas and desmoid tumours of the abdominal wall. The extracolonic manifestations of the syndrome may predate the colonic adenomas by some years. The risk of cancer is similar to that in familial polyposis. Radical resection is indicated.

Carcinoma of the colon and rectum

Adenocarcinoma of the colon and rectum is one of the most common cancers occurring in the western world (Fig. 32.7). It occurs in both sexes but is somewhat more common in men. Almost half of these tumours occur in the rectum and almost three-quarters are within reach of the flexible sigmoidoscope (60 cm from the anal margin). Hereditary factors, such as familial polyposis coli, are

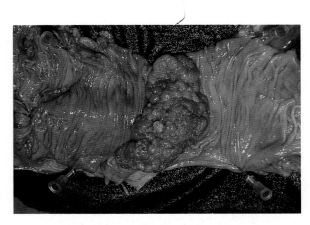

Figure 32.7 Pathology specimen showing circumferential colon cancer.

responsible for its development in some cases. Other aetiological factors include ulcerative colitis, colonic polyps and excess bile salts. The high incidence in western countries is attributed to the low-fibre, high-fat diet common in industrialized societies.

Pathology

Carcinoma of the colon or rectum is an adenocarcinoma with a fibrous stroma that may progress in different ways:
- as an exophytic cauliflower-type of growth;
- as an ulcerating lesion penetrating through the bowel wall;
- as an annular constricting growth;
- as a diffuse infiltrating tumour;
- as the rare colloidal mucus-secreting tumour.

Colorectal carcinoma metastasizes to regional lymph nodes and via the bloodstream to the liver. Figure 32.8 shows a skin deposit from a primary bowel cancer.

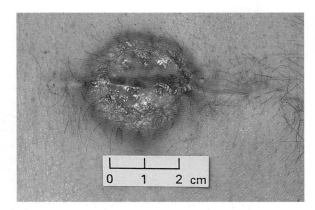

Figure 32.8 Skin deposit from a primary colon cancer.

Clinical features

The clinical presentation reflects the location of the tumour.

● A carcinoma in the caecum progresses silently, the only manifestation being occult blood in the stools and persistent anaemia due to chronic blood loss. This is sometimes mistaken for an appendix mass but its persistence despite treatment invites further investigation, and identification at barium enema or colonoscopy follows.

● A tumour in the ascending colon is likely to behave similarly to caecal carcinoma but may give rise to dyspeptic symptoms or colicky abdominal pain.

● The latter is a constant feature of carcinoma in the transverse or descending colon due to the partial obstruction of an annular constricting lesion. Alteration in bowel habit is also a consequence of a constricting lesion, with periods of constipation followed by episodes of diarrhoea. Blood and mucus can be identified in the stool.

● Tumours in the rectum secrete mucus and bleed from the ulcerated surface. The accumulated blood and mucus are passed accompanied by tenesmus as an early morning bloody diarrhoea.

● A significant percentage present as large-bowel obstruction.

Investigation

Digital rectal examination is essential and many rectal tumours can be identified as a craggy ulcerated mass during this procedure. More proximal tumours are identified at sigmoidoscopy or colonoscopy. The rigid sigmoidoscope affords only a limited examination to 30 cm but the flexible sigmoidoscope enables the distal 60 cm of bowel to be examined, which should identify 70% of tumours. Access to the remainder requires full colonoscopy or double-contrast barium enema. Biopsy of any lesion visualized is essential. Even if a tumour is seen and confirmed at biopsy, a full colonic examination should always be carried out as 3% of tumours are synchronous. Metachronous tumours occur in 3% of cases also, so follow-up of previously treated tumours should include full investigation.

The appearance of a tumour on barium enema is of a constricting filling defect, characteristically an 'apple-core' deformity (Fig. 32.9a). Double-contrast enema will identify smaller tumours and suspicious polyps (Fig. 32.9b).

Treatment

Resection of the tumour with adequate margins and including the regional glands is indicated when the diagnosis has been confirmed. It is advisable to arrange an intravenous urogram prior to operation to exclude involvement of the ureters and bladder. Bowel preparation is undertaken prior to resection of lesions on the left side of the colon. No preparation is required for right-sided lesions. Appropriate antibiotics should be given perioperatively to cover Gram-positive aerobes (e.g. *Streptococcus faecalis*), Gram-negative aerobes (e.g. *Escherichia coli*, *Klebsiella*, *Proteus*) and Gram-negative anaerobes (e.g. *Bacteroides*).

Surgical procedures

General principles include early ligation of the vascular pedicle, no-touch technique and avoidance of contamina-

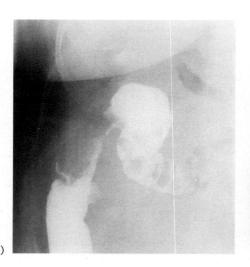

(a)

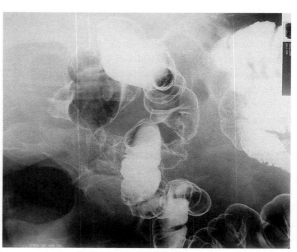

(b)

Figure 32.9 Barium enema showing 'apple-core' lesion at (a) the splenic flexure and (b) the sigmoid colon.

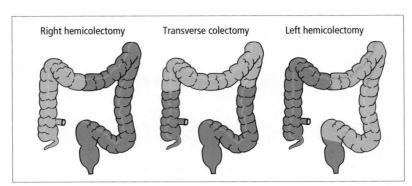

Figure 32.10 Surgery for colonic tumours. The area of resection for right hemicolectomy, left hemicolectomy and transverse colectomy is shown.

Table 32.2 Modified Dukes classification for staging colorectal cancer.

Dukes stage	Extent of pathology	5-year survival (%)
A	Tumour confined to bowel mucosa	90
B1	Tumour involves the muscle wall but not completely	70
B2	Involves the serosa	60
C1	Tumour involves the muscle wall but not completely Local lymph nodes involved	30
C2	Involves the serosa Local lymph nodes involved	

tion by bowel content. The procedure varies with the site of the lesion. Right hemicolectomy with end-to-end ileocolic anastomosis is indicated for carcinoma of the caecum or ascending colon. Wide resection, including hepatic and splenic flexure, is indicated in tumours of the transverse colon. In tumours of the descending or sigmoid colon the splenic flexure should be included in the resection (Fig. 32.10).

Low anterior resection is now the standard operation for most rectal tumours. Formerly, the belief that 5 cm distal clearance was necessary and that 5 cm of distal rectum had to be preserved to ensure normal sphincter function meant that if the tumour was within 10 cm of the anal margin, an abdominoperineal resection was mandatory. The subsequent realization that rectal tumours drained proximally and that 2 cm distal clearance was adequate, plus the realization that sphincter control could be maintained with less than 5 cm of rectum, enabled very low anterior resections to be carried out. The advent of circular stapling instruments was of enormous benefit in overcoming the technical difficulties of very low anastomoses. However, abdominoperineal resection with an end-colostomy in the left iliac fossa is still necessary occasionally.

When a patient presents with colonic obstruction or perforation secondary to a carcinoma, a laparotomy is performed and the carcinoma-bearing segment of bowel excised. However, primary anastomosis is inadvisable in this situation. Preliminary defunctioning colostomy may be carried out for obstruction and Hartmann's procedure is appropriate in the presence of perforation, with excision of the perforated segment, proximal colostomy and closure of the rectal stump.

Prognosis

The outcome of resection for carcinoma of the colon and rectum depends on the stage of the tumour. Dukes classification, although originally described for carcinoma of the rectum, can be applied to the colon also. A modified Dukes classification is in wide usage (Table 32.2).

Radiotherapy and chemotherapy have a limited role in the management of patients with colorectal cancer, although most patients with Dukes stage C disease now receive adjunctive chemotherapy. Studies have shown that fluorouracil and levamisole given 3–5 weeks after surgery reduce the recurrence rate by about 40% and mortality by 30% in patients followed for a median of 5 years. Liver metastases can be resected with a good prospect of survival if there are fewer than five metastases or the metastases are confined to a lobe of the liver. About 25% of such patients survive for 5 years.

04

Colorectal cancer at a glance

Definition

Colorectal carcinoma: the occurrence of malignant lesions in the mucosa of the colon or rectum

Epidemiology
- Male/female ratio 1.3 : 1
- Age 50+ years
- Incidence has increased in western world over last 50 years

Aetiology
Predisposing factors in decreasing importance:
- Prior colorectal carcinoma or adenomatous polyps
- Hereditary polyposis syndromes
- Family history of colorectal carcinoma
- Chronic active ulcerative colitis
- Diet (low in indigestible fibre, high in animal fat)
- Increased faecal bile salts, selenium deficiency

Pathology
Macroscopic
- Polypoid, ulcerating, annular, infiltrative
- 75% of lesions are within 60 cm of the anal margin (rectum, sigmoid, left colon)
- 3% are synchronous (i.e. a second lesion will be found at the same time) and 3% are metachronous (i.e. a second lesion will be found later)

Histology
- Adenocarcinoma (10–15% are mucinous adenocarcinoma)
- Staging: Dukes classification and TNM
- Spread: lymphatic, haematogenous (via veins to liver), peritoneal

Clinical features
- Anaemia: caecal cancers often present with anaemia
- Colicky abdominal pain: tumours causing partial obstruction, e.g. transverse or descending colonic lesions
- Alteration in bowel habit: either constipation or diarrhoea
- Bleeding or passage of mucus per rectum
- Tenesmus (frequent or continuous desire to defecate): rectal lesions

Investigations
- Digital rectal examination and faecal occult blood

- Full blood count: anaemia
- Urea and electrolytes: hypokalaemia
- Liver function tests: liver metastases
- Sigmoidoscopy (rigid to 30 cm/flexible to 60 cm) and colonoscopy (whole colon): observe lesion, obtain biopsy (virtual colonoscopy may have a role in future)
- Double-contrast barium enema: 'apple-core' lesion, polyp
- Carcinoembryonic antigen is often raised in advanced disease

Management
Surgery (potentially curative)
- Resection of the tumour with adequate margins to include regional lymph nodes
- Resection possible for liver metastases if fewer than five are present

Procedures
- Right hemicolectomy (no bowel preparation) for lesions from caecum to splenic flexure
- Left hemicolectomy (bowel preparation) for lesions of descending and sigmoid colon
- Anterior resection for rectal tumours
- Abdominoperineal resection and colostomy for very low rectal lesions
- Hartmann's procedure for emergency surgery to left colon

Surgery/interventions (palliative)
- Open resection of tumour (with anastomosis or stoma) for obstructing or symptomatic cancers despite metastases
- Surgical bypass for obstructing inoperable cancers
- Transanal resection for inoperable rectal cancer
- Intraluminal stents for obstructing cancers

Other treatment
- Radiotherapy may be used to shrink rectal cancers preoperatively or palliate inoperable rectal cancer
- Adjuvant chemotherapy (5-fluorouracil ± levamisole) to reduce risk of systemic recurrence (Dukes stage C and some Dukes stage B) or to palliate liver metastases

Prognosis
- 5-year survival depends on staging: A, 80%; B, 60%; C, 35%; D, 5%

04

Rectal bleeding at a glance

Definition

Rectal bleeding: the passage of blood from the anus. It may occur at any age, may be small or large in volume and may be bright red or dark in colour, and should always be investigated

Causes

Small intestine
- Meckel's diverticulum: young adults, painless bleeding, dark red/melaena common
- Intussusception: young children, colicky abdominal pain, retching, bright red/mucus stool
- Enteritis: infection, radiation, Crohn's
- Ischaemic: severe abdominal pain, physical examination shows few signs, often atrial fibrillation (AF), later collapse and shock
- Tumours (leiomyoma/lymphoma): rare, intermittent history, often modest volumes lost

Proximal colon
- Angiodysplasia: common in the elderly, painless, no warning, often large volumes, fresh and mixed with clots
- Carcinoma of the caecum: causes anaemia rather than frank rectal bleeding

Colon
- Polyps/carcinoma: may be large or small volume. May be associated with altered bowel habit. Blood often mixed with stool

- Diverticular disease: elderly, spontaneous onset, painless, large volumes, mostly fresh blood, history of constipation. Difficult to differentiate from angiodysplasia
- Ulcerative colitis: blood mixed with mucus, associated with systemic upset and abdominal pain, long history, intermittent course, severe diarrhoea
- Ischaemic colitis: elderly, severe abdominal pain, AF, bloody diarrhoea, collapse and shock later

Rectum
- Carcinoma of the rectum: change in bowel habit, associated mucus, small volumes of blood
- Proctitis: bloody mucus, purulent diarrhoea in infected proctitis, perianal irritation common
- Solitary rectal ulcer: bleeding post defecation, small volumes, feeling of 'lump' in anus, mucus discharge

Anus
- Haemorrhoids: common cause of rectal bleeding. Bright-red bleeding post defecation, stops spontaneously, perianal irritation, sometimes patient feels 'something coming down' from anal canal depending on degree of haemorrhoids
- Fissure *in ano*: extreme pain on defecation, bright-red blood on toilet paper. Common cause of rectal bleeding in children
- Carcinoma of the anus: elderly, mass in anus, small volumes, bloody discharge, anal pain, non-healing ulcer.
- Perianal Crohn's disease: small amounts of blood, perianal sepsis and fistula tracks

Management and investigation

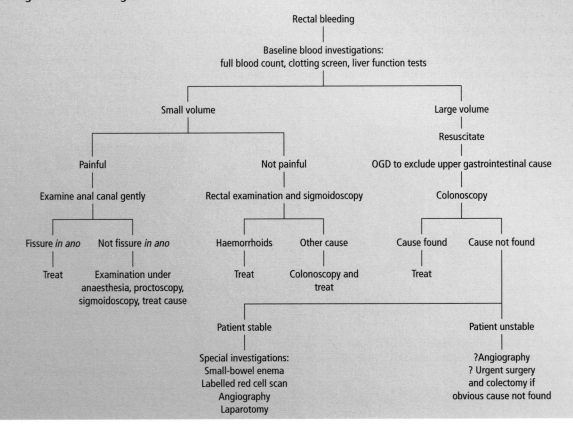

Carcinoma of the anus

Anal carcinoma is uncommon. The carcinoma arises from the squamous epithelium of the lower half of the anal canal. It is a disease of the elderly that presents with rectal bleeding, anal pain, discharge and ulceration. The diagnosis is confirmed by biopsy and metastases are to the inguinal nodes. Treatment now is by combined local radiotherapy and chemotherapy, which has displaced abdominoperineal resection. Rarely, malignant melanoma presents as an anal lesion. Early metastases are frequent and this lesion has a well-deserved notoriety (see Chapter 36).

Benign anal and perianal disorders

Perirectal abscess

A basic knowledge of rectal anatomy is fundamental to understanding perirectal disease (Fig. 32.11). The rectum is the distal 15 cm of the large intestine. The anal canal, the terminal end of the alimentary tract, measures approximately 4 cm. The rectal wall consists of the mucosa, submucosa and two complete muscle layers: the inner circular and the outer longitudinal. In the anal canal the internal sphincter is the continuation of the inner circular smooth muscle layer. The external sphincter, the continuation of the outer longitudinal skeletal muscle layer, consists of three parts: subcutaneous, superficial and deep muscle. The superior border of the external sphincter fuses with the puborectalis muscle and forms a sling originating at the pubis and joining behind the rectum. The intersphincteric plane, the space between the internal and external sphincters, is a fibrous continuation of the longitudinal smooth muscle of the rectum. Normally, six to ten anal glands lie in the intersphincteric space. Each gland has a duct and discharges into the anal crypt of the dentate line. Infection originating in these glands is the primary cause of perirectal abscess and fistula *in ano*.

The dentate line is an important surgical landmark at the union of the embryonic ectoderm with the gut endoderm. The line is recognizable as the line demarcating the transitional epithelium below and the rectal mucosa above. The columns of Morgagni begin at this line and extend cephalad. The dentate line divides the nervous, vascular and lymphatic supply of the anal canal into two routes.

Symptoms and signs

Pain is the most common symptom, and swelling is present in 95% of patients. However, only 12% of patients have perianal discharge and only 18% have fever. The male to female ratio is approximately 2 : 1. Peak incidence is in the third and fourth decades.

Types of abscess (Fig. 32.12)

● Intersphincteric abscess results from infection in the anal glands between the internal and external sphincters. Faecal coliforms are typically the offending organisms. As the abscess enlarges within the intersphincteric plane, it can spread in any of several directions.

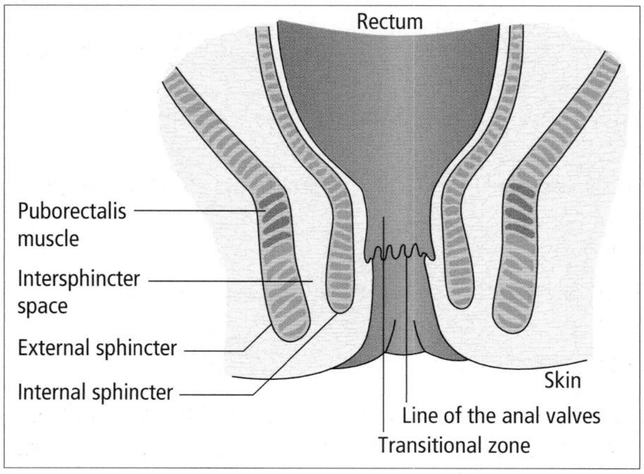

Figure 32.11 Cross-section through the anal canal and lower rectum showing the important anatomical relations of the region.

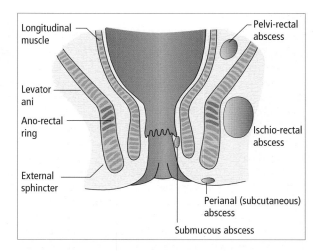

Figure 32.12 Common sites of anorectal suppuration.

- Perianal abscess results when pus spreads downwards between the two sphincters. It manifests as a tender swelling of the anal verge.
- Ischiorectal abscess is formed if a growing intersphincteric abscess penetrates the external sphincter below the puborectalis. Infection can spread into the fat of the ischiorectal fossa and the abscess can become quite large.
- Supralevator abscess develops when an intersphincteric abscess expands upwards between the internal and external sphincters.

Differential diagnosis

The differential diagnosis includes pilonidal abscess, hydradenitis suppurativa, folliculitis, periprostatic abscess, Bartholin gland abscess, inflammatory bowel disease, actinomycosis and tuberculosis.

Management and treatment

For most patients, particularly those with perianal abscess, incision and drainage alone are adequate. The primary opening of the anal crypt is rarely identified (the rate of identification was only 34% in one series). Intersphincteric abscess is treated by using the proctoscope to observe the bulging area and then performing an internal sphincterotomy over the abscess. Supralevator abscesses are drained through the appropriate ischiorectal space or through the rectum. Horseshoe abscesses (those that surround the rectum) are drained through the rectum, with corner drains placed in each ischiorectal abscess.

Fistula *in ano*

A fistula is an abnormal communication between two epithelial/endothelial-lined surfaces. A fistula *in ano* has its external opening in the perirectal skin and its internal opening in the anal canal at the dentate line. Pain is rare with fistula *in ano*, patients more commonly complaining of perirectal itching, irritation and discharge.

A fistula *in ano* forms during the chronic stage of an acute inflammatory process that begins in the intersphincteric anal glands. As previously discussed, extension of the acute inflammation can result in a supralevator, ischiorectal or perianal abscess. With chronic inflammation, the abscess communicates with the external surface, forming supralevator trans-sphincteric or intersphincteric fistulae. Approximately 40% of patients develop fistula *in ano* after the treatment of perirectal abscess (Fig. 32.13).

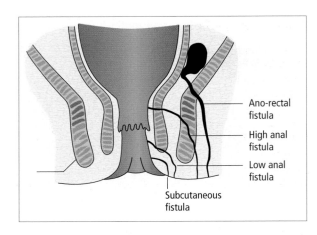

Figure 32.13 Classification of fistula *in ano*.

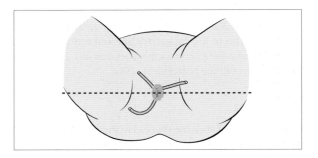

Figure 32.14 Goodsall's rule.

Other disease processes that can cause fistula *in ano* include:
- Crohn's disease;
- diverticulitis with perforation and fistula to the perineum;
- hydroadinitis suppurativa;
- pilonidal sinus;
- malignancies of the distal rectum, anal canal or perianal skin;
- tuberculosis;
- actinomycosis.

Goodsall's rule

Goodsall's rule relates to the location of the internal and external openings of a fistula *in ano* (Fig. 32.14). If the anus is bisected by a line in the frontal plane, an external opening inferior to that line connects to the internal opening via a short direct tract. However, if the external opening is posterior to this imaginary line, the fistula

04

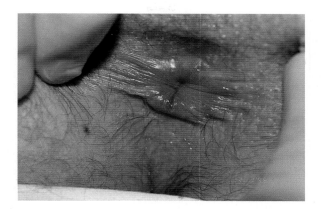

Figure 32.15 Fissure *in ano* in the classical position (midline posteriorly).

tract follows a curved route to the internal opening in the posterior midline. An exception is an external opening that is anterior to this imaginary line and more than 3 cm from the anus, in which case the tract may be curve posteriorly and end in the posterior midline.

Treatment

The mainstay of treatment is to lay the fistula tract open; thus internal sphincterotomy is the treatment for an inter-sphincteric fistula. Deep or high fistulae may require a two-stage operation to prevent incontinence. In the first stage, a seton suture is placed around the sphincter to stimulate fibrosis adjacent to the sphincter muscle. In the second stage, performed 6–8 weeks later, the intersphincteric portion of the fistual tract is laid open.

Anal fissures

An anal fissure is a tear in the anal canal, frequently associated with sudden pain or bleeding during defecation (Fig. 32.15). The fissure occurs in the posterior midline and may be associated with skin tags or a sentinel pile. Stool softeners prevent recurrence. Chronic anal fissures may require a lateral sphincterotomy, although there are a number of new medical treatments, e.g. nitrates in the form of 0.2% glyceryl trinitrate (GTN) ointment.

Haemorrhoids

The anal canal is lined by the anal cushions, which consist of three thick vascular submucosal bundles that always lie in the left lateral, right posterior lateral and right anterior lateral positions. The function of these cushions is not entirely clear, but they aid continence and engorge during defecation to protect the anal canal from abrasions. 'Haemorrhoid' is the pathological term for a downward displacement of the anal cushions, which produces dilatation of the venules. Haemorrhoids thus consist of a dilated venous plexus, a small artery and areolar tissue.

Presenting symptoms

The most common manifestation of internal haemorrhoids is painless rectal bleeding, often during a bowel movement. Patients often notice bright red blood in the stool, on the toilet seat or in the toilet. Prolapse of internal haemorrhoids may produce moisture in the anal region or mucus discharge that causes itching (Fig. 32.16a,b). Pain is not a common symptom of internal haemorrhoids unless infection is also present. The standard classification of haemorrhoidal disease is described in Table 32.3.

Diagnosis

Although internal haemorrhoids are the most common cause of rectal bleeding, it is prudent to exclude other causes of bleeding. Haemorrhoids are easily visualized using a proctoscope. Endoscopy is the procedure of choice to rule out other sources of rectal bleeding, such as cancer and inflammatory bowel disease. All patients, including those with atypical symptoms, require a complete colonic evaluation to exclude colonic disease.

Treatment

External haemorrhoids are best treated with analgesia and warm soaks. However, if the pain is severe, the thrombosed haemorrhoid must be excised. Mild bleeding and protrusion of external haemorrhoids can be controlled with conservative treatment that includes avoidance of constipating foods, increasing the fibre content of the diet and using bulk-forming stool agents. These measures alone can often resolve all symptoms. Rubber-band ligation, a simple outpatient procedure, can be used to treat first- and second-degree haemorrhoids; injection with phenol and almond oil could play a similar role. Third- and fourth-degree haemorrhoids and mixed internal/external haemorrhoids require haemorrhoidectomy.

Pilonidal sinus

A pilonidal sinus is a hair-containing sinus or abscess that usually involves the skin and adjacent tissues in the intergluteal region. Most patients have pain, swelling and drainage when these sinuses become infected (Fig. 32.17).

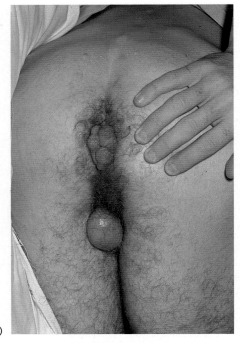

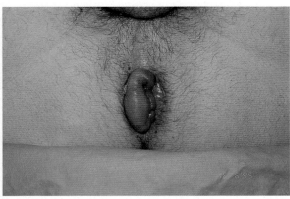

(a)

(b)

Figure 32.16 (a) Third-degree haemorrhoids. (b) Prolapsed thrombosed piles are extremely painful and usually require surgical treatment.

Most investigators believe that this condition is caused by ingrowth of hair, although whether it is acquired or congenital is not known. Pilonidal disease can occur at any age but is most prevalent between adolescence and the third decade of life. Recurrent infections are common.

The treatment depends on the phase of the disease at

Table 32.3 Classification of haemorrhoidal disease.

First degree	Does not protrude
Second degree	Protrudes on straining, reduces either spontaneously or digitally
Third degree	Protrudes, requires manual reduction

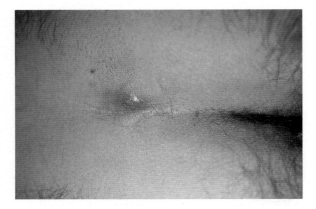

Figure 32.17 Pilonidal sinus and abscess.

presentation. Pilonidal abscess is best treated by incision and drainage. However, for a pilonidal cyst, results of treatment remain imperfect, although numerous methods have been reported. The simplest methods of treatment are incision and drainage, and curettage with secondary healing or cyst excision and closure.

Anorectal warts (condylomata acuminata)

Condyloma acuminatum is a disease caused by human papilloma virus and anal intercourse is the most common means of transmission. Condyloma acuminatum is often associated with other sexually transmitted disease, and therefore examination and testing for herpes or chlamydia infection, gonococcal proctitis, anorectal syphilis and HIV/AIDS is prudent. If the warts are small and few, they are treated with Podophyllin Paint. For numerous and large anal warts, excision with electrocautery is effective. The successful use of adjuvant interferons has been reported for severe cases. Infection with human papilloma virus type 16 and 18 is associated with malignant degeneration.

04

Benign anal and perianal disorders at a glance

Haemorrhoids ('piles')

Definition

A submucosal swelling in the anal canal arising from the anal cushions and consisting of a dilated venous plexus, a small artery and areolar tissue. Internal haemorrhoids only involve tissues of upper anal canal; external haemorrhoids involve tissues of lower anal canal

Aetiology

● Increased venous pressure from straining (low-fibre diet) or altered haemodynamics (e.g. during pregnancy) causes chronic dilation of submucosal venous plexus
● Found at the 3, 7 and 11 o'clock positions in the anal canal

Clinical features

● First degree: bleeding/itching only
● Second degree: prolapse during defecation, spontaneous reduction
● Third degree: prolapses and requires manual reduction
● Fourth degree: prolapses but cannot be reduced manually, often requires urgent surgery

Treatment

● Simple: bulk laxatives and high-fibre diet
● Bleeding internal piles; injection sclerotherapy, Barron's bands, cryosurgery
● Prolapsing external: haemorrhoidectomy (complications: bleeding, anal stenosis)

Rectal prolapse

Definition

Protrusion from the anus to a variable degree of the rectal mucosa (partial) or rectal wall (full thickness)

Aetiology

● Rectal intussusception
● Poor sphincter tone
● Chronic straining
● Pelvic floor injury

Clinical features

● Mucous discharge, bleeding, tenesmus, obvious prolapse

Treatment

● Stool manipulation and biofeedback
● Delorme's peranal mucosal resection

● Abdominal rectopexy (rectum is 'hitched up' on to sacrum)

Perianal haematoma

● Very painful subcutaneous haematoma caused by rupture of small blood vessel in the perianal area
● Evacuation of the clot provides instant relief

Anal fissure

Definition

Longitudinal tear in the mucosa of the anal canal, in the midline posteriorly (90%) or anteriorly (10%)

Aetiology

● 90% caused by local trauma during passage of constipated stool and potentiated by spasm of internal anal sphincter
● Other causes: pregnancy/delivery, Crohn's disease, sexually transmitted infections (often lateral position)

Clinical features

● Exquisitely painful on passing bowel motion
● Small amount of bright-red blood on toilet tissue
● Severe sphincter spasm
● Skin tag at distal end of tear ('sentinel pile')

Treatment

● First line: stool softeners/bulking agents, local anaesthetic gels, 0.2% GTN ointment
● Second line: botulinum toxin injection, lateral internal sphincterotomy
● Examination under anaesthesia and biopsy for atypical/suspicious abnormal fissures

Perianal abscess

Aetiology

Focus of infection starts in anal glands ('cryptoglandular sepsis') and spreads into perianal tissues to cause:
● Perianal abscess: adjacent to anal margin
● Ischiorectal abscess: in ischiorectal fossa
● Pararectal abscess: above levator ani

Clinical features

● Painful, red, tender, swollen mass
● Fever, rigors, sweating, tachycardia

Treatment

● Incision and drainage
● Antibiotics

Fistula *in ano*

Definition/aetiology
- Abnormal communication between perianal skin and anal canal established that persists following drainage of a perianal abscess
- May be associated with Crohn's disease (multiple fistulae), ulcerative colitis or tuberculosis
- Low: below 50% of the external anal sphincter
- High: crossing 50% or more of the external anal sphincter

Clinical features
- Chronic perianal discharge
- External orifice of track with granulation tissue seen perianally

Treatment
- Low: probing and laying open the track (fistulotomy)
- High: seton insertion, core removal of the fistula track

Pilonidal sinus

Definition
A blind-ending track containing hairs in the skin of the natal cleft

Aetiology
- Movement of buttocks promotes hair migration into a (?congenital) sinus

Clinical features
May present as:
- Natal cleft abscess
- Discharging sinus in midline posterior to anal margin with hair protruding from orifice
- Natal cleft itch/pain

Treatment
- Good personal hygiene
- Incision and drainage of abscesses, excision of sinus network

Anorectal warts
- Anorectal warts (condylomata acuminata) are caused by human papilloma virus and are sexually transmitted
- Consider presence of other sexually transmitted disease (chlamydia, gonorrhoea, syphilis, HIV/AIDS)
- Treatment: Podophyllin Paint (if warts are small and few) or electrocautery under general anaesthesia (if warts are large and numerous)

04

Disorders of the Breast

33

Must know Must do

Must know
Symptomatology of breast disorders
How to conduct an examination of the breasts
Management and diagnosis of common benign breast disorders
Management and diagnosis of breast cancer
Principles underlying breast screening
Methods of investigation of patients with breast disorders

Must do
Attend breast clinics
Examine patients presenting with breast lumps (under supervision)
Learn how to interpret mammograms
Observe fine-needle aspiration cytology of a breast lump
Observe Trucut biopsy of a breast lump
Talk to breast care and McMillan nurses
Observe a breast operation including axillary sentinel node(s) biopsy
Follow a patient undergoing treatment for carcinoma of the breast

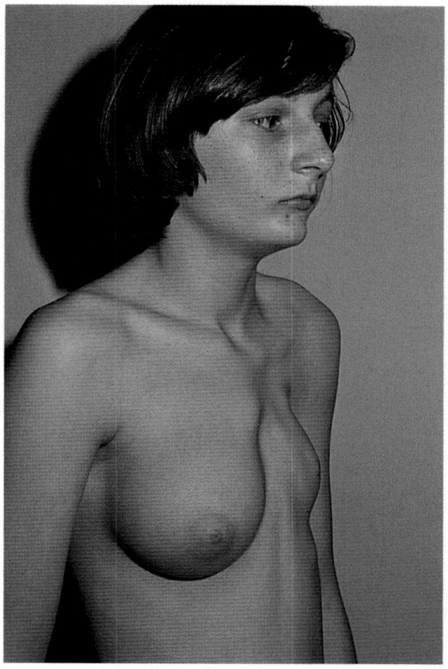

Figure 33.1 Congenital absence of breast (Poland's syndrome).

Breast anatomy and physiology

The adult breast lies between the second and sixth ribs and extends from the sternal edge to the midaxillary line. Its size and shape varies from one individual to the next but is characterized by fullness in the lower area and ptosis or drooping, which becomes pronounced with increasing age. The breast develops from an intrauterine milk ridge that extends from the axilla to the groin and coalesces in the pubertal breast bud. Occasional anomalies arise, such as total lack of breast development (Poland's syndrome, Fig. 33.1) or occasional development of a second breast or nipple along the milk line or massive breat hypertrophy (Fig. 33.2).

The functional unit in the breast is the terminal duct lobular unit. These units are capable of milk production and drain into branching ducts that coalesce to form the main ducts (usually less than 20) which open into the nipple. Each duct drains a segment of breast tissue and investigation such as ductography reveals that each such segment spreads over a fairly diffuse area towards the periphery of the breast. This has implications for the surgical management of conditions such as ductal carcinoma *in situ*, which tends to follow the distribution of a duct. As well as the epithelial/ductal structures, the breast is composed of support structures comprising fibrous elements, muscle, fat and fascia.

Blood supply and lymphatic drainage

The arterial blood supply to the breast comes from the surrounding area: perforating branches of the internal

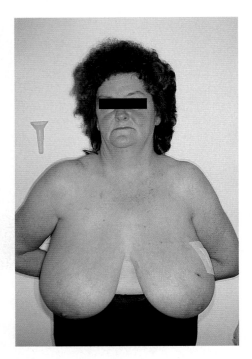

Figure 33.2 Massive breast hypertrophy.

mammary artery, intercostal arteries and branches of the lateral thoracic and acromiothoracic arteries in the axillary tail. Venous drainage follows the arterial supply. In addition, superficially the venous drainage can cross to the contralateral breast.

The lymphatic drainage of the breast is mainly to the axilla, although in the medial quadrants it may also drain to the internal mammary chain. The axillary nodal basin is divided into three levels depending on the relationship to pectoralis minor muscle, level 1 being below, level 2 behind and level 3 above the insertion of pectoralis minor.

Congenital anomalies

These can be understood from the earlier description of breast development. It is extremely unusual for a second breast pair to be found in humans but an accessory nipple can be found anywhere along the milk line and accessory breast tissue in the axillary tail area is not at all unusual.

Usually, differences in size and shape of an individual's breasts are small but may be apparent on examination. Complete absence of breast development (amazia) can occur and is usually found in association with lack of development of the pectoralis major muscle (Poland's syndrome). Other causes for absence of a breast include inadvertent excision of the breast bud (breast lumps

should not be excised in children) or radiotherapy to the chest wall in children.

Benign breast disease

The cause of a breast lump depends on the age of the patient. Young women commonly present with fibroadenomas (so-called 'breast mouse' because of its mobility), while middle-aged women (30–50 years old) usually present with breast cysts. In postmenopausal women, all new lumps are due to breast cancer until proven otherwise.

Breast lumps can be divided into those that are discrete (usually fibroadenomas or cysts) and those that represent a prominent area on a background of general lumpiness (fibroadenosis). These benign conditions are very common and are best considered as abnormalities of the normal development and involution of the breast. Benign breast lumps commonly occur at two stages in the life of normal women: (i) during puberty and early adulthood and (ii) in the premenopausal and perimenopausal periods.

In early adulthood the most common presenting feature is a discrete lump, while later in life the presenting feature may be a large cyst or fibrosis causing generalized lumpiness. Neither of these conditions are premalignant and both are very common. In the intervening years the breast is subjected to the normal cyclical changes associated with each menstrual cycle and benign breast conditions may present clinically as cyclical mastalgia, premenstrual breast tenderness, etc.

Nowadays the majority of patients with benign breast lumps can be spared the trauma of anaesthesia and surgery and be reassured that they do not have breast cancer. A quality assurance parameter in all breast units is the number of patients undergoing surgery for benign disease, which should be about the same number as those undergoing surgery for malignancy.

Assessment

All patients presenting with a breast lump should have a clinical, radiological and pathological assessment (known as triple assessment) carried out during their first visit to the clinic (Table 33.1).

Clinical assessment

Clinical assessment consists of history and physical examination. Important points in the history include the patient's age, age at menarche (and menopause if applicable), family history of breast cancer (number of affected first- and second-degree relatives, age at disease onset), number of children, age at childbirth and drug history (oral contraceptive pill/hormone replacement therapy).

04

Table 33.1 Triple assessment.

Physical examination
Radiological assessment
    Ultrasound in patients under 35 years old
    Mammography in patients over 35 years old
Pathological assessment
    Fine-needle aspiration cytology
    Trucut biopsy

The length of time since onset of the lump (whether enlarging or reducing) and date of last menstrual period (if applicable) are then documented.

Both breasts should be inspected for skin changes, tethering or dimpling in a good light. The breasts should first be inspected with the patient sitting upright and the arms to the side. Distortions can be assessed by asking the patient to raise her arms over her head and then return them to her side. Then each separate quadrant should be palpated to ensure no lumps are present. The nodal basin (axilla and supraclavicular fossa) should also be examined.

Radiological assessment

In women under 35 years of age ultrasound is the preferred technique, whereas in women over 35 mammography is usually performed. Ultrasound is particularly useful in assessing whether a lump is solid or cystic. With mammography, benign lumps are usually very well defined and may have a surrounding halo, whereas breast cancers are commonly associated with spiculation, architectural distortion or malignant microcalcification.

Pathological assessment

Fine-needle aspiration allows cells to be taken from the lump. A fine needle attached to a syringe is inserted into the lump and cells are withdrawn by making several passes through the lump with negative pressure (6 mL). A major advantage of this technique is that it allows drainage of a cyst (if fluid is present, then the diagnosis is invariably benign). If the fluid withdrawn is bloody or the lump persists, then further investigation is necessary. Occasionally a breast cyst can be associated with the presence of an intracystic papilloma (rarely carcinoma) and in these cases excision of the cyst is necessary. Clinically, these cysts recur and an intracystic abnormality is visible on ultrasound.

Once cells are withdrawn from a breast lump they can be either fixed and air-dried on a slide immediately or drawn into a transport medium and sent to the laboratory,

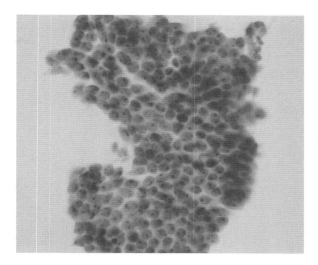

Figure 33.3 Benign cytology.

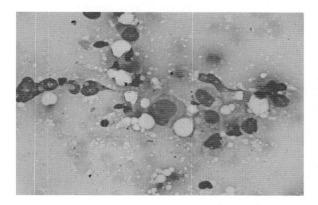

Figure 33.4 Malignant cytology.

where they are centrifuged and plated on a glass slide, fixed and stained with either haematoxylin and eosin or Papanicolaou stain. The cells are classified as follows:
C1, inadequate;
C2, normal/benign (Fig. 33.3);
C3, atypia probably benign;
C4, atypia probably malignant;
C5, malignant (Fig. 33.4).
A C5 diagnosis on cytology that is congruous with the clinical and radiological features is sufficient to allow the surgeon carry out a definitive surgical procedure for breast cancer (Fig. 33.4).

When cytology is inadequate or unhelpful the next step in diagnosis is core biopsy. This is a minimally invasive procedure where, under local anaesthesia, a sliver of

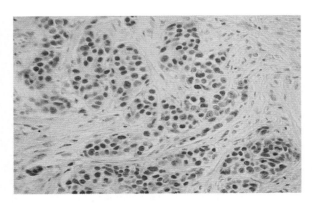

Figure 33.5 Immunohistochemistry showing oestrogen receptor positive staining.

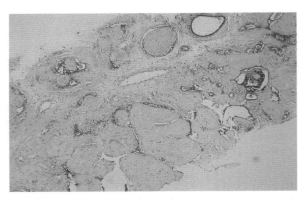

Figure 33.6 Core biopsy histology showing a benign fibroadenoma.

breast tissue is obtained from the breast lump. This carries some advantages over fine-needle aspiration cytology in that a histological assessment of tumour grade (when a lump is malignant) can be made and oestrogen receptor status can also be assessed (Fig. 33.5).

> **Breast lumps**
>
> - Likely diagnosis varies with age
> - Fibroadenomas common in young women
> - Cysts are common in women aged 30–50 years
> - All new lumps in women over 50 years old are cancer until proven otherwise

Fibroadenoma

Fibroadenomas are the most common breast lumps in young women but can occur at any time during the reproductive years. Although traditionally thought to be benign neoplasms, they are so common that they are probably best considered an aberration of normal development. Support for this hypothesis comes from the fact that they develop from the whole lobule (unlike cancers) and their epithelium is normal. In addition they are subject to the same hormonal control as the rest of the breast and often enlarge in pregnancy and involute during the menopause (Fig. 33.6).

Giant fibroadenomas (usually > 5 cm) can occur and can be difficult to distinguish from phylloides tumours both clinically and on core biopsy. In contrast to fibroadenomas, phylloides tumours (previously known as cystosarcoma phylloides) can recur locally and should be surgically removed with wide excision. In exceptional cases phylloides tumours can metastasize and behave in a malignant fashion; an indication of their malignant potential can be obtained from the number of mitoses per high power field seen on microscopic examination.

Management

Like all breast lumps, the investigation of a fibroadenoma involves triple assessment and it is perfectly acceptable to leave small fibroadenomas (< 2 cm) in the breast unless the patient requests excision. The natural history of these lesions is that 20% involute, 20% increase in size and 60% remain the same. However, it is worth emphasizing that a discrete breast lump even in a woman in her early twenties should not be considered a fibroadenoma until all relevant investigations are complete. All large fibroadenomas should be excised, as should clinically apparent lesions in the postmenopausal period (uncommon).

Fibroadenosis

This term refers to a spectrum of conditions that commonly present as lumpiness or discomfort on a background of generally lumpy breasts. As previously outlined, it represents an abnormality of normal breast involution rather than a disease process and is very common in women in their forties and during the perimenopausal period. Breast involution causes changes at the microscopic level, including fibrosis (increase in fibrous tissue), adenosis (increase in glandular elements) and apocrine change (the normal epithelium lining the ducts becomes sweat gland-type epithelium). In addition, minimal hyperplasia of the epithelial cells lining the ducts occurs and small breast cysts may develop. None of these changes are in any way premalignant but sometimes present as lumps due to either macrocyst formation or excessive palpable fibrous tissue.

04

Clinically, women in the 35–50 age group commonly present with breast cysts or a lump that represents either focal nodularity or a prominent area on a background of generalized nodularity. Investigation of these lumps should always involve triple assessment, i.e. clinical examination and risk factor analysis, radiology (usually mammography with ultrasound if the lump is solid) and fine-needle aspiration cytology. Fine-needle aspiration cytology is especially useful as a cyst will disappear and allows cells from a solid lump to be examined.

Breast cysts

The development of breast cysts is so common as to be part of the normal process of involution of the breast in women in the premenopausal years. Debate exists as to whether women with persistent or recurrent cysts have an increased risk of breast cancer, with some studies showing that the risk of developing cancer is 1.5–4 times higher in women with cysts particularly in those under 45 years old. Cysts require no treatment unless they are associated with a persistent lump, recur repeatedly in the same area or the cyst fluid is blood-stained. Ultrasound can sometimes identify an intracystic papilloma that causes recurrence of the cyst and this merits excision. In these cases the cyst and a small amount of surrounding tissue can be excised.

Nipple discharge

Nipple discharge is a very common complaint in the breast clinic and requires investigation if it is blood-stained. It is important to determine if the discharge is from a single duct or multiple ducts and whether it is unilateral or bilateral (see box below).

Nipple discharge

- Single duct or multiple ducts involved
- Blood or no blood
- Cosmetically disfiguring or not
- Non-cosmetically disfiguring, non-bloodstained discharge from multiple ducts requires no intervention

The majority of patients have a physiological discharge that varies in colour from clear to greenish/brown. Provided it does not contain blood and is discharged from multiple ducts, no further intervention is necessary. Duct ectasia is a physiological condition in which the large terminal duct dilates and retains secretions, causing a physiological discharge as patients get older.

Milky discharge from a single duct is usually physiological and requires no treatment. However, in patients with bilateral milky discharge a serum prolactin estimation should be assessed to rule out a pituitary microadenoma (prolactinoma).

A unilateral blood-stained nipple discharge is usually due to an intraductal papilloma, although an intraductal carcinoma must of course be ruled out. These patients must have a full triple assessment, with ultrasound of the retroareolar area being useful. It is helpful to confirm the presence of blood in the discharge by a dipstick test and ductography may be helpful in showing a space-occupying lesion in the duct. The patient should undergo microdochectomy (surgical excision of the duct) performed via a periareolar incision. This allows full assessment of the cause of the discharge. Patients who have troublesome bilateral benign discharge from several ducts can have bilateral major duct excision (Hadfield's procedure). This carries significant risk of rendering the nipple insensate.

Breast pain

Breast pain is very common and is not usually associated with breast cancer. Several underlying conditions can cause referred pain to the breast, including angina, pneumonia, pleurisy, intercostal neuralgia, oesophagitis and costochondritis. These should be obvious from a good history and clinical evaluation. Breast pain (mastalgia) can be divided into cyclical and non-cyclical.

Cyclical mastalgia

Cyclical mastalgia is extremely common: most women suffer from some form of premenstrual mastalgia. When this discomfort is severe or prolonged beyond the usual 3–5 days, it requires intervention. It is not due to an increase in fluid retention and therefore diuretics have no role in its management.

Management of cylical mastalgia involves firstly reassurance that it is a physiological condition and not associated with an increased risk of breast cancer. Evening primrose oil (which contains free fatty acids, particularly γ-linoleic acid) has been shown to greatly improve cyclical mastalgia in the majority of women. Its exact mechanism of action is poorly understood but it is thought to influence lipid metabolism and improve transport across the intercellular membranes. The recommendation is 1000 mg of evening primrose oil or a definitive preparation of γ-linoleic acid for 3 months only. In about 50% of cases the mastalgia will not recur; if it does, the regimen can be repeated. In severe or non-responding cases, several other medications have been tried with some benefit. Tamoxifen (usually 20 mg daily for 3 months) can be tried, although its use is not supported by randomized trials as yet.

04

Drugs acting on the pituitary–ovarian axis have a role in the management of cyclical mastalgia. Danazol, commencing on the first day of the menstrual cycle, induces amenorrhoea and should be combined with appropriate contraceptives. Unfortunately it is often poorly tolerated because of its adverse effects, which include androgenic actions on the voice, hirsutism and weight gain. Bromocriptine, a synthetic dopamine agonist, has also been used. The dose is titrated to about 2.5 mg b.d. but like danazol is often poorly tolerated due to its adverse effects.

Non-cyclical mastalgia

This is less common than cyclical mastalgia but is more difficult to treat as a response to free fatty acids is unusual.

Common chest wall disorders such as costochondritis (Tietze's syndrome) must be ruled out. This is a common condition that tends to be self-limiting within 6–8 weeks and responds to non-steroidal anti-inflammatory drugs (NSAIDs). It is characterized by pain induced by pressure on the costochondral junction where the ribs join the sternum.

Benign breast disorders such as periductal fibrosis, fat necrosis (local trauma) and sclerosing adenosis can cause tender spots in the breast. While these conditions tend to be localized, surgery is rarely of any value as the condition usually recurs. A combination of evening primrose oil, NSAIDs and massage of NSAID cream into the area of tenderness is usually the therapeutic strategy.

Benign breast disease at a glance

Definitions

Abnormalities of the normal development and involution of the breast (ANDI): a broad term covering benign conditions of the breast, many of which have overlapping features. ANDI are common in younger premenopausal women and often cause considerable anxiety. Any breast lump should be evaluated by triple assessment for risk of malignancy whatever the likely diagnosis

Breast lump: any palpable mass in the breast. It is the most common way for benign and malignant disease to present

Gynaecomastia: diffuse enlargement of one or both breasts in the male

Mastalgia: any pain felt in the breast. Cyclical mastalgia is breast pain that varies with the menstrual cycle. Non-cyclical mastalgia is pain that follows no particular pattern or is intermittent

Nipple discharge: any fluid, which may be physiological or pathological, emanating from the breast

Triple assessment: a breast lump is examined by clinical, radiological (< 35 years, ultrasound; > 35 years, mammography) and cytological examination, usually during the first visit to a breast clinic. Reassurance, counselling and/or planning for definitive treatment can then be done jointly with the patient, nurse, surgeon, radiologist, oncologist and pathologist

ANDI – Abnormalities of development
Fibroadenoma
● Benign breast lump caused by overgrowth of single breast lobule. Manifests as one or more firm, mobile, painless lumps usually in women under 30 years of age
● Investigation: triple assessment

● Treatment:
  (a) Age < 30: either observe or excise if worried
  (b) Age > 30: excise to exclude malignancy

Abnormalities of cycles: fibrocystic disease
● Usually presents at age 25–45 years. May present as breast pain, tenderness, breast lump(s), breast cyst(s), especially during the second half of the menstrual cycle
● Investigation: triple assessment of all lumps
● Treatment: patient reassurance, analgesics, γ-linoleic acid, hormone manipulation, cyst aspiration, excision of persistent localized masses after aspiration. Avoid xanthine-containing substances (coffee)

Abnormalities of involution: breast cysts
● May be single or multiple. Firm, round discrete lump(s)
● Investigation: aspiration ± mammography. Triple assessment for any discrete associated lumps
● Treatment: reassurance, aspiration (repeated), hormone manipulation

Other benign conditions
Breast abscess
● Usually infection of the pregnant or lactating breast with *Staphylococcus aureus*. Patient presents with redness, swelling, heat and pain in the breast
● Treatment: antibiotics (flucloxacillin) initially but, if an abscess develops, incision and drainage will be required. Lactation/breast-feeding does not need to be suppressed while the abscess is being treated

Mammary duct ectasia
● Dilated subareolar ducts are filled with cellular debris that causes a periductal inflammatory response. Associated with smoking and recurrent non-lactational abscesses.

04

Usual presentation is a green nipple discharge and a subareolar lump
- Treatment: subareolar excision of the involved ducts

Duct papilloma
- Small papillomas arise in the major breast ducts. They cause a bloody or serous nipple discharge
- Treatment: excision of the affected duct by microdochectomy

Fat necrosis
- Fibrous scar in the breast tissue caused by injury, haematoma and necrosis of breast fat with subsequent scarring. History of trauma to the breast in 50% of cases. May be associated superficial ecchymoses
- Histology: periductal cellular infiltrate and fibrosis
- Investigation: triple assessment
- Treatment: usually surgical excision to exclude malignancy

Gynaecomastia
- Presence of breasts in the male resembling those of the sexually mature female
- Usually physiological but often needs to be investigated for hormonal causes:

(a) Oestrogen or steroid therapy
(b) Liver disease
(c) Pituitary gland tumour
(d) Testicular tumour
(e) Use of spirinolactone
- Treatment in severe cases is by excision of breast tissue

Mastalgia
Non-breast pathology
- Costochondritis (Tietze's disease)
- Pleurisy
- Atypical angina pectoris
- Bornholm's disease

Breast pathology
- Breast abscess/mastitis
- Infected sebaceous cyst
- Fibrocystic disease

No obvious breast pathology
- Cyclical mastalgia: γ-linoleic acid (evening primose oil), danazol, tamoxifen, bromocriptine
- Non-cyclical mastalgia: NSAIDs, γ-linoleic acid

Breast cancer

Breast cancer is a major health problem. It is the most common cancer in women and the most common cause of death in middle-aged women. It is a very common disease in the western world. Breast cancer is a rare disease in women under 35 years old but its incidence doubles every 5 years until the age of 50, when it affects 1 in 400 women per year. This incidence continues to increase very slightly through to the eighth and ninth decades.

Apart from the western lifestyle, several factors have been implicated in the development of breast cancer (Table 33.2). Genetic influences alone account for the development of the disease in about 5–8% of cases. The genes *BRCA1* and *BRCA2* carry an approximately 80% lifetime risk for breast cancer. *BRCA1*, located on chromosome 17 and about 4000 bp in size, and was first described in Ashkenazi Jews. A mutation in any of the base pairs causes a predisposition to breast cancer and ovarian cancer. Families who carry a *BRCA1* or *BRCA2* abnormality usually have a history of at least four affected relatives with the disease, breast cancer at a young age (under 40), bilateral breast cancer, breast and ovarian cancer in the same individual (*BRCA1*) or male breast cancer (*BRCA2*). A third major genetic defect associated with breast cancer is Li–Fraumeni syndrome (caused by mutation in the *P53* gene on chromosome 17), where female members develop

Table 33.2 Breast cancer predisposing factors.

Genetic
BRCA1, BRCA2, P53, HNPCC, AT

Hormonal
Early mearche
Late menopause
Hormone replacement therapy (> 10 years)
Nulliparity
Late first birth

Familial
As yet unknown genetic factors that cause individual to have up to 30% lifetime risk of developing breast cancer include:
  First-degree relative with breast cancer under 40 years old
  Two first-degree relatives with breast cancer under 60 years old
  Three first-degree relatives with breast cancer at any age
  First-degree relative with breast and ovarian cancer
  First-degree relative with bilateral breast cancer

breast cancer at a very young age. Other genetic abnormalities predisposing to breast cancer are associated with the ataxia telangiectasia and hereditary non-polyposis coli genes.

Hormonal factors are also implicated in the development of breast cancer. Prolonged exposure of the breast to oestrogens predisposes to breast cancer, e.g. early menarche, late menopause, hormone replacement therapy and nulliparity or late first birth.

Histological types

The majority (85%) of breast cancer is invasive ductal cancer (Fig. 33.7). Tubular cancer is very low grade and represents very little long-term risk to patients. Ductal carcinoma can be graded from 1 to 3 (1, well differentiated, low grade; 3, poorly differentiated, high grade) on the basis of a grading system originally described by Bloom and Richardson and modified by Elston and Ellis from Nottingham. This grading system is based on tubule formation, mitotic index and differentiation/nuclear pleomorphism and correlates with tumour outcome.

Lobular carcinoma accounts for about 10% of breast cancers. It is characterized by small round cells infiltrating the lobule and is often missed on cytology, where the appearance of the cells can be difficult to differentiate

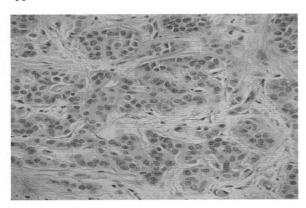

Figure 33.7 Invasive ductal carcinoma.

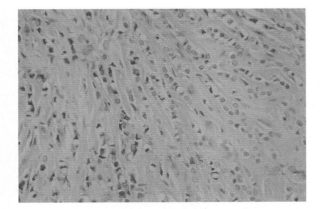

Figure 33.8 Invasive lobular carcinoma.

from normal epithelial cells (Fig. 33.8). Clinically, lobular cancer tends to be multifocal within the breast and may also be bilateral. These features mean that it is more frequently treated by mastectomy.

A small percentage of breast cancers belong to special types, including medullary (lymphocytic infiltration, better prognosis), colloid or mucinous, and tubular. These are usually towards the well-differentiated end of the spectrum and consequently have a better prognosis.

Carcinoma *in situ*

Ductal carcinoma *in situ* is a premalignant condition of the breast where the cells have taken on a malignant phenotype but invasion through the basement membrane has not yet taken place. Prior to mammographic screening this entity accounted for less than 3% of breast cancers but within screening programmes it now accounts for nearly 20% of all malignant abnormalities. The reason for this is that it is represented by microcalcification on mammography.

Ductal carcinoma *in situ* carries a high risk for the development of breast cancer in the area of the breast in which it occurs, the risk being proportional to the grade of ductal carcinoma *in situ*. Treatment is similar to invasive breast cancer and usually consists of wide excision of the area with a rim (1 cm) of normal breast tissue around the abnormality. In patients with high-grade ductal carcinoma *in situ*, radiotherapy may be used to reduce the risk of local recurrence. When the area of ductal carcinoma *in situ* is greater than 4 cm, mastectomy is usually required as therapy.

Lobular carcinoma *in situ* is characterized by lobules filled with malignant-type cells but the risk of invasion is less than that associated with ductal carcinoma *in situ*. Lobular carcinoma *in situ* increases the risk of development of breast cancer but the risk is considerably less than that associated with ductal carcinoma *in situ*. In addition, breast cancer when it occurs is often in a different quadrant or indeed in the contralateral breast. Patients with this condition are usually managed by close surveillance rather than surgery.

Clinical assessment

The clinical features of breast cancer are:
- breast lump (in postmenopausal women almost all new lumps represent breast cancer);
- bloody nipple discharge;
- skin changes such as tethering or nipple eczema (Paget's disease) (Fig. 33.9); or
- mammographic screening abnormalities. If neglected breast cancer may ulcerate through the skin of the breast (Fig. 33.10).

04

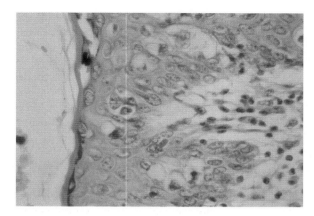

Figure 33.9 Pagets disease.

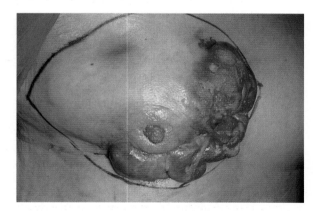

Figure 33.10 Advanced carcinoma of the breast.

Staging

Breast cancer is staged according to the TNM classification (T, tumour size; N, nodes; M, metastases) (Fig. 33.10; Table 33.3). The TNM classification is based on clinical assessment of the breast. Nowadays, we tend to classify tumours according to histological assessment following definitive surgery. In screening programmes a high proportion of patients with breast cancer have tumours less than 2 cm that are node negative. These patients are subdivided into those whose tumour is less than 5 mm (T1a), 5–10 mm (T1b) or 10–15 mm (T1c).

Breast cancer commonly metastasizes to the liver, bones, brain or lungs and a breast secondary at a distant site can occur in any woman with a history of breast cancer.

Patients with tumours less than 3 cm and clinically node negative have operable breast cancer. In these patients preoperative scanning for metastases is not necessary. In more advanced cases, the following investigations should be performed:
- liver ultrasound;
- bone scan;

Table 33.3 TNM classification.

T0	Carcinoma *in situ* or microinvasion
T1	Tumour < 2 cm
T2	Tumour 2–5 cm
T3	Tumour > 5 cm
T4	Overlying skin or underlying muscle attachment
N0	No axillary nodal involvement
N1	Free axillary nodes (histologically less than three involved nodes)
N2	More than three involved nodes or fixed axillary nodes
N3	Supraclavicular nodes involved
M0	No metastases
M1	Metastatic disease present

- blood tests, e.g. full blood count, liver function tests, carcinoembryonic antigen, Ca15.3 (a relatively specific breast cancer tumour marker).

Management/treatment

Surgery remains the cornerstone of breast cancer management. Radical surgery for breast cancer, including mastectomy with excision of the pectoral muscles (radical mastectomy, Halsted), was in vogue in the early years of the last century. During the second half of the 20th century the most commonly performed operation was a modified radical (Patey) mastectomy, where the muscle was spared and all the axillary lymph nodes were removed. Over the past 25 years, trials from Milan and the National Surgical Adjuvant Breast and Bowel Project (Fisher) have shown that in early breast cancer wide excision of the tumour (lumpectomy or segmentectomy) gives as good long-term results as mastectomy. Conservative breast surgery followed by radiotherapy is now the accepted surgical practice for early breast cancer. Some indications for mastectomy still exist:
- large tumour/breast size;
- multifocal tumours;
- extensive premalignant change;
- tumours in pregnancy (particularly first trimester);
- recurrence of breast cancer following previous breast conservation.

Surgery

There is now well-established evidence that conservative breast surgery and radiotherapy is as useful as more radical surgery for breast cancer. Conservative breast surgery consists of wide local excision of the tumour. In some situations mastectomy is still necessary:
- large tumours in a small breast;
- centrally placed tumours;

- multifocal disease where more than one tumour exists;
- previously treated carcinomas and cases where radiotherapy is contraindicated, e.g. connective tissue disorders/scleroderma or in the first trimester of pregnancy.

Axillary surgery

Axillary nodal status is the single most important prognostic indicator in breast cancer. Patients who have no involved nodes have an almost 80% chance of long-term survival. The most effective means of staging the axilla is at least a level 2 clearance, as in lesser procedures there is a risk of understaging the disease. However, sectional node biopsy is being used increasingly as the primary means of staging the axilla; with clearance or radiotherapy being reserved for patients who have a positive axillary sentinel node. Some clinicians believe a four-node sample to be sufficient to stage the axilla; again radiotherapy must be used in the presence of positive nodes, which may increase the risk of lymphoedema.

There is a direct correlation between the risk of nodal disease and the size of the primary tumour. In recent years the concept of sentinel node biopsy has evolved. Originally described in penile cancer and used in malignant melanoma, the sentinel node concept is that lymph flows in an orderly direction from the primary site to a single gatekeeper or sentinel node and then migrates to other nodes. If the sentinel node could be found to be benign, then no other nodes need be removed. In breast cancer the sentinel node may be identified by the use of an intraoperative gamma probe following the injection of ^{99}Tc-labelled sulfacolloid around the primary tumour site or by the use of patent blue V dye or lymphosurin, which can travel in the lymphatics and colour the lymph node blue. A drawback of the technique is that even in the best hands there seems to be a 5% false-negative rate and there is a definitive learning curve.

Local recurrence

Local recurrence can be a problem after conservative breast surgery. It is very important to ensure negative margins and some patients may require a mastectomy if they have an extensive intraductal component around the tumour (ductal carcinoma *in situ*), are younger than 35 years of age or the tumour exhibits extensive lymphovascular invasion. Following conservative breast surgery, local recurrence occurs in about 8% of cases by 5 years and 13% by 10 years.

Radiotherapy

All patients who have breast conservation for invasive cancer should have postoperative external beam radiation to minimize local recurrence rates. The usual dose is 50 Gy in 25 fractions and local brachytherapy or electron boost to the tumour bed may be useful in selected cases. Following mastectomy, radiotherapy is indicated in patients with large tumours (T3, > 5 cm) and in those who have more than four positive axillary nodes.

Mammographic screening programmes

Evidence from several trials has shown that screening mammography leads to earlier detection of breast cancer. The principal trials were carried out in the 1960s and 1970s (Health Insurance Plan in New York, Dutch trials in Nijmegen, DOM project in Utrecht, Swedish two-county trials). All these trials suggest that even without modern mammography a survival benefit of about 25% occurs from screening.

It is now accepted that screening with two-dimensional mammography read by two radiologists at 2-yearly intervals in women aged between 50 and 70 is appropriate. The incidence of screen-detected cancer varies from about 8 per 1000 women screened in the initial (prevalent) round to about 5 per 1000 in subsequent (incident) rounds. Approximately 20–25% of cancers are detected in the premalignant phase (ductal carcinoma *in situ*) becuase they present with microcalcification.

Classically, the appearance of breast cancer on a mammogram is as a stellate density (Fig. 33.11). It can also present as architectural distortion or microcalcification. A radial scar is a radiologically suspicious lesson that carries about a 15% risk of associated early cancer and merits excision.

04

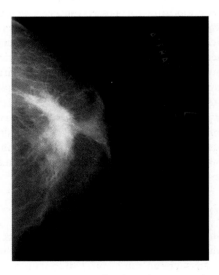

Figure 33.11 Mammogram showing a large central cancer.

Adjuvant therapy

Adjuvant therapy is treatment given following complete excision of the tumour in order to improve prognosis for the patient. It is thought to work by inhibiting the growth of micrometastases or circulating tumour cells at distant sites. In breast cancer the common adjuvant treatments are hormone therapy or chemotherapy.

Hormone therapy

Adjuvant hormone therapy is given to all patients with hormone-sensitive tumours. This is assessed by measuring oestrogen and progesterone receptor status by immunohistochemistry of the resected tumour. Tamoxifen is the best known and most widely used hormone therapy. It is an oestrogen receptor antagonist and reduces the risk of metastases by about 15% in all oestrogen/ progesterone receptor-positive patients regardless of age. Apart from reducing metastatic potential, it also has a pro-oestrogenic effect that reduces bone loss/osteoporotic potential and improves the circulatory lipid profile. Its drawbacks include increased risk of carcinoma of the womb, postmenopausal bleeding and thromboembolic phenomena.

Over the past few years a newer group of drugs called aromatase inhibitors have been used. Aromatase is an enzyme involved in the steroid hormone cascade; inhibitors of aromatase thus reduce oestrogen to very low levels. There is emerging evidence that these products may be at least as effective as tamoxifen against breast cancer with a more acceptable adverse effect profile. However, more experience is required before the long-term adverse effects, particularly with regard to bone, are known.

Chemotherapy

Adjuvant chemotherapy is the second major systemic treatment modality for breast cancer. Chemotherapy significantly diminishes the risk of metastatic spread but this decrease is greater in the premenopausal period and in patients at higher risk, i.e. node-positive patients. All chemotherapy regimens use combinations of drugs; the standard regimen (Bonadonna) uses cyclophosphamide, methotrexate and 5-fluorouracil and there is evidence that anthracycline-containing regimens may improve the outlook further. Recently, paclitaxel (Taxol) and docetaxel (Taxotere) have been used but the most efficacious chemotherapy regime remains controversial and is still open to question.

Breast reconstruction

Following mastectomy, a breast reconstruction can be done either immediately or as a delayed procedure. The tissue used can be an autologous flap containing skin and muscle from the patient or prosthetic material such as silicone. The commonly used autologous flaps are either the latissimus dorsi flap from the back or a transverse rectus abdominis muscle flap (TRAM) from the abdomen. TRAM flaps may be used as a pedicled flap or a free flap, in which case the inferior epigastric vessels are anastomosed to either the internal mammary or thoracodorsal vessels.

The simplest form of reconstruction involves placing a submuscular prosthetic expander at the time of mastectomy and inflating the expander slowly in the postoperative period. It can then be removed and replaced by a permanent prosthesis. Complications include infection, haematoma, pain and capsular contracture.

The aim of breast reconstruction is to restore the patient's shape; sometimes the native contralateral breast may need to be lifted or reduced to match the shape of the reconstructed breast.

Management of breast cancer

- Radical surgery does not benefit patients with early breast cancer
- All patients who have conservative breast surgery for cancer should have postoperative radiotherapy
- Tamoxifen (or some other antioestrogen, e.g. aromatose inhibitor) should be given to all patients with oestrogen or progesterone receptor-positive tumours
- Chemotherapy benefits patients with breast cancer and the benefits are greater for young women and those with aggressive tumours
- Axillary nodal status is the most important prognostic indicator in breast cancer

---

Key points

- Breast disease is very common and is usually benign
- Lumps in young women are usually fibroadenomas
- Breast cysts are common in the 30–50 age group
- Diagnosis of breast disease is now minimally invasive and involves either fine-needle aspiration or core biopsy
- Breast cancer is the most common malignancy in women and the most common cause of death in middle-aged women
- The prognosis of breast cancer depends on the size and grade of the tumour and especially the axillary nodal status
- All patients with oestrogen or progesterone receptor-positive tumours should receive antioestrogen therapy (tamoxifen or an aromatose inhibitor)
- Combination chemotherapy benefits women; benefits are greater in young women
- Screening mammography involves screening women in the 50–64 age group with two-view mammography at 2–3 year intervals

04

Breast cancer at a glance

Definition

Breast cancer: malignant lesion of (predominantly) the female breast

Epidemiology
- Male/female ratio 1 : 100
- Any age (usually > 30 years)
- High incidence in western world and in white people more than black people

Aetiology
- Strong family history of breast cancer (genetic factors)
- Breast cancer genes: *BRCA1*, *BRCA2*, *P53*, *HNPCC*, *AT*
- Early menarche and late menopause especially in nulliparous women
- Nulliparity
- Late first birth
- Hormone replacement therapy for > 10 years
- Social class I and II

Pathology
- Histology: adenocarcinomas arising from the glandular epithelium. Common types are invasive ductal or lobular carcinoma. Paget's disease is ductal carcinoma involving the nipple
- Spread: lymphatics, vascular invasion, direct extension; spreads to lung, liver, bone, brain, adrenal, ovary
- Staging: TNM classification important for treatment and prognosis

Clinical features
- Palpable, hard, irregular, fixed breast lump, usually painless
- Nipple retraction and skin dimpling
- Nipple eczema in Paget's disease
- *Peau d'orange* (cutaneous oedema secondary to lymphatic obstruction)
- Palpable axillary nodes

Investigations
- Triple assessment: clinical, radiological, cytological
- Radiological assessment: mammography (ultrasound in young women with dense or large breasts). Features on mammography: irregular, spiculated, radiopaque mass with microcalcification
- Cytological assessment: fine-needle aspiration cytology or core biopsy
- Breast biopsy: excision biopsy occasionally required for diagnosis

- Staging investigations for proven cancer:
  (a) All: chest X-ray, full blood count, serum alkaline phosphatase, γ-glutamyltransferase, serum calcium (suggest liver or bone metastases)
  (b) If clinically indicated: isotope bone scan, ultrasound scan of liver, brain CT scan
- Breast tissue for hormone receptor status (oestrogen receptor +/–): important for treatment and prognosis

Screening
- Screening mammography leads to earlier detection of breast cancer
- Incidence of screen-detected cancer is 5–8 per 1000 women screened
- Two-dimensional mammography read by two radiologists at 2-yearly intervals in women aged 50–70 years is appropriate

Management
Early breast cancer (no evidence of distant spread at time of diagnosis)
- Early breast cancer can be effectively treated in many cases
- Treatment is aimed at local control/lymph node treatment and prevention of systemic relapse
- Local treatment is usually either:
  (a) Lumpectomy + radiotherapy to breast or
  (b) Simple mastectomy
- Treatment for axillary lymph nodes is usually either:
  (a) Axillary dissection (at time of surgery) and removal or
  (b) Radiotherapy to axilla
- Prevention of systemic spread is usually:
  (a) Hormonal therapy (e.g. tamoxifen)
  (b) Adjuvant chemotherapy (cyclophosphamide, methotrexate, 5-fluorouracil) if high risk (positive lymph nodes, bad histological features)
- Prognosis depends on lymph node status, tumour size and histological grade: overall 80% 10-year survival rate

Late breast cancer (distant spread at time of diagnosis)
- Treatment of late breast cancer is usually palliative and mostly medical
- Local treatment is directed at controlling local recurrence: lumpectomy/mastectomy/radiotherapy
- Distant metastases: radiotherapy to relieve pain from bony metastases; chemotherapy (tamoxifen, cytotoxics, aminoglutethimide) to control tumour load
- Prognosis: poor, only 30–40% respond to treatment with mean survival of 2 years, by which time the non-responders have usually died

04

Evidence-based medicine

Early Breast Cancer Trialists' Collaborative Group (1996) Ovarian ablation in early breast cancer: overview of the randomised trials. *Lancet* **348**, 1189–67.

Early Breast Cancer Trialists' Collaborative Group (1998) Tamoxifen for early breast cancer: an overview of the randomised trials. *Lancet* **351**, 1451–67.

Early Breast Cancer Trialists' Collaborative Group (1998) Polychemotherapy for early breast cancer: an overview of the randomised trials. *Lancet* **352**, 930–42.

Early Breast Cancer Trialists' Collaborative Group (2000) Favourable and unfavourable effects on long-term survival of radiotherapy for early breast cancer: an overview of the randomised trials. *Lancet* **355**, 1757–70.

Harris, J.R., Lippman, M.E., Morrow, M. & Hellman, S. (2001) *Diseases of the Breast*. Lippincott-Raven, Philadelphia, New York.

Roses, D.F. (1999) *Breast Cancer*. Churchill Livingstone, Philadelphia.

Winer, E., Morrow, M., Osborne, K. & Harris, J.R. (2001) Cancer of the breast. In: V de Vita, S. Hellman & S.A. Rosenberg (eds) *Cancer Principles and Practice of Oncology*, pp. 1651–716.

04

Disorders of the Endocrine Glands

34

Must know Must do

Must know

How to examine the neck and diagnose thyroid
  enlargement from other neck lumps

Clinical presentations of hyperthyroidism and
  hypothyroidism

Meaning and interpretation of thyroid function tests

How to investigate and manage a patient with solitary
  thyroid nodule

Clinical features, diagnosis and management of
  thyroid neoplasms

Causes of hypercalcaemia

Types, clinical features and management of
  hyperparathyroidism

Clinical features and management of Cushing's
  syndrome

Diagnosis and management of pituitary and adrenal
  insufficiency

Clinical features and principles of management of
  adrenal cortical tumours

Clinical features and management of
  phaeochromocytomas

Must do

Examine patients with neck lumps

Examine patients with non-toxic goitre

Examine patients with untreated primary
  hyperthyroidism

Attend endocrine outpatient clinic

Follow up a patient admitted with medically controlled
  thyrotoxicosis for elective subtotal thyroidectomy
  (including obtaining consent, drug premedication,
  the operation and postoperative period)

Similarly, follow a patient admitted for elective
  surgical treatment of primary hyperparathyroidism

Thyroid

Anatomy and pathophysiology

The thyroid gland consists of two lobes joined by an isthmus, with occasionally an embryological extension of the
isthmus superiorly called the pyramidal lobe. The thyroid
is supplied by two arteries (superior thyroid from the
external carotid, inferior thyroid from the subclavian) and
is drained by three veins (superior and middle thyroid to
the internal jugular, inferior thyroid to the innominate;
Fig. 34.1). It is invested in pretracheal fascia, which is
attached to the larynx, thus causing the thyroid to move
on swallowing. This important clinical finding helps to
discriminate thyroid swellings from other causes of
swellings in the neck. The thyroid gland originates from
the foramen caecum at the base of the tongue and
descends into the neck, anterior to the hyoid bone, to lie in
front of the trachea (Fig. 34.2). The tract left behind (the
thyroglossal tract) usually closes, although a portion of the
epithelial lining may persist and form a cyst (*thyroglossal
cyst*), usually in the late adolescent. The connection to the
tongue means that the cyst will move on protrusion of the
tongue (Fig. 34.3). The cyst may become infected, occasionally leading to a cutaneous fistula (*thyroglossal fistula*).

The causes of midline swellings of the neck include the
following.

- Thyroid (by far the most common): moves on
swallowing.
- Thyroglossal cyst: moves on swallowing and on protrusion of the tongue.
- Dermoid cyst (embryological skin cyst): does not move
on swallowing or protrusion of the tongue.

The causes of midline swellings of the neck can therefore
be differentiated by first asking the patient to swallow and
then to stick out the tongue.

Intimate anatomical relationships exist between the
thyroid and the recurrent laryngeal nerve (supplying the
intrinsic muscles of the larynx and vocal cords) and
the external branch of the superior laryngeal nerve (supplying the cricothyroid muscle, a tensor of the vocal
cords). In addition, the four parathyroid glands (two
superior, two inferior) are situated on the lateral surface of
the thyroid lobes and can be damaged during thyroid
surgery (see Complications of thyroid surgery).

The thyroid gland consists predominantly of follicular
cells, with some calcitonin-secreting parafollicular cells.
The follicular cells are controlled by the anterior pituitary

04

441

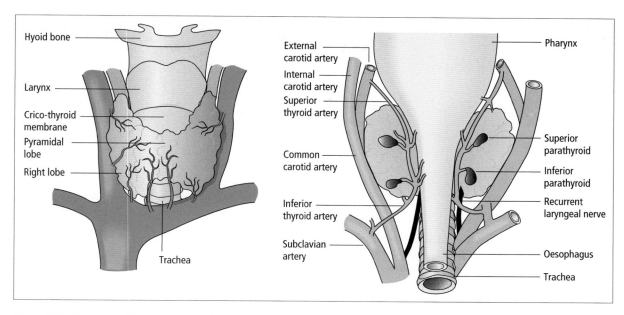

Figure 34.1 Anatomy of the thyroid gland.

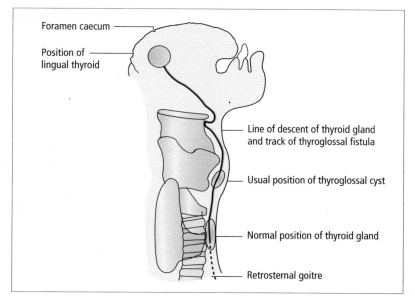

Figure 34.2 Thyroglossal tract.

secretion of thyroid-stimulating hormone (TSH), which stimulates the thyroid gland to take up iodine to form T_4 (thyroxine) and the more active T_3 (triiodothyronine), which are stored by binding to thyroglobulin in the follicles. In the circulation, most of the T_4 is bound to albumin and thyroid-binding globulins; a small proportion (0.05%) is unbound (free T_4), which is the functional constituent. At tissue level, deiodinase enzymes convert T_4 to T_3, which is the physiologically active hormone. Production of T_4 and T_3 is involved in the maintenance of the basal metabolic rate. Disorders of the formation of follicles in the thyroid are relatively common and lead to clinically palpable nodules, which may be single (solitary thyroid nodule) or multiple (multinodular goitre).

Clinical examination of the thyroid has been dealt with in Chapter 1. Essentially, it is important to describe the

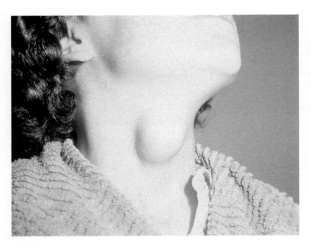

Figure 34.3 Patient with a thyroglossal cyst.

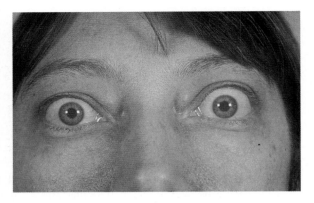

Figure 34.4 Patient with exophthalmus.

nature of the thyroid swelling, i.e. whether there is a smooth uniform enlargement, a single nodule or multiple palpable nodules. In addition, it is important to check for any associated cervical lymphadenopathy or hoarseness, suggesting recurrent nerve palsy; the latter two features are highly suggestive of thyroid malignancy.

Disorders of the thyroid

Hypothyroidism

This is a common condition, affecting about 5% of the female population (female/male ratio 10 : 1). It is usually due to an autoimmune disorder (also called *Hashimoto's thyroiditis*), with antibodies raised against the enzyme thyroid peroxidase (TPO), which is important for the production of thyroid hormones, and against thyroglobulin (antithyroglobulin antibodies). The symptoms and signs are shown in the Endocrine disorders at a glance box. Examination will usually reveal a small firm goitre. If a nodule is present, then this should be investigated as for a solitary thyroid nodule in order to exclude malignancy. Thyroid lymphoma usually develops on a background of autoimmune hypothyroidism. Extreme hypothyroidism can present as myxoedema madness, with confusion leading to coma.

Investigations
- TSH: elevated in hypothyroidism, with decreased free T_4 and/or T_3.
- Antibodies: TPO, antithyroglobulin

Treatment
Patients are rendered euthyroid by treatment with thyroxine. In the elderly patient with ischaemic heart disease, thyroxine should be introduced cautiously, starting at 25 µg and increasing the dose every fortnight in order to avoid precipitating tachyarrhythmias and cardiac failure. The normal dose required is usually between 75 and 150 µg. Patients should have their TSH checked every 12–18 months thereafter to ensure correct thyroxine dosage. For some patients, liothyronine (T_3) is an alternative.

Hyperthyroidism

Hyperthyroidism is a clinical state in which there is excess circulating thyroid hormones, leading to an alteration in the basal metabolic rate. It may be caused by:
- Graves' disease (autoimmune thyrotoxicosis);
- toxic multinodular goitre;
- solitary toxic adenoma.

Graves' disease
Autoimmune thyrotoxicosis is caused by an antibody raised against the TSH receptor (TSH receptor antibody, TRAb). The condition has a genetic predisposition and affects mostly females (female/male ratio 8 : 1). The symptoms and signs are shown in the Endocrine disorders at a glance box. Examination of the patient will in addition usually show a moderate firm goitre, which in severe thyrotoxicosis may have a vascular thrill and bruit. Some patients may develop dysthyroid eye disease (only seen with Graves' disease). This may manifest itself as lower eyelid retraction, lid lag, periorbital oedema, chemosis or, if severe, proptosis and exophthalmus (Fig. 34.4).

04

INVESTIGATION
- Suppressed TSH, with raised free T_4 and/or T_3.
- 90% of patients will have a raised TRAb.
- 70% of patients will have a raised TPO (see earlier).

TREATMENT

Initial treatment consists of thyroid uptake blocking drugs, such as carbimazole (or methimazole in the USA) and propylthiouracil, to render the patient euthyroid. Important adverse effects include neutropenia (which may present as sore throat), profuse diarrhoea or hepato-cellular failure (which initially presents as jaundice). All patients should be warned about these life-threatening complications. Other adverse effects include skin rashes, nausea and joint pains. If adverse effects occur, then propylthiouracil may be used, although there may be some cross-reactivity. In addition, a β-blocker (e.g. pro-pranolol) may be used if the patient is particularly symp-tomatic with sweating, tremor or tachycardia.

Control of thyrotoxicosis usually takes about 6 weeks, but maintenance is required for at least 18 months before cessation of carbimazole. Alternatively, higher doses of carbimazole can be taken in conjunction with thyroxine for about 12 months. If the patient relapses after this then definitive long-term treatment is required: either radioac-tive iodine or, if this is inappropriate (e.g. young children at home), surgery. Some patients choose to take radio-iodine early and often do not require pretreatment with carbimazole, but most patients treated with radioiodine develop long-term hypothyroidism. If surgery is the pre-ferred option, then previously a subtotal thyroidectomy was performed to render the patient 'euthyroid'. How-ever, 10% of these patients developed recurrent thyro-toxicosis and 70% developed hypothyroidism in the long term. In view of this, the current surgical treatment of choice is total thyroidectomy and long-term thyroxine postoperatively.

Multinodular goitre

While the majority of multinodular goitres are non-toxic, over a period of time the presence of large functioning nodules may render the patient hyperthyroid, leading to toxic multinodular goitre (MNG) (Plummer's disease). The large goitre may extend retrosternally and cause tra-cheal deviation and compression, occasionally leading to stridor (a low-pitched crowing noise on inspiration caused by narrowing of the trachea). Examination will reveal multiple nodules, either bilaterally or unilaterally (Fig. 34.5). If there is a dominant nodule within the gland, then this should be investigated as for solitary thyroid nodule (see later) as the risk of malignancy in this nodule is about 10%. Elevation of the patient's arms may lead to venous congestion and stridor if there is retrosternal

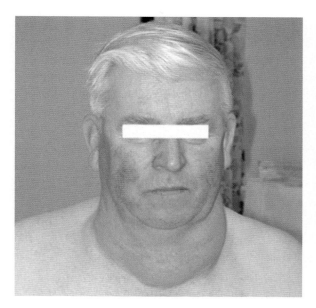

Figure 34.5 Patient with multinodular goitre.

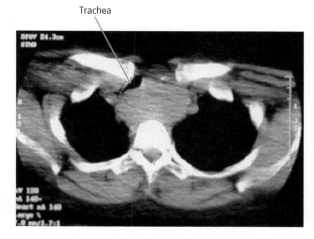

Figure 34.6 CT scan demonstrating tracheal deviation and compression by multinodular goitre.

extension of the goitre (Pemberton's sign). The position of the trachea should be checked for possible tracheal deviation. Dysthyroid eye disease is *not* associated with MNG.

INVESTIGATION
- TSH: reduced if toxic MNG.
- Fine-needle aspiration of dominant nodule, if present.
- Ultrasound may confirm multiple nodules.
- X-ray of thoracic inlet and computed tomography (CT) will delineate the extent of retrosternal extension and the degree of tracheal deviation and compression (Fig. 34.6).

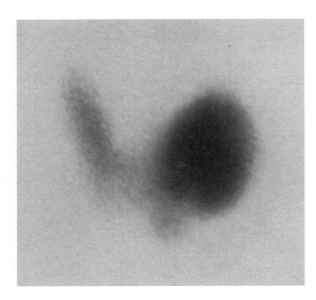

Figure 34.7 'Hot' nodule on thyroid isotope scan.

TREATMENT

Total thyroidectomy should be performed for non-toxic MNG if there is retrosternal extension of the goitre, tracheal compression or if the patient finds the goitre cosmetically unacceptable. A toxic MNG should be treated with carbimazole initially and then either total thyroidectomy or radioiodine, depending on the suitability of the patient.

Solitary toxic adenoma

Occasionally, a single thyroid adenoma may be active enough to render the patient hyperthyroid. The patient normally presents with a solitary thyroid nodule (see below) and should be investigated as such in order to exclude malignancy. In patients with solitary toxic adenoma, TSH is suppressed and a $^{99m}TcO_4$ thyroid isotope scan will show a solitary 'hot' nodule (Fig. 34.7). Treatment is initially with carbimazole, followed by either thyroid lobectomy or radioactive iodine depending on preference.

Solitary thyroid nodule

Solitary thyroid nodule (STN) is a common condition. It affects 5% of the female population but only 5% of STNs are malignant. Investigations are therefore required to discriminate between a benign and malignant thyroid nodule, as usually surgery is not required for benign STN.

The causes of STN include:
- thyroid cyst;
- degenerative thyroid nodule;
- benign follicular adenoma (including solitary toxic adenoma);
- differentiated thyroid carcinoma.

History

Features that suggest malignancy include a previous history of neck irradiation (e.g. as a child), hoarseness (potentially caused by infiltration of the recurrent laryngeal nerve) and a family history of thyroid carcinoma (there can be a genetic predisposition to papillary thyroid carcinoma). Enquiries should be made about any hyperthyroid symptoms and obstructive symptoms (e.g. stridor, dysphagia).

Investigations

It is important to exclude solitary toxic adenoma (where TSH is suppressed) and malignancy in the investigation of STN. The two most important investigations are therefore measurement of TSH and fine-needle aspiration (FNA).

FNA is the single most useful investigative tool in the management of STN. A 21G needle, attached to a syringe flushed with saline, is passed several times through the nodule while suction is maintained on the syringe. The aspirated cells are then smeared on to slides and wet and/or dry fixed. Results of cytology show benign cells, suspicious cells, malignant cells or the specimen is inadequate and consists of red cells only (about 10–20% of thyroid FNAs). If FNA reports suspicious cells, then the nodule should be removed as 30% of these are malignant. A treatment algorithm is shown in Fig. 34.8.

Other investigations may include thyroid ultrasound and $^{99m}TcO_4$ thyroid isotope scan. Ultrasound can discriminate between solid nodules and thyroid cysts and determine whether the STN is a dominant nodule within an MNG (50% of clinically diagnosed STN are in fact the dominant nodule within an MNG). Ultrasound control is also useful for performing FNA, especially if the initial aspiration is inadequate. Thyroid isotope scan can give an idea of the function of the nodule: if there is increased uptake of the isotope, it is a 'hot' nodule (and if TSH is suppressed, the nodule is a solitary toxic adenoma); if there is decreased uptake of the isotope, the nodule is described as 'cold'. There is a slight increased risk of malignancy in a cold nodule (10% vs. 5% for a hot nodule) but neither thyroid ultrasound nor isotope scanning are reliable indicators for malignancy and are not routinely required for investigation of the majority of STNs.

Treatment

A benign thyroid nodule does not require treatment unless symptomatic or cosmetically unacceptable. Suppression of TSH by thyroxine therapy is generally unhelpful in trying to reduce the size of a benign nodule. FNA should be repeated after 1 year and if this remains benign then no further treatment is required. Patients with suspicious nodules on FNA should undergo thyroid lobectomy as 30% of these nodules are malignant. Frozen section is

04

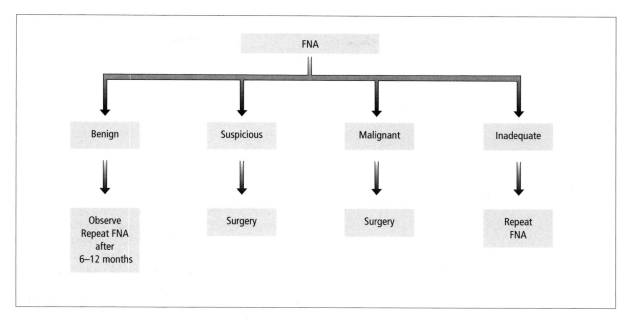

Figure 34.8 Algorithm for results of fine-needle aspiration (FNA).

of little value at surgery as the degree of capsular invasion, required to differentiate between benign follicular adenoma and carcinoma, cannot be assessed. Patients with malignant nodules should undergo surgery as outlined below.

Thyroid malignancy
Differentiated thyroid carcinoma
PAPILLARY THYROID CARCINOMA
This is the most common thyroid carcinoma (70%) and is more common in females. It presents in a young age group (20–40 years) and metastasizes to the regional lymph nodes. It most commonly presents as STN but can occasionally present as a cervical lymph node metastasis with a non-palpable thyroid primary. The majority (80%) of papillary thyroid carcinomas are multifocal throughout the thyroid gland. Papillary thyroid carcinoma has an excellent prognosis (90% 20-year survival rate).

FOLLICULAR THYROID CARCINOMA
This occurs in an older age group (40–50 years), is slow-growing and eventually spreads by the haematogenous route. Most present as STN and the prognosis of these tumours depends on the degree of capsular and vascular invasion. Patients with minimal capsular invasion can be treated by thyroid lobectomy and TSH suppression with thyroxine (differentiated thyroid carcinomas are TSH responsive and it is therefore important to keep TSH suppressed by administering thyroxine). If there is significant capsular or vascular invasion, the patient is best served by total thyroidectomy and subsequent radioiodine and thyroxine therapy.

TREATMENT OF DIFFERENTIATED
THYROID CARCINOMA
Treatment of differentiated thyroid carcinoma is best served by either thyroid lobectomy or total thyroidectomy. Because of the excellent survival rate, it is difficult to identify the best treatment modality. There are several grading systems for differentiated thyroid carcinoma. These grading systems allow a treatment protocol for patients with differentiated thyroid carcinoma to be formulated, dividing the patients into groups with good and poor prognosis (Table 34.1).

Patients with a good prognosis may be treated by thyroid lobectomy with subsequent TSH suppression. Patients with a poor prognosis may be treated by total thyroidectomy. Following surgery, these patients may be treated with high-dose radioiodine (^{131}I) to deal with any occult distant metastases. They are also given TSH suppression therapy with thyroxine. Thyroglobulin (a protein within the thyroid follicle) is a useful tumour cell marker for differentiated thyroid carcinoma and can be used to monitor patients following total thyroidectomy.

Undifferentiated thyroid carcinoma (anaplastic)
This usually occurs in elderly females and represents less than 5% of all thyroid malignancies. Patients present with

Table 34.1 Grading system for differentiated thyroid carcinoma.

Good prognosis
Female < 45 years
Male < 40 years
Tumour < 5 cm
Minimally invasive follicular carcinoma

Poor prognosis
Female > 45 years
Male > 40 years
Tumour > 5 cm
Any patient with distant metastasis
Extrathyroidal invasion

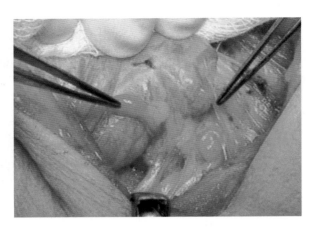

Figure 34.9 Normal parathyroid glands.

a rapidly enlarging thyroid mass (occasionally within a long-standing MNG); symptoms of stridor or dysphagia occur early. Surgery has only a limited role (usually to relieve airway obstruction), as the tumours are generally fixed and irresectable by the time of presentation. External beam radiotherapy and/or chemotherapy are mostly palliative and the vast majority of patients die within 12 months.

Medullary thyroid carcinoma

Medullary thyroid carcinoma is a rare but interesting tumour of the parafollicular calcitonin-secreting cells of the thyroid. It usually presents as a thyroid nodule in a sporadic form (70% of cases) but can be familial or associated with multiple endocrine neoplasia (see later). Patients with medullary thyroid carcinoma are best treated by total thyroidectomy with central lymph node clearance. Postoperatively, patients are given thyroxine replacement (but not TSH suppression); postoperative calcitonin measurement is a useful tumour cell marker and can be used as a method of follow-up. The prognosis is approximately 60% 5-year survival.

Thyroid lymphoma

This rare tumour usually presents in the elderly female with a background history of autoimmune (Hashimoto's) thyroiditis as a rapidly growing thyroid nodule. It may be diagnosed by FNA or Trucut biopsy. As for all lymphomas, it should be staged with a bone marrow aspirate and CT scan of the chest and abdomen. If confined to the thyroid alone, it may be treated by thyroid lobectomy with subsequent adjuvant radiotherapy and chemotherapy; otherwise it is treated by chemoradiation alone.

Complications of thyroid surgery

- Damage to the recurrent laryngeal nerve, leading to palsy (~ 2% of thyroidectomies) and causing hoarseness.

- Damage to the external branch of the superior laryngeal nerve, leading to palsy and causing hoarseness.
- Hypocalcaemia caused by damage to the parathyroids (~ 5% of thyroidectomies).
- Haemorrhage, potentially causing laryngeal oedema and respiratory compromise.

Parathyroid

Anatomy and physiology

The four parathyroid glands arise embryologically from the fourth (superior parathyroids) and third (inferior parathyroids with the thymus) pharyngeal pouches. The four glands are situated adjacent to the lateral portion of the thyroid lobes and have an intimate relationship to the thyroid (Fig. 34.9). They secrete parathormone (PTH), which plays an important role in the homeostasis of calcium by acting on the small intestine, kidneys and bone (Fig. 34.10). Disorders of the parathyroid glands result from overactivity (hyperparathyroidism) or underactivity (hypoparathyroidism). Hyperparathyroidism leads to an increase in the serum corrected calcium and is an important cause of hypercalcaemia (Table 34.2).

Primary hyperparathyroidism

Symptoms and signs

Classically, the symptoms are bone pain, renal stones, constipation, abdominal pain (related to pancreatitis or duodenal ulcer), and psychiatric symptoms of lassitude and depression (typically remembered as 'bones, stones, groans and moans'). Nowadays, however, these symptoms are rare and most patients present asymptomatically (with a raised corrected calcium found incidentally) or

04

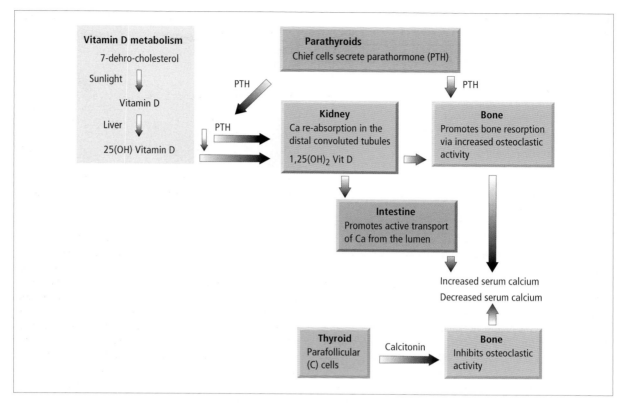

Figure 34.10 Calcium metabolism.

Table 34.2 Causes of hypercalcaemia.

Primary hyperparathyroidism
Malignancy
Familial hypocalciuric hypercalcaemia*
Drugs (e.g. thiazides, lithium)
Sarcoidosis
Vitamin D excess
Thyrotoxicosis
Prolonged immobilization

* Familial hypocalciuric hypercalcaemia is a rare autosomal dominant disorder in which a mutation in the calcium receptor of the parathyroid cell leads to an elevation in the set-point in the suppression of PTH, leading to mild hypercalcaemia with a mildly elevated PTH. It can easily be misinterpreted as primary hyperparathyroidism. However, the urinary excretion of calcium is reduced compared with primary hyperparathyroidism, which helps differentiate the two conditions. There are no long-term health consequences of familial hypocalciuric hypercalcaemia.

these symptoms appear in patients with recurrent renal stones or profound osteoporosis.

Diagnosis

The diagnosis is made biochemically: there is an elevated corrected and ionized calcium in association with elevated PTH levels and increased 24-h urinary calcium excretion. Serum phosphate may be reduced but alkaline phosphatase is usually normal. Several measurements of PTH together with the corrected calcium are usually required. The cause of primary hyperparathyroidism is predominantly a single parathyroid gland adenoma (95%), with four-gland hyperplasia seen much less frequently (5%).

Hyperparathyroidism may be associated with multiple endocrine neoplasia (MEN) (see below).

Treatment

Surgery is indicated in symptomatic patients (e.g. with significant osteoporosis) and in asymptomatic patients aged under 70 years who are otherwise fit, as these patients have an increased mortality from cardiovascular or cere-

brovascular disease compared with normal controls. Surgery consists of excision of a single gland if an adenoma is present. In patients with parathyroid hyperplasia, subtotal parathyroidectomy (removal of three-and-a-half glands) is performed, together with excision of the cervical portion of the thymus as this may contain parathyroid rest cells due to the embryological association. Half a gland is left *in situ* in an attempt to preserve normocalcaemia.

Secondary/tertiary hyperparathyroidism

Secondary hyperparathyroidism occurs in patients with chronic renal failure. An inability to excrete phosphate in the urine (leading to hyperphosphataemia) and to absorb calcium from the gut (caused by low levels of 1,25-dihydroxycholecalciferol) leads to relative hypocalcaemia, with consequent stimulation of the parathyroid glands. Of patients with secondary hyperparathyroidism, 95% can be treated medically with oral calcium supplements, oral phosphate binders to reduce the absorption of phosphate, and vitamin D. If the patient develops symptoms or significant reduced bone density, then subtotal parathyroidectomy may be required.

Tertiary hyperparathyroidism is an autonomous condition in a patient who has had prolonged secondary hyperparathyroidism. This can occur after renal transplant, when despite an improvement in renal function hyperparathyroidism still persists. If the hyperparathyroidism remains for at least a year after renal transplant, then subtotal parathyroidectomy may be required.

Hypoparathyroidism

Hypoparathyroidism most commonly occurs after total thyroidectomy and is caused by inadvertent damage to the parathyroid glands during surgery, leading to hypocalcaemia. This may occur in about 5% of all thyroidectomies. Patients may show symptoms of hypocalcaemia, including perioral paraesthesiae, digital paraesthesiae, tetany and even fits. Clinical examination may reveal two signs.
● Chovstek's sign: tapping over the facial nerve anterior to the ear with the mouth partially open induces facial muscle twitching and contraction.
● Trousseau's sign: inflating a sphygmomanometer cuff on the arm to above systolic pressure induces carpopedal spasm with the classical *main d'accoucheur* (literally, the shape of the hand used when performing an obstetric delivery: thumb apposition, wrist flexion and extension at the metacarpophalangeal joints).

Acute hypocalcaemia is treated with 10 mL of 10% calcium gluconate or chloride, given as a slow intravenous injection over 10 min, with the patient monitored by elec-

trocardiography. Oral calcium supplements and vitamin D may be given.

Adrenal

Anatomy and physiology

The two adrenal glands are situated superomedially to the kidneys (Fig. 34.11). They are supplied by three arteries (adrenal artery direct from the aorta, and a branch from the inferior phrenic artery and renal artery) and drained by a single vein (left adrenal vein draining into the renal vein, right adrenal vein draining directly into the inferior vena cava). The adrenal gland consists of two distinct parts: the outer cortex and the inner medulla. The cortex is derived from the mesoderm of the urogenital ridge and consists of three distinct layers: the outer zona glomerulosa, which produces mineralocorticoids (aldosterone), and the zona fasciculata and reticularis, which produce the glucocorticoids cortisol and testosterone. The production of mineralocorticoids is controlled by the renin–angiotensin system and the production of glucocorticoids by adrenocorticotrophic hormone (ACTH). The medulla is derived from the neural crest and is thus similar in origin to the sympathetic nervous system. The medulla produces the catecholamines adrenaline and to a lesser extent noradrenaline.

Disorders of the adrenal

Cushing's syndrome

Cushing's syndrome is a disorder of the adrenal cortex that results in excessive secretion of cortisol. The causes of Cushing's syndrome include:
● chronic steroid therapy;
● ACTH-producing tumour of the pituitary gland (Cushing's disease);
● ectopic ACTH-producing tumour (e.g. oat-cell carcinoma of the lung);
● adrenocortical adenoma (or more rarely carcinoma).
The features of hypercortisolism include:
● skin thinning with spontaneous purpura;
● proximal muscle wasting and weakness;
● osteoporosis;
● hypokalaemia;
● central obesity, usually affecting the face (facial mooning, Fig. 34.12) and the trunk (buffalo hump);
● hypertension.
The investigation of the patient with Cushing's syndrome needs to differentiate between the potential causes, i.e. adrenal adenoma/carcinoma, anterior pituitary adenoma or ectopic ACTH-secreting tumour.

04

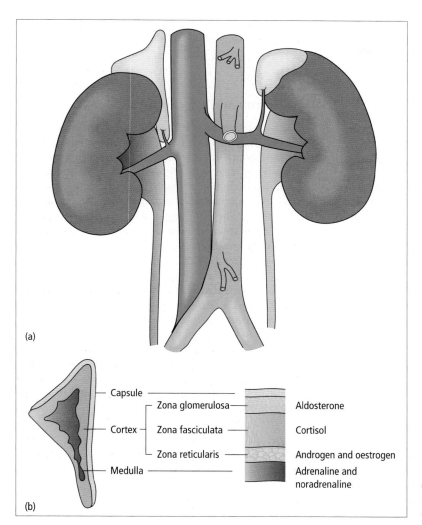

(a)

(b)

Capsule

Cortex — Zona glomerulosa — Aldosterone

Zona fasciculata — Cortisol

Zona reticularis — Androgen and oestrogen

Medulla — Adrenaline and noradrenaline

Figure 34.11 (a) Surgical anatomy of the adrenal glands showing their position in relation to the kidneys and (b) the various zones of the gland.

Screening test

The best screening test is the 1-mg overnight dexamethasone suppression test. The patient takes 1 mg oral dexamethasone at midnight and the serum cortisol is measured at 8 a.m. the following morning. The serum cortisol should be less than 50 nmol/L in a healthy individual. A 24-h urinary free cortisol is another option but may be slightly less sensitive. If these tests are positive, further investigations with low-dose and high-dose dexamethasone tests, corticotrophin-releasing hormone tests and ACTH assays may be warranted. CT or magnetic resonance imaging (MRI) will help to identify the pituitary or adrenal adenoma.

Treatment

A pituitary adenoma is treated by either surgical excision or external beam radiotherapy. An adrenocortical adenoma is treated by excision of the affected adrenal gland (adrenalectomy). Ectopic ACTH production is best treated by metyrapone (an inhibitor of steroid biosynthesis) or bilateral adrenalectomy. Following bilateral adrenalectomy, ACTH levels are unsuppressed and grossly elevated, occasionally leading to Nelson's syndrome (hyperpigmentation of the skin, particularly scars).

Conn's syndrome (primary hyperaldosteronism)

Conn's syndrome is caused by an adrenocortical adenoma (of the zona glomerulosa) that secretes aldosterone. This results in suppression of renin activity, with resultant hypertension in the presence of hypokalaemia. Around

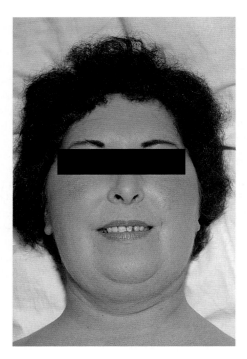

Figure 34.12 Facial appearance in Cushing's syndrome.

5% of essential hypertension may be caused by primary hyperaldosteronism. Investigations reveal a raised aldosterone/renin ratio, usually associated with a low serum potassium. CT or MRI locates the adenoma (usually < 1 cm). Occasionally, primary hyperaldosteronism is caused by bilateral micronodular hyperplasia of the adrenal glands, which is best treated with spironolactone (an antialdosterone diuretic) or amiloride.

Phaeochromocytoma

This is a tumour of the neural crest tissues that secretes excess catecholamines. The tumour may arise anywhere within the neural crest tissue (e.g. cervical sympathetic ganglia, thoracic paraganglionoma, organ of Zuckerkandl at the aortic bifurcation) but 90% originate in the adrenal gland; 10% may affect both adrenal glands (bilateral phaeochromocytoma) and about 10% are malignant. Phaeochromocytomas are also associated with MEN syndromes (see below). The symptoms of phaeochromocytoma are notoriously difficult to pinpoint and a significant number can present as a crisis, either during labour or during anaesthesia for an unrelated problem. Intermittent headaches, hypertensive episodes, panic attacks, palpitations and attacks of sweating and flushing may all be ascribed to surges of catecholamines.

The tumour may produce adrenaline, noradrenaline or dopamine. Extra-adrenal phaeochromocytomas do not produce adrenaline because it is only produced in the adrenal gland (by conversion from noradrenaline via the enzyme phenylethanolamine-N-methyltransferase). Raised levels of dopamine are suggestive of a malignant phaeochromocytoma.

Investigation
The most useful test is the measurement of 24-h urinary excretion of catecholamines. False-positive results may occur if the patient is physically stressed or has taken large quantities of alcohol. Once a high urinary output of catecholamines is confirmed, the tumour can be located by CT, MRI and the radioisotope meta-iodobenzylguanidine (MIBG), which is taken up by the chromaffin cells.

Preparation and treatment
Treatment of a phaeochromocytoma is by surgical excision, but prior to this the patient must be prepared for anaesthesia. This is accomplished by administering an α-blocker (phenoxybenzamine) in the first place; a β-blocker (such as propranolol) is sometimes required later. Following the introduction of phenoxybenzamine, the intravascular space may be depleted (following release of the vasoconstrictive effect of catecholamines) and the patient may require significant volume replacement with Gelofusine. After surgery, the α- and β-blockers may be discontinued and the patient monitored for life with annual measurements of 24-h urinary catecholamines in case the phaeochromocytoma recurs.

Adrenal incidentaloma

Of all abdominal CT scans, 2% will show an incidental mass in the adrenal gland, the so-called adrenal incidentaloma. The vast majority of these are benign and non-secreting, although all patients with an adrenal mass should be investigated to exclude phaeochromocytoma (24-h urinary catecholamines), Conn's syndrome (serum potassium and blood pressure) and Cushing's syndrome (1-mg overnight dexamethasone test). If the incidentaloma is non-secreting and less than 6 cm in size, then it can be followed with annual CT scans to check that it is not increasing in size. If the incidentaloma is larger than 6 cm, then it is advisable for these masses to be removed as about 30% are malignant (adrenocortical carcinoma).

Multiple endocrine neoplasia

These are rare syndromes with associated diseases involving the adrenal, parathyroid, thyroid, pancreas and pituitary glands.

04

MEN1 is an autosomal dominant disorder characterized by the following:
- Parathyroid: four-gland hyperplasia (90–100% of cases).
- Pancreas: multiple endocrine adenomas, usually gastrinomas (75% of cases).
- Pituitary: usually a prolactinoma (30% of cases).

MEN2a and MEN2b syndromes are characterized by the following:
- Medullary thyroid carcinoma (invariable).
- Phaeochromocytoma (50% of cases).
- Parathyroid adenoma causing hyperparathyroidism (25% of cases).

Patients with MEN2b syndrome also have a marfanoid habitus, with mucosal neuroganglionomas on the lips and tongues. They have a high mortality rate due to an aggressive form of medullary thyroid carcinoma.

Pituitary

The pituitary gland is situated in the pituitary fossa at the base of the skull and consists of an anterior lobe and a posterior lobe, both of which secrete hormones (Table 34.3). The production of hormones is controlled by the hypothalamus and by feedback mechanisms from their target glands. The pituitary gland is immediately inferior to the optic chiasma and if tumours are large enough may impinge on the chiasma, causing bilateral temporal hemianopia (Fig. 34.13).

Disorders of the pituitary gland are related to the overproduction of hormones by tumours; if tumours are non-functioning, they may cause underproduction of the surrounding hormones due to pressure effects, resulting in panhypopituitarism.

Table 34.3 Hormones of the pituitary gland.

Anterior pituitary
Adrenocorticotrophic hormone
Luteinizing hormone/follicle-stimulating hormone
Thyroid-stimulating hormone
Prolactin
Growth hormone
Melanocyte-stimulating hormone

Posterior pituitary
Vasopressin
Oxytocin

Panhypopituitarism (Simmond's disease)

This usually results from serious infection or ischaemia of the gland; rarely, postpartum ischaemia of the anterior lobe can occur (Sheehan's syndrome). It may be diagnosed by assay of the relevant hormones and treatment consists of replacement with hydrocortisone, thyroxine, sex hormones, growth hormone and desmopressin where applicable.

Tumours of the anterior pituitary

Many anterior pituitary tumours secrete prolactin (prolactinoma), growth hormone (acromegaly) or ACTH (Cushing's disease, see earlier). Tumours of other hormone-secreting cells in the pituitary are very rare. The symptoms caused by these tumours are manifest by local pressure effects of the tumour on the optic chiasma, pressure effects causing hypopituitarism or endocrine effects of the hormones produced.

Investigation

- MRI of the pituitary fossa.
- Visual field assessment.
- Pituitary function tests.

Prolactinoma

Prolactin is responsible for the initiation and maintenance of lactation. Women with a prolactinoma usually present with unilateral or bilateral milk discharge from the nipple (galactorrhoea), amenorrhoea and infertility. Men usually present with impotence, infertility or occasionally gynaecomastia. The prolactin level is grossly elevated (> 4500 mU/L, 180 μg/L). As opposed to other anterior pituitary adenomas, which are best treated by surgery, the treatment of choice is medical, using a dopamine agonist such as bromocriptine, cabergoline or quinagolide.

Growth hormone excess

An adenoma secreting growth hormone presents either in childhood as gigantism (when the long bone epiphyses have not yet fused) or in adulthood as acromegaly (prognathism with overgrowth of the hands and feet). The patient may also have hypertension, headaches, sweating, diabetes and cardiomyopathy. The serum growth hormone levels are grossly elevated and the condition is preferentially treated by surgical removal of the pituitary tumour. Medical treatment is with somatostatin analogues (e.g. octreotide) or growth hormone receptor antagonists (e.g. pegvisomant). Additional radiotherapy may be required.

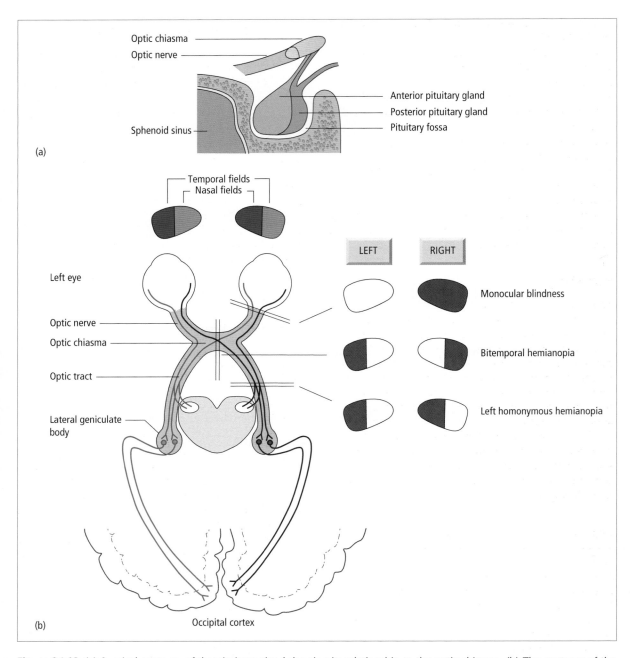

Figure 34.13 (a) Surgical anatomy of the pituitary gland showing its relationship to the optic chiasma. (b) The anatomy of the visual pathway showing how lesions at different points along the pathway produce different eye signs. Classically, pituitary lesions which affect the optic chiasma cause bitemporal hemianopia.

Endocrine disorders at a glance

Hyperthyroidism
Symptoms
- Excessive sweating
- Increased appetite/weight loss
- Irritability, insomnia, anxiety
- Palpitations
- Loose bowel motions

Signs
- Tachycardia/atrial fibrillation
- Tremor/sweaty palms
- Goitre
- Dysthyroid eye disease (Graves' disease)

Causes
- Graves' disease
- Toxic multinodular goitre
- Solitary toxic adenoma

Investigations
- TSH, free T_4, T_3
- TRAb: raised in Graves' disease
- TPO antibodies
- Thyroid isotope scan (useful to diagnose solitary toxic adenoma) or ultrasound

Initial treatment
- Carbimazole/propylthiouracil
- Propranolol if symptomatic

Definitive treatment
- Radioactive iodine
- Total thyroidectomy
- Thyroid lobectomy for solitary toxic adenoma

Thyroid malignancies
Predisposing factors
- Family history of thyroid malignancy
- Previous neck irradiation

Pathology
- Differentiated thyroid carcinoma:
  (a) Papillary
  (b) Follicular
- Undifferentiated thyroid carcinoma (anaplastic)
- Medullary thyroid carcinoma
- Lymphoma

Clinical features
Differentiated thyroid carcinoma
- Solitary thyroid nodule
- Dominant nodule in multinodular goitre
- Cervical lymphadenopathy
- Hoarseness

Undifferentiated thyroid carcinoma
- Rapidly growing thyroid mass
- Stridor or dysphagia

Investigations
- TSH
- Fine-needle aspiration
- Vocal cord check if hoarse

Treatment
Differentiated thyroid carcinoma
- Total thyroidectomy or thyroid lobectomy
- Radioiodine
- TSH suppression with postoperative thyroxine
- Excellent prognosis

Undifferentiated thyroid carcinoma
- Radiotherapy or chemotherapy
- Poor prognosis

Hyperparathyroidism
Causes
- Single parathyroid adenoma (95%)
- Hyperplasia of all four glands (5%)
- Parathyroid carcinoma (< 1%)

Biochemistry
- Raised serum corrected calcium
- Raised PTH
- Raised urinary excretion of calcium
- Reduced serum phosphate

Investigations
- Sestamibi isotope scan (to localize the parathyroid adenoma)

Treatment
- Parathyroidectomy:
  (a) Excision of single gland if adenoma
  (b) Excision of $3^1/_2$ glands if hyperplasia (subtotal parathyroidectomy)

Adrenal disorders
Anatomy
- Adrenal cortex: produces glucocorticoids and mineralocorticoids
- Adrenal medulla: produces catecholamines

Disorders of the adrenal cortex
Primary hyperaldosteronism
- Excess production of aldosterone caused by adenoma (Conn's syndrome) or bilateral hyperplasia
- Diagnosis: raised aldosterone/reduced renin, CT/MRI of the adrenals
- Treatment: surgical excision of the adenoma (Conn's syndrome) or spironolactone (hyperplasia)

Hypercortisolism (Cushing's syndrome)
● Excess production of glucocorticoids caused by cortical adenoma or carcinoma
● Diagnosis: raised diurnal cortisol and no suppression with low- or high-dose dexamethasone, CT/MRI of the adrenals
● Treatment: surgical excision of the adenoma or carcinoma

Disorders of the adrenal medulla
Phaeochromocytoma
● Excess production of catecholamines (noradrenaline, adrenaline or dopamine) leading to intermittent hypertension (occasionally hypotension), flushing attacks, palpitations or headaches
● Diagnosis: increased 24-h urinary catecholamine excretion and CT/MIBG isotope scan
● Treatment: preoperative preparation with phenoxybenzamine followed by surgery

04

Salivary Glands

35

Must know Must do

Must know
Location of the parotid and submandibular glands and their ducts
Course of the facial nerve
Classification of salivary tumours

Must do
Clinical examination of a parotid tumour
Bimanual oral examination
Examination of the mouth for the orifices of the parotid and submandibular ducts
Examine a lower motor neurone lesion facial palsy

Introduction

The salivary tissues comprise the paired parotid, submandibular and sublingual glands as well as tiny accessory salivary glands scattered over the buccal membrane. The normal function of the salivary glands is to produce saliva, approximately 1500 mL each day. Saliva has several important physiological functions:
- facilitates swallowing;
- keeps the mouth moist and aids speech;
- serves as a solvent for molecules that stimulate the taste buds;
- cleanses the mouth, gums and teeth;
- contains an enzyme, salivary amylase, that breaks down starch.

The glands most often involved in pathological processes are the submandibular and parotid glands. Rarely do the sublingual or accessory glands cause trouble.

Submandibular gland

Anatomy

The submandibular gland, which is about the size of a walnut, lies beneath and in front of the angle of the jaw. The gland envelops the posterior margin of the myelohyoid muscle, which separates it into a superficial and a deep part. The submandibular duct (Wharton's duct) passes forwards for 5 cm from the deep part of the gland to the floor of the mouth, where it has its orifice just lateral to the frenulum of the tongue (Fig. 35.1). Most of the problems with the submandibular gland arise because of duct obstruction.

Clinical assessment

Symptoms

The symptom of submandibular pathology is a history of swelling beneath and in front of the angle of the jaw, usually associated with pain. A history that the pain and swelling are induced or exacerbated by eating is indicative of submandibular duct obstruction. Painless swelling is more suggestive of a salivary gland tumour.

Physical examination

Normally, the submandibular gland is not palpable. When the gland is enlarged it is palpable 2–3 cm in front of the sternomastoid muscle just beneath the horizontal ramus of the mandible. The submandibular gland is rubbery in consistency and may be difficult to distinguish from enlarged cervical lymph nodes. The orifices of both ducts should be inspected with the aid of a torch. The patient opens the mouth and lifts the tongue to the roof of the mouth, thus displaying the orifices of the two ducts on either side of the frenulum of the tongue. The presence of inflammation or a bead of pus at the orifice should be noted and sometimes a bulge indicating the presence of a stone in the duct may be seen in the floor of the mouth. Submandibular swellings should be palpable bimanually between the index finger of one hand inside the mouth and the fingers of the other hand over the outer surface of the lump in the neck. Finally, the duct should be palpated for the presence of a stone.

04

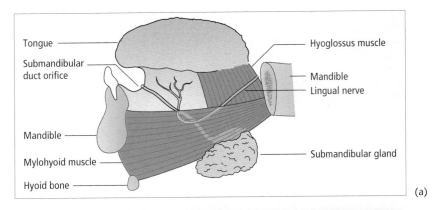

(a)

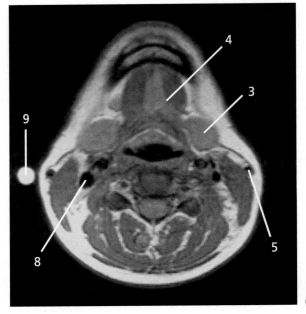

(b)

Figure 35.1 (a) Surgical anatomy of the submandibular gland. (b) Computed tomography of normal submandibular glands.

04

Investigations

Generally, a plain radiograph of the jaw area is all that is required to demonstrate a calculus, which is invariably radiopaque, in the submandibular duct. In equivocal cases, sialography may be performed by injecting a small amount of contrast into the opening of the duct (Fig. 35.2).

Parotid gland

Anatomy

The parotid gland is an irregular structure that lies *below* the external auditory meatus between the vertical ramus of the mandible and the mastoid process. Swellings of the parotid are seen in this area and not in front of the ear, a common mistake made by students. The confusion arises because a small portion of the gland (the accessory part) projects forwards on to the masseter muscle, but the bulk of the gland lies deep in the space between the mandible and the mastoid. Other preauricular and postauricular swellings are not uncommon in children and are usually due to enlarged lymph nodes. The 5-cm long parotid duct passes forwards from the gland across the masseter muscle (where it may be palpated) to gain entry to the mouth via a small papilla on the buccal membrane opposite the crown of the second upper molar tooth. An important anatomical feature of the parotid gland is that the facial nerve passes through the gland quite superficially and divides into its branches as it does so (Fig. 35.3).

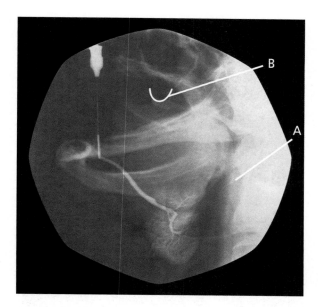

Figure 35.2 Sialogram demonstrating normal submandibular duct (Wharton's duct) and gland.

Clinical assessment

Symptoms

The symptoms of parotid disease are a history of swelling of the gland that may or may not be associated with pain, depending on the underlying pathology.

Physical examination

Examination of the parotid consists of inspection and palpation of the swelling. If the patient has parotitis, then signs of inflammation will be present. Tumours present as painless swellings. The anterior part of the parotid duct can be palpated as it crosses the anterior border of the masseter muscle one finger-breadth below the inferior border of the zygomatic bone. Rarely, a calculus may be palpated in this part of the duct. The orifice of the duct in the mouth (opposite the second upper molar) should also be inspected by retracting the cheek with a spatula. Pressure applied to the body of the gland may cause a bead of pus to appear at the orifice in patients with parotitis.

Investigations

Baseline haematological and biochemical investigations are indicated if salivary pathology is part of a systemic disease, such as Sjögren's syndrome, sarcoidosis or leukaemia; more specific investigations may be required depending on the nature of the systemic problem. Imaging of the parotid ducts can be performed by sialography, which demonstrates obstructions, dilatations and narrowings of the duct. It is particularly useful in the diagnosis of sialectasis (see later).

Disorders of the salivary glands

Salivary manifestations of systemic disease

Xerostomia

Xerostomia is defined as decreased salivary flow and it may result from many causes. These include mumps, Sjögren's syndrome, sarcoidosis, radiation-induced atrophy (e.g. following radiation therapy to oral cancer) and drugs (antihistamines, phenothiazines, antimuscarinics).

Sialorrhoea

Sialorrhoea is defined as increased salivary flow and is associated with many conditions, such as aphthous stomatitis, rabies, unrelieved oesophageal obstruction.

Specific salivary gland pathology

Salivary calculi

Sialolithiasis is common in the submandibular gland and Wharton's duct and, more rarely, in the parotid gland. The aetiology of salivary stones is unknown but they are more common in countries with a hot climate. The stones are composed of mucus, cellular debris and calcium and magnesium phosphates. The most important consequence of stone formation is obstruction of the salivary duct, which may lead to inflammation characterized by swelling of the gland. Calculi in the submandibular duct may be removed via an incision into the duct in the floor of the mouth, while stones in the substance of the submandibular gland are removed by gland excision. Anteriorly placed parotid duct stones may also be removed through the mouth, while symptomatic stones in the gland require formal exploration.

Inflammation
Mumps
Mumps (endemic parotitis) is an infectious viral disease caused by a paramyxovirus with an incubation period of 17–21 days. It has become uncommon since the introduction of an effective vaccine given to infants. It usually affects the parotid glands bilaterally, although the sub-

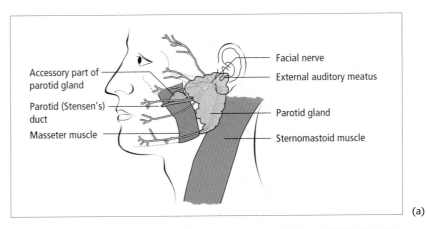

(a)

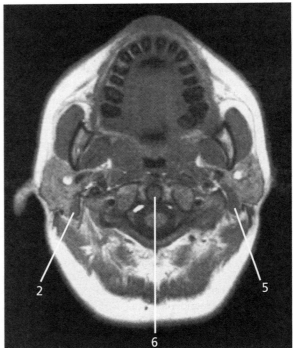

(b)

Figure 35.3 (a) Surgical anatomy of the parotid gland. (b) Computed tomography of normal parotid glands.

04

mandibular and sublingual glands may also be affected. Viral-induced pancreatitis and orchitis are not uncommon in adults affected by mumps. The disease is self-limiting without serious sequelae in most patients. Rarely, however, bilateral orchitis can lead to sterility or failure of testosterone production.

Acute suppurative (postoperative) parotitis
Suppurative parotitis is caused by ascending infection from the oral cavity with reduced salivary flow. *Staphylococcus aureus* is the usual causative agent. This condition was once commonly seen in debilitated or postoperative patients (hence the name) in whom there was dehydration, dental sepsis and poor oral hygiene, but has become uncommon in modern surgical practice. It is still sometimes seen in patients with poorly fitting dentures. Clinically, one or both glands may be enlarged and painful and there may be a purulent discharge from the duct. Prophylaxis is achieved by removing the aetiological factors and maintaining good hydration and mouth care preoperatively. Established cases require antibiotics and surgical drainage if an abscess develops.

	Major glands	Minor glands	Table 35.1 Pathological classification of salivary tumours (percentage of all salivary tumours).
Adenomas			
Pleomorphic adenoma	70%	50%	
Monomorphic adenoma	5–10%	5–10%	
Adenolymphoma (Warthin's tumour)			
Oncocytoma (oxyphilic adenoma)			
Carcinomas			
Mucoepidermoid	5–10%	10%	
Adenoid cystic	5%	20%	
Carcinoma in pleomorphic adenoma	Rare	Rare	
Adenocarcinoma	Rare	Rare	
Undifferentiated carcinoma	Rare	Rare	
Secondary malignancy	Rare	Rare	

Chronic parotitis

Chronic inflammation of the parotid gland is often associated with obstruction and infection of the gland leading to *sialectasia*, i.e. dilatation of the duct system analogous to bronchiectasis. Sialography demonstrates these changes in the duct system. Treatment involves removal of any duct obstruction (calculi or strictures) and promotion of salivary flow. Occasionally gland excision is required.

Sjögren's syndrome

Sjögren's syndrome is an autoimmune chronic inflammatory disease characterized by keratoconjunctivitis sicca (dry eyes; Latin *siccus*, dry), xerostomia, parotid swelling and rheumatoid arthritis. Sjögren's syndrome may be accompanied by other autoimmune disorders, e.g. scleroderma, systemic lupus erythematosus, primary biliary cirrhosis, and is found mostly in postmenopausal women. *Mikulicz's disease* is a symmetrical enlargement of the salivary and lacrimal glands caused by the benign inflammatory infiltrate characteristic of Sjögren's syndrome but also of sarcoidosis, lymphoma and leukaemia. Treatment is difficult and is mostly symptomatic. Good oral hygiene is to be encouraged. Closure of the lacrimal punctum and regular instillation of 1% methylcellulose (artificial) tears helps to relieve the ocular symptoms. The prognosis is that of the associated disease.

Tumours

Tumours of the salivary glands are classified on the basis of their clinical and pathological features (Table 35.1). They affect males and females about equally (except for adenolymphoma, see later) and occur usually in middle-aged to elderly patients. The vast majority are benign; however, the smaller the salivary gland affected, the more likely a tumour is to be malignant. Thus 70–80% of parotid tumours are benign, whereas only 50% of submandibular gland tumours are benign. Tumours are usually painless, although malignant tumours may cause pain or facial muscle paralysis through involvement of the facial nerve. Painless swellings may be dealt with directly by surgical excision. The use of ultrasonography, computed tomography or enhanced magnetic resonance imaging is becoming more widespread and may differentiate benign from malignant tumours and facilitate better preoperative planning. Fine-needle aspiration cytology is useful in cases of suspected malignancy in order to facilitate preoperative counselling, as resection of the facial nerve may be necessary. The types of tumours that may affect the salivary gland are quite diverse. Only the common tumours are discussed here.

Pleomorphic adenoma

This is the most common tumour of the salivary glands, occurring more frequently in the parotid than in the submandibular gland and usually in the superficial portion of the parotid (Fig. 35.4). It presents in middle age as a slow-growing, painless, smooth mass in the parotid. Histologically, pleomorphic adenomas consist of epithelial cells mixed with myxoid, mucoid and chondroid elements and the tumour is surrounded by a fibrous capsule. The tumour also has projections that protrude beyond the fibrous capsule into the surrounding parotid gland. Failure to remove these projections at surgery may result in tumour recurrence. Parotid tumours are treated by resection, ensuring that a rim of normal parotid gland is taken around the fibrous tumour capsule. Great care must be taken not to damage the facial nerve. If a salivary tumour involves a gland other than the parotid, complete

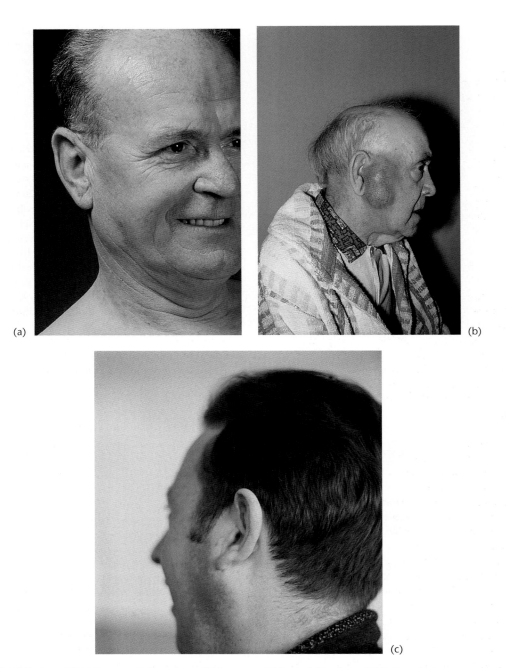

Figure 35.4 (a) Early and (b) late presentation of parotid tumours. (c) Typical site of parotid tumour between angle of mandible and mastoid process. Note the way the tumour distorts the ear lobe.

excision of that gland is indicated. Complete removal of the tumour carries an excellent prognosis. *Frey's syndrome* is a curious postoperative phenomenon characterized by facial sweating and flushing while eating. It is due to the aberrant regeneration of secretomotor parasympathetic nerves through the nerve sheaths of sympathetic fibres

that supply the sweat glands of the skin overlying the parotid.

Adenolymphoma (Warthin's tumour)
These account for about 10% of parotid tumours. They present as soft cystic masses in men over 50 years of age. It

04

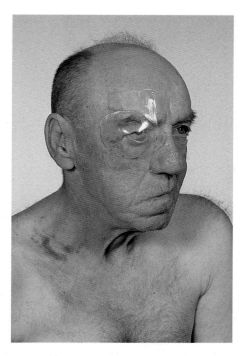

Figure 35.5 Facial nerve palsy following surgery for carcinoma of the parotid gland.

is the only salivary tumour more common in men than women. Histologically, the tumour is composed of cystic glandular spaces with papillary projections, surrounded by lymphoid tissue. Treatment is by surgical excision and the prognosis is very good.

Carcinomas

Several histological types are recognized (Table 35.1) but these tumours usually present as a hard, rapidly growing, infiltrating parotid mass in a middle-aged or elderly patient. Malignant transformation may occur in benign pleomorphic adenomas present for 10–20 years. Secondary tumours may rarely affect the major salivary glands.

The mass may be painful and the facial nerve may be involved. These features may also be present in inflammatory processes such as sarcoidosis and histological confirmation is mandatory. Spread is to local lymph nodes and, if left untreated, ulceration of the tumour through the skin will occur.

Treatment consists of radical parotidectomy with sacrifice of the facial nerve (Fig. 35.5), block dissection of the regional lymph nodes and radiotherapy. Carcinomas of the submandibular glands are similarly treated by radical resection. Prognosis is poor for this tumour.

Salivary glands at a glance

Definitions

Salivary glands: the paired parotid, submandibular and sublingual glands as well as tiny accessory salivary glands scattered over the buccal membrane that produce 1500 mL of saliva daily

Xerostomia: decreased salivary flow

Sialorrhoea: increased salivary flow

Functions of saliva
- Facilitates swallowing
- Keeps the mouth moist and aids speech
- Solvent for molecules that stimulate the taste buds
- Cleanses the oral cavity
- Contains α-amylase, which breaks down starch

Pathology
Salivary calculi (sialolithiasis)
- Common in the submandibular gland and Wharton's duct
- Rare in the parotid gland
- Treatment: surgical removal

Inflammation
Mumps (paramyxovirus)
- Bilateral parotid swelling
- Sometimes pancreatitis ± orchitis in adults
- Vaccination during infancy

Acute suppurative (postoperative) parotitis
- Staphylococcal infection of parotid in debilitated patients with poor oral hygiene (rare now)

Chronic parotitis
- Chronic inflammation of the parotid gland
- Often associated with obstruction and infection of the gland leading to sialectasia

Sjögren's syndrome
- Autoimmune chronic inflammatory disease characterized by keratoconjunctivitis sicca (dry eyes), xerostomia, parotid swelling and rheumatoid arthritis
- May be accompanied by other autoimmune disorders, e.g. scleroderma, systemic lupus erythematosus, primary biliary cirrhosis
- Seen mostly in postmenopausal women

Mikulicz's disease
● Symmetrical enlargement of the salivary and lacrimal glands caused by the benign inflammatory infiltrate

characteristic of Sjögren's syndrome but also of sarcoidosis, lymphoma and leukaemia

Tumours

Type	Gland	Sex	Age (years)	Presentation	Treatment	Prognosis
Pleomorphic adenoma (benign*)	Parotid > submanbibular	M = F	50+	Slow-growing, painless, smooth mass	Excision with rim of normal tissue outside tumour capsule	Excellent
Adenolymphoma (Warthin's tumour) (benign)	Parotid	M > F	50+	Cystic mass	Excision	Very good
Carcinoma						
Primary	Parotid	M = F	70	Rapidly growing infiltrating parotid mass	Radical resection	Poor
Secondary (malignant)	Parotid or submandibular	M = F	50+		Block dissection Radiotherapy	

* Malignant transformation may occur.

Evidence-based medicine

Vaughan, E.D. (2001) Management of malignant salivary gland tumours. *Hosp Med* **62**, 400–5.

http://www.nlm.nih.gov/medlineplus/salivaryglanddis-orders.html   National Library of Medicine website for salivary gland disorders. Provides very good links to other websites on specific aspects of salivary gland disease.

04

Must know Must do

Must know

Main features and risk factors for skin malignancies
Pathology, diagnosis and principles of treatment of
malignant melanoma

Must do

Learn to recognize common benign skin lesions, basal
cell carcinoma and melanoma
Observe excision of a minor skin lesion

Skin

Cysts

Sebaceous cyst

Sebaceous cysts are more correctly called *epidermal inclusion cysts* as they are composed of thin layers of epidermis and contain epidermal debris. They are retention cysts produced by obstruction to the mouth of a sebaceous gland. They commonly occur on the face, neck, scalp, scrotum and vulva (Fig. 36.1). They cannot occur on gland-free areas such as the palm of the hand or the sole of the foot. Clinically, they are smooth, soft or firm and are attached to the skin. A pathognomonic punctum is often

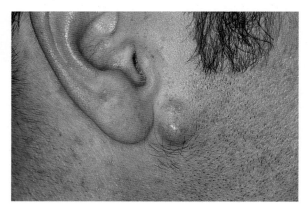

Figure 36.1 Sebaceous cyst on the side of the face.

visible in the overlying skin. They contain soft cheesy material and occasionally become infected. Sebaceous cysts may be complicated by infection, ulceration (Cock's peculiar tumour), calcification and horn formation. For these and cosmetic reasons they are best treated by surgical excision, which is performed under local anaesthetic.

Hyperplasia of the sebaceous glands at the tip of the nose leads to the development of a protruberant mass called a rhinophyma. This is treated by shaving the mass down to a reasonable size. Skin regeneration occurs rapidly.

Dermoid cyst

Congenital dermoid cysts lie deep to the skin and are not attached to it. They arise from epidermal cells separated from the skin during fusion of the embryological lines in the face and are found at the junctions of lines of fusion of facial skin. External angular (Fig. 36.2a) and midline angular (Fig. 36.2b) dermoids are the most common examples seen. They usually present as a pea-sized swelling under the skin but fixed to the underlying bone. Occasionally a dermoid (usually a midline dermoid) may extend through bone to communicate with a cyst in the anterior fossa of the skull. Skull X-ray or computed tomography (CT) may be necessary to exclude this.

An *implantation dermoid* is a cystic lesion that develops following a puncture injury in which epithelial cells are implanted into the subcutaneous tissue. They are often found on the fingers. Excision is the treatment for these cysts (Fig. 36.3).

Ganglion

A ganglion is a unilocular synovial fluid-filled cyst arising from synovial tissue in relation to joints or tendons. A ganglion is not a pouch from the joint space but arises from other synovial tissues near the wrist, ankle or digits. The most frequent location for a ganglion is the dorsum of the wrist and patients usually present with a hard lump that may or may not cause discomfort. On examination they are 1–2 cm in diameter, smooth, firm and slightly fluctuant, and not attached to the overlying skin. Treatment is by formal surgical excision.

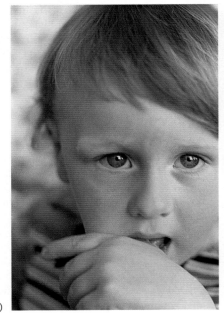 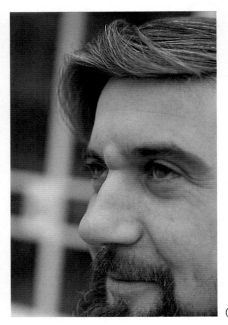

(a)   (b)

Figure 36.2 (a) External and (b) internal angular dermoids.

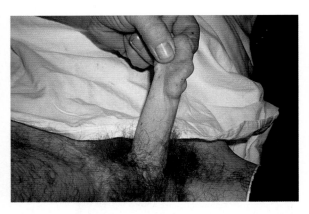

Figure 36.3 Implantation dermoid of the penile skin following 'zipper' injury.

Vascular lesions of the skin

Vascular malformations can be categorized as arterial, venous, capillary, lymphatic or mixed. Vascular malformations are the most common of all malformations and occur in 10% of the normal population, being somewhat higher in premature infants.

Strawberry naevus

A strawberry mark or naevus (capillary–cavernous angioma) characteristically appears as small red marks at a week to 10 days after birth and rapidly enlarges over a few weeks to several centimetres in diameter. They are raised, fleshy, compressible vascular lesions (Fig. 36.4). These regress spontaneously over 5 years, leaving either no mark at all or occasionally a small whitish scar that may need excision. Treatment of strawberry naevi is therefore conservative.

Lesions involving the eyelids may impair vision and lead to sympathetic ophthalmoplegia. Treatment of such lesions must be by early surgery (Fig. 36.5).

Capillary haemangioma (portwine stain)

Capillary haemangiomas may occur at any site. However, they often conform to sensory dermatomes, especially when seen on the face (Fig. 36.6). Ipsilateral meningeal involvement may occur in conjunction with hemifacial haemangiomas (Sturge–Weber syndrome). Treatment is usually not required for portwine stains as attempts to remove the haemangioma often result in unsightly scarring. The Klippel–Trenaunay syndrome is a triad of varicose veins, limb hypertrophy and portwine staining (see Chapter 37).

Cavernous haemangioma

Cavernous haemangiomas (localized collections of dilated

04

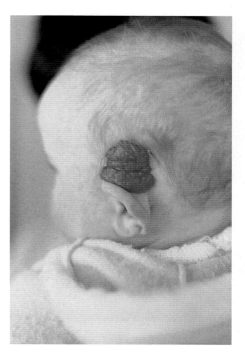

Figure 36.4 Strawberry naevus adjacent to the left ear. In the vast majority of patients these lesions are treated conservatively and eventually disappear or leave only a small blemish.

veins) are commonly found on the limbs and trunk. They are usually asymptomatic but may be associated with arteriovenous fistula, which may cause either local gigantism because of the increased local blood flow or high-output cardiac failure. After excision they are prone to recurrence.

Lymphangioma

The *linear naevus* is the most common form of lymphangioma, comprising small vesicles often arranged in a linear fashion as a skin naevus. These vesicles contain lymphatic channels with clear fluid within them. The larger and much rarer form of lymphangioma is the highly transilluminable *cystic hygroma*, often found in the neck (see Fig. 1.8).

Glomus body tumour

A *glomangioma* is a tumour of the glomus body, a convoluted arteriovenous formation that is sensitive to temperature and controls local arterial blood flow. Glomus bodies are distributed widely through the skin, with a preference for the fingers and toes. Glomangiomas are small (< 1 cm), rounded, firm, purple tumours frequently found beneath the nail. Their outstanding feature is that

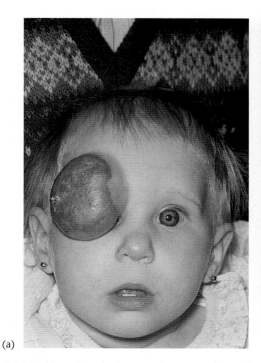

(a)

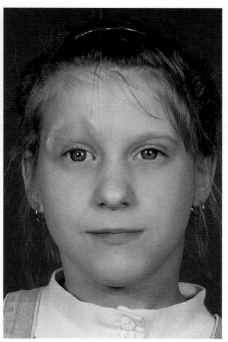

(b)

Figure 36.5 (a) In this patient the haemangioma was obstructing vision and hence surgery was required to prevent amblyopia. (b) Late postoperative appearance in the early teens.

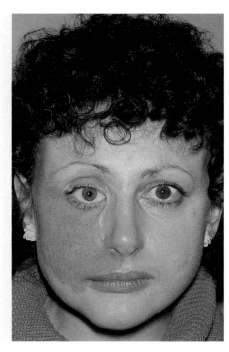

Figure 36.6 Portwine stain affecting the right cheek in the distribution of the maxillary division of the trigeminal nerve.

they are exquisitely tender, and for this reason they should be excised.

Spider naevus

Spider naevi are subcutaneous endarterioles and therefore when emptied by compression fill from the centre outwards (centripetally). They appear in the distribution of the superior vena cava and are found in patients with liver disease.

Campbell de Morgan spots

These are small (1–2 mm) bright-red spots that occur in the skin of the trunk in middle-aged and elderly patients. They are localized capillary proliferations. At one time they were thought to indicate deep-seated malignancy but in fact they have no clinical significance.

Skin appendages

Sweat gland tumours

The most common tumour to arise from sweat gland tissue is the cylindroma, named after the histological appearance of the cellular component of the lesion. The common

sites of origin are the scalp and the hair-bearing skin of the axilla, groin and pubis. Excision biopsy is usually necessary to establish the diagnosis.

Benign skin tumours

Benign papilloma (skin tag)

A benign papilloma is an overgrowth of the skin that presents as a sessile or pedunculated polyp. They may occur at any age but usually in adult life. They are completely harmless but should be removed if cosmetically unacceptable or liable to trauma.

Warts (verruca vulgaris)

Warts are a very common problem and not really a skin tumour but an infection of the epidermis. They are caused by viruses and pathologically consist of papillary hyperplasia of the epidermis and excessive keratinization. Warts are common on the fingers and hands; when they occur on the sole of the foot they are called plantar warts or verrucas. Verrucas are commonly transmitted in swimming pools and may occur in epidemics in schools. Warts occurring on the genitalia, in the perineum and perianally are spread by sexual contact. These are caused by human papilloma viruses and are also referred to as venereal warts or *condylomata acuminata*.

Warts often disappear spontaneously. This phenomenon probably explains the efficacy of the myriad folk cures that have been used to treat warts over the centuries. However, sometimes they require treatment because they are cosmetically unacceptable or cause pain or discomfort. Several treatments exist, including applications of podophyllin and salicylic acid or silver nitrate, curettage or excision with diathermy or cryosurgery. Plantar warts should be curetted if they cause a lot of pain on walking.

Keloid scar

Keloid (Greek κελοιδ, crab claw) scar formation is a complication of wound healing caused by excessive deposition of extracellular matrix at the wound site. Histologically, there is excessive production of collagen, fibroblasts and capillaries in the healing wound. Typically, keloids are raised pink deforming lesions along the course of the wound. They commonly occur on the skin of the head and neck and upper trunk (Fig. 36.7). Unfortunately, keloid formation frequently follows piercing of the earlobes for earrings. It is much more frequent in blacks and orientals than in Caucasians. Treatment is difficult but low-dose radiotherapy and local steroid injections have been effective in some cases.

04

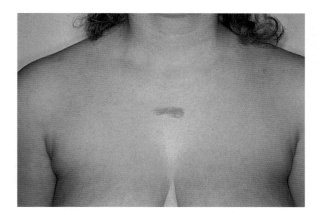

Figure 36.7 Presternal keloid scar.

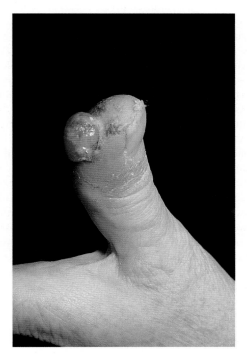

Figure 36.8 Pyogenic granuloma of the thumb following an injury.

04

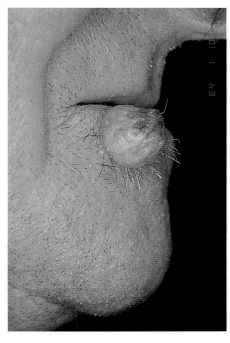

Figure 36.9 Keratoacanthoma of the lip in an elderly man.

Pyogenic granuloma

A pyogenic granuloma is a mass of vigorously growing granulation tissue that arises in relation to an area of minor skin trauma. The patient notices a rapidly growing reddish/pink lump on the skin which bleeds easily. Pyogenic granulomas usually occur in areas most likely to be traumatized, e.g. hands, feet, face and lips. They are not painful. Treatment is by excision and curettage (Fig. 36.8).

Histiocytoma

Histiocytomas are benign skin nodules caused by infiltration of lipid-filled macrophages (histiocytes). They are firm hemispherical nodules about 1 cm in diameter. They occur singly in adults and are found slightly more often on the limbs. While they are benign, treatment is by excision to confirm the diagnosis.

Keratoacanthoma

Keratoacanthomas are thought to arise from hair follicles and are frequently misdiagnosed clinically as squamous carcinomas. They commonly occur on the face or hand in older adults (Fig. 36.9). The patient complains of a rapidly growing lump that may measure up to 2 cm in 6 weeks. The centre then ulcerates and the lesion begins to regress and will eventually heal in 2–3 months. Keratoacanthomas are not painful. Treatment should be excision for cosmetic reasons and to confirm that the lesion is not a squamous carcinoma.

Keratoses

Keratoses are lesions caused by hypertrophy of the epidermis. They are very common and solar keratoses may undergo malignant change. Two types are recognized.

Solar keratosis

This is a well-demarcated premalignant lesion caused by solar damage, and histologically is an area of hyperkeratosis. Solar keratoses usually occur on the back of the hands or on the face or ears (all areas exposed to the sun) and are commoner in the elderly and outdoor workers and in fair-skinned people living in the tropics and subtropics. Clinically, solar keratoses develop as an adherent scale that can be removed with difficulty to reveal a hyperaemic base. Often a small keratotic horn develops. As they are precancerous, isolated lesions should be removed (by excision or cryotherapy) and the patient advised to avoid exposure to the sun and to use appropriate protection (e.g. hats and sunscreen creams) when exposure is inevitable.

Seborrhoeic keratosis

This occurs as multiple, raised, frequently pigmented lesions that develop on the trunk in middle-aged or elderly people (Fig. 36.10). They are extremely common and their aetiology is unknown. Histologically, they consist of cords of stratified squamous epithelium with keratin cysts. They are benign and generally require no treatment.

Bowen's disease

Bowen's disease is squamous cell carcinoma *in situ* and is a premalignant lesion. This is a rare condition characterized by a red, raised, hyperkeratotic plaque with well-defined margins. Exposure to arsenic compounds is an aetiological factor in some patients. Local cytotoxic therapy (e.g. 5-fluorouracil) and cryotherapy has been employed to treat it but local recurrence is frequent after such therapy and surgical excision gives the best results. Bowen's disease involving the glans penis bears the exotic name *erythroplasia of Queyrat*.

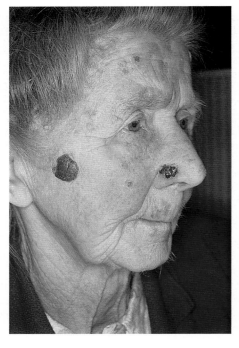

Figure 36.10 Seborrhoeic keratosis on the face. (Note that this lady also has a basal cell carcinoma on the side of the nose.)

Malignant skin tumours

Aetiological factors

Several aetiological factors for skin malignancies have been identified, the most important of which are summarized in Table 36.1.

04

Benign skin and adnexal lesions at a glance

Definitions

Skin or integumentum (also integument and integumentum commune): the protecting layer that envelops the whole body comprising the epidermis and dermis, as well as all of the appendages such as hair, nails, sweat and sebaceous glands, and the mammary glands

Adnexa (Latin 'things bound to'): the appendages or accessory parts adjoining the skin, e.g. the nails and subcutaneous tissue

Benign skin lesions

Cysts
Sebaceous cyst
- Retention cysts caused by obstruction to the mouth of a sebaceous gland
- Has a pathognomonic punctum
- Occurs on face, neck, scalp scrotum and vulva

Dermoid cyst
- Congenital: arise from epidermal cells separated from skin during fusion of embryological lines in the face

- Implantation: cystic lesion (often on fingers or hand) that develops following puncture wound in which epithelial cells are implanted into the subcutaneous tissue

Ganglion
- Unilocular synovial fluid-filled cyst arising from synovial tissue in relation to joints or tendons

Vascular skin lesions
Strawberry naevus
- Capillary–cavernous angioma that appears as a red mark at about 10 days after birth
- Enlarge rapidly and then regress and disappear by age 5 years
- Treatment: observation

Capillary haemangioma
- Portwine stain: conforms to sensory dermatomes. No treatment required
- Sturge–Weber syndrome: hemifacial haemangioma + ipsilateral meningeal involvement
- Klippel–Trenaunay syndrome: portwine stain + varicose veins + limb hypertrophy

Cavernous haemangioma
- Localized collections of dilated veins found on limbs and trunk

Lymphangioma
- Linear naevus: linear vesicles containing lymphatic channels
- Cystic hygroma: large cystic swelling containing lymph, often found on the neck and always brilliantly transilluminable

Glomus body tumour
- Glomangiomas are small, rounded, firm, purple tumours frequently found under the nails
- Exquisitely tender

Spider naevus
- Subcutaneous endarterioles found in the distribution of the superior vena cava in patients with liver disease
- Fill from the centre outwards

Campbell de Morgan spots
- Localized capillary proliferations that appear as small bright-red spots on the trunk of older people
- They have no significance (other than as questions in clinical examinations!)

Skin appendages
Sweat gland tumours
- Cylindromas are sweat gland tumours that may be found on scalp, axilla, groin and pubis

Benign skin tumours
Papilloma (skin tag)
- Overgrowth of skin presenting as a sessile or pedunculated polyp

Verruca vulgaris (warts)
- Infection of the epidermis caused by viruses
- Common on fingers and hands and soles of feet
- Genital warts (caused by human papilloma virus) are spread by sexual contact

Keloid scar
- Complication of wound healing caused by excessive deposition of collagen, fibroblasts and capillaries in the wound
- Most frequent on upper trunk, head and neck
- Commoner in black and oriental peoples
- Treatment: steroid injection, low-dose radiotherapy

Pyogenic granuloma
- Mass of granulation tissue following a minor wound

Histiocytoma
- Benign skin nodule caused by infiltration of lipid-filled macrophages

Keratoacanthoma
- Arise from hair follicles but look like squamous carcinomas

Keratoses
- Solar keratosis:
  (a) *Premalignant* hypertrophy of the epidermis
  (b) Adherent scale can be removed with difficulty to reveal a hyperaemic base
  (c) Occur on areas exposed to sun (hands, face, ears)
- Seborrhoeic keratosis:
  (a) Multiple raised often pigmented lesions on the trunk of older people
  (b) Contain squamous epithelium with keratin cysts and are *not* premalignant

Premalignant skin lesions
Bowen's disease
- Squamous carcinoma *in situ*
- Premalignant
- Red, raised, hyperkeratotic plaque

Erythroplasia of Queyrat
- Bowen's disease involving the glans penis

Treatment
Treatment of all benign skin lesions is excision, usually under local anaesthetic

Table 36.1 Aetiological factors implicated in skin malignancy.

Factor	Evidence
Exposure to sunlight	Keratinocytes are damaged by ultraviolet light
	Majority (90%) of cancers occur in exposed sites
	Skin cancer is common in outdoor workers
	Incidence increases in fair-skinned races
	Increased incidence in areas of high annual sunshine (e.g. Australia, southern USA)
Immunosuppression	Increased incidence in patients on immunosuppressive therapy (e.g. after renal transplantation) and in patients with AIDS
Radiation exposure	Increased incidence following radiotherapy and among radiologists
Chemical carcinogens	Hydrocarbons, arsenic, coal tar, oils, soot (chimney sweeps' scrotal carcinoma was described by Percival Pott in 1775)
Inherited disorders	Very high occurrence of skin cancer in albinism and xeroderma pigmentosum
Chronic irritation	Carcinoma may develop in scars or in relation to a chronic ulcer (Marjolin's ulcer)

Basal cell carcinoma

Basal cell carcinoma (BCC) is a malignant tumour of the skin arising from basal cells in the epidermis. BCCs are very common tumours, particularly in those exposed to ultraviolet light. They usually appear after the age of 50 and 90% are found on the forehead, face and hair margin. Clinically, BCCs present as small nodules that soon become ulcerated centrally, producing an umbilicated lesion (Fig. 36.11a). A history of a lesion that apparently heals only to recur soon after is not unusual. As the lesion progresses large areas of ulceration with slightly raised pearly coloured edges develop and, untreated, large areas of the face may be eaten away with invasion of bone and cartilage (rodent ulcer; Fig. 36.12). BCCs do not, however, metastasize.

The diagnosis is made clinically but if there is any doubt a biopsy may be obtained prior to definite treatment. Five methods of treatment are available for BCC.

- *Curettage and cautery*: effective for small lesions but leaves an open wound.
- *Cryotherapy*: no tissue for histology and clearance of margins is uncertain.
- *Surgical excision*: clean closed wound, provides specimen for histology and proof that margins are clear. Larger lesions may require skin grafting (Fig. 36.11b) and more extensive lesions may even require reconstructive surgery (see Chapter 42).
- *Radiotherapy*: produces excellent results. No tissue for histology and should be avoided near cartilage, which may undergo necrosis. The usual dose is 40–60 Gy given over 2–3 weeks.
- *Topical chemotherapy*: not as effective as the other methods. The most frequently used agent is 5-fluorouracil.

Squamous cell carcinoma

Squamous cell carcinoma (SCC) of the skin arises from the keratinocytes in the epidermis. It grows rapidly with anaplasia, local invasion and metastases. Solar keratoses and Bowen's disease are precursors of SCC of the skin (see earlier). SCC also occurs mostly on the exposed areas of the body (75% on the head, 15% on the hands) and may present with a variety of lesions, ranging from a superficial skin ulcer to a fungating lesion or extensive ulceration with heaped-up edges. These are aggressive tumours that will invade the structures deep to the dermis with metastases to regional lymph nodes (Fig. 36.13).

Establishing the diagnosis is the first step in the management of SCC. This is done by obtaining a biopsy for histological diagnosis. The main forms of treatment are surgical excision and radiotherapy, although occasionally cryotherapy or curettage and cautery are used for small lesions. In general, results of treatment are very good but patients should be followed for 5 years after treatment.

Malignant melanoma

See section below.

Kaposi's sarcoma

Kaposi's sarcoma is a multicentric angiosarcoma affecting the skin characterized by purple-brown tumour nodules that vary from 1 mm to 1 cm in diameter. The tumour occurs most often on the hands and feet. Classically, Kaposi's sarcoma occurred in elderly men and was rare in the UK though common in parts of Central Africa. Recently, however, this condition has been recognized as one of the diagnostic presentations of acquired

04

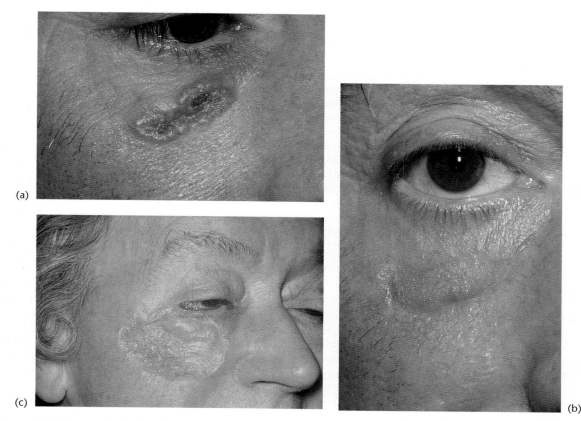

Figure 36.11 Surgery for basal cell carcinoma. (a) Basal cell carcinoma just below the right eye. Note the rolled edge and pearly colour. (b) Early postoperative result following excision of the lesion and full-thickness skin grafting of the defect (Wolfe graft). (c) A split-skin graft would contract and cause ectropion of the eyelid.

04

immunodeficiency syndrome (AIDS). In non-AIDS patients, treatment of individual lesions is by excision, although this is not always possible when large numbers of tumours are present.

Pigmented skin lesions

Naevi

Naevi are benign pigmented lesions of the skin that arise from increased numbers of melanocytes. A number of different types are recognized depending on the site of melanocyte accumulation (Fig. 36.14).
- *Lentigo*: accumulation of melanocytes within the basal layer of the epidermis. Usually found as pigmented lesions on the face and hands of the elderly (Fig. 36.15).
- *Junctional*: proliferation of melanocytes at the dermal–epidermal junction. Clinically present as smooth, flat and often irregularly pigmented lesions. They arise most commonly at or before puberty.

- *Dermal*: melanocytes entirely within the dermis. These are elevated fleshy to brown-coloured, sometimes pedunculated and may contain hair. They usually occur in adults.
- *Compound*: melanocytes lie both at the dermal–epidermal junction and within the dermis and display clinical features of both junctional and dermal naevi. These may develop into malignant melanomas.
- *Blue*: melanocytes lie deep within the dermis. Clinically they are small, sharply defined, dark blue or blue-grey lesions found anywhere on the body but most commonly on the head and neck. It is the depth of the cells in the dermis that accounts for the blue rather than brown appearance of these lesions.

Management of pigmented lesions
Most pigmented lesions are benign and do not require any treatment. A proportion require treatment for aesthetic reasons and a number are treated because of suspicion of malignant change. Treatment is by excision and lesions that should be removed include:

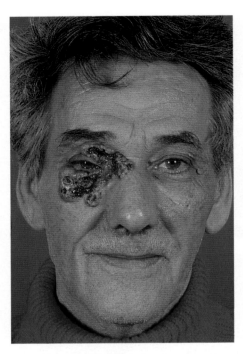

Figure 36.12 A neglected basal cell carcinoma around the left orbit. This patient required extensive reconstructive surgery.

- newly discovered pigmented lesions in an adult;
- lesions that have undergone a change in colour, shape or size;
- lesions which bleed;
- lesions subject to chronic irritation;
- lesions on the sole of the foot or palm of the hand;
- any lesion about which the patient is concerned.

The majority of these lesions will turn out to be naevi of various sorts but a few will be malignant melanoma.

Malignant melanoma

Malignant melanoma is a malignant tumour arising from the melanocytes. The incidence of the most common type of malignant melanoma (superficial spreading type) is increasing more rapidly than any other human cancer and it has been estimated that approximately 1% of all children born today will develop this condition. Since 1979 the incidence of malignant melanoma has been rising at a rate of 6% per annum and it causes about 1000 deaths annually in the UK. Approximately 50% of all melanomas arise in pre-existing naevi and exposure to intense ultraviolet radiation from sunlight is the most important aetiological factor (see Table 36.1). Fair-skinned people are affected most often.

Pathology

Pathologically, the two most common forms of malignant melanoma are:
- superficial spreading (Fig. 36.16a);
- nodular (Fig. 36.16b);

while less frequently encountered varieties include:
- lentigo maligna melanoma (Hutchinson's freckle, Fig. 36.16c);
- acral lentiginous melanoma.

Two phases of tumour progression occur in malignant melanoma. First, the malignant cells grow in all directions; this is referred to as the *radial growth phase*. It is important to recognize this phase as tumours treated at this stage do not metastasize. After 1–2 years a change occurs in some of the malignant cells, which grow as spheroidal nodules and expand more rapidly than the rest of the cells. The direction of this rapid growth is vertical and this phase is called the *vertical growth phase*. The tumour now has the potential to metastasize. Spread to regional lymph nodes occurs early. Haematogenous spread is to liver, bone and brain.

Local staging of malignant melanoma is usually determined by Breslow's tumour thickness. In Breslow's method the tumour thickness in millimetres is used to predict outcome (Table 36.2).

Other prognostic factors include the following.
- Ulceration of the lesion: prognosis is worse if ulceration is present.
- Sex of patient: men do worse than women.
- Anatomical location: extremities do better than the trunk.
- Age of onset of lesion: prognosis is better with lesions that arise before puberty or in the elderly.

Clinical features

Malignant melanomas are found most commonly on the lower limbs, feet, head and neck. They are usually pigmented but a small number lack pigment (amelanotic melanoma; Fig. 36.17). Usually the patient presents with a history of a *change* in a pigmented lesion. Such changes include:
- increasing size;
- increasing pigmentation;
- bleeding;
- pain or itching;
- ulceration;
- development of satellite lesions.

The appearance of a melanoma varies considerably. Most are brown/black irregular lesions on the skin, approximately 1 cm in diameter. The colour is not uniform and there may be evidence of bleeding or ulceration. Satellite lesions are like a number of small moons surrounding a planet represented by the melanoma.

04

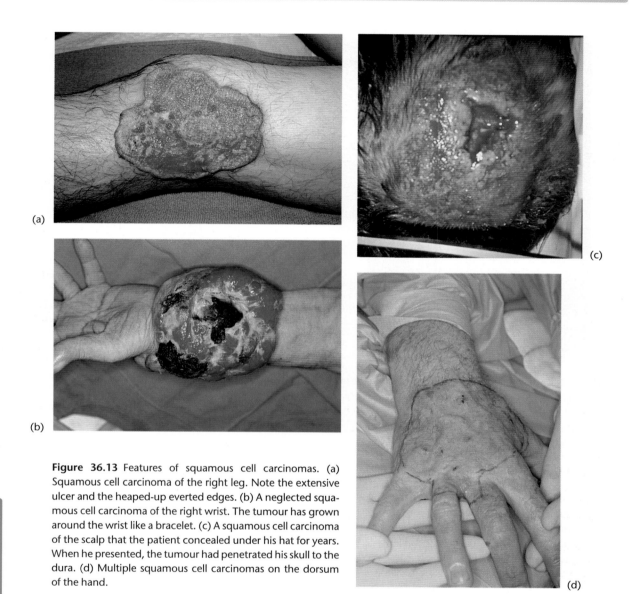

(a)

(b)

(c)

Figure 36.13 Features of squamous cell carcinomas. (a) Squamous cell carcinoma of the right leg. Note the extensive ulcer and the heaped-up everted edges. (b) A neglected squamous cell carcinoma of the right wrist. The tumour has grown around the wrist like a bracelet. (c) A squamous cell carcinoma of the scalp that the patient concealed under his hat for years. When he presented, the tumour had penetrated his skull to the dura. (d) Multiple squamous cell carcinomas on the dorsum of the hand.

(d)

04

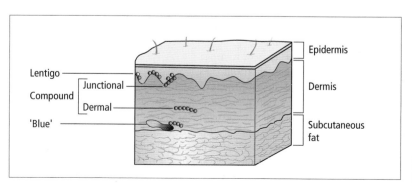

Figure 36.14 Sites of melanocyte accumulation in different types of naevi.

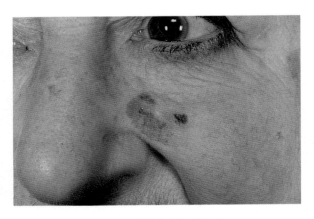

Figure 36.15 Lentigo on the left side of the face.

Management

Surgical excision is the treatment of choice for almost all melanomas. Definitive surgery as the primary procedure may be undertaken providing the diagnosis is strongly suspected or following a biopsy. In the past, very wide margins of excision (> 5 cm) were recommended but it is now recognized that lateral margins of 2–3 cm are adequate. Usually, the subcutaneous tissue is excised with the lesion but it is not necessary to excise fascia or muscle underneath the lesion. These smaller excisions allow primary closure of the wounds in the majority of patients.

Controversy exists regarding the surgical management of regional lymph nodes. In a patient in whom there is clinical evidence of regional node involvement, a lymph node dissection of that area is appropriate. Some surgeons also advocate node dissections prophylactically with intermediate-stage primary lesions (i.e. Clarke levels III and IV and Breslow's 0.76–3.99 mm thickness).

Other forms of treatment include immunotherapy, chemotherapy (both systemic and local perfusion, e.g. of a limb) and radiotherapy. However, survival rates have not been drastically altered by any of several innovative treatments. Occasionally, spontaneous remission of a primary malignant melanoma occurs.

Table 36.2 Survival after surgery for malignant melanoma according to tumour thickness.

Tumour thickness (mm)	5-year survival (%)
< 0.76	98
0.76–1.49	95
1.50–2.49	80
2.50–3.99	75
4.00–7.00	60
> 8.00	40

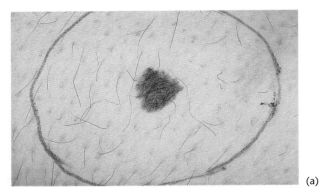

(a)

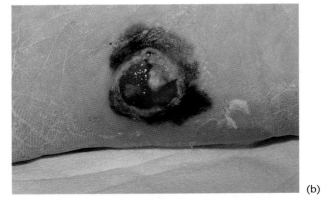

(b)

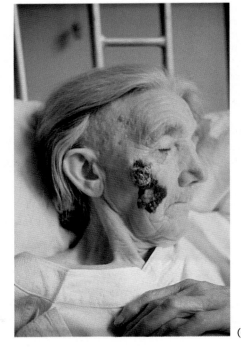

(c)

Figure 36.16 Patterns of malignant melanoma: (a) superficial spreading malignant melanoma; (b) nodular malignant melanoma of the sole of the foot; (c) lentigo maligna melanoma.

04

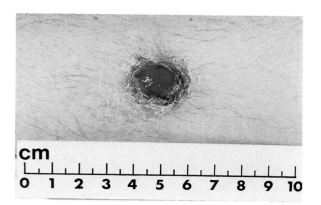

Figure 36.17 Amelanotic melanoma.

Subcutaneous tissue

Lipoma

Lipomas are multilobular benign tumours of fat usually arising in the superficial subcutaneous tissues of the trunk and limbs but may also be found in the peritoneal cavity and within muscles. Lipomas present as soft, fluctuant, painless, subcutaneous lumps measuring from 2 to 20 cm in diameter. Most lipomas are excised for cosmetic reasons. Usually an incision in the skin over the lump allows the lipoma to be enucleated. *Liposarcomas* are rare and tend to occur in the body cavities rather than subcutaneously.

Skin cancer at a glance

Definition

Skin cancer: malignant lesions of the epidermis of the skin, principally BCC, SCC and malignant melanoma

Epidemiology
- Male/female ratio 2 : 1 for BCC and SCC
- Elderly males
- Equal sex distribution and all adults for malignant melanoma
- All tumours common in areas of high annual sunshine (e.g. Australia, southern USA)

Aetiology
- Exposure to sunlight (especially in fair-skinned races)
- Immunosuppression (high incidence after renal transplant)
- Radiation exposure (radiotherapy, among radiologists)
- Chemical carcinogens (hydrocarbons, arsenic, coal tar)
- Inherited disorders (albinism, xeroderma pigmentosum)
- Chronic irritation (Marjolin's ulcer)
- Naevi (50% of malignant melanomas arise in pre-existing benign pigmented lesions)
- Bowen's disease and erythroplasia of Queyrat

Pathology
BCC
- Arises from basal cells of epidermis
- Aggressive local spread but do not metastasize

SCC
- Arises from keratinocytes in the epidermis
- Spreads by local invasion and metastases

Malignant melanoma
- Arises from melanocytes often in pre-existing naevi
- Superficial spreading and nodular types
- Radial and vertical growth phases
- Lymphatic spread is to regional lymph nodes and haematogenous spread to liver, bone and brain

Staging
- Clarke's levels I–V, Breslow's tumour thickness

Clinical features
BCC
- Recurring, ulcerated, umbilicated skin lesion on forehead or face
- Ulcer has a raised pearl-coloured edge
- Untreated, large areas of the face may be eroded (rodent ulcer)

SCC
- Lesions (ulcers, fungating lesions with heaped-up edges) on exposed areas of the body

Malignant melanoma
- Pigmented lesions (occasionally not pigmented, i.e. amelanotic) l cm in diameter on lower limbs, feet, head and neck
- Usually present as a change in a pigmented lesion: increasing size or pigmentation/bleeding/pain or itching/ulceration/satellite lesions

Investigations
- Biopsy (usually excisional) of the lesion unless clinically certain (definitive surgery)

- For malignant melanoma:
  (a) Helical CT scan for involved draining nodes
  (b) Fine-needle aspiration cytology for palpable draining nodes
  (c) ?Peroperative sentinel node biopsy using dye injection mapping

Management
Prophylaxis
- Protection from sun exposure reduces the risk of all forms of skin cancer dramatically (*Slip, Slap, Slop!*)
- All 'moles' with suspicious features should have *excision* biopsy

BCC
- Curettage, cautery, cryotherapy or topical chemotherapy (5-fluorouracil): these treatments are suitable for small lesions
- Surgical excision/radiotherapy

SCC
- Surgical excision/radiotherapy

Malignant melanoma
- Surgical excision with 2–3 cm margin
- Lymph node dissection if CT, fine-needle aspiration cytology or sentinel node biopsy positive for metastases with no systemic disease

- Immunotherapy, chemotherapy (systemic and local limb perfusion), radiotherapy disseminated disease (poor response)

Prognosis
- BCC, SCC: prognosis is usually excellent but patients with SCC should be followed for 5 years
- Prognosis for early malignant melanoma is excellent with surgery but late disease is usually fatal
- Prognosis for malignant melanoma depends on staging:

	5-year survival (%)
Clarke's level	
I (epidermis)	100
II (papillary dermis)	90–100
III (papillary/reticular dermis)	80–90
IV (reticular dermis)	60–70
V (subcutaneous fat)	15–30
Tumour thickness (mm)	
< 0.76	98
0.76–1.49	95
1.50–2.49	80
2.50–3.99	75
4.00–7.99	60
> 8.00	40

Neurofibroma

Benign nerve sheath tumours may be either schwannomas (neurilemmomas) or neurofibromas. *Schwannomas* are benign slow-growing neoplasms of Schwann cells and may arise in any nerve. They are oval well-demarcated tumours ranging in size from a few millimetres to several centimetres and are often solitary. *Neurofibromas* are also thought to arise from Schwann cells and should be differentiated from schwannomas because of their potential for sarcomatous degeneration. Neurofibromas present as small, firm, smooth, mobile, subcutaneous masses of variable size.

Neurofibromatosis (also called von Recklinghausen's disease) is an autosomal dominant inherited disorder of the ectoderm characterized by multiple neurofibromas and *café-au-lait* spots. Some members of affected families may only have cutaneous pigmentation while others have a fuller clinical picture, including the following features.
- Cutaneous pigmentation: brownish spots or areas invariably present.
- Cutaneous fibromas: soft pinkish sessile or pedunculated swellings, usually on the trunk.

- Neurofibromas: usually along the course of the superficial cutaneous nerves.
- Plexiform neuroma: diffuse neurofibromatosis of nerve trunks associated with hypertrophy of the skin and subcutaneous tissue (Fig. 36.18).
- Acoustic neuroma: often bilateral. Presents in middle age with tinnitus and progressive deafness.

Nails

Nails in systemic disease

Abnormalities of the nails often indicate the presence of systemic disease and examination of the nails is an important part of the physical examination of a patient. Such abnormalities include the following.

Clubbing

This is swelling of the finger (or toe) tips such that there is loss of the normal angle between the nail and the skin covering the nail bed or, more simply, the depression

04

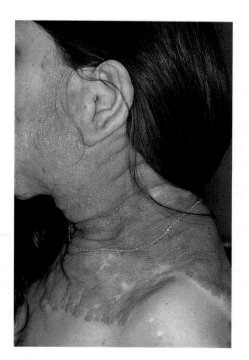

Figure 36.18 Plexiform neurofibroma of the neck.

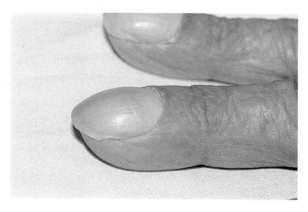

Figure 36.19 Clubbing of the nails of the hands. This patient also had clubbing of his toenails.

at the base of the nail is replaced with a convexity (Fig. 36.19). Clubbing is associated with:
- bronchogenic carcinoma;
- bronchiectasis;
- cyanotic congenital heart disease;
- cirrhosis of the liver.

Koilonychia

Thin, brittle, concave nails are referred to as koilonychia (Greek κοιλοσ, concave; ονψχ, nail). This physical sign is associated with iron-deficiency anaemia and may also be found after trauma to the nail and in the skin disease lichen planus.

Leuconychia

White patches or discoloration of the fingernails are referred to as leuconychia. It is sometimes seen with cirrhosis of the liver.

Splinter haemorrhages

These are small linear streaks of blood under and in the long axis of the nail caused by small haemorrhages from the vessels of the nail bed. They are caused by micro-embolic disease and classically are found in patients with bacterial endocarditis.

Paronychia (whitlow)

Paronychia is an infection of the soft tissue at the margin of the nail. The diagnosis is easily made. The margin of the nail is red, hot, tender and swollen and a small collection of pus may be visible. Treatment usually involves drainage of the collection of pus under local anaesthetic through an incision into the affected part. As with all hand infections, antibiotics and elevation of the hand are also required. Extensive infection may require avulsion of the nail. (Infection of the pulp space of a fingertip is called a *felon* and these frequently require surgical drainage via an incision placed at the periphery of the pulp space.)

Onychogryphosis

Onychogryphosis is a deformity of the toenail that usually affects the big toe (Fig. 36.20). It is referred to as a 'ram's horn' deformity because there is exuberant growth of the nail resulting in a nail that looks like a ram's horn. It is usually seen in the elderly but may also occur after trauma. Clipping and filing the nail may keep it under control. Avulsion of the nail does not cure the condition as the new nail will also be onychogryphotic. If a cure is desired, then ablation of the nail bed is necessary.

Ingrowing toenail

An ingrowing toenail is a common problem in adolescents and young adults (Fig. 36.21). It most commonly affects the hallux but other toenails may be affected. One should be wary of making this diagnosis in the elderly as a toe problem in this age group is often a manifestation of peripheral vascular disease.

An ingrowing toenail is caused by the lateral edge of the toenail cutting and growing into the adjacent soft tissue of the nail fold. Superimposed infection (bacterial or fungal)

04

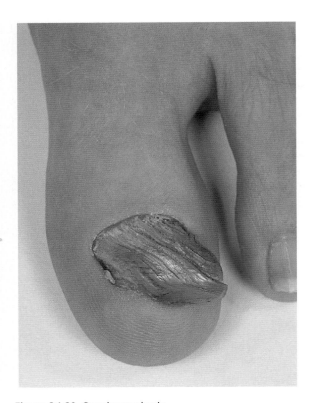

Figure 36.20 Onychogryphosis.

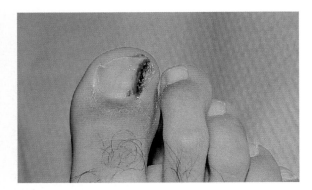

Figure 36.21 Ingrowing toenail.

causes inflammation and attempted tissue repair results in exuberant granulation tissue formation. A combination of factors leads to ingrowing toenails:

- tight-fitting shoes (e.g. winkle pickers, beloved of the teddy-boys of the 1950s);
- cutting (or picking!) the nail down into the nail fold rather than transversely;
- sweaty feet and poor hygiene.

Clinically, the patient may present with features ranging from the nail fold riding up on to the nail to a grossly infected, painful nail fold with cellulitis and weeping granulation tissue. One side, rarely both sides, of a nail may be affected.

Management

If seen in the early stages, an ingrowing toenail may be treated conservatively by:

- regular soaking and washing of the feet;
- carefully drying the feet after washing;
- wearing clean socks and wide-fitting shoes;
- avoiding trauma;
- cutting toenails properly (i.e. transversely);
- using a cotton-wool pledget placed under the corner of the nail to help it grow out from the nail fold.

With perseverence these measures are very successful in many cases.

With more severe cases surgery is necessary. The aim of surgery in the acute situation is to remove the ingrowing nail from the nail fold, thus allowing the wound to heal. This can be achieved by avulsion of the whole nail or avulsion of the side of the nail that is ingrowing. Following avulsion the nail will regrow and if the conservative measures listed above are followed the new nail should grow normally.

In the event of recurrence more drastic measures are undertaken.

- *Wedge resection*: removes about 25% of the width of the nail *and the nail bed* on the affected side. Ablation of the nail bed is achieved by a combination of surgery and phenolization (i.e. a small amount of liquid phenol is left in contact with the nail bed wound for a minute or two). If the nail bed has not been completely ablated, little spikes of nail regenerate and can be a considerable nuisance.
- *Zadek's operation*: the entire nail bed is removed surgically so that the patient is left without a toenail. This is reserved for the severest cases.

Subungual haematoma

Trauma to a fingertip frequently results in a haematoma under the nail. This is an extremely painful condition as there is no room for the haematoma to expand in the confined space under the nail. Drilling a small hole through the nail with a sterile needle produces a small quantity of old blood and instant relief. Frequently, the nail separates after a few days. Occasionally, a malignant melanoma presents under a nail (*subungual melanoma*) and may be mistaken for a subungual haematoma. Lesions under the nail should be biopsied.

Evidence-based medicine

http://www.cancerindex.org/clinks2s.htm   Skin cancer resources directory website.

04

Key points

- Keloid scars are common in coloured races and have a strong tendency to recur after excision
- Some vascular cutaneous lesions are markers for a more generalized vascular condition or some congenital syndromes
- Solar radiation skin damage is the single most common cause of skin malignancies of all types, particularly in fair-skinned people
- Basal cell carcinomas should be treated with local ablation or excision only
- Suspect malignant change in a pigmented lesion if there is a change in size, shape or colour or if there is associated bleeding, itching or pain
- Suspected malignant melanomas must be biopsied by *excision* to established the diagnosis
- Deep penetration or distant spread in malignant melanoma carries a very poor prognosis
- Malignant change is extremely rare in isolated lipomas
- Most neurofibromas are isolated and not part of a neurofibromatosis syndrome
- Most in-growing toenails can be managed conservatively without recourse to surgery

04

Cardiovascular Disorders

37

Must know Must do

Must know

Pathophysiology of atherosclerosis
Clinical features and management of chronic and acute peripheral occlusive vascular disease
Differences between ischaemic and neuropathic foot ulcers
Clinical features and management of abdominal aortic aneurysm
Clinical features and management of carotid artery disease
Clinical features and management of deep vein thrombosis and pulmonary embolism
Pathophysiology and clinical features of a venous ulcer
Clinical features and management of coronary artery disease
Common valvular heart conditions

Must do

Attend a vascular laboratory and see segmental pressures being measured and the ankle–brachial pressure indices being calculated; speak to patients with a history of intermittent claudication and/or rest pain
Examine a patient with an abdominal aortic aneurysm and inspect an ultrasound or computed tomography (CT) scan of an aneurysm
Inspect a carotid duplex scan and speak to a patient with a history of transient ischaemic attacks
Attend a nuclear medicine department and understand how a ventilation–perfusion scan is performed
Watch a compression bandage being applied to a venous ulcer
Wear graduated compression stockings for a day
Attend an operation for varicose veins
Observe electrocardiography, echocardiography and cardiac catheterization being performed
Inspect a cardiopulmonary bypass circuit

Introduction

Disorders of the circulation are common and can be conveniently considered under four headings: cardiac problems, arterial problems, venous problems and lymphatic problems. Coronary artery disease and peripheral vascular disease are serious problems and the leading causes of death in the western world today. Venous thromboembolism may cause death by pulmonary embolism while other venous disorders, such as varicose veins, are a major cause of morbidity worldwide. Lymphatic disease is uncommon but causes considerable distress in those unfortunate enough to be afflicted by it. This chapter considers the causes, clinical manifestations and management of the common cardiac and vascular problems encountered in clinical practice (and examinations!).

Pathophysiology

The primary function of the circulation is the delivery of oxygen and nutrients to maintain the viability of the cells. This is achieved by the heart pumping oxygenated blood through a series of viscoelastic tubes to the periphery. Inadequate blood supply is the single most important determinant in the pathogenesis of cellular injury in human disease. This inadequacy, called *ischaemia*, arises from either a failure of the pumping action of the heart or from local interference with the circulation as a result of disease of blood vessels, or a combination of both.

The consequences of circulatory failure depend on the severity of circulatory disruption, the acuteness of the event and the vulnerability of the tissue to ischaemia. A range of cellular injury may occur, from rapidly reversible anaerobic metabolism, loss of membrane integrity and cellular swelling to cell death and death of tissue en masse. In addition, restoration of normal blood flow after a

05

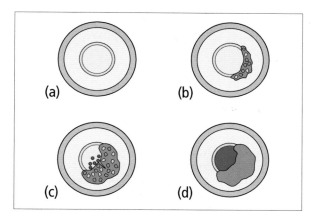

Figure 37.1 Arterial wall changes in atherosclerosis. (a) The earliest changes are increased endothelial permeability to low-density lipoproteins and upregulation of leukocyte adhesion molecules. (b) A fatty streak forms when lipids accumulate in the intimal wall, accompanied by lipid-laden macrophages, T cells and smooth muscle cells, with an overlying fibrous cap. (c) Plaque rupture or ulceration may occur due to release of proteolytic enzymes and metalloproteinases that cause thinning of the fibrous cap. This leads to thrombus formation. (d) Arterial occlusion leads to a clinical syndrome of acute or chronic symptoms, depending on the development of collateral vessels.

Table 37.1 Risk factors for atherosclerosis.*

Cigarette smoking
Hypertension
Raised serum cholesterol
Diabetes mellitus
Age and sex

* Any factor associated with 100% increase in the incidence of atherosclerosis.

the influence of HDL in preventing LDL oxidation. The initial changes probably occur in the endothelium, with increased permeability to lipoproteins and upregulation of leukocyte adhesion molecules. This allows lipid-laden macrophages to form an atheromatous plaque with an overlying fibrous cap. Expansion and ulceration of this intimal lesion (plaque) leads to narrowing of the lumen of the artery, thrombosis and occlusion of a distributing artery. The established risk factors for atherosclerosis are shown in Table 37.1. The effects of smoking, which is the most important (and most preventable) risk factor, are additive to those of other risk factors. In addition, biochemical abnormalities have been sought in high-risk populations. For example, high levels of plasma homocysteine are associated with an increased risk of atherosclerosis. This risk is as yet unquantified; however, homocysteine-lowering therapy with folic acid and vitamin B_6 may be of benefit in susceptible individuals. Family history is very important and genetic predisposition to atherosclerosis is likely to be multifactorial.

Rarer causes of arterial disease are inflammatory conditions such as thromboangiitis obliterans or Buerger's disease. Vasculitis is defined as inflammation and necrosis of blood vessels and may be caused by infectious agents (e.g. syphilis), trauma (e.g. frostbite, radiation) and altered immunology (e.g. temporal arteritis). Whatever the cause of the arterial lesion, the resulting clinical picture depends on the site and speed of onset of arterial occlusion or arterial rupture.

Less severe occlusion, in which blood flow is restricted by a gradual narrowing of the arterial lumen, produces ischaemia on exercise. During exercise the blood supply to the tissues is not adequate for increasing energy demands and the byproducts of anaerobic metabolism (lactic acid and potassium) accumulate and cause pain. Long-recognized symptoms of this process are angina pectoris in the heart and intermittent claudication in the limbs. Sudden occlusion of an artery usually results in death of the tissues supplied by that artery and, if it is an important vessel (e.g. anterior descending branch of the left coronary artery), death of the individual.

period of ischaemia results in *reperfusion injury*, i.e. further tissue injury occurs locally and systemically when the products of ischaemia are carried into the systemic circulation. Thus reperfusion may cause cardiac, renal and pulmonary dysfunction.

Interference with arterial blood flow may result from external compression of the artery (trauma), disease in the arterial wall (atherosclerosis), intraluminal obstruction (thromboembolism) and variations in arterial tone (vasospastic disorders). Each of these events may cause endothelial damage with subsequent activation of the clotting mechanism.

The human body contains one arterial system and the symptoms and signs of coronary, cerebral and peripheral arterial disease simply reflect underlying arterial pathology in those areas. The most important disease to affect arteries is atherosclerosis (Fig. 37.1), an acquired condition, the complications of which account for more than half of the entire annual mortality of the USA. The main sites of atherosclerosis in the human body are shown in Fig. 37.2. Atherosclerosis is characterized by the proliferation of intimal smooth muscle cells and the accumulation of lipids such as oxidized low-density lipoprotein (LDL). The inverse relationship between high-density lipoprotein (HDL) and atherosclerosis is probably explained by

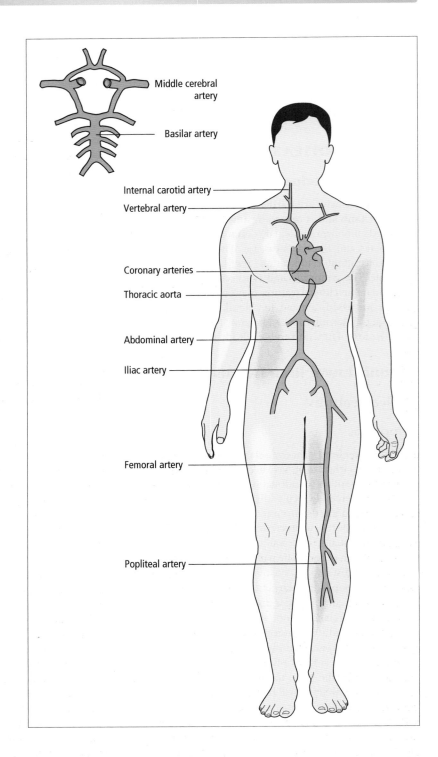

Labels on figure:
Middle cerebral artery
Basilar artery
Internal carotid artery
Vertebral artery
Coronary arteries
Thoracic aorta
Abdominal artery
Iliac artery
Femoral artery
Popliteal artery

Figure 37.2 Common sites of atherosclerosis in the human body.

Occasionally, an artery is occluded by an embolus, usually a thrombus that has migrated from the heart or a larger proximal vessel. For example, small emboli from plaques at the origin of the internal carotid artery migrate into the brain and cause strokes or, if the neurological deficit is temporary, transient ischaemic attacks (TIAs).

Atherosclerosis (or other factors) may also weaken the wall of an artery so that the artery expands and becomes an

05

aneurysm. The tension on the wall of the aneurysm is directly related to the blood pressure and the diameter of the lumen (law of Laplace); as the lumen increases, the tension on the wall increases and, like a balloon, the aneurysm will eventually burst; if it is an abdominal aortic aneurysm, it will kill the patient.

ARTERIAL DISEASE

Peripheral occlusive arterial disease

Peripheral occlusive arterial disease predominantly affects the lower limb and is caused by atherosclerosis (thrombosis and embolism), vascular trauma, the complications of diabetes and Buerger's disease. The patient presents with intermittent claudication, rest pain, ulceration or gangrene. The symptoms and signs reflect the severity of ischaemia; thus clinical features may only be present when there is increased demand for blood supply, e.g. when exercising (intermittent claudication), or there may be complete loss of function and cell death at rest (gangrene).

Chronic lower limb ischaemia

Clinical features

Symptoms

Chronic lower limb ischaemia classically occurs in elderly male patients who are or have been cigarette smokers and who may have other manifestations of atherosclerosis, e.g. coronary or cerebral vascular disease. Intermittent claudication is the mildest symptom of arterial insufficiency to the lower limb. It is characterized by pain or discomfort on walking, usually in the calf or buttocks, but occasionally in the thigh or foot. The pain will always appear in the segment just distal to the site of obstruction of the artery. Thus femoropopliteal obstruction will produce calf claudication while common iliac disease will produce buttock as well as calf claudication. Aortic occlusion produces buttock pain and loss of erection in the male (Leriche's syndrome). The pain steadily increases until the patient is compelled to stop. Resting in the upright position rapidly relieves the pain, usually within a few minutes. Resumption of walking will reproduce the pain at exactly the same distance as before; this is called the claudication distance. Some patients will also report coldness, numbness or paraesthesia of the foot with muscle pain. This is thought to be due to shunting of blood from the skin to the ischaemic muscle. The majority of patients with claudication will never progress to develop critical ischaemia in the affected limb. It may be sometimes difficult to distinguish ischaemic claudication from 'spinal' claudica-

Table 37.2 Examination of the legs in a patient with peripheral vascular disease.

Inspection
Colour
Buerger's test
Posture of the limb
Venous guttering
Gangrene
Ulceration

Palpation
Temperature
Capillary refilling
Pulses
Sensation and movement

Auscultation
Bruits

tion, which is caused by stenosis of the spinal canal due to degenerative disease of the lumbosacral spine. This latter pain does not usually disappear rapidly on standing.

Rest pain is characterized by a continuous aching severe pain and is indicative of critical ischaemia, i.e. arterial insufficiency severe enough to threaten the viability of the foot or leg. Elderly smoking men are the usual sufferers and often a history of intermittent claudication can be elicited. In general, patients with rest pain are older and less active than typical claudicants. Rest pain usually occurs in the most distal part of the limb, i.e. the toes and forefoot, and is often associated with tissue destruction, either ulceration or gangrene. The pain is worse at night in bed, when the blood supply to the foot is reduced because of loss of hydrostatic pressure due to gravity that is present in the upright position; thus the patient seeks relief by hanging the leg over the side of the bed or sleeping in a chair. Rest pain is of far greater significance than claudication, as it indicates limb-threatening ischaemia.

Physical examination

The clinical examination should be performed in a warm room. The entire cardiovascular system should be examined, including the heart and abdominal aorta, with measurement of blood pressure and auscultation of the carotid arteries. The main points to be considered in physical examination of the legs are given in Table 37.2.

Inspection
In the early stages of the disease the leg will look remarkably normal. With more severe disease the leg may look pale at or on elevation from the horizontal and a dusky

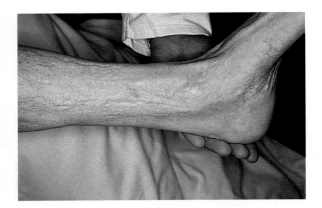

Figure 37.3 Venous guttering in a patient with arterial disease. Because of poor inflow there is not enough blood to fill the veins when the limb is elevated.

reddish purple when it hangs down. This observation is the basis of Buerger's test. The limb is raised for a minute or two. With a normal peripheral circulation the toes should remain pink at 90°. In an ischaemic limb, because arterial pressure is unable to overcome gravity, the elevated leg becomes a waxy, cadaveric, white colour, best seen on the sole of the foot. In the raised position, a visible vein may be emptied of blood by running a finger along it, leaving a 'gutter' appearance. The time it takes for the vein to refill with blood from the arterial side when the limb is lowered again is a good indicator of the degree of ischaemia. The normal venous refilling time is less than 15 s (Fig. 37.3). The angle to which the leg must be raised before it becomes white is the vascular angle or Buerger's angle, usually less than 30° in an ischaemic limb. When the limb is hung down it gradually becomes a bluish-red colour due to reactive hyperaemia. If the patient has been sitting with the knee flexed in an attempt to relieve the pain of severe ischaemia, there may be a fixed flexion deformity of the hip or knee.

Gangrene is the digestion of dead tissue by saprophytic bacteria, i.e. bacteria incapable of invading and multiplying in living tissue. In severe peripheral vascular disease, tissue death is produced by ischaemia and gangrene results from subsequent saprophytic invasion. This is usually dry gangrene or mummification initially. Clinically, dead tissue looks brown or black and contracts into a shrunken crinkled mass. The junction between gangrenous and living tissue is often distinct and is known as the line of demarcation. If left alone the dry dead tissue may fall off. However, if the gangrenous area develops invasive infection (wet gangrene) the tissues become boggy and ulcerated, the gangrene spreads proximally and the patient becomes toxic. An urgent amputation is required in this situation. Gangrene may affect patches of

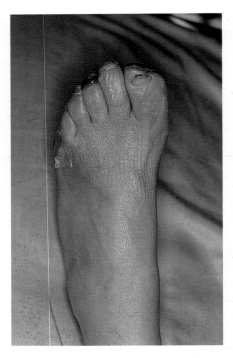

Figure 37.4 Patches of dry gangrene over pressure points in the foot.

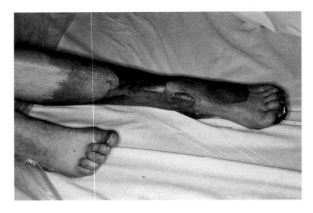

Figure 37.5 Gangrene of the lower limb following a neglected arterial embolus. This patient requires an urgent above-knee amputation.

skin (think of microemboli; Fig. 37.4), a digit, the foot or the distal limb (Fig. 37.5).

Ischaemic ulcers are often present in severe peripheral vascular disease and may be caused by very minimal local trauma. They are usually very painful and are found over pressure areas (heel, heads of the first and fifth metatarsals) and the toes. They vary in size from a few millimetres to several centimetres in diameter; they are

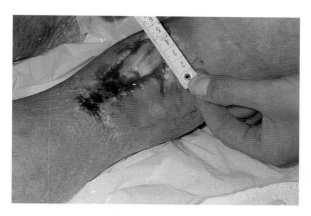

Figure 37.6 Arterial ulcer on the lower limb with gangrene and an exposed tendon in a patient with diabetes mellitus. This patient's ulcer healed following a bypass operation, débridement of the ulcer and skin grafting.

punched out, there is usually no evidence of healing and often tendons or bone are exposed in the base of the ulcer (Fig. 37.6).

Palpation

The severely ischaemic leg, regardless of its colour, feels cold. It is always surprising to find that a red dependent foot is stone cold. To assess the temperature properly, both legs should be exposed for 5 min. The capillary refilling time gives a crude estimation of capillary blood flow. Press the tip of a toenail or the pulp of a toe for 2–3 s and observe the time taken for the blanched area to return to its normal pink colour after releasing pressure. Capillary refilling should be almost instantaneous with a normal circulation but will be retarded in an ischaemic limb.

Examination of the peripheral pulses reveals the anatomical site of arterial obstruction. The pulses will be present proximal to and absent distal to the site of obstruction. The first pulse sought should always be that of the abdominal aorta, as the presence of an aneurysm may signify embolic disease. The peripheral pulses to be examined are the femoral, popliteal, dorsalis pedis and posterior tibial. The femoral pulse lies midway between the symphysis pubis and the anterior superior iliac spine and is easily felt if present, except in very obese patients who should be examined flat with the hip externally rotated. The popliteal pulse is more difficult to feel (Fig. 37.7).

The dorsalis pedis pulse is found in the middle third of a line drawn from the midpoint of the malleoli to the cleft between the first and second toes and just lateral to the extensor hallucis longus tendon. This artery is congenitally absent from its usual position in 10% of patients. The posterior tibial artery lies halfway between the posterior

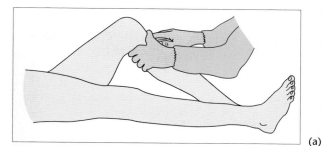

(a)

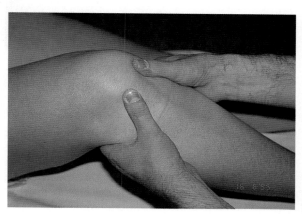

(b)

Figure 37.7 (a, b) Palpation of the popliteal pulse. The usual method of palpating this pulse is to flex the knee partially, to about 140°. With your thumbs on the tibial tuberosity and your fingers over the lower part of the popliteal fossa, compress the artery between your thumbs and the upper end of the tibia. Occasionally, you will have to place the patient prone and feel along the course of the artery. If the popliteal pulse is very easily palpable, the patient may have a popliteal aneurysm.

margin of the medial malleolus and the medial border of the tendo Achilles. The peroneal artery is occasionally palpable (and usually audible with Doppler) and should be sought 1 cm anterior to the lateral malleolus.

Auscultation

Turbulent flow over a roughened artery wall produces vibration, which can be heard as a bruit on auscultation. For a bruit to occur, there must be sufficient flow through a roughened vessel. The loudness of a bruit does not grade a stenosis. It is convenient to record the pulses and bruits in diagrammatic form (Fig. 37.8).

Non-invasive tests of peripheral vascular disease

Non-invasive tests are part of the clinical evaluation and should be undertaken after history and physical examination. They can be classified as indirect tests, which

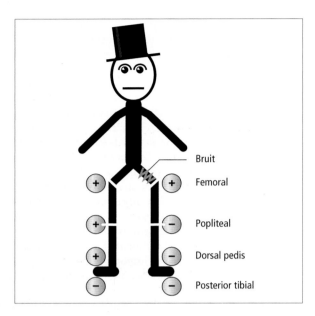

Figure 37.8 'A picture is worth a thousand words'. It is convenient to record the peripheral pulses and bruits in diagrammatic form.

Table 37.3 Non-invasive tests for assessment of peripheral vascular disease.

Indirect tests
Doppler velocimetry
   Ankle pressure measurement
   Segmental pressure measurement
   Waveform analysis
   Exercise response
Plethysmography
   Pulse volume recording
   Digital plethysmography

Direct tests
Duplex colour ultrasonography

measure the haemodynamic characteristics of the disease, and direct tests, which evaluate the artery and define precisely the location of the atherosclerotic lesions. These tests are listed in Table 37.3. However, only Doppler velocimetry and digital plethysmography are currently widely used in the assessment of peripheral vascular disease. Duplex colour ultrasonography is used extensively in the assessment of carotid disease.

The simplest non-invasive test to perform is ankle pressure measurement. A pneumatic cuff, attached to a sphygmomanometer, is applied immediately above the malleoli and the posterior tibial arterial signal is located with a Doppler probe. The cuff is inflated and the pressure at

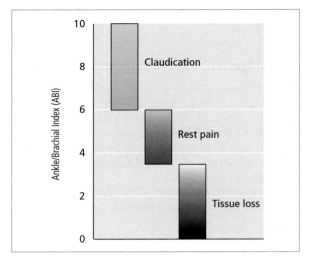

Figure 37.9 Relationship between the ankle/brachial index and the clinical features of peripheral occlusive arterial disease.

which the signal disappears is noted. The cuff is then deflated and the pressure at which the signal reappears is also noted. The mean of the two readings is the ankle pressure. The dorsalis pedis pressure should also be measured and the highest ankle measurement taken as the reference. Because systemic arterial pressure varies from patient to patient, the ankle pressure is expressed as a percentage of the brachial systolic pressure (ankle/brachial index or ABI). The relationship between ABI and the clinical symptoms of peripheral occlusive disease is shown in Fig. 37.9.

Segmental pressures record the arterial systolic pressure along the length of the limb and give a more precise determination of the anatomy of the occlusion. The sites of measurement are high thigh, above knee, below knee and above the ankle. In the normal arterial tree pressures should decrease by about 10 mmHg (1.3 kPa) from one segment to the next. A gradient of more than 20 mmHg (2.6 kPa) is considered an abnormal finding. If the patient's symptoms are present only on exercise, then measurements at rest may not show any abnormality. It is therefore important to repeat the ABI and segmental pressures after exercise. Such a stress test is best achieved with a treadmill. Walking at 3 kph with a 10% gradient usually yields an abnormal result in most claudicants.

Doppler waveform analysis and pulse volume recordings are useful adjuncts to ABI and segmental pressure measurement and give more information in patients with rigid arteries and proximal aortoiliac disease. Digital plethysmography, which measures the increase in volume of the digit that occurs with systole, is useful in the evaluation of diabetic patients in whom abnormally

05

high ankle pressures may be recorded due to medial calcification.

Investigation and management

The management of chronic lower limb ischaemia ranges from simple advice about smoking and exercise to detailed assessment of the vascular tree prior to reconstructive surgery. The management plan is based on the clinical assessment, having regard for the severity of the disease and the impact it has on a given patient's lifestyle. Three groups are recognized:

- patients with non-disabling claudication;
- patients whose lifestyle is seriously curtailed by claudication; and
- patients with critical ischaemia.

Non-disabling intermittent claudication

The natural history of patients with intermittent claudication is that one-third will get better, one-third will remain about the same and one-third will progress to rest pain and critical ischaemia. Thus, over 60% of claudicants improve or remain stable and only about 7% come to amputation after 5 years. Patients with intermittent claudication that does not seriously interfere with their lifestyle should have simple non-invasive tests (ABI and segmental pressures) to quantify their disease and then be given a trial of non-operative therapy (Table 37.4).

A full blood count should be performed to exclude polycythaemia and thrombocythaemia, both of which will exacerbate the symptoms of peripheral occlusive disease. The β-adrenergic blocking agents may also worsen intermittent claudication by their negative inotropic and peripheral vasoconstrictor effects.

Non-operative treatment of chronic lower limb ischaemia consists of cessation of smoking, exercise and drug therapy. Cessation of all tobacco use is the foundation of

Table 37.4 Management of non-disabling claudication.

Investigation
History (β-blockers)
Physical examination
Ankle/brachial index and segmental pressures
Full blood count (exclude polycythaemia and thrombocythaemia)

Treatment
Stop smoking completely
Exercise programme
Aspirin
Pentoxifylline(?)

non-operative therapy of chronic lower limb ischaemia and this must be emphasized to the patient at every opportunity. Most smokers are aware of an increased risk of lung cancer and heart disease with smoking but are ignorant of the connection between smoking and peripheral vascular disease. Patients who stop smoking usually experience a doubling of their walking distance and do better than patients who continue to smoke. A walking exercise programme should also be initiated. Patients should be advised to walk for 1 h each day, repeatedly approaching the point of claudication. Attempts to walk through the claudication are misguided and may induce arrhythmias. Exercise does not, as was previously thought, enhance collateral circulation but, analogous to athletic training, probably results in more efficient oxygen extraction from the limited blood supply. Treatment of hypertension and hypercholesterolaemia is also important in order to prevent progression of what is a systemic disease process.

Numerous pharmacological agents have been evaluated for possible benefit in chronic lower limb ischaemia with generally mixed results. Pentoxifylline, which reduces blood viscosity, gives a modest improvement in walking distance and recently cilostazol has been shown to improve walking distance in patients with intermittent claudication. However, patients with peripheral occlusive arterial disease should receive aspirin 75 mg/day because of its general beneficial effects on survival in patients with atherosclerotic disease. Recently, it has been suggested that clopidogrel, a thienopyridine derivative that inhibits platelet activation by adenosine diphosphate, may be better than aspirin in reducing some of the complications of atherosclerosis, including stroke, myocardial infarction and vascular death. In addition, the cholesterol-lowering statins have been shown to reduce cardiac events in arteriopaths, even if serum cholesterol is normal.

Disabling claudication and critical ischaemia

Claudication that is rapidly worsening despite good non-operative therapy or which produces marked exercise restriction in young people is defined as disabling claudication. In addition to non-invasive assessment, these patients should undergo arteriography prior to surgical or radiological intervention. Patients with critical ischaemia require similar investigation prior to surgical treatment.

Arteriography

This provides a two-dimensional map of the arterial system indicating the site and severity of the vessel occlusions and stenoses. It does not measure blood flow or circulatory dynamics and should only be used in patients in whom interventional radiology or surgery is being considered. Where possible, the safer per-femoral approach

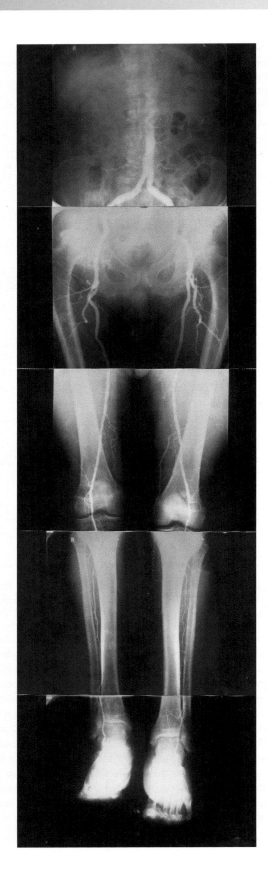

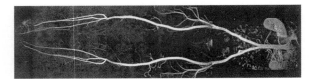

Figure 37.11 Magnetic resonance arteriogram demonstrating the arterial tree.

should be used and the arterial tree from the renal arteries to the pedal arches should be demonstrated (Fig. 37.10). Where both femoral pulses are absent, it may be necessary to gain direct access to the abdominal aorta via a translumbar approach. Digital subtraction arteriography (DSA) is a technique which 'subtracts' the bony image and enhances the arteriographic profile. DSA also permits the use of much smaller doses of contrast than in standard arteriography (Fig. 37.12a).

The direct treatment of the critically ischaemic limb consists of percutaneous catheter procedures and surgical treatment (Table 37.5).

Parenteral drug therapy for rest pain or tissue loss

Most limbs with ischaemic rest pain and tissue loss will be lost unless arterial inflow can be restored either radiologically or surgically. However, temporary relief of symptoms and possibly improved ulcer healing can be achieved in some patients by a small improvement in tissue perfusion and oxygenation. The agents showing most promise in achieving this goal are pentoxifylline, which decreases plasma viscosity, diminishes platelet aggregation and increases extremity blood flow, and prostanoids (PGI_2, PGE_1 and prostacyclin analogues), which cause vasodilation and inhibit platelet aggregation. However, none of the drugs investigated to date has shown a significant benefit.

Percutaneous transluminal angioplasty

This is a technique where under fluoroscopy a balloon catheter is introduced over a guidewire into the lumen of an artery. The balloon is advanced over the guidewire until it lies across the stenosis or occlusion. The balloon is then inflated to a high pressure, crushing the atheroma into the arterial wall. The technique is most effective for short (≤ 5 cm) proximal stenoses but total occlusion can also be recanalized. On average there is a greater than 85% initial success rate with balloon angioplasty and a 1-year patency rate of 70% (Fig. 37.12b). Newer techniques include the placement of metal expandable stents across the stenosis/occlusion after angioplasty and subintimal

Figure 37.10 (*left*) A standard arteriogram demonstrating the arterial tree from the renal to the pedal arteries.

05

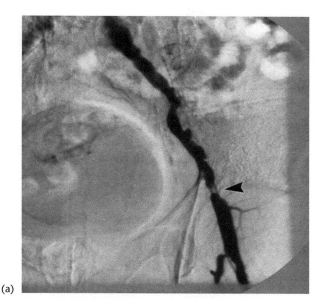

(a)

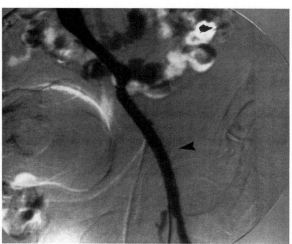

(b)

Figure 37.12 (a) Digital subtraction angiogram demonstrating a diseased left iliac arterial tree with a tight stenosis (arrow) in the external iliac artery. Note the absence of the internal iliac artery and the 'ghost' outline of the pelvic bones and hip joint. (b) The same patient following percutaneous transluminal angioplasty. The strictured areas have been completely dilated.

Table 37.5 Direct treatment of the critically ischaemic leg.

Intravenous pharmacotherapy
Pentoxifylline
Prostanoids

Percutaneous catheter procedures
Balloon angioplasty
Expandable stent placement

Surgery
Reconstructive operations
 Bypass grafting
 Endarterectomy
Amputation

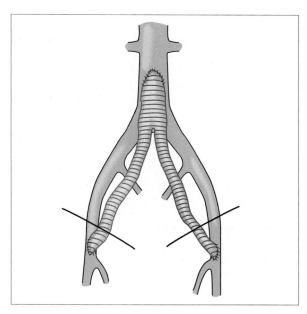

Figure 37.13 A bifurcated tube-graft has been inserted from the aorta to the femoral arteries, bypassing the diseased lower aorta and iliac arteries.

05

angioplasty where an intentional dissection of the vessel is ballooned in order to create a new lumen.

Surgical procedures

Reconstructive surgery, including bypass grafting and occasionally endarterectomy, is the usual treatment for patients with critical limb ischaemia. Endarterectomy is a procedure whereby an atheromatous plaque is removed by direct operation on the artery. Its use is now almost confined to carotid artery stenosis but occasionally it is performed for an isolated peripheral lesion, e.g. an iliac stenosis. However, most patients require some form of bypass procedure.

Aortoiliac occlusive disease is treated by inserting a synthetic polyester (Dacron) bifurcated graft from the aorta to the femoral arteries (Fig. 37.13), bypassing the diseased lower aorta and iliac arteries. If the patient is not fit for an aortic procedure, then blood flow to the legs can be restored by placing a bifurcated graft subcutaneously from one axillary artery to the femoral arteries. This is an example of an extra-anatomical bypass procedure.

Table 37.6 Patency rates of surgical bypass procedures for lower limb ischaemia.

Bypass operation	Patency at 1 year (%)
Aortobifemoral	90
Above-knee femoropopliteal (vein)	75
Above-knee femoropopliteal (synthetic)	65
Below-knee femoropopliteal (vein)	70
Below-knee femoropopliteal (synthetic)	60

Femoropopliteal occlusion is relieved by using the patient's own saphenous vein to bypass the obstruction. Duplex ultrasonography may be helpful in evaluating the suitability of a vein before operation. The vein is removed completely, reversed so that the valves do not obstruct the flow, and then anastomosed to the femoral artery above the obstruction and the popliteal artery below the obstruction. Alternatively, the vein may be left *in situ* so that a more distal bypass, e.g. to the tibial arteries, can be performed. The diameter of the distal saphenous vein matches that of the small tibial arteries, facilitating anastomosis. However, with this technique the valves have to be destroyed with a valvulotome. If the ipsilateral saphenous vein is not satisfactory, a vein may be harvested from the other leg or arm and, if all else fails, a synthetic polytetrafluoroethylene (PTFE) or Dacron graft may be used. However, the best results will be obtained with the patient's own saphenous vein (Table 37.6).

Lumbar sympathectomy

This can be performed surgically or chemically (by injecting phenol or absolute alcohol) in patients with peripheral vascular disease. The rationale behind the procedure is that sympathetic blockade may improve the blood flow to the skin, thereby relieving pain and promoting ulcer healing. A sympathectomy may be performed in patients in whom there is no possibility of reconstruction and in some patients with thromboangiitis obliterans (see later). In some patients it may lead to warming of the foot and subjective improvement but there is no evidence that sympathectomy significantly alters the outcome for the patient.

Amputation

While the majority of patients with peripheral vascular disease are amenable to limb salvage procedures, an amputation will be required in patients with critical ischaemia in whom reconstruction fails or is not possible and who do not respond to maximum medical therapy, e.g. iloprost infusions. An amputation should be per-

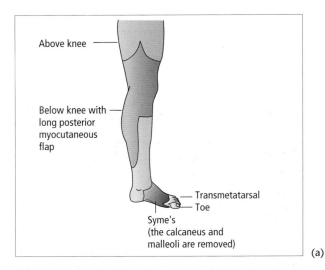

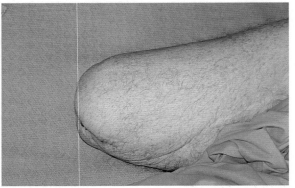

(a)

(b)

Figure 37.14 (a) Sites of commonly performed amputations of the lower limb. (b) An above-knee amputation stump.

formed through healthy tissue and the stump should facilitate early fitting of a prosthesis and rehabilitation. The most frequently performed amputations are toe, transmetatarsal, Syme's, below knee and above knee (Fig. 37.14). Amputees have a very poor prognosis for survival and 40% will die within 2 years of amputation. A major amputation of the other leg is required in 30% of patients and full mobility is achieved in only 50% of below-knee and 25% of above-knee amputees.

Acute lower limb ischaemia

Pathophysiology

Embolism, thrombosis and vascular injury are the causes of acute lower limb ischaemia. The usual sources of arterial embolus are given in Table 37.7.

Emboli usually impact at branching points in the arterial tree, particularly at the bifurcation of the aorta

05

Table 37.7 Sources of arterial emboli.

Heart (90%)
Arrhythmias (e.g. atrial fibrillation)
Valvular heart disease
Prosthetic heart valves
Mural thrombus post myocardial infarction
Ventricular aneurysm
Atrial myxoma

Great vessels (9%)
Atherosclerotic aorta
Aortic aneurysm
Popliteal artery aneurysm
Internal carotid artery plaque

Other (1%)
Paradoxical
Malignant tumour emboli

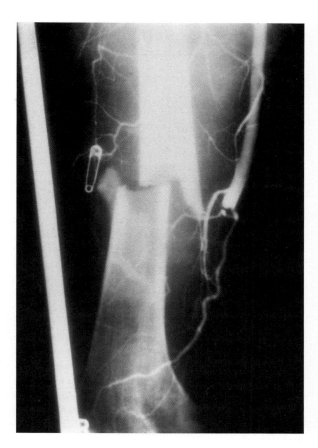

Figure 37.15 Complete disruption of the superficial femoral artery at the adductor canal in association with a comminuted fracture of the femur following a road traffic accident.

(saddle embolus), the common femoral bifurcation and the popliteal trifurcation. *Thrombosis* of a pre-existing atherosclerotic lesion may also cause acute ischaemia. Occasionally, thrombosis in a relatively normal artery can occur in patients with hypercoagulable states, e.g. patients with malignancy, polycythaemia or those taking high doses of oestrogen. *Vascular injury* can be caused by penetrating or blunt trauma (Fig. 37.15). Trauma may cause complete disruption of an artery or only fracture the intima. The blood flow may dissect the torn intima from the media, creating a small flap that impedes flow. Even if no flap develops, a thrombus forms over the torn intima, causing an acute occlusion of the artery.

Regardless of the cause, sudden interruption of the blood supply to the lower limbs causes acute ischaemia. Two phases of cellular injury are recognized. Acute ischaemia alone rapidly causes cell damage but further injury occurs if and when the blood supply is restored to the ischaemic tissues. This second phase of injury is called reperfusion injury. It is caused by the production of toxic oxygen radicals (superoxide, O_2^-; hydrogen peroxide, H_2O_2; hydroxyl radical, OH^-) in the tissues when blood flow is re-established. Some drugs, e.g. mannitol and allopurinol, help to protect the cell from reperfusion injury by inhibiting the production of oxygen radicals or scavenging them as they are produced.

Compartment syndromes are also a consequence of acute ischaemia. The muscles of the lower limb are in osseofascial compartments (i.e. compartments bounded by bone and fascia). Ischaemia (and reperfusion) cause the muscles to swell within these rigid compartments. The result is an increase in pressure in the compartment greater than the capillary perfusion pressure; thus the blood supply to the muscle is interrupted and further

ischaemia and swelling occur. The muscle cells break down and release myoglobin, which in turn causes renal damage and myoglobinuria; this can be recognized clinically by a characteristic black/brown urine. To break this cycle of injury the muscle compartment has to be opened surgically by dividing the fascia and allowing the muscle to expand; this operation is called a fasciotomy (Fig. 37.16).

Clinical features

The classical manifestations of acute ischaemia are pain, paraesthesia, pallor, paralysis, pulselessness and a perishing cold foot (the six Ps). Pain is the most frequent manifestation of acute arterial occlusion. Its onset is sudden, it is severe and progressive and affects the most distal part of the limb first. As the nerves become ischaemic, pain is replaced by a feeling of numbness. The presence of paraesthesia demands immediate treatment as it indicates severe ischaemia. Loss of two-point discrimination is a significant prognostic sign. Pallor is

05

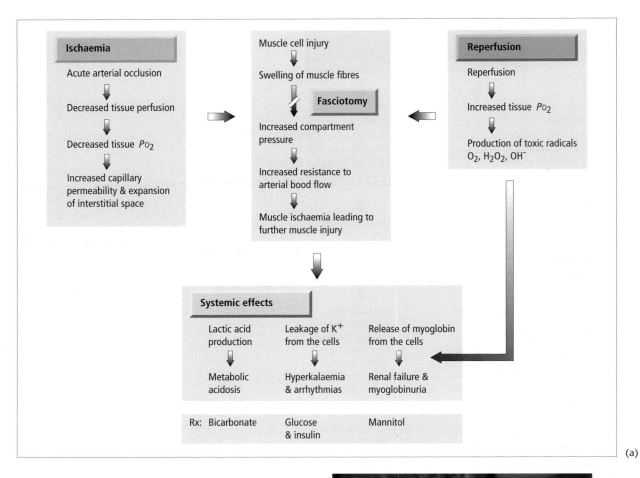

Figure 37.16 (a) Pathophysiology of compartment syndrome and the systemic consequences that may follow reperfusion of an ischaemic limb. Fasciotomy may break the cycle, preventing further muscle cell injury and thereby decreasing the systemic consequences of reperfusion, i.e. myonephropathic metabolic syndrome (metabolic acidosis, arrhythmias, renal and respiratory failure). (b) Fasciotomy of the forearm and the hand in a patient following a gunshot injury to the axillary artery. Note that the separation of the skin edges is entirely due to the degree of swelling that occurred in the muscle compartment.

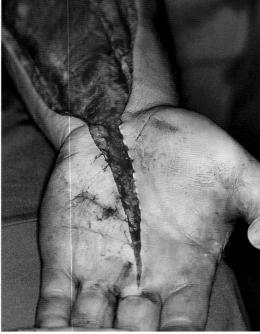

(b)

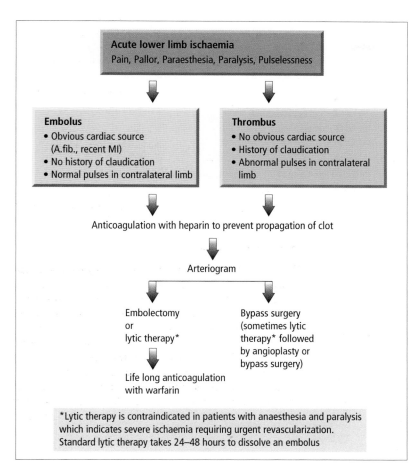

Acute lower limb ischaemia
Pain, Pallor, Paraesthesia, Paralysis, Pulselessness

Embolus
- Obvious cardiac source (A.fib., recent MI)
- No history of claudication
- Normal pulses in contralateral limb

Thrombus
- No obvious cardiac source
- History of claudication
- Abnormal pulses in contralateral limb

Anticoagulation with heparin to prevent propagation of clot

Arteriogram

Embolectomy or lytic therapy*

Bypass surgery (sometimes lytic therapy* followed by angioplasty or bypass surgery)

Life long anticoagulation with warfarin

*Lytic therapy is contraindicated in patients with anaesthesia and paralysis which indicates severe ischaemia requiring urgent revascularization. Standard lytic therapy takes 24–48 hours to dissolve an embolus

Figure 37.17 Clinical differentiation between an embolus and acute thrombosis is important as it has therapeutic implications.

manifested as a white waxy colour and is seen early with acute ischaemia. Stagnant capillary circulation leads to mottling, which is the herald of blistering and gangrene. Paralysis and sensory deficits are late findings in acute ischaemia and indicate severe ischaemia. Diffuse muscle rigidity usually indicates an unsalvageable limb. On examination there is often tenderness over the femoral artery and the pulses will be absent in the embolized limb.

Clinical assessment can usually establish whether acute ischaemia is due to an embolus or a thrombus and this differentiation has therapeutic implications (Fig. 37.17). If a history of previous claudication can be elicited in a patient with no obvious cardiac source of embolus, thrombosis of a pre-existing atherosclerotic plaque is most likely. These patients will require bypass surgery. However, if the patient has atrial fibrillation or a recent myocardial infarction, has no prior history of claudication and has normal pulses in the opposite limb, then a diagnosis of embolus can be made with confidence. These patients will do well with embolectomy or in some cases lytic therapy.

Investigation and management

The outcome of acute arterial occlusion depends on the medical condition of the patient, the degree of ischaemia of the limb and the promptness of revascularization. The aim of therapy is early revascularization of the limb after stabilization and control of coexisting medical problems. In patients with a recent myocardial infarct or atrial fibrillation, assessment of haemodynamics is important and adequate urinary output should be established. Patients with acute ischaemia should be anticoagulated with unfractionated heparin as soon as the diagnosis is made. This prevents propagation of thrombus and distal thrombosis and is achieved by giving a bolus of 10,000 units of unfractionated heparin intravenously and an infusion of about 1000 units/h of heparin after that.

Patients in whom thrombosis is thought to be the diagnosis should be considered for arteriography in order to define the extent of the problem before revascularization. To avoid delay in revascularization this can be performed peroperatively.

Table 37.8 Agents currently used for thrombolytic therapy.

	Streptokinase	Tissue plasminogen activator	Urokinase
Discovered	1933	1940s	1947
Source	Haemolytic *Streptococcus*	Vascular endothelium	Urine
Speed of lysis	++	+++	++
Risk of haemorrhage	+	+	+
Allergic reactions	+	−	−
Cost	+	+++	+++

Patients who are found to have an embolus should be investigated to establish its source; investigations should include electrocardiogram (ECG), cardiac enzymes, Holter monitoring, echocardiography and abdominal ultrasonography for aneurysm.

Surgical management

Embolectomy
Since 1963 the standard approach to a peripheral embolus has been embolectomy. This operation is usually performed under local anaesthesia as patients often have a medical problem that precludes general anaesthesia, e.g. recent myocardial infarction. A groin incision is made and the common femoral artery is opened. Often clot is found in the artery at the site of arteriotomy. A Fogarty balloon catheter is passed in turn into the proximal and distal arteries, the balloon is inflated and the catheter is withdrawn, removing the clot. An arteriogram should be done to ensure that the distal circulation is clear. If it is not, then a more distal arteriotomy and further embolectomy may be required with or without thrombolytic therapy, or an immediate bypass operation if one is dealing with an acute atherosclerotic thrombus. *Percutaneous aspiration embolectomy* is a technique where a percutaneous catheter is advanced into the embolus and the embolus is aspirated through the catheter. A small number of patients present having had an embolus a number of days or weeks previously. Their symptoms are obviously mild and they have a viable limb. These patients can be treated electively by *delayed embolectomy*.

Thrombolytic therapy

Percutaneous intra-arterial thrombolytic therapy may be used to manage some patients with non-limb-threatening ischaemia. Systemic thrombolytic therapy is not used because of the risks of bleeding. The agents available are streptokinase, urokinase and tissue plasminogen activator (t-PA) (Table 37.8). All of these agents activate the body's own fibrinolytic system; they convert plasminogen to plasmin, which is the active lytic agent. Lytic therapy takes approximately 12–72 h to dissolve the clot and patients require careful monitoring during therapy (Fig. 37.18).

Ischaemia–reperfusion injury

This is a systemic process characterized by metabolic acidosis, hyperkalaemia, myoglobinaemia and pulmonary dysfunction. It is caused by the outpouring of the products of anaerobic metabolism into the venous circulation following revascularization of an ischaemic limb. It is a potentially lethal condition; patients may die from severe acidosis (lactic acid), arrhythmias (hyperkalaemia), renal failure (myoglobinaemia) or respiratory failure (activated white cells). Patients with clearly non-viable extremities (such as the patient shown in Fig. 37.5) should have early amputation to avoid this devastating complication (see Fig. 37.16a).

Results

Early aggressive treatment of acute limb ischaemia and its complications is associated with limb salvage rates of 85–90% and mortality rates of 10–15%.

The diabetic foot

Pathophysiology

Vascular disease in the patient with diabetes takes two forms. *Macroangiopathy* is atherosclerosis affecting the larger arteries, while *microangiopathy* is a thickening of the basement membrane of smaller vessels and affects the arterioles and capillaries. Microangiopathy is responsible for the renal, ophthalmic and neural complications of diabetes. There are three distinct processes involved in the aetiology of what is called the diabetic foot: ischaemia (caused by both microangiopathy and macroangiopathy), neuropathy (sensory, motor and autonomic) and sepsis (the glucose-rich environment favours bacterial growth). Undetected repeated trauma is the usual cause of ulceration in the diabetic foot. Foot problems account for 20%

05

Peripheral occlusive arterial disease at a glance

Definition

Peripheral occlusive arterial disease: a common disorder caused by acute or chronic interruption of the blood supply to the limbs, usually due to atherosclerosis

Epidemiology

- M > F before age 65
- Increasing risk with increasing age

Aetiology

- Atherosclerosis and thrombosis
- Embolism
- Vascular trauma
- Buerger's disease

Risk factors

- Cigarette smoking
- Hypertension
- Hyperlipidaemia
- Diabetes mellitus

Pathology

- Reduction in blood flow to the peripheral tissues results in ischaemia, which may be acute or chronic
- *Critical ischaemia* is present when the reduction of blood flow is such that tissue viability cannot be sustained

Clinical features

Chronic ischaemia
- Intermittent claudication in calf (femoral), thigh (iliac) or buttock (aortic occlusion)
- Cold peripheries
- Prolonged capillary refill time
- Rest pain, especially at night
- Venous guttering
- Absent pulses
- Arterial ulcers
- Gangrene over pressure points
- Knee contractures

Acute ischaemia
- Pain
- Pallor
- Pulselessness
- Paraesthesia
- Paralysis
- 'Perishing' cold
- Pistol-shot onset
- Mottling (late sign)
- Muscle rigidity (late sign)

Investigations

Chronic ischaemia
- ABI measurement (normal > 1.0) at rest and post exercise on treadmill
- Full blood count (exclude polycythaemia)
- Doppler waveform analysis
- Digital plethysmography (in diabetes)
- Per-femoral angiography

Acute ischaemia
- ECG, cardiac enzymes
- Angiography (?), may be performed peroperatively
- Find source of embolism:
    (a) Holter monitoring
    (b) Echocardiography
    (c) Ultrasound of aorta for abdominal aortic aneurysm

Management

Non-disabling claudication
- Stop smoking
- Exercise programme
- Avoid β-blockers
- Aspirin 75 mg/day
- Pentoxifylline (?)

Disabling claudication/critical ischaemia
- Balloon angioplasty ± intravascular stent
- Bypass surgery
- Amputation
- Intravenous therapy: iloprost

Acute ischaemia
- Heparin anticoagulation
- Surgical embolectomy
- Thrombolytic therapy (streptokinase, t-PA, urokinase)

Prognosis

Non-disabling claudication
- Over 65% respond to conservative management. The rest require more aggressive treatment

Disabling claudication/critical ischaemia
- Angioplasty and bypass surgery overall give good results. The more distal the anastomosis, the poorer the result

Acute ischaemia
- Limb salvage 85%
- Mortality 10–15%

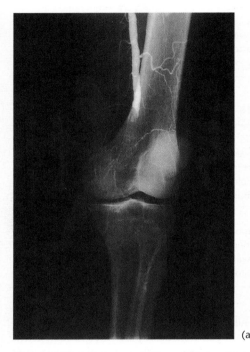
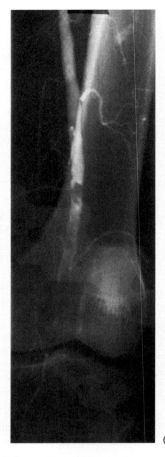
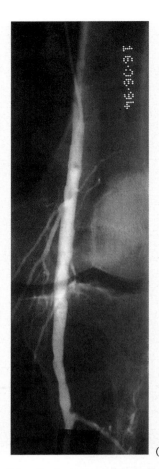

(a)   (b)   (c)

Figure 37.18 (a) Intra-arterial thrombolysis with streptokinase 500 units/h was commenced in this patient who presented with an acutely ischaemic limb due to an arterial embolus. (b) After 24 h the embolus is beginning to lyse and some contrast is seen flowing around the embolus. (c) At 72 h there is complete clot lysis with recanalization of the popliteal artery.

of all hospitalizations of diabetics and patients with diabetic foot problems are incapacitated for an average of 16 weeks.

Clinical features

The diabetic foot usually presents with predominantly neuropathic features or a combination of neuropathic and ischaemic features. Diabetic neuropathy presents with sensory disturbances, trophic skin lesions, plantar ulceration and degenerative arthropathy (Charcot's joints; Fig. 37.19). Neuropathic ulcers are deep and painless and situated on the plantar aspect of the foot or big toe. The pedal pulses are present and an obvious sensory deficit will be found in the foot. Autonomic neuropathy is manifested by a warm foot (Table 37.9).

Ischaemic diabetic foot problems present with rest pain and usually there is a history of intermittent claudication.

Ischaemic ulcers are painful and are present over the toes or pressure areas, e.g. the medial aspect of first and fifth metatarsals. The foot may be cold. Both neuropathic and ischaemic ulcers may be complicated by sepsis, characterized by cellulitis, deep tissue abscesses, osteomyelitis and, if unchecked, gangrene. Often sepsis begins as a fungal (mycotic) infection, which leads to maceration and ulceration between the toes and secondary bacterial infection. The usual organisms found are staphylococci, streptococci, colonic organisms and anaerobic bacteria. Gas gangrene may occasionally occur.

Investigation and management

The presence of a palpable pedal pulse in a warm pink foot is a good indicator of adequate perfusion and ulcers in this situation will probably heal with local treatment. Non-invasive vascular tests, including ABI, segmental pressures

05

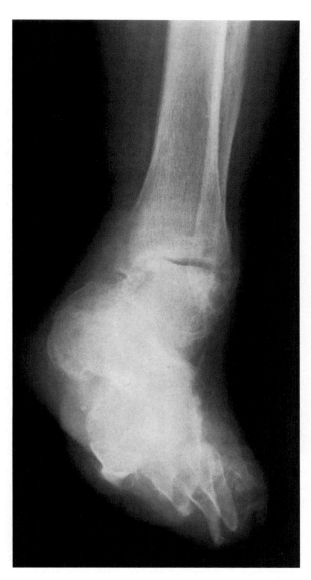

Figure 37.19 A Charcot's joint. This patient's ankle joint was completely destroyed as a consequence of diabetes.

Table 37.9 Features of neuropathic and ischaemic diabetic ulcers.

Neuropathic ulcer	Ischaemic ulcer
Painless	Painful
Normal arterial pulses	Reduced or absent pulses
Loss of sensation	Variable sensory findings
Warm foot	May be cold foot
Plantar ulceration	Toe ulceration
No intermittent claudication	Intermittent claudication
Treated by local measures	Requires reconstructive surgery

Table 37.10 Advice on foot care for diabetic patients.

Do
Carefully wash and dry feet daily
Inspect feet for injury daily
Take meticulous care of toenails
Apply antifungal powder to feet daily

Don't
Walk barefoot
Wear ill-fitting shoes
Use a hot-water bottle
Ignore any foot injury

and digital pressure, are helpful. Because of medial calcification, the arteries in diabetes mellitus are relatively incompressible, leading to falsely elevated segmental pressures, usually 20 mmHg (2.6 kPa) higher than in the non-diabetic patient. Thus, most diabetic patients require an ankle pressure of at least 80–90 mmHg (10.6–12 kPa) to heal minor amputations. Because digital blood vessels are frequently spared from medial calcification, a better estimate of foot blood flow is obtained by measuring digital blood pressure by Doppler ultrasound or plethysmography. A digital pressure of 30–40 mmHg (4–5.3 kPa) is required to heal wounds.

When non-invasive tests indicate inadequate perfusion, an arteriogram should be performed to demonstrate the entire vascular tree from the aorta to the pedal vessels. Patients with diabetes have an increased risk of contrast nephrotoxicity and they should be well hydrated before arteriography and a DSA technique should be performed.

Prevention

The old adage that prevention is better than cure is better illustrated in the management of the diabetic foot than anywhere else in medicine. A large percentage of patients with established disease ultimately have some form of amputation. Patients with diabetes should be given detailed advice on foot care (Table 37.10) and they should have rapid access to specialist care for even minor lesions.

Neuropathic disease can usually be treated by controlling infection and local removal of necrotic tissue. Plain X-rays of the foot may show gas in the tissues indicative of severe anaerobic infection, or bony destruction indicative of osteomyelitis. Intravenous antibiotics are required to control infection and the choice depends on the results of culture. Several organisms are often isolated and aerobic and anaerobic antibiotic cover has to be given, e.g. metronidazole, ampicillin and an aminoglycoside or third-

05

generation cephalosporin if there is renal impairment. Deep infection in the foot is not uncommon and should be managed by wide incision, drainage and débridement, which will often include amputation of toes or the fore-foot. These measures usually result in complete healing.

If ischaemic disease is present, an arterial bypass using autogenous saphenous vein should be performed either prior to or in conjunction with local treatment. Often a distal bypass is required, sometimes to the pedal arch, before healing of an ischaemic ulcer can occur. It should be remembered that sepsis may precipitate ketoacidosis in diabetic patients. The patient with a diabetic foot should therefore be managed jointly by surgeons and specialist physicians in diabetes mellitus.

Thromboangiitis obliterans (Buerger's disease)

Pathophysiology

Thromboangiitis obliterans is a clinical syndrome charac-terized by segmental thrombotic occlusions of small and medium-sized arteries in the lower and often the upper limb, accompanied by a dense inflammatory infiltrate that affects the arterial wall and often the adjacent veins and nerves as well. Its exact aetiology is unknown but it occurs mostly in men (90%) and there is a clear association with smoking. It is particularly prevalent in Mediterranean, East European and oriental countries.

The diabetic foot at a glance

Definition

Diabetic foot: a spectrum of foot disorders ranging from ulceration to gangrene occurring in diabetics as a result of peripheral neuropathy or ischaemia or both

Pathophysiology

Three distinct processes lead to the problem of the diabetic foot
- *Ischaemia*: caused by macroangiopathy and microangiopathy
- *Neuropathy*: sensory, motor and autonomic
- *Sepsis*: glucose-saturated tissue promotes bacterial growth

Clinical features
Neuropathic features
- Sensory disturbances
- Trophic skin changes
- Plantar ulceration
- Degenerative arthropathy (Charcot's joints)
- Pulses often present
- Sepsis (bacterial/fungal)

Ischaemic features
- Rest pain
- Painful ulcers over pressure areas
- History of intermittent claudication
- Absent pulses
- Sepsis (bacterial/fungal)

Investigations
- Non-invasive vascular tests:
  (a) ABI, segmental pressure, digital pressure
  (b) ABI may be falsely elevated due to medial sclerosis

- X-ray of foot may show osteomyelitis
- Arteriography

Management
Should be undertaken jointly by surgeon and physician as diabetic foot may precipitate diabetic ketoacidosis

Prevention
Do
- Carefully wash and dry feet daily
- Inspect feet daily
- Take meticulous care of toenails
- Use antifungal powder

Don't
- Walk barefoot
- Wear ill-fitting shoes
- Use a hot-water bottle
- Ignore any foot injury

Neuropathic disease
- Control infection with antibiotics effective against both aerobes and anaerobes
- Carry out wide local excision and drainage of necrotic tissue
- These measures usually result in healing

Ischaemic disease
- Formal assessment of the vascular tree by angiography and reconstitution of the blood supply to the foot (either by angioplasty or bypass surgery) has to be achieved before local measures will work
- After restoration of blood supply, treat as for neuropathic disease

Table 37.11 Features of thromboangiitis obliterans.

Clinical
Males under 45 years old at onset of disease
Upper and lower limb involvement
Heavy smokers
Absence of embolic source, trauma, autoimmune disease, diabetes or hyperlipidaemia

Arteriogram
Normal proximal arteries
Distal occlusions
Corkscrew collaterals

Table 37.12 Disorders associated with Raynaud's syndrome.

Abnormal circulating globulins, e.g. cold agglutinin
Arteritis, e.g. polyarteritis nodosa
Autoimmune connective tissue diseases, e.g. rheumatoid arthritis
Malignancy
Myeloproliferative disorders, e.g. leukaemia
Peripheral embolization, e.g. proximal subclavian disease
Trauma, e.g. vibrating tools

Clinical features

The symptoms and signs of thromboangiitis obliterans are those of peripheral occlusive arterial disease, but the upper limb may be involved and frequently there is superficial venous thrombosis and thrombophlebitis migrans. However, the specific criteria listed in Table 37.11 have been proposed for the diagnosis of thromboangiitis obliterans.

Investigation and management

Digital plethysmography may yield some useful information but arteriography is indicated in patients with threatened limb loss. The cornerstone of treatment is *complete cessation* of all tobacco use. No further tissue loss will occur if the patient stops smoking completely. Various drugs, including aspirin, prostacyclin analogues, nifedipine and pentoxifylline, have been tried but at present no drug is of proven benefit. Lumbar sympathectomy may occasionally be helpful but reconstructive surgery is rarely possible. Thromboangiitis obliterans is associated with a 30% major amputation rate over 5–10 years.

Raynaud's syndrome

Raynaud's syndrome is defined as episodic digital vasospasm occurring in response to cold or emotional stimulus. It usually affects the digits of the hand and is characterized by sequential colour changes in the fingers: white (ischaemia), blue (cyanosis) and red (hyperaemia). There may also be associated pain and paraesthesia.

Pathophysiology

There are two mechanisms of inducing Raynaud's syndrome in patients. *Vasospastic Raynaud's syndrome* is an exaggerated digital artery contraction in response to cold or an emotional stimulus. This contraction overcomes digital perfusion pressure, causing ischaemia. This is

the basis of the syndrome in 40% of patients. In *vaso-obstructive Raynaud's syndrome*, digital perfusion is already compromised by obstructive disease. This form of the syndrome may be associated with a long list of disorders, a small sample of which is listed in Table 37.12. However, collagen vascular disease is eventually found in about 30% of patients. Ischaemia is produced when the normal arterial contraction response to cold overcomes the compromised digital arterial perfusion pressure.

Clinical features

Vasospastic disease typically occurs in young females with a long history of cold sensitivity. There may be a positive family history and usually it is the hands rather than the feet which are affected. All or only some of the fingers may be involved. Tissue loss rarely occurs in this group and the symptoms are more of a nuisance than disabling.

Patients with vaso-obstructive disease are older and do not have a long history of cold sensitivity. The digital involvement is asymmetrical and trophic changes or tissue loss may be present in the involved digits. The patient may have other manifestations of the underlying disease.

Investigation and management

If the history and examination give a clue to the underlying pathology, then the patient should be investigated appropriately, e.g. unilateral Raynaud's syndrome should make one consider subclavian embolic disease and the patient should have arteriography. However, routine bloods should be drawn for erythrocyte sedimentation rate (ESR), serum rheumatoid factor and antinuclear antibody titre in order to screen for collagen vascular disease. If the antinuclear antibody is negative, it is most unlikely that the patient has an underlying collagen disorder such as scleroderma.

Non-invasive testing, including measurement of digital systolic pressure and plethysmographic waveform analysis, is useful for detecting vaso-obstructive disease. Abnormal vasospastic activity can be elicited by cold challenge (i.e. immersion of hands in ice water for 30 s) and

measuring the digital temperature recovery time (normally 5 min) with a thermistor.

Treatment consists of education and reassurance, especially about tissue loss and amputation. As with all other vascular disorders, patients should *stop smoking*. Cold should be avoided and the hands should be protected when cold exposure is unavoidable. Mittens should be worn in preference to gloves. Fewer than 50% of patients will require drug therapy and then only during the cold months. Several sympatholytic agents that produce vasodilatation have been used with variable results. However, many are associated with unpleasant adverse effects at the doses required to provide relief of vasospasm. The calcium channel blocking agent nifedipine, which produces vasodilatation by inhibiting calcium ingress into cells, gives good relief of symptoms at a dose of 10 mg twice or three times daily depending on the severity of symptoms. To date, nifedipine has proved the most successful drug therapy for Raynaud's syndrome. For severe prolonged attacks a course of intravenous prostacyclin analogue (iloprost) is very effective. This drug inhibits platelet aggregation, increases red cell deformability, decreases blood viscosity and affects neutrophil function. Its effect can last for up to 16 weeks. Surgical sympathectomy has little or no role in the modern management of Raynaud's syndrome.

Aneurysms

An aneurysm can be defined as a permanent localized dilatation of an artery to the extent that the affected artery is 1.5 times its normal diameter. Aneurysms commonly affect the abdominal aorta and the iliac, femoral and popliteal arteries. Cerebral and thoracic aortic aneurysms are less common and occasionally patients present with false (pseudo) aneurysms following penetrating trauma or iatrogenic trauma after arterial puncture. The majority of abdominal aortic aneurysms extend from just below the renal arteries to the bifurcation of the aorta. The incidence of abdominal aortic aneurysm (AAA) in the western world is rising and is now about 2–3% in men aged between 65 and 80 years. This increase appears to be real and not merely a reflection of increased longevity and improved methods of diagnosis. Multiple aneurysms are common in the same individual and patients with popliteal or femoral aneurysms have a 50% incidence of AAA.

Pathophysiology

AAAs are fusiform in shape and their aetiology is probably multifactorial. The traditional view is that AAA is caused by atherosclerosis and there is a higher incidence of AAA in patients with atherosclerosis and in smokers. However,

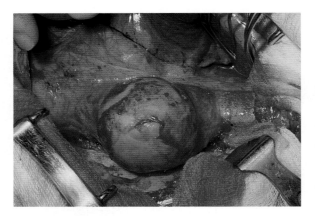

Figure 37.20 Thoracic aortic aneurysm. These aneurysms were often caused by syphilis in the past.

biochemical studies have shown that there are decreased quantities of elastin and collagen in the wall of aneurysms, suggesting abnormal collagenase or elastase activity, and there is a marked familial tendency for aneurysmal disease (an AAA will be found in 10–20% of first-degree relatives of patients with AAA).

● *Thoracic aneurysms* tend to be saccular (Fig. 37.20) and were commonly caused by syphilis.
● *Cerebral aneurysms* (*berry aneurysms*) occur usually at the circle of Willis and are due to a congenital weakness of the arterial wall.
● *Mycotic aneurysms* are caused by a bacterial aortitis secondary to septic emboli, usually from bacterial endocarditis.
● *Pseudo* or *false aneurysm* develops after penetrating trauma and is an expanding pulsating haematoma in contact with an arterial lumen (Fig. 37.21).

Once an aneurysm develops, regardless of its cause, its enlargement is governed by a simple physical law: the law of Laplace ($T = RP$). This quite simply states that the tension on the wall of an artery (T) is proportional to the radius of the artery (R) and the blood pressure (P). Put another way, the higher the blood pressure and the wider the lumen, the more likely an aneurysm is to rupture. While control of blood pressure, especially with β-blockers, may be helpful, serial ultrasound examination shows that AAAs increase in size by 0.3–0.5 cm per annum; it is only a matter of time before most aneurysms rupture. Thrombus developing within an abdominal aortic aneurysmal sac may act as a source of peripheral embolus and frequently popliteal aneurysms undergo complete thrombosis and the patient presents with an acutely ischaemic limb.

Autopsy studies indicate that 64% of patients with ruptured aneurysms die at home. These are probably patients who have free intraperitoneal rupture. Most patients who arrive at hospital have a contained leak, i.e. the aneurysm

05

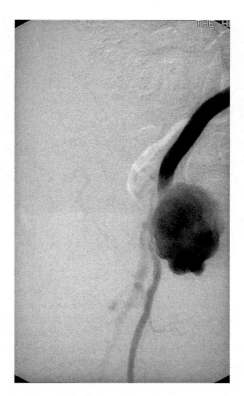

Figure 37.21 A pseudo aneurysm at the right distal anastomosis of an aortobifemoral graft bypass, such as shown in Fig. 37.13.

has ruptured through its left posterolateral wall into the retroperitoneum. The leak is tamponaded in the retroperitoneum for up to 6–10 h. This is the explanation for survival in patients with a ruptured/leaking aneurysm transferred over long distances to a vascular unit.

Screening for AAA

The arguments for screening for AAA are compelling. There is an increasing incidence of aneurysms in identifiable groups (e.g. males over 65 years old, patients with other vascular disease and first-degree relatives of patients with AAA). The mortality following ruptured AAA is 85%, while elective repair carries a 5% mortality and is followed by good quality of life. A simple non-invasive screening test is available in B-mode ultrasonography (see later).

Clinical features

Asymptomatic

The vast majority of AAAs (75%) are asymptomatic when discovered. Often they are detected at routine physical examination or during an ultrasonographic or radiological procedure for other reasons. The distinctive feature of an aneurysm on physical examination is expansile epigastric pulsation, i.e. it expands outwards when digital pressure is applied gently to each side of the mass. This finding differentiates it from transmitted pulsation such as might occur with a stomach neoplasm. It is usually possible to palpate between the upper border of the aneurysm and the costal margin and this finding indicates that the AAA is infrarenal, an important surgical consideration.

Symptomatic

AAA can cause symptoms as a result of pressure on adjacent structures, expansion, rupture or embolization. Back pain is a common symptom as the aneurysm presses on and in some cases erodes the spine. However, compression on adjacent viscera may produce abdominal or flank pain and sometimes nausea.

Rapid expansion (but not rupture) of aneurysms occurs in a small number of patients, producing severe flank or back pain. Expansion is usually the herald of rupture. Pain typical of renal colic occurring in an elderly male should be suspected to be due to an AAA until proven otherwise. Free intraperitoneal rupture is characterized by sudden abdominal pain, collapse and rapid death. Patients with ruptured/leaking aneurysms typically present with severe back or flank pain, shock and an ill-defined left-sided mass, which may or may not be pulsating.

More rarely, an aneurysm may erode into the inferior vena cava, producing a characteristic clinical picture: congestive cardiac failure, a loud abdominal bruit, lower limb ischaemia and gross oedema. An aneurysm may also erode into the duodenum, although this is more often seen as a long-term complication of aneurysm repair but it can occur primarily. These patients have a minor herald gastrointestinal bleed initially, followed 24–48 h later by exsanguinating haemorrhage.

Investigation and management

AAAs increase in size until they rupture. Two-thirds of patients with ruptured AAAs die at home; of those who reach hospital, 50% die. Thus the overall mortality for ruptured AAA is in excess of 85%. By contrast, the operative mortality for elective AAA repair is less than 5%. Therefore, elective repair of AAA should be performed. There is some argument over the size an AAA should have reached before it is repaired but most vascular surgeons now agree that an AAA of 5.5 cm should be repaired (Table 37.13). However, before elective repair the diagnosis has to be confirmed and the patient assessed for fitness for operation.

Table 37.13 Risk of rupture of abdominal aortic aneurysm related to size.

Size of aneurysm (cm)	5-year rate of rupture (%)
≥ 7.0	> 75
6.0	35
5.0–5.9	25
≤ 5.0	~ 10

Diagnostic methods

● *Physical examination* is not a very exact method of detecting or determining the size of an AAA. A plain abdominal and lateral spine X-ray may show the calcified rim of an aneurysm but it is only useful in 50% of patients (Fig. 37.22). The diagnostic methods currently used to confirm the diagnosis of AAA are ultrasonography, CT and magnetic resonance imaging (MRI).

● *Real-time or B-mode ultrasonography* is a non-invasive investigation that gives anatomical detail of the vessel wall and provides an accurate measurement of aneurysm size (Fig. 37.23). It is the modality of choice for initial evaluation of pulsatile abdominal masses and for screening of AAA. It is less reliable for evaluation of the renal and iliac arteries.

● *CT* with or without contrast enhancement provides more information than ultrasonography; in particular,

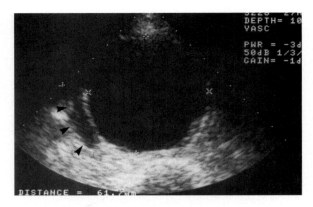

Figure 37.23 Real-time or B-mode ultrasound scan demonstrating an abdominal aortic aneurysm that measures 6.17 cm in diameter. Note the small compressed inferior vena cava to the right of the aneurysm (arrow).

the relationship between the renal arteries and the AAA can be established. This modality is also useful for detecting retroperitoneal haematoma and contained rupture (Fig. 37.24). Disadvantages are expense and radiation exposure.

● *MRI* employs radiofrequency energy and a strong magnetic field to produce images. It is probably better than CT in demonstrating involvement of branch arteries and it does not expose the patient to radiation. MRI angiography uses better signal acquisition and computerized

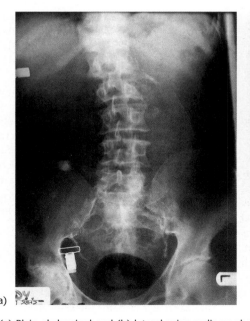

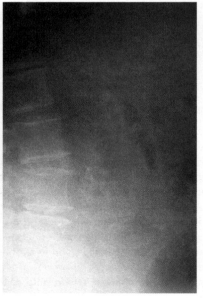

(a)

(b)

Figure 37.22 (a) Plain abdominal and (b) lateral spine radiographs may demonstrate calcification in the wall of an abdominal aortic aneurysm.

05

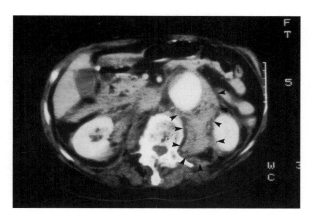

Figure 37.24 Contrast-enhanced computed tomography scan demonstrating a contained left posterior rupture of an abdominal aortic aneursym (arrows).

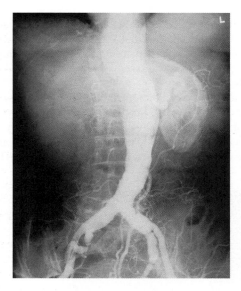

Figure 37.25 Suprarenal abdominal aortic aneurysm seen on angiography.

analysis to provide images similar to conventional angiograms. However, it is expensive and the presence of metal in the patient (e.g. metallic surgical clips) precludes its use.
● Because AAAs are often filled with layers of mural thrombus, the lumen through which the blood flows is often much smaller than the true lumen of the aneurysm. *Aortography* therefore cannot be relied upon to establish the presence or the size of an AAA. However, *arteriography* is useful for determining the relationship of the renal arteries to the AAA (Fig. 37.25) and it may be indicated if a correctable occlusive lesion is suspected, e.g. occlusive iliofemoral disease.

Table 37.14 Problems that increase mortality during elective repair of abdominal aortic aneurysm.

Cardiac
Unstable angina
Angina at rest
Congestive cardiac failure
Ejection fraction < 30%

Pulmonary
$Po_2 < 8.0$ kPa

Renal
Serum creatinine > 260 µmol/L

Preoperative assessment

Thorough preoperative evaluation is important prior to elective repair of AAA. High-risk patients are those with cardiac disease, pulmonary disease and renal disease and it is imperative to detect these patients and optimize the function of these systems prior to operation (Table 37.14).

Coronary artery disease, which may be completely asymptomatic, is prevalent in patients with AAA and most deaths occurring with elective AAA repair are due to ischaemic heart disease. Echocardiography can be used to estimate left ventricular ejection fraction at rest but stress testing (either by radionuclide scanning or dobutamine echocardiography) is probably a better means of preoperative functional cardiac assessment. If a reversible myocardial defect is detected, then coronary angiography and bypass grafting should be undertaken prior to or simultaneously with AAA repair. Similarly, patients with symptomatic carotid artery disease should be treated prior to AAA repair.

Pulmonary complications are common after aortic surgery and preoperative pulmonary function tests (especially FEV_1 and vital capacity) should be obtained. Preoperative and postoperative physiotherapy and epidural analgesia help to reduce pulmonary complications. A raised creatinine preoperatively is a risk factor for mortality after aortic surgery. In these patients maintenance of haemodynamic stability and meticulous care with fluid balance are essential. Mannitol may be needed in some patients.

Principles of aneurysm surgery
Elective repair of AAA
ENDOVASCULAR REPAIR
Surgical repair remains the standard method of treating AAA. In the last 10 years, however, there has been a huge interest in endovascular repair of AAA. In this technique a

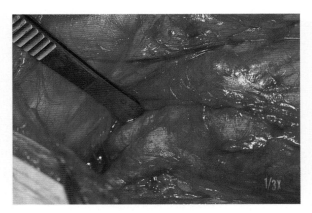

Figure 37.26 Retroperitoneal exposure of aortic and iliac artery aneurysms.

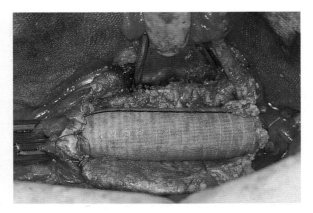

Figure 37.27 A Dacron tube graft that has been inlaid into an opened abdominal aortic aneurysm sac.

stent-graft is introduced over a guidewire into the femoral artery and, under fluoroscopic guidance, is advanced up the aorta and deployed so that the graft lies within the lumen of the aneurysm. The graft is held in position by proximal and distal attachments that are held in place by outward pressure of the stent against the aortic wall. While this technique is very attractive as it is less traumatic for the patient than the standard surgical AAA repair, there are problems with blood leaking into the aneurysm sac (*endoleaks*) and patients have to be monitored for this complication for the rest of their lives. There are many different endovascular stent designs currently available and the ideal design is yet to be determined. In addition, there are concerns that long-term follow-up may reveal problems due to deformation of the graft as the aneurysm sac shrinks. Results of randomized trials of endovascular repair vs. conventional open repair are awaited with interest.

SURGICAL REPAIR

Extensive monitoring is required during aortic surgery, as clamping and unclamping the aorta are associated with profound haemodynamic changes. Thus it is necessary to insert large-bore intravenous cannulae, urinary catheter, rectal temperature probe and central venous catheter to measure central venous pressure (CVP). Arterial pressure is also monitored by placing a catheter in the radial artery. An epidural catheter can be useful in blood pressure control during surgery as well as pain control postoperatively. Autotransfusion techniques minimize the need for blood transfusion during the operation.

The aorta can be approached through the peritoneal cavity via a midline longitudinal incision or extraperitoneally via a retroperitoneal incision (Fig. 37.26). The aim of the operation is to open the aneurysm along its

length, remove any contained thrombus and inlay a synthetic graft (Dacron) into the aorta (Fig. 37.27). The native aneurysm sac is then closed back over the graft. Occasionally, as with aortoiliac occlusive disease, a bifurcated graft has to be placed. A number of surgeons have repaired aneurysms using laparoscopic techniques or a combination of laparoscopic and open surgery with good results.

Repair of ruptured AAA

A ruptured/leaking AAA is the quintessential surgical emergency. As soon as the diagnosis is established (usually on clinical grounds but occasionally by ultrasound or CT) and blood has been sent for cross-matching, the patient is taken to the operating theatre where resuscitation continues while the monitoring lines are being inserted. The patient is not anaesthetized until the surgeons are ready to make the incision as the administration of muscle relaxant will remove the tamponading effect of the anterior abdominal wall; the aneurysm/haematoma will expand rapidly and the patient may die. The operative approach is through a midline abdominal transperitoneal incision. Once a clamp has been placed on the aorta, the operation continues as for an elective repair.

Complications of aneurysm surgery

The most frequent complications following AAA repair are cardiac, pulmonary and renal, as discussed above. However, there are some other specific problems that may occur and these are presented in Table 37.15. While a long list of complications may occur, most patients do well following elective aneurysm repair and have a good quality of life.

05

Aneurysms at a glance

Definition

Aneurysm: a permanent localized dilatation of an artery to the extent that the affected artery is 1.5 times its normal diameter. A *pseudo* or *false* aneurysm is an expanding pulsating haematoma in continuity with a vessel lumen. It does not have an epithelial lining

Sites
- Abdominal aorta and iliac, femoral and popliteal arteries
- Cerebral and thoracic aneurysms are less common

Aetiology
- Atherosclerosis
- Familial (abnormal collagenase or elastase activity)
- Congenital (cerebral or berry aneurysm)
- Bacterial aortitis (mycotic aneurysm)
- Syphilitic aortitis (thoracic aneurysm)

Risk factors
- Cigarette smoking
- Hypertension
- Hyperlipidaemia

Pathology
- Aneurysms increase in size according to law of Laplace ($T = RP$, where T is tension on the arterial wall, R is radius of artery and P is blood pressure). Increasing tension leads to rupture
- Thrombus from within an aneurysm may be a source for peripheral emboli
- Popliteal aneurysm may undergo complete thrombosis
- Aneurysms may be fusiform (AAA, popliteal) or saccular (thoracic, cerebral)

Clinical features of AAA
Asymptomatic
- Vast majority have no symptoms and are found incidentally. This has led to the description of an AAA as a 'U-boat in the belly'

Symptomatic
- Back pain from pressure on the vertebral column
- Rapid expansion causes flank or back pain
- Rupture causes collapse, back pain and an ill-defined mass
- Erosion into IVC causes congestive cardiac failure, loud abdominal bruit, lower limb ischaemia and gross oedema

Investigations
Detection of AAA
- Physical examination (not accurate)
- Plain abdominal X-ray (aortic calcification)
- Ultrasonography: best way of detecting and measuring aneurysm size
- CT: provides good information regarding relationship between AAA and renal arteries
- Angiography: not routine for AAA

Determination of fitness for surgery
- History and examination
- ECG ± stress testing
- Radionuclide cardiac scanning: multiple gated acquisition (MUGA) or stress thallium scan
- Pulmonary function tests
- Urea and electrolytes and creatinine for renal assessment

Management
- Surgical repair is the treatment of choice for AAA
- AAAs ≥ 5 cm should be repaired *electively* as they have a high rate of rupture (perioperative mortality for elective AAA repair is 5%)
- Surgical repair with inlay of a synthetic graft is the standard method of repair
- Endovascular repair with graft/stent devices is indicated in selected patients
- *Ruptured AAAs* require immediate surgical repair (perioperative mortality 50% but 70% of patients die before they get to hospital so that overall mortality is 85%)

Prognosis
- Most patients do well after AAA repair and have an excellent quality of life

05

Extracranial arterial disease

Stroke continues to be a major worldwide health problem. In the USA, approximately 500,000 people suffer from stroke annually and at any given time there are about 1,000,000 disabled stroke victims needing care, at a cost of billions of dollars. The causes of stroke are cerebral haemorrhage, lacunar infarcts, emboli from cardiac sources and extracranial arterial disease.

Pathophysiology

The carotid arterial system is the most frequent site of extracranial arterial pathology, followed by the vertebral arteries and the great vessels. Pathological lesions produce symptoms as a result of emboli or, much more rarely, flow restriction. By far the most common extracranial lesion is an atherosclerotic plaque at the bifurcation of the carotid artery. Turbulence over an irregular plaque stimulates

Table 37.15 Specific complications of abdominal aortic aneurysm (AAA) surgery.

Early complications

Bleeding
Peroperative bleeding from veins can be very troublesome but arterial bleeding is the most common reason for re-exploration in the early postoperative period

Clotting abnormalities
May develop as a consequence of bleeding, especially after repair of a ruptured AAA

Acute limb ischaemia
Usually caused by embolism of thrombus from the aneurysmal sac. The fragments enter the small distal vessel, producing the characteristic 'trash foot'

Colonic ischaemia
Occurs in 5% of patients but is usually subclinical. However, one of the internal iliac arteries or the inferior mesenteric artery should be preserved

Spinal cord ischaemia
Rarely seen after infrarenal AAA repair. It is much more likely following suprarenal or thoracoabdominal aneurysmal repair

Late complications

Graft infection
A devastating complication that occurs in 1–2% of patients. Prevention is by controlling infection preoperatively and careful antiseptic technique and prophylactic antibiotics peroperatively. Bowel surgery at the same time as aortic surgery should be avoided. Treatment of an established graft infection may require graft removal and axillobifemoral grafting. Aortic graft infection is a lethal condition

Aortoenteric fistula
The most common cause of gastrointestinal haemorrhage after an aortic graft. A minor 'sentinel' bleed may be followed by massive haemorrhage. Infection is probably the underlying cause and this complication carries a poor prognosis

Anastomotic aneurysm
A false aneurysm that develops at the site of a graft/artery anastomosis. It is most frequently seen in the groin following aortobifemoral anastomoses. Fortunately, most can be managed successfully by a local interposition graft

Sexual dysfunction
Not uncommon with aortic surgery due to damage to the autonomic nerves or the pelvic blood supply through the internal iliac arteries

platelet aggregation and cerebral or ocular symptoms develop, with embolization of the platelet aggregates into the brain or eye respectively. Bleeding into the plaque may lead to intraluminal rupture and discharge of the plaque contents (e.g. cholesterol, fibrin and atheromatous debris) as emboli into the bloodstream. Sometimes cholesterol emboli will be detected in the retinal vessel on fundoscopy. If the emboli break up quickly, then symptoms will be transient but failure of the embolic material to disperse leads to a focal infarct. TIAs often precede a major stroke.

Flow-related symptoms are rare because of the excellent collateral circulation to the brain via the circle of Willis. This explains how complete occlusion of both internal carotid arteries can occur without any symptoms in some patients. However, posture-related basilar artery insufficiency may be present in patients with diseased vertebral arteries, e.g. neck extension produces cerebellar symptoms. In the subclavian steal syndrome, the origin of the subclavian artery is occluded and the arm is perfused by reversed blood flow from the vertebral artery into the distal subclavian artery, thus 'stealing' from the posterior cerebral circulation. Symptoms may be present only when the arm is exercised.

Clinical features

Patients with carotid disease may be asymptomatic or present with TIAs or stroke. TIAs are temporary focal neurological or ocular deficits lasting not more than 24 h with complete recovery. An embolus from a carotid source will produce ischaemia of the ipsilateral cerebral hemisphere, resulting in neurological deficits on the contralateral side of the body. Symptoms may be motor (weakness, clumsiness, paralysis), sensory (numbness, paraesthesia) or speech related (receptive or expressive dysphasia). Transient visual loss is usually described by the patient as a curtain coming down over the visual field. This symptom is called *amaurosis fugax* and in contrast to the contralateral symptoms from a hemispheric deficit is due to an embolus from an ipsilateral carotid source.

Careful physical examination of the patient is very important as demonstration of a neurological deficit indicates the presence of a cerebral infarct and early cerebral reperfusion (by carotid endarterectomy) could precipitate a haemorrhage into the infarct. A bruit may be heard on auscultation over the carotid arteries but this finding is not helpful. Significant lesions can occur in the absence of a bruit and a bruit can occur in the absence of significant lesions. A bruit may even be heard in the presence of internal carotid occlusion, due to turbulent flow in a patent external carotid artery.

05

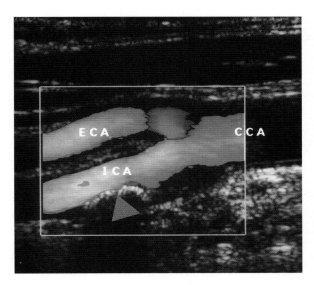

Figure 37.28 Duplex scan demonstrating a 95% stenosis at the origin of the left internal carotid artery. The acoustic shadow indicates the presence of calcification in the plaque.

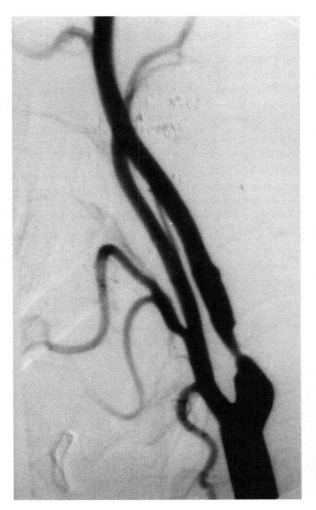

Figure 37.29 Digital subtraction carotid angiogram showing a tight stenosis at the origin of the internal carotid artery.

Investigation

Patients with TIAs, stroke and some asymptomatic patients (e.g. those undergoing coronary artery bypass surgery) should have non-invasive assessment of their carotid arteries. This is best achieved by duplex ultra-sonography or colour ultrasonography. This has replaced routine preoperative arteriography in many centres. Patients being considered for surgery may sometimes require CT brain scanning or MRI of the brain as well as carotid angiography.

● *Duplex scanning* incorporates real-time B-mode scanning, which provides anatomical detail of the structures being scanned, and Doppler ultrasonic velocimetry, which assesses blood flow through the vessel being examined (Fig. 37.28). Colour has been added to this system so that blood flowing in one direction appears red while blood flowing in the opposite direction appears blue. Duplex scanning is an excellent test for detecting and grading stenoses at the carotid bifurcation. The result is usually expressed as percentage stenosis: < 50%, 50–79%, 80–99%. Detection of a complete occlusion, i.e. 100% stenosis, can sometimes be difficult but is important to distinguish from a 99% stenosis as surgery is not indicated for complete occlusion.

● *Carotid angiography* is an invasive technique to demonstrate pathology in the carotid arterial tree (Fig. 37.29). It carries a small risk of stroke and should therefore be reserved for patients in whom surgery is contemplated; some vascular surgeons have dispensed with angiography prior to carotid endarterectomy. DSA is now the preferred angiographic technique for imaging the carotid arteries.

● *CT or MRI brain scanning* will differentiate between a haemorrhagic and an ischaemic cerebral infarct (Fig. 37.30).

Management

The management of extracranial carotid disease includes medical (antiplatelet drugs) and surgical (carotid endarterectomy) therapy. The indications for carotid endarterectomy have been clarified recently and depend

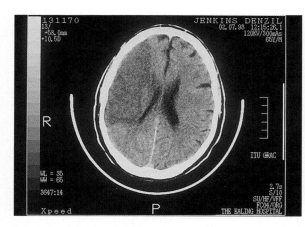

Figure 37.30 Computed tomography scan showing large infarct in right hemisphere.

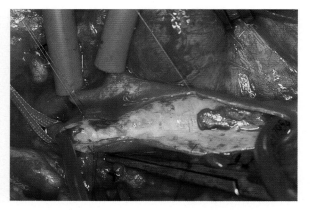

Figure 37.31 A large loose plaque in the common carotid artery seen during carotid endarterectomy.

Table 37.16 Indications for carotid endarterectomy.

Carotid distribution transient ischaemic attacks
> 70% ipsilateral stenosis
> 50% ipsilateral stenosis with ulceration

Stroke with good recovery after 1-month delay
> 70% ipsilateral stenosis
> 50% ipsilateral stenosis with ulceration

Controversial indications
Asymptomatic carotid stenosis
Vertebrobasilar symptoms with combined vertebral and
    carotid disease
Acute stroke within first few hours of occurrence

on symptoms and the degree of narrowing in the artery (Table 37.16).

Medical therapy

Medical therapy has centred on drugs that inhibit platelet aggregation for the treatment of carotid disease and full anticoagulation for cardiac sources of embolus.

Aspirin has its therapeutic action by the irreversible inactivation of platelet cyclooxygenase, preventing the production of thromboxane A_2 and thus inhibiting platelet aggregation for the duration of the life of the platelets, i.e. 7–10 days. Aspirin results in a 20–30% decrease in stroke after TIA. Doses ranging from 75 to 1300 mg/day have been given but it seems prudent to prescribe smaller doses. Dipyridamole is ineffective in preventing TIAs or strokes and its use in combination with aspirin is no better than aspirin alone. Clopidogrel is a new drug that inhibits platelet activity without interfering with the synthesis of prostaglandins or cyclooxygenase. Initial studies are promising and this drug may have a major role in the management of cerebrovascular disease. Anticoagulation with heparin and warfarin is indicated in patients who have cerebral symptoms as a result of cardiac embolic disease. The presence of a haemorrhagic infarct has to be excluded by CT before initiating therapy.

Surgical therapy

Surgical therapy consists of carotid endarterectomy (Fig. 37.31) and this has been shown to be superior to medical therapy in the management of patients with symptomatic high-grade (> 70%) carotid stenoses. The best available evidence suggests that six operations will prevent one stroke. Randomized trials have also shown the benefit of surgery for asymptomatic patients with high-grade stenosis; however, the advantage over medical therapy is marginal and 50 operations are required to prevent one stroke. The operation consists of opening the carotid bifurcation longitudinally and scooping out the atheromatous plaque from the arterial wall. The blood supply to the brain is obviously interrupted during this procedure and if there is not adequate collateral blood flow, a shunt (a simple plastic tube) has to be placed to maintain cerebral perfusion. Cerebral function is usually monitored during the operation by electroencephalography or transcranial Doppler monitoring. Carotid endarterectomy is a very successful operation but it does have a small mortality (1%) and morbidity (5%).

Similar to endovascular management of AAAs, technological advances have made possible the introduction of *carotid artery stenting*. It is yet to be proven conclusively that this technique can be safely performed with the same low morbidity rates as open surgery.

05

Extracranial arterial disease at a glance

Definition

Extracranial arterial disease: a common disorder characterized by atherosclerosis of the carotid or vertebral arteries resulting in cerebral–ocular (stroke, TIA, amaurosis fugax) or cerebellar (vertigo, ataxia, drop attacks) ischaemic symptoms

Epidemiology
- M > F before age 65
- Increasing risk with increasing age

Aetiology
- Atherosclerosis and thrombosis
- Thromboemboli
- Fibromuscular dysplasia

Risk factors
- Cigarette smoking
- Hypertension
- Hyperlipidaemia

Pathophysiology
- Most common extracranial lesion is an atherosclerotic plaque at the carotid bifurcation. Platelet aggregation and subsequent *platelet embolization* cause ocular or cerebral symptoms
- Symptoms due to *flow reduction* are rare in the carotid territory but vertebrobasilar symptoms are usually flow-related. Reserved flow in the vertebral artery in the presence of ipsilateral subclavian occlusion leads to cerebral symptoms as the arm 'steals' blood from the cerebellum (subclavian steal syndrome)

Clinical features
- Cerebral symptoms (contralateral):
  - (a) Motor (weakness, clumsiness or paralysis of a limb)
  - (b) Sensory (numbness, paraesthesia)
  - (c) Speech-related (receptive or expressive dysphasia)
- Ocular symptoms (ipsilateral): amaurosis fugax (transient loss of vision described as a veil coming down over the visual field)
- Cerebral (or ocular) symptoms may be transitory (TIA is a focal neurological or ocular deficit lasting not more than 24 h) or permanent (stroke)
- Vertebrobasilar symptoms: vertigo, ataxia, dizziness, syncope, bilateral paraesthesiae, visual hallucinations
- A bruit may be heard over a carotid artery but is an unreliable indicator of pathology

Investigations
- Duplex scanning: B-mode scan and Doppler ultrasonic velocimetry; method of choice for assessing degree of carotid stenosis
- Carotid angiography: not essential any more prior to surgery
- CT or MR brain scan: demonstrates the presence of a cerebral infarct

Management
Medical therapy
- Aspirin (75 mg/day) inhibits platelet aggregation for the life of the platelet
- Ticlopidine and clopidogrel have similar actions to aspirin
- Anticoagulation is indicated in patients with cardiac embolic disease

Surgical therapy
- Carotid endarterectomy (+ aspirin)

Indications for carotid endarterectomy
- Carotid distribution TIA or stroke with good recovery after 1-month delay:
  - (a) > 70% ipsilateral stenosis
  - (b) > 50% ipsilateral stenosis with ulceration
- Asymptomatic carotid stenosis > 80%
- Carotid endarterectomy has about 5% morbidity and mortality

Arterial miscellany

Renovascular hypertension

Renovascular hypertension (RVH) is the cause of hypertension in approximately 5–10% of all hypertensive patients and is commoner in patients with severe hypertension. The essential lesion in RVH is a stenosis of one or both renal arteries. RVH affecting children and young women is often caused by fibromuscular dysplasia, while RVH in the elderly is usually due to atherosclerosis.

Hypertension results from activation of the renin–angiotensin system in unilateral disease and, in addition, expansion of plasma volume in bilateral disease. A renal artery bruit may be heard but the diagnosis is made by isotope renography, angiography and renal vein renin assays.

Treatment consists of dilating, removing or bypassing the stenosed segment of renal artery. Percutaneous transluminal angioplasty is successful for some lesions, particularly fibromuscular dysplasia. The surgical approaches to RVH are thromboendarterectomy or aortorenal bypass. Improved renal function and beneficial blood pressure

05

response can be expected in most patients and some, especially those with fibromuscular dysplasia, will be cured following surgical therapy.

Mesenteric ischaemia

Acute mesenteric ischaemia is caused by sudden occlusion of the superior mesenteric artery due to thrombosis or embolism, or an acute thrombosis of the mesenteric veins. Non-occlusive mesenteric ischaemia occurs when there is splanchnic vasoconstriction in response to hypotension. Clinically the patient presents with abdominal pain, which is very severe and often disproportionate to the degree of tenderness on examination. Initially there is a paucity of abdominal findings but later the signs of an acute abdomen will develop and there may be gastrointestinal bleeding. Most patients have a leukocytosis and severe metabolic acidosis. These are very ill patients. Therapy is directed at resuscitating the patient, treating the underlying cause, e.g. cardiac failure, and revascularizing or resecting the ischaemic bowel. Despite aggressive management, the mortality from acute mesenteric ischaemia is still over 70%.

Chronic mesenteric ischaemia is 'intermittent claudication' or 'angina' of the bowel. Symptoms develop after meals, when the increased energy demands of the bowel for digestion cannot be met by an impoverished blood supply. The result is postprandial abdominal pain. Atherosclerotic involvement of the mesenteric vessels is almost always the cause. The anatomical diagnosis is made by angiography. Symptoms can be relieved by an aorto-superior mesenteric artery bypass in properly selected patients.

Thoracic outlet compression syndrome

The subclavian artery passes out of the chest through a crowded narrow space over the first rib and under the clavicle. The artery is surrounded by the brachial plexus and passes over the first rib between the attachments of the anterior scalene muscle (in front) and the middle scalene muscle (behind). Narrowing of this space results in compression of the artery and the brachial plexus. This may be caused by a cervical rib, an extra rib cephalad to the first rib, or more commonly by congenital fibrocartilaginous bands. Long-standing compression on the artery may lead to poststenotic dilatation and aneurysm formation.

Symptoms are often neurological and are made worse when the arms are abducted and externally rotated ('hands-up' position). The first presentation may be a digital embolus from a subclavian aneurysm. An Adson manoeuvre (assessment of the radial pulse during hyperabduction and external rotation of the arm) and an elevated arm stress test (rapid opening and closing of the fists while the arms are held overhead) are the two most useful clinical tests. Objective investigations include cervical spine X-ray for detection of arthritic/degenerative vertical spine changes, thoracic inlet X-ray for the presence of a cervical rib, chest X-ray to detect apical lung pathology, nerve conduction studies, duplex ultrasonography and arteriography of the abducted externally rotated arm. Relief of symptoms can be obtained by scalenotomy or scalenectomy and resection of a cervical rib if present. If a subclavian aneurysm is present, resection is mandatory.

VENOUS DISEASE

While congenital abnormalities of veins exist (Klippel–Trenaunay syndrome; Fig. 37.32) and occasionally veins are involved by inflammation (thrombophlebitis), by far the greatest venous problem is thrombosis (phlebothrombosis) and its sequelae. Acute thrombosis manifests clinically as deep vein thrombosis (DVT) or, more seriously, iliofemoral thrombosis (Fig. 37.33). Migration of the thrombus to the lungs (pulmonary embolism) may be fatal, while local destruction of the valves in the deep venous system of the leg results in venous hypertension and ulceration (postphlebitic limb; Fig. 37.34). Chronic venous insufficiency is a source of considerable morbidity

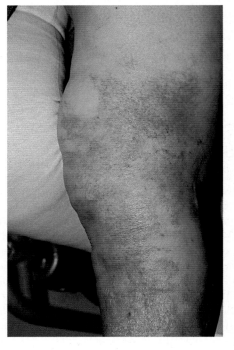

Figure 37.32 Skin changes seen in a patient with Klippel–Trenaunay syndrome.

05

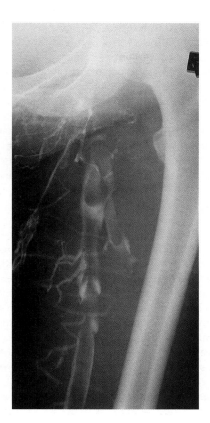

Figure 37.33 Ascending venogram demonstrating filling defects in the femoral vein due to thrombus.

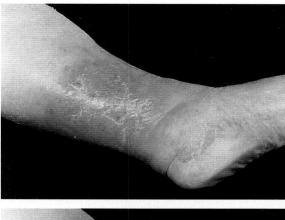

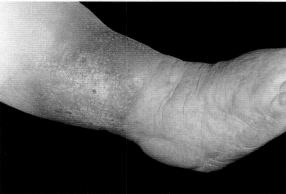

Figure 37.34 Typical changes seen in a postphlebitic limb.

and is a major healthcare problem. Finally, varicose veins continue to plague humanity as they have done for centuries.

Venous thrombosis

Pathophysiology

Blood is maintained in its normal state by the interaction of several processes that prevent bleeding (haemostasis) and, simultaneously, prevent the accumulation of clot within the circulation (anticoagulation/fibrinolysis). Haemostasis is achieved by contraction of the blood vessel wall, platelet adhesion and aggregation, and coagulation, which may be activated by the intrinsic and extrinsic pathways. The major naturally occurring anticoagulant is antithrombin III; others of less importance are proteins C and S. Fibrinolysis is achieved by the action of plasmin, which is activated by plasminogen activators, the most important of which is t-PA (Fig. 37.35).

Virchow suggested that venous thrombosis resulted from a triad of factors: stasis, endothelial injury and hypercoagulability of the blood. Venous thrombosis usually begins with aggregation of platelets in vein valve pockets, where maximum stasis occurs, or on a damaged vein wall. Activation of the clotting cascade (e.g. by surgical trauma) produces fibrin at a rate that cannot be controlled by the anticoagulant/fibrinolytic system and a venous thrombus develops.

Risk factors for venous thrombosis include increasing age, trauma, immobilization, sepsis, obesity, heart disease, malignancy, pregnancy and oestrogen therapy, and previous history or family history of venous thromboembolic disease (Table 37.17). A number of congenital deficiencies of anticoagulant proteins have been recognized. Antithrombin III deficiency is the most common of these, with an incidence of 1 in 2000–5000 of the general population. Heparin resistance may be the first manifestation of this disorder. Fibrinolytic deficiencies also occur.

DVT, which is very common in both medical and surgical patients, can have devastating consequences. An analysis by the National Hospital Discharge Survey suggests that DVT accounts for 10,000 deaths per annum in the USA. The natural history of DVT includes:

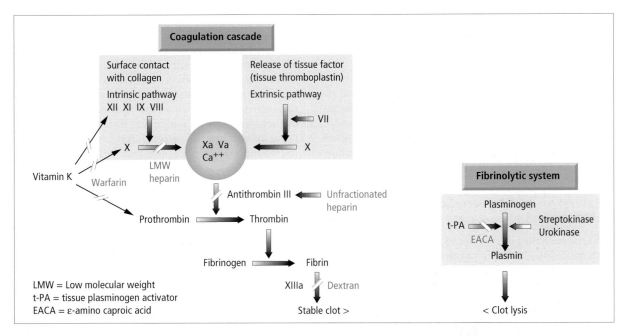

Figure 37.35 Schematic representation of the clotting and lytic systems and the sites of action of the commonly used anticoagulants and thrombolytic agents. Low-molecular-weight heparin acts on factor Xa; unfractionated heparin acts on antithrombin III).

Table 37.17 Risk factors for deep vein thrombosis.

Age (> 40 years)
Prior history of deep vein thrombosis
Surgery
Trauma
Sepsis (particularly with endotoxin)
Recumbency/immobilization
Obesity
Malignancy
Heart disease
Pregnancy
Oestrogen administration
Inflammatory bowel disease
Blood disorders
   Thrombocytosis
   Polycythaemia
   Antithrombin III deficiency
   Fibrinolytic deficiencies

● complete resolution (the vein recanalizes and the valves remain competent);
● pulmonary embolism (clot migrates and causes a pulmonary infarct);
● development of chronic venous insufficiency (either the vein does not recanalize at all or the valves are destroyed when recanalization occurs).

The importance of DVT as a cause of mortality and morbidity cannot be overstated.

Clinical features

DVT in the lower limbs is often silent and is clinically apparent in only 40% of cases. Moreover, only 50% of patients with clinical suspicion of DVT actually have venous thrombosis. However, when symptoms and signs are present two groups can be defined:

1 Patients with DVT in the calf veins may have calf tenderness, ankle oedema, low-grade pyrexia and increase in leg temperature. Calf pain on passive dorsiflexion (Homan's sign) is a well-known but dangerous physical sign. Attempting to elicit it may cause a pulmonary embolus.

2 Iliofemoral thrombosis, which occurs predominantly on the left side, produces pain, extensive pitting oedema and blanching of the limb. This is called *phlegmasia alba dolens* and because it was often seen in puerperal women it was also called the 'milk leg of pregnancy'. Progression of thrombosis impedes most of the venous return, producing a painful blue leg (*phlegmasia caerulea dolens*). Without aggressive treatment this will lead to venous gangrene.

Investigation

Because the clinical diagnosis of DVT is so inexact and its

05

complications so serious, considerable effort has gone into the development of diagnostic tests for DVT.

D-dimers

D-dimers are breakdown products of coagulation and are invariably raised in DVT. The limitation of this investigation is that it is very non-selective, i.e. it will have raised values in many conditions other than DVT. Nevertheless it is a useful adjunct because if the D-dimers level is normal, it effectively rules out a diagnosis of DVT.

Bilateral ascending venography (phlebography)

This has been the gold standard for the diagnosis of DVT. The patient is tilted to an angle of 45–60° with the feet down. A dorsal vein in the foot is cannulated and 200 mL of dilute contrast is injected. Venous tourniquets are placed at the knee and ankle to direct the contrast preferentially into the deep venous system. The result will give information about the site, size and extent of thrombosis and its propensity for embolization. Disadvantages are that venography is expensive and invasive (see Fig. 37.33). Duplex scanning is now the investigation of choice in many centres.

Doppler ultrasound

Venous obstruction distorts blood flow and this can be detected using a Doppler velocimeter probe. A normal vein gives a phasic signal with respiration. Compression of the vein distal to the probe causes flow augmentation, while compression proximally stops flow and abolishes the signal. With DVT the respiratory variation is lost and there is no flow augmentation on distal compression. While this test can be very accurate, it is very dependent on the operator.

Duplex imaging

The combination of Doppler ultrasound velocimetry and B-mode ultrasound images (i.e. duplex imaging) is a very accurate non-invasive method for diagnosing DVT, especially in the proximal veins. The anatomy of each segment of the deep venous system is defined by B-mode imaging and thrombus can be detected by altered echogenicity. Doppler evaluation is performed as before. Both Doppler ultrasound and duplex imaging are very useful in pregnancy where venography is contraindicated. Duplex scanning may eventually displace venography as the gold standard for the diagnosis of DVT.

^{125}I-Fibrinogen scanning

The incorporation of radioactive fibrinogen into a forming thrombus is the basis of this test. An injection of ^{125}I-fibrinogen is given and counts are obtained from marked locations on the legs and expressed as a percentage of the radioactivity measured over the heart. An increase of 20% or more indicates an underlying thrombus. Thrombi in pelvic veins cannot be detected. It is useful as a screening test and in assessment of methods of DVT prophylaxis, but is of little value in the clinical setting.

Impedance plethysmography

This test assesses the change in volume in a limb by measuring changes in electrical resistance. Two pairs of electrodes are placed on the calf and a pneumatic veno-occlusive tourniquet is placed around the thigh. The normal leg will rapidly swell when the tourniquet is inflated and rapidly return to normal when the occlusive tourniquet is released. Both responses are abolished or considerably slowed if DVT is present. Disadvantages are that it is cumbersome to use and it cannot detect small non-occlusive thrombi. More recently, photoplethysmography and air plethysmography have been used to assess deep vein function.

Management

Prophylaxis (see Chapter 5)

Treatment of established DVT

The aims of management of an established DVT are to minimize the risk of pulmonary embolism, limit further thrombosis, facilitate complete resolution of the DVT and avoid a postphlebitic limb. The availability of low-molecular-weight heparins has prompted a number of recent clinical trials that have changed the management of DVT dramatically. Specific measures are anticoagulation, thrombolysis and thrombectomy.

Anticoagulation

The mainstay of therapy for DVT is adequate anticoagulation. This is achieved initially with low-molecular-weight heparin, which prevents clot propagation, and subsequently warfarin, which protects against recurrent thrombosis. In the past, initial therapy with intravenous heparin was undertaken in hospital with bedrest for 4–5 days. This has been superseded by outpatient treatment with low-molecular-weight heparin at a dose adjusted according to patient weight, which has been shown to be both safe and

effective. An added advantage of low-molecular-weight heparin is that laboratory monitoring of activated partial thromboplastin time (APTT) is unnecessary. Complications of heparin therapy include bleeding, hypersensitivity and thrombocytopenia. Bleeding should be managed by cessation of heparin. Rarely is the specific antagonist protamine sulphate required. Heparin-induced thrombocytopenia is due to an immune reaction and is rapidly reversed by stopping the drug. Patients on heparin should have regular platelet counts performed.

Oral anticoagulation with warfarin is begun as soon as the diagnosis is confirmed, and concurrently with subcutaneous heparin. It usually takes several days to achieve the optimal antithrombotic effect, i.e. a prothrombin time (PT) of 1.5–2 times the control value. Complications of warfarin therapy include bleeding, dermatitis and skin necrosis and several commonly used drugs (e.g. analgesics, alcohol) interact with warfarin. Most problems resolve with discontinuation of the drug and, if necessary, vitamin K or fresh frozen plasma (contains clotting factors) can be administered to restore the PT. After an episode of uncomplicated DVT, anticoagulant therapy should be continued for 6 months.

Thrombolysis

While the use of thrombolytic agents (streptokinase, urokinase and t-PA) to dissolve intravenous thrombus is theoretically attractive, in practice these agents have very little role in the management of venous thrombosis. Their use does not give better results than adequate anticoagulation with heparin and haemorrhage is a major complication. Only in patients with phlegmasia alba/caerulea dolens should their use be considered, and then only in consultation with a haematologist. Streptokinase is associated with allergic reactions in 10% of patients.

Thrombectomy

This is achieved by a direct operation on the common femoral vein and the removal of thrombus with a Fogarty catheter. There is a high incidence of rethrombosis and, as with thrombolysis, removal of the thrombus does not improve the outlook for valve function. The procedure is seldom performed today and is reserved for patients with impending gangrene.

Pulmonary embolism

Pulmonary embolism is the most serious complication of venous thrombosis. Approximately 1 in 5 patients with a DVT will develop pulmonary embolism and 50% of those will be fatal. If no prophylaxis is given, 0.5–3.4% of patients will have a fatal pulmonary embolism following major surgery of any kind. Pharmacological prophylaxis (see earlier) with heparin or dextran reduces the incidence of fatal pulmonary embolism by 50%.

Pathophysiology

The lower limb is the source of embolus in 85% of patients; in 10% the embolus arises in the right atrium, while in the remaining 5% it arises in the pelvic veins and vena cava. Thrombi that become detached from their site of origin migrate through the great veins, through the chambers of the right heart and lodge in the pulmonary arteries. The result depends on the extent of the obstruction of the pulmonary circulation. Thus a large embolus which blocks the major pulmonary arteries interrupts the circulation and causes death. A massive pulmonary embolus has been defined as embolic obstruction of 40–50% of the pulmonary vasculature. Smaller emboli interrupt the circulation to isolated areas of lung tissue and produce infarction of those areas. As the infarcted lung tissue rubs against the parietal pleura, pleuritic pain is produced and clinically pleural rub can be detected on auscultation. An exudate from the infarct may collect in the pleural cavity and be detected as a pleural effusion. Bleeding into and destruction of the infarct lead to haemoptysis and superimposed infection may result in a lung abscess. Multiple small emboli may cause sufficient destruction to produce pulmonary hypertension and, as a consequence, right heart failure (cor pulmonale).

Clinical features

Symptoms

The classical presentation of massive pulmonary embolism is crushing substernal chest pain, dyspnoea, circulatory arrest and death. Pulmonary embolism was said to occur at 7–10 days postoperatively but in reality it may occur at any time in the postoperative period. Non-fatal emboli also present with sudden chest pain (occasionally epigastric pain) and dyspnoea. The chest pain is classically pleuritic (i.e. made worse by deep inspiration) and is followed by haemoptysis in only about 15% of patients. Less obvious presentations include unexplained pyrexia, tachycardia or tachypnoea in the postoperative or postpartum period.

Physical examination

Signs of DVT may be present but usually examination of the legs is unrewarding. Tachycardia and tachypnoea are frequently observed and the patient may be cyanosed if

05

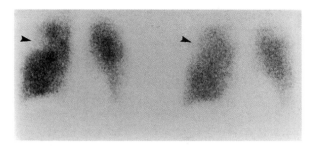

Figure 37.36 Ventilation–perfusion scan showing a perfusion defect (left) in the absence of a ventilation defect (right) in the right upper lobe, indicating a pulmonary embolism.

there is a large embolus. A pleural friction rub (which has been likened to the sound of a finger being slid hard over a pane of glass) may be present with peripheral emboli. Rales may be heard over the infarcted area and a pleural effusion may be detected in some patients.

Investigations

The ECG and chest X-ray may provide useful pointers to the diagnosis of pulmonary embolism. The classical ECG (S wave in lead I and Q waves and inverted T waves in lead III; S1QT3) is found in only 10–20% of patients. Decreased vascularity, dilated pulmonary veins or a pleural effusion may be seen on the chest film. If infarction is present, wedge-shaped infiltrates may be detected. However, the chest radiograph rarely shows specific changes. Most laboratory tests are unhelpful but a low Pao_2 (< 10.4 kPa, 80 mmHg) with hypocarbia ($Paco_2$ < 4.6 kPa, 36 mmHg) and alkalosis (pH > 7.44) may indicate embolism. A firm diagnosis of pulmonary embolism requires more specific investigation.

Ventilation–perfusion (V/Q) lung scan

Ventilation–perfusion scanning is an isotope study designed to identify ventilation–perfusion mismatch in lung tissue. In the normal lung the perfusion pattern should match the ventilation pattern exactly. Two isotopes are used. Technetium-labelled microspheres or macroaggregates are injected intravenously into the patient and its distribution throughout the lung detected by a gamma-camera. As there is no circulation through the area of lung tissue blocked by a pulmonary embolus, no radioactivity will be emitted from that area and it will appear as a filling defect on the perfusion scan (Fig. 37.36). The patient then inhales a radioactive gas (krypton, xenon) or aerosol (technetium-labelled diethylenetriaminepentaacetic acid or DTPA) and its distribution

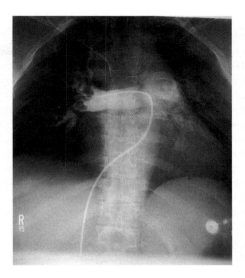

Figure 37.37 Pulmonary angiogram in a patient with a pulmonary embolus. Note the filling defect at the bifurcation of the right pulmonary artery.

throughout the airways is again detected by a gamma-camera. The ventilation scan in acute pulmonary embolism is usually normal. In areas of atelectasis or pneumonia the perfusion scan is normal, while the ventilation scan will demonstrate filling defects.

Pulmonary angiography

Pulmonary angiography provides the most effective means of diagnosing pulmonary embolism and is most helpful in diagnosing the presence and extent of massive pulmonary embolus. It is indicated if the diagnosis cannot be established by any other means and is essential prior to embolectomy or thrombolytic therapy. Pulmonary arteriography is achieved by inserting a catheter through the right heart into the pulmonary artery and injecting contrast directly into the pulmonary circulation (Fig. 37.37). Pressure measurements in the pulmonary circulation can be obtained simultaneously and haemodynamic monitoring established. Recently, spiral CT has been shown to be very effective in diagnosing pulmonary embolism, is non-invasive and has already replaced pulmonary angiography in many centres (Fig. 37.38).

Management

The therapeutic approaches to pulmonary embolism include anticoagulation, thrombolysis and physical removal of the embolus by open operation or embolectomy.

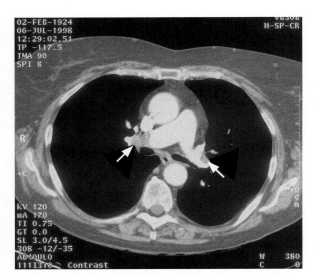

Figure 37.38 Spiral computed tomography scan of a patient with a pulmonary embolus.

Table 37.18 Contraindications to thrombolytic therapy.

Intracranial or spinal cord pathology
Recent brain, eye or spinal cord injury
Malignant hypertension
Recent major surgery or trauma
Active internal bleeding
Active peptic ulcer
Recent childbirth
Pregnancy

Streptokinase, urokinase and t-PA are the three agents used for thrombolysis. Allergic reactions may occur with streptokinase and it should be avoided if the patient has had a recent streptococcal infection or has received streptokinase within 6 months.

Anticoagulation

The majority of patients with pulmonary embolism are treated with anticoagulation therapy alone. The lung has the highest concentration of t-PA in the body and thus the capacity for spontaneous thrombolysis of pulmonary emboli is high. A large bolus dose of heparin (10,000–15,000 units) should be administered initially and thereafter heparin is administered as a continuous infusion at a dose to maintain the APTT between 50 and 80 s. Continuous infusion is associated with fewer bleeding complications than intermittent bolus injections, although infusion of up to 1500 units/h may have to be given. Uncomplicated pulmonary emboli may be safely treated with subcutaneous low-molecular-weight heparin, administered once or twice daily. Warfarin therapy can be instituted early and there is no advantage in continuing heparin therapy for 7 or 10 days. Warfarin therapy is continued for 6 months but in patients who have idiopathic pulmonary embolism or those who suffer recurrent pulmonary embolism lifelong anticoagulation is indicated.

Thrombolytic therapy

Thrombolytic therapy results in greater improvement and normalization of the haemodynamic responses to pulmonary emboli than heparin alone. Thrombolytic therapy should be considered in all patients with an established diagnosis of pulmonary embolism with haemodynamic compromise. However, there are many contraindications to its use (Table 37.18).

Pulmonary embolectomy

Attempts to remove pulmonary emboli by thoracotomy and direct operation on the pulmonary arteries (Trendelenburg procedure), with or without bypass, are associated with a high mortality from uncontrollable pulmonary parenchymal haemorrhage. More recently, pulmonary emboli have been aspirated from the pulmonary arteries using a special steerable cup catheter introduced via the femoral vein and steered through the right heart into the pulmonary artery. The embolus is suctioned into the cup and the whole apparatus is withdrawn through the femoral venotomy. Several passages may be required to clear an embolus and a filter (see later) should be left in the vena cava at the end of the procedure to prevent recurrent embolism. This technique should be considered in haemodynamically unstable patients in whom thrombolytic therapy is contraindicated. With improved skill and advances in interventional radiology, better outcomes from massive pulmonary emboli are reported.

Recurrent pulmonary embolism

Adequate anticoagulation is usually effective in managing pulmonary embolism and usually prevents further embolization from a DVT. However, if recurrent embolization occurs during *adequate* anticoagulation or there is a contraindication to anticoagulation, then surgical prophylaxis is indicated. The operative placement of clips (e.g. De Weese clip) on the inferior vena cava (IVC) has been superseded by the transvenous placement of filters (e.g. Greenfield filter; Fig. 37.39), which are positioned in the IVC below the level of the renal veins. The filter traps migrating thrombus and protects the pulmonary circulation from embolism.

05

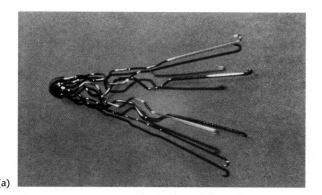

(a)

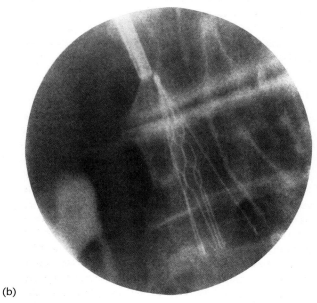

(b)

Figure 37.39 (a) Greenfield filter. (b) This Greenfield filter has just been placed into the inferior vena cava to prevent migration of thrombus from the leg veins to the pulmonary circulation.

Post-thrombotic (postphlebitic) limb

The post-thrombotic limb is a common sequel to DVT and is a major source of morbidity and expense worldwide. A knowledge of venous anatomy and physiology is essential to understand this condition.

Venous anatomy of the lower limb

Venous blood is drained from the lower limb by deep and superficial vein systems. The deep system consists of the soleal plexus of veins in the soleal muscle, and the popliteal and femoral veins. The long and short saphenous veins make up the superficial system and they drain into the femoral and popliteal veins respectively. The superficial system also communicates with the deep system through a series of perforating veins along the medial side of the leg at the mid-thigh and at 5, 10 and 15 cm above the medial malleolus. Normal venous flow is unidirectional from the foot to the groin and from the superficial to the deep venous systems. Contraction of the soleal and gastrocnemius muscles during walking compresses the blood and pumps it towards the heart. Reverse flow is prevented by the action of numerous valves throughout both systems. One of the most important is at the junction of the saphenous and femoral veins. Trouble begins when the valves are destroyed or become incompetent.

Pathophysiology of post-thrombotic limb

The venous pressure at the ankle while standing is approximately 125 cmH$_2$O, which corresponds with the distance from the diaphragm to the ankle (125 cm). On walking, this pressure falls to 30% of the resting pressure. This response is dependent on calf muscle contraction and competent valves to prevent blood regurgitating into the deep system. If the deep valves are incompetent or, worse, if the deep system is occluded as a sequela to DVT, venous ankle pressure will remain elevated and will actually rise with calf compression, producing venous hypertension. Continued back-pressure on the valves in the perforator veins renders them incompetent, resulting in inefficient drainage of blood from the superficial system. This may manifest as secondary varicose veins.

It has been suggested that venous hypertension results in loss of plasma protein (especially fibrin) from the capillaries in the tissues around the ankle; pericapillary fibrin cuffs develop that interfere with the transfer of oxygen to the tissues, leading to hypoxic injury. A second theory suggests that trapping of white cells and release of cytokines may be the underlying cause of tissue injury. A reduction in fibrinolytic activity in the tissues and blood has also been observed in patients with venous hypertension. Whatever the exact mechanism of injury, the result is the same: varicose eczema, lipodermatosclerosis and, eventually, venous ulceration.

Clinical features

The typical post-thrombotic sequelae appear at 2–30 years after the thrombotic episode. Consequently, many patients do not remember that they had a thrombus and many patients may have had a silent DVT in any case. The patient may complain of an aching sensation in the limb. The post-thrombotic leg is typically chronically swollen and may have secondary varicose veins with incompetent perforators. Usually there is varicose eczema above the medial malleolus (see Fig. 37.34). This is due to haemosiderin

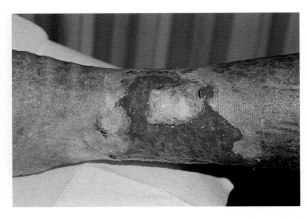

Figure 37.40 A typical venous ulcer (the term 'varicose ulcer' is incorrect).

deposition and indicates chronic venous stasis and red cell destruction in the tissues. The subcutaneous tissues may be thickened and contracted around the ankle (lipodermatosclerosis), giving the characteristic inverted champagne-bottle appearance to the leg. The most serious problem associated with the post-thrombotic leg is venous ulceration (Fig. 37.40). The term 'varicose ulcer' is a misnomer as many patients do not have varicose veins.

Venous ulceration is most commonly seen in elderly female patients. The ulcer is usually on the medial side of the leg just above the ankle. They can be of any shape and size but are commonly shallow with a sloping edge. A raised or thickened edge in a chronic venous ulcer should raise the suspicion of malignant change (Marjolin's ulcer). The base of the ulcer is usually covered with strawberry red granulation tissue covered by a variable amount of slough and often the surrounding tissues are indurated and pigmented. Occasionally, cellulitis may be present.

Investigation

Modalities used are venography, duplex scanning and plethysmography. Proper investigation of a patient with a suspected post-thrombotic limb is important as treatment will depend on the findings.

- *Ascending venography* has been the gold standard against which other non-invasive techniques are measured. It will demonstrate the anatomy of the deep venous system, determine the site of any obstruction that may be present and, if the veins are patent, determine the competence of the deep and perforating valves.
- *Doppler ultrasound* can be used to assess the deep venous system. If an obstruction is present, the same findings are elicited as in acute DVT (see earlier). However, if the deep system is patent but incompetent, then compression distal to the probe produces minimal flow

augmentation and compression proximally produces flow augmentation as the blood regurgitates down the leg. Perforator vein competence can easily be assessed by placing the probe over the perforator, occluding the superficial vein above and below the probe and compressing the leg. Flow augmentation indicates an incompetent perforator.

- *Duplex scanning* provides additional anatomical information and has replaced venography as the investigation of choice in many centres.
- *Photoplethysmography*, in which changes in the volume of the microcirculation are detected by the transmission of light through the superficial layers of the skin, indicates the overall effect of venous insufficiency.
- *Ambulatory venous pressure* at the ankle can also be measured using direct cannulation. High venous pressure during calf exercise is typical of a post-thrombotic limb.

Management

Patient education is important and time is well spent in explaining the disease process to the patient. Patients will then understand why there is no 'quick-fix' operation for their disease, why they should elevate their legs above the level of the heart when sitting or reclining and why they must put on elastic compression stockings before they get out of bed in the morning. Compression is the mainstay of non-operative treatment and elastic graduated compression stockings and compression bandaging are the principal methods of applying compression (Fig. 37.41). A graduated stocking is one that applies the greatest pressure at the ankle and progressively less pressure up the limb. Elevation reduces venous pressure, promotes reabsorption of oedema fluid, and prevents the action of the calf muscle pump and thus the development of ambulatory venous hypertension.

Leg ulcers

When managing a patient with a presumed venous ulcer, it is important first to exclude other causes of leg ulcer, including arterial disease, vasculitis and diabetes mellitus. In some patients there may be a combination of pathology (e.g. venous hypertension and arterial insufficiency) and all elements will require treatment. However, an established venous ulcer can be healed with careful treatment. Surrounding cellulitis should be treated with a course of systemic antibiotics and after gentle débridement the ulcer should be treated with a mild antiseptic solution until clean, when saline dressings should be used. Elevation and compression bandaging are essential in the management of venous ulcers. An effective bandaging regimen known as four-layer bandaging has revolutionized the management of this difficult problem

05

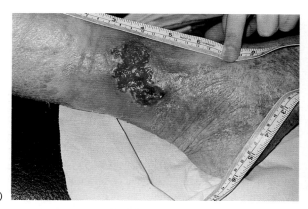

(a)

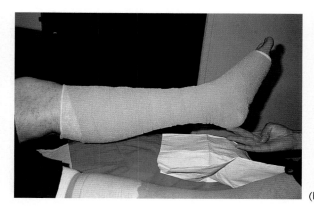

(b)

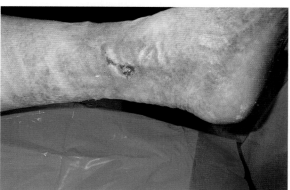

(c)

Figure 37.41 Four-layer compression bandaging has revolutionized the management of venous ulcers: (a) typical venous ulcer prior to treatment; (b) four-layer bandage in place; (c) the ulcer after 12 weeks of bandaging.

(Fig. 37.41b). In the USA a gauze boot (Unna's boot) impregnated with zinc oxide, gelatin and glycerin, wrapped around the lower leg, is frequently used to treat venous ulceration. The boot has to be changed twice weekly.

Several drugs have been used in the treatment of venous ulceration. Stanozolol, an anabolic steroid that enhances fibrinolysis, helps to reduce lipodermatosclerosis but does not improve ulcer healing. Defibrotide, a new antithrombotic and profibrinolytic agent, improves ulcer healing in combination with compression therapy. Prostaglandin E$_1$, which has to be given parenterally, and pentoxifylline (400 mg t.d.s.) have both improved ulcer healing in combination with compression therapy.

Surgical intervention is indicated if a large varicose vein is seen draining from the ulcer. Before ligating it, however, it has to be established that the deep system is patent. If it is not, then ligating the varicose vein may disrupt the only venous drainage of the limb. Occasionally, perforating veins under the ulcer are ligated and, even more rarely, attempts at deep vein valve reconstruction or valve transplantation from the axillary vein are undertaken. A recent advance is the development of subfascial endoscopic perforator surgery where an endoscopic camera is inserted into the plane between the muscle compartments and the overlying fascia in the leg. This allows the identification and ligation of perforator veins with surgical clips by a minimally invasive method. However, the role of this technique in the management of venous ulcers is uncertain.

05

Deep vein thrombosis at a glance

Definition

Deep vein thrombosis: a condition in which the blood in the deep veins of the legs or pelvis clots. Embolization of the thrombus results in a *pulmonary embolus* (PE), while local venous damage may lead to chronic venous hypertension and the *postphlebitic limb* (PPL)

Epidemiology

- DVT is extremely common among medical and surgical patients, affecting 10–30% of all general surgical patients over 40 years who undergo a major operation
- PE is a common cause of sudden death in hospital patients (0.5–3% of patients die from PE)

Aetiology
Risk factors
- Increasing age > 40 years
- Immobilization
- Obesity
- Malignancy
- Inflammatory bowel disease
- Anticoagulant protein (e.g. antithrombin III, protein C, protein S) deficiency
- Trauma
- Sepsis
- Heart disease
- Pregnancy/oestrogens

Virchow's triad
- Stasis
- Endothelial injury
- Hypercoagulability

Pathology
- Aggregation of platelets in valve pockets (areas of maximum stasis or injury)
- Activation of clotting cascade producing fibrin
- Fibrin production overwhelms the natural anticoagulation (fibrinolytic) system
- Natural history: complete resolution, PE or PPL

Clinical features
DVT
- Asymptomatic
- Calf tenderness
- Ankle oedema
- Mild pyrexia
- Phlegmasia alba/caerulea dolens

PE
- Substernal chest pain
- Dyspnoea
- Circulatory arrest
- Pleuritic chest pain
- Haemoptysis

PPL
- History of DVT
- Aching limb
- Leg swelling
- Venous eczema
- Venous ulceration
- Inverted-bottle-shaped leg

Investigations
DVT
- Duplex imaging
- Ascending venography

PE
- ECG (S1QT3)
- Chest X-ray
- Blood gases
- Ventilation–perfusion lung scan
- Spiral CT scanning
- Pulmonary angiography

PPL
- Ascending ± descending venography
- Duplex scanning
- Plethysmography
- Ambulatory venous pressure

Management
Prophylaxis against DVT
Indications
- Presence of risk factors (see above)

Methods
- Mechanical: compression (TED) stockings
- Pharmacological: subcutaneous low-molecular-weight heparin, warfarin 1 mg/day, dextran 70,500 mL/day i.v.

Definitive treatment
DVT
- Anticoagulation for 6 months:
    (a) Low-molecular-weight heparin
    (b) Warfarin (check efficacy with PT)
- (Thrombolysis)
- (Thrombectomy)

PE
- Anticoagulation for 6 months:
    (a) Low-molecular-weight heparin
    (b) Warfarin (check efficacy with PT)
- Thrombolysis
- Pulmonary embolectomy
- IVC filters for recurrent PE

PPL
- Limb elevation
- Compression
- Four-layer bandaging to achieve ulcer healing
- Graduated compression stockings to maintain limb compression
- (Venous valve reconstruction)

05

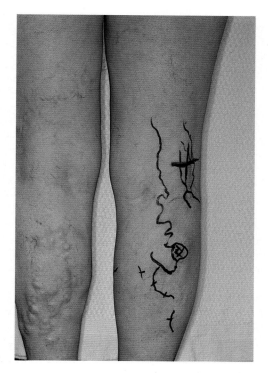

Figure 37.42 Varicose veins.

Varicose veins

Varicose veins are tortuous, dilated, prominent superficial veins in the lower limb, often in the anatomical distribution of the long and short saphenous veins. Descriptions of varicose veins exist from the earliest medical writings. They are exceedingly common and in the western world are found in half of the adult male and two-thirds of the adult female population. However, only 10–15% of those affected have symptoms or complications (Fig. 37.42).

Pathophysiology

While the exact aetiology of varicose veins remains elusive, various types have been recognized:
- primary or familial (most common type);
- secondary or post-thrombotic (see earlier);
- congenital malformations of veins alone (Klippel–Trenaunay syndrome) comprising varicose veins, limb hypertrophy and portwine staining (see Fig. 37.32);
- congenital malformations of veins in combination with arteriovenous malformations (Parkes Weber syndrome);
- varicosities deliberately created by arteriovenous fistulae in patients with renal failure in order to facilitate repeated cannulation for haemodialysis.

Primary or familial varicose veins usually appear early in life and more than one family member is affected. Preg-

nancy is often the precipitating event. Progesterone, the principal hormone of pregnancy, causes passive dilatation of veins, facilitating the development of varicose veins. Secondary varicose veins occur with the post-phlebitic limb and are usually caused by perforator valve failure.

Venous valve failure is the essential factor in development of varicose veins. In most patients with primary disease the process begins with failure of the valve at the saphenofemoral junction. The pressure in the femoral vein is then transmitted into the proximal long saphenous vein, causing dilatation and progressive distal valvular incompetence. As with the post-thrombotic limb, an incompetent long saphenous vein disrupts the capillary circulation around the ankle, which may lead to varicose eczema, lipodermatosclerosis and sometimes ulceration. However, unlike the post-thrombotic limb, surgical removal of the varicose vein reverses the microcirculatory changes and allows the ulcer to heal.

Clinical features

Varicose veins may be totally asymptomatic but common symptoms include dull aching leg pain and a sensation of heaviness in the leg. The symptoms are absent in the early morning and are most severe in the evening. They are exacerbated by long periods of standing and relieved by lying down, leg elevation and elastic support stockings. Cutaneous itching and night cramps may also occur. Patients frequently seek treatment because of poor cosmetic appearance and occasionally they may give a history of repeated superficial thrombophlebitis. The complications of varicose eczema, venous ulceration or haemorrhage may also be presenting features. Haemorrhage caused by local trauma to large varicosities may result in spectacular blood loss. In this situation, initial management consists of simply eliminating hydrostatic pressure by lying the patient supine and elevation of the affected limb.

The patient should be examined standing up. On inspection, obvious varicose veins are seen usually, but not exclusively, associated with the tributaries of the long and short saphenous systems. Pigmentation or ulceration may be present around the ankle. Many patients have unsightly spidery vascular markings composed of small clumps of dilated superficial venules. These are not really varicose veins and camouflage is the best policy in their management as no therapy is satisfactory.

Varicose veins feel tense on palpation and a cough impulse may be elicited at the saphenofemoral junction. A *saphena varix* is a soft compressible dilatation of the saphenous vein just adjacent to the saphenofemoral junction. A thrill may be elicted over a saphena varix on coughing (Cruveilhier's sign) and an impulse will be felt if the saphenous vein distally is percussed. Palpation along the

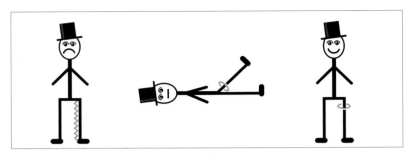

Figure 37.43 Trendelenburg test. A tourniquet is applied to the elevated limb just below the groin. The patient stands up. If there is no filling of the veins below the tourniquet, then the incompetence is above the tourniquet, i.e. at the saphenofemoral junction.

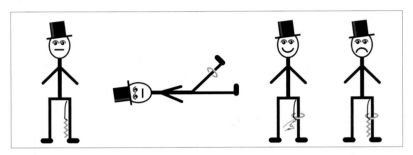

Figure 37.44 To identify an incompetent perforator in the lower leg, a tourniquet is placed on the elevated limb just above the suspected incompetent perforator. Digital pressure directly over the perforator with the tourniquet in place prevents reflux. However, the vein fills immediately on removal of the digit.

medial side of the leg may reveal defects in the deep fascia at the site of perforating veins.

Tourniquet tests identify clinically the sites of reflux from the deep to the superficial vein systems. A tourniquet is applied to the elevated limb just below the groin. The patient stands up. If there is no filling of the veins below the tourniquet, as in the vast majority of patients with varicose veins, then the incompetence is above the tourniquet (i.e. at the saphenofemoral junction; Fig. 37.43), while rapid filling of the veins below the tourniquet indicates short saphenous vein incompetence or an incompetent perforator distally. To identify such an incompetent perforator a tourniquet is placed on the elevated limb just above the suspected incompetent perforating vein. Digital pressure directly over the perforator with the tourniquet in place prevents reflux. However, the vein fills immediately on removal of the digit (Fig. 37.44). Direct digital pressure over the saphenofemoral junction preventing retrograde filling of the saphenous vein is called the Trendelenburg test. Assessment of varicose veins has become much more precise with the advent of hand-held Doppler probes and, in complex cases, plethysmography and duplex scanning. Regurgitation following calf compression can easily be detected over the saphenofemoral junction using a hand-held Doppler probe.

Investigation

While most patients with simple varicose veins do not need elaborate investigation, any suggestion that they have a post-thrombotic limb warrants full investigation, as described previously. However, because autogenous vein should be preserved for peripheral or coronary artery bypass grafting, it is important to evaluate patients who have equivocal clinical findings. The most useful methods to determine whether there is saphenofemoral or perforator incompetence are duplex scanning and photoplethysmography. Detection of reflux with a Valsalva manoeuvre is a very specific test for venous valvular insufficiency. Rarely, varicography is used to detect incompetent perforators. With more precise diagnosis, more precise treatment can be planned and valuable venous segments can be preserved.

Management

Many patients simply need to be advised to elevate their legs when sitting and to wear elastic stockings. The indications for more specific treatment, i.e. sclerotherapy or surgery, are appearance, pain and heaviness, superficial thrombophlebitis and external bleeding. Impending or established ulceration in association with varicose veins is an indication for ablative treatment provided the patient does not have a postphlebitic limb.

Sclerotherapy

Injection sclerotherapy is useful for treating small varicose veins below the knee but is not suitable for large varicosities, particularly above the knee. The principle of the technique is that sclerosant (sodium tetradecyl) injected into a vein produces a superficial thrombophlebitis and obliteration of the vein. Compression with a foam pad has to be applied over the injection site and compression bandaging has to be maintained for 3–6 weeks. Patients are also

advised to walk several miles per day. Anaphylaxis and local ulceration are complications of sclerotherapy, and recurrence is common.

Surgical ablation

This is quite a successful treatment for varicose veins. Prior to surgery, with the patient standing up, the varicose veins to be removed should be marked with an indelible marker by the surgeon who is going to perform the operation. Long saphenous incompetence is present in the majority of cases. A formal exploration of the saphenofemoral junction has to be made and the long saphenous vein (and all its tributaries) disconnected from the deep system. If a long segment of vein is varicose, it may be stripped out (from above downwards to avoid lymphatic and cutaneous nerve damage) and the best results are achieved by stripping the above-knee segment of the long saphenous vein. The veins below the knee are removed by making a small stab incision of only 2–3 mm over the vein. A hook or fine artery forceps is used to hook the vein out through the wound, where it is avulsed. Steri-strips or fine sutures are used to close the skin. If short saphenous incompetence is present, it is useful to identify and mark the skin over the saphenopopliteal junction by duplex scanning preoperatively. Postoperatively, the leg is bandaged firmly from the toes to the groin and an elastic support stocking is applied at 24 h. The bandages may be removed at a week, when stitches are removed, but the stocking should be worn for several weeks. Patients are encouraged to walk a little every day and should keep their legs elevated when sitting.

Varicose veins at a glance

Definition

Varicose veins: tortuous, dilated, prominent superficial veins in the lower limbs, often in the anatomical distribution of the long and short saphenous veins

Epidemiology
- Very common in the western world, affecting about 50% of the adult population

Pathophysiology
- *Venous valve failure*, usually at the saphenofemoral junction (and sometimes in perforating veins), results in increased venous pressure in the long saphenous vein with progressive vein dilatation and further valve disruption

Aetiology
- Primary or familial varicose veins
- Pregnancy (progesterone causes passive dilatation of veins)
- Secondary to postphlebitic limb (perforator failure)
- Congenital: Klippel–Trenaunay syndrome, Parkes Weber syndrome
- Iatrogenic: following creation of an arteriovenous fistula

Clinical features
- Asymptomatic
- Cosmetic appearance
- Dull aching leg pain ⎫ symptoms worse in the evening
- Heaviness in the leg ⎭ or on standing for long periods
- Itching and eczema
- Superficial thrombophlebitis
- Bleeding
- Saphena varix
- Ulceration

Investigations
- Clinical assessment by Trendelenburg tourniquet tests
- Doppler velocimetry
- Duplex scanning

Management
Symptomatic veins should be treated

General
- Avoid long periods of standing
- Elevate limbs
- Wear support hosiery

Specific
Injection sclerotherapy with sodium tetradecyl
- Suitable for small veins and usually only below the knee
- Patients are encouraged to walk several miles per day
- Anaphylaxis and local ulceration may occur

Surgical ablation
- With the patient standing, the dilated veins are carefully marked with an indelible marker
- Saphenous vein is surgically disconnected from the femoral vein and the perforators are also ablated
- The elongated veins are removed via multiple stab incisions and long segments above the knee are removed using a vein stripper
- Postoperatively, compression stockings are worn for several weeks and exercise is encouraged
- Surgery is the most effective treatment for large varicose veins but recurrence rates are high

Venous miscellany

Superficial thrombophlebitis

Superficial thrombophlebitis is characterized by local inflammation of a segment of superficial vein. It may occur in a segment of varicosed long saphenous vein and is usually non-infective. A common iatrogenic cause is prolonged cannulation (< 72 h) of a forearm vein for intravenous administration of fluids or drugs. Administration of acidic fluids (e.g. dextrose and some antibiotics) predisposes to thrombophlebitis. It may also follow injection of contrast material into a vein. Thrombophlebitis migrans is a condition of recurrent episodes of superficial thrombophlebitis and is associated with malignancy and collagen vascular disease. With thrombophlebitis the vein feels like a cord and the surrounding skin is red and tender. Aseptic thrombophlebitis, which is common, does not require antibiotic therapy and rest but instead local compression, analgesia and gentle mobilization. Occasionally, thrombophlebitis of the long saphenous vein in the upper thigh may extend towards the saphenofemoral junction and in this circumstance it is necessary to perform a saphenofemoral ligation to prevent DVT occurring. Iatrogenic thrombophlebitis usually resolves following removal of the cannula. However, septic thrombophlebitis, either bacterial or fungal, seen commonly in intravenous drug addicts, can be a serious condition requiring antibiotics and excision of the infected peripheral vein.

Subclavian or axillary vein thrombosis

Subclavian vein thrombosis is most likely to be due to cannulation of the vein for diagnostic or therapeutic purposes (e.g. cardiac catheterization or indwelling cannula). Subclavian or axillary vein thrombosis can occur as a primary event in a fit athletic person following prolonged arm exercise (effort thrombosis). Repetitive intermittent venous compression is thought to be the precipitating cause. The patient presents with aching arm pain, swelling and bluish discoloration of the arm. Prominent superficial collateral veins are seen over the shoulder, arm and chest wall. Treatment consists of arm elevation and anticoagulation and an underlying cause, e.g. a cervical rib, should be sought. There is a 10% incidence of pulmonary emboli with subclavian vein thrombosis.

Superior vena cava thrombosis

Superior vena cava (SVC) obstruction may be secondary to a neoplastic process in the mediastinum, usually bronchogenic carcinoma. In the past, mediastinal saccular syphilitic aneurysms were a common cause of SVC obstruction and occasionally fibrosing mediastinitis is a cause. Symptoms include headache, swelling of the face and eyelids and chemosis. Lying down exacerbates the symptoms. Prominent neck veins, cyanosis and oedema are frequent findings. The diagnosis is usually obvious from the clinical findings but venography is sometimes required. Patients with SVC obstruction due to malignancy usually have a very poor prognosis but palliation can sometimes be achieved with radiotherapy and, more recently, self-expanding stents have been inserted transvenously into the obstructed SVC.

LYMPHATIC DISEASE

The lymphatic system consists of a network of capillary-like vessels that coalesce to form collecting lymphatics which, like veins, have valves and drain via the lymph node groups, the cysterna chyli and thoracic duct into the venous circulation. The functions of the lymphatic system are:
- to drain some of the macromolecular protein (mostly albumin) lost from the capillary circulation;
- to remove bacterial and foreign material from tissues;
- to transport specific materials (e.g. vitamin K and long-chain fatty acids) from the gut.

The spectrum of lymphatic disease consists of inflammatory conditions (e.g. lymphangitis), failure of lymph drainage (lymphoedema) and tumours of the lymphatic system. Lymphangitis is usually caused by streptococcal infection and often follows cellulitis.

Lymphoedema

Lymphoedema results from the accumulation of protein-rich fluid in the tissues and is caused by failure of lymph transport. Lymphangitis is a frequent complication and produces fibrosis, which makes the oedema worse. Lymphoedema may be primary, for which no obvious cause can be discerned (Fig. 37.45), or secondary, when lymphoedema follows a well-defined event (Table 37.19).

Primary lymphoedema

This type of oedema is congenital in origin but three distinct times of onset are recognized.
- *Congenital lymphoedema* presents at birth. Milroy's disease is a specific subgroup of congenital oedema characterized by hypoplasia of the lymphatic trunks and a familial sex-linked incidence.
- *Lymphoedema praecox* presents in adolescence and accounts for 80% of all patients with primary lymphoedema. It is not known why this congenital condition presents in a delayed fashion.

05

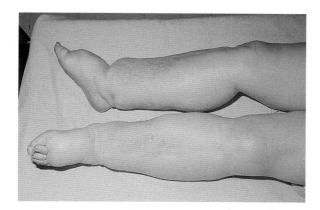

Figure 37.45 Primary lymphoedema.

Table 37.19 Classification of lymphoedema.

Lymphoedema	Lymphatic defect
Primary	
Congenital (Milroy's disease)	Aplasia
Praecox	Hypoplastic
Tarda	Hyperplastic/varicose
Secondary	
Infection*	
Surgery	Hyperplastic/varicose
Radiation therapy	
Trauma	

* Filariasis, tuberculosis, lymphogranuloma, actinomycosis, chronic lymphangitis.

- *Lymphoedema tarda* presents in middle age.

  Patients with primary lymphoedema have three different congenital lymphatic abnormalities:
- aplasia (15%), in which there are no lymphatic trunks;
- hypoplasia (70%), in which there are only a few rudimentary trunks;
- hyperplastic (15%) or varicose, in which there are several dilated lymphatic trunks secondary to lymphatic valve incompetence.

Secondary lymphoedema

The removal or destruction of inguinal or axillary nodes by surgery, radiation therapy, infection or tumour infiltration results in secondary lymphoedema. The most common worldwide cause of secondary lymphoedema is infestation of the lymph nodes by the filarial worm *Wuchereria bancrofti*. Anatomically, secondary lymphoedema has a hyperplastic (varicose) pattern.

Clinical features

Lymphoedema usually starts at the ankle and ascends the leg over a period of months, giving a characteristic 'tree-trunk' appearance. Lymphoedema can be differentiated from venous oedema by the absence of pigmentatory changes. Pitting can occur with lymphoedema but is related to the degree of fibrosis present. The diagnosis can be established clinically and detailed investigations such as lymphangiography should be reserved for those patients where surgery is being considered.

Management

There is no cure for lymphoedema and the chronic nature of this condition should be explained to the patient. The aims of therapy are to preserve skin quality, soften subcutaneous tissue, prevent lymphangitis and reduce limb size. The key elements of treatment are limb elevation, graduated compression hosiery (which needs to be renewed every 3 months) and external pneumatic compression (e.g. Flowtron pump).

Surgical therapy is only considered in a small number of patients for recurrent lymphangitis, functional impairment and cosmesis. Attempts to anastomose lymphatic channels to veins have not been very successful and most surgery now involves excision of subcutaneous tissue and redundant skin.

Tumours of lymphatics

Lymphangioma

Lymphangiomas are benign tumours of lymphatics that are usually present at birth. These are sequestered portions of the lymphatic system that can produce lymph. The most common is cystic hygroma (see Fig. 1.8), which is found typically around the head and neck and presents as a soft, non-tender, cystic mass that transilluminates. Treatment is by surgical excision.

Lymphangiosarcoma

Lymphangiosarcoma is an aggressive malignant tumour of the lymphatics that is associated with lymphoedema. It generally appears 10 years after the onset of lymphoedema and has an average survival rate of 19 months. Lymphangiosarcoma presents as a reddish-purple discoloration or nodule and early radical amputation remains the mainstay of therapy.

CARDIAC SURGERY

The successful use of cardiopulmonary bypass in the

1950s revolutionized cardiac surgery. While the heart was paralysed, the patient's blood could be moved around the circulation and oxygenated. For the first time the heart became amenable to surgical treatment, just like any other organ. Heart surgery has continued to expand, to the extent that now many cardiac operations are regarded as routine and carry acceptably low risks. In this section, the more common aquired cardiac surgical problems and the principles underlying their treatment are presented with special reference to basic pathophysiology.

Evaluation of the patient

Despite the development of sophisticated invasive and non-invasive techniques by which the heart and its pathology may be investigated, a highly important means of evaluation, both before and after operation, remains the clinical history and examination. It should be remembered that investigations demonstrate the patient's haemodynamics at only one point in time, often extending to no more than a few heart beats. A better understanding of the patient's ability to function may be obtained from a careful history and detailed physical examination.

Clinical assessment

General medical history and risk factors

Routine cardiac surgery is now commonplace, and the mortality for operations such as coronary artery bypass graft is about 1–4%. Nonetheless, it is still a major undertaking and the low mortality is a reflection of improved surgical techniques, technological advances in cardiopulmonary bypass, myocardial preservation techniques and, at least in part, identification of risk factors for morbidity and mortality. These are of paramount importance if complications are to be avoided and adequate prophylaxis and early institution of therapy are to be carried out (Table 37.20).

Symptoms

The common symptoms of cardiac disease are listed in Table 37.21. For the patient with cardiac disease these symptoms should be specifically sought; at the same time, assessment should also be made of the duration of symptoms and whether they are stable or have recently undergone a deterioration.

Chest pain (Table 37.22)
Chest pain is a common feature of cardiac surgical disease. *Angina pectoris* is pain derived from the heart itself when the oxygen demand of the myocardium exceeds supply.

Table 37.20 Important questions to ask the patient about to undergo cardiac surgery.

General
Family history of coronary artery disease
Smoking, calculated as number of pack-years (see Chapter 38)
Hypercholesterolaemia (> 6.5 mmol/L or treated)
Advancing age
Alcoholism
Ankylosing spondylitis, Marfan's syndrome, osteogenesis imperfecta, Ehlers–Danlos syndrome

Endocrine
Diabetes (diet-controlled, oral therapy or insulin)
Hypothyroidism

Gastrointestinal tract
History of peptic ulcer, hiatus hernia, gallstones
Diverticular and inflammatory bowel disease
Previous abdominal surgery

Respiratory
Clinical chronic obstructive airways disease
Asthma
History of tuberculosis

Cardiac
Hypertension (140/90 mmHg or treated)
Previous myocardial infarction
Previous cardiac or thoracic surgery
History of rheumatic fever/scarlet fever
History of bacterial endocarditis
Known congenital valve abnormality

Vascular
Carotid bruit, previous transient ischaemic attack or cerebrovascular accident
Peripheral vascular disease
Previous deep vein thrombosis or pulmonary embolus
Varicose veins

Renal
Functioning transplant
Acute or chronic renal failure: dialysis
Creatinine ≥ 200 μmol/L

Table 37.21 Symptoms of cardiac disease.

Chest pain
Dyspnoea
Syncope
Palpitations
Fatigue
Haemoptysis
Oedema

05

NYHA 1	No limitation of ordinary physical activity
NYHA 2	Ordinary physical activity causes discomfort
NYHA 3	Moderate to great limitation of ordinary physical activity
NYHA 4	Unable to perform any physical activity without discomfort

Table 37.22 New York Heart Association (NYHA) grading of cardiac symptoms.

In the assessment of a patient whose predominant features are *angina* or *dyspnoea*, a system of grading by severity of symptom occurrence has been instituted by the NYHA. It represents a means by which subsequent improvement or deterioration may be measured

The causes are given below but it is not uncommon for these factors to coexist.
● Commonly, angina results from coronary artery stenosis due to atheroma.
● However, angina may also occur when the oxygen supply is insufficient to meet the demands of an increase in cardiac muscle mass as a result of aortic stenosis or systemic hypertension. In these cases the increased bulk of the myocardium is due to left ventricular hypertrophy.
● A low cardiac output, which may occur as a result of ischaemic damage or cardiomyopathy, may also cause angina.

Angina is a strangulating pain felt substernally that may radiate to the arm, jaw or neck. The pain is often described as 'tight' or 'crushing'. It is commonly exacerbated by exercise and cold weather and relieved by rest and sublingual nitrates. It may also occur at night and wake the patient from sleep, and it may occur after eating. The clinician should always be vigilant because angina may often manifest itself atypically, for example as epigastric pain and thus mimic the pain of a peptic ulcer or biliary colic. An episode of pain lasting longer than a few minutes and associated with nausea or vomiting may signify that the angina has become unstable or that the patient has sustained a myocardial infarction. Any new episode of chest pain, particularly in an individual with risk factors for atherosclerosis, should be considered due to cardiac ischaemia until proven otherwise.

Severe constant pain felt in the anterior chest with radiation through to the back is characteristic of an acute dissection of the thoracic aorta and is often associated with hypertension.

Dyspnoea (see Table 37.22)

In the cardiac patient, dyspnoea results from loss of elasticity of the lungs secondary to passive congestion. This may be due to left ventricular failure or valvular obstruction. In such cases congestion is passive, in contrast to active congestion seen with increased pulmonary blood flow (from a left-to-right shunt) in congenital heart disease. Congested lungs become turgid and stiff and increased effort is required to inflate them.

● *Orthopnoea* is defined as breathlessness on lying flat. When a patient adopts a recumbent position there is an increase in venous return to the heart that cannot be adequately dealt with by a failing or obstructed heart. In addition, in the supine position, there is 'splinting' of the diaphragm by the abdominal viscera and the volume of potential lung expansion is reduced. It is useful to enquire how many pillows a patient sleeps with, as this helps to reduce the splinting effect.
● *Paroxysmal nocturnal dyspnoea* is breathlessness that wakes the patient from sleep. Typically, the patient describes 'gasping for air' and may open a window to try to ease the distress. The mechanism is similar to orthopnoea but because sensory awareness is reduced during sleep, severe interstitial and alveolar oedema can accumulate.
● *Wheezing* may occur in association with the above due to bronchial endothelial oedema (cardiac asthma), and the sputum may be tinged with blood.

Syncope

Syncope of cardiac origin is sudden and of brief duration.
● Aortic stenosis causes syncope on exercise. It may be due to decrease in cerebral blood flow, as peripheral resistance falls secondary to exercise, or to high intraventricular pressures generated within the left ventricle.
● Pulmonary and mitral stenosis (when associated with pulmonary hypertension) may also cause syncope on exercise. The fixed low cardiac output that results from these conditions is unable to increase to accommodate the demands of exercise.
● Arrhythmias and atrioventricular block, themselves caused by ischaemic heart disease, may also cause syncope. Syncope due to heart block is known as Stokes–Adams syndrome.
● Rarely, tumour or clot within the left atrium may cause a low cardiac output that secondarily leads to diminished ventricular filling and may present with syncope on exercise.

Palpitations

A palpitation is an increased awareness of the heart beat. It may be the result of extrasystoles or tachyarrhythmia; an

example of the latter is atrial fibrillation, which often occurs in patients with mitral stenosis due to enlargement of the left atrium. Atrial fibrillation may be a further manifestation of ischaemic heart disease. Palpitations may also be due to an increased force of contraction, as occurs in aortic regurgitation, due to volume loading of the left ventricle.

Fatigue

Fatigue consists of tiredness and lethargy. As an indicator of heart disease *per se*, the symptom is of little use. However, commonly in patients with severe heart disease, fatigue is experienced as a result of a poor cardiac output leading to reduced cerebral and peripheral perfusion. β-Blockers used in the treatment of hypertension or angina may also cause fatigue.

Haemoptysis

A variety of underlying pathological processes may cause haemoptysis (see Chapter 38). Cardiac causes include those listed below.
● Mitral stenosis may cause haemoptysis due to rupture of congested bronchial capillaries or pulmonary hypertension causing pulmonary congestion.
● Pulmonary apoplexy is the effortless sudden coughing of a large volume of bright-red blood. It occurs in cases of pulmonary venous hypertension and the event acts as a physiological venesection.
● The pink blood-stained frothy sputum of pulmonary oedema is a common feature of cardiac failure and of sinister significance.
● Pulmonary infarction, which may occur as a result of pulmonary embolism, is another cause of haemoptysis. Pulmonary venous or arterial thrombosis as a result of a large left-to-right shunt is a rarer cause.

Oedema

This is the result of salt and water retention consequent upon heart failure. Retained fluid will accumulate in the feet and ankles of ambulant patients, and over the sacrum in bedridden patients. It generally worsens during the day and may be absent on initial rising as the fluid is resorbed on lying down. In severe cases, ascites, pleural effusions, leg and thigh oedema may occur.

General physical examination

A general assessment of the patient is made first. This should include an assessment of whether the patient is well or unwell and whether the patient is anaemic, jaundiced, obese or cachectic. The patient's pulse rate, blood pressure, temperature and respiratory rate should be noted. Examination of a patient's teeth is important when implanting a new heart valve as poor dental hygiene is a common source of valve infection. The liver should be palpated to see if it is enlarged, tender and, in the case of tricuspid regurgitation, pulsatile. The spine and limbs should be examined for pitting oedema of the sacrum and ankles, and the lung bases should be auscultated for crackles after the patient has coughed.

Physical examination of the cardiovascular system

Clubbing

The common cardiac causes of clubbing are subacute infective endocarditis and cyanotic congenital heart disease. Clubbing takes many months to develop and is therefore not seen in infants or neonates, or in acute endocarditis. The mechanism remains obscure; clubbing might be due to hepatic impairment or occur as part of the condition of hypertrophic pulmonary osteoarthropathy. Another possible mechanism is that clubbing is due to a blood-borne factor either produced in or not deactivated by the lungs; this would explain clubbing in right-to-left shunts where a portion of the blood effectively bypasses the pulmonary circulation. Clubbing appears first in the thumb and the great toe (see Fig. 38.1).

Cyanosis

The dusky blue discoloration of the skin and mucous membranes is due to the presence of unoxygenated haemoglobin (at least 5 g/dL). It is uncommon in the anaemic patient and is more common in the polycythaemic patient. Cyanosis may be central or peripheral. *Central cyanosis* occurs when the tongue, lips and conjunctivae are cyanosed. Its presence indicates the mixing of venous and arterial blood. It is improved by breathing oxygen. *Peripheral cyanosis* is observed in the extremities and is due to vasoconstriction and stasis of blood in these areas, with a concomitant increased oxygen extraction. It will occur when there is inadequate peripheral circulation, as in shock, exposure to cold and severe low cardiac output (e.g. cardiac failure).

Arterial pulse

The rate, rhythm, character and volume of the arterial pulse should be examined.

RATE
The radial pulse should be examined for not less than 30 s. *Bradycardia*, a pulse rate of less than 60 beats/min, could be physiological or due to heart block or drugs, e.g. β-blockade or digitalis overdosage. *Tachycardia*, a pulse rate of over 100 beats/min, may signify hypovolaemia or sepsis but may also be caused by emotion, fever, thyrotoxicosis

05

or an abnormal rhythm. In cases of atrial fibrillation, the rate counted at the wrist does not indicate the true rate of ventricular contraction. In this case the actual heart rate should be counted by auscultation at the apex, and the difference between this and the rate at the wrist is recorded as the *pulse deficit*. This phenomenon is the result of the variable length of diastole in patients with atrial fibrillation. When diastole is short, the heart barely fills and consequently the stroke volume will be small and as such will not be felt at the wrist, although the heart will have contracted.

RHYTHM

The examiner should next decide whether the rhythm is regular or irregular. If it is irregular, the next decision is whether it is regularly irregular (usually the result of ectopic beats) or irregularly irregular (atrial fibrillation). In normal patients the pulse may be felt to quicken slightly in inspiration and to slow slightly in expiration, so-called *sinus arrhythmia*.

CHARACTER

This is best determined by palpation of the carotid pulse. The normal pulse has a moderately rapid upstroke coinciding with left ventricular ejection. As left ventricular pressure falls, aortic and ventricular pressure fall to their different diastolic levels. In certain situations the character of the pulse is detectably abnormal.

Slow-rising 'plateau' pulse is typically found in aortic stenosis. It is small in volume and slow in rising to a peak as a result of the prolonged ejection phase of the left ventricle.

Collapsing, 'water-hammer' or Corrigan's pulse is typically found in aortic regurgitation; it is characterized by a rapid upstroke and rapid descent of the arterial pressure wave. The rapid upstroke is due to an increased stroke volume consequent upon a leaking or regurgitant valve. The rapid decline in pressure is due to the leak back into the left ventricle and also to a reduced systemic vascular resistance.

Bisferiens pulse is a combination of the slow-rising and collapsing pulse and is found in mixed aortic valve disease (stenosis and incompetence) and hypertrophic obstructive cardiomyopathy. This is in fact a 'double pulse'. When the left ventricle is obstructed or empties slowly, the elastic recoil of the peripheral vascular bed that normally occurs in diastole (and produces the dicrotic notch) occurs in late systole and is felt as a double pulse. In the case of mixed aortic valve disease, it is the increased volume loading produced by a regurgitant aortic valve that causes prolonged emptying, and it is this together with an obstructed aortic valve that cause a double waveform.

Bigeminal pulse or 'pulsus bigeminus' occurs as a result of a premature ectopic beat following a sinus beat. There is a compensatory pause following the extrasystole that makes the sinus beat larger than normal.

Pulsus paradoxus is an exaggerated normal response. Deep inspiration causes a reduction in intrathoracic pressure. This has a twofold effect: right ventricular volume increases and pooling of blood occurs within the pulmonary circulation. The overall result is that with inspiration there is diminished return to the left ventricle, resulting in lower stroke volume and decreased pulse volume. Pulsus paradoxus is an exaggeration of this response.

In patients with cardiac tamponade, the fluid within the pericardium exerts its own pressure and the normal physiological response is exaggerated by further compromising the volume of the left ventricle. It is also an important sign in patients with severe asthma; in this situation severe airflow limitation produces a sudden and increased negative intrathoracic pressure that exacerbates the normal physiological response. The paradox is that the heart may still be auscultated even though there may be no pulse palpable at the wrist.

VOLUME

With pulsus alternans, the pulse volume alternates between strong and weak with successive beats; its presence is an indication that there is severe damage to the left ventricular muscle mass.

Jugular venous pulse

A measure of right atrial pressure may be obtained from the jugular venous pulse (JVP). It does not measure volume but its level may give the observer an indication of the 'filling' of the cardiovascular system. It is an indicator of the competence of the right heart to accept and deliver blood (Fig. 37.46). The *a* wave is distinguished from the *v* wave by palpation of the carotid artery. The *a* wave occurs immediately before the carotid pulsation.

MEASUREMENT OF JVP

The patient should recline at an angle of 45° with the head supported and the neck muscles relaxed. In the normal subject, the peaks of the JVP waves are just visible in the internal jugular vein. Without distinguishing the three separate waves, there is a mean level that corresponds to the perpendicular height of the blood column above the right atrium. The JVP is measured as the vertical distance between the manubrial sternal angle and the top of the venous column. It is usually less than 3 cmH$_2$O.

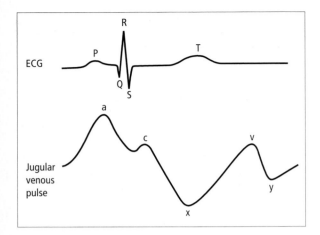

Figure 37.46 Jugular venous pulse in relation to the electro-cardiogram: *a* wave, produced by atrial systole; *x* descent, occurs when atrial contraction finishes; *c* wave, interrupts the *x* descent and is caused by displacement of the tricuspid annulus into the right atrium as right ventricular pressure rises — it is synchronous with ventricular systole; *v* wave, results from continued filling of right atrium during ventricular systole; *y* descent, represents the fall in right atrial pressure when the tricuspid valve opens and enters the right ventricle.

VARIATIONS IN JVP
Low JVP occurs in hypovolaemic states. It cannot be measured clinically, but it is possible to measure CVP by pressure transduction of the internal jugular vein. The JVP is defined by three waves (*a*, *c*, *v*) and two negative descents (*x* and *y*).

Raised JVP is seen in:
• heart failure;
• cardiac tamponade;
• fluid retention, including fluid overload;
• constrictive pericarditis;
• SVC obstruction.
Kussmaul's sign is an elevation of JVP on inspiration, seen in patients with cardiac tamponade or constrictive pericarditis in whom ventricular filling is impeded.

Changes in wave pattern: *a* waves are absent in atrial fibrillation because there is no atrial contraction, while frequent *a* waves are seen with atrial flutter. Large *a* waves occur when there is increased resistance to ventricular filling, e.g. tricuspid stenosis, pulmonary stenosis, pulmonary hypertension, all of which result in right ventricular hypertrophy. Commonly in tricuspid stenosis the patient is in atrial fibrillation and therefore the waves are not noticed. *Cannon waves* occur when the right atrium contracts against a closed tricuspid valve in complete

heart block. Large *v* waves result from tricuspid regurgitation, as the ventricular contraction is transmitted directly to the internal jugular veins.

Examination of the precordium
INSPECTION
Deformities of the chest wall should be noted, e.g. pectus excavatum (funnel chest), pectus carinatum (pigeon chest). Attention should also be paid to spinal curvature, e.g. kyphoscoliosis. Gross thoracic skeletal deformities may produce functional embarrassment of the heart as well as making surgery and anaesthesia more difficult.

PALPATION
The apex beat is the most lateral and inferior point of cardiac pulsation. It is normally felt in the midclavicular line at the level of the left fifth intercostal space. The position of the apex beat is subject to great variability and it may be displaced as a result of thoracic cage deformities or lung disease. In many cases palpation of the left and right ventricles may be of greater value. This will yield information as to which ventricle is under strain and whether the load is due to an increased stroke volume or is obstructive in nature.

Left ventricular impulse. The examiner's palm locates the apex beat. As mentioned previously, it is the nature of this impulse which is of greater value than its position. In aortic stenosis, the left ventricle is obstructed and hence the myocardium hypertrophies. This will be felt as a powerful heaving impulse. In aortic regurgitation, the ventricle deals with increased volumes of blood and the resulting impulse will be turbulent and hyperdynamic. The left ventricular enlargement will produce a rather more diffuse impulse.

Right ventricular impulse is palpable to the left of the sternum. If the right ventricle is hypertrophied, e.g. in atrial septal defect or pulmonary stenosis, a definite 'lift' may be felt.

Thrills. These are palpable murmurs felt with the flat of the hand. They are caused by turbulent flow produced by blood flowing through stenosed valves or large volumes of blood passing through normal valves. Thrills indicate a definite abnormality. Systolic thrills in the aortic area are commonly due to aortic stenosis, and at the apex to mitral regurgitation. A diastolic thrill at the apex is usually due to mitral stenosis. A thrill from aortic regurgitation is uncommon.

AUSCULTATION
By the time the examiner uses a stethoscope there should

05

be well-founded clinical suspicion of the diagnosis. It should thus be regarded as a confirmatory diagnostic tool. However, once the mechanics underlying the heart sound are understood, further information may be elicited.

There are four areas where the normal heart sounds and added sounds (including murmurs) are most easily heard.
- Aortic area: second right intercostal space just to the right of the sternum.
- Pulmonary area: second left intercostal space just to the left of the sternum.
- Tricuspid area: fourth intercostal space to the left of the sternum (left sternal edge).
- Mitral area: point at which apex beat is heard.
The heart should be auscultated in all areas (aortic, pulmonary, mitral and left sternal edge) as well as the neck and axilla. The patient is turned on to the left side to listen for mitral stenosis, and sat forward on expiration to listen for aortic regurgitation. Listen for the first and second heart sounds, then added sounds and finally murmurs. The bell picks up low-pitched sounds, e.g. third and fourth sounds and murmur of mitral stenosis. The diaphragm picks up high-pitched sounds, e.g. first and second heart sounds and most murmurs. The heart sound and any murmurs should always be timed with the carotid pulse.

Heart sounds

1 The first heart sound is caused by closure of mitral (M1) and tricuspid (T1) valves. The cessation of mitral valve flow might also contribute to the sound. Electrical and mechanical events on the left side of the heart slightly precede those on the right. Therefore mitral valve closure slightly precedes tricuspid closure. However, the observer may not hear this split. It is best heard over the mitral and tricuspid areas.

2 The second heart sound is due to closure of the aortic and pulmonary valves. The second sound is also normally split and is best heard in the corresponding aortic and pulmonary areas. The presence of two distinct components indicates that both valves are present and working. The aortic (A2) components slightly precede the pulmonary component (P2). The gap between the first and second heart sounds represents the systolic phase of the cardiac cycle.

3 The third heart sound is due to rapid expansion of the left ventricle in early diastole and therefore closely follows the second sound. It is a normal finding in patients with hyperdynamic states and in individuals under 30 years of age. Later in life a dilated left ventricle, mitral and aortic regurgitation will give rise to a third heart sound.

4 The fourth heart sound is also due to ventricular filling and results from atrial contraction and hence immediately precedes the first heart sound. It occurs when the ventricle is non-compliant as in cardiac hypertrophy secondary to

Table 37.23 Heart murmurs.

Systolic murmurs
Ejection systolic murmurs
Aortic stenosis
Aortic sclerosis
Pulmonary stenosis
Atrial septal defect

Pansystolic regurgitant murmurs
Mitral regurgitation
Tricuspid regurgitation
Ventricular septal defect

Diastolic murmurs
Mid-diastolic murmurs
Mitral stenosis
Tricuspid stenosis
Austin Flint murmur

Early diastolic murmurs
Aortic regurgitation
Pulmonary regurgitation
Graham Steell murmur

systemic hypertension or aortic stenosis. It has been observed as a normal finding in young athletes but is much more commonly associated with underlying pathology.

Additional sounds

- An opening snap of the mitral valve strongly suggests that the valve is thickened and fibrotic. It is heard just after the second sound and indicates mitral stenosis. It is heard best just medial to the apex beat. In surgical terms it signifies pliability of the valve, which may be suitable for a valve conservation procedure known as valvotomy (division of fused leaflets). This does not occur with a heavily calcified valve.
- Friction rubs are scratching/crunching noises produced by movement of the inflamed pericardium. As they are high-pitched sounds, they are best heard with the diaphragm in systole.

Murmurs

Turbulent flow causes heart murmurs. Turbulence may be produced when there is high flow through a normal valve or normal flow through an abnormal valve. The murmurs that may be heard in the heart are listed in Table 37.23.

- *Grading* should be carried out to indicate the intensity of the murmur in question. This is arbitrary, on a scale of 1–4 or 1–6. A grade of 1 is very soft and heard only in good circumstances. The top end of the range indicates a very loud murmur associated with a palpable thrill.

Table 37.24 Cardiac enzymes.

Enzyme	Time of peak level after myocardial infarction
Creatine phosphokinase (CPK) (CK-MB isoenzyme is more specific for myocardial infarction)	Within 24 h
Aspartate aminotransferase (AST)	24–48 h
Alanine aminotransferase (ALT)	24–48 h
Lactate dehydrogenase (LDH)	3–4 days
Troponin T	Up to 1 week

- *Loudness and length* are proportional to the pressure gradient along which the blood passes. They are not good indicators of severity of the lesion. This is because, with a severely stenotic valve, the blood flow will be so little that no murmur will result.
- *Character*
  (a) Mitral/tricuspid murmurs in diastole: low-pitched and rumbling.
  (b) Aortic/pulmonary murmurs in diastole: high-frequency, decrescendo.
  (c) Mitral/tricuspid murmurs in systole: blowing quality.
  (d) Aortic/pulmonary murmurs in systole: harsher, rushing.
- *Ejection systolic murmurs.* Aortic stenotic murmurs are harsh and radiate to the neck. They are best heard over the aortic area. Pulmonary stenosis and atrial septal defect are best heard at the left sternal edge on inspiration.
- *Pansystolic regurgitant murmurs.* Mitral regurgitation is best heard at the apex, and radiates to the axilla. Tricuspid regurgitation and ventricular septal defect (VSD) are best heard at the left sternal edge.
- *Mid-diastolic murmurs.* Mitral stenosis is best heard at the apex. There is a loud mitral first sound, opening snap and low-pitched rumbling diastolic murmur. The patient should be rolled to the left side, and the murmur is accentuated on exertion. A presystolic murmur may also be heard. The latter is caused by the cusps almost closing together at the end of diastole. Tricuspid stenosis is best heard at the left sternal edge. The Austin Flint murmur is sometimes heard in aortic regurgitation (incompetence); it is produced where the flow of blood back into the left ventricle partially closes and obstructs the mitral valve.
- *Early diastolic murmur.* Aortic regurgitation is best heard at the left sternal edge and apex with the patient sitting forward and in expiration. Pulmonary regurgitation is best heard to the right of the sternum and is louder on inspiration. The Graham Steell murmur is heard in pulmonary hypertension when it is due to mitral stenosis that leads to pulmonary regurgitation.

Investigations

Cardiac enzymes

When myocardial muscle cells are damaged, a number of enzymes escape into the circulation. These can be detected in the serum and their presence used to confirm that tissue damage (e.g. myocardial infarction) has occurred. The commonly used enzymes are listed in Table 37.24.

Chest radiography (see Chapter 38)

Attention should be paid to the bony outline, cardiac contour, areas of calcification and lungs. The size of the heart is compared with the diameter of the chest; the ratio should be no more than 50%.

Electrocardiography

The ECG records the electrical activity generated by the myocardium. It is of value because it can identify myocardial ischaemia and infarction, ventricular hypertrophy and disturbances of rhythm. *Exercise electrocardiography* is a technique used to assess the cardiac response to exercise. The ECG is recorded while the patient is walking or running on a treadmill, and the work rate is gradually increased. The test is terminated if the patient complains of chest pain or dyspnoea or if there are significant ST changes or the emergence of an arrhythmia. Myocardial ischaemia provoked by exertion results in ST-segment depression of greater than 1 mm in the leads facing the affected area. During the exercise test, full resuscitation equipment should be available. Some patients may be unable to complete a conventional treadmill stress test because of intermittent claudication or osteoarthritis for example. In these cases it is useful to administer an inotropic drug such as dobutamine, which increases cardiac work in the same way as exercise and can be used as a pharmacological stress test.

Holter monitoring is a technique where a 24-h record of a patient's ECG is obtained. The ECG leads are placed on the patient and the ECG is recorded on a tape in a small

05

recorder that the patient wears on a belt at the waist. The recording is analysed later, specifically looking for runs of arrhythmias.

Echocardiography and Doppler ultrasound

In this technique, ultrasound waves are used to map the heart and study its function.

M-mode echocardiography
This utilizes a single ultrasound beam directed towards the heart in order to detect movement of structures within the heart (hence M-mode). These tracings are limited by the small area that can be visualized at any given time. M-mode images require considerable expertise to interpret correctly.

Cross-sectional or two-dimensinal echocardiography
This method visualizes a wedge, from which the relationships of various cardiac structures can be observed. Multiple ultrasound beams convey a moving image that is more easily recognized as an anatomical representation of a slice through the heart. It is well suited to demonstrating malformation of the cardiac valves, septal defects, size of cardiac chambers and the presence of fluid or blood within the pericardium.

Doppler echocardiography
This provides knowledge about the velocity and direction of blood flow within the heart by utilizing the Doppler principle: if sound is reflected from a moving object, its frequency increases if the object is moving towards the observer and decreases if the object is moving away. In Doppler echocardiography, ultrasonic beams are reflected from the red blood cells with a frequency that is proportional to the velocity of blood flow. It is thus possible to detect a jet of blood passing across a regurgitant or leaking valve. In addition, further information may be obtained by applying the Bernoulli equation in order to estimate the pressure difference that generated the measured velocity. It is therefore possible to estimate the pressure differences across the heart valves, as well as estimating left ventricular ejection fraction (LVEF):
- normal ($\geq 60\%$);
- depressed ($40-50\%$);
- severely depressed ($< 30\%$).

A deterioration on pharmacological stressing with inotropic drugs is suggestive of coronary disease or an abnormality of the myocardium.

Transoesophageal echocardiography
In transoesophageal echocardiography (TOE), M-mode and cross-sectional imaging transducers as well as Doppler transducers are incorporated into the end of a flexible endoscope. The procedure is performed as per gastroscopy: the pharynx is sprayed with local anaesthetic and the patient is given a small amount of sedative intravenously. As the oesophagus is traversed by the endoscope, the heart is seen anteriorly and the descending thoracic aorta posteriorly. Although this procedure takes a long time and requires operator skill, the images obtained are of very high quality as the heart is imaged with little intervening tissue and its important structures are near the transducer. TOE is very valuable in the diagnosis of infective endocarditis because of its ability to detect very small vegetations. It also enables the detection of unstable atheroma in the ascending and descending aorta as a source of cerebral or peripheral emboli, as well as regurgitation through a mitral valve prosthesis. Hyperinflated lungs do not interfere with the images obtained by TOE and the technique may be used to image the heart during cardiac surgery.

Nuclear imaging

These techniques are primarily used in the assessment of ischaemic heart disease.

Thallium imaging
Thallium behaves like potassium, with healthy myocardium taking it up and ischaemia or infarction producing a 'cold spot'. A cold spot that appears on exercise and which is reversed by rest implies ischaemia on exertion, whereas a persistent cold spot implies infarction.

Pyrophosphate imaging
Pyrophosphate labelled with technetium will produce a 'hot spot' in an infarcted area. Disadvantages include uptake into other tissue, and complete occlusion of the artery causing the infarction will not distribute the isotope.

Radionuclide imaging
*Mu*ltiple *g*ated *a*cquisition (MUGA) is obtained by the injection of technetium-99. This radioisotope attaches to the erythrocytes of the patient and can therefore outline the ventricle and estimate the volume of ventricular ejection (LVEF).

Computed tomography and magnetic resonance imaging

CT will show clearly the size and shape of the cardiac chambers as well as the thoracic aorta and mediastinum. The development of MRI has lagged behind its other applications due to the movement of the heart and because

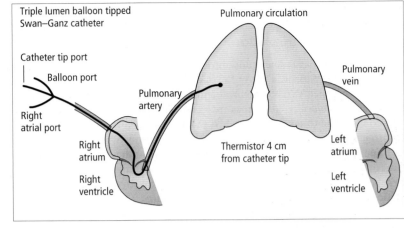

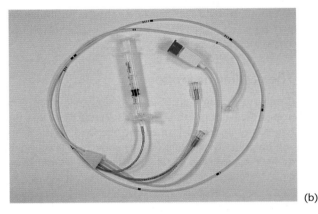

(a)

(b)

Figure 37.47 (a) Schematic representation of a Swan–Ganz catheter. The catheter is passed via the superior vena cava through the right atrium and ventricle into the pulmonary artery. Right atrial pressure (= central venous pressure) is measured via the right atrial port. Pulmonary artery pressure is measured via the catheter tip port when the balloon at the tip of the catheter is deflated. Inflating the balloon occludes the peripheral branch of the pulmonary artery and measures pulmonary capillary wedge pressure, which reflects left atrial pressure. Cardiac output can be measured using a thermodilution technique. A 10-mL bolus of saline at 0°C is injected via the right atrial port and the temperature change is detected by the thermistor at the catheter tip. From this dilution, cardiac output can be calculated. (b) Swan–Ganz catheter.

of the continued development of CT and echocardiography. The significant development of ECG-synchronized images has led to wider application by producing images in systole and diastole. MRI is particularly useful in the investigation of pericardial disease, cardiac tumours, prosthetic valve pathology and thoracic aortic disease.

Cardiac catheterization and angiography

This technique is performed to measure intracardiac pressures, blood oxygen content in the various heart chambers and cardiac output.

The right heart is catheterized by introducing the catheter into a peripheral vein and advancing it through the right atrium and ventricle to the pulmonary artery. The left heart is catheterized via the brachial or femoral artery. The catheter then traverses the aortic valve to enter the left ventricle. Direct-pressure measurements may be made of the right heart chambers, aorta, left ventricle and pulmonary artery. Left atrial pressure may be measured by indirect means, carried out by wedging the catheter into the distal pulmonary artery. The pressure from the right

ventricle is obstructed by the catheter and only the pulmonary venous and left atrial pressures are measured. This value is the pulmonary capillary wedge pressure (PCWP). A simplified version of this manoeuvre, in which a balloon-tipped (Swan–Ganz) catheter is floated into the pulmonary circulation and the balloon is inflated to obtain a wedge pressure, has widespread application in the monitoring of patients with heart failure in the intensive care unit (ICU) (Fig. 37.47).

Cardiac catheterization allows the selective injection of radiopaque contrast material so that patterns of blood flow can be observed and recorded. The dye may be injected down the orifices of the left and right coronary arteries to identify abnormalities within these arteries. This process is called angiography and is an essential prerequisite for coronary bypass surgery by identifying the coronary anatomy and distribution of the disease. Different views are taken to provide a three-dimensional impression of the coronary arterial circulation. Angiography is not entirely without risk and as such should only be performed when other non-invasive investigative techniques are unable to provide the information required.

05

Perioperative care

Preoperative preparation

Following clinical assessment and informed consent, the cardiac surgical patient is ready for operation. Blood is drawn for preoperative biochemical and haematological investigations; blood is also cross-matched. The patient should continue to take all prescribed medications prior to surgery, except aspirin which should be discontinued 7–10 days beforehand. If a patient is taking aspirin at the time of operation, there might be a problem with bleeding peroperatively because of its antiplatelet effects. Prophylactic antibiotic cover is mandatory in all procedures. The antibiotics of choice differ between cardiothoracic units but should cover *Streptococcus* and *Staphylococcus* species. Antibiotics should be continued into the postoperative period for 2 days or until central lines are removed, whichever is longer.

The cardiac operation

Cardiac operations differ from other types of surgery in that the heart has to be stopped (arrested) so that the operation may be performed and the work of the heart and lungs has to be taken over by a machine (cardiopulmonary bypass; Fig. 37.48). Furthermore, as the heart itself is not being perfused during the operation it becomes ischaemic and must therefore be protected (myocardial protection).

Cardiopulmonary bypass

It is necessary to support the circulation during a variety of cardiac surgical procedures. This is because the heart has to remain motionless for accurate placement of sutures and also because, in many cases, the heart has to be disturbed from its normal functional position. The elements of a cardiopulmonary bypass circuit are:

- venous reservoir;
- heat exchanger;
- oxygenator;
- roller pump;
- arterial filter.

The circuit is maintained and operated by a trained *perfusionist*. Blood is drained from the right atrium under the force of gravity. It passes to an oxygenator, which takes over the function of the lungs and so ventilation can be discontinued. The blood is returned to the systemic circulation by roller pumps, having passed through a heat exchanger for cooling and rewarming and an arterial filter to remove any microemboli. Venous drainage is accomplished by either one cannula placed into the right atrium or two cannulae placed into the SVC and IVC. Arterial

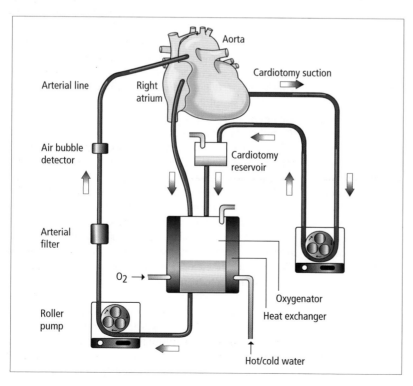

Figure 37.48 Cardiopulmonary bypass circuit.

05

return is by a cannula placed within the ascending aorta. The bypass circuit will activate the patient's clotting cascade and in order to prevent this the patient is heparinized (3 mg/kg).

Complications

Adverse effects may occur even after short-term use of cardiopulmonary bypass.

- *Clotting factor activation and consumption* occur when blood comes into contact with foreign surfaces. Heparin prevents this but has to be reversed with protamine at the end of the procedure to prevent excessive bleeding. If a coagulopathy persists, then additional clotting factors may be necessary.
- *Destruction of blood components*: haemolysis and platelet destruction occur as a result of the shearing forces encountered during bypass.
- *Immunological derangements*: all components of the cellular and humoral divisions of the immune system are depressed during cardiopulmonary bypass. Of particular importance is the additional activation of the complement system, which results in vasoconstriction, whole-body inflammation and capillary leakage.
- *Oedema*: the combination of haemodilution and decrease in plasma colloid osmotic pressure, together with the fluid-conserving response to surgery, results in postoperative oedema.
- *Cerebral dysfunction*: stroke occurs in 1–2% of patients. However, neuropsychological tests will show minor abnormalities in a high proportion of patients. These tend to disappear within the first few months following surgery. These effects may be partly explained by microemboli of air and formed elements within the bloodstream, as well as the presence of pre-existing extracranial or intracranial vascular disease.

Myocardial protection

To prevent the heart from beating, a cross-clamp is applied between the aortic valve and the arterial cannula. This renders the heart ischaemic, and two methods have evolved to limit ischaemic damage.

Defibrillation

Following application of the aortic cross-clamp, the heart is fibrillated using an electrical fibrillator. This arrests the pulsatile movement of the heart; however, the 'safe' period of ischaemia is only about 15 min. Following the removal of the cross-clamp the heart is allowed to reperfuse in sinus rhythm, which is obtained by defibrillation. This method is used by some surgeons when performing the distal anastomosis of a coronary bypass graft.

Cardioplegia

This method has superseded the former for the majority of cardiac operations. Following application of the aortic cross-clamp, an infusion of a cold hyperkalaemic solution is made via a small cannula in the aortic root (below the cross-clamp). The fluid flows into the ostia of the left and right coronary arteries. The high potassium content produces rapid diastolic arrest and the cold temperature gives reliable protection to the myocardium for long periods of ischaemia. Cooling via the heat exchanger to 28–32°C provides additional myocardial protection by slowing the metabolic rate.

Postoperative management

Transfer from the operating theatre to the ICU is a dangerous period. Mechanical ventilation and monitoring are maintained and sedation, inotropes and vasodilators are continued by infusion pumps. As a general rule most patients are ventilated overnight, although routine noncomplex cases are increasingly being extubated earlier. Premature extubation will provide additional stresses to the myocardium. In the immediate postoperative period, continuing diuresis, rewarming and blood loss will require volume expansion using either blood or plasma expanders. This depends on the haematocrit of the patient's blood, which should ideally be kept at 0.3–0.35. There may be a large requirement for electrolytes, particularly potassium, as a result of the postoperative diuresis, large infused volumes of crystalloid and preoperative status. Postassium should be maintained in the range 4.5–5.0 mmol/L. Following extubation the patient is transferred to a high-dependency unit where invasive monitoring continues for another 24 h in uncomplicated cases.

Cardiac physiology

An understanding of circulatory physiology is essential for the management of the cardiac surgical patient. Changes induced by disease or surgery will not be appreciated unless the principles that govern cardiovascular responses in the normal individual are understood. Table 37.25 highlights the haemodynamic parameters commonly used to assess circulatory function and provides some understanding of their derivation. Most of the parameters listed are measured routinely in cardiac patients postoperatively.

Invasive monitoring

The routine measurements performed in the ICU are urinary output, CVP, arterial blood pressure and arterial blood gases. Measurement of hourly urine output is a

05

Table 37.25 Some commonly used haemodynamic parameters.

Parameter	How derived	Normal value
Direct measurements		
Heart rate	Direct measurement, usually from ECG	72–88 beats/min
Arterial pressure	Direct measurement via radial artery cannula	120/80 mmHg
Mean arterial pressure	Diastolic blood pressure + one-third (pulse pressure)	70–105 mmHg
Central venous pressure	Direct measurement via central venous line	0–9 cmH_2O
Mean pulmonary arterial pressure	Direct measurement via Swan–Ganz catheter	9–16 mmHg
Pulmonary capillary wedge pressure (PCWP)	Direct measurement via Swan–Ganz catheter	8–12 mmHg
Derived measurements		
Pulse pressure	Systolic blood pressure — diastolic blood pressure	40–60 mmHg
Stroke volume	End-diastolic volume — end-systolic volume	75–80 mL/beat
Cardiac output	Stroke volume × heart rate	5.5–6.0 L/min
Cardiac index	Cardiac output/body surface area	3.0 L/min per m^2
Systemic vascular resistance	(Mean arterial pressure — right atrial pressure)/cardiac output	900–1400 dyn/s per cm^5
Pulmonary vascular resistance	(Pulmonary arterial pressure — PCWP)/cardiac output	150–250 dyn/s per cm^5

simple way to assess that the kidneys and, by inference, the rest of the peripheral tissues are being adequately perfused. A urine output of 0.5 mL/kg per h (i.e. > 30 mL/h for most people) indicates adequate perfusion. Frequently, more sophisticated assessment of cardiac function is required and for this a Swan–Ganz catheter has to be placed.

Pulmonary and systemic vascular resistance are calculated by computer with a knowledge of the measured cardiac output and the patient's body surface area, venous and arterial pressures and heart rate.

Specific problems following cardiac surgery

Bleeding may be due to a coagulopathy as a result of cardiopulmonary bypass or to inadequate control of bleeding at the time of surgery. The patient should be returned to theatre if the bleeding is not arrested by additional clotting factors.

Low cardiac output state is manifested by hypotension, cool extremities, tachycardia, oliguria and obtundation. The cause may be primary cardiac failure, which may be due to intraoperative myocardial infarction, poor revascularization (in the case of coronary artery bypass) and poor myocardial protection. In addition, compression of the heart by blood within the pericardial cavity will cause tamponade. In this case, CVP will usually be high. Other causes include hypoxia, hypovolaemia or the development of arrhythmias. In most cases pharmacological treatment is directed at the cause. Surgical reopening may be necessary in some cases to exclude the presence of a tamponade.

Hypertension is common in patients with pre-existing hypertension and good left ventricles. Before treatment is commenced, pain, hypoxia and hypercarbia should be excluded.

Arrhythmias: the development of an arrhythmia requires prompt treatment. The most common arrhythmia is atrial fibrillation. Hypoxia, hypercarbia and electrolyte abnormalities should be sought and treated, although commonly no cause is found.

Hypoxia: it is essential that the patient remains adequately oxygenated. As well as oxygen therapy, a cause should be sought, e.g. pneumothorax, lobar collapse, consolidation, atelectasis, position of endotracheal tube and pulmonary oedema. A postoperative chest X-ray is mandatory.

Hypothermia: the patient is frequently cooled in theatre. Hypothermia is deleterious as it may lead to hypertension, myocardial irritability and shivering, with increased oxygen requirements. Humidified ventilation, space blankets and warmed intravenous fluid should be used.

Renal failure: a diuresis is common following cardiopulmonary bypass. It may be due to pre-existing disease, haemolysis, hypoperfusion, renal vasoconstriction, long cardiopulmonary bypass and toxins. Treatment is along conventional lines.

Neurological deficits: investigations include CT or MRI plus Doppler studies of the internal carotid arteries. Treatment may include heparinization but is usually expectant and supportive.

05

New developments in cardiac surgery

The expansion in minimally invasive surgical techniques in other areas of surgery has also led to advances in cardiac surgery. It is now possible to perform major cardiac surgery via four small stab incisions using an endoscopic camera and instruments, so-called minimally invasive coronary artery bypass. Perhaps the most exciting, but as yet unproven, innovation is in the area of robotics. The da Vinci telemanipulation system uses three-dimensional videoscopic images to allow tremor-free and up-scaled remote control of endoscopic surgical instruments. This can even be performed on the beating heart by using an endoscopic stabilizer, so-called off-pump coronary artery bypass.

Cardiac surgery for specific diseases of the heart

Surgery for ischaemic heart disease

Coronary artery disease

Ischaemic heart disease is the most common cause of death in the western world, claiming more than 3000 deaths per million each year in the UK. It results from atheromatous narrowing of the coronary arteries and may present as sudden death or as acute myocardial infarction, but more commonly presents as angina pectoris. This is typically provoked by exertion and relieved by rest.

Physical examination is frequently normal, although the stigmata of hypercholesterolaemia or diabetes may be present. The auscultation of a heart murmur or carotid bruit will require further investigation.

Investigations
● Resting and exercise ECGs will demonstrate evidence of exercise-induced ischaemia, previous infarction or arrhythmias. This test provides objective evidence so that medical therapy may be instituted, monitored and the need for further intervention assessed.
● Coronary angiography is performed when it is felt that patients need revascularization, whether this is by angioplasty or coronary bypass surgery.

Indications for surgery
Medical therapy is recommended when the ischaemia is prevented by anti-ischaemic drugs that are well tolerated. With one- or two-vessel disease not involving the left anterior descending artery, medical therapy (or angioplasty) is recommended first, with coronary artery bypass grafting (CABG) being reserved for refractory ischaemia. With limited coronary artery disease refractory to medical

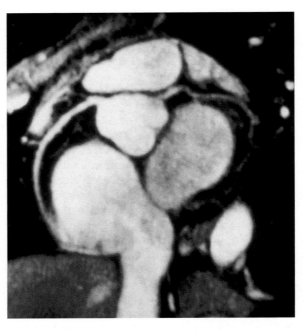

Figure 37.49 Computed tomography image of the heart showing the right and left coronary arteries.

therapy, angioplasty should be considered before recommending surgery, unless there is a compelling reason such as left main artery disease. If angioplasty is high risk or the lesions are technically unsuitable, CABG is the correct way to proceed.

Coronary artery surgery may benefit the patient by providing symptomatic relief and in many cases is of prognostic benefit. Data accumulated from three large, prospective, randomized trials have shown that surgery is better than medical therapy for improving survival in left main stem or triple-vessel disease (i.e. stenosis in each of the three main arteries: right, left anterior descending and circumflex), double-vessel disease involving the left anterior descending artery (Fig. 37.49), and chronic ischaemia leading to left ventricular dysfunction.

Surgical procedure
1 Following the institution of cardiopulmonary bypass and application of the aortic cross-clamp, the heart is arrested in diastole and protected from ischaemic damage by the administration of cardioplegia. Usually 1 L is infused in the first instance, followed by further infusions at further time intervals thereafter. Topical cooling in the form of ice is applied to the myocardial surface, and the patient is also systemically cooled by the heat exchanger on the bypass machine.
2 The graft of choice is the *internal mammary* (*internal*

05

thoracic) artery. It is anastomosed (joined with sutures) most commonly to the left anterior descending artery. In this situation it confers greater protection from subsequent cardiac events (angina, myocardial infarction and sudden death). Its patency rates are superior to long saphenous vein (95% and 85% patency at 5 and 10 years, respectively, can be expected).

3 Reversed long saphenous vein is also used extensively as a conduit. However, vein grafts are prone to occlusion at a rate of 10–20% in the first year, with an occlusion rate of 2–3% per year thereafter. Treatment with low-dose aspirin following the operation enhances patency.

4 An arteriotomy is made distal to the coronary artery stenosis. The reversed saphenous vein is then anastomosed using a fine polypropylene suture. All distal anastomoses are performed in this fashion; if the internal mammary artery is being used, it is anastomosed last. When all distal anastomoses have been performed, the aortic cross-clamp is removed, allowing the heart to reperfuse and beat. As the patient rewarms, the proximal anastomoses to the aorta are performed.

5 Following completion of all anastomoses and warming of the patient, ventilation is recommenced and, providing the patient is in stable rhythm, cardiopulmonary bypass is discontinued. Following removal of venous and arterial cannulae, protamine is given to reverse the anticoagulant effects of heparin.

Outcome

The hospital mortality following CABG is 1–4% and this is likely to be a reflection of operating on older patients and those with impaired left ventricular function. Although the majority of patients obtain relief from angina, recurrent angina is most likely to occur within the first year following surgery. This is usually due to graft failure as a result of poor anastomotic technique, or an inadequate distal vessel. Only 50% of vein grafts are patent at 10 years. The internal mammary artery has a superior patency rate. Approximately 10% of patients will have a second operation within the ensuing 10 years. Reoperation is associated with an increased operative mortality and is reserved for patients with severe symptoms refractory to maximal medical therapy.

Complications of myocardial infarction

Most complications of acute myocardial infarction occur in the period immediately after the infarction. The patient is frequently in cardiogenic shock. The aetiology of the circulatory collapse must be ascertained before a management plan can be formulated. As a general rule the earlier the occurrence of the complication, the higher the overall mortality.

The surgically correctable complications of myocardial infarction are:

- VSD;
- mitral regurgitation;
- left ventricular aneurysm;
- ventricular arrhythmias;
- ruptured ventricle.

The patient is normally profoundly unwell and is admitted directly to the ICU. Full invasive monitoring, including the insertion of a Swan–Ganz catheter (which may demonstrate an interventricular shunt), will be necessary. Cardiogenic shock is treated by inotropic drugs, vasodilators and diuretics. Shock refractory to these therapies will frequently require a mechanical device to assist the failing heart. Such a device is known as an intra-aortic balloon pump, which is positioned in the descending aorta via the femoral artery and provides synchronized alterations in left ventricular afterload to improve cardiac output. If arrhythmias are the cause of heart failure they should be treated by the use of antiarrhythmics, pacing or direct current (DC) cardioversion.

An ECG will demonstrate the presence and extent of an infarct, and associated arrhythmias. Echocardiography will demonstrate mitral regurgitation, VSD, left ventricular aneurysm, left ventricular dysfunction and a ruptured left ventricle.

If the patient is stable, then angiography can proceed so that revascularization may be performed in association with any other corrective procedure. This is often not possible as the risks of catheterization may be prohibitive.

Transplantation should be considered for some patients with poor left ventricular function and heart failure refractory to medical or surgical therapy.

Surgery for valvular heart disease

The number of operations for valvular heart disease has not risen as dramatically as those for coronary artery disease. The function of the heart valves is to maintain the forward flow of blood through the chambers of the heart. Disease may affect a valve by making the orifice smaller (*stenosis*) or by allowing back-flow or leakage through the valve (*regurgitation* or *incompetence*). Both stenosis and incompetence may coexist.

A stenotic valve produces a *pressure load* on the cardiac chamber immediately proximal to it. This chamber responds by becoming hypertrophied. Back-pressure on other chambers and vessels may follow. An incompetent valve produces a *volume load*, which has effects both upstream and downstream from the valve. The proximal heart chamber will enlarge predominantly by dilatation but also to some extent by hypertrophy.

05

Ischaemic heart disease at a glance

Definition

Ischaemic heart disease: a common disorder caused by acute or chronic interruption of the blood supply to the myocardium, usually due to atherosclerosis of the coronary arteries, i.e. *coronary artery disease*

Epidemiology
- M > F before age 65
- Increasing risk with increasing age up to 80 years
- Most common cause of death in the western world

Aetiology
- Atherosclerosis and thrombosis
- Thromboemboli
- Arteritis (e.g. periarteritis nodosa)
- Coronary artery spasm
- Extension of aortic dissecting aneurysm
- Syphilitic aortitis

Risk factors
- Cigarette smoking
- Hypertension
- Hyperlipidaemia
- Type A personality
- Obesity

Pathology
- Reduction in coronary blood flow is critical when lumen is decreased by 90%
- Angina pectoris results when the supply of oxygen to the heart muscle is unable to meet the increased demands for oxygen, e.g. during exercise, cold, after a meal
- Thrombotic occlusion of the narrowed lumen precipitates acute ischaemia
- Heart muscle in the territory of the occluded vessel dies (myocardial infarction). May be subendocardial or transmural

Clinical features
Angina pectoris
- Central chest pain on exertion, especially in cold weather, lasts 1–15 min
- Radiates to neck, jaw, arms
- Relieved by glyceryl trinitrate (GTN)
- Usually no signs

Myocardial infarction
- Severe central chest pain for > 30 min duration
- Radiates to neck, jaw, arms

- Not relieved by GTN
- Signs of cardiogenic shock
- Arrhythmias

Investigations
Angina pectoris
- Full blood count for anaemia
- Thyroid function tests
- Chest X-ray: heart size
- ECG: ST-segment changes
- Exercise ECG
- Coronary angiography

Myocardial infarction
- ECG: Q waves, ST-segment and T-wave changes
- Cardiac enzymes: LDH/CPK, CPK-MB
- Chest X-ray
- Full blood count, urea and elctrolytes

Management
Angina pectoris
- Lose weight
- Avoid precipitating factors (e.g. cold)
- GTN (sublingual)
- Calcium channel blockers
- β-Blockers, nitrates, aspirin
- Treat hypertension and hyperlipidaemias
- Coronary angioplasty or CABG

Indications for CABG
- Left main stem disease
- Triple-vessel disease
- Two-vessel disease involving left anterior descending
- Chronic ischaemia + left ventricular dysfunction

Myocardial infarction
- Bedrest, oxygen, analgesia
- Thrombolysis
- Aspirin
- Treat heart failure (diuretics)
- Treat arrhythmias

Complications of myocardial infarction
- Arrhythmias
- Cardiogenic shock
- Myocardial rupture
- Papillary muscle rupture causing mitral incompetence
- Ventricular aneurysm
- Pericarditis
- Mural thrombosis and peripheral embolism

05

Aetiology of heart valve disease
Rheumatic fever

In the UK rheumatic fever has largely disappeared. However, in developing countries its incidence is still high. The pathology of rheumatic fever is an immune-mediated acute inflammatory reaction that affects predominantly the heart valves (although the epicardium and myocardium may also be involved). It is due to cross-reaction between surface antigens of group A β-haemolytic streptococci and certain cardiac proteins. In the acute phase a valvulitis occurs that is followed by further haemodynamic trauma, resulting in progressive valve failure with fibrosis and calcification. The initial valvulitis may be diagnosed by detecting the presence of a murmur. Stenosis results when there is fusion of the valve leaflets and regurgitation occurs when there is retraction and shortening of the scar tissue.

Congenital valve abnormalities

Several valve abnormalities may occur as part of the spectrum of congenital heart disease, e.g. Fallot's tetralogy (Fig. 37.50) but detailed discussion of the various congenital abnormalities is beyond the scope of this book.

The aortic valve is normally tricuspid but in 1–2% of individuals it has only two cusps. A functional disturbance presents in middle adult life related to long-term turbulent flow associated with the bicuspid valve. The disturbance is related to progressive calcification of the valve, which leads to stenosis and incompetence.

Degenerative valve disease

Degenerative valve disease is caused by progressive 'wear and tear' of the valvular apparatus. It is being increasingly recognized as a feature of the elderly population. A syndrome described as the mitral floppy valve syndrome is a particular form of degenerative valve disease. Not only is there cystic change within the mitral valve leaflets but the chordal apparatus becomes increasingly elongated. It leads to mitral regurgitation.

Infective endocarditis (see p. 545)

Pathophysiology of heart valve abnormalities
Aortic valve
AORTIC STENOSIS

A narrowed aortic orifice results in increased pressure in the left ventricle. Because the valve is stenosed, the pressure in the ventricle will be higher than the pressure in the root of the aorta during systole, i.e. a gradient exists across the valve. Because the ventricle has to work harder to overcome the obstruction, it hypertrophies. As the size of the ventricle increases, there is a corresponding increase in

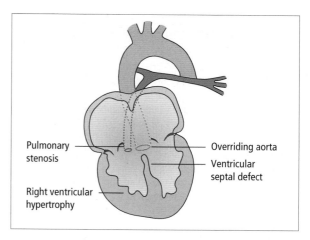

Figure 37.50 Tetralogy of Fallot is the most common type of cyanotic congenital heart disease in older children and adults. Because of the pulmonary stenosis the shunt is from right to left and the patient is cyanotic. These patients often have marked finger clubbing.

myocardial oxygen requirements. When supply exceeds demand the patient experiences angina. Syncopal attacks may also occur, particularly on exertion. Syncope occurs because the left ventricle is unable to increase its output in response to exercise-induced systemic vasodilatation. Left ventricular hypertrophy is a compensatory mechanism. However, there is a limit to the amount of compensation that can be achieved and as the stenosis becomes tighter the compensatory mechanisms begin to fail, resulting in progressive ventricular dilatation and heart failure. Operation is performed to improve prognosis and to relieve symptoms, particularly if the aortic valve gradient is in excess of 60 mmHg (8 kPa).

AORTIC REGURGITATION

When the aortic valve is incompetent blood floods back into the ventricle during diastole. Thus the ventricle has to deal with an increased volume load, which it does by dilatation. Aortic regurgitation is usually better tolerated than aortic stenosis but will progressively lead to left ventricular failure.

Mitral valve
MITRAL STENOSIS

A pressure load is placed on the left atrium. This is transmitted to the pulmonary circulation, which responds by progressive pulmonary hypertension. The left atrium is not usually dilated. As pulmonary arterial pressure increases there is an increasing load on the right ventricle. In due course the tricuspid valve, right atrium and liver

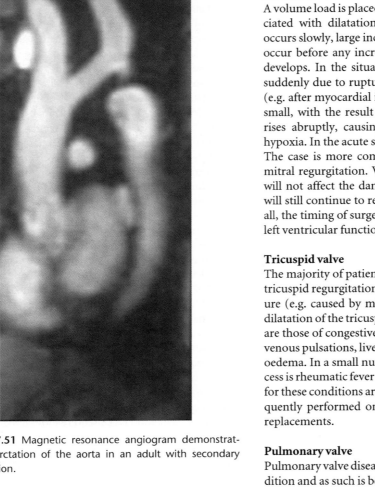

Figure 37.51 Magnetic resonance angiogram demonstrating a coarctation of the aorta in an adult with secondary hypertension.

tion, particularly New York Heart Association (NHYA) class III or IV. A valve area of less than 1 cm is a further indication for operation. The left atrium may contain thrombus, which makes systemic embolization particularly likely, especially if atrial fibrillation has developed. This constitutes a further reason for operation.

MITRAL REGURGITATION

A volume load is placed on the left atrium and is also associated with dilatation of the left ventricle. When this occurs slowly, large increases in cardiac chamber size may occur before any increase in pulmonary artery pressure develops. In the situation where regurgitation develops suddenly due to rupture of a papillary muscle or chorda (e.g. after myocardial infarction), the left atrial volume is small, with the result that pulmonary vascular pressure rises abruptly, causing pulmonary oedema and severe hypoxia. In the acute situation surgery may be life-saving. The case is more complex for the patient with chronic mitral regurgitation. Valve replacement in this situation will not affect the damaged and dilated ventricle, which will still continue to require a high filling pressure. Overall, the timing of surgery should be judged on the basis of left ventricular function as well as symptoms.

Tricuspid valve

The majority of patients with tricuspid valve disease have tricuspid regurgitation secondary to right ventricular failure (e.g. caused by mitral valve disease) with long-term dilatation of the tricuspid valve annulus. The clinical signs are those of congestive cardiac failure: prominent jugular venous pulsations, liver congestion, ascites and peripheral oedema. In a small number of cases the pathological process is rheumatic fever or carcinoid syndrome. Operations for these conditions are uncommon in the UK and are frequently performed only in association with other valve replacements.

Pulmonary valve

Pulmonary valve disease is almost always a paediatric condition and as such is beyond the scope of this chapter.

Investigations of patients with heart valve disease

As has been stressed earlier in this chapter, the history and clinical examination of the patient are of great importance. While the symptoms and physical signs of mitral valve disease frequently mirror the severity of the valvular defect, the symptoms of aortic valve disease may present at a later state when the point of optimal surgical intervention has been passed.

suffer the effects of back-pressure (congestive cardiac failure). In the early stages of mitral stenosis acute pulmonary oedema may occur, often as paroxysmal nocturnal dyspnoea. This will occur when left atrial pressure exceeds oncotic pressure in the pulmonary circulation. In some cases this may be precipitated by the development of an atrial arrhythmia, characteristically atrial fibrillation. In long-established cases, pulmonary oedema occurs less frequently. Surgery is performed for symptomatic deteriora-

05

● *ECG*: defines the cardiac rhythm and gives an indication of heart hypertrophy.
● *Chest radiography*: demonstrates cardiac size and heart chamber size (in some cases) and provides evidence of pulmonary oedema.
● *Echocardiography* (*transthoracic* and *transoesophageal*): used increasingly to provide evidence of chamber enlargement, imaging of the heart valve and calcification.
● *Doppler techniques*: provide a measure of valve gradients and of regurgitation.
These assessments negate in many circumstances the need for cardiac catheterization.

In certain situations, cardiac catheterization may be required. It allows imaging of the coronary arteries, which is important in elderly patients, particularly with the symptoms of angina. It also allows direct measurement of transvalvular gradients and visualization and quantification of the degree of valvular regurgitation.

Surgery for heart valve disease

The vast majority of operations are performed with cardiopulmonary bypass and cardioplegia. The heart chambers are opened, allowing the surgeon to see the valves. Minimally invasive techniques are gaining in popularity with technological advances but are not currently standard practice.

Valve replacement vs. valve conservation
Artificial heart valves are non-physiological. Therefore, if possible, the patient's diseased valve should be remodelled. This is usually only possible with the mitral and sometimes the tricuspid valve. The criteria for valve repair are as follows:
● valve damage is minimal;
● valve leaflets are mobile; and
● there is no calcification.

Artificial heart valves
There are three main groups of artificial heart valves.

PROSTHETIC VALVES
Prosthetic valves are the most popular choice for the majority of patients. These valves are either of the ball-and-cage variety or use a tilting disc occluder or bileaflet mechanism. The initial use of metal alloys and plastics is now being superseded by pyrolytic carbon. A sewing ring made of Dacron allows suture of the valve to the native valve annulus. Patients with prosthetic valves implanted are at risk from thromboembolism, endocarditis (which may also produce septic emboli) and valve 'wear-out'.

Because of the risk of thromboembolism, lifelong anticoagulation is required in patients with prosthetic heart valves. Warfarin is commenced within 48 h of operation. In the UK, the currently recommended range for the international normalized ratio (INR) has been arbitrarily set at 3–4.5. Any interventional procedures on patients with prosthetic heart valves, including dentistry, should be performed with antibiotic cover to prevent valve endocarditis occurring (see later).

BIOPROSTHETIC VALVES
Animal tissue is mounted on a synthetic frame or stent. A common tissue used is porcine aortic valve, which is treated with glutaraldehyde to reduce antigenicity. For patients with bioprosthetic valves, anticoagulation is carried on for 3 months until the valve has become epithelialized.

BIOLOGICAL VALVES
These contain only biological tissue. Cadaveric tissue is used to create a homograft valve. In the hands of enthusiastic proponents they give excellent haemodynamic performance and are relatively free from thromboembolic risk. Anticoagulation is not required for biological valves.

Valvular heart disease at a glance

Definition

Valvular heart disease: a group of conditions characterized by damage to one or more of the heart valves, resulting in deranged blood flow through the heart chambers

Epidemiology
● Rheumatic fever is still a major problem in developing countries
● Congenital heart disease occurs in 8–10 per 1000 live births worldwide

Aetiology
● Congenital valve abnormalities
● Infective endocarditis
● Rheumatic fever
● Degenerative valve disease

Pathology
● *Rheumatic fever*: immune-mediated acute inflammation affecting the heart valves due to a cross-reaction between antigens of group A β-haemolytic streptococci and cardiac proteins

- Disease may make the valve orifice smaller (*stenosis*) or unable to close properly (*incompetence* or *regurgitation*) or both
- Stenosis causes a *pressure load*, while regurgitation places a *volume load* on the heart chamber immediately proximal to it with upstream and downstream effects

Clinical features

Aortic stenosis
- Angina pectoris
- Syncope
- Left heart failure
- Slow upstroke arterial pulse
- Precordial systolic thrill (second right intercostal space)
- Harsh midsystolic ejection murmur (second right intercostal space)

Aortic regurgitation
- Congestive cardiac failure
- Increased pulse pressure
- Water-hammer pulse
- Decrescendo diastolic murmur (lower left sternal edge)

Mitral stenosis
- Pulmonary hypertension
- Paroxysmal nocturnal dyspnoea
- Atrial fibrillation
- Loud first heart sound and opening snap
- Low-pitched diastolic murmur with presystolic accentuation at the apex

Mitral regurgitation
- Chronic fatigue
- Pulmonary oedema
- Apex laterally displaced
- Hyperdynamic precordium
- Apical pansystolic murmur radiating to axilla

Tricuspid stenosis
- Fatigue
- Peripheral oedema
- Liver enlargement/ascites
- Prominent JVP with large *a* waves
- Lung fields are clear
- Rumbling diastolic murmur (lower left sternal border)

Tricuspid regurgitation
- Chronic fatigue
- Hepatomegaly/ascites
- Right ventricular heave
- Prominent JVP with large *v* waves
- Pansystolic murmur (subxiphoid area)

Investigations
- ECG
- Chest X-ray
- Echocardiography and colour Doppler techniques
- Cardiac catheterization with measurement of transvalvular gradients

Management

Medical
- Treat cardiac failure, diuretics, restrict salt intake, reduce exercise, digitalis for rapid atrial fibrillation and anticoagulation for peripheral embolization

Surgical
- Repair (possible in mitral and tricuspid valve only) or replace diseased valve
- Artificial valves available:
  (a) Prosthetic (lifelong anticoagulation)
  (b) Bioprosthetic (animal tissue on prosthetic frame, 3 months' anticoagulation)
  (c) Biological (cadaveric homografts, no anticoagulation)

Infective endocarditis

Infective endocarditis affects 6–7 per 100,000 annually in the UK, with a male to female ratio of 2 : 1. It usually results from a bacterial infection originating on the endocardium or vascular endothelium, although infection may be caused by rickettsiae and fungi. The use of prophylactic antibiotics in patients with known valve lesions is of extreme importance in negating the bacteraemic effect of potential sources of infection, e.g. dental procedures, urinary infections or prostatectomy. The disease may occur as a fulminating or acute infection but more commonly runs an insidious and protracted course known as sub-acute (bacterial) endocarditis. Infective endocarditis is typically associated with a preceding valvular or intracardiac abnormality. However, patients with normal valves (especially those with impaired immunity) may be affected by highly virulent organisms.

Before the advent of antibiotics, bacterial endocarditis was uniformly fatal; with the introduction of penicillin the mortality was reduced to 30–40%.

Aetiology

The most common organisms responsible for infective endocarditis are listed below.

05

- *Streptococcus viridans* forms part of the bacterial flora of the pharynx and upper respiratory tract. Any instrumentation of these areas (e.g. dental procedures, tonsillectomy) is liable to cause a transient bacteraemia that will initiate the infection.
- *Streptococcus faecalis* is found in faecal and perineal flora. As a consequence, manipulation of the genitourinary tract may predispose to infection.
- *Staphylococcus aureus* is an organism of high virulence. Cellulitis or skin abscesses often provide the source of the infection. Patients with intravenous lines (particularly central lines), feeding lines, temporary pacemaker electrodes and catheters are at risk.

Pathophysiology

Continuous bacteraemia combined with local pathological change are the prerequisites for endocarditis. A pre-existing valve lesion produces an abnormal blood flow with turbulence and jet effects. This traumatizes the endocardium and a platelet and fibrin thrombus (vegetation) is formed that acts as a nidus for colonization. Deposition of microorganisms from the bloodstream on the thrombus initiates the infection. Injection of particulate matter by drug abusers will also cause endothelial damage, usually on the tricuspid valve, which may subsequently become colonized. The valve most commonly affected is the tricuspid valve. Infection may also occur on normal valves, particularly by organisms of high virulence.

Clinical presentation

The patient will frequently demonstrate the clinical features of sepsis: fever, rigors, malaise, anorexia, weight loss, myalgia and arthralgia. This may lead to anaemia and splenomegaly. A heart murmur is common but is not a prerequisite for diagnosis. Other manifestations include the following.
- Heart failure secondary to regurgitation due to perforation of a valve leaflet or fistula into another cardiac chamber.
- Complete heart block or pericarditis secondary to an annular or myocardial abscess.
- Disordered haemodynamics secondary to further valve distortion due to vegetations.
- Pulmonary or peripheral arterial emboli. Well-recognized clinical manifestations of peripheral emboli include splinter haemorrhages, Roth's spots, Janeway lesions and Osler's nodes. Emboli may also produce ischaemia of the peripheral or mesenteric circulation, mycotic abscesses and neurological syndromes. Renal infarction and infection may also occur, as may pneumonia from septic pulmonary emboli.

Investigation and evaluation

Blood cultures are of extreme importance, not only in achieving a diagnosis but also in monitoring the effect of antibiotic therapy. Cultures may be negative in up to 20% of patients; this may reflect prior antibiotic therapy. False-negative cultures may result from *Chlamydia* and fungi.

A normochromic normocytic anaemia is a common feature, in association with mild elevation of the white cell count and a moderately raised ESR and high C-reactive protein. Red blood cell casts and protein may be found in the urine. The ECG may be non-specific or show a prolonged PR interval or complete heart block. The latter is an ominous occurrence. Chest radiology may demonstrate heart failure, a pericardial effusion or evidence of septic pulmonary emboli. Echocardiography is able to demonstrate vegetations, regurgitation and the presence of an abscess.

Role of surgery

Surgery should follow a standard 4–6 weeks of antibiotic therapy with two synergistic antibiotics. Ideally, the patient should receive antibiotics for at least 1 week prior to surgery but if there is evidence of haemodynamic deterioration or severe sepsis, urgent surgery is indicated.

Other indications for surgical intervention include:
- moderate to severe congestive heart failure;
- persistent sepsis;
- abscess, conduction disturbance, fistulae;
- systemic emboli;
- progressive renal dysfunction;
- enlarging vegetations or persistence following an embolic event;
- prosthetic valve endocarditis.

At operation all the infected valve tissue is excised and any abscess cavities are drained and débrided. Damaged valves are repaired or replaced along with any associated pathology, e.g. septal defects. The operative mortality is high (20%), with a 4% incidence of developing infection on the newly replaced valve. This is higher if the operation is performed during active endocarditis.

Following operation the patient should be maintained on intravenous antibiotics until all investigations, both radiological and serological, show no evidence of continuing sepsis. This is commonly for a period of 6 weeks and is followed by a longer period of oral antibiotic therapy.

Aortic dissection

Pathophysiology

Aortic dissection usually occurs in the region of the aortic arch and is caused by an intimal tear; blood then enters the

media, which is cleaved proximally and distally into its inner two-thirds and outer third. The tear is the result of shear stress forces generated by the left ventricular ejection velocity and systemic arterial pressure. These forces cause fractional movement of aortic intima over media. Medial degeneration from hypertension, eccentric jet of blood from a bicuspid aortic valve or ageing predisposes to aortic dissection. Risk factors include hypertension, Marfan's syndrome, bicuspid aortic valve, pregnancy and surgery to the ascending aorta (as in aortic valve replacement). Traumatic aortic transection following blunt injury to the chest is a well-recognized but usually fatal event. It is often associated with a left first rib fracture and the usual site of transection is in the descending aorta just distal to the left subclavian artery. It is caused by rapid deceleration such as occurs in a restrained occupant of a high-speed road traffic accident or a fall from a height.

A diastolic murmur may indicate aortic annulus involvement, leading to severe incompetence of the aortic valve, in which case a valve replacement or resuspension procedure will be required. The dissection may extend into or shear off aortic side branches. Rupture may occur of the false lumen through the thin outer media and adventitia. Death is due to rupture or ischaemia of viscera.

Stanford classification

● Type A: ascending aorta involved, regardless of whether descending aorta is involved.
● Type B: dissection confined to the descending thoracic aorta.

Clinical presentation and investigation

Patients usually present with sudden severe chest pain radiating into the back, neck or arms. They may also be shocked, either from external rupture or severe aortic incompetence. If the latter, a diastolic murmur will be heard. The chest radiograph will usually show widening of the mediastinum. Further investigation should aim to provide confirmatory evidence of an aortic dissection, identify whether the ascending aorta is involved, and whether the dissection has disrupted other arterial branches.

For many years aortography was the only accurate diagnostic procedure for the evaluation of patients with suspected aortic dissection. More recently, CT, MRI, TOE, and transthoracic echocardiography have also been shown to be useful. For patients who are haemodynamically stable, CT or MRI should be the investigation of choice, with echocardiography reserved for patients who are haemodynamically unstable as it can be performed at the bedside.

Management
Type B dissections
Conservative management should be instituted for type B dissections as surgery confers no additional benefit in the absence of complications. Complications requiring operative intervention include bleeding, visceral ischaemia, uncontrollable hypertension, neurological deficits, persistent pain, arterial compromise, expansion or rupture. The main features of conservative management are careful monitoring of the patient, provision of haemodynamic support and control of blood pressure. Of paramount importance is the lowering of the arterial pressure of a hypertensive patient and the velocity of ventricular ejection. Sodium nitroprusside is an arterial vasodilator but increases the velocity of ventricular ejection as a result of reflex tachycardia. However, it may be combined with a β-adrenergic blocker, which will decrease ejection velocity, and a heart rate of 60 beats/min may be used as an endpoint. Intravenous β-blockers should be used. Labetalol is a combined α- and β-blocker that effectively lowers arterial blood pressure as well as reducing the velocity of left ventricular ejection due to negative chronotropic and inotropic effects.

Type A dissections
Type A dissections require surgery with use of cardiopulmonary bypass. The patient should be monitored in a high-dependency unit or ICU until transfer to a cardiothoracic unit can be made. Blood pressure should be controlled as above.

The ascending aorta (with or without the aortic valve) is replaced using a Dacron graft; the arch of the aorta may also have to be replaced if flow into the carotid or subclavian vessels has been compromised or if rupture is likely. Early diagnosis and rapid emergency transfer and surgery has reduced in-hospital mortality of acute type A dissection to 20%.

Evidence-based medicine

Akbari, C.M. & LoGerfo, F.W. (1999) Pathogenesis of the diabetic foot: diabetes and peripheral vascular disease. *J Vasc Surg* **30**, 373–84.
Ross, R. (1999) Pathogenesis of atherosclerosis: atherosclerosis an inflammatory disease. *N Engl J Med* **340**, 115–26.
http://www.esvs.org/international/eurostar.htm Evidence for endovascular aneurysm repair, EUROSTAR registry of endovascular aneurysm repair.

05

Pulmonary Disorders

38

Must know Must do

Must know

Clinical assessment and examination of patients with acute and chronic pulmonary disorders
How to inspect chest radiographs (posteroanterior and lateral) for lung, pleural and mediastinal disease
Pulmonary function tests and blood gas analysis
Pulmonary collapse and pneumonia
Types and management of respiratory failure
Aspiration syndromes
Principles underlying oxygen therapy
Core knowledge of common disorders of the pleura
Pathology and management of bronchial neoplasms
Core knowledge of mediastinal lesions

Must do

Examine chest radiographs showing collapse, pneumothorax, effusion, pneumonia, lung abscess, bronchial neoplasms, acute respiratory distress syndrome (ARDS)
Observe spirometry
Observe insertion of chest drain
Administer oxygen to patients (under supervision)
Visit the intensive care unit (ICU) to see patients with ARDS on ventilatory support
Observe a flexible bronchoscopy
Clerk and follow the management of a patient with bronchial carcinoma

Introduction

Diseases of the respiratory system are a major cause of illness and are frequently encountered in surgical practice. Many patients require detailed assessment of their pulmonary function prior to surgery and postoperative respiratory complications are not uncommon. Bronchial carcinoma is the most common fatal cancer and the lung is often the site of secondary deposits from tumours elsewhere in the body, e.g. renal carcinoma. The complications of 'benign' pulmonary disease sometimes require surgical treatment (e.g. drainage or decortication of the lung for empyema, resection of emphysematous bullae for persistent pneumothorax), and chest injury (see Chapter 20) is also a serious problem that requires skilful management.

Evaluation of the patient

Patients with acute or chronic disorders of the chest have specific symptoms and signs. The elucidation of the underlying problem is achieved by good history-taking, followed by complete physical examination and the performance of certain specific investigations. Some investigations are needed in all patients with chest problems, while others are dictated by details of the individual case.

Clinical assessment

Symptoms

The history often provides the most important piece of information leading to the diagnosis of a pulmonary disorder. General points to be considered in the history are listed below.

- *Smoking*: an attempt should be made to quantify the number of cigarettes smoked by calculating the 'pack-year' history. Smoking 20 cigarettes per day for 1 year represents 1 pack-year. Smoking 40 cigarettes per day for 1 year represents 2 pack-years.
- *Foreign travel*: tuberculosis is still common in certain parts of the world.
- *Exposure to asbestos*: bronchial carcinoma or pleural mesothelioma may develop years after exposure to asbestos.
- *Risk factors for human immunodeficiency virus (HIV) infection*: pneumonia is often the first indication of HIV infection.

Table 38.1 Symptoms of chest disorders.

Cough
Sputum production
Chest pain
Dyspnoea
Wheezing
Fever/rigors
Weight loss
Hoarseness
Dysphagia
Joint and bone pain

The important symptoms of chest disease are outlined in Table 38.1 and described below.

Cough. This may be dry or productive of sputum. It may occur in the morning only, as in chronic smokers, or be nocturnal (asthma, heart disease). In some disorders, the patient develops attacks of coughing when lying supine. This is encountered in patients with oesophageal disease and in those suffering from lung abscess. A 'bovine' cough suggests left recurrent laryngeal nerve palsy, often secondary to bronchial carcinoma.

Sputum. In patients suffering from chronic bronchitis the sputum is white and tenacious. A purulent nature is indicative of acute infections. In patients with bronchial carcinoma the sputum is often both purulent and blood-stained, while bronchiectasis results in copious amounts of yellow or green sputum.

Chest pain. This may originate from disorders of the chest, oesophagus (reflux disease and motility disorders) or ischaemic heart disease. The exact location, distribution, radiation and precipitating factors must be determined in the individual patient. Pulmonary pain is usually deep-seated and dull, whereas pleuritic pain encountered in pulmonary embolism and infection of the pleural space is sharp, synchronous with respiration and often accompanied by a pleural rub.

Dyspnoea. Breathlessness may be acute (e.g. pneumonia, pulmonary embolism, pneumothorax, pulmonary oedema, asthma) or chronic (e.g. obstructive airways disease, emphysema, fibrosing alveolitis). Breathlessness on lying flat is called orthopnoea and occurs with pulmonary oedema and asthma. Paroxysmal nocturnal dyspnoea is characteristic of left ventricular failure and is relieved by sitting up. Dyspnoea may be accompanied by wheezing in patients with asthma and it is painful in patients suffering from lobar pneumonia.

Wheeze and stridor. A wheeze is a high-pitched noise produced when the patient exhales. It denotes intrathoracic airway obstruction. It may be unilateral (bronchial foreign body, bronchial adenoma) or bilateral, as in patients suffering an asthmatic attack and those who develop pulmonary embolism. Stridor is a low-pitched noise produced on inspiration and usually indicates obstruction to the trachea or a major bronchus.

Fever/rigors. These are indicative of pulmonary sepsis such as pneumonia, bronchiectasis, tuberculosis (patients characteristically have night sweats) and lung abscess, which may be caused by aspiration, postpulmonary infarction or bronchial occlusion from carcinoma of the lung.

Weight loss. This is encountered in chronic pulmonary sepsis and bronchial carcinoma.

Hoarseness and dysphagia. These symptoms may be encountered in patients with intrathoracic malignancy (bronchial carcinoma or secondary mediastinal node involvement) and always signify advanced disease. The hoarseness is due to involvement of the recurrent laryngeal nerve. The dysphagia is caused by compression or invasion of the oesophagus and may progress to malignant tracheo-oesophageal fistula. The patient then develops significant respiratory problems due to flooding of the bronchial tree by saliva and ingested liquids. Involvement of the phrenic nerve leading to unilateral diaphragmatic paralysis is also a sign of advanced inoperable intrathoracic tumour.

Joint and bone pain. Patients with bronchial carcinoma most commonly experience bone pain as a result of osseous metastases. Less frequently, some patients develop a syndrome of hypertrophic pulmonary osteoarthropathy that causes persistent bone and joint (wrists and ankles) pain and marked finger clubbing. In this condition (which is quite unrelated to metastatic disease) there is thickening of the bones near the affected joints due to subperiosteal deposition of osteoid tissue.

Haemoptysis. This is always significant and may be due to neoplasms (bronchial carcinoma), infections (pneumonia, lung abscess, tuberculosis, bronchiectasis, fungal, parasitic) or cardiovascular disorders. Pulmonary embolic disease and pulmonary infarction also cause haemoptysis.

Physical examination

The important physical signs of pulmonary disease are cyanosis, finger clubbing (Fig. 38.1), pyrexia, altered respiratory pattern and rate, supraclavicular lymph node

05

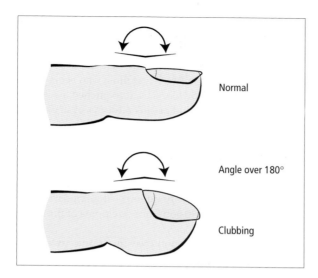

Normal

Angle over 180°

Clubbing

Figure 38.1 Finger clubbing: there is an increase in the nail bed angle, increased curvature of the nail and swelling of the tip of the finger.

enlargement and the specific chest signs elicited by inspection, palpation, auscultation and percussion (Table 38.2). Cyanosis is present when about 5 g/dL of haemoglobin is in the reduced state within the skin blood vessels. Peripheral cyanosis is usually due to local circulatory slowing and the part (e.g. hand) is generally cold. Central cyanosis is associated with hypoxaemia ($Pao_2 < 6$ kPa or 45 mmHg). However, cyanosis may not be detectable clinically if the patient is anaemic with a haemoglobin of less than 5 g/dL. In contrast, the patient may appear to be cyanotic if he or she is polycythaemic. The latter may be secondary to chronic hypoxia or develop as a primary disease (polycythaemia rubra vera). Cyanosis may also be due to the presence of significant amounts of circulating altered haemoglobin, e.g. methaemoglobinaemia and sulphaemoglobinaemia. Inspection of the sputum should be part of the clinical examination. The amount of sputum produced, the colour (white, yellow or green) and the presence or absence of blood should all be noted.

Investigations

The investigations commonly used for assessing patients with pulmonary disease are described in Table 38.3. The initial essential investigations for patients with pulmonary disease include chest X-ray (posteroanterior and lateral films), full blood count (FBC) and erythrocyte sedimentation rate (ESR). Radiographs should be examined for the specific features listed in Table 38.4. The FBC may show secondary polycythaemia in response to chronic hypoxia and a raised ESR may indicate infection. If the patient has a productive cough, sputum culture and cytology are also performed routinely. An electrocardiogram (ECG) is indicated to detect underlying heart disease.

Imaging

Other imaging tests such as computed tomography (CT) are carried out to obtain better definition of pulmonary and mediastinal lesions encountered on the chest radiograph. Ventilation–perfusion scanning (V/Q scan) is used in the diagnosis of pulmonary embolism. A gamma-camera is used to compare the distribution of radioactivity

Table 38.2 Examination of a patient with a suspected pulmonary disorder.

Inspection	Palpation	Percussion	Auscultation
Hands Nicotine staining Clubbing Peripheral cyanosis Tremor or flap	Pulse		
Face and neck Conjunctiva (anaemia) Lips and tongue (central cyanosis) Accessory muscles of respiration Jugular venous pressure	Lymph nodes	Supraclavicular fossae	Supraclavicular fossae
Chest Deformities Breathing rate and pattern Accessory muscles of respiration	Ribs Trachea Apex beat	Compare two sides of chest wall Note hepatic and cardiac dullness	Nature of sounds Added sounds Vocal resonance

05

Table 38.3 Investigations available for assessment of patients with pulmonary disease.

Haematology
Full blood count: secondary polycythaemia

Microbiology
Sputum culture and direct staining: Ziehl–Neelsen staining
   for tuberculosis

Imaging
Chest radiography: both posteroanterior and lateral films
Computed tomography of the thorax: identifies small lesions
Bronchography: used now only for bronchiectasis
Ventilation–perfusion scan: diagnosis of pulmonary embolus

Endoscopy
Indirect laryngoscopy: assess vocal cords
Bronchoscopy: visualize and biopsy bronchial tree
Mediastinoscopy: assess lymph node status in bronchial
   carcinoma
Thoracoscopy: examine pleural cavity

Pulmonary function tests
Detect and define abnormal lung function

Biochemistry
Arterial blood gas analysis: respiratory failure

Biopsy for histopathology
Bronchoscopy: biopsy of bronchial tree to fourth or fifth
   divisions
Bronchoalveolar lavage: collects fluid for cytology and culture
Percutaneous fine-needle biopsy: for discrete lung lesions
   beyond bronchoscopic range and pleural biopsy
Thoracocentesis: drains pleural effusion and provides cells for
   cytology
Open or thoracoscopic lung biopsy: lung tissue is removed
   via thoracotomy or thoracoscopy

Table 38.4 Specific features to look for on a chest radiograph.

Penetration and rotation
Overpenetrated films are very dark
Underpenetrated films are white
Vertebral spines should be midway between the
   costoclavicular joints

Bony skeleton
Collapse or secondary deposits in the vertebrae
Fractures or metastases in ribs

Heart
Size, shape and cardiothoracic ratio (< 0.5 normally)

Trachea and major bronchi
Position of trachea and bronchi

Hilar regions
Abnormal configuration may indicate lymphadenopathy

Lung fields
Pneumothorax
Collapse
Consolidation
Shadows
Effusion

Diaphragm and pleura
Position of diaphragms
Costophrenic angles for fluid
Air under diaphragm
Pleural thickening

in the lung when the patient breathes radiolabelled xenon gas (ventilation scan) and after injection of radiolabelled albumin (perfusion scan). Normally, the two scans should match perfectly and the test is most reliable when normal in excluding pulmonary embolism. It may be highly suggestive of pulmonary embolism if the ventilation scan is normal and the perfusion scan abnormal (no filling) in several segments (see Chapter 37). Otherwise the test is indeterminate because perfusion defects may be caused by a variety of chest disorders.

Endoscopy

Endoscopic visualization of the bronchial tree includes indirect laryngoscopy, which assesses vocal cord function, bronchoscopy and mediastinoscopy. Bronchoscopy allows

visualization of the endobronchial tree down to the fourth or fifth divisions. It is performed using a fine flexible endoscope (Fig. 38.2), which has now replaced the rigid bronchoscope. Bronchoscopy can be diagnostic, when the entire tracheobronchial tree is inspected and any lesions encountered are biopsied, or therapeutic when used for the removal of thick retained secretions and extraction of foreign bodies. Mediastinoscopy is performed under general anaesthesia and is used to sample mediastinal lymph nodes prior to surgery for bronchial carcinoma. Thoracoscopy is a technique where a rigid scope is passed into the pleural cavity. A number of operative procedures may be performed using this technique, e.g. transthoracic sympathectomy for hyperhidrosis, pulmonary biopsy and even pulmonary lobectomy.

Pulmonary function tests

In the elective situation, a good indication of global pulmonary function is obtained by assessing the exercise tolerance of the patient, i.e. distance walked before development of breathlessness and ability to climb a flight

05

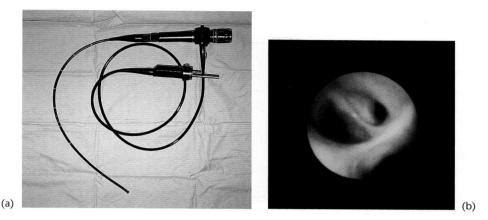

(a)   (b)

Figure 38.2 (a) Flexible bronchoscope. (b) A view of the right upper lobe obtained at bronchoscopy.

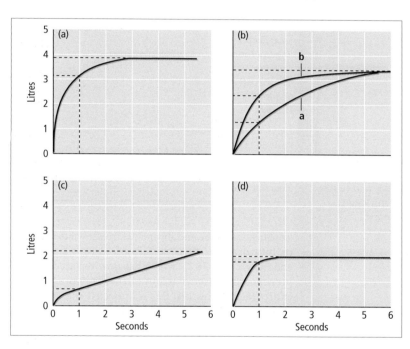

Figure 38.3 Spirogram tracings obtained from a vitalograph. (a) Normal: forced expiratory volume in 1 s (FEV_1) 3.1 L, forced vital capacity (FVC) 3.8 L, FEV_1/FVC 82%. (b) Obstructive reversible defect (asthma): **a**, before bronchodilator: FEV_1 1.4 L, FVC 3.5 L, FEV_1/FVC 40%; **b**, after bronchodilator: FEV_1 2.5 L, FVC 3.5 L, FEV_1/FVC 71%. (c) Obstructive irreversible defect (chronic bronchitis and emphysema): unchanged with bronchodilator, FEV_1 0.5 L, FVC 2.2 L, FEV_1/FVC 23%. (d) Restrictive defect (fibrosing alveolitis): unchanged with bronchodilator, FEV_1 1.8 L, FVC 2.0 L, FEV_1/FVC 90%.

of stairs. Dyspnoea at rest always indicates severe compromise of pulmonary function.

Peak expiratory flow rate (PEFR) can easily be measured with a peak expiratory flow meter and is the flow over the first 10 ms on maximal expiration after a maximum inspiration. It correlates well with forced expiratory volume in 1 s (FEV_1) and is reduced by airway narrowing (asthma, bronchitis) or muscle weakness (Fig. 38.3). Measurements of lung volume (Fig. 38.4) are used to estimate functional lung volumes. The best parameters for detection and quantification of airflow obstruction in chronic obstructive disease (e.g. chronic bronchitis) are FEV_1 and forced vital capacity (FVC). The ratio FEV_1/FVC (70–80%

normally) can be used to distinguish between obstructive (decreased ratio < 60%) and restrictive (increased ratio > 80%) lung disease (Fig. 38.3). However, the best indicators for restrictive lung disease (e.g. interstitial pulmonary fibrosis) are vital capacity (VC) and total lung capacity (TLC). Transfer factor (T_{LCO}), also called diffusing capacity (D_{LCO}), is a measurement that uses small amounts of inert gases or carbon monoxide to test the diffusion capacity of the alveolar–capillary membrane.

Blood gas analysis

This is performed on a sample of arterial blood (usually

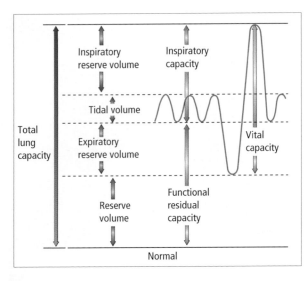

Figure 38.4 Subdivisions of total lung capacity.

obtained by a femoral stab). The analysis gives valuable information on the state of oxygenation, presence of pulmonary injury or disease, acid–base balance and the cause of acidosis or alkalosis. The Pao_2 reflects the amount of oxygen dissolved in the blood at sea level. Hypoxaemia is said to be present when this falls below 10.4 kPa (80 mmHg). However, oxygen in solution only represents 1–2% of the blood's total oxygen content, 98% of which is carried by haemoglobin. It is more important to realize that adequate oxygenation of the blood does not ensure adequate tissue oxygenation to the vital organs. This necessitates efficient transport to (by nutrient flow) and extraction by the tissues. The difference between oxygen tension in the alveolar space (Pao_2) and the arterial tree (Pao_2) is used to distinguish the pulmonary origin of the hypoxaemia from extrapulmonary causes (e.g. hypoventilation and low inspired oxygen tension). This difference ($Pa–ao_2$) is increased in pulmonary disease from any cause and is normal in patients with extrapulmonary impairment. Pao_2 can be calculated by the alveolar air equation:

$$Pao_2 = \text{inspired } Po_2 - (Paco_2/0.8)$$

A $Paco_2$ greater than 7.1 kPa (55 mmHg) is always indicative of severe respiratory impairment. The relationship between pH, bicarbonate and $Paco_2$ is outlined in Chapter 13.

Biopsies for histopathology or cytology

These may be obtained by thoracoscopy, thoracocentesis, percutaneous techniques or, in the last restort, thoracotomy.

Thoracocentesis is a technique that entails aspiration of pleural fluid to relieve dyspnoea and to obtain samples of pleural fluid for bacteriology and cytology. Percutaneous lung or pleural biopsies are obtained using conventional or CT imaging to guide the needle to the correct site for the diagnosis of primary pleural disorders (e.g. mesothelioma) or solitary accessible lung lesions (on the periphery of the pulmonary parenchyma). Nowadays, most wedge lung biopsies are performed via the thoracoscopic approach, which has replaced open thoracotomy for this purpose.

Pulmonary embolism, collapse and infections

Pulmonary embolism (see Chapter 37)

The types of emboli that may lodge in the main pulmonary trunk or pulmonary arteries or their branches include thromboemboli, tumour emboli, foreign-body emboli (venous cannulae), air emboli (exogenous air inadvertently introduced into the venous system) and fat emboli (after multiple fractures). Of these, by far the most common is thromboembolism and this is the condition commonly referred to as pulmonary embolism. It can be immediately fatal and is often accompanied by significant morbidity. The complications of pulmonary embolism consist of pulmonary infarction and pneumonia. Both are serious and may contribute to death of the patient. Pulmonary infarction tends to occur if the obstruction occurs in a peripheral branch and is associated with hypotension or heart failure. Pulmonary embolism is fully discussed in Chapter 37.

Pulmonary collapse

Pulmonary collapse results from alveolar hypoventilation such that the alveolar walls collapse and become de-aerated. The term is often used synonymously with atelectasis which, strictly speaking, is incorrect; pathologically, atelectasis refers to alveoli that have never been filled with inspired air. Pulmonary collapse is due to proximal bronchial occlusion, which may be organic or secretional in origin. Examples of the former include obstruction by bronchogenic carcinoma. Secretional airway obstruction leading to collapse is the most common cause in the postoperative period and is encountered predominantly in chronic smokers and patients with chronic bronchitis (Fig. 38.5). Aside from increased airway resistance, these patients develop bronchorrhoea after surgery and general anaesthesia. This consists of thick viscid mucus that plugs various segments of the bronchopulmonary tree leading to patchy segmental or lobar collapse. In addition, ciliary

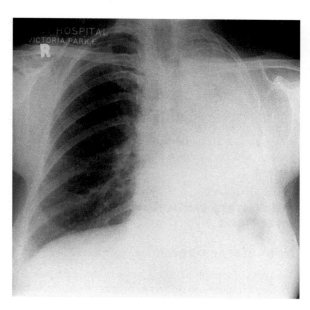

Figure 38.5 Complete collapse of the left lung due to a mucus plug in the main bronchus.

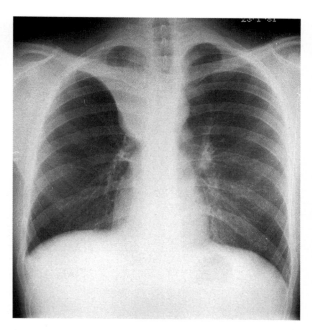

Figure 38.6 Right upper lobe collapse. Note the elevation of the right hilum and spreading of the right lower zone blood vessels.

activity is impaired so that movement of the secretion into the upper reaches of the bronchial tree where it can be expectorated is impaired. Following bronchial obstruction, the residual air trapped in the alveoli is absorbed and the resulting de-aerated area becomes prone to infection (bronchopneumonia). This is the most common type of postoperative chest infection.

Diagnosis

The collapse of a pulmonary segment is associated with pyrexia and the clinical manifestations of chest infection: tachypnoea, productive sputum, diminished air entry and bronchial breathing. A more severe ventilatory disturbance is exhibited by patients who develop lobar or pulmonary collapse, when respiratory difficulty and significant hypoxaemia are present. The diagnosis of pulmonary collapse is confirmed by a chest X-ray (Fig. 38.6).

Treatment

As in pulmonary embolism, prophylaxis is important. This consists of deep-breathing exercises started preoperatively, adequate pain relief and early ambulation. The treatment of established pulmonary collapse is by intensive physiotherapy. Antibiotics are administered in the presence of infection. If the secretional airway obstruction is major (as in the patient shown in Fig. 38.5), broncho-

scopic suction is necessary. Patients with severe disease with persistence of excessive bronchial secretion are nowadays managed by minitracheostomy.

Pulmonary infections

Pneumonia

Pneumonia is an infective consolidation of the pulmonary parenchyma and may be caused by bacterial (Table 38.5), viral (influenza, cytomegalovirus, varicella), fungal (*Candida*, *Aspergillus*, *Cryptococcus*) and protozoal (*Pneumocystis*, *Toxoplasma*) infections. The most common variety of pneumonia is bacterial, due to *Streptococcus pneumoniae* (Fig. 38.7). When serious, it carries a high mortality from acute pulmonary failure.

Certain groups of people are especially prone to develop life-threatening pneumonia (Table 38.6). Pneumonia can be acquired in the community or subsequent to admission to hospital (*hospital-acquired pneumonia*). There are important differences between the two, especially with regard to aetiology. Hospital-acquired pneumonia is an infective consolidation developing more than 3 days after admission to hospital. It affects approximately 2–5% of patients postoperatively and shows the highest

Table 38.5 Microorganisms causing bacterial pneumonia.

Streptococcus pneumoniae (most common)
Staphylococcus aureus (children and elderly)
Haemophilus influenzae (children, chronic lung disease, alcoholism)
Gram-negative organisms (severely ill and immunocompromised patients)
Acinetobacter spp., methicillin-resistant *Staph. aureus* (ventilator pneumonia)
Legionella spp.
Myobacteria (malnutrition, poor social conditions)

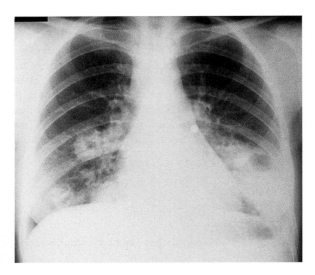

Figure 38.8 Bilateral cavitating pneumonia due to staphylococcal pneumonia.

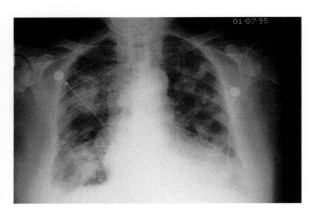

Figure 38.7 Bronchopneumonia that developed postoperatively in a patient after laparotomy.

Table 38.6 Patient groups prone to severe pneumonia.

Elderly
Patients with chronic lung and heart disease
Heavy smokers
Chronic alcoholics
Debilitated individuals
Diabetics
Immunodeficiency from any cause
Asplenic state
Patients on mechanical ventilation
Cerebrovascular accident victims

incidence in patients admitted to the ICU. When it develops in patients on mechanical ventilation it is called ventilator-associated pneumonia. Whereas community-acquired pneumonia is most commonly caused by *Strep. pneumoniae*, *Haemophilus influenzae*, influenza virus, etc., hospital-acquired pneumonia is due to infection with Gram-negative organisms such as *Pseudomonas aerugin-*

osa, *Enterobacter* spp., *Klebsiella pneumoniae*, *Proteus mirabilis*, *Acinetobacter* spp.

Pneumonia causes obvious respiratory distress with dyspnoea, which is painful, and tachypnoea. In addition, breathing is laboured with recruitment of the accessory muscles of respiration. If the resulting hypoxia is profound, the patient becomes confused or stuporous. Coughing is usually productive and purulent and haemoptysis may occur. Physical signs include pyrexia, cyanosis, tachycardia and hypotension (in severe pneumonia). The chest signs are those of diminished air entry and consolidation over a lobe or whole lung. The chest X-ray is usually diagnostic. Aside from the consolidation, pleural effusion, interstitial infiltrates and air–fluid cysts may be present (Fig. 38.8). Sputum culture is essential for effective antibiotic therapy.

Treatment

The management of streptococcal pneumonia entails respiratory support and specific medication. Respiratory support consists of oxygen therapy, ensuring adequate tissue perfusion by administration of crystalloid solutions and physiotherapy. If hypoxaemia is severe with obvious acute pulmonary failure, endotracheal intubation with mechanical ventilation becomes essential.

In the absence of the results of sputum culture, microscopic examination of the sputum with Gram staining can yield valuable information on the nature of the infecting organism and hence guide the selection of the appropriate antibiotic regimen. Penicillin remains the antibiotic

05

of choice for streptococcal pneumonia, while vancomycin is used for staphylococcal disease and ampicillin for *H. influenzae* infection. Most hospital-acquired pneumonias are due to Gram-negative organisms and for these the best-guess antibiotic regimen is a combination of an aminoglycoside and a cephalosporin. An aerosol β-adrenergic bronchodilator or intravenous aminophylline is administered in patients with chronic obstructive airways disease and those who have associated acute bronchospasm.

Lung abscess

The causes of lung abscess include:
- aspiration;
- secondary to specific pneumonias (*Staphylococcus, Klebsiella*);
- metastatic;
- malignant;
- post pulmonary infarction;
- specific (amoebic, tuberculous).

Aspiration lung abscess is most commonly located in the apical segment of the left lower lobe because the left bronchus is more in line with the trachea and this segment is in the dependent position when the patient is supine. It is due to aspiration and infection by organisms from the oropharynx during episodes of loss of consciousness, e.g. epileptic fit, alcoholic stupor. Lung abscess may develop as a complication of specific pneumonias, e.g. staphylococcal pneumonia, or be metastatic when the infection is carried to the lung from a focus of sepsis elsewhere in the body. Malignant lung abscess may arise in two ways: from bronchial obstruction by the tumour or as a result of central necrosis with superadded infection. An abscess may burst and discharge its contents into the bronchial tree (e.g. patient coughs up 'anchovy sauce' in amoebic lung abscess) or into a branch of the pulmonary artery (e.g. tuberculous abscess), when it may cause fatal exsanguination and drowning. Fungal (*Aspergillus*) infection of an abscess cavity may occur and can be very difficult to eradicate.

Suppurative pulmonary infections are caused by infection with *Klebsiella* and *Staphylococcus* with pulmonary abscess formation. Staphylococcal bronchopneumonia occurs predominantly in the elderly and may follow influenza, when it carries a high mortality. There are multiple small peribronchial abscesses. Children develop staphylococcal lobar pneumonia with abscess formation. These abscess cavities become inflated during coughing and crying, resulting in tension pneumatoceles through a check-valve mechanism. As these expand, they may compress the lung, causing respiratory embarrassment or rupture into the pleural space forming a tension pyopneu-

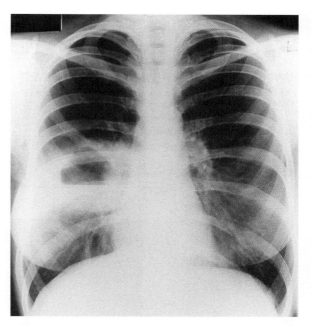

Figure 38.9 Lung abscess in the right lower lobe. Note the air–fluid level in the cavity.

mothorax. Suppurative *Klebsiella* pneumonias usually start in the right upper lobe and unless treated aggressively rapidly spread to the remaining lung, producing extensive destruction, abscess formation and fibrosis. Elderly males are principally affected. If the destroyed lobes become the site of persistent or recurrent infection, resection may be necessary.

The symptoms of lung abscess include malaise, intermittent fever and sweating, weight loss and cough. The diagnosis is usually established by chest X-ray (Fig. 38.9). An associated pleural effusion is common. An abscess may resolve with antibiotic therapy but when it becomes chronic, drainage is essential.

Pulmonary tuberculosis

Most tuberculous infections involve only the lungs or occur in association with extrapulmonary lesions such as tuberculosis of the skin (once known as scrofula), lymph nodes, bones and joints, genitourinary system, abdomen, intestines and central nervous system. In the western hemisphere the disease is rare as a result of improved nutrition and housing, pasteurization of milk, tuberculin testing in cattle and eradication of positive reactors, and human bacillus Calmette–Guérin (BCG) vaccination. Most of the infections in these countries are caused by *Mycobacterium tuberculosis*. They are acquired by

05

inhalation of organisms present in fresh droplets or dust contaminated with dried sputum from a patient with open pulmonary tuberculosis, i.e. a patient with myobacteria in the sputum. In economically deprived countries, infections caused by *M. bovis* are common. These are acquired by both ingestion and inhalation.

Pulmonary tuberculosis in childhood is characterized by marked involvement of the regional lymph nodes which, together with the solid pulmonary focus usually in the lung midzone (Ghon focus), is referred to as the primary complex. Particularly in malnourished individuals the disease may spread to both lungs in miliary fashion.

In adults, pulmonary tuberculosis extends locally by caseation (coagulative necrosis) with cavitation; healing is by fibrosis (Fig. 38.10). Apart from the chest symptoms and signs, pulmonary tuberculosis is accompanied by malaise, asthenia, weight loss, fever and night sweats. Diagnosis is made by identifying the tubercle bacillus; the presence of alcohol- and acid-fast bacilli on Ziehl–Neelsen staining of a sputum smear indicates tuberculosis. Frequently, surgeons are asked to biopsy lymph nodes to confirm the diagnosis. Tuberculosis is curable by modern chemotherapy, which has eliminated the need for sanatorium management. Drugs available include streptomycin, para-aminosalicylic acid, isoniazid, rifampicin, pyrazinamide and ethambutol.

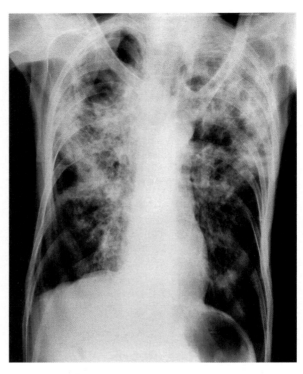

Figure 38.10 Extensive bilateral cavitating tuberculosis. This patient died despite aggressive and appropriate antituberculous chemotherapy.

Pulmonary collapse and postoperative pneumonia at a glance

Definitions

Pulmonary collapse (atelectasis): results from alveolar hypoventilation such that the alveolar walls collapse and become de-aerated. Pneumonia is an infection with consolidation of the pulmonary parenchyma

Aetiology/pathophysiology

Postoperatively, patients frequently develop atelectasis, which may develop into pneumonia

Pulmonary collapse
- Proximal bronchial obstruction
- Trapped alveolar air absorbed
- Common in smokers
- Common with chronic bronchitis

Predisposing factors
- Secretional airway obstruction:
  (a) Bronchorrhoea post surgery
  (b) Mucus plugs block bronchi
  (c) Impaired ciliary action

(d) Postoperative pain prevents effective coughing (especially thoracotomy and upper laparotomies)
- Organic airway obstruction: bronchial neoplasm

Pneumonia
Infection with microorganisms:
- Bacterial: *Streptococcus pneumoniae*, *Staphylococcus*, *Haemophilus influenzae*
- Viral: influenza, cytomegalovirus
- Fungal: *Candida*, *Aspergillus*
- Protozoal: *Pneumocystis*, *Toxoplasma*

Patients prone to severe pneumonia
- The elderly
- Alcoholics
- Chronic lung and heart disease
- Debilitated patients
- Diabetes
- Post cerebrovascular accident
- Immunodeficiency states
- Post splenectomy
- Atelectasis post surgery

05

Clinical features
Pulmonary collapse
- Pyrexia
- Tachypnoea
- Diminished air entry
- Bronchial breathing

Pneumonia
- Respiratory distress
- Painful dyspnoea
- Tachypnoea
- Productive cough ± haemoptysis
- Hypoxia (confusion)
- Diminished air entry
- Consolidation
- Pleural rub
- Cyanosis

Investigations
- Chest X-ray: consolidation, pleural effusion, interstitial infiltrates, air–fluid cysts

- Sputum culture: essential for correct antibiotic treatment
- Blood gas analysis: diagnosis of respiratory failure

Management
Prophylaxis
- Preoperative deep-breathing exercises
- Incentive spirometry
- Adequate analgesia postoperatively
- Early ambulation

Treatment
- Intensive chest physiotherapy
- Respiratory support:
  (a) Humidified oxygen therapy
  (b) Adequate hydration
  (c) Bronchodilators if bronchospasm is present
- Specific antimicrobial therapy

Complications
- Respiratory failure
- Lung abscess

Disorders of the pleura

The pleural space is outlined by the pleural membrane, which covers the inner chest wall (parietal pleura), the mediastinum and the lung surface (visceral pleura). In the normal state intrapleural pressure is negative such that only a thin film of fluid separates the two opposing pleural surfaces. Various pathological states result in abnormalities of the pleural lining and these are accompanied by accumulation of fluid, blood or air within the pleural cavity itself.

Traumatic disorders of the pleura

The traumatic disorders are pneumothorax (air in the pleural cavity), haemothorax (blood in the pleural cavity) and haemopneumothorax. The cause is most commonly fracture of the ribs. The fragments may lacerate the intercostal vessels as well as the subjacent lung. Rarely, open chest wounds can result in air entering the pleural cavity through the wound itself. This is referred to as sucking pneumothorax. Pneumothorax is also encountered in patients with rupture of the bronchi (see Chapter 20).

Pneumothorax
Pathophysiology
When the pressure inside a pneumothorax is static, the condition is called a *simple pneumothorax* and although this condition requires treatment, it is not usually serious (Fig. 38.11). In contrast, a *tension pneumothorax* is always

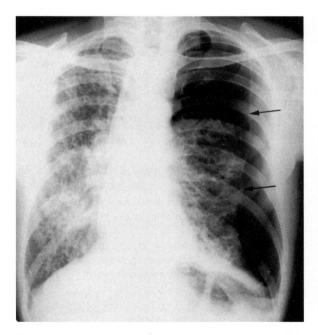

Figure 38.11 Left-sided pneumothorax in a patient with extensive bilateral pulmonary fibrosis following a percutaneous drill biopsy.

life-threatening. In these patients, the pulmonary laceration acts as a one-way valve, admitting inspired air into the pleural cavity with each inspiration but closing during expiration. The consequence is a progressive build-up of

05

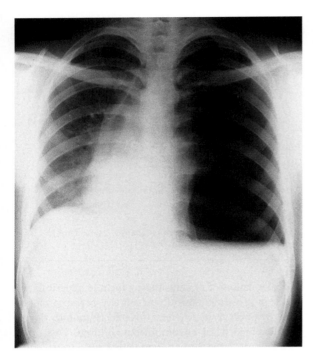

Figure 38.12 Left tension hydropneumothorax. Note the absence of lung markings on that side. The heart and trachea are shifted to the right. This patient requires urgent treatment to release the pneumothorax.

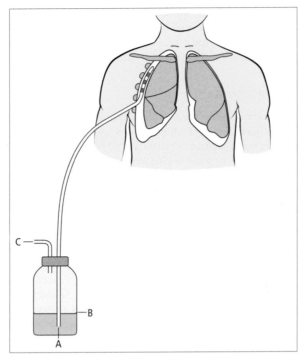

Figure 38.13 Principle of underwater seal drainage. A, the drainage point situated underwater; B, water level separating pleural pressure from the atmosphere; C, exit tube exposed to atmospheric pressure and to which low-pressure suction may be applied.

air with rising pleural pressure on the affected side. The result is total lung collapse and a shift of the mediastinum, including the heart and great vessels, to the contralateral side. Thus, in addition to respiratory distress and hypoxaemia, the patient may develop cardiovascular collapse (Fig. 38.12).

Symptoms

The symptoms of pneumothorax are anxiety, breathlessness and cyanosis. The trachea may be deviated. Percussion of the chest wall reveals hyperresonance and on auscultation air entry is diminished or absent. The diagnosis is confirmed by a portable chest X-ray.

Treatment

The treatment of a patient with tension pneumothorax must be immediate. If the patient is very distressed, a large-bore hypodermic needle is inserted into the second or third interspace anteriorly to decompress the pleural cavity until the equipment for underwater seal drainage becomes available.

The principle of underwater seal drainage is that a liquid trap is interposed between the tube exiting the pleural cavity and the atmosphere. If the pressure in the

pleural cavity is greater than atmospheric pressure, air, fluid or blood will drain out through the water-immersed tube (A in Fig. 38.13). On the other hand, when pleural pressure becomes negative, atmospheric air is prevented from being sucked into the pleural space by the water level (B in Fig. 38.13). The underwater seal bottle or disposable equivalent (such as Pleurivac) must always be kept at a lower level than the chest, and during changes or emptying of the bottle the exit tubing from the chest cavity must be clamped.

For treatment of a pneumothorax, the chest drain is inserted into the apex of the pleural cavity, either anteriorly through the second intercostal space in the midclavicular line or, preferably, through the fourth interspace in the midaxillary line. A basal drain is necessary for drainage of blood or fluid. This is inserted posterolaterally through the fifth interspace. Patients with haemopneumothorax require both apical and basal chest drains.

The chest drain is maintained until there is full lung expansion and any blood or fluid has drained away. A persistent air leak is easily recognized as bubbling through the water of the underwater seal drain. Lung expansion is signified by cessation of movement of the fluid column

but this must be confirmed by chest X-ray. The tube is then clamped for several hours and if repeat radiography shows that the lung remains expanded, the drain is removed and the chest wound sutured and dressed.

Haemothorax

This is the accumulation of blood in the pleural space and is a frequent result of either blunt or penetrating trauma. A plain radiograph of the chest should be obtained as early as possible during the resuscitation of the injured patient. Despite the diverse nature of chest injuries, many of these patients present initially with either haemothorax or pneumothorax, or haemopneumothorax (both air and blood). Treatment of haemothorax or pneumothorax is often the sole intervention required in patients with chest trauma. The bleeding may range from minimal to massive life-threatening haemorrhage depending on the nature of the injury (intercostal vessels, pulmonary laceration, laceration of major pulmonary vessels, etc.). Initial treatment of haemothorax requires placement of a chest tube (underwater seal thoracostomy) large enough to ensure evacuation of the accumulated blood, volume replacement and close observation of vital signs. The majority of lacerations to the pulmonary parenchyma involve low-pressure vessels of the pulmonary circulation. Such bleeding can be expected to stop after placement of the chest tube and re-expansion of the lung. Injuries to systemic arteries, including the intercostal arteries and internal mammary arteries, can lead to massive haemorrhage, especially if the vessels are only partially transected. Most cases of haemothorax can be treated by intercostal tube drainage alone. Surgery is required if:

- initial drainage > 1000 mL when chest drain placed;
- there is significant continued bleeding in excess of 200–300 mL/h.

Spontaneous pneumothorax

The causes of pneumothorax are listed in Table 38.7. Spontaneous pneumothorax arises in the absence of trauma. There are two groups of patients most at risk. The first consists of fit young adults (often tall thin young men) in whom apical blebs, often bilateral, rupture and cause pneumothorax. In this group pneumothorax is often recurrent unless specific surgical treatment is undertaken. These blebs were once thought to result from childhood tuberculosis but they are now considered to be due to congenital defects in the alveolar wall. The other group of patients who commonly develop spontaneous pneumothorax are those suffering from emphysema with air trapping and bullae formation. Due to impaired pulmonary reserve, pneumothorax induces severe respiratory distress in these patients.

Table 38.7 Causes of pneumothorax.

Spontaneous rupture of a congenital pleural bleb
Rupture of an emphysematous bulla
Trauma
   Penetrating injury
   Fractured ribs
   Iatrogenic (e.g. following central line insertion or after lung biopsy)
Rupture of intrapulmonary cavity (e.g. staphylococcal pneumonia)
Positive-pressure ventilation
Resuscitation and ventilation of the newborn
Asthma
Cystic fibrosis
Rare connective tissue disorders (Marfan's syndrome, Ehlers–Danlos syndrome)

Other causes of pneumothorax include hyperinflation of the lung during intermittent positive-pressure ventilation, α_1-antitrypsin deficiency-related pulmonary disease and staphylococcal pneumonia in children. This pneumonia leads to the formation of tense cystic spaces within the area of consolidation. These cystic lesions may rupture and cause a pyopneumothorax.

Initially, the management of spontaneous pneumothorax is with intercostal drainage as described above. Lung expansion may be expedited by low negative suction to the outlet of the underwater seal (C in Fig. 38.13). If the lung does not expand or the pneumothorax is recurrent, surgical treatment designed to obliterate the bullae and excise or abrade the parietal pleura is required. Pleurectomy or pleural abrasion is undertaken to encourage the formation of adhesions between the lung surface and the chest wall. This is now performed via the thoracoscopic approach.

Pleural effusions

A pleural effusion is an abnormal amount of fluid within the pleural space. A collection in excess of 100 mL can be detected radiologically but for clinical detection (by physical examination) the collection has to exceed 500 mL. The mechanisms involved include the following.

- Increased capillary hydrostatic pressure: left heart failure, congestive heart failure, etc.
- Decreased colloid osmotic pressure: hypoproteinaemia from any cause if severe enough.
- Increased capillary permeability due to inflammation of the pleura, e.g. pneumonia, pulmonary infarction, pulmonary tuberculosis. When the primary focus of infection/inflammation is in the subphrenic region, the term *sympathetic effusion* is often used, e.g. acute necrotizing pancreatitis.

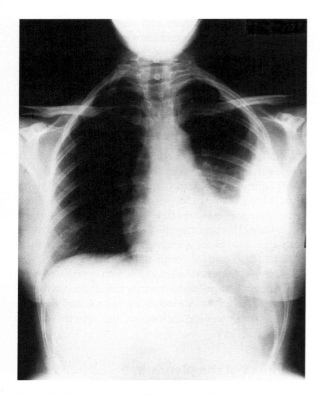

Figure 38.14 Medium-sized left pleural effusion.

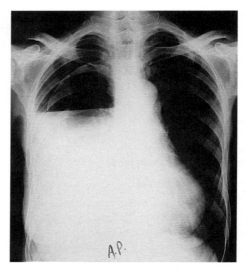

Figure 38.15 Air–fluid level in a patient with haematopneu-mothorax.

• Impaired lymphatic drainage: blockage of the lymphatics by lymph node infiltration by tumour.

• Damage to the thoracic duct during oesophagectomy or spontaneous rupture from malignant occlusion may result in accumulation of pure lymph in the thorax (chylothorax).

Clinically, a pleural effusion is detected by stony dullness on percussion and diminished breath sounds on auscultation. Radiologically, effusions appear as basal areas of uniform shadowing without distinct margins (Fig. 38.14) unless the effusion is loculated. An air–fluid level signifies either a leak from the lung or exogenous air introduced during chest aspiration (Fig. 38.15). If massive, the patient will experience breathlessness at rest.

The management of pleural effusion consists of treating the underlying cause and relieving symptoms caused by the effusion. Aspiration of a little fluid from an area of maximal dullness confirms the diagnosis and the macroscopic appearance often gives a clue to the probable diagnosis.

• Clear light straw-coloured fluid that does not clot (transudate): heart failure, hypoproteinaemia, etc.

• Dark-yellow fluid that clots on standing (exudate): local pulmonary cause such as tumour or infection.

• Blood-stained (old/altered blood): malignancy, pulmonary infarction, tuberculosis, necrotizing pancreatitis.

• Frank blood: haemothorax from chest trauma
• Turbid: pneumonic effusions.
• Frank pus: empyema.
• Milky white: chylothorax due to malignant involvement/iatrogenic damage to large lymphatic ducts.

Further information is obtained by cytology, culture and biochemical analysis of the pleural aspirate. If the pleural effusion is massive and symptomatic, evacuation by aspiration (thoracocentesis) is performed to relieve the dyspnoea. Malignant pleural effusions are caused by secondary involvement of the pleural lining or by primary pleural tumours. They often require aspiration. Reaccumulation may be prevented by intrapleural instillation of a pleural sclerosing agent such as tetracycline, bleomycin or *Corynebacterium parvum*.

Empyema

Empyema is defined as an infection within the pleural cavity with formation of purulent exudate or frank pus. It is always secondary to spreading infection from the underlying lung or elsewhere. The causes of empyema are shown in Table 38.8. A neglected empyema may burst through the chest wall and discharge externally (empyema necessitatis).

Irrespective of cause, pleural inflammation results in the formation of fluid rich in fibrin and polymorphonuclear leukocytes. The fibrin is continually deposited on the pleural surfaces, which become progressively thickened. The deeper layers of this pyogenic membrane become fibrotic and contract down, trapping the lung parenchyma and preventing expansion of the alveoli.

05

Table 38.8 Causes of empyema.

Pulmonary infections
Pneumonia
Lung abscess
Bronchiectasis
Tuberculosis

Trauma and postoperative
Chest injuries
Oesophageal perforations
Leaking intrathoracic anastomosis

Subdiaphragmatic infections
Subphrenic abscess
Hepatic abscess

Osteomyelitis
Ribs and vertebrae

Metastatic infection
Septicaemia

Untreated, the process continues until the empyema becomes chronic and the underlying lung totally collapsed. The transition from acute to chronic empyema takes 6–12 weeks from the onset of the disease. A chronic empyema may become calcified.

Clinical features

The usual clinical picture is that of a patient who develops a chest infection which fails to respond to treatment or relapses soon after. The situation following oesophageal perforation or leaking intrathoracic anastomosis is more dramatic and the patient rapidly becomes acutely ill. The symptoms of empyema include toxicity with fever, malaise and dyspnoea. The physical findings are similar to those of a pleural effusion, except in patients with perforated/leaking oesophagus who exhibit a pyopneumothorax. This may also be encountered in victims of staphylococcal pneumonia. Radiologically, an empyema resembles a pleural effusion and, if large, the entire hemithorax may become opaque. A marked leukocytosis is invariably present.

Treatment

An acute empyema is treated with appropriate antibiotics, repeated chest aspirations and vigorous physiotherapy. If the fluid is or becomes too thick for aspiration, an intercostal underwater seal drain is inserted. Failure of such treatment or the presence of chronic empyema are indications for surgical treatment, i.e. decortication. Decortication is an operation whereby the chest cavity is opened via a thoracotomy and the thickened inflamed pleura is stripped off the surface of the lung, thus allowing the lung to expand. Antibiotics are continued until the infection has been eradicated. During surgery, any underlying lung pathology is also dealt with. This often involves resection of the affected lung parenchyma.

Chylothorax

Chylothorax signifies the presence of lymph fluid in the pleural space. The condition is readily diagnosed by chest aspiration, when the nature of the opalescent milky fluid becomes apparent. Chylothorax most commonly arises from trauma to the thoracic duct or right lymphatic duct during thoracic operations such as oesophagectomy. Other causes include malignant obstruction of the thoracic duct by metastatic lymph nodes.

Although conservative measures such as repeated chest aspiration with instillation of intrapleural sclerosants may be employed, these are often ineffective and open or thoracoscopic surgical ligation of the affected duct is usually necessary.

Tumours of the pleura

The primary tumour that affects the pleural membrane arises from mesothelial tissue and is therefore known as a mesothelioma. Histologically, the tumour consists of a mixture of epithelial and connective tissue components in varying proportions. The important aetiological factor is exposure to asbestos, usually 20–40 years prior to the development of the tumour. There are two macroscopic types of mesothelioma: localized and diffuse lesions. Malignant diffuse mesothelioma is a prescribed industrial disease and should be reported to the appropriate authorities for compensation.

Localized lesions

These are well-encapsulated tumours and may affect the visceral or parietal pleura. They usually form thickened plaques but occasionally may be nodular or even pedunculated. They are often of low-grade malignancy and some are benign.

Diffuse malignant mesothelioma

This tumour carries a poor prognosis. It forms a thick spreading sheet of tumour tissue which infiltrates the underlying lung, chest wall, mediastinum, opposite pleura and even the peritoneum by direct extension. A bloodstained pleural effusion may be present initially, but in time the entire pleural space becomes completely obliterated by

tumour. Spread to the regional mediastinal lymph nodes is present in the majority of patients at the time of diagnosis.

Treatment

Localized disease is readily amenable to surgical excision, with good results in terms of long-term survival. Diffuse mesothelioma may be operable when a radical pleuro-pneumonectomy is performed. Often, however, the disease is inoperable. There is little that can be done aside from analgesia and terminal care in these patients as the tumour does not respond to radiotherapy or chemotherapy.

Pleural disorders at a glance

Definitions

Pleura: membrane that lines the inside of the chest wall (*parietal pleura*), mediastinum and lung (*visceral pleura*). The pleural space is a potential space between the two layers of the pleural membrane and contains a thin film of fluid. Normally the intrapleural pressure is negative

Pneumothorax: presence of air in the pleural cavity

Haemothorax: presence of blood in the pleural cavity

Haemopneumothorax: presence of blood and air in the pleural cavity

Pleural effusion: accumulation of an abnormal amount of fluid (> 100 mL) in the pleural space

Empyema: infection within the pleural cavity with the formation of purulent exudates or frank pus

Pneumothorax
Causes
Trauma
- Penetrating injury
- Fractured ribs
- Iatrogenic (central line insertion, lung biopsy)

Spontaneous rupture of an emphysematous bulla
- Young males (often tall and thin) with congenital apical blebs
- Older patients with emphysema

Rare causes
- Positive-pressure ventilation
- Rupture of intrapulmonary cavity
- Asthma
- Cystic fibrosis
- Connective tissue disorders

Classification
- *Simple pneumothorax*: pressure is stable
- *Tension pneumothorax*: pressure is rising on affected side, causing mediastinal shift to contralateral side, compression of the great veins, reduced venous return, cardiac arrest and death. It is a medical emergency

Diagnosis
Clinical
- Dyspnoea
- Hyperresonant on percussion
- Shift of apex beat and trachea if tension pneumothorax

Radiological
- Loss of lung markings out to chest wall
- May be fractured ribs

Treatment
- Immediate needle decompression of thoracic cavity via second intercostal space, midclavicular line for tension pneumothorax
- Chest drain via fourth intercostal space, midaxillary line with underwater seal drainage
- Chest drain maintained until full expansion of lung, i.e. cessation of movement of fluid column in drain

Haemothorax
Causes
Trauma
- Blunt
- Penetrating

Source of bleeding
- Intercostal vessel injury
- Lung parenchymal lacerations
- Laceration of major pulmonary vessels or heart

Diagnosis
Clinical
- History of trauma
- Dyspnoea
- Dull on percussion

Radiological
- Pleural effusion
- May be fractured ribs

Treatment
- Large chest drain in dependent area, e.g. fourth intercostal space, midaxillary line with underwater seal drainage

05

- Surgery usually not required for most haemothoraces
- Indications for surgery:

    (a) Initial drainage > 1000 mL when chest drain placed
    (b) Continued discharge from chest drain of > 200–300 mL/h

Pleural effusion
Aetiology

Mechanism	Causes
Increased capillary hydrostatic pressure	Left heart failure, congestive cardiac failure
Decreased colloid osmotic pressure	Hypoproteinaemia
Increased capillary permeability due to inflammation of pleura	Pneumonia, pulmonary infarction, pulmonary tuberculosis, sympatheic effusion from subdiaphragmatic inflammatory process
Impaired lymphatic drainage	Blockage of lymphatics or lymph nodes by tumour
Injury to thoracic duct leading to chylothorax rupture	Iatrogenic (e.g. during oesophagectomy), spontaneous

Diagnosis
Clinical

- Dyspnoea
- Stony dullness on percussion
- Reduced breath sounds on auscultation

Radiological

- Basal areas of shadowing with meniscus on radiograph

Aspirate
Confirms diagnosis and may give clue to cause:
- Clear, straw-coloured, does not clot (transudate): heart failure, hypoproteinaemia
- Dark yellow, clots on standing (exudate): tumour or infection
- Blood-stained: malignancy, infarction, tuberculosis, pancreatitis
- Frank blood: haemothorax
- Turbid: pneumonia
- Pus: empyema
- Chyle (milky white): chylothorax

Treatment
- Treat cause but if massive and patient is distressed then drainage may be required by thoracentesis

Empyema
Causes
Pulmonary infections
- Pneumonia
- Lung abscess
- Bronchiectasis
- Tuberculosis

Trauma
- Chest injuries (inadequately drained haemothorax)
- Oesophageal perforations
- Leaking anastomosis

Subdiaphragmatic infections
- Subphrenic abscess
- Hepatic abscess

Osteomyelitis
- Ribs and vertebrae

Metastatic infection
- Septicaemia

Diagnosis
Clinical
- Unresolving or relapsing chest infection
- Toxicity
- Malaise
- High swinging fever
- Dyspnoea
- Leukocytosis

Radiological
- Pleural effusion

Aspiration
- Pus

Treatment
- Antibiotics, drainage and physiotherapy
- Surgical decortication: thickened pleura is stripped off the surface of the lung allowing it to expand

Bronchial neoplasms

Although the most common pulmonary tumours are secondary deposits, primary bronchial neoplasms are frequent, with an incidence of 40–110 per 100,000 of the population above the age of 45 years. Primary pulmonary lymphomas are rare, although secondary involvement from Hodgkin's and non-Hodgkin's disease is common. Benign lung tumours (e.g. hamartoma, chondroma, angioma) are uncommon and produce symptoms by local effects. Bronchial adenomas are also uncommon and cause bronchial obstruction and distal collapse. They present with cough and haemoptysis. Histologically, the majority are bronchial carcinoids but carcinoid syndrome is rare and suggests the presence of metastases. These tumours are slow-growing and locally invasive, but 10% show malignant features. Treatment is by surgical excision.

Secondary pulmonary deposits

The extensive capillary bed of the pulmonary parenchyma is the main reason for the common occurrence of pulmonary metastases from a variety of malignant neoplasms. Although virtually any malignant tumour may metastasize to the lungs, some tumours have a special predilection for this site. These include breast cancer, hypernephroma, melanoma, neuroblastoma and osteogenic sarcoma. The pulmonary deposits are usually multiple and bilateral (Fig. 38.16). Less frequently, a solitary metastasis is encountered and this may be amenable to surgical resection. When the secondary nodules involve the pleura, malignant pleural effusion occurs. Pulmonary deposits indicate advanced incurable disease, although modern chemotherapy may result in significant regression in some patients.

Primary bronchial neoplasm

Bronchial carcinoma remains one of the major killer diseases and 80% of victims die within 1 year of diagnosis. The mean age at presentation is in the seventh decade, with men affected four to five times more frequently than women. The important aetiological factor is cigarette smoking, which increases the risk of death from bronchial carcinoma by a factor of 10. Other aetiological factors include atmospheric pollution and industrial exposure to uranium, chromium, arsenic, haematite and asbestos. The various histological types of bronchial tumours are shown in Table 38.9.

Squamous cell lesions are the most common and now account for 35% of all bronchial carcinomas in the UK. They occur centrally in the main bronchi and have a tendency to undergo central necrosis. Small-cell carcinomas

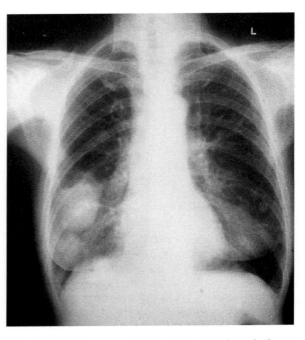

Figure 38.16 Two cannonball metastases in the right lower lobe.

Table 38.9 Histological types of bronchial carcinomas.

Epithelial
Squamous cell carcinoma
Adenocarcinoma
Large-cell carcinoma
Adenosquamous carcinoma
Epithelial of salivary gland type
Adenoidcystic carcinoma
Epithelial with neuroendocrine features
Small-cell carcinoma
Carcinoid tumour

include oat-cell tumours and other cell types. These lesions are responsive to chemotherapy. Adenocarcinomas tend to be peripheral tumours and may arise in relation to scars. They carry the best prognosis after resection. The most common sites for metastases from bronchial carcinomas are brain, bone, liver and contralateral lung.

Clinical features

The early symptoms are non-specific and include tiredness, cough, anorexia and weight loss. The cough may be productive and the sputum is often purulent due to secondary infection. Haemoptysis is usually minor but

05

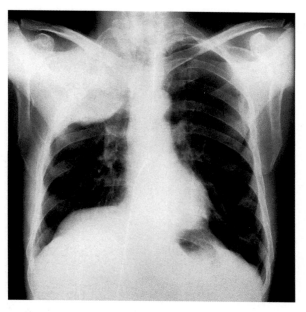

Figure 38.17 Carcinoma of the right upper lobe. This is the type of lesion that produces Pancoast syndrome (lower brachial plexus lesion, Horner's syndrome, rib erosion and an apical lung shadow).

persistent. Often the presentation is with an acute chest illness, i.e. bronchopneumonia due to infection within the collapsed lung parenchyma following bronchial occlusion by the tumour. Pleuritic pain may be secondary to the infection or result from invasion of the chest wall. Other manifestations include neuropathy and myopathy, hypertrophic osteoarthropathy and endocrine syndromes. The latter are usually caused by oat-cell tumours, which may secrete adrenocorticotrophic hormone (ACTH) causing adrenocortical hyperplasia, parathormone (hypercalcaemia) and antidiuretic hormone.

Other symptoms and signs are produced by direct invasion and these signify inoperability. Invasion of the cervical sympathetic chain causes Horner's syndrome. Hoarseness is due to involvement of the left recurrent laryngeal nerve and breathlessness may be caused by paralysis of the diaphragm following invasion of the phrenic nerve. Pancoast syndrome is particularly distressing. It results from an apical tumour that invades the sympathetic trunk and brachial plexus, causing Horner's syndrome, severe brachial neuralgia and paralysis of the upper limb (Fig. 38.17). Dysphagia signifies invasion of the oesophagus and this may progress to a malignant broncho-oesophageal fistula. Finally, mediastinal involvement, particularly of the lymph nodes, results in superior vena caval obstruction. In the physical examination of patients with bronchial carcinoma, the neck must be examined for supraclavicular lymph node enlargement and the abdomen for hepatomegaly.

Investigations

The essential investigations for establishing the diagnosis of bronchial carcinoma are chest X-ray, sputum cytology and bronchoscopy with biopsy. Other tests, such as CT of the thorax and abdomen and liver ultrasound, are used to stage the disease and detect inoperability (Fig. 38.18). Lung function tests are performed to establish whether the patient has enough pulmonary reserve to tolerate lung resection.

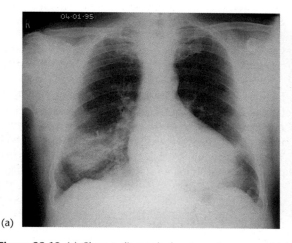

(a)

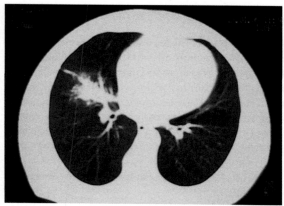

(b)

Figure 38.18 (a) Chest radiograph showing a large bronchial neoplasm in the right lower lobe. (b) CT scan of the same lesion. This was a squamous carcinoma and as there was no evidence of metastatic disease the patient underwent a right lower lobe lobectomy.

Treatment

The best results follow excision via thoracotomy. The extent of the resection depends on the size and location of the tumour. It may involve a lobe (lobectomy) or a whole lung (pneumonectomy). Adjuvant (additional) treatment with chemotherapy, especially for small (oat)-cell tumours, and radiotherapy is used in some centres.

Surgery is contraindicated for advanced inoperable disease and in patients with poor respiratory function. These patients are treated by supervoltage radiotherapy and combination chemotherapy. Small-cell carcinomas are the most radiosensitive, whereas adenocarcinomas respond poorly to this treatment. The best results with combination chemotherapy (vincristine, methotrexate and cyclophosphamide) are obtained in patients with small-cell carcinomas.

Palliation of symptoms such as breathlessness caused by narrowing of a major bronchus can be achieved by destroying the tumour with laser therapy applied via a bronchoscope. Superior vena caval obstruction may be helped by steroids; more recently, it has been relieved by endovascular stenting. Pain control and relief of distressing symptoms such as cough and breathlessness are important and dedicated care either in a hospice or at home should be provided for all terminally ill patients with cancer.

Prognosis

The prognosis for lung cancer is grim. Most patients will be dead within 12 months of diagnosis. Following 'curative' resection, 5-year survival rates are approximately 20–30% but overall 5-year survival is only about 6%. Chemotherapy may produce a response in 60–80% of patients with small-cell carcinoma but survival is not

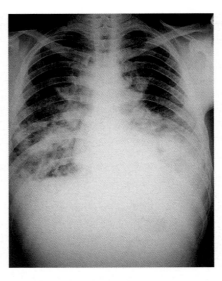

Figure 38.19 Primary non-Hodgkin's lymphoma of the lung.

greatly improved, although 10% remain disease-free at 2 years.

Lymphomas

Secondary involvement of the lung from primary extrapulmonary lymphomas (Hodgkin's and non-Hodgkin's) is more common than primary disease. Primary pulmonary Hodgkin's disease arises in peribronchial lymph nodes, usually in young patients. The symptoms include pyrexia, cough, asthenia, haemoptysis and itching. The lesion appears as a well-circumscribed shadow. If the diagnosis is established, treatment is by radiotherapy and chemotherapy. When the diagnosis remains in doubt, thoracotomy and excision of the lobe containing the lesion are performed (Fig. 38.19).

Bronchial carcinoma at a glance

Definition

Bronchial carcinoma: malignant lesion of the respiratory epithelium

Epidemiology
- Male/female ratio 5 : 1
- Uncommon before age 50, most patients are in their sixties
- Accounts for 40,000 deaths per annum in the UK

Aetiology
- Cigarette smoking
- Air pollution

- Exposure to uranium, chromium, arsenic, haematite and asbestos

Pathology
Histology
- Squamous carcinoma: 50%
- Small (oat)-cell carcinoma: 35%
- Adenocarcinoma: 15%

Spread
- Direct to pleura, recurrent laryngeal nerve, pericardium, oesophagus, brachial plexus
- Lymphatic to mediastinal and cervical nodes

05

- Haematogenous to liver, bone, brain, adrenals
- Transcoelomic pleural seedlings and effusion

Clinical features
- Symptoms may be masked by coexistent lung pathology: chronic obstructive pulmonary disease (COPD)
- History of tiredness, cough, anorexia, weight loss
- Productive cough with purulent sputum
- Haemoptysis
- Finger clubbing
- Bronchopneumonia (secondary infection of collapsed lung segment distal to malignant bronchial obstruction)
- Pleuritic pain
- Neuropathy, myopathy, hypertrophic osteoarthropathy
- Endocrine syndromes: ACTH secreted by oat-cell tumours, parathormone by squamous cell carcinoma (hypercalcaemia)
- Pancoast tumour (apical tumour invading sympathetic trunk and brachial plexus): Horner's syndrome, brachial neuralgia, paralysis of upper limb
- Dysphagia and broncho-oesophageal fistula
- Superior vena caval obstruction

Investigations
Diagnostic
- Chest X-ray (posteroanterior and lateral): lung opacity, hilar lymphadenopathy
- CT-guided lung biopsy
- Sputum cytology
- Bronchoscopy and cytology of brushings or lavage fluid

Assessment of operability
- Helical CT of thorax/abdomen: involvement of adjacent structures, hepatic metastases, multiple primary lesions
- Bone scan: metastases
- Liver ultrasound: metastases
- Mediastinoscopy: involvement of mediastinal nodes
- Lung function tests: likely patient tolerance of pulmonary resection

Management
Bronchial carcinoma often presents late and most are not resectable

Surgery
- Indicated only for non-small-cell tumours when tumour is confined to one lobe or lung, no evidence of secondary deposits, carina is tumour-free on bronchoscopy
- Operation: lobectomy or pneumonectomy

Palliation
- Radiotherapy (small-cell carcinoma most radiosensitive): stop haemoptysis, relieve bone pain from secondaries, relieve superior vena caval obstruction

Prognosis
- Following 'curative' resection, 5-year survival rates are approximately 20–30% but overall 5-year survival is only about 6%

Mediastinal lesions

The mediastinum, the intrathoracic space between the two lungs, is anatomically divided into four regions (Fig. 38.20). The mediastinum contains the heart and great vessels; the oesophagus, trachea and main bronchi; the thymus; the azygous system of veins; the thoracic and right lymphatic ducts and lymph nodes; and nerves (recurrent laryngeal, vagal, phrenic and autonomic).

The disorders of the mediastinum are classified as:
- infection (mediastinitis);
- syndromes arising from ectopic endocrine tissue;
- tumours;
- idiopathic mediastinal fibrosis.

Mediastinitis

This is a suppurative inflammation of the mediastinal space and is usually encountered as a complication of oesophageal perforation (see Chapter 25). Much less commonly, it occurs secondary to infection of the medi- astinal lymph nodes (from a focus in the lungs) or ver- tebral osteomyelitis. The condition is always serious. The clinical features include chest pain, rigors, pyrexia and dyspnoea. When secondary to oesophageal perforation, it is accompanied by surgical emphysema in the neck and mediastinal air on the chest radiograph. Treatment is surgical with measures to deal with the underlying per- foration, drainage and broad-spectrum antibiotic therapy.

Syndromes arising from ectopic endocrine tissue

Truly ectopic thyroid tissue that derives its blood supply from the mediastinum is exceedingly rare and is usually a chance radiological finding. Symptomatic mediastinal thyroid tissue is the result of retrosternal extension of a large multinodular goitre which derives its blood supply from the neck. The rounded mediastinal extension is best visualized by the lateral film.

In some 5% of patients with hyperparathyroidism (see Chapter 34), the adenoma causing the disease arises from

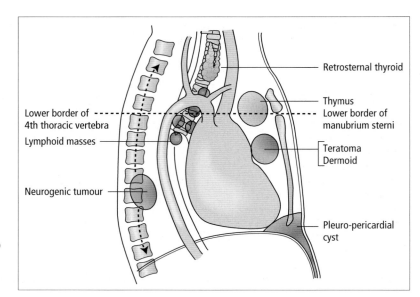

Figure 38.20 Diagrammatic representation of the mediastinum. For diagnostic purposes the mediastinum is divided into four regions: (i) superior; (ii) anterior; (iii) middle; and (iv) posterior. The sites of the commoner mediastinal tumours are also shown.

a genuinely ectopic gland. These patients usually come to light after neck exploration performed by an expert fails to reveal the tumour.

Tumours of the mediastinum

These are shown in Table 38.10. It is important to stress that the important common tumours are secondary deposits in the mediastinal lymph nodes (usually from lung, oesophagus, stomach and breast) and primary lym-

Table 38.10 Tumours of the mediastinum.

Secondary deposits in mediastinal lymph nodes

Primary lymphomas

Primary tumours of
Oesophagus
Trachea and main bronchi
Heart and great vessels

Specific mediastinal tumours
Thymic cysts and tumours
Teratomas and extragonadal germ-cell tumours
Neurogenic tumours
Thoracic meningocele
Pleuropericardial cysts (coelomic, spring-water cysts)
Cystic duplications of the foregut
    Bronchogenic cysts
    Enterogenous cysts

phomas. Thus, mediastinal involvement occurs in 50% of patients with Hodgkin's disease and in 10–20% of patients with non-Hodgkin's lymphoma. Both secondary nodal deposits and mediastinal lymphomas may present with compression of the superior vena cava, oesophagus and trachea that requires urgent treatment.

Thymomas

These are the most common anteriorly situated specific mediastinal tumours. Their histology is often very difficult to interpret, especially in terms of whether the tumour is benign or malignant. They are composed of a mixture of epithelial and lymphocytic components, often with one of these elements predominating. These tumours have a propensity to recur after excision irrespective of their histological appearance.

Thymomas may be clinically silent (detected on a chest film) or cause non-specific symptoms if large (chest pain, cough, breathlessness) or be accompanied by myasthenia gravis. In myasthenia gravis, an antibody is present that blocks the effect of acetylcholine at the motor end-plate. Although the thymus is often abnormal in these patients, thymic tumours are only found in 10–20%. Thymic tumours should be removed whether symptomatic or not. About 75% of patients with myasthenia gravis derive some benefit from thymectomy (irrespective of the presence or absence of thymic tumour) and half obtain a satisfactory remission. Radiotherapy is administered after resection of thymic tumours to reduce the risk of recurrence and in patients with irresectable lesions.

05

Table 38.11 Neurogenic mediastinal tumours.

Benign
Neurilemmoma
Neurofibroma
Ganglioneuroma (dumb-bell)
Phaeochromocytoma

Malignant
Malignant schwannoma
Neurogenic sarcoma
Neuroblastoma
Ganglioneuroblastoma
Phaeochromocytoma

Teratomas

Teratomas are developmental tumours composed of tissue elements from all the germinal layers. They are always situated in the anterior mediastinum and may be cystic or solid. Although benign, teratomas may undergo malignant change, particularly those that are solid. About one-third of these lesions are calcified at the time of diagnosis, which is usually made by chest X-ray. Some may exhibit recognizable teeth and the cystic variety may communicate with the tracheobronchial tree, when a fluid level is visible on the chest film. Symptoms, when they arise, are largely due to compression. The treatment of teratomas is excision via a median sternotomy or postero-lateral thoracotomy.

Extragonadal germ-cell tumours

These are similar in nature to the germ-cell tumours that affect the testis and, like their testicular counterparts, they secrete tumour surface antigens that are used as tumour markers (see Chapter 39). They are always malignant and may be seminomas or teratomas. Treatment is by excision, radiotherapy and chemotherapy.

Neurogenic tumours

Neurogenic tumours occur in the posterior mediastinum and are often associated with rib and vertebral abnormalities.

They are classified in accordance with the neural tissue of origin (Table 38.11). The benign nerve sheath tumours are neurilemmoma and neurofibroma, with malignant schwannoma and neurogenic sarcoma being, respectively, their malignant counterparts. Ganglioneuromas are benign tumours arising from the autonomic ganglia and have the propensity to extend to the spinal canal via the intervertebral foramina (dumb-bell tumours). Neuro-

blastoma is a malignant tumour of ganglionic tissue that occurs in children, usually in the upper posterior mediastinum, and is not encapsulated and infiltrative. It secretes catecholamines and a specific tumour antigen (neurone-specific enolase), which are used for establishing the diagnosis preoperatively. The equivalent malignant tumour in adults is ganglioneuroblastoma. This has a better prognosis and is encapsulated. For this reason it is also known as differentiated neuroblastoma. Phaeochromocytoma occurs very rarely in the mediastinum (see Chapter 34).

All neural tumours should be removed surgically. Children suffering from neuroblastomas receive pre-operative radiotherapy. In addition, following excision pulsed chemotherapy using *cis*-platinum-based regimens is administered.

Idiopathic mediastinal fibrosis

This is a condition of unknown aetiology (currently thought to be immunological) and is related to retroperitoneal fibrosis and Riedel's thyroiditis. It is characterized by dense fibrous infiltration of the mediastinum (especially the superior), eventually leading to obstruction of the trachea, vena cava, oesophagus and pulmonary vessels.

Aspiration syndromes

The aspiration of liquids or solids into the tracheobronchial tree is always serious and may have a fatal outcome. Although aspiration can occur in any individual, the risks are significantly increased in the presence of the following.
- Impaired conscious level from any cause: anaesthesia, head injury, hypoxia and hypercarbia, drug overdose, alcohol intoxication, cerebrovascular accidents, etc.
- Impaired protective reflexes (cough and gag): immediately after extubation of endotracheal tube, neurological disease (e.g. myasthenia, motor neurone disease), facial, neck and pharyngeal injury/surgery.
- In the presence of disease/conditions that result in passive regurgitation of gastric contents: gastro-oesophageal reflux, nasogastric tube, achalasia, intestinal obstruction, oesophageal obstruction, after oesophagectomy.

Aspiration of liquids

The outcome depends on:
- nature of the fluid (pH, corrosive nature and bacterial content);
- amount aspirated.
Aspiration accounts for 25% of ARDS. The most severe injury to the respiratory epithelium is caused by an acid

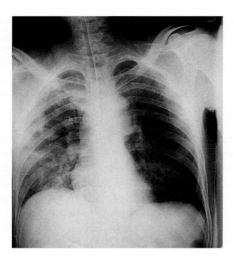

Figure 38.21 Areas of consolidation in the right lung are due to inhaled vomitus. Regurgitation of gastric contents and aspiration during general anaesthesia resulting in bronchospasm, atelectasis, oedema and hypoxia is called Mendelson's syndrome.

attempts at breathing by the victim result in paradoxical chest wall movements, with indrawing of the intercostal spaces. Unrelieved the acute hypoxia causes rapid loss of consciousness, bradycardia and death within minutes. The Heimlich manoeuvre aims to dislodge the foreign body and may be life-saving. The manoeuvre involves gripping the victim from behind with the right fist clasped by the left hand over the upper abdomen. Vigorous inward and upward thrusts are applied to raise intra-bronchial pressure in an effort to dislodge the foreign body. If dislodgement of the foreign body proves unsuccessful, life-saving measures include:
- direct laryngoscopy, with suction of oropharynx and manual dislodgement of any supraglottic foreign body;
- orotracheal intubation and ventilation;
- immediate cricothyroidotomy or transtracheal jet ventilation if orotracheal intubation fails.

Smaller objects cause partial obstruction, with choking and spluttering. If not expectorated, they lead to obstruction of distal bronchi/bronchioles with lobar/segmental collapse, consolidation, abscess formation and ultimately bronchiectasis.

Respiratory (ventilatory) failure

Ventilatory failure is defined as the inability of the respiratory system to oxygenate the blood and remove carbon dioxide. More specifically, it is defined as a Pao_2 at sea level of less than 8.0 kPa (60 mmHg), i.e. hypoxia due to inadequate gas exchange within the lung. A Pao_2 of 8.0 kPa lies close to the critical point on the oxygen dissociation curve below which further small changes in Pao_2 are associated with large falls in arterial oxygen tension and hence significant reduction in the oxygen available to the tissues.

Clinically, respiratory failure may assume several forms: it may be acute, where the dominant feature is severe life-threatening hypoxaemia ($Pao_2 < 6.5$ kPa or 50 mmHg; see Chapter 11) or chronic. The $Paco_2$ is used to subdivide respiratory failure into two categories.
- Type I: $Paco_2 < 6.6$ kPa, i.e. hypoxia with normal or low $Paco_2$.
- Type II: $Paco_2 > 7.2$ kPa, i.e. hypoxia with hypercapnia.

However, during the course of an illness, a patient may pass from type I to type II failure and vice versa. Type I respiratory failure is associated with pulmonary and cardiac causes where *alveolar hyperventilation* maintains a normal or low Pco_2. Type II respiratory failure is linked to disorders of the central and peripheral nervous system and skeletal abnormalities where *alveolar hypoventilation* predominates. COPD may present as either type I or type II failure, in which case ventilation–perfusion (V/Q) imbalance rather than alveolar hypoventilation accounts for the type II failure.

aspirate, which has a very high mortality. Aspiration of acidic fluid (usually gastric contents, when it is referred to as Mendelson's syndrome) is immediately followed by a vagally mediated marked and diffuse bronchospasm; this precedes the loss of surfactant function and the direct corrosive damage to the respiratory epithelium that induces fluid and protein leakage into the alveolar space (pulmonary oedema) within 1 h of the aspiration (Fig. 38.21). This almost invariably progresses to ARDS.

Aspiration of neutral fluid such as blood or isotonic solutions is much less harmful unless the volume aspirated is large, when the 'near-drowning' effect results in severe pulmonary dysfunction with loss of surfactant function, alveolar collapse and pulmonary oedema. Aspiration of infected liquid/secretions following colonization of the oropharynx by Gram-negative organisms is the underlying cause for hospital acquired-pneumonia, including ventilator pneumonia in the ICU.

Aspiration of solids

The clinical picture and pathology depend on the nature of the foreign body and the level and degree of occlusion of the airway. The group at greatest risk of accidental death from aspiration of solid foreign bodies are infants but no age is immune, especially the elderly and individuals with dentures. Complete upper airway obstruction results in inability to breath, cough and articulate. The patient becomes agitated and rapidly cyanotic. The vigorous

05

Type I respiratory failure

Three mechanisms underlie the development of type I respiratory failure:
- ventilation–perfusion imbalance;
- physiological venous shunting;
- alveolar capillary block.

The imbalance between ventilation and perfusion of the pulmonary alveoli becomes very marked as a result of lung disorders. The $Paco_2$ of blood leaving poorly ventilated lung is raised to levels similar to that in venous blood. The rise in CO_2 stimulates brainstem chemoreceptors, increasing ventilation rate and causing expulsion of CO_2 from well-ventilated areas, thus maintaining a normal or low arterial. However, the hyperventilation cannot increase the extraction of oxygen by the pulmonary capillary blood in the best-ventilated alveoli. Thus the maximum Pao_2 from well-ventilated areas is 13.3 kPa (100 mmHg) but is diluted by blood from the poorly ventilated areas, thus reducing overall Pao_2. In pneumonia or left ventricular failure, many alveoli may be perfused but are poorly ventilated because of alveolar fluid. Again should the $Paco_2$ rise, the respiratory centre responds by initiating hyperventilation thus expelling the excess CO_2. Any thickening of the alveolar–capillary membrane impairs the diffusion of oxygen from the alveolar space to the capillary blood, although in practice this is rarely sufficient to produce hypoxia but becomes significant with concomitant ventilation–perfusion imbalance. If the $Paco_2$ remains normal or low, type I respiratory failure is treated with high concentrations of oxygen via an appropriate mask or by high-flow oxygen in a tent.

Type II respiratory failure

In many cases of type II respiratory failure, alveolar hypoventilation is responsible for the breakdown in adequate gas exchange within the lung. The main causes are depressed respiratory drive and increased impedance. Depression of the respiratory centre may be caused by drugs, head injury or central nervous system disease. As the lungs themselves are usually normal, the term 'extrapulmonary ventilatory failure' (EPVF) is sometimes used for the disorders caused by increased impedance. The causes of type II respiratory failure due to increased impedance include:
- morbid obesity;
- chest trauma with large haemothorax/pneumothorax or tension pneumothorax;
- ruptured diaphragm with extensive herniation of abdominal contents;
- massive pleural effusion;
- massive ascites;
- ankylosing spondylitis;
- kyphoscoliosis.

In the acute situation, oxygen therapy alone is insufficient and ventilatory support by intermittent positive-pressure ventilation is usually needed. In surgical practice, morbid obesity is the most common cause of EPVF after surgery.

Type II respiratory failure can occur in patients with chronic obstructive airways disease when it is caused by gross ventilation–perfusion imbalance. Brainstem chemoreceptor insensitivity to $Paco_2$ and arterial hydrogen ion concentration plays a part in some patients, who are then dependent on stimulation from the aortic and carotid oxygen chemoreceptors for their respiratory (hypoxic) drive. These patients have a Po_2 set at much lower levels than normal individuals. In patients dependent on hypoxic drive, efforts to raise Pao_2 to levels above 10 kPa are dangerous since the patient may stop breathing, with a rapid increase in $Paco_2$ and hydrogen ion concentration. Thus in these patients controlled oxygen therapy is usually administered by a Venturi-type mask in a concentration that must not exceed 24% and blood gases are monitored 1 h later. If the rise in $Paco_2$ is small (< 1.3 kPa) and $Paco_2$ is below 10 kPa, Fio_2 is increased to 30%. If $Paco_2$ rises despite these measures, a doxapram (Dopram) drip is started to stimulate the brainstem chemoreceptors. Failure to maintain adequate Pao_2 without a rising $Paco_2$ or hydrogen ion concentration is an indication for respiratory support by intermittent positive-pressure ventilation.

Acute pulmonary failure

Acute pulmonary failure is caused by either ARDS or severe lobar pneumonia. The change in nomenclature from 'adult respiratory distress syndrome' to 'acute respiratory distress syndrome' is due to the fact that this life-threatening condition also occurs in children. The syndrome has a multiple aetiology (Table 38.12).

ARDS due to massive blood transfusion is less common nowadays because of blood warming and improved transfusion practice. It may complicate cardiopulmonary bypass and is common in fat and air embolism, smoke inhalation, poisoning (paraquat and other inhaled toxins) and oxygen toxicity.

The pathogenesis of the acute lung injury is now thought to result from excess sequestration and activation of neutrophils in the lung following activation of the complement system. The neutrophils induce parenchymal damage by the release of reactive oxygen species, proteolytic enzymes (especially elastase) and eicosanoids (thromboxane, leukotrienes and prostaglandins) that cause extensive damage to both the endothelium of the pulmonary capillaries and the epithelium of the alveolar

Table 38.12 Causes of acute respiratory distress syndrome.

Common causes
Shock (of any type)
Pulmonary infections
Severe sepsis
Severe pancreatitis
Severe trauma
Drug overdose
Aspiration (gastric juice, drowning; see Fig. 38.21)

Other causes
Massive blood transfusion
Cardiopulmonary bypass
Fat and air embolism
Smoke inhalation
Poisoning: paraquat and inhaled toxins
Oxygen toxicity
Neurogenic

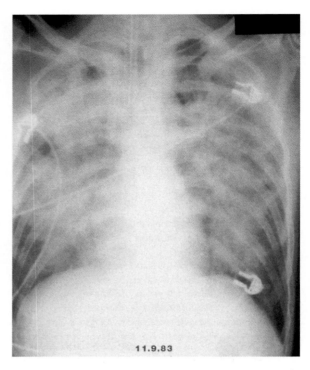

Figure 38.22 Non-cardiogenic pulmonary oedema in a patient with acute respiratory distress syndrome.

membrane. This results in increased permeability of the alveolar–capillary membrane, with the development of gross non-cardiogenic pulmonary oedema (in the first instance) and impaired gas exchange. Aerated lung volume is reduced to less than half the total lung volume. Proliferation of the alveolar epithelial cells occurs as a result of the injury and this is accompanied by increased fibroblastic activity and collagen formation in the interstitial tissues of the lung. Thus pulmonary compliance is greatly reduced.

In contrast to cardiogenic oedema, ARDS is usually sudden in onset. The physical signs in the chest are minimal, despite obvious respiratory distress (tachypnoea and laboured breathing) and refractory hypoxaemia. Initially, the chest radiograph may be normal or show an interstitial infiltrate, but as the condition progresses diffuse alveolar infiltrates become evident ('white-out', Fig. 38.22). The cardiac shadow is normal in shape and size, and pleural effusion is absent. Cardiac output in ARDS is normal at the onset but often falls during the course of the disease. Blood gas analysis shows a severe hypoxaemia ($Pao_2 < 6.5$ kPa) with a low $Paco_2$ and low pH (mixed respiratory alkalosis and metabolic acidosis).

Treatment

All patients with ARDS require ventilatory support and intensive care. The hypoxaemia is often refractory to high Fio_2 due to intrapulmonary shunting. Recovery from ARDS depends on correction of the underling condition and good pulmonary and cardiac support in the ICU. Infection control is very important but prophylactic use of antibiotics is not indicated. Careful intravenous fluid management with crystalloid solutions is essential to maintain adequate circulation without overload. Often, diuretics are needed to prevent the latter complication. When cardiac output is reduced, inotropic agents (e.g. dopamine) are administered. Antacids or histamine H_2 blockers are given by some as prophylaxis against stress-induced erosive gastritis. Lung recovery depends to a large extent on correction of the underlying condition. This applies especially to the treatment of intra-abdominal sepsis. Antibiotics are used for suspected or established infection.

Extracorporeal lung assistance is used in some centres but controlled clinical trials have not demonstrated a survival advantage over conventional management. There is no evidence that corticosteroids are useful.

Death (overall mortality 50–60%) usually occurs within 2–4 weeks of onset of the disease, either from infection or multiorgan failure. Surviving patients usually achieve good pulmonary function, although weaning from ventilatory support may be prolonged. However, some sustain permanent pulmonary dysfunction.

Fat embolism

This is a rare cause of respiratory insufficiency including full-blown ARDS. It is encountered most commonly after

05

Respiratory (ventilatory) failure at a glance

Definition

Respiratory failure: inability of the respiratory system to oxygenate the blood and remove carbon dioxide. More specifically, it is defined as a Pao_2 at sea level of < 8.0 kPa (60 mmHg)

Type I respiratory failure

Defined as $Paco_2$ < 6.6 kPa, hypoxia with normal or low $Paco_2$

Pathophysiology
- Ventilation–perfusion imbalance
- Physiological venous shunting
- Alveolar capillary block
- Because of ventilation–perfusion imbalance (e.g. pulmonary embolism) or because the alveoli are filled with fluid (e.g. pneumonia, left ventricular failure), $Paco_2$ begins to rise thus stimulating brainstem chemoreceptors, with resultant increased ventilation and reduction in $Paco_2$. The $Paco_2$ is therefore normal or low in type I respiratory failure

Treatment
- High concentrations of oxygen given by an appropriate mask

Type II respiratory failure

Defined as $Paco_2$ > 7.2 kPa, hypoxia with hypercapnia

Pathophysiology of alveolar hypoventilation
Depression in respiratory drive
- Drugs
- Head injury
- CNS pathology

Increased pulmonary impedence (EPVF)
- Morbid obesity
- Haemothorax/pneumothorax
- Ruptured diaphragm with herniation of abdominal contents into chest
- Massive pleural effusion
- Massive ascites
- Ankylosing spondylitis
- Kyphoscoliosis

Treatment
- Ventilatory support by intermittent positive-pressure ventilation. Oxygen therapy alone is not enough
- Type II failure (i.e. $Paco_2$ > 7.2 kPa, hypoxia with

hypercapnia) can also occur in patients with COPD whose brainstem chemoreceptors are insensitive to rising $Paco_2$ levels. Administering high concentrations of oxygen to these patients is dangerous as it abolishes their hypoxic drive and they stop breathing. Controlled therapy is given via a Venturi mask (24% oxygen) and blood gases checked 1 h later

Acute pulmonary failure
Causes
- ARDS
- Lobar pneumonia

Pathophysiology
- Increased permeability of the alveolar capillary membrane, with leakage of fluid into the alveoli, impaired gas exchange and increased pulmonary compliance

Diagnosis
- Sudden onset of breathlessness
- Few chest signs
- Refractory hypoxaemia
- Diffuse alveolar infiltrates ('white-out') on radiograph

Treatment
- Ventilatory support and management in ICU
- Requires positive end-expiratory pressure ventilation
- Treat underlying cause and other manifestations of multiorgan dysfunction syndrome if present

ARDS
Common causes
- Shock of any type
- Pulmonary infections
- Severe sepsis
- Severe pancreatitis
- Severe trauma
- Drug overdosage
- Aspiration
- Lower torso ischaemia–reperfusion injury

Other causes
- Massive blood transfusion
- Cardiopulmonary bypass
- Fat and air embolism
- Smoke inhalation
- Poisons (paraquat)
- Oxygen toxicity
- Neurogenic

major orthopaedic trauma but has been documented as a complication of pancreatitis, parenteral nutrition, cardiac massage, liposuction and bone marrow transplantation. The fat globules are thought to arise from the bone marrow and adipose tissue. These enter the venous circulation and cause occlusion of the pulmonary capillaries, although some pass through into the systemic circulation to embolize in the skin (causing petechial haemorrhages) and other organs (kidney, brain, retinal capillaries, etc.). Within the lung the globules of neutral fat are hydrolysed by lung lipase, producing highly toxic free fatty acids that are responsible for the acute lung damage. The triad of mental confusion, respiratory failure and petechial skin haemorrhages should suggest the diagnosis, which may be difficult to confirm. Treatment is supportive.

Evidence-based medicine

Arms, R., Dines, D. & Tinstman, T. (1997) Aspiration pneumonia. *Chest* **65**, 136–9.

Bernard, G.R., Artigas, A., Brigham, K.L. *et al.* (1994) Report of the American–European consensus conference on ARDS: definitions, mechanisms, relevant outcomes and clinical trial coordination. *Intensive Care Med* **20**, 225–32.

Dal Nogare, A.R. (1994) Nosocomial pneumonia in the medical and surgical patient. *Med Clin North Am* **78**, 1081–90.

Elpern, E., Scott, M., Petro, L. & Ries, M. (1994) Pulmonary aspiration in mechanically ventilated patients with tracheostomies. *Chest* **105**, 563–6.

Genitourinary Disorders

39

Must know Must do

Must know

How to evaluate, examine and investigate patients
    with genitourinary disorders

Clinical features and principles of management of
    infections and stones (calculi) of the urinary tract

Clinical features and principles of management of
    tumours of the kidneys, bladder and testis

Diagnosis, pathology and management of acute and
    chronic retention of urine

Clinical features, diagnosis, types and principles of
    management of incontinence of urine

Common benign disorders of the male external
    genitalia

Must do

Examine the genitourinary system including a digital
    rectal examination

Examine urine specimen for protein and microscopic
    haematuria

Clerk a patient admitted with renal colic due to stones
    and follow the management

Observe a flexible cystoscopy

Attend a urology outpatient clinic

Follow the management of a patient with retention
    of urine caused by benign prostatic enlargement,
    including the operation of transurethral resection

Observe extracorporeal shock-wave lithotripsy for
    stones

05

Introduction

Disorders of the genitourinary system are very common
and encompass a huge spectrum of pathology, including
congenital anomalies, infections, stone disease, benign
and malignant tumours and disorders of sexual function.

The consequences of disorders of the kidney and urinary
tract range from local discomfort (e.g. a quiescent renal
calculus) to life-threatening situations (e.g. septicaemia).
The management of patients with genitourinary problems
also ranges from very simple treatments to extremely
complicated and sophisticated management strategies.
These treatments are undertaken by a wide range of physicians, including general practitioners, paediatricians
and paediatric surgeons, radiologists, general surgeons,
gynaecologists, nephrologists and urologists.

Clinical assessment

Symptoms

There are a number of important symptoms that should
be recorded in the clinical history (Table 39.1). A number
of general points also need to be considered in a patient
presenting with a genitourinary problem.

- In women, the obstetric history, with special reference
to difficult deliveries, is crucial; previous gynaecological
procedures are also relevant.

- The occupational history of the patient is especially
relevant in patients suspected of having urothelial cancer.
Employment in the dye, rubber, cable or sewage industries
exposes the patient to industrial carcinogens. There is a
long latent period (15–20 years) between exposure and
development of cancer.

- Similarly, a smoking history is important as certain
by-products of cigarette smoke have been implicated in
the pathogenesis of urothelial tumours.

- Allergies and drug history are also relevant as a large
number of drugs affect the urinary tract.

Physical examination

Physical examination follows the standard sequence of
abdominal examination (see Chapter 3) (Table 39.2).

Table 39.1 Symptoms of genitourinary disease.

Symptoms related to micturition
Frequency (number of episodes)
Nocturia (number of episodes at night)
Hesitancy (delay in starting micturition)
Force and calibre of the stream
Postmicturition dribble
Dysuria (pain or burning on micturition)
Pneumaturia (bubbles of gas in the urine)
Faecaluria (faecal debris in the urine)

Incontinence
Continuous (often called passive) or intermittent
Stress (related to coughing, sneezing, etc.)
Urge (related to urgency and inability to control the flow)
Enuresis (voiding at night)

Haematuria
Painful or painless
Gross (visible to the naked eye) or microscopic
Initial (only at the start of the stream)
Terminal (only at the end of the stream)
Clots present
Haemospermia (blood also in the semen)

Pain
Site, radiation and periodicity
Acute or chronic
Relieving, aggravating or precipitating factors

Non-specific symptoms
Headache and visual disturbance (suggestive of
  hypertension)
Sweating and rigors (suggestive of infection)
Oedema, dyspnoea, orthopnoea (suggestive of intrinsic renal
  disease)
Malaise, nausea, vomiting (suggestive of uraemia)
Weight loss

Table 39.2 Physical examination of the genitourinary system.

General
Anaemia, jaundice, cachexia
Pulse, blood pressure

Abdomen (looking for)
Renal mass
  Arising in the loin
  Palpable bimanually
  Ballottable
Distended bladder
  Mass arising from pelvis
  Dull to percussion suprapubically

External genitalia
Prepuce (size, retractability, signs of infection)
Urethral meatus (position and size)
Scrotum (testis, cord, skin and coverings)

Rectal
Anal tone (sacral innervation)
Prostate
  Size
  Contour (presence of median sulcus, smooth or craggy)
  Consistency (solid, hard, isolated nodule, tender)

Perineum
Sensation (sacral innervation)

Investigations (Table 39.3)

Urinalysis

The most appropriate urine specimen for laboratory analysis is a freshly voided midstream specimen of urine. This urine sample can be tested using dipsticks, which are strips coated with chemicals that indicate urine pH and the presence of glucose, protein, blood, bilirubin, ketones and nitrates. If the dipstick test is positive, full urinalysis is necessary. However, for patients presenting with urinary symptoms, it is better to proceed to a formal analysis of the urine specimen in the hospital laboratory by microscopy, culture and sensitivity testing.

Microscopy is performed on the urinary sediment after centrifugation. Specifically, the urine is examined for red blood cells, white blood cells, casts, crystals and bacteria. The presence of more than three red blood cells per high-power field examined is a significant finding that warrants further investigation. The presence of more than five white blood cells per high-power field (pyuria) is also a significant finding. Bacteria may also be noted and should be examined by Gram stain to aid identification. In addition, the urine should be cultured. If pyuria exists without bacteria (sterile pyuria), tuberculosis should be considered and the urine stained by the Ziehl–Neelsen technique. If sterile pyuria is noted, urine should be obtained for culture of *Mycobacterium tuberculosis*. Three early-morning urine samples are examined. The presence of casts in the urine, which are formed in the distal tubules and collecting ducts, may indicate renal disease.

The presence of bacteria in the urine may indicate urinary tract infection (UTI) but may result from an improperly collected urine sample. To confirm a diagnosis of infection, urine culture is necessary. A significant infection exists if the culture reveals more than 100,000 single-type organisms per millilitre.

05

Table 39.3 Investigations for assessment of the urinary tract.

Urinalysis		
Dipsticks	pH, glucose, protein, blood, bilirubin, ketones, nitrates	Useful screening test for diabetes and renal and hepatic disease
Microscopy and Gram stain	RBCs, WBCs, casts, crystals, bacteria	May indicate infection or renal disease
Urine culture	Number and type of bacteria	Diagnosis of urinary tract infection
Blood analysis		
	Haemoglobin, WBCs, platelets	May detect anaemia or polycythaemia
	Urea, creatinine, electrolytes	Raised in patients with renal failure
	Calcium, phosphates, uric acid, albumin	Used for screening for metabolic disorders in patients with renal calculi
	Prostate-specific antigen, α-fetoprotein and human chorionic gonadotrophin	Tumour markers for prostatic cancer and testicular cancer
Imaging		
Structure	Abdominal radiograph (KUB)	Detects bony metastases, Paget's disease, soft-tissue masses, abnormal calcification
	Intravenous urogram	Delineates the entire urinary tract
	Ultrasonography	Assessment of renal and scrotal masses and bladder emptying
	Transrectal ultrasound	Useful in assessing prostatic disease
	Contrast-enhanced computed tomography	Preoperative staging of renal carcinoma
Function	Radioisotope renography (DTPA, DMSA)	Assesses function of each kidney independently
Urodynamics		
	Urine flow rates	Useful in assessing degree of obstruction to micturition, e.g. benign prostatic hyperplasia
	Cystometry (static and ambulant)	Differentiates between urge and stress incontinence
Endoscopy		
	Cystoscopy	Assessment of urinary tract for neoplastic or stone disease
	Ureteroscopy	
	Ureterorenoscopy	

DMSA, dimercaptosuccinic acid; DTPA, diethylenetriaminepentaacetic acid; KUB, kidney, ureter, bladder; RBCs, red blood cells; WBCs, white blood cells.

Blood investigation

A full blood count may show anaemia, polycythaemia, a raised white cell count, abnormal erythrocyte sedimentation rate (ESR) and platelet abnormalities. Renal function is assessed by measurement of serum urea, creatinine and electrolytes. In patients with stone disease, serum calcium, phosphates, uric acid and albumin should also be estimated. In patients with suspected prostate cancer, serum prostate-specific antigen (PSA) is measured as a tumour marker. In patients suspected of having testicular neoplasia, α-fetoprotein (AFP) and β-human chorionic gonadotrophin (HCG) are measured as tumour markers.

Imaging

The basic urological radiological investigation is the plain film of abdomen, frequently referred to as a KUB (kidneys, ureter and bladder). Examination of this radiograph consists of evaluation of the bony skeleton for areas of increased density (osteoblastic prostatic metastases, Paget's disease), soft-tissue masses and abnormal calcification (stones, phleboliths, calcified mesenteric nodes, gallstones).

An intravenous urogram (IVU) is performed by injecting intravenously an iodine-containing contrast medium that is excreted by the kidneys (Fig. 39.1). Serial radiographs are taken to show passage of the contrast through the glomeruli and tubules (nephrogram); passage through the collecting system outlines the calyces, renal pelvis and ureters. Films are taken before and after bladder emptying. In patients with iodine allergies a renal ultrasound may be performed instead. In patients with a suspected kidney lesion, renal ultrasound is particularly helpful and will distinguish between solid and cystic lesions.

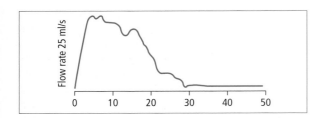

Figure 39.1 Intravenous urogram showing normal urine flow.

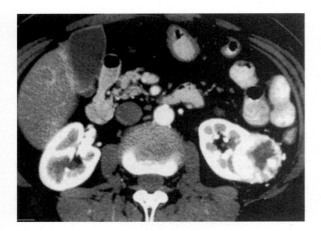

Figure 39.2 Computed tomography of renal tumour mass.

Ultrasound examination is also helpful in the evaluation of scrotal masses. Computed tomography (CT) combined with contrast injection gives great detail and is an essential part of staging tumours prior to surgery (Fig. 39.2).

The above investigations give information about structure, but for detailed assessment of function radioisotope renography is required (Fig. 39.3). Renal scanning is simple to perform and can give detailed information on the function of each kidney. Technetium-labelled diethylenetriaminepentaacetic acid (DTPA) is excreted in the urine like contrast material. DTPA scans provide information on renal perfusion, function and the presence of obstruction. Renal scanning with technetium-labelled dimercaptosuccinic acid (DMSA) allows assessment of renal size and function. Radioisotope scanning with technetium-labelled methylene diphosphonate can be used to detect bony secondaries.

Urodynamics

Urodynamics is a dynamic assessment of the storage and voiding functions of the urinary tract. The simplest test is urine flow rate, which assesses the rate and pattern of voiding. Another easily obtained test is the measurement of residual volume after catheterization. Ranges of normal values for age and sex aid in the interpretation of results. Cystometry involves the measurement of intravesical pressure during filling and voiding and is useful in differentiating between stress and urge incontinence. By filling the bladder with contrast medium during cystometry it is possible to watch bladder activity on a fluoroscope during the filling and voiding phases (videocystometry). Ambulatory measurements of bladder function are now possible.

Endoscopy

Almost the entire urinary tract can be visualized using various endoscopes. The urethra and bladder can be examined with a cystoscope, which may be either rigid or flexible. Traditionally, rigid scopes were used but flexible scopes have the advantage that the examination can be performed with minimal anaesthesia. The ureters can be examined by ureteroscopy and a flexible ureterorenoscope can be used to examine the ureter and renal pelvis.

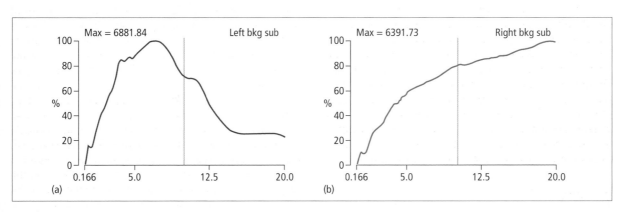

Figure 39.3 Radioisotope renogram.

Infection of the genitourinary tract

Many factors play a role in genitourinary infection (e.g. age, sex, location of infection, infective agent, state of the patient's immune system and the presence or absence of obstruction). Bacteriuria is defined as the presence of bacteria in the urine. Although colony counts greater than 100,000/mL are considered significant, counts less than this do not rule out infection.

Laboratory diagnosis

The laboratory diagnosis of a UTI relies on proper collection of the urine specimen, avoidance of contamination and prompt culturing of the urine. Refrigeration of the specimen will enable accurate results to be obtained when immediate culturing is not possible. The method of collection of urine samples is also important to ensure reliable results. In adult males, urine should be collected prior to prostatic examination and the clean-catch midstream method should be used. Uncircumcised men must retract the foreskin and clean the meatus with an antiseptic solution to avoid contamination. After the first 25–50 mL has passed, a sterile container is used to collect the specimen. A similar technique is used for women, with attention to separating the labia and cleansing the meatus. If difficulty arises in obtaining an uncontaminated specimen, sterile catheterization of the bladder must be used. In young children, urine is usually collected by applying a sterile bag over the cleansed penis or vulva. If this method appears unreliable, suprapubic needle aspiration of the bladder is often employed.

It is often difficult to distinguish urinary infection isolated to the lower tract from that of the upper tract. Several non-invasive tests have been developed to make this distinction, including the presence of antibody-coated bacteria, urinary α_2-microglobulin and lactate dehydrogenase levels. However, these tests are non-specific and of limited clinical value. Blood cultures are of good diagnostic sensitivity, although cystoscopy with catheterization of each ureter to collect urine and percutaneous needle aspiration of urine in the renal pelvis may occasionally be necessary.

Urinalysis and Gram-stain techniques can provide immediate information regarding the presence of UTI. This is particularly helpful in acute symptomatic infections when early antibiotic treatment is necessary while awaiting urine culture results. Interpreting urine culture results depends on several factors: method of collection, type of organisms isolated, patient's symptoms and the number of colony-forming units per millilitre of urine. The organism *Escherichia coli* has been cultured in over 80% of urine samples received from patients with uncomplicated cystitis or pyelonephritis. *Enterobacter* and *Klebsiella* are more likely to be found with nosocomial (hospital-acquired) infections. *Pseudomonas* and *Candida* UTIs often appear in patients with lowered host resistance or those who have been receiving antibiotics. *Staphylococcus aureus* can be a urine pathogen, usually in the presence of obstruction, while *Proteus* infection (a urea-splitting organism) suggests the existence of urinary calculi (struvite stones). Multiple organisms are cultured from urine in only about 5% of true infections, usually indicating contamination of the specimen in asymptomatic patients.

Classification

- A UTI is a documented episode of significant bacteriuria.
- *Unresolved bacteriuria* refers to an infection that is never totally eliminated from the urine during and after treatment.
- *Bacterial persistence* refers to urine that is sterilized by treatment although a persistent source of infection remains in the urinary tract (e.g. foreign bodies, infected stones, bladder or urethral diverticula, renal abscess).
- *Reinfection* refers to urine that is sterilized by initial treatment but a new infection with a new organism has developed (most recurrent UTIs).

Bacteraemia and sepsis

The mortality rate from Gram-negative bacteraemia approaches 15%. Septic shock develops in 25% of bacteraemic patients and carries a mortality of 50% (see Chapter 16). Gram-negative sepsis commonly occurs in hospitalized patients after instrumentation of the genitourinary tract or from a primary focus in the genitourinary tract. Aerobic Gram-negative bacteria (*E. coli*, *Klebsiella*, *Enterobacter*, *Serratia*, *Pseudomonas* and *Proteus*) are the usual causes of sepsis originating from the genitourinary tract. Anaerobic bacteria can also produce sepsis as a result of transrectal biopsy of the prostate, while Gram-positive sepsis can result from enterococcal infection. Any patient with bacteriuria is at risk for sepsis if obstruction of the genitourinary tract exists or if the patient undergoes instrumentation.

The diagnosis of bacteraemia can be made on symptoms, signs and laboratory data. The development of pyrexia, especially with rigors, is evidence of bacteraemia in any patient after recent instrumentation. However, bacteraemia must be ruled out in a patient who is found to be ill after instrumentation, as 10% of patients will be hypothermic initially, while another 5% will be unable to mount a febrile response.

The clinical signs of bacteraemia include the following.

- Early: tachycardia, tachypnoea, oliguria and hypotension
- Established: confusion, agitation or other changes in mental status
- Late: lethargy, coma, cardiovascular 'collapse'.
  Laboratory findings commonly include:
- leukocytosis;
- thrombocytopenia;
- disseminated intravascular coagulation;
- hypoxia;
- azotaemia and jaundice.

Treatment measures should be implemented immediately upon suspicion of bacteraemia or septic shock. Both urine and blood cultures should be obtained, with Gram staining of urine to determine whether Gram-negative or Gram-positive bacteria are present. Serum determinations of white blood cell count, platelets, creatinine, electrolytes and coagulation status should be made as well as arterial blood gas analysis. If sensitivities of specific bacteria to antibiotics are known, the appropriate drugs should be delivered intravenously immediately. However, as is usually the situation, if the offending organism is not immediately known, empirical antibiotic therapy should commence until specific sensitivities are revealed. Coverage should include antibiotics effective against Gram-negative, Gram-positive and anaerobic bacteria and must be administered intravenously. Once the organism is isolated and treated, intravenous therapy should continue for at least 5 days after the patient is apyrexial. The management of established septic shock follows the broad principles of cardiovascular and respiratory support (see Chapter 16). These may need to include invasive monitoring and advanced cardiovascular or respiratory support.

Renal infection

Acute pyelonephritis

Acute pyelonephritis is a bacterial infection causing acute inflammation of one or sometimes both kidneys. The process involves the renal parenchyma but may also involve the calyces, renal pelvis and ureter. The most common causative agents are aerobic Gram-negative bacteria, with infection of the kidney occurring generally by ascending infection from the lower urinary tract. *Escherichia coli* is the most common organism cultured in acute pyelonephritis. *Proteus mirabilis* and *Klebsiella* are urease-splitting organisms that create an alkaline urine secondary to release of ammonia, a condition that allows the precipitation of struvite stones in the renal pelvis and calyces. Gram-positive bacteria are a rare cause of acute pyelonephritis.

Several underlying conditions can predispose a patient to acute pyelonephritis (Table 39.4). Vesicoureteral reflux

Table 39.4 Factors that predispose to pyelonephritis.

Vesicoureteric reflux
Obstruction
Congenital, e.g. pelviureteric obstruction
Acquired, e.g. urethral stricture, stone disease
Anatomical, e.g. short urethra in females
Neurogenic bladder
Haematogenous spread from skin or gastrointestinal tract
Diabetes mellitus

is associated with an increased risk of pyelonephritis. Obstruction anywhere in the urinary tract will lead to stasis of urine with subsequent pyelonephritis. Obstruction can have multiple aetiologies, including congenital causes (such as pelviureteric junction obstruction) or acquired causes, as in ureteral stricture or calculous disease. Anatomical factors can predispose patients to pyelonephritis: the condition is more common in females because of the shorter length of the urethra and increased incidence of bacterial colonization of the lower urinary tract. Patients with neurogenic bladder dysfunction may develop chronically increased intravesical pressures that are transmitted to the upper tracts, leading to functional obstruction and pyelonephritis. Although a less common cause, haematogenous spread of infection to the kidney can occur from bacteria of the gastrointestinal tract or skin, especially in the face of kidney obstruction. Another common condition that may increase the risk of pyelonephritis is diabetes mellitus. Contributing factors include decreased host resistance, obstruction from sloughed papillae and bladder dysfunction. An uncommon but potentially fatal form of this disease seen in diabetic patients is termed 'emphysematous pyelonephritis' and is caused by gas-forming organisms.

Pyrexia, rigors, flank pain and dysuria are the clinical features of acute pyelonephritis. Patients may also complain of generalized malaise and anorexia. Physical examination will often elicit significant costovertebral angle tenderness as well as abdominal pain. Laboratory findings include a marked leukocytosis, urinalysis showing pyuria, bacteriuria and microscopic haematuria. Urine culture almost always reveals greater than 100,000 colonies per millilitre of the bacteria causing infection. Acute pyelonephritis can mimic other disease processes. Included in the differential diagnosis are acute appendicitis, acute pancreatitis, acute cholecystitis and pelvic inflammatory disease in women.

Critical to the investigation of a patient with suspected pyelonephritis is the radiological work-up, which is often diagnostic. An excretory urogram will usually show renal enlargement and a somewhat decreased nephrogram,

both of which return to normal with resolution of the infection. An ultrasound study of the kidney may reveal a dilated collecting system from obstruction, the presence of urinary stones or renal abscess. Lobar nephronia, a form of pyelonephritis limited to a focal area within the kidney, can also be seen with ultrasound.

In the absence of complicating factors such as obstruction or infected stones, acute pyelonephritis is treated by intravenous antibiotic therapy (determined by urine culture and sensitivity) until the patient is apyrexial and clinically improved. This is followed by a 2-week course of oral antibiotics. If no significant improvement is seen after 2–3 days of therapy, the diagnosis of abscess or obstruction with pyelonephrosis must be considered and if necessary treated, e.g. by percutaneous nephrostomy placement.

Chronic pyelonephritis

Chronic pyelonephritis is a condition in which active infection is not usually demonstrated; however, parenchymal scarring of the kidney is featured along with generalized chronic inflammation and glomerular fibrosis. The condition is often the result of childhood infection of the kidney, especially in the face of vesicoureteral reflux. The presentation of adults with bilateral chronic pyelonephritis is frequently that of azotaemia or hypertension rather than evidence of infection. Findings on both excretory urography and ultrasonography include polar renal scarring, typically with underlying dilated calyces. If a single kidney is involved, the contralateral normal kidney will usually show evidence of compensatory hypertrophy, while in bilateral disease both kidneys are small.

Xanthogranulomatous pyelonephritis

A form of chronic pyelonephritis known as xanthogranulomatous pyelonephritis is usually unilateral and characterized by multiple renal parenchymal abscesses, pyelonephrosis and poor renal function. It is characterized by an inflammatory response with the presence of xanthogranulomas containing lipid-laden macrophages, which can be difficult to distinguish from the clear cell appearance of renal adenocarcinoma. Pyuria and bacteriuria with *E. coli* or *P. mirabilis* are usually present and IVU often reveals renal calculi and a non-visualizing kidney. The treatment of xanthogranulomatous pyelonephritis is usually nephrectomy.

Renal abscess

A renal abscess may develop by several mechanisms: it may arise as a direct result of pyelonephritis or occur by haematogenous spread from a distant site. A perinephric abscess is caused by rupture of a renal abscess into the

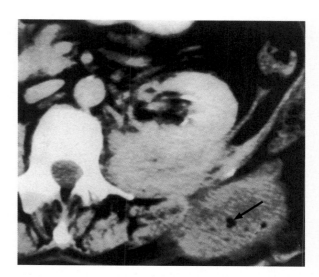

Figure 39.4 Perinephric abscess demonstrated on computed tomography.

perirenal space. The clinical findings include pyrexia, rigors and flank pain. Patients with an abscess secondary to pyelonephritis will usually have a history of previous urinary infection, obstruction or stones and are generally found to have bacteriuria.

Abscess caused by haematogenous infection usually arises from skin lesions or intravenous drug use, with *Staph. aureus* being the predominant causative organism, usually affecting the cortex of the kidney. The intrarenal abscess resulting from pyelonephritis, sometimes referred to as medullary abscess, will involve both medulla and cortex and be multifocal in nature. Underlying obstruction often exists, with Gram-negative bacteria as the cause. Several radiological modalities are useful in diagnosing renal abscesses. Ultrasound will often reveal a well-circumscribed fluid collection differing in density from that of the surrounding parenchyma or of a simple renal cyst. IVU may show a poorly functioning kidney if an abscess is large or multifocal. A large perinephric abscess may obscure the renal outline and psoas shadow, making diagnosis difficult. When diagnosis is unclear or when it is necessary to distinguish renal abscess from solid masses, CT and magnetic resonance imaging (MRI) may be required (Fig. 39.4).

Treatment of renal abscess usually centres on draining the fluid collection. Localized abscesses can be drained by percutaneous or surgical means and should be accompanied by appropriate intravenous antibiotic therapy. Small abscesses, renal carbuncles and those seen in the paediatric population can often be adequately treated with antibiotic therapy alone. Prompt therapy is necessary to try to minimize damage to the kidney.

Infections of the bladder

Acute cystitis

Acute bacterial cystitis refers to infection of the urinary bladder and is usually caused by coliform bacteria that ascend from the urethra to the bladder. Females are especially susceptible to ascending infections because of the short female urethra and the tendency of the rectal flora to colonize the perineum and vaginal vestibule. Sexual intercourse is also a major precipitating factor for urinary infection in women. Gram-positive bacteria and viruses are a less common cause of cystitis, although adenovirus infection can cause haemorrhagic cystitis in children.

Patients generally present with irritative voiding symptoms (dysuria, frequency and urgency). Suprapubic pain and low back pain occur commonly, as do haematuria and urge incontinence. Pyrexia occurs infrequently. Urinalysis usually shows pyuria and bacteriuria with microhaematuria. Urine cultures will reveal the infecting organism. A full blood count is often normal but occasionally leukocytosis may be present. Radiological investigation is limited to cases where renal infection is suspected. Patients found to have *Proteus* infections unresponsive to antibiotic therapy should have radiography to exclude infection (struvite) stones. Cystoscopic evaluation is generally reserved for situations where haematuria is prominent but should be performed after the infection has been treated.

Complications of acute cystitis include ascending infections of the kidneys, to which pregnant women and children with vesicoureteral reflux are most susceptible. The differential diagnosis of acute bacterial cystitis varies widely but can usually be distinguished from other processes by proper examination and laboratory findings. In women, the urethral syndrome will cause frequency and dysuria but cultures generally show no growth. Vulvovaginitis can be distinguished by pelvic examination, looking for vaginal discharge. In males, acute cystitis can be differentiated from infections of the prostate, urethra and kidney by careful physical examination and specific laboratory testing. Non-infectious causes include cystitis secondary to radiation therapy, chemotherapy, bladder cancer and carcinoma *in situ*, eosinophilic cystitis and interstitial cystitis.

Acute uncomplicated bacterial cystitis generally responds rapidly to antimicrobial therapy. In women, short-term treatment with appropriate oral antibiotics is effective, ranging from a single dose to 1–2 days' therapy. *Escherichia coli* causes 80% of uncomplicated, non-hospital-acquired infections and is usually sensitive to a wide array of antibiotics. Infections that do not respond appropriately to this treatment should be further investigated by urological and radiological means.

Urethral syndrome

Acute urethral syndrome is characterized by frequency, urgency and dysuria in women, with urine cultures showing no growth or low bacterial counts. The urethral syndrome can vary in cause.
● Women with low bacterial counts but acute symptoms should be treated appropriately with the antibiotic to which the organism is sensitive.
● Some will have sexually transmitted organisms such as *Chlamydia trachomatis* or *Neisseria gonorrhoeae*.
● Some women will have no identifiable organism but many still respond to antimicrobial therapy.

Infections of the prostate

Acute bacterial prostatitis

This form of prostatitis is a bacterial infection characterized by pyrexia, rigors, low back pain, perineal discomfort, dysuria, urinary frequency and urgency. The major cause is aerobic Gram-negative bacilli, of which *E. coli* is seen in 80% of patients. *Pseudomonas* and enterococcus are also commonly found.

Possible routes of infection of the prostate include ascending organisms from the urethra, reflux of infected urine into prostatic ducts, lymphatic spread from the rectum or haematogenous spread. Acute bacterial prostatitis will often result in acute urinary retention but this usually resolves after the infection has been treated.

Rectal examination reveals an extremely tender prostate that is swollen, warm and firm. Acute cystitis will often accompany the disease, causing pyuria, bacteriuria and microhaematuria. Urine culture will usually reveal the causative bacteria and in addition prostatic massage will express pus and bacteria; however, this is generally avoided in the acute setting because of pain and risk of bacteraemia. Microabscesses may occur early in the disease process and develop into large abscesses if treatment is not implemented rapidly. Patients with acute bacterial prostatitis generally respond well to antimicrobial agents directed at the specific organism. Initial therapy usually includes intravenous antibiotics for acute pyrexic episodes, changing to oral agents after about 1 week. Subsequent oral therapy should continue for 1 month to prevent progression to chronic bacterial prostatitis or prostatic abscess formation.

Chronic bacterial prostatitis

Chronic bacterial prostatitis is an indolent non-acute infection of the prostatic ducts and glands. It is the most common cause of relapsing urinary tract infection in men.

05

The causative agents are similar to those of acute bacterial prostatitis, i.e. Gram-negative aerobes. Enterococcus has been found on occasion to cause this condition; however, other Gram-positive bacteria are unusual causes. The mechanism and routes of infection are the same for acute and chronic bacterial prostatitis and in some situations chronic infection can be seen to evolve from previous acute episodes. However, it is often the case that no preceding history of acute prostatitis is found.

Symptoms vary widely; some patients are completely asymptomatic and are diagnosed only on the basis of bacteriuria found incidentally on urinalysis. However, most patients have differing degrees or irritative voiding symptoms, including dysuria, frequency and urgency, along with complaints of perineal discomfort and low back pain. Examination of the prostate may also be quite variable, with its consistency ranging from normal to boggy or at times indurated. If urine is sterile, sequential collections of specimens from the urethra, midstream urine and prostatic secretions should be performed. The first 10 mL of voided urine represents a urethral specimen, a midstream urine sample represents a bladder specimen, and the first 10 mL of urine voided after prostatic massage represents a prostatic specimen.

The differential diagnosis of chronic prostatitis includes cystitis, haemorrhoids and anal fissures.

Treatment of chronic bacterial prostatitis is directed at eradicating the prostatic focus of infection. Trimethoprim is recommended for patients with normal renal function. Long-term oral antibiotic therapy for 12 weeks has been shown to be more successful than short-term therapy and combinations such as trimethoprim and sulfamethoxazole have the best success rates.

Prostatic abscess

Most cases of prostatic abscess are progressions or complications of acute bacterial prostatitis and signs and symptoms will often mimic this. Physical examination of the prostate usually reveals a swollen tender gland and fluctuation may be present. Coliform bacteria, typically *E. coli*, are the most common infecting organisms in prostatic abscesses. Transrectal ultrasound (TRUS) is useful in confirming or excluding an uncertain diagnosis. Treatment consists of surgical drainage together with appropriate therapy. Drainage options include TRUS-guided transrectal drainage, transperineal needle aspiration, transurethral resection or open perineal incision.

Non-bacterial prostatitis

Non-bacterial prostatitis often presents with dysuria, perineal discomfort or low back pain, although repeated cultures fail to reveal an infectious agent. Treatment usually starts with antibiotics, but if unsuccessful symptomatic treatment can be tried with anti-inflammatory and anticholinergic agents and α-adrenergic antagonists.

Infection of the testes and epididymis

Acute orchitis

In the absence of epididymitis, most cases of acute orchitis are due to haematogenous spread of a systemic bacterial or viral infection.

Mumps orchitis is a serious complication of mumps parotitis that typically affects adolescent boys or young men. Some 20–35% of adolescent patients with mumps will develop orchitis and, of these, 10% will be bilateral. Presentation generally occurs 3–4 days after onset of parotitis with acute testicular pain and swelling noted. The scrotum becomes erythematous and oedematous. Significant pyrexia is common but urinary symptoms generally do not occur. Hydrocele can develop as a result of the inflammation.

The differential diagnosis includes acute epididymitis, torsion of the spermatic cord, trauma, tumour and granulomatous diseases, including tuberculosis. The serious complication of irreversible loss of spermatogenesis occurs in about 30% of the affected testes. Treatment of mumps orchitis centres on relief of symptoms as no specific therapy is available. Infiltration of the spermatic cord with 1% lidocaine will give rapid pain relief and may protect the testis from further damage by improving blood supply.

Acute epididymitis

Most cases of acute epididymitis develop from retrograde contamination of the epididymis by urethral contents via the vas deferens. Infection starts at the distal portion or tail of the epididymis but may progress to involve the entire structure and the testis (epididymo-orchitis).

The aetiology of epididymitis may be either sexually transmitted due to *C. trachomatis*, *N. gonorrhoeae* or both (most commonly seen in men under the age of 35 years) or due to a bacterial genitourinary infection (most common cause in men over 40 years of age).

Clinical findings include sudden pain in the scrotum radiating along the spermatic cord while the epididymis is exquisitely tender. Scrotal swelling occurs rapidly, with erythema, oedema and occasionally reactive hydrocele. Generalized swelling may cause differentiation between the epididymis and testis to be difficult. High pyrexia is usually noted, while symptoms of cystitis or prostatitis may be present. Laboratory findings include a leukocytosis.

Pyuria is often seen as well as bacteraemia in cases of epididymitis due to bacterial infection.

All causes of scrotal swelling are included in the differential diagnosis. In situations where urinalysis is unrevealing, elevating the scrotum may relieve pain due to epididymitis while increasing the pain due to torsion (Prehn's sign). Doppler flow studies and radionuclide scans may aid in diagnosis but none of these methods

Urinary tract infection at a glance

Definition

Urinary tract infection: a documented episode of significant bacteriuria (i.e. an infection with a colony count of > 100,000 organisms per millilitre) that may affect the upper urinary tract (pyelonephritis, renal abscess) or lower urinary tract (cystitis), or both

Epidemiology
- UTI is a very common condition in general practice (usually *E. coli*)
- Accounts for 40% of hospital-acquired (nosocomial) infections (often *Enterobacter* or *Klebsiella*)

Risk factors
- Urinary tract obstruction
- Instrumentation of urinary tract (e.g. indwelling catheter)
- Neurogenic bladder
- Diabetes mellitus
- Vesicoureteric reflux
- Immunosuppression
- Pregnancy

Pathology
- Ascending infection: most UTI is caused in this way (bacteria from gastrointestinal tract colonize lower urinary tract)
- Haematogenous spread: infrequent cause of UTI (seen in intravenous drug users, bacterial endocarditis and tuberculosis)

Clinical features
Upper urinary tract infection
- Fever
- Rigors/chill
- Flank pain
- Malaise
- Anorexia
- Costovertebral angle and abdominal tenderness

Lower urinary tract infection
- Dysuria
- Frequency
- Urgency
- Suprapubic pain
- Haematuria

- Scrotal pain (epididymo-orchitis) or perineal pain (prostatitis)

Investigations
- Gram stain and culture of 'clean-catch' urine specimen before antibiotics have been given. Usual organisms are *E. coli, Enterobacter, Klebsiella, Proteus* (suggests presence of urinary calculi)

Upper urinary tract infection
- Full blood count, urea and electrolytes
- Serum creatinine
- Renal ultrasound
- Intravenous urogram
- CT scan
- Isotope scan (DTPA, DMSA)

Lower urinary tract infection
- Full blod count
- Cystoscopy only if haematuria
- If obstruction is present, ultrasound, IVU and cystoscopy may be needed

Management
- Principles of management are to treat the infection with an appropriate antibiotic based on urine culture results and deal with any underlying cause (e.g. relieve obstruction). High fluid intake should be encouraged and potassium citrate may relieve dysuria
- Upper-tract UTIs, epididymo-orchitis and prostatitis require intravenous antibiotic therapy. Agents commonly used: gentamicin, cephalosporin or co-trimoxazole
- Cystitis and uncomplicated lower UTIs can be managed with oral antibiotics. Agents commonly used: trimethroprim, ampicillin, nitrofurantoin, cephalosporin
- An abscess will require drainage either radiologically or surgically
- If there is a poor response to treatment, consider unusual urinary infections: tuberculosis (sterile pyuria), candiduria, schistosomiasis, *C. trachomatis, N. gonorrhoeae*

Complications
- Bacteraemia and septic shock
- Chronic and xanthogranulomatous pyelonephritis
- Renal and perinephric abscesses

05

should cause delay in surgical exploration of potential torsion. Torsion of testicular or epididymal appendages can mimic epididymitis and torsion of the spermatic cord. Testicular tumours are generally non-tender and testicular trauma is usually diagnosed by history and lack of findings on urinalysis.

If torsion of the testis is excluded, treatment centres on the suspected or isolated organism. Sexually transmitted cases caused by *Chlamydia* are treated with a tetracycline or erythromycin, gonorrhoeal causes by penicillin, tetracycline or quinolone. Bacterial causes of acute epididymitis generally respond to prompt treatment with oral antibiotics chosen on the basis of culture and sensitivities. Severe cases with significant pyrexia may require hospitalization and intravenous antibiotics.

Sexually transmitted diseases in males

Sexually transmitted diseases (STDs) form a constantly changing group of diseases influenced by mode of transmission, contraceptive practices and antibiotic treatment. Before the Second World War, syphilis was the most common STD but has now become somewhat rare. Gonorrhoeal infection was also quite common but its incidence is declining, while that of non-gonococcal urethritis (NGU) is increasing. Genital herpes is a disease of great concern as its prevalence has increased in both men and women. In general, male patients with STDs present with variable complaints of urethral discharge, dysuria or an ulcerative lesion of the genital skin.

Gonococcal urethritis

Gonococcal urethritis is caused by the bacterium *N. gonorrhoeae*. In men, the urethra is the most common site of infection but other sites may be involved, including the oropharynx and the rectum.

In males, the most common presentation is acute purulent urethritis and dysuria. Symptoms generally begin 3–10 days following sexual contact but the incubation period can vary from 1 day to 3 months. The urethral discharge is diffuse and usually yellow or brown with meatal erythema and oedema. Laboratory diagnosis is based on Gram stain and culture of the urethra.

Treatment of gonococcal urethritis has been influenced by the existence of β-lactamase-producing and other resistant strains of *N. gonorrhoeae*. Patients should refrain from sexual intercourse until cure is established. Complications of gonococcal infection include periurethritis, which can lead to the formation of periurethral abscess, urethral fibrosis and stricture. Prostatitis and epididymitis also develop if not treated expeditiously. Systemic infection is uncommon.

Non-gonococcal urethritis

NGU is a syndrome with multiple microbial aetiology and is diagnosed when *N. gonorrhoeae* cannot be isolated. The most common organisms are *C. trachomatis* and *Ureaplasma urealyticum*. The typical presentation of NGU includes a thin mucoid urethral discharge, dysuria and pruritus at the meatus. Asymptomatic infections can occur. When suspected, patients should be examined several hours after last voiding to demonstrate discharge reliably. Gram stain of a urethral swab will reveal numerous polymorphonuclear leukocytes. Other causes of NGU include *Trichomonas vaginalis* and herpes infection.

Results of treatment for NGU are inconsistent as the syndrome can be caused by various organisms that respond to differing therapy. Patients with *C. trachomatis* infections respond best because tetracycline resistance has not been documented. *Ureaplasma* will also respond to tetracyclines but are much less sensitive than chlamydiae. Sexual partners should be treated with the same regimen. Complications of NGU include epididymitis, prostatitis, proctitis and Reiter's syndrome, a disorder characterized by urethritis, conjunctivitis, arthritis and mucocutaneous lesions and associated with *C. trachomatis* infection.

Genital ulcers

Genital ulcers include several disease entities that most commonly affect younger, sexually active men. It is difficult to make the diagnosis based solely on the appearance of the lesion, which can present as a papule, vesicle or pustule before developing into a true ulcer. Laboratory tests are necessary to make the diagnosis, while other factors, including the presence of inguinal adenopathy and incubation time, must be taken into account.

Primary syphilis
The primary genital ulcer of syphilis generally develops as a painless lesion, termed a chancre, 2–4 weeks after sexual exposure. The ulcer commonly appears on the glans penis but may form on the foreskin, shaft, suprapubic or scrotal areas and is typically a deep non-tender ulcer with indurated edges and a clean base. Inguinal lymph nodes are often enlarged but also non-tender. The diagnosis can be made by observing spirochaetes on dark-field examination of scrapings from the base of the ulcer or laboratory testing, e.g. the fluorescent *Treponema* antibody absorption test. Treatment for primary syphilis consists of penicillin, although tetracycline or erythromycin may be used for patients with penicillin allergies.

Chancroid
Chancroid is a genital lesion caused by the organism

05

Haemophilus ducreyi. The ulcer is generally soft with erythematous borders and often has purulent secretions and may be painful. Many patients may develop constitutional symptoms of pyrexia, malaise and headache. Painful inguinal adenopathy is often seen. The ulcer usually appears within a few days of sexual exposure. Diagnosis can be made with Gram stain or culture for *H. ducreyi.* Treatment includes erythromycin or tetracycline.

Granuloma inguinale

This is a chronic infection of the skin and subcutaneous tissue of the genitalia, perineum and inguinal areas caused by *Calymmatobacterium granulomatis.* The genital ulcer is firm, indurated and non-tender with an erythematous border. Subcutaneous inguinal granulomas cause inguinal swelling rather than true adenopathy. Chronic inguinal inflammation may produce lymphatic obstruction.

Lymphogranuloma venereum

This is caused by immunotypes of *C. trachomatis.* The genital lesion is generally small, superficial and transient but painful lymphadenitis usually ensues and lymph nodes may become matted and suppurative. Treatment includes tetracycline or trimethoprim.

Genital herpes

Most cases of genital herpes infections are caused by type 2 virus. The herpesvirus may also cause persistent or latent infections in both men and women.

Although symptoms vary depending on prior exposure to the herpesvirus, the first clinical episode is usually most severe. Grouped vesicles on an erythematous base are pathognomonic for genital herpes. The lesions are painful and do not follow a neural distribution. Lymphadenopathy is often present and painful, with most patients developing pyrexia and malaise. Dysuria is often seen in men. The laboratory diagnosis is made on cytological techniques and viral culture.

The treatment of genital herpes is with aciclovir, available in topical, oral and intravenous forms. However, topical treatment will not decrease dysuria, vaginal discharge or systemic symptoms. The oral and intravenous forms are effective in reducing recurrences and decreasing systemic symptoms, dysuria and vaginal discharge.

Genital warts (condyloma acuminata)

These are due to the DNA-containing papillomavirus. Several subtypes exist, with visible genital warts caused by types 6 and 11. Other subtypes seen in the anogenital areas, such as 16, 18 and 31, are associated with epithelial dysplasia and predispose to squamous carcinoma formation. Lesions in males are typically found on the glans penis, foreskin or shaft, although intraurethral lesions can

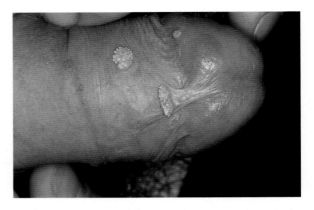

Figure 39.5 Penile warts.

develop (Fig. 39.5). Involvement at the urethral meatus or persistent dysuria are indications for endoscopic evaluation. Although no treatment has been shown to eliminate the virus completely, several therapies are available. Topical podophyllin can be applied at weekly intervals. Cryosurgery or laser therapy is also effective in removing visible lesions. However, recurrences are common with all forms of treatment.

Urinary tract obstruction

Obstruction of the urinary tract may occur at any level from the external urinary meatus to the ureteropelvic junction. Obstruction may be classified according to site as lower urinary tract obstruction (i.e. distal to the bladder) and obstruction of the upper urinary tract (i.e. bladder and upwards). Within each type of obstruction further subclassification according to aetiology (congenital or acquired), duration (acute or chronic) and degree of obstruction (partial or complete) is possible.

Lower urinary tract obstruction

Outflow obstruction of the lower urinary tract remains one of the most prevalent and clinically significant diseases in urology. Symptoms referable to the lower urinary tract are categorized into obstructive and irritative (Table 39.5).

Obstructive symptoms include weak stream, hesitancy, intermittency, dribbling and straining to void. Irritative symptoms typically include urinary frequency, urgency, nocturia, dysuria and urge incontinence. The term 'prostatism' refers to a combination of these symptoms, including frequency, urgency, hesitancy and weak stream. While the name implies that prostatic obstruction is the cause, this is not always the case as bladder instability in

05

Table 39.5 Symptoms of lower urinary tract obstruction.

Obstructive	Irritative
Weak stream	Frequency
Hesitancy	Urgency
Intermittency	Nocturia
Dribbling	Dysuria
Straining to void	Urge incontinence

patients with no evidence of obstruction can present in an identical fashion.

Differential diagnosis

The differential diagnosis of lower urinary tract obstruction varies widely and can be classified on the basis of structural or functional causes (Fig. 39.6).

Obstruction of the distal urethra can result from meatal stenosis, typically seen in newborn or infant males. There is usually a congenital web of epithelial tissue permitting only a pinpoint opening at the meatus. In adults this may be the result of inflammatory processes of the glans penis (balanitis). In uncircumcised males, chronic inflammation and scarring of the prepuce or foreskin can lead to an inability to retract the prepuce (phimosis) and occasionally cause obstruction of urine. The condition of urethral stenosis in females is rare and may be related to trauma or inflammation. Urethral stricture is a frequent problem seen in adult males. Although a common sequel to gonococcal urethritis in the past, the majority of strictures now seen are the result of trauma to the urethra from instrumentation or catheterization.

Posterior urethral valves, i.e. congenital mucosal folds in the area of the membranous urethra, are the most common cause of proximal urethral obstruction in male infants. In adults, obstruction in this region can be both functional and anatomical. Failure of the external urethral sphincter to relax secondary to spasm during micturition will impede flow. Several neurological diseases, including spinal cord injury and multiple sclerosis, as well as psychogenic causes will result in this type of obstruction. The most common anatomical obstructive lesion in adult males is benign prostatic hyperplasia (see later). Carcinoma of the prostate is a less common cause of obstruction as most cancers occur in the peripheral regions of the prostate while benign prostatic hyperplasia tends to occur in the periurethral transition zone. Infectious processes of the prostate can also lead to obstructive symptoms owing to surrounding inflammation and oedema and include acute prostatitis and prostatic abscesses.

Obstruction at the level of the bladder neck can occur under several circumstances. Contracture of the bladder neck is a common cause and typically seen secondary to surgery or trauma. Neurological and idiopathic dysfunction are less common causes and are characterized by failure of the vesical neck to open completely during micturition without anatomical cause. This may mimic benign prostatic hyperplasia but usually occurs in a younger age group. In female patients who have had vaginal deliveries or pelvic surgery, cystocele may develop, causing a range of symptoms from obstruction and retention to urinary incontinence.

Several neuromuscular aetiologies of vesical dysfunction exist and can present with obstructive urinary symptoms or complete retention. Peripheral neuropathies may adversely affect detrusor muscle contraction by involving the autonomic nerve supply. Causes include diabetes mellitus, chronic alcoholism, uraemia, Guillain–Barré syndrome and trauma. Many pharmocological agents have been shown to exacerbate obstructive symptoms and precipitate retention. Drugs with anticholinergic activity such as phenothiazines and certain antianxiety medications act by inhibiting detrusor contractility. The commonly used α-adrenergic agonists pseudoephedrine, ephedrine and phenylpropanolamine increase sympathetic tone of the bladder neck and prostatic urethra. Both temporary and permanent detrusor dysfunction can be seen from prolonged overdistension or ischaemia of the bladder muscle, so-called myogenic failure.

Benign prostatic hypertrophy
Pathophysiology
The initial change in benign prostatic hypertrophy (BPH) is the development of microscopic stromal nodules around the periurethral glands. Around these nodules,

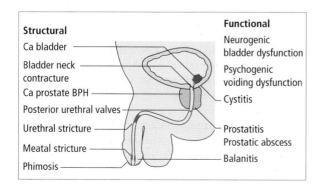

Figure 39.6 Differential diagnosis of lower urinary tract obstruction.

glandular hyperplasia originates. A review of ageing in otherwise normal males revealed the incidence of BPH to be slightly over 50% in men between 60 and 90 years of age. Early changes probably occur between the ages of 30 and 40 years. The aetiology of BPH is uncertain, although it is probably multifactorial with a hormonal element present.

Clinical findings
BPH induces gradual changes in the urinary tract, which result from the interactions between prostatic urethral resistance and intravesical pressure. The symptoms of BPH are a combination of the obstructive and irritative symptoms discussed earlier (see Table 39.5). Urethral compression from the enlarging prostate will result in a decreased force of stream, while hesitancy is due to the prolonged time required for the detrusor muscle to overcome the increased urethral resistance. Intermittency, terminal dribbling and incomplete emptying arise when the detrusor muscle can no longer maintain the increased pressure required to empty the bladder. Irritative symptoms, including frequency and nocturia, result from incomplete bladder emptying. Thus there are shortened intervals between voids, as well as increased excitability of the hypertrophied detrusor muscle leading to bladder instability. When patients are asleep, cortical inhibition is decreased, as is urethral tone, leading to nocturia. Incontinence is generally a late finding with BPH, when large volumes of residual urine accumulate in the bladder and overcome urethral resistance, often called overflow incontinence. Acute urinary retention may develop as a result of a precipitating factor aggravating existing BPH. Such factors include pharmacological agents (α-adrenergic drugs, anticholinergics and psychotropic agents), alcohol, cold temperatures and infection.

Physical signs attributable to BPH tend to occur late in the disease. Examination of the abdomen may reveal a distended bladder or occasionally a palpable kidney and flank tenderness from hydronephrosis or pyelonephritis. Rectal examination of patients with BPH usually reveals an enlarged prostate with a smooth surface. Right and left lobes are often not discernible although asymmetry is common, while the consistency of the gland may be either soft or firm, depending on whether there are more glandular or fibromuscular elements. Seminal vesicles are usually not palpable with enlarged glands. If irregularities of the prostate are felt on digital rectal examination, including firm nodules, induration or a generally hard prostate, carcinoma is more likely and further investigation including biopsy should ensue. In advanced cases signs of uraemia secondary to renal failure may be present: hypertension, tachycardia and tachypnoea from metabolic acidosis and anaemia as well as neurological changes and uraemic fetor.

Investigations
The investigation of a patient with BPH should start with urinalysis to look for evidence of infection and haematuria. If haematuria exists, other causes referable to the urinary tract should be excluded. Serum levels of electrolytes, creatinine and blood urea nitrogen should be tested. Objective signs of BPH can be evaluated using uroflowmetry and determining postvoid residual volume. Diminished flow rates indicate prostatic outlet obstruction, while residual urine volumes greater than 100 mL would indicate significant failure to empty the bladder completely.

Radiological and imaging studies have an important role in evaluation as they can assess the volume of BPH and of residual urine and exclude other urinary tract pathology. Studies typically used include ultrasonography to evaluate the kidneys and bladder, while TRUS more accurately assesses the prostate for size and evidence of cancer. IVU is a more invasive technique that will study the entire urinary tract.

Cystoscopy is an important modality for evaluating BPH and is often done prior to transurethral resection of the prostate (TURP). Bladder capacity can be evaluated, as well as the presence of trabeculations and diverticula. This inspection also includes evaluation of the ureteric orifices, the possible presence of bladder tumours or stones, size and length of the prostate, and condition of the urethra.

Treatment
SURGICAL TREATMENT
BPH is most effectively treated by surgical removal of the adenomatous portion of the prostate. Surgical indications for prostatectomy vary among urologists but a number of conditions that develop as a result of BPH are widely accepted as indications for surgery. Included in this group are uraemia, hydronephrosis, acute or chronic urinary retention, bladder calculi, urinary sepsis and symptoms extremely bothersome to the patient.

TURP is the most common surgical treatment of BPH. Methods for open prostatectomy are limited to patients with extremely large glands that are not suitable for TURP because of gland size and time required for resection. Open prostatectomy is associated with greater blood loss and higher morbidity and mortality. During TURP, the adenomatous portion of the prostate is removed via a resectoscope using electrocautery from within the prostatic urethra.

COMPLICATIONS OF TURP
During TURP, irrigation fluid containing sorbitol or

glycine is used. An average of 900 mL of fluid is absorbed into the extravascular and intravascular space through open venous sinuses in the prostatic capsule. This fluid is electrolyte-free and although absorption of these volumes is generally well tolerated by patients, occasionally a hyponatraemic, hypochloraemic metabolic acidosis can develop (TURP syndrome). Other immediate complications include failure to void, postoperative haemorrhage, urinary retention due to clots and UTI. Late complications include impotence, incontinence and bladder neck contractures.

NON-SURGICAL TREATMENT

Alternative treatment options to prostatectomy are gaining acceptance. Non-surgical therapies include:
- α-adrenergic blockers;
- agents that inhibit the conversion of testosterone to dihydrotestosterone by blocking the enzyme 5α-reductase;
- intermittent self-catheterization;
- transurethral balloon dilatation of the prostate;
- microwave hyperthermic prostatic therapy;
- prostatic urethral stents;
- transurethral needle ablation;
- high-intensity focused ultrasound.

Benign prostatic hypertrophy at a glance

Definition

Benign prostatic hypertrophy: a condition of unknown aetiology characterized by an increase in size of the inner zone of the prostate gland

Epidemiology
- Benign prostatic hypertrophy is present in 50% of 60–90-year-old men

Pathophysiology
- Microscopic stromal nodules develop around the periurethral glands
- Glandular hyperplasia originates around these nodules
- As the gland increases in size it compresses the urethra, leading to urinary tract obstruction

Clinical features
- Weak stream
- Frequency
- Hesitancy
- Urgency
- Intermittency
- Nocturia
- Dribbling
- Dysuria
- Straining to void
- Urge incontinence
- Acute urinary retention
- Overflow incontinence
- Palpable (or percussable) bladder
- Enlarged smooth prostate on digital rectal examination

Investigations
- Urinalysis for evidence of infection or haematuria
- Urine culture
- Full blood count, urea and electrolytes, serum creatinine
- Uroflowmetry
- Pressure–flow studies
- Residual volume measurement (normal < 100 mL)
- Ultrasonography of kidneys and bladder
- TRUS to determine prostate size
- IVU
- Cystoscopy

Management
Medical
- α-Adrenergic blockers (e.g. phenoxybenzamine, prazosin)
- Antiandrogens acting selectively at prostatic cellular level (e.g. finasteride)
- Intermittent self-catheterization
- Balloon dilatation and stenting of prostate

Surgical
- Majority of patients are treated surgically
- Surgical removal of the adenomatous portion of the prostate
- TURP with electrocautery or laser
- Open prostatectomy, which may be transvesical or retropubic

Complications of surgical treatment
- TURP syndrome: in 2% of patients, absorption of irrigation fluid via venous sinuses in the prostate causes hyponatraemia and metabolic acidosis
- Postoperative haemorrhage and clot retention
- UTI
- Retrograde ejaculation
- Incontinence
- Urethral stricture

Prognosis
- Majority of patients have very good quality of life after prostatectomy

Upper urinary tract obstruction

Upper urinary tract obstruction may result in renal impairment, especially if the obstruction is prolonged. The kidney responds to distal obstruction, partial or complete, by a decrease in ipsilateral renal blood flow with a concomitant increase in contralateral renal blood flow. Other protective mechanisms include ureteric dilatation, which dissipates the increased pressure to some extent, urine reabsorption through the renal lymphatics and collecting ducts (pyelointerstitial back-flow), and papillary shutdown. However, continued unrelieved obstruction produces renal impairment due to a combination of pressure and ischaemic atrophy. Acute obstruction is symptomatic with low pain but chronic obstruction may be asymptomatic or produce vague symptoms. Diagnosis of obstruction depends mainly on IVU, with judicious application of specialized radiographic techniques such as isotopic renography, ascending ureterography and perfusion studies (Whitaker test). On the basis of clinical and radiological findings, obstruction may be found to be unilateral or bilateral, complete or partial, acute or chronic.

Unilateral upper tract obstruction

The causes of unilateral upper tract obstruction are summarized in Fig. 39.7. Such obstruction may be due to lesions within the ureteric lumen, lesions within the ureteric wall or lesions outside the wall of the ureter compressing it.

Intraluminal obstruction

The most common cause is a calculus. Ureteric calculi usually present with acute ureteric colic with associated haematuria. A plain abdominal film will demonstrate the calculus in 90% of patients and IVU will confirm the diagnosis and indicate the degree of obstruction (for treatment of ureteric calculi, see p. 594).

Clots from bleeding in the renal pelvis or kidney (transitional cell carcinoma, renal cell carcinoma) may mimic ureteric colic but the findings on X-ray of a filling defect in the renal pelvis or distorted calyces gives a clue to the correct diagnosis.

Renal papillary necrosis is uncommon but the sloughed papilla may obstruct the ureter, mimicking the clinical picture of ureteric stone. Causes include sickle-cell disease, diabetes mellitus and chronic use of non-steroidal anti-inflammatory drugs (NSAIDs). The symptoms are pain associated with haematuria and sterile pyuria. A typical IVU shows defects in the medulla where the papillae were and a non-calcified obstructing ureteric lesion. Sloughed papillae are managed as for ureteric calculi.

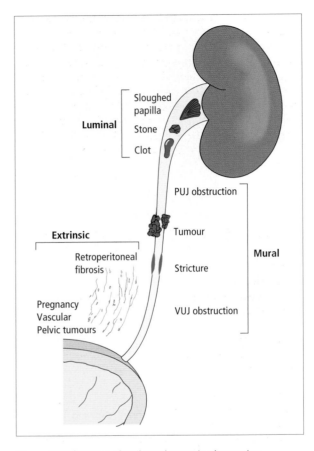

Figure 39.7 Causes of unilateral ureteric obstruction.

Intramural obstruction
CONGENITAL OBSTRUCTION OF THE PELVIURETERIC JUNCTION

Congenital obstruction of the pelviureteric junction (PUJ) is a common ureteric abnormality caused by a failure of transmission of peristalsis from the pelvis to the ureter. As a result of this block intrapelvic pressure rises and the renal pelvis and calyces dilate. Gradual deterioration of renal function on the affected side is the rule. This condition may be asymptomatic or it may produce loin pain, especially after an increased fluid load (Dietl's crisis). IVU will show dilated calyces and pelvis with obstruction at the level of the PUJ (Fig. 39.8). The ureter is not visible; if it can be seen on IVU, then the diagnosis of PUJ obstruction is incorrect. A renogram with diuretic will confirm the obstructive nature of the lesion and give a rough estimate of renal function on the obstructed side. Treatment is surgical. If renal function is poor, nephrectomy is the most appropriate treatment provided the condition is not bilateral. If renal function is good, then a reconstructive operation (pyeloplasty) is undertaken.

05

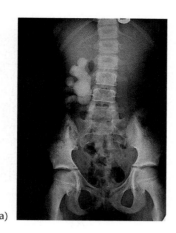

(a)

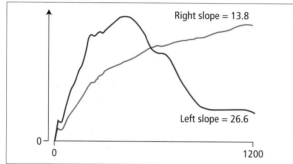

(b)

Right slope = 13.8

Left slope = 26.6

0

0   1200

Figure 39.8 (a) Intravenous urogram showing right pelvi-ureteric junction (PUJ) obstruction. (b) Renogram demonstrating the presence of PUJ obstruction on the right side. There is a normal trace on the left and a rising trace on the right, confirming the presence of obstruction on that side.

OBSTRUCTION OF THE URETEROVESICAL JUNCTION

Obstruction may also occur at the ureterovesical junction (obstructed megaureter) and failure of transmission of peristalsis at the junction is believed to be the mechanism. Pain, haematuria and infection are the usual presenting symptoms. IVU will show a dilated ureter with less dilatation proximally and blunting of the calyces. A diuretic renogram to confirm obstruction is indicated. Treatment consists of reimplantation of the ureter after excision of the diseased distal portion.

URETERIC STRICTURES

Ureteric strictures may occur after ureteroscopy and stone manipulation, pelvic surgery, irradiation (for carcinoma of the prostate, cervix or bladder) or chronic inflammatory conditions (tuberculosis or schistosomiasis).

URETERIC TUMOURS

Ureteric tumours account for approximately 1% of all urothelial tumours and may present as ureteric pain with haematuria mimicking a stone. Diagnosis depends on urine for cytology and IVU. Treatment consists of nephroureterectomy and regular follow-up cystoscopy, as recurrences in the bladder are common.

Extramural obstruction

Extramural causes of ureteric obstruction are rare.

Bilateral upper tract obstruction

The common causes of bilateral upper tract obstruction are shown in Fig. 39.9.

Tumours of the pelvis and retroperitoneum

Tumours of the pelvis and retroperitoneum may also obstruct both ureters. Most tumours in the retroperitoneum are malignant, invasion arising from the cervix, prostate, bladder, breast, colon, ovary or uterus. The remainder are primary retroperitoneal tumours such as lymphoma or sarcoma. When treatment of the underlying tumour is feasible, the ureters may be reimplanted or urinary diversion may be considered.

Retroperitoneal fibrosis

Retroperitoneal fibrosis is usually idiopathic, although some cases are secondary to malignant disease of the retroperitoneum, irradiation-induced fibrosis or drugs such as methysergide or β-blockers. As the fibrotic plaque develops, the ureters are pulled towards the midline and progressively obstructed. This may present as backache and gradual renal impairment. Hypertension and signs of distal venous occlusion are frequently associated features. Renal failure occurs in a small proportion of cases. Men are affected more often than women and the disease usually presents in middle age. Laboratory investigation may reveal impaired renal function, anaemia and a raised ESR. An IVU will show deviation of the ureters towards the midline and hydronephrosis. CT-guided biopsy of the plaque is necessary to rule out underlying malignancy. Initial treatment consists of relieving the ureteric obstruction, although freeing the ureters from the fibrous plaque (ureterolysis) and wrapping the ureters in omental tubes to prevent recurrence may occasionally be undertaken.

Urolithiasis

The prevalence of urinary tract stones among Europeans is 3%, with an estimated incidence of new stone formation of between 45 and 80 per 100,000 of the population. Calculi are especially common in Europe, North America and Japan. A diet rich in refined carbohydrate and animal protein with a low intake of crude fibre is thought to predispose to stone formation. Urinary calculi are more

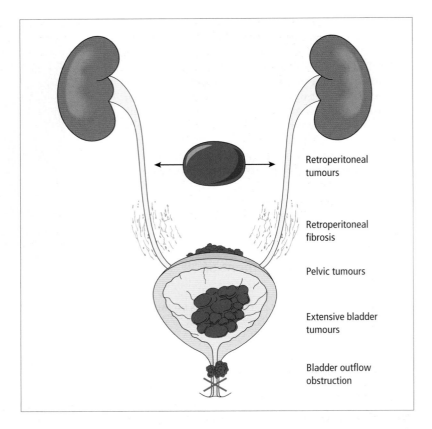

Retroperitoneal
tumours

Retroperitoneal
fibrosis

Pelvic tumours

Extensive bladder
tumours

Bladder outflow
obstruction

Figure 39.9 Causes of bilateral ureteric
obstruction.

common in people with sedentary occupations such as
doctors. Urinary calculi usually present in early adult
life and are more common in males. The exception to
this is infective stones, which are more common in
women, who are frequently middle-aged at the time of
presentation.

The exact mechanism of stone formation is unclear and
probably involves several mechanisms acting in concert.

- Nucleation theory: a crystal or foreign body acts as
the nucleus for deposition of further crystals in a urine
supersaturated with crystallizing salts. These crystals may
form on the basement membrane of the collecting tubules
or the surface of the renal papillae or within the renal
lymphatics.
- Stone matrix theory: crystals form in a supersaturated
urine and become embedded in a protein matrix secreted
by the renal tubular cells.
- Stone-forming patients may have reduced urinary
levels of naturally occurring inhibitors of crystallization
such as glycosaminoglycans.
- Some patients will have inherited renal diseases, such as
renal tubular acidosis, medullary sponge kidney and
cystinuria, that predispose them to stone formation.
- Other risk factors include hypercalcaemia, inflammatory bowel disease, gout, prolonged immobilization

or recurrent UTI and certain medications (e.g.
hydrochlorothiazide).

However, in the majority of patients with urinary stones
there are no associated predisposing causes but urine
metabolic abnormalities can be identified in most patients. Of these, idiopathic hypercalciuria, urine infection
and hyperparathyroidism are the most important.

Assessment of a patient presenting with urinary calculi
should include a detailed history, seeking evidence of familial renal disease, associated diseases and medications.
Laboratory investigation should include serum analysis of
creatinine, urea, electrolytes, calcium and phosphates,
urates, serum proteins (especially albumin) and alkaline
phosphatase. Blood for serum calcium estimation should
be taken after an overnight fast, with the patient resting
and without a tourniquet. If hypercalcaemia is found, it
should be confirmed on a second sample prior to sending
blood for parathormone estimation. Urine microscopy
for haematuria and crystals, as well as urine for culture, is
a basic part of the initial assessment. Special kits are available to test for cystinuria. At least one 24-h urine collection should be performed, preferably when the patient is
in his or her normal environment at home. Any stone
passed by the patient, or removed surgically, should be
tested for its constituents.

05

Radiological investigation is essential to confirm the diagnosis and aid management decisions. A plain abdominal film, which is the preliminary radiograph of an IVU, will reveal 90% of urinary calculi because they contain either calcium or cystine (which are radiopaque). Approximately 70% of stones contain calcium oxalate or phosphate, while infective stones (20%) contain calcium, magnesium and ammonium phosphate, so-called triple-phosphate stones. The films taken after injection of contrast will confirm that the opacity seen on the plain film lies within the genitourinary tract and show what level the stone is at and whether it is causing obstruction. A radio-lucent stone will appear as a filling defect but so will a tumour, so that CT may be needed to help in the differential diagnosis.

Diagnosis and management of urinary calculi

The management of urinary calculi depends on their site, size and the degree of trouble they are causing.

Renal and ureteric stones
Diagnosis
Caliceal stones are usually asymptomatic and are found incidentally, but they may cause haematuria. Occasionally, these stones may obstruct the infundibulum leading from the calyx to the pelvis, causing pain.

Stones in the renal pelvis may be asymptomatic or may pass down the ureter causing ureteric colic. If the stone is too large to pass through the PUJ, it may cause obstruction with colic. Pain due to a stone at the PUJ or in the ureter is severe, colicky in nature and radiates from the groin towards the loin. The pain may radiate to the testis in males or the labium majus in females. Haematuria, gross or microscopic, is present in almost all patients with colic. If obstruction occurs and is complicated by infection, pyrexias and rigors will also be experienced. As the stone moves down the ureter, the site of pain follows the route of the stone. When the stone reaches the intramural ureter, trigonal irritation with frequency may be noted. Physical examination is usually non-contributory unless there is gross hydronephrosis (palpable kidney) or pyelonephritis (tender kidney). The plain abdominal radiograph may not be diagnostic and IVU will confirm the diagnosis and reveal the size and site of the stone as well as the degree of obstruction (Fig. 39.10).

Management
The first priority in renal or ureteric colic is pain relief. Voltarol (a NSAID) is highly effective. The role of high fluid intake is questionable. Patients with stones in the

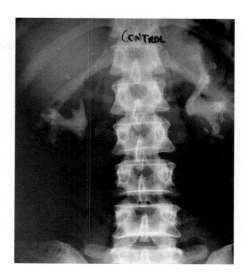

Figure 39.10 Plain abdominal radiograph showing staghorn calculi.

Table 39.6 Indications for intervention in a patient with a urinary calculus.

Site of stone	Indication for intervention
Kidney	Symptomatic (pain, haematuria) Obstruction (pelviureteric junction) Staghorn
Ureter	Failure to pass Large stones Obstruction Infection
Bladder	All stones

ureter can be managed expectantly in the first instance because as many as 80% of these stones will pass, usually within the first 48 h. The indications for intervention include failure of conservative management, obstruction and infection. The size and site of the stone help in predicting the outcome of conservative management. Stones less than 4 mm in diameter almost always pass. Stones of 4–6 mm are more likely to pass if situated in the lower ureter, while stones greater than 6 mm are unlikely to pass. Renal stones causing pain or obstruction of the PUJ also require intervention (Table 39.6).

Interventional techniques
RENAL STONES
- *Extracorporeal shock-wave lithotripsy* (ESWL) is a technique whereby shock waves generated outside the body

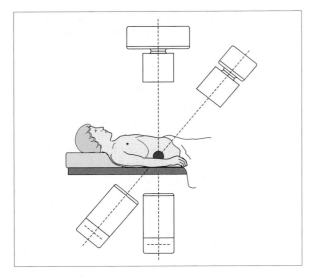

Figure 39.11 Diagram of a lithotriptor. A shock wave generated outside the body (extracorporeal) is focused on the stone in the kidney. Repeated shocks cause the stone to disintegrate (lithotripsy), hence extracorporeal shock-wave lithotripsy.

are focused on stones within the body; repeated application of shock energy to a stone causes internal stress in the stone, leading to fragmentation (Fig. 39.11). The fragments are then passed in the urine. For larger renal stones a ureteric stent is often inserted to prevent larger fragments obstructing the ureter (Fig. 39.12). Almost all patients have haematuria after ESWL. Some patients experience

colic, which may be due to fragments obstructing the ureter. Larger stones may require multiple treatments.

- For stones that fail to break or are considered too large, *percutaneous nephrolithotomy* may be considered. In this technique a guidewire is placed percutaneously into the renal pelvis and the tract is dilated to accommodate a nephroscope. The stone can be grasped with a forceps and extracted or fragmented and the remnants extracted. The kidney is drained with a nephrostomy tube postoperatively for 48 h. If the patient is stone-free and a nephrostogram shows normal drainage down the ureter, the tube may be removed.
- If these modalities fail, then open surgery may be necessary. The kidney is exposed through a loin incision and the stone is removed through an incision in the renal pelvis (pyelolithotomy).

URETERIC STONES
- *ESWL*: this may be possible for ureteric stones but stones that lie over the bony pelvis or vertebral transverse processes on the radiograph are generally not suitable.
- *Endoscopy*: if ESWL is unavailable or the stone is not suitable because of its position, endoscopy is required. Stones in the ureter above the pelvic brim may be pushed back to the renal pelvis, a stent inserted and the patient referred for lithotripsy. Alternatively, the stone may be disintegrated *in situ* using ureteroscopic instruments. For stones in the lower ureter, the stone may be snared in a basket and gently removed down the ureter using a ureteroscope, or disintegrated *in situ*. If these options fail, then open surgery (ureterolithotomy) is required.

05

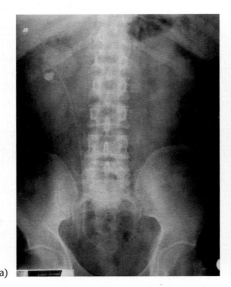
(a)

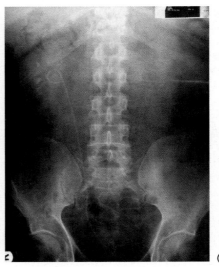
(b)

Figure 39.12 (a) A double-J stent has been placed into the right ureter prior to extracorporeal shock-wave lithotripsy (ESWL). (b) The stone has completely fragmented following one treatment with ESWL (approximately 1500 shocks in this case).

Staghorn calculi

These are so called because the outline on the abdominal radiograph resembles a stag's horn. A complete staghorn fills the renal pelvis and collecting system, while an incomplete staghorn calculus fills the pelvis and one or two of the calyces. These stones are triple-phosphate (calcium, ammonium, magnesium phosphate) stones of infective origin. Women are infected more often than men. These stones are formed by the action of bacteria found between the stone crystals, and because of these organisms the infection is very difficult to eradicate. Because of persistent infection the recurrence rate is very high.

Pain is unusual but loin ache may be present. Recurrent infection (pyelonephritis) is the usual presentation. Diagnosis is obvious from a plain abdominal radiograph. However, because renal damage can frequently occur as a result of recurrent infections and obstruction by the stone mass, an IVU and renogram should be performed.

Management

If the stone is unilateral and the renogram shows very poor function, a nephrectomy is the best option. However, if the disease is bilateral, then nephrectomy should be avoided. In this instance the poorer of the two kidneys is treated first and its function reassessed before treating the other kidney. If kidney function is reasonable in a patient with a staghorn calculus, every effort should be made to make the patient stone-free while conserving the remaining functioning renal tissue.

● *ESWL*: because of the stone size, there is a risk of ureteric obstruction from large fragments so that a double-J stent should be passed prior to commencing lithotripsy. The results with lithotripsy are disappointing even with multiple treatment sessions.

● *Percutaneous nephrolithotomy*: the stone may be fragmented using this method and the fragments remaining dealt with by ESWL.

● *Nephrolithotomy*: for complete staghorn calculi open surgical removal remains the best option.

Bladder calculi

While the incidence of renal calculi is increasing worldwide, the incidence of bladder calculi is diminishing, except in those areas where schistosomiasis is endemic. Although some bladder calculi were originally renal calculi that have lodged and enlarged in the bladder, most originate in the bladder. Bladder calculi usually result from bladder outflow obstruction but can occur due to the presence of foreign bodies in the bladder, such as urethral catheters. Bladder calculi may also form in diverticula or in neuropathic bladders.

Coexistent UTI is common and may give rise to dysuria, frequency and haematuria. In patients with bladder outflow obstruction, nocturia, hesitancy and poor flow will also be present. The classic symptom ascribed to a bladder calculus is a sudden cessation of flow with pain in the perineum and tip of the penis due to the stone obstructing the bladder neck on voiding. Diagnosis may be made on the plain film, when an opacity is noted in the bladder. An IVU will show a filling defect in the bladder with the stigmata of outflow obstruction: detrusor hypertrophy, diverticula (possibly), a raised bladder base and residual urine. Treatment consists of removal of the stone and relief of the underlying cause. Most bladder calculi may be dealt with endoscopically but very large stones will require open surgery (cystolithotomy).

Management of recurrent stone disease

Patients with recurrent stone disease require a more indepth evaluation in conjunction with a metabolic physician to determine predisposing abnormalities. Based on the findings of these investigations, dietary manipulation and medications may be used to lessen the chance of further recurrence.

Renal calculi at a glance

Definition

Renal stones: concretions formed by precipitation of various urinary solutes in the urinary tract. They contain calcium oxalate (60%), a mixture of calcium, ammonium and magnesium phosphate (triple-phosphate stones are infective in origin; 30%), uric acid (5%) and cystine (1%)

Epidemiology

● M > F
● Age: early adult life
● Among Europeans, prevalence is 3%

Pathogenesis

● *Hypercalciuria*: 65% of patients have idiopathic hypercalciuria
● *Nucleation theory*: a crystal or foreign body acts as a nucleus for crystallization of supersaturated urine
● *Stone matrix theory*: a protein matrix secreted by renal tubular cells acts as a scaffold for crystallization of supersaturated urine
● *Reduced inhibition theory*: reduced urinary levels of naturally occurring inhibitors of crystallization, e.g. glycosaminoglycans

- *Infection*: staghorn triple-phosphate calculi are formed by the action of urease-producing organisms (*Proteus*, *Klebsiella*) that produce ammonia and render the urine alkaline. Schistosomiasis predisposes to bladder calculi (and cancer)

Pathology
- Staghorn calculi are large, fill the renal pelvis and calyces and lead to recurring pyelonephritis and renal parenchymal damage
- Other stones are smaller, ranging in size from a few millimetres to 1–2 cm
- They cause problems by obstructing the urinary tract, usually the ureter
- Calyceal stones may cause haematuria and bladder stones may cause infection. Chronic bladder stones predispose to the unusual squamous carcinoma of the bladder

Clinical features
- Calyceal stones may be asymptomatic
- Staghorn calculi present with loin pain and upper tract UTI
- Ureteric colic: severe colicky pain radiating from the loin to the groin and into the testes or labia associated with gross or microscopic haematuria
- Bladder calculi present with sudden interruption of urinary stream, perineal pain and pain at the tip of the penis

Investigations
- Full blood count, urea and electrolytes, serum creatine, calcium, phosphate, urate, proteins and alkaline phosphatase
- Urine microscopy for haematuria and crystals
- Urine culture

- Plain abdominal X-ray (90% of renal calculi are radiopaque)
- IVU confirms the presence and identifies the position of the stone in the genitourinary tract
- A renogram may be indicated with staghorn calculi to assess renal function
- 24-h urine collection when patient is home in normal environment
- Stone analysis

Management
- Pain relief for ureteric colic: pethidine, Voltarol
- High fluid intake
- 80% of ureteric stones pass spontaneously: stones < 4 mm in diameter almost always pass; stones > 6 mm almost never

Indications for intervention
- Kidney stones: symptomatic, obstruction, staghorn
- Ureteric stones: failure to pass, large stone, obstruction, infection
- Bladder: all stones

Interventional procedures
- ESWL for small/medium kidney stones
- Percutaneous nephrolithotomy for large kidney stones and staghorn calculi
- ESWL or contact lithotripsy for upper ureteric stones (above pelvic brim)
- Contact lithotripsy or extraction with a dormia basket for lower ureteric stones
- Open surgery: ureterolithotomy or nephrolithotomy
- Mechanical lithotripsy or open surgery for bladder stones

Urological malignancies

Malignancy may develop in almost any part of the urinogenital tract and a variety of tumours may be present. The most common tumours of the urinary tract are prostate tumours and transitional cell carcinomas of the bladder.

Renal carcinoma

Incidence

Renal carcinoma (hypernephroma or Grawitz tumour) is most common in males over the age of 40 years. It accounts for 2–3% of all tumours in adults and 85% of all renal tumours.

Aetiology

The cause of renal carcinoma is unknown. A number of factors are associated with an increased incidence of the disease.
- Diet: a high consumption of fat, oils and milk.
- Toxic agents: exposure to lead, cadmium, asbestos, petroleum byproducts and tobacco smoke.
- Genetic factors: oncogenes localized to the short arm of chromosome 3 and human leukocyte antigen (HLA) types BW-44 and DR-8.
- Associated diseases: there is an association between renal carcinoma and von Hippel–Lindau syndrome, adult polycystic renal disease and acquired renal cystic disease due to chronic renal failure.

Pathology

The preferred name for the condition is renal cell carcinoma. The tumour is an adenocarcinoma, arising from the proximal convoluted tubular cell. The tumours are grossly orange or yellow because of the high lipid content.

05

Histologically, there are many subtypes including 'clear cell' and 'granular cell'.

Renal carcinoma may spread locally into the renal vein, extending as high as the right atrium in some cases. It may also spread through the pseudocapsule that surrounds the tumour. The tumour may metastasize to lymph nodes, most commonly the hilar nodes and the interaortocaval nodes. Distant visceral metastases may occur, most commonly to the lung and bones (usually vertebrae and ribs) with the contralateral kidney being involved occasionally.

Staging

A number of staging methods exist and the most commonly used in Europe is the TMN classification. This is wide-based but to describe the tumour fully it must be divided into five sublevels, in addition to a presurgical and postsurgical classification. The basic T classification is as follows.

- T1: < 7 cm in size.
- T2: > 7 cm limited to the kidney.
- T3: spread into perinephric fat, adrenal, renal vein or vena cava.
- T4: invasion beyond Gerota's fascia.

The original staging system of Flocks and Kadesky, which was introduced in the USA in 1958, is still satisfactory and in some ways preferable.

- Stage I: tumour confined to the kidney.
- Stage II: tumour extends through capsule.
- Stage III: tumour extends into renal vein or spreads to lymph nodes, or through Gerota's fascia.
- Stage IV: distant metastases or invasion of adjacent organs.

Clinical features

Renal carcinoma is well known for its association with many different symptoms and signs. There is a classic triad of haematuria, flank pain and a palpable mass, but these three features are only seen together in a small percentage of cases. Individually, they constitute the most common presentations of renal carcinoma:

- haematuria in 50–60%;
- flank pain in 35–40%;
- abdominal mass in 25–45%.

Renal carcinoma may also present in a number of different ways which indirectly point to the diagnosis. The effects of malignancy, e.g. anaemia, weight loss, pyrexia of unknown origin or raised ESR, or a combination of these, may indicate an underlying renal tumour. Renal carcinoma may also present with endocrine effects such as hypertension or erythrocytosis. Hypercalcaemia or elevation of adrenocorticotrophic hormone (ACTH), antidiuretic hormone (ADH), prolactin, gonadotrophins, insulin or glucagon is much less common.

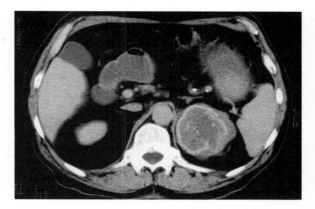

Figure 39.13 Computed tomography scan showing large renal mass.

In 10% of patients, hepatic dysfunction (e.g. raised alkaline phosphatase, γ-glutamyltransferase and bilirubin and prolonged prothrombin time) may be present even in the absence of metastatic disease. Sometimes this tumour may present with evidence of widespread disease or a left-sided varicocele may be present due to left renal vein spread, which blocks the insertion of the gonadal vein. Haemoptysis, with or without a pleural effusion, may indicate pulmonary metastases, and pain in the posterior region of the chest or the lumbar area of the back should suggest that bony deposits may be present.

Investigations

Routine blood and urine investigations should be performed. It is essential that these be used not only to help in diagnosis but also as a preoperative baseline so that all postoperative events may be viewed with this in mind. These investigations are also important because patients are often sick and anaemic before surgery and will therefore need careful preoperative management. Liver function tests may on occasion be abnormal, even in the absence of metastatic disease, and this can be suggestive of a poor prognosis. Imaging of the kidneys must be performed. On some occasions the lesion is discovered routinely on upper abdominal ultrasound. In this instance, not only must the lesion be imaged carefully but also the opposite normal kidney must be shown to be present and functioning. It is sufficient to proceed to CT where intravenous contrast has been administered (Fig. 39.13). This will enhance both kidneys in the form of a step-section IVU. CT will show the size of the mass, its fixity to adjacent organs, the presence of enlarged lymph nodes, and may give an indication as to whether there is renal vein and/or vena caval involvement.

The inferior vena cava may also be imaged if there is a suspicion of vena caval extension of the tumour. In cases

where vena caval extension of the tumour thrombus has gone as far as the right atrium, echocardiography may be required.

Management

Radical surgery offers the best chance for patients with renal carcinoma. This entails removal of the affected kidney and upper ureter with the renal vessels in addition to the adrenal gland and Gerota's fascia.

Management of metastases

A number of strategies are available for the management of metastatic renal carcinoma.

● *Surgery*: in patients with a single pulmonary metastasis, resection of the metastasis may be possible. If several metastases are present at the time of diagnosis, it is probably unjustified to perform a radical nephrectomy. It could only be justified if the patient is in danger of bleeding to death (a very unusual situation) or if some form of adjuvant chemotherapy or immunotherapy is proposed. Spontaneous regression of metastases after surgery may occur but is very uncommon.

● *Renal artery embolization*: this may be an alternative to surgery for the primary lesion in patients who have multiple metastases and who may also be bleeding from their tumour.

● *Chemotherapy*: has been largely unsuccessful in the management of renal carcinoma.

● *Hormone therapy*: hormonal agents have been trialled but none has been of great success.

● *Immunotherapy*: the following therapies may have a future role in treatment:
  (a) interferon;
  (b) lymphokine-activated killer cells;
  (c) tumour-infiltrating lymphocytes.

These methods of treatment are currently under evaluation and are encouraging in their early response rates. They are associated with a high morbidity, and this of necessity means that their use is confined to specialized units.

Renal cell carcinoma at a glance

Definition

Renal cell carcinoma (also known as hypernephroma and Grawitz tumour): malignant lesion (adenocarcinoma) of the kidney

Epidemiology
● M/F ratio 2 : 1
● Uncommon before age 40 years
● Accounts for 2–3% of all tumours in adults and 85% of all renal tumours (the other renal tumours are urothelial tumour, Wilms' tumour and sarcoma)

Aetiology
● Diet: high intake of fat, oil and milk
● Toxic agents: lead, cadmium, asbestos, petroleum byproducts
● Smoking
● Genetic factors: oncogene on short arm of chromosome 3; HLA BW-44 and DR-8
● Other diseases: von Hippel–Lindau syndrome, adult polycystic disease

Pathology
Histology
● Adenocarcinoma (cell of origin is the proximal convoluted tubular cell)

Staging
● TNM staging
● Flocks and Kadesky stages I–IV

(a) Stage I: tumour confined to kidney
(b) Stage II: tumour extends through capsule
(c) Stage III: tumour to renal vein, nodes or through Gerota's fascia
(d) Stage IV: distant metastases or invasion of adjacent organs

Spread
● Direct into renal vein and perirenal tissue
● Lymphatic to periaortic and hilar nodes
● Haematogenous to lung, bone and contralateral kidney

Clinical features
● Triad of haematuria (50–60%), flank pain (35–40%), palpable abdominal mass (25–45%). All three are present in < 10% of patients
● Anaemia, weight loss, pyrexia of unknown origin
● Hypertension, erythrocytosis
● Hypercalcaemia, ectopic hormone production (ACTH, ADH)
● Liver dysfunction (raised enzymes and prolonged prothrombin time) in absence of metastatic disease
● Renal carcinoma is one of the 'great mimics' of medicine

Investigations
● Full blood count, ESR, urea and electrolytes, liver function test
● Urine culture
● Abdominal ultrasound: assess renal mass and inferior vena cava

05

- Contrast-enhanced CT: assess renal mass, fixity, nodes
- IVU: image renal outline
- Cavogram and echocardiogram: assess inferior vena cava and right atrium

Management
Surgery
- Offers best chance for patients with renal carcinoma
- Remove kidney, renal vessels, upper ureter, adrenal and Gerota's fascia

- Isolated lung metastases should also be removed surgically

Palliation
- Renal artery embolization (may stop haematuria)
- Chemotherapy (only 10% response rate)
- Hormone therapy (only 5% response rate)
- Immunotherapy (currently under review)

Prognosis
- Overall survival is 40% at 5 years

Nephroblastoma (Wilms' tumour)

Nephroblastoma is a malignant mixed renal tumour that occurs predominantly in children and usually appears at about 3 years of age. Approximately one-third are hereditary. The tumours are usually solitary, soft, lobulated and tan or grey in colour. Histologically, they are composed of a mixture of epithelial, stromal and immature mesenchymal elements. Direct spread via capsular invasion occurs and the tumour also metastasizes via lymphatics and the renal vein. The lung is the most common site for metastases.

The tumour may present with pain but many are detected serendipitously during a well-baby examination. An abdominal mass is the usual physical finding. Ultrasonography and enhanced CT scanning support the diagnosis and treatment is a combination of surgery, radiotherapy and chemotherapy. The outlook for patients with Wilms' tumour has improved remarkably in recent years and an 80% cure rate can now be achieved with combination therapy.

Tumours of the renal pelvis and ureter

Incidence

Tumours of the renal pelvis and ureter are uncommon. Patients who develop a transitional cell carcinoma of the pelvis or ureter have a 30–50% chance of developing a transitional cell tumour of the bladder in the future. The presence of a transitional cell carcinoma of the bladder is associated with only a 2–3% chance of future development of a tumour in the upper urinary tract.

Clinical features

The most common presenting symptom is painless intermittent haematuria. Other patients may present with clot colic, loin pain, anorexia and weight loss. These tumours may be found incidentally in up to 10% of patients. Physical examination may be unhelpful, with an abdominal mass palpable in only 5% of patients.

Investigations

The following investigations may be helpful in establishing the diagnosis:
- urine cytology;
- IVU;
- ultrasonography;
- retrograde ureterography;
- antegrade pyelography;
- CT;
- chest X-ray;
- cystoscopy;
- ureteroscopy.

Management

Patients with tumours of the renal pelvis or ureter should be managed by nephroureterectomy and partial cystectomy. In the presence of lymph node metastases, the same chemotherapy as is given for bladder cancer is helpful.

Carcinoma of the bladder

Incidence

Carcinoma of the bladder is usually not seen before the age of 50 years. The incidence begins to rise in the fifth decade and continues thereafter. Over the last number of years in the UK there has been an increase every year in the incidence of bladder cancer and the death rate from bladder cancer is 7.6 per 100,000.

Aetiology

Transitional cell carcinoma is the most common type of

Table 39.7 Staging of bladder tumours.

		TIS	Carcinoma *in situ*
Superficial tumours		Ta	Tumour confined to the urothelium
		T1	Involvement of the lamina propria
Invasive tumours		T2	Superficial muscle invasion
		T3a	Deep muscle invasion
		T3b	Serosal involvement
Fixed tumours		T4a	Invasion of prostate, uterus or vagina
		T4b	Fixation to pelvic wall

bladder cancer in the western world and is known to be associated with certain types of occupation. Aetiological agents include:

- urothelial carcinogens related to the chemical, rubber and cable industries (1- and 2-naphthylamine, benzidine, aminobiphenyl);
- smoking;
- tryptophan metabolites;
- phenacetin.

In areas where schistosomiasis is endemic, squamous cell carcinoma of the bladder occurs frequently. In other parts of the world, squamous cell carcinoma is uncommon and may result from prolonged irritation by infection or stones. Adenocarcinoma of the bladder may occur but is very uncommon. It virtually always develops in a urachal remnant at the dome of the bladder.

Pathology

In the UK, by far the most common type of bladder tumour is the transitional cell carcinoma, with squamous cell carcinoma and adenocarcinoma being very uncommon. Transitional cell carcinoma may be divided into three types, which aids in staging (Table 39.7).

Carcinoma *in situ*

Malignant changes take place in transitional cells with no involvement of the deeper layers. These malignant changes are subtle and are sometimes difficult to distinguish from severe dysplasia of the bladder. It is a very important condition as up to 60% of patients with flat carcinoma *in situ* may subsequently develop invasive bladder cancer.

Superficial bladder cancer

This term is applied to papillary tumours that have remained confined to the urothelial layer (Ta) and to tumours that have penetrated the basement membrane into the lamina propria (T1). Although the latter are classified as being superficial, they have an increased tendency to recur and to become truly invasive.

Invasive bladder cancer

These are most often solid, although on some occasions they have papillary areas. The tumour invades muscle either superficially (T2) or deeply (T3a) or through the wall to invade the serosa (T3b). It may also invade prostate, uterus or vaginal wall (T4a) or be fixed to the wall of the pelvis (T4b). Metastases occur in the internal iliac lymph nodes and then spread to the para-aortic lymph nodes. More distant spread may occur to the liver, lungs and, less commonly, the brain. Local spread may occlude one or both of the ureters, leading to uraemia. Not only is the stage of the tumour important but also the grade. Tumours are graded from 1 to 3. Higher-grade tumours (grade 3 or poorly differentiated) have a worse prognosis than well-differentiated tumours (grade 1).

Clinical features

The most common symptom of bladder carcinoma is painless intermittent haematuria; it is present in up to 95% of patients. In addition, 20% of patients with bladder cancer may have dysuria or frequency without haematuria. Microscopic haematuria is of significance if there is in excess of eight red cells per high-power field; 10% of patients with asymptomatic microscopic haematuria have been found to have bladder carcinoma.

Investigations

The essential investigations are:
- IVU (Fig. 39.14);
- cystourethroscopy; and
- urine cytology.

If a superficial papillary tumour is found, the resected specimen and multiple random bladder biopsies should be sent for histology. If an invasive tumour is found and surgery is contemplated, a chest X-ray and CT scan of the abdomen and pelvis will be required. Transvesical ultrasound may be helpful in assessing depth of invasion, but deep resection of the tumours will be required to confirm this histologically.

05

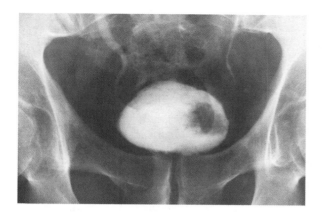

Figure 39.14 Intravenous urogram showing bladder-filling defect secondary to tumour in the left side of the bladder.

Management

The treatment of bladder cancer is dictated by the stage of the tumour.

Superficial tumours (Ta, T1)

Initial treatment is by transurethral resection of the tumour and follow-up cystoscopy. Regular cystoscopic examination should be performed when following up these patients. The overall incidence of recurrence is in the region of 50–60% and the development of invasion is low. Risk factors for recurrence and invasion include:

- smoking;
- presence of large tumours;
- multiple tumours;
- severe dysplasia or carcinoma *in situ* in random biopsies and high-grade superficial tumours.

Any patient who is in the high-risk category or who has had a number of recurrences should be considered for treatment with intravesical chemotherapy. Several agents have been used, including thiotepa, ethoglucid, doxorubicin, mitomycin C and bacillus Calmette–Guérin (BCG).

Invasive tumours (T2, T3)

When muscle has been invaded, local treatment by transurethral resection must be supplemented by a more radical form of treatment. In some patients, partial cystectomy may be indicated, but most tumours require either radical radiotherapy or radical surgery.

- Radical radiotherapy gives a 35–40% 5-year survival rate and leaves the patient with the bladder and without an appliance. The disadvantage is that troublesome symptoms of radiation cystitis and proctitis may occur. If the patient fails to respond to radiotherapy, savage cystectomy may be difficult and associated with significant morbidity.

- Radical cystectomy is also associated with a 35–40% 5-year survival rate in patients with T3 tumours. Usually a urinary diversion such as an ileal conduit is required in these patients. Preoperative radiotherapy and preoperative neoadjuvant chemotherapy have been tried.

Fixed and metastatic tumours

Patients in whom the bladder tumour is fixed to either organs or the pelvic side wall, or in whom metastases to lymph nodes or distant viscera have developed, have a short life expectancy. Recently, chemotherapy regimens have been introduced and early results have been encouraging.

Carcinoma *in situ*

This condition can present clinically with frequency, urgency and severe dysuria. Bladder capacity is markedly reduced and haematuria is generally not a presenting symptom. This will usually respond to intravesical chemotherapy, particularly intravesical BCG, but resistant cases are likely to require radical cystourethrectomy.

Prostatic cancer

Prostate cancer is the most common malignancy of the genitourinary tract in the male. In the USA it is the most common malignancy of all types in the male and the second most frequent cause of cancer deaths. In the recent past, many new developments have taken place in the diagnosis and staging of this disease, as well as the introduction of new therapeutic modalities.

Aetiology

The presence of latent prostatic carcinoma in the aged male is a well-known autopsy finding. The disease is usually found in patients over 60 years of age but can present in patients much younger than this, particularly in the black population. The following have been suggested as possible aetiological factors in the development of prostatic carcinoma:

- age;
- race;
- environmental factors;
- diet;
- nationality;
- endocrine environment;
- viral infection.

Pathology

The most common type of prostatic tumour is the adenocarcinoma, which arises from the glandular epithelium;

05

this comprises 95% of tumours. An adenocarcinoma arises in the outer part of the prostate gland or peripheral zone. As the tumour enlarges, it spreads medially into the remainder of the gland and outwardly to the surrounding tissues, particularly the seminal vesicles. Invasion of the rectum is uncommon, as it is protected by the fascia of Denonvilliers. The tethering of the rectal mucosa that may occur does not indicate invasion of the rectum but rather of the fascia beneath it.

Tumours are graded using the Gleason grading system: a tumour is assigned a single grade on a scale of 2–10, where a score of 8–10 indicates a poorly differentiated tumour and a score of 2–4 a well-differentiated tumour.

Clinical features

Most patients will present with symptoms of bladder outflow obstruction, such as poor stream, hesitancy, nocturia and incomplete bladder emptying. Sometimes the tumour may present as acute urinary retention. About 40% of patients may present with symptoms of advanced prostatic carcinoma, caused by either ureteric obstruction or bony metastasis. The pain associated with bony metastasis occurs classically at night, waking the patient from sleep. The pain may be relieved by getting out of bed and walking for a while.

On physical examination the prostate may feel normal. In the case of localized prostatic carcinoma, there may be a hard nodule in one of the lobes or a hard area which has spread into the opposite lobe but with no evidence of spread outside the gland. If digital rectal examination of the prostate reveals the presence of locally invasive prostate cancer, there may be a hard mass spreading outside the boundaries of the prostate and involving the seminal vesicles or the side wall of the pelvis. In this instance, the examining finger may feel a hard flat prostate that may be irregular, and associated with a fixed gland and sometimes tethering of the rectal mucosa.

Investigations

These should include:
- full blood count and renal profile;
- liver function tests;
- PSA;
- chest X-ray.
  Imaging investigations may involve:
- TRUS (including guided needle biopsy of the prostate);
- isotope bone scan for the presence of bony metastases (Fig. 39.15);
- MRI to evaluate local invasion and regional lymphadenopathy.

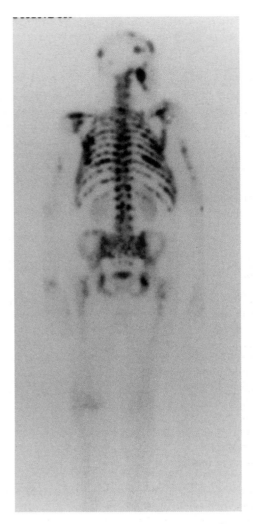

Figure 39.15 Bone scan showing multiple metastases secondary to prostatic cancer.

Management

If a carcinoma of the prostate is suspected, tissue must be removed for histological examination and confirmation of the diagnosis. This can be performed by:
- TURP (especially with outflow tract obstruction present);
- TRUS-guided needle biopsy.

Unsuspected carcinoma of the prostate (stage T0)
If the prostate feels normal on examination but the specimen from TURP has revealed well-differentiated tumour in some of the removed tissue, the recommended method of treating the patient is by observation, with regular digital rectal examination of the prostate and assessment of serum PSA.

05

Localized prostatic carcinoma (stages T1 and T2)
There are three treatment options in this type of prostatic tumour:

- radical prostatectomy;
- radical radiotherapy;
- interstitial irradiation with ^{125}I or ^{198}Au.

Radical prostatectomy is associated with a very low incidence of urinary incontinence and a low rate of impotence. Radical radiotherapy may be associated with cystitis and proctitis. The long-term survival of patients treated by irradiation or radical surgery is comparable.

Local spread (stages T3 and T4)
The treatment of choice is almost certainly external-beam radiotherapy. In some cases, particularly those with incipient ureteric obstruction, endocrine therapy may be required (as described below) in addition to irradiation.

Metastatic disease (stages T1–T4, M1)
The treatment options for metastatic disease centre on androgen deprivation because the prostate gland is very sensitive to androgen. Methods of therapy include:

- luteinizing hormone-releasing hormone (LHRH) agonists;
- antiandrogens (cyproterone or flutamide);
- bilateral orchidectomy;
- diethylstilbestrol;
- progestational agents.

Carcinoma of the prostate at a glance

Definition

Carcinoma of the prostate: malignant lesion of the prostate gland

Epidemiology
- Uncommon before age 60 years
- 80% of prostate cancers are clinically undetected (latent carcinoma) and are only discovered at autopsy
- True incidence of this disease is considerably higher than clinical experience would indicate

Aetiology
- Increasing age
- Commoner in black men
- Hormonal factors: prostate cancer growth is enhanced by testosterone and inhibited by oestrogens or antiandrogens

Pathology
Prostatic tumours are multicentric and located in the periphery of the gland

Histology
- Adenocarcinoma arising from glandular epithelium; Gleason grading (2–10) is used to grade differentiation

Staging

T0	Unsuspected
Localized	T1: localized to one lobe of prostate T2: spread within prostate
Local spread	T3: spread to seminal vesicles T4: spread to pelvic wall
T1–4, M1	Metastatic disease

Spread
- Direct into remainder of gland and seminal vesicles
- Lymphatic to iliac and periaortic nodes
- Haematogenous to bone (usually osteosclerotic lesions), liver, lung

Clinical features
- Bladder outflow obstruction (poor stream, hesitancy, nocturia)
- Symptoms of advanced disease (ureteric obstruction and hydronephrosis or bone pain from metastases, classically worse at night)
- Nodule or mass detected on rectal examination

Investigations
- Full blood count, urea and electrolytes, creatinine
- Specific markers: PSA, alkaline and acid phosphatase
- TRUS
- Needle biopsy of the prostate
- Bone scan

Management
- Depends on stage of tumour
- Stage T0: observation, repeated digital (or ultrasound) examination and PSA
- Stages T1 + T2: radical prostatectomy or radical radiotherapy or interstitial radiation with ^{125}I or ^{198}Au
- Stages T3 + T4: external-beam radiation ± hormonal therapy
- Metastatic: hormonal manipulation
  (a) Bilateral orchidectomy, diethylstilbestrol
  (b) LHRH agonists, antiandrogens (cyproterone acetate)

Prognosis
- Localized tumours: 80% 5-year survival
- Local spread: 40% 5-year survival
- Metastases: 20% 5-year survival

Table 39.8 Classification of tumours of the testis.

Germ-cell tumours
Seminoma
Non-seminomatous germ-cell tumour
    Embryonal carcinoma
    Teratocarcinoma
    Choriocarcinoma

Stromal tumours
Leydig cell
Sertoli cell
Granulosa cell

Metastatic tumours

Testicular cancer

The vast majority of tumours found in the testis are primary testicular tumours (Table 39.8). Germ-cell tumours are by far the most common tumours of the testis and constitute the most common solid tumour in males aged between 20 and 40 years. Metastatic tumours may occur, particularly in the older age group, including lymphoma and leukaemia. Predisposing factors include abnormal testicular descent (cryptorchidism) and previous testicular surgery.

Germ-cell tumours of the testis

Germ-cell tumours of the testicle can be divided into two types: seminoma and non-seminomatous germ-cell tumours (see Table 39.8). These are important tumours that occur mainly between the ages of 20 and 40 years. Because of the vastly improved cure rates that can be achieved with this form of tumour, early diagnosis, aggressive treatment, and close and careful follow-up are essential. Germ-cell tumours of the testicle metastasize directly to the para-aortic lymph nodes. Subsequent spread takes place to the supradiaphragmatic lymph nodes and to viscera such as the lungs or brain.

Clinical features

Common presentations for a germ-cell tumour of the testis include:
- a painless swelling in the testis often noted incidentally;
- traumatic 'predetermination' (minor trauma reveals an otherwise incidental mass that is initially ascribed to trauma);
- vague testicular discomfort;
- rarely, symptoms of metastatic disease or hormonal effects (e.g. gynaecomastia).

On physical examination there is generally a hard, irregular, non-tender mass occupying a part of the testis or the testis in its entirety. Transillumination of the scrotum will not show any evidence of fluid.

Tumour markers

If a germ-cell tumour of the testis is suspected, then the tumour markers AFP and HCG should be estimated. These markers are essential in the staging and follow-up of patients with germ-cell tumours of the testis. Elevation of one or both of these markers will occur in 75–80% of non-seminomatous germ-cell tumours. Serum should be drawn before and after surgery. It is important to remember that the half-life of AFP is 5–7 days, so elevation of this marker for up to 1 week after surgery may not be significant; persistent elevation at 2 weeks raises the suspicion of metastatic disease.

Imaging

- Scrotal ultrasonography is helpful in excluding cystic lesions of the intrascrotal contents and in ruling out infective lesions of the testicle.
- Chest X-ray must be performed in order to assess the lungs and mediastinum. If a suspicion of metastatic lesions in these areas exists, CT scanning of the chest should be performed.
- Abdominal CT will identify the presence of enlarged para-aortic lymph nodes within the abdomen. It will also show any evidence of obstruction of the ureters by a mass of lymph nodes.

Pathology

Histological examination of the tumour gives the diagnosis. Once the clinical suspicion of a testicular tumour is confirmed by elevated tumour markers and scrotal imaging, surgical removal of the testicle is undertaken. Trans-scrotal approaches to the testis, by either needle aspiration or incision, must be avoided because of the danger of involving the scrotal lymphatics, which drain to the inguinal lymph nodes.

STAGING

Staging includes testicular histology, serum tumour markers, abdominal CT and chest X-ray. A CT scan of the chest and brain may be performed if suspicion of metastatic disease exists. Staging of testis tumours is related to whether disease is localized to the testicle, whether there is spread to the abdominal lymph nodes, or whether there is spread to the supradiaphragmatic lymph nodes or distant viscera (Table 39.9).

Management

The primary treatment of testis tumours is removal of the affected testicle. Further treatment depends on histological identification of the tumour and adequate staging.

05

Table 39.9 Staging and treatment of testicular tumours (Royal Marsden staging).

	Staging	Treatment of seminoma	Treatment of non-seminomatous germ-cell tumours
Stage I	Disease confined to the testis	DXT to abdominal nodes	Observation or RPLND
Stage II	Retroperitoneal lymph node involvement		
	IIa: nodes < 2 cm in size	DXT to abdominal nodes	Chemotherapy and RPLND for residual disease
	IIb: nodes 2–5 cm in size	DXT to abdominal nodes	Chemotherapy and RPLND for residual disease
	IIc: nodes > 5 cm in size (bulky disease)	Chemotherapy	Chemotherapy and RPLND for residual disease
Stage III	Nodal disease above the diaphragm	DXT to abdominal nodes and thoracic nodes or chemotherapy	Chemotherapy
Stage IV	Visceral metastases	Chemotherapy	Chemotherapy

DXT, deep X-ray therapy; RPLND, retroperitoneal lymph node dissection.

SEMINOMA

This tumour is highly radiosensitive, although large tumour bulks are less radiosensitive and thus chemotherapy has a significant role to play in treating large tumours. The current treatment of seminoma is summarized in Table 39.9. For patients with abdominal lymphadenopathy in stages IIc and III or thoracic lymphadenpoathy in stage III, chemotherapy should be considered.

NON-SEMINOMATOUS GERM-CELL TUMOUR

This tumour is not radiosensitive but has been found to be highly chemosensitive. There has been controversy as to whether the correct form of management for stage I disease is careful observation or 'prophylactic' retroperitoneal lymph node dissection (RPLND). It is essential that careful and regular follow-up by chest X-ray, serum markers and CT is carried out. In stage II disease, chemotherapy is the treatment of choice. Any residual nodal enlargement following a full course of chemotherapy should be treated by RPLND.

CHEMOTHERAPY

The exact form of chemotherapy used varies from department to department, but one of the most effective regimens comprises bleomycin, etoposide and cisplatin (BEP).

Testicular cancer at a glance

Definition

Testicular cancer: malignant lesion of the testis

Epidemiology
- Age 20–40 years
- Most common solid tumours in young males

Aetiology
- Cryptorchidism: 50-fold increase in risk of developing testicular cancer
- Risk is unaffected by orchidopexy
- Higher incidence in whites

Pathology
Classification of testicular tumours
Germ-cell tumours (90%) (secrete AFP and HCG)
- Seminoma

- Non-seminoma
  - (a) Embryonal carcinoma
  - (b) Teratocarcinoma
  - (c) Choriocarcinoma

Stromal tumours
- Leydig cell
- Sertoli cell
- Granulosa cell

Metastatic tumours
Staging
- Stage I: confined to scrotum
- Stage II: spread to retroperitoneal lymph nodes below the diaphragm
- Stage III: distant metastases

Spread
- Germ-cell tumours metastasize to the para-aortic nodes, lung and brain
- Stromal tumours rarely metastasize

Clinical features
- Painless swelling of the testis, often discovered incidentally or after trauma
- Vague testicular discomfort
- Rarely, evidence of metastatic disease or gynaecomastia
- Examination reveals a hard, irregular, non-tender testicular mass

Investigations
- Blood for tumour markers, i.e. AFP and HCG
- AFP is elevated in 75% of embryonal carcinomas and 65% of teratocarcinomas
- AFP is *not* elevated in pure seminoma or choriocarcinoma
- HCG is elevated in 100% of choriocarcinomas, 60% of embryonal carcinomas, 60% of teratocarcinomas and 10% of pure seminomas
- Scrotal ultrasound

- Chest X-ray to assess lungs and mediastinum
- CT of chest and abdomen to detect lymph nodes
- Laparoscopy (retroperitonoscopy) to assess abdominal nodes

Management
- Orchidectomy (via groin incision) and histological diagnosis, further treatment depends on histology and staging

Seminoma
- Stage I: radiotherapy to abdominal nodes
- Stage II: radiotherapy to abdominal nodes
- Stage III: chemotherapy (bleomycin, etoposide, cisplatin)

Non-seminoma germ cell
- Stage I: RPLND
- Stage II: chemotherapy + RPLND
- Stage III: chemotherapy

Prognosis
- Overall cure rates are over 90% and node-negative disease has almost 100% 5-year survival

Cancer of the penis

Incidence

Carcinoma of the penis is uncommon in the UK, occurring in only 1 per 100,000 males. It rarely occurs in patients who have been circumcised or in patients under the age of 45 years. It most commonly occurs in the sixth and seventh decades, and in patients over 75 years of age the incidence is 8.9 per 100,000 males.

Aetiology

The aetiology of cancer of the penis is uncertain but a number of factors associated with its development have been described, including age, oriental origin, long-standing phimosis and poor penile hygiene (related to non-circumcision and STDs).

Pathology

In nearly every case, tumours of the penis are squamous cell carcinomas that exhibit keratinization, epithelial pearl formation and mitotic activity. The tumours are usually low grade and on microscopic examination are usually papillary or ulcerating lesions. Spread occurs most commonly to the inguinal lymph nodes, with distant visceral metastatic spread being uncommon.

Clinical features

An ulcerating or papillary lesion of the penis may be found; this may be painful. It may present as a painful swelling underneath a tight foreskin, with a foul-smelling purulent and haemorrhagic discharge. Palpable lymph nodes in the inguinal region may be found, although these may be associated with infection of the tumour. If this is the case, they will disappear shortly after treatment of the primary tumour.

Management
Treatment of the primary lesion
- If the lesion is localized to the prepuce, circumcision is likely to be all that is required.
- If the glans alone is affected, especially if the tumour is 1 cm or less in size, local radiotherapy gives excellent results.
- Where the shaft of the penis is involved, partial amputation is the preferred treatment.
- Where extensive involvement of the shaft has taken place, total amputation of the penis would probably be required, although partial amputation is possible if a 2-cm margin of normal tissue can be removed proximal to the tumour.

Management of inguinal lymph nodes
- Impalpable nodes: careful follow-up is required. If

05

treatments fail, an artificial urinary sphincter or urinary diversion may be necessary. Incontinence after pelvic fracture may be treated by sphincter insertion or very occasionally by urethral sphincter reconstruction.

Overflow incontinence

Overflow incontinence due to outflow obstruction as a result of BPH or urethral stricture is treated by TURP or urethrotomy respectively. Bladder emptying after surgery may be initially poor due to overstretching of the detrusor muscle, in which case temporary catheter drainage or drugs that stimulate detrusor contraction (e.g. bethanechol or distigmine) may be used. If all else fails the patient may need to commence clean intermittent self-catheterization (CISC) or may require a long-term indwelling urethral catheter. Overflow incontinence secondary to neuropathic atonic bladder is best managed by CISC.

Nocturnal enuresis

As children grow older an increasing number achieve continence. Daytime continence should be achieved by 2 years, although night-time continence takes a little longer and is more variable. About two-thirds of children are dry at night by the age of 3 years. At least half the remainder will be dry by 10 years of age. By the age of 15 years only 2% of children are incontinent at night. Investigation of enuresis includes a detailed history and physical examination, urine microscopy and culture, an IVU and urodynamics.

Management consists of bladder training during the day, gradually increasing the interval between voiding, combined with voiding last thing at night. In younger children the parents should lift the child before they retire at night. Enuresis alarms triggered by small amounts of leakage may also be used. These alarms probably condition the patient to wake when the bladder becomes full. In addition, pharmacological manipulation using a variety of agents has met with good success.

The most commonly employed drug is imipramine (Tofranil), a tricyclic antidepressant that acts by inhibiting detrusor contractions and reducing the depth of sleep so that bladder distension is appreciated and the patient wakes to void. Anticholinergic agents (propantheline, oxybutynin) may also be used to inhibit unstable detrusor contractions. Desmopressin is an ADH analogue that decreases urine output overnight and may help some patients. A daily diary should be kept to assess the success of treatment.

Failure of medical treatment with persistent bed-wetting is often associated with daytime frequency and urgency also. For these patients, augmentation cystoplasty may be the only solution.

Incontinence secondary to fistula

Surgical intervention is the best treatment for vesicovaginal fistula. There are a number of possible approaches to repair the defect and prevent leakage.

Incontinence in the elderly

Approximately 15% of elderly patients experience incontinence. The percentage of nursing-home or hospital-dwelling elderly who suffer with incontinence is even higher. Treatment is determined by the cause. However, incontinence in the elderly is usually multifactorial, with decreased mobility and altered mental status having a significant impact on treatment options and outcomes. Regular toileting is an important part of the treatment. Specific abnormalities are treated as indicated.

Neuropathic bladder disorders

Anatomy and physiology

As the bladder fills with urine, the bladder muscle (detrusor) is stretched. There is an awareness of filling at a volume of 150–250 mL and a desire to void when normal bladder capacity (400–500 mL) is reached. Micturition is achieved by relaxation of the pelvic floor musculature, including the voluntary sphincter. The trigone contracts, opening the bladder neck and closing the ureteric orifices, thus preventing urine reflux during voiding. The detrusor then contracts, expelling the stored urine. The pelvic nerves supplying the bladder and urethra with motor and sensory fibres synapse in the micturition centre located in the S2–4 segments of the spinal cord, which corresponds with the T2–L1 vertebral level. This centre is connected to centres in the pons and cerebrum (especially frontal lobes) which exert an inhibitory effect that is central to voluntary control. Disease or injury at any of these levels may result in abnormal bladder or urethral function.

Classification

Traditionally, neuropathic bladder disorders have been described according to the site of neurological injury as upper or lower motor neurone injuries.
- Lesions above the micturition centre are characterized by detrusor overactivity, which is frequently associated with uncoordinated increased urethral sphincter activity.
- Lesions at the level of the micturition centre (S2–4) or lower are characterized by decreased activity of the detrusor and sphincter.

However, in individual patients a mixed pattern of injury is not uncommon and the clinical picture may

Table 39.10 Classification of neuropathic disorders.

Detrusor activity	Urethral sphincter activity	Sensation
Normal	Normal	Normal
Overactive (hyperreflexic)	Overactive	Hypersensitive
Underactive (areflexic)	Incompetent	Hyposensitive

not fit one or other neurological pattern exactly. For this reason the International Continence Society has classified neuropathic disorders according to urodynamic findings on assessment of detrusor and urethral function (Table 39.10).

Causes

A large number of diseases that affect the nervous system from the cerebral cortex to the pelvic nerves may result in neuropathic bladder (Table 39.11).

Investigation

Diagnosis of neuropathic bladder disorders depends on a complete history and physical examination with an extensive neurological assessment. Special features in the history include the voiding pattern (which should be described in detail with reference to daytime and nighttime frequency), urgency, incontinence, pain on urination, hesitancy, poor stream, straining to void, dribbling and incomplete emptying. In males sexual function should be documented, with special attention to the presence or absence of erections and ejaculation. In both sexes any disturbance of bowel function should be noted. Associated medical disorders such as diabetes mellitus and present medication should also be noted. More generalized neurological symptoms, such as disturbed cerebral function, weakness, sensory loss or altered coordination, should also be ascertained. Visual disturbances may occur in patients with diabetic retinopathy or with multiple sclerosis (retrobulbar neuritis).

A full physical examination, with special reference to urological and neurological examination, should be performed. Urological examination involves assessment of the kidneys for hydronephrosis, the bladder for urine retention and the scrotum for epididymitis. Neurological examination involves assessment of cerebral function, sensory level, muscular tone, power and reflex activity.

Investigation should include urinalysis to rule out infection and assessment of renal function. IVU is necessary to document upper-tract (i.e. kidneys and ureter) status. Urodynamic assessment is the key to accurate diagnosis and is essential in the follow-up of any treatment regimen.

Table 39.11 Causes of neuropathic bladder.

Cerebral
Cerebrovascular accident
Dementia
Frontal lobe tumours
Parkinson's disease

Spinal
Trauma
Multiple sclerosis
Amyotrophic lateral sclerosis
Compression (tumour, abscess, disc prolapse)
Spina bifida

Peripheral nerves
Diabetes mellitus
Surgical injury (pelvic surgery)

Urodynamics
- *Uroflowmetry*: this is the study of the flow of urine from the urethra. The flow rate, volume voided, time of voiding, pattern on voiding and residual volume all give valuable information about lower urinary tract function.
- *Cystometry*: this test evaluates the reservoir function of the lower urinary tract. Cystometry evaluates bladder capacity, intravesical pressure during filling, bladder pressure during voiding and the presence of premature unstable contractions. In addition, the patient's ability to perceive filling is tested.
- *Urethral pressure profilometry*: this technique involves measurement of urethral pressure with the bladder at rest and during voiding. The technique is reserved for difficult cases where a combination of uroflowmetry and cystometry has not produced a clear assessment of the neuropathic abnormality.

Management of incontinence

The goals of treatment are to reverse the pathological abnormality where possible, alleviate the symptoms and preserve renal function. Treatment is dependent on the functional disorder produced by the disease or injury.

05

Detrusor overactivity

Detrusor hyperreflexia may be treated by drugs that have an anticholinergic and/or smooth-muscle relaxant effect, e.g. oxybutynin, flavoxate hydrochloride or emepronium carageenate. Adverse effects such as dry mouth and blurred vision are common. Failure of pharmacological manipulation is an indication for surgical intervention. Phenol injection into the vesical nerves under the trigone and division of the anterior sacral nerve roots (presacral neurectomy) may be tried. Augmentation cystoplasty (bladder enlargement) or substitution cystoplasty (bladder substitution) may be used.

Management of retention

Urine retention is most commonly due to an underactive detrusor muscle.

Underactive detrusor

It is important to establish proper bladder emptying in order to avoid infection, stone formation and renal impairment. Patients may empty their bladders simply by a combination of abdominal straining and manual pressure suprapubically (Credé manoeuvre). This is not a very efficient manoeuvre. Drugs that stimulate smooth muscle contraction such as bethanechol or distigmine may also be used. It is important when using these drugs to ensure that there is no outflow obstruction, otherwise bladder rupture is a real possibility. A more widely applied alternative is the technique of CISC. Complications such as infections or stricture are uncommon. For those patients unable to manage this technique, an indwelling catheter or a urinary diversion may be necessary.

Management of specific causes of neuropathic bladder

Spinal cord injury

After the initial injury there is a period of 'spinal shock' that lasts on average 2–3 months. This results in paralysis of the detrusor muscle with retention of urine. It is important to avoid overdistension of the bladder in order to prevent permanent bladder dysfunction. A urethral catheter should be inserted when the patient presents with a spinal injury. To avoid the complications associated with long-term urethral catheterization (stricture), subsequent bladder emptying can be achieved by intermittent catheterization or a suprapubic catheter. When the period of spinal shock passes, bladder or urethral function is assessed by urodynamics and definitive therapy commenced based on the findings of this investigation. Regular follow-up with urinalysis, blood urea nitrogen, IVU and urodynamics is necessary.

Spina bifida

Bladder dysfunction is common in patients with spina bifida cystica (see Chapter 40). The first priority is to ensure adequate bladder emptying in order to prevent upper-tract deterioration. In infants, the parents may need to perform intermittent catheterization; alternatively, a temporary vesicostomy may be formed. As the child grows older, control of incontinence becomes an important objective. Urodynamic assessment of bladder and urethral function will indicate the treatment options.

Diabetes mellitus

Peripheral neuropathy is a significant complication of diabetes mellitus, involving both the sensory and motor nerves. Decreased detrusor activity leading to retention is the usual bladder abnormality. CISC is the most attractive treatment option.

Multiple sclerosis

Bladder dysfunction is a common complication of multiple sclerosis. Treatment is difficult because of the fluctuating nature of the disease. As the demyelination usually affects the spinal cord above the micturition centre (S2–4), an upper motor neurone-type lesion is the usual presentation. If the nerve supply to the sphincter is also involved, detrusor sphincter dyssynergia may result. Less commonly the pelvic nerves are involved, with an atonic detrusor and retention of urine. Urodynamic assessment will indicate the appropriate treatment. Where possible, a conservative approach is advocated as the bladder abnormality may change in nature as the disease progresses.

Cerebral disorders

Bladder dysfunction can occur with a variety of cerebral disorders, such as stroke, Parkinson's disease, dementia and frontal lobe tumours. These disorders are characterized by loss of cerebral inhibition of micturition leading to incontinence. Treatment is difficult and consists of regular toileting and urine collection devices if necessary.

Complications

The complications of neuropathic bladder include:
- recurrent urinary infections;
- stone formation due to stasis;
- renal dysfunction;
- hydronephrosis due to chronic back-pressure.

Prognosis

The greatest threat to the patient with neuropathic bladder is progressive renal damage leading to renal failure, which may be caused by hydronephrosis, infection or

stone disease. Careful management of bladder function with regular follow-up has significantly improved long-term survival in these patients.

Disorders of the testis and scrotum

Torsion of the testis

Torsion of the testis may occur at any age but most commonly affects adolescent males. In most cases the underlying cause is a high insertion of the tunica vaginalis on the spermatic cord, which allows the testis to rotate within the tunica. This abnormality is described as a 'bell clapper' deformity. Less commonly, a long mesentery may separate the epididymis and testis, allowing torsion of the testis on this long 'mesorchium'. Undescended testes are more prone to torsion. In neonates torsion of the testis and the tunica vaginalis may occur. Torsion is more common at night.

The clinical features are sudden onset of severe scrotal pain, which may radiate to the lower abdomen. Nausea and vomiting may occur with the pain. In at least half such patients a preceding history of sudden-onset, short-duration scrotal pain can be elicited. These testes have twisted and untwisted (intermittent torsion). Patients with a history of intermittent torsion may be noted to have an abnormal horizontal lie of the testis when examined in the standing position. Because of the risk of acute torsion, urgent elective (i.e. next operating list) fixation of the testes is recommended. Examination of the patient with acute torsion may reveal a testis that lies higher in the scrotum than the opposite testis. This is due to shortening of the cord by twisting. The overlying skin may be reddened and the testis is extremely tender. The spermatic cord may be thickened and shortened.

The diagnosis is a clinical one and any difficulty in deciding whether the patient has torsion is best resolved at exploration. The diagnosis may be effectively excluded by colour Doppler ultrasonography showing a normal testicular blood supply, although any delay in obtaining a scan may compromise the viability of the testis. Therefore, patients with a suspected torsion usually require immediate exploration.

Exploration is carried out through a midline scrotal incision which will reveal a congested ischaemic testis with a twisted spermatic cord (Fig. 39.16). Broadly, if the testis is infarcted, it should be removed. If it is viable and the duration of torsion is short, it should be preserved and fixed to the scrotum to prevent recurrent torsion. With longer duration of torsion, the testis may atrophy and be hypofunctional but should be preserved if viable. Because there is a 10% risk of torsion in the unaffected side it should also be fixed at the first operation.

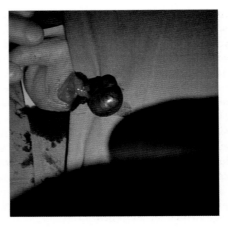

Figure 39.16 Torsion showing ischaemic testis and twisted spermatic cord.

The differential diagnosis of torsion of the spermatic cord includes the following.
- Acute epididymitis: may be bacterial or viral in nature and has similar presenting symptoms but signs of systemic upset such as pyrexia and rigors may be present. However, acute epididymitis is uncommon in adolescent males.
- Torsion of the testicular appendages: the symptoms are those of acute torsion but differentiation may be possible at an early stage, when a normal testis is noted with an exquisitely tender upper pole and a blue dot visible through the scrotal skin. As the condition progresses, the tenderness becomes more generalized and differentiation from acute torsion is impossible. The diagnosis is best made at exploration. If the pain is due to torsion of the hydatid of Morgagni, the appendages should be excised.

Undescended testis

When a testis is missing from the scrotum, several explanations are possible. The testis may be retractile, ectopic in position, undescended or absent.
- A *retractile testis* can be coaxed to the bottom of the scrotum and does not require intervention. However, retractile testes should be monitored to ensure that they eventually achieve their correct position in the scrotum. If the testis cannot be brought down to the bottom of the scrotum but only as far as mid or high scrotum, then it is not retractile.
- An *ectopic testis* is one which has strayed from the path of normal descent. Most commonly the testis lies in the superficial inguinal pouch. Other ectopic sites include the femoral triangle, perineum and the root of the penis. It is thought that ectopy results from an abnormal connection to the gubernaculum testis which leads the gonad to the

05

abnormal position. Treatment is by orchidopexy to place the testis in the scrotum.

• An *undescended testis* is one that has stopped in the normal path of descent and may be intra-abdominal, inguinal, at the superficial ring or high in the scrotum.

• An *absent testis*: approximately 5% of missing testes are truly absent but this diagnosis can only be made after CT has ensured that the testis is not intra-abdominal.

Several theories have been proposed to explain maldescent (ectopic and undescended testis). These include an abnormality of the gubernaculum such as shortness or complete absence, an intrinsically abnormal (dysgenetic) testis and deficiency of gonadotrophins required for descent. If a testis remains undescended, the seminiferous tubules become progressively damaged; thus early orchidopexy is necessary to preserve spermatogenesis. However, as many as 10% of undescended testes are intrinsically abnormal and may never attain normal spermatogenesis despite early orchidopexy.

Undescended testis is noted in 20% of premature boys, although most testes descend to the scrotum within the first month of life. An incidence of roughly 4% is noted in full-term boys and half of these will have attained a normal scrotal position by the end of the first month of life. By the end of the first year of life 99% of testes should be descended and the remaining 1% require surgical correction (orchidopexy). Surgical correction should be undertaken at this time as delay serves no purpose. The reasons for surgical intervention are:

• to preserve fertility;

• to deal with the coexistent hernial sac present in 90% of patients;

• to reduce the risk of torsion or traumatic injury;

• orchidopexy may also decrease the risk of malignant change.

The risk of malignant change in an undescended testis is probably 30 times greater than in a normally descended testis. Seminoma is the most common tumour of undescended testes. Orchidopexy before the age of 8 years reduces the risk of malignant change but does not decrease it to the level of a normally descended testis. If a patient is aged 10 years or greater, orchidectomy is preferred to orchidopexy unless the maldescent is bilateral, in which case one testis is removed and the other brought down. Despite early orchidopexy, as many as 20% of patients with unilateral undescent will be infertile, while the remainder will produce sperm of poor quality. Bilateral undescent almost invariably results in infertility.

Scrotal masses

A mass in the scrotum may arise from the scrotum or its contents or may be due to an inguinoscrotal hernia. If one can get above the mass at the neck of the scrotum, then it is scrotal in origin. Scrotal masses may be solid (tumour, chronic epididymo-orchitis) or cystic (hydrocele, epididymal cyst). Varicoceles may also present as a scrotal mass.

Hydrocele*

A hydrocele is a collection of fluid within the tunica vaginalis and may be congenital (infantile hydrocele) or acquired. Infantile hydrocele is due to a patent processus vaginalis, which allows fluid from the abdominal cavity to collect in the scrotum. If the communication is wider, a hernia results. Most of these hydroceles will close spontaneously by the end of the first year of life. Persistent hydroceles require ligation of the patent processus vaginalis at the deep inguinal ring.

Adult hydroceles are non-communicating, i.e. there is no patent processus vaginalis. These hydroceles may be idiopathic or secondary to intrascrotal pathology such as tumour, torsion, trauma or infection. Hydroceles secondary to underlying disease tend to be acute, while those that are idiopathic in nature are chronic. Hydroceles are fluctuant, unless very tense, and they transilluminate. The swelling lies anterior to the testis. However, the testes may be impalpable within a tense hydrocele. Hydroceles should not be tapped because of the risk of introducing infection or causing haemorrhage into the hydrocele by inadvertently stabbing a vein.

Hydroceles are dealt with by excision of the hydrocele sac or plication of the sac (Lord's procedure).

(*Note: the etymology of *-cele* and *-coele*. There is some confusion as to the spelling of words such as hydrocele, varicocele, etc. Some think that the British English suffix is *-coele* and that the *-cele* version is American English. Not so. In fact both derive from Greek, κελε (*-cele*) meaning 'tumour' and κοιλοσ (*-coele*) meaning 'hollow'.)

Epididymal cyst

Cystic swellings of the epididymis are located above and behind the testis and separate from it. If the cyst contains spermatozoa it is called a spermatocele. These cysts may be multilocular and/or multiple and may replace much of the epididymis. Epididymal cysts are usually asymptomatic but may cause discomfort. If symptoms are troublesome, these cysts may be excised but the patient must be warned that the epididymis may also have to be excised if extensively involved. Bilateral cyst excision poses a very significant risk to fertility.

Varicocele

A varicocele is a scrotal mass due to varicosities of the pampiniform plexus of veins above the testis. It is present in 10% of men and is uncommon before adolescence. The majority of varicoceles (95%) are left-sided and are due to incompetence, or absence, of the valve at the termination of the left testicular vein before its insertion into the renal vein. On examination with the patient in the standing position it feels like a bag of worms. A varicocele of recent onset, especially one which does not empty on lying down, may be due to venous occlusion by a renal or retroperitoneal tumour and should be investigated by renal ultrasound. Varicoceles are believed to raise the temperature around the ipsilateral testis and some reports suggest that sperm count and motility are significantly decreased in 65–70% of patients. This is the usual indication for surgical intervention. The gonadal veins may be ligated within the inguinal canal (low tie) or in the retroperitoneum above the deep ring (high tie).

Disorders of the scrotal skin

Fournier's gangrene is an infection of the scrotal skin caused by the synergistic action of aerobic and anaerobic bacteria. It is predisposed to by diabetes mellitus, perianal sepsis or periurethral abscess. It causes gangrene of the scrotal and penile skin and may be life-threatening. Treatment is by intensive antibiotic therapy combined with extensive débridement of devitalized tissue with later plastic reconstruction. Idiopathic scrotal oedema is an acute oedematous swelling of the skin that occurs in young boys and may be infective in nature. Treatment is conservative.

Scrotal skin tumours are now rare. In the past they arose from occupational exposure to soot (chimney sweeps' cancer, first described by Percival Pott in 1775), tars, oil and other petroleum products. Poor hygiene and chronic inflammation are predisposing factors today. Scrotal cancers are nearly always squamous carcinomas. Treatment is by wide excision and groin dissection if there is a suspicion of lymph node metastases. Prognosis is fairly good (60% cure) if the tumour is confined to the scrotum but poor (< 25% cure) if metastases are present.

Benign disorders of the foreskin and penis

Balanitis

Balanitis is an infection of the foreskin (prepuce), usually seen in young boys and usually caused by staphylococci.

The patient complains of a sore penis and on examination the foreskin is swollen and red with a purulent discharge. It is treated by bathing and penicillin and usually settles rapidly. If, when the infection settles, the foreskin is very adherent to the glans and cannot be retracted easily, then circumcision should be recommended.

Phimosis

Phimosis is defined as a tightness of the foreskin of such a degree as to prevent retraction. It may be congenital or secondary to infection. Ballooning of the foreskin may occur on micturition. On examination it is possible to retract the foreskin and there may only be a small contracted orifice. Treatment is by circumcision.

Paraphimosis

Paraphimosis occurs when the foreskin retracts behind the corona of the glans penis, producing a tourniquet effect. The foreskin and glans become oedematous, making it impossible to pull the foreskin forwards without great difficulty. As the oedema progresses the constriction becomes tighter and, if not treated, the foreskin will become ulcerated. Treatment consists of reduction of the paraphimosis under anaesthesia. Occasionally, the constricting ring of foreskin has to be divided on the dorsal aspect to facilitate reduction. This is called a dorsal slit. Paraphimosis is an indication for circumcision, which may be undertaken as part of the emergency treatment if the tissues are not too oedematous. An iatrogenic cause of paraphimosis is failure to retract the foreskin following insertion of a urinary catheter.

Hypospadias

Hypospadias is a condition where the urethral orifice opens in an abnormal proximal position on the ventral surface of the penis or scrotum (Fig. 39.17). It occurs in about 1 in 800 live births. The majority (80%) are glandular, with the urethral meatus lying at the base of the glans penis. In penile hypospadias the meatus is somewhere along the shaft of the penis and is always associated with ventral flexion deformity of the penis (referred to as chordee). The most severe and rarest form of hypospadias is perineal, in which the urinary meatus is found behind a cleft scrotum. It is important to differentiate this condition from an intersex problem.

Minor degrees of hypospadias require no treatment, while there are several complicated surgical procedures available for the management of more severe forms.

05

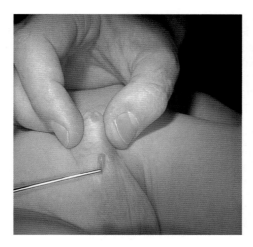

Figure 39.17 Hypospadias: the urethral orifice is on the ventral surface at the base of the shaft of the penis.

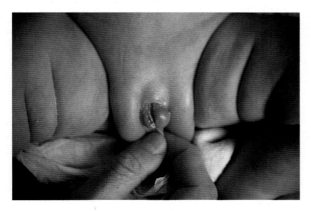

Figure 39.18 Epispadias: the urethral orifice is on the dorsal surface of the penis.

Epispadias

Epispadias is a condition in which the penile urethra opens on to the dorsum of the penile shaft (Fig. 39.18). It is very rare and in its extreme form may be associated with ectopia vesicae or exstrophy of the bladder (i.e. the bladder is exposed on a poorly developed lower anterior abdominal wall). If epispadias is not associated with incontinence, surgical treatment is similar to that for hypospadias. The presence of incontinence makes management much more difficult.

Impotence

Impotence or erectile dysfunction describes the persistent inability to obtain and sustain an erection sufficient for sexual intercourse. Primary impotence refers to impotence throughout a patient's lifetime, while secondary impotence refers to loss of previously normal erections. Psychogenic impotence is caused by psychiatric illness or emotional stress. This is in contrast to organic impotence, which may result from physical causes such as vascular, neurological or endocrine dysfunction.

Erectile physiology

Erection is governed by smooth muscle in the pudendal artery branches to the corpora cavernosa. When the smooth muscle is contracted, blood is not able to enter the spaces of the corpora cavernosa and thus blood is shunted to the venous side. When the muscle is in a relaxed state, blood can enter the corporal spaces and the penis becomes distended. Detumescence results from decreased smooth muscle tone and increased corporal venous drainage.

The sensory pathway of erection is mediated by the dorsal penile nerve, a branch of the pudendal nerve. The motor limb is mediated by the sacral outflow of the parasympathetic nervous system via the pelvic nerves. Pelvic nerve stimulation produces an increase in pudendal arterial flow into the cavernosal spaces. Detumescence is mediated by both activation of sympathetic nerves and decreased parasympathetic outflow.

Aetiology

Although most cases (> 60%) have an organic basis, a large number of patients will have a psychological element contributing to the problem.

Vascular

Atherosclerosis is responsible for the majority of cases of erectile dysfunction in men over 60 years of age. Approximately half of men afflicted with peripheral vascular disease note some degree of impotence. Impotence may also result from disruption of the venous mechanism involved in erection. Causes include atherosclerosis, trauma and Peyronie's disease.

Diabetes mellitus

Diabetes is the second most important cause of erectile dysfunction. Impotence is known to occur 10–15 years prior to the general population and in up to 60% of men with the disease. Both vascular and neurological factors, due to small-vessel disease and peripheral neuropathic changes respectively, contribute to the dysfunction.

Neurological

Men who have spinal cord lesions will have varying

degrees of erectile dysfunction based on the level of the lesion. Approximately 50% of men with lumbar lesions will have erections, while 70% of those with thoracic and 90% with cervical lesions are able to have erections. In addition to spinal cord trauma, other neurological causes of impotence include myelodysplasia, multiple sclerosis, tabes dorsalis and all peripheral neuropathies.

Endocrine

Endocrine disorders are a rare cause of impotence, accounting for fewer than 5% of cases. Syndromes of hypogonadism are associated with erectile dysfunction, including hypogonadotrophic hypogonadism seen in Klinefelter's syndrome or surgical orchidectomy. Prolactin-producing tumours will lead to low testosterone levels and possible impotence. Isolated deficiencies of testosterone are uncommon.

Trauma

Traumatic rupture of the posterior urethra and perineal trauma, including straddle injuries, can lead to impotence. Pelvic fracture is also associated with impotence as a result of arterial injury in up to one-third of patients.

Uraemic

Uraemic patients on chronic dialysis have a high incidence of impotence. However, half of these patients recover erectile ability after renal transplantation, secondary to reversal of uraemic neuropathy.

Iatrogenic

Many surgical procedures may lead to vascular or neurological impairment and hence impotence. Radical prostatectomy or cystoprostatectomy were long associated with impotence. However, new techniques using an anatomical nerve-sparing approach have dramatically improved this. Aortic and peripheral vascular surgery may disrupt hypogastric arterial inflow. Neurological surgical procedures may produce impotence as a complication. Transurethral endoscopic procedures may cause thermal injuries leading to erectile dysfunction. Therapeutic measures such as pelvic irradiation are associated with an increased incidence of impotence.

Medications

Many commonly used drugs have long been known to cause impotence. The patient's history must include a thorough list of all medications used, both prescription

Table 39.12 Medications that may cause impotence. From Siroky, M.B. & Krane, R.J. (eds) (1990) *Manual of Urology Diagnosis and Therapy*. Boston: Little, Brown, with permission.

Centrally acting agents	*Hyperprolactinaemic agents*
Phenothiazines	Oestrogens
Tricyclic antidepressants	Phenothiazines
Chronic ethanol abuse	Haloperidol
Narcotic abuse	Cimetidine
Marijuana abuse	Metoclopramide
Reserpine	Reserpine
	α-Methyldopa
Anticholinergic agents	Opiates
Tricyclic antidepressants	
Phenothiazines	*Sympatholytic agents*
Antimuscarinic agents	Clonidine
Guanethidine	Bretylium
	α-Methyldopa
Antiandrogenic agents	β-Adrenergic antagonists
Spironolactone	α-Adrenergic antagonists
Oestrogens	
Cyproterone	*Agents with unknown mechanisms*
Digoxin	ε-Aminocaproic acid
Ketoconazole	Naproxen
Cimetidine	Thiazide diuretics
Disopyramide	

and recreational. As is often the case, adjusting the dose or type of medication may correct a patient's erectile dysfunction. Table 39.12 lists some of the potentially causative agents.

Diagnosis

Central to the diagnosis of impotence is a careful and detailed history. Questions related to onset, duration, degree and circumstances of erectile dysfunction are important. Past history should focus on those causes outlined in the section on aetiology. Psychological assessment by trained professionals will allow identification and treatment of those patients with psychogenic impotence.

Physical examination should start with the evaluation of male secondary sexual characteristics. The penis is examined for length, plaques or deformity of the corporal bodies. Peripheral pulses must be evaluated, as absent pulse is indicative of peripheral vascular disease. The testes should be examined in order to assess presence or absence, size and consistency. Patients with androgen deficiency may have gynaecomastia. Neurological assessment should include sensory testing of the penile and perineal skin and the bulbocavernosus reflex to evaluate sacral reflexes.

Nocturnal penile tumescence testing will note changes in penis size during sleep. This test is based on the

05

knowledge that in normal postpubertal males the stage of rapid eye movement (REM) sleep is associated with the development of erection. Several techniques are available to measure circumferential changes in penile size during sleep that indicate the presence of erection. The penile brachial index is a technique used to assess penile blood pressure. Ratios of less than 75% of systemic pressure are indicative of vascular impotence. Biothesiometry is a method to test sensation of the penis by placing vibrations of differing intensity directly on the penis. Loss of vibratory sensation is an early sign of peripheral neuropathy.

Dynamic infusion cavernosometry and cavernosography is a technique used to assess the presence of venous leak or corporal leak as a contributing factor in impotence. Intracavernosal pressures are measured during infusion of saline after administration of intracavernosal papaverine. This agent produces arteriolar dilatation and erection ensues. The inability to maintain normal intracavernosal pressures while infusing saline at a constant rate is indicative of venous leak impotence. Arteriography is reserved for cases of impotence felt to be secondary to arterial insufficiency but only when penile revascularization surgery is proposed.

Treatment

As discussed above, psychogenic impotence should be evaluated and treated by a trained psychotherapist or sex therapist.

Medical therapy

Medical therapy varies widely in both the proposed mechanism of action and effectiveness.

● Sildenafil (Viagra) is an orally administered, peripherally acting phosphodiesterase inhibitor that promotes vasodilatation, but is unsuitable for patients taking nitrates for ischaemic heart disease.

● Apomorphine (Uprima) acts centrally on dopaminergic receptors to increase neuronal stimulation, but may be associated with nausea.

● Intracorporal administration of vasoactive substances has proven efficacy. Papaverine hydrochloride is the mainstay of therapy and causes prolonged corporal arterial dilatation and venous compression. This drug may be combined with other vasodilators, including phentolamine. Prostaglandin E_1 is also used extensively. Complications of intracorporal pharmacological therapy include local haematoma at the site of injection and induration from repeated injections. Priapism or prolonged painful erections can develop and potentially lead to permanent corporal fibrosis. Persistent erections due to this therapy can be treated by corporal aspiration and infusion of α-adrenergic agents such as adrenaline to bring about detumescence.

● Androgen replacement therapy with testosterone has been used with some efficacy in men with documented androgen deficiency. It is not indicated in patients with normal androgen levels and should not be given empirically.

● Vacuum suction devices rely on negative pressure within the vacuum to allow the corpora to fill with blood, producing an erection. A constrictive band is placed at the base of the penis following removal of the vacuum cylinder in order to reduce venous outflow. Many patients are able to achieve and maintain erections adequate for sexual intercourse. Complications following the use of vacuum suction include penile pain, ejaculatory difficulty and ecchymosis.

Surgical therapy

Surgical therapy for impotence includes the placement of intracorporal penile prostheses and, more recently, vascular surgical techniques in isolated cases of vasculogenic impotence.

● Penile prostheses are safe and effective but the therapy requires patient motivation. There are currently many prostheses available, including both non-inflatable and inflatable devices. Inflatable prostheses consist of paired intracorporal cylinders attached to a reservoir and pump mechanism. The patient can inflate and deflate the device, which has excellent cosmetic and functional results.

● Vascular surgical techniques have met with varied success for arteriogenic impotence. Penile revascularization involves the microsurgical anastomosis of the inferior epigastric artery to the dorsal penile artery.

Evidence-based medicine

Working Party on Lithiasis, European Association of Urology (2001) Guidelines on urolithiasis. *Eur Urol* **40**, 362–71.

http://www.doh.gov.uk/cancer/prostate.htm Department of Health prostate cancer programme website.

http://www.cancerindex.org/clinks1.htm Cancer resources directory website.

http://bmj.com/cgi/content/full/322/7302/1583 *British Medical Journal* review of testicular cancer management.

Patient information on urinary diversion, Urostomy Association (UA), Buckland, Beaumont Park, Danbury, Essex CM3 4DE.

05

Neurosurgical Disorders

40

Must know Must do

Must know

How to evaluate patients presenting with neurological
    symptoms
Glasgow Coma Scale
How to care for an unconscious/paralysed patient
Different types of intracranial tumour
Different types of intracranial haemorrhage
Presentation, diagnosis and management of
    hydrocephalus
Common spinal disorders

Must do

Observe an unconscious patient being managed in the
    intensive care unit
Observe a lumbar puncture being performed
Examine the fundi and look at the optic disc
Examine computed tomography/magnetic resonance
    scans of brain tumours and intracranial
    haemorrhage
See patients with spinal disc problems
See patients with peripheral nerve injuries
See a patient with hydrocephalus

Introduction

Neurosurgery is concerned with disorders of the brain, spinal cord, peripheral nerves and their surrounding structures. Neurosurgical problems can be classified as follows.

● Congenital anomalies: neural tube defects (spina bifida, meningoencephalocele), congenital hydrocephalus, craniofacial anomalies.
● Traumatic injuries: head injuries, spinal injuries, peripheral nerve injuries.
● Tumours: primary malignant tumours (e.g. gliomas), secondary spinal and cerebral tumours (metastases from bronchial neoplasm), benign tumours (e.g. meningiomas).

● Vascular disorders: subarachnoid haemorrhage, intracerebral haemorrhage, carotid artery disease.
● Infection: cerebral abscess, meningitis.
● Degenerative diseases: spinal degenerative diseases (e.g. disc prolapse), functional degenerative diseases (e.g. Parkinson's disease).
● Hydrocephalus: congenital, acquired (e.g. post meningitis).
● Pain.

The management of head injury is probably the commonest neurosurgical problem encountered by most doctors but only a small percentage of these require specialist neurosurgical care.

Evaluation of patients with neurosurgical disorders

Clinical assessment

Symptoms

Careful, detailed, chronological history-taking is essential for all neurosurgical patients. It needs to include a general history and family history and, when assessing paediatric neurosurgical problems, pregnancy and delivery history. History-taking will be difficult if the patient is confused or in a coma, but talking to relatives, friends, police and ambulance crews can be valuable. If the patient has come from another hospital, a close and critical review of the notes may be rewarding.

Neurological histories are usually:
● immediate, as in trauma or intracranial haemorrhage;
● progressive, as in tumours;
● intermittent, as in multiple sclerosis.
Sometimes an immediate event can be a feature of a progressive condition, e.g. a tumour can cause both a progressive deterioration and epilepsy.

Some important symptoms of neurosurgical disorders are listed in Table 40.1 and described below.

Table 40.1 Symptoms of neurosurgical disorders.

Headache
Weakness
Numbness
Dizziness
Visual disturbance
Blackouts

Headache

Headache may have extracranial or intracranial causes. *Stress* or *tension headache* arising from the muscles or fascia of the neck and scalp is probably the most common extracranial headache encountered. It may be chronic and is usually helped by resting. Sinusitis is another common non-neurological cause of headache. A *migraine headache*, which is associated with prodromal visual symptoms, is severe and often unilateral and is accompanied by photophobia, nausea, vomiting and prostration. Unilateral headache may also occur with *giant cell arteritis* and may also be accompanied by visual loss. Headache as a result of intracranial causes is usually due to *raised intracranial pressure*. Characteristically, the headache is intermittent, severe on waking and disappears after an hour or two. Usually supratentorial lesions produce frontal headache while posterior fossa lesions induce occipital headache. Headache resulting from loss of cerebrospinal fluid, e.g. after spinal anaesthesia, is relieved by lying down and exacerbated by standing or sitting up. Sudden-onset headache, especially accompanied by a stiff neck, is usually due to intracranial haemorrhage.

Weakness

Weakness may be described as general or specific. A general feeling of weakness may be indicative of a systemic disease (e.g. hypokalaemia, Parkinson's disease) but specific muscle group weakness is caused by upper or lower motor neurone lesions. With upper motor neurone lesions, e.g. following a stroke, the patient may complain of dragging or heaviness in a limb. With lower motor neurone lesions, the patient will usually recognize loss of power in the muscle group supplied by the nerve, e.g. quadriceps weakness following femoral nerve injury.

Numbness

Numbness means loss of cutaneous sensation and is seen with lesions of the peripheral nerves, e.g. the ulnar one-and-a-half fingers will be numb following transection of the ulnar nerve. Loss of sensation may also occur with cerebral pathology, e.g. during a transient ischaemic attack. Paraesthesiae or tingling may be encountered in patients with peripheral neuropathy (extremities), spinal cord lesions (from feet to waist), peripheral nerve lesion (unilateral), migraine, brainstem ischaemia, hypoglycaemia and hypocalcaemia (circumoral).

Dizziness and unsteadiness

These symptoms can mean different things to different people. It is important to establish whether there are any precipitating factors, e.g. unsteadiness on standing up suddenly may indicate orthostatic hypotension, dizziness on looking upwards may signify cerebrobasilar vascular insufficiency. A rotational element in the description of dizziness usually indicates vertigo. A history of continually veering to one side while walking may point to a cerebellar lesion.

Visual disturbance

There are many visual symptoms which may occur and patients may have difficulty describing them. Blurring or loss of vision in some or all of the fields of vision produces a confusing array of symptoms. It is very difficult for a patient who does not know the anatomy of the visual tracts to distinguish between hemianopia and monocular blindness. Therefore specific visual symptoms such as diplopia (seeing two of an object on moving the eye in one or more directions) or amaurosis fugax (transient blurring of vision in one eye) must be sought. It can be very difficult to determine visual loss in children and it may be profound before the child complains.

Blackouts

A blackout is a spontaneous loss of consciousness. The common causes are epilepsy or syncope. A major epileptic fit is characterized by aura, tongue biting, incontinence and convulsive movements, followed by headache and drowsiness, although lesser attacks may manifest themselves as short absences. Syncope is produced when there is reduced oxygen supply to the brain. The common causes of syncope are postural hypotension (the soldier who faints while standing rigidly to attention on a summer's day), Stokes–Adams attack (hypotension induced by heart block) and idiopathic orthostatic hypotension (caused by degeneration of the sympathetic autonomic nervous system or following drug treatment, e.g. antihypertensives). Unusual causes of syncope are micturition syncope and cough syncope.

Physical examination

Physical examination of a patient with a suspected neurosurgical disorder must include a thorough general examination, as the nervous system is commonly involved in cancer. For example, sciatica is usually caused by a prolapsed lumbar disc but can occasionally be the first

Table 40.2 Mnemonic for remembering the sequence of neurological examination of the limbs.

Member	Muscle tone and power
Royal	Reflexes
College	Coordination
Surgeons	Sensation
Glasgow	Gait

Table 40.3 Adult Glasgow Coma Scale.

	Score
Eye opening	
Spontaneous	4
To voice	3
To pain	2
No eye opening	1
Voice response	
Alert and orientated	5
Confused	4
Inappropriate	3
Incomprehensible	2
No voice response	1
Best motor response	
Obeys commands	6
Localizes pain	5
Flexes to pain	4
Abnormal flexion to pain	3
Extends to pain	2
No response to pain	1

manifestation of pelvic secondaries from rectal or gynaecological cancer. Always examine the abdomen of any patient with sciatica.

Neurological examination should be detailed and logical. One method is to assess higher mental function and level of consciousness while taking the history, and then to examine the cranial nerves in order from I to XII, the upper limbs and the lower limbs. When examining the limbs, test muscle tone and power first, then the reflexes, followed by coordination, sensation and gait (only for the lower limbs!). A useful mnemonic for the order of neurological examination is given in Table 40.2. Throughout the examination look carefully for any wasting, fasciculation or abnormal movement. In addition, compare right with left and upper limbs with lower limbs as differences can be important. For example, brisk lower limb reflexes in isolation suggest spinal cord pathology but if accompanied by brisk upper limb reflexes and flexor plantars, these may be features of a nervous patient. Always examine the patient's complaint thoroughly. For example, if the patient is complaining of difficulty with vision, measure and document visual acuity. If difficulty with walking is the problem, ask the patient to stand up and take some steps.

Examination of the unconscious patient

Unconscious patients need special care. Every effort must be made to obtain a history of events leading up to the coma. Occasionally, however, no helpful history is available. A low body temperature suggests that the coma is of at least 12 h duration, though this depends on the weather and where the patient is found. Before performing a detailed examination of any unconscious patient, first check that the airway is protected and that breathing, blood pressure and blood sugar do not need immediate attention. Look very closely at the whole body for signs of trauma and needle marks. At the same time someone else should examine the patient's possessions for drugs and relevant medical information. Such a search may reveal that the patient is a diabetic or has epilepsy.

Glasgow Coma Scale
Terms such as 'semiconscious', 'very confused' or 'drowsy'

give no meaningful information about a patient's state of consciousness as they can mean different things to different people. Therefore, reproducible scales based on objective criteria have been developed to record accurately the level of consciousness of a patient at any particular time. The most popular scale used today is the Glasgow Coma Scale. This scale is based on the measurement of three features that change with the level of consciousness: the stimulus needed to cause eye opening, the voice response and the best motor response (Table 40.3).

A fully conscious person will have a Glasgow Coma Scale score of 15, while the deepest level of coma will score 3. Although not absolutely defined, a score of 8 or less is generally considered to indicate coma. As this scale is reproducible, any changes in a patient's condition can be easily detected and communicated. The Glasgow Coma Scale must be used with some care and thought, however, as there are circumstances when responses can be wrongly interpreted. Such circumstances should be carefully noted and include the following.
● Swollen eyelids: if a patient's eyelids are swollen, he or she will be unable to open the eyes.
● Intubation or tracheostomy: if a patient is intubated or has a tracheostomy, he or she will not be able to speak.
● Difficulty differentiating between a confused and inappropriate voice response. The difference between confused and inappropriate is a matter of degree: patients may be confused about what hospital or city they are in or

05

what day it is, but thinking they are at home or in a different country or year is inappropriate.

• Foreign language-speaker or aphasia: a patient may be alert and orientated in his or her own foreign tongue but be incomprehensible to the observer. Likewise, a patient may be fully conscious yet aphasic and unable to speak.

• Best motor response in hemiplegia and paraplegia: for assessment of best motor response, the emphasis is on 'best'; a patient may be fully conscious and obeying commands yet hemiplegic or paraplegic.

Some Glasgow Coma Scales omit the abnormal flexion category of the best motor response as there can be difficulty differentiating between a flexion withdrawal response and an abnormal spastic flexion. The maximum score a patient can reach is then 14 not 15. When recording the Glasgow Coma Scale score, the maximum score should be split into its component parts, for example:

Eyes open to voice	3
No voice response	1
Best motor response localizes to pain	5
Total	9/15

The pain stimulus should be sufficient to stimulate the patient and not leave unsightly bruises. The most appropriate pain stimulus is pressure on the nail beds with a pen.

Paediatric modifications. The language development of children under 5 years of age makes the use of the adult Glasgow Coma Scale unreliable, although paediatric modifications are available, with rising levels of total score with increasing age.

Relevant neurological signs

Having assessed and recorded the level of consciousness, it is essential to examine quickly for relevant neurological signs. In practice, for the patient in coma this means:

• checking that life-protecting cranial nerve reflexes are present (e.g. gag and cough reflexes);

• examining pupil size, equality and responses;

• looking for any localizing signs (e.g. conjugate or dysconjugate eye deviation, blink reflexes, facial palsy, hemiparesis, etc.).

This assessment should allow an estimate of the depth of the coma and its source, which may be general (i.e. metabolic or drug-induced), supratentorial, infratentorial or in the brainstem.

Investigations

The pace of investigation will depend on the clinical circumstances. There are situations, e.g. deteriorating

undiagnosed coma, when the clinical team may have to take a history and examine at the same time as treating (i.e. securing an airway, raising blood pressure, giving anticonvulsants) and investigating (blood sugar) the patient. Whatever the situation, it is of no value to investigate to the detriment of a patient, e.g. subjecting a comatose patient to computed tomography (CT) before securing the airway and resuscitation. All too often, inadequately stabilized patients with a head injury or subarachnoid haemorrhage deteriorate during transit to the scanner or to a neurosurgical centre. Appropriate intubation, ventilation and transfusion may have saved them. The investigations commonly used in the management of neurosurgical patients are given in Table 40.4.

General investigations

A decreased level of consciousness can be caused or compounded by abnormal serum levels of sodium, glucose, calcium and urea, as well as by hypoxia and acid–base abnormalities. These must all be excluded. Haemoglobin and clotting screen should be routine. Because of the close association between the chest and intracranial problems chest radiography is essential, especially when an intracranial tumour is suspected as metastases are common.

Specific investigations
Lumbar puncture

Lumbar puncture is a useful investigation. It allows measurement of cerebrospinal fluid (CSF) pressure in the cranial–spinal axis and examination of the CSF is important in diagnosing subarachnoid haemorrhage, meningitis, encephalitis, Guillain–Barré syndrome, multiple sclerosis and other less common conditions. In communicating hydrocephalus, lumbar puncture allows therapeutic drainage of large volumes of CSF. Lumbar puncture is essential for myelography.

Lumbar puncture is a dangerous investigation if the patient has an intracranial mass and must not be performed if there is:

• a history suggesting an intracranial mass (e.g. progressive morning headache, epilepsy, a combination of frontal sinusitis and headache that may be due to an abscess);

• depressed level of consciousness;

• any focal neurological sign (e.g. hemiparesis, third cranial nerve palsy, nystagmus);

• papilloedema.

If any of these circumstances apply, obtain an urgent CT scan before performing a lumbar puncture even if meningitis is suspected. Lumbar puncture before scanning has no place in the diagnosis of coma.

Table 40.4 Investigations available for assessment of patients with neurosurgical disease.

General investigations

Haematology
Full blood count: baseline investigation
Clotting screen: promotes intracranial bleeding if abnormal

Biochemistry
Urea, sodium, calcium, glucose, blood gas analysis: if abnormal may cause or exacerbate coma

Imaging
Chest radiograph: cerebral secondaries are frequent from a primary lung tumour

Specific investigations

Lumbar puncture
Measures cerebrospinal fluid pressure
Useful in diagnosis of subarachnoid haemorrhage, meningitis, encephalitis, Guillain–Barré syndrome, multiple sclerosis

Imaging
Skull radiography: diagnosis of skull fracture
Computed tomography: diagnosis of intracranial lesions, e.g. tumour, haemorrhage, infarct
Magnetic resonance imaging: more sensitive than computed tomography, imaging of choice for many neurosurgical disorders
Myelography: invasive method of assessing spinal cord
Angiography, magnetic resonance angiography: used to demonstrate intracerebral circulation and therapeutic embolization
Positron emission tomography: dynamic scan of brain function

Neurophysiological studies
Electroencephalography: used in diagnosis of epilepsy
Somatosensory evoked potential: used to assess sensory pathways
Nerve conduction studies: used to assess peripheral nerves
Electromyography: used to assess peripheral nerves

Imaging

PLAIN RADIOGRAPHY

With the development of more sophisticated radiological investigations such as CT and magnetic resonance imaging (MRI) there is now little need for plain radiographs in the investigation of neurological disease. In spinal disease plain radiographs are mandatory:

- in the management of suspected spinal trauma;
- in the management of cord compression from malignant disease;
- to assess spinal instability using flexion and extension views.

COMPUTED TOMOGRAPHY

CT has revolutionized neurosurgical practice in the last 25 years. Multiple X-rays generated on a rotating gantry that encircles the part of the patient being investigated show tissues of differing density on a screen or X-ray plate so that the image resembles a picture of the structures (see Chapter 3). However, CT scans are only representations of X-ray density. It is due to computer graphics that the slices appear as if they are actual slices of the body. Skill and experience are therefore needed to interpret CT scans accurately, and appearances must be considered in conjunction with the clinical picture.

On a CT head scan, denser tissues (e.g. blood, bone) appear white, water and CSF black and the brain a mottled grey. Intravenous contrast (Omnipaque, Niopam) will be taken up by vascular tissue, tumours and areas of blood–brain barrier breakdown, and contrast enhancement is therefore useful in the diagnosis of these conditions.

There is no standard system for printing the pictures: some scanners print the left side of the patient on the right side of the film and vice versa. Make sure you check which side is which. It is usually written somewhere on the scan but may be in surprisingly small type. CT can be used for head and spinal scans. Reconstruction in coronal and sagittal planes, special views and three-dimensional effects can provide considerable information.

MAGNETIC RESONANCE IMAGING

MRI is a more modern scanning system than CT (Fig. 40.1). MRI works on the basis that if a magnetic field is applied across a patient, different molecules have different rates of realignment if the field is altered (see Chapter 3). The energy released in these realignments can be detected and presented by computer graphics so that the image resembles a photograph of the tissue being scanned. MRI scans tend to be more sensitive than CT scans. However, the increased scanning time, cost and the claustrophobic nature of the machine (the patient lies in a long tube) mean that MRI will not replace CT at present. However, MRI is now the investigation of choice in imaging most cerebral tumours and spinal disorders. With increased use of image-guided surgery and magnetic resonance angiography (MRA), MRI is becoming an essential preoperative investigation for elective intracranial surgery. It is essential when treating paediatric tumours, although general anaesthesia is usually required.

MYELOGRAPHY

Myelography involves placing contrast, nowadays water-soluble contrast (e.g. Niopam, metrizamide), in the subarachnoid space by lumbar puncture or, rarely, cervical puncture. As MRI has become widely available,

05

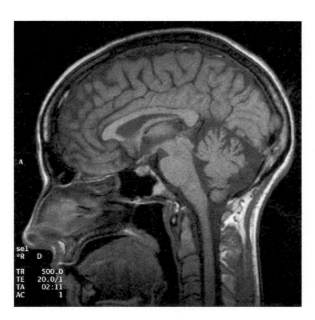

Figure 40.1 Magnetic resonance image (sagittal section) demonstrating normal anatomy of the brain and upper spinal cord.

myelography is following air encephalography and ventriculography into the history books.

ANGIOGRAPHY

Angiography is used to demonstrate the blood supply of the brain or spinal cord. This is usually achieved by direct injection of contrast into the blood vessels and the acquisition of multiplanar radiographs. Digital subtraction angiography is a technique whereby the soft-tissue images are subtracted from the angiogram, leaving a clear image of the blood vessels unobscured by the bones of the skull or vertebral column. Smaller amounts of contrast may be used with this technique. A newer technique is MRA, with which the direction and velocity of blood flow can be determined without need for any contrast injection. Duplex scanning is a useful screening investigation for extracranial vascular disease. Cerebral aneurysms, arteriovenous malformations (AVMs) and tumour circulations can currently only be accurately demonstrated by direct arterial puncture via a transfemoral catheter. Skilled neuroradiologists can extend these diagnostic pictures therapeutically by embolizing tumour vessels and AVMs, or occluding some aneurysms with balloons or platinum coils.

Neurophysiological investigations

Neurosurgeons rarely carry out neurophysiological investigations themselves; instead they are performed by a neurophysiologist. Electroencephalography (EEG), somatosensory evoked potential (SSEP), nerve conduction studies and electromyography (EMG) all help locate the exact site of a lesion.

Most investigations used routinely in neurosurgery have been discussed above. However, a number of very specialized investigations may occasionally be used, often in a research setting. These include cerebral blood flow monitoring, positron emission tomography (PET), single-photon emission computed tomography (SPECT) and cerebral metabolic studies.

Principles of management of neurosurgical patients

Having taken a history, examined the patient and performed the appropriate investigations, a plan of management can then be decided. As well as treating the condition, consider the effects the condition may have on the general well-being of the patient. Specifically for neurosurgery, this requires familiarity with the care of unconscious and paraplegic patients, whatever the underlying cause.

Care of the unconscious patient

In everyday life we protect ourselves without being aware of it: a cough clears our chest, a yawn opens up collapsed alveoli, a shuffle on our seats prevents a pressure sore, moving prevents contractures, and blinking protects our corneas from foreign bodies. We also take care of ourselves by deliberate actions, which include urination, defecation, feeding and washing. The unconscious patient is unable to do any of these things. The carers of an unconscious patient therefore need to anticipate and perform these activities on a regular basis. This requires much time and effort. Slapdash care, either through ignorance or overwork, can lead to secondary complications such as chest infections, pressure sores and corneal ulceration, all of which may ruin otherwise effective treatment (Fig. 40.2).

Chest care

The airway must be protected at all times. Oral or nasal airway intubation or tracheostomy may be necessary depending on the depth of coma. The advantage of either intubation or tracheostomy is that it allows easy access to the bronchi with suction catheters to help clear secretions. Physiotherapists are a fundamental requirement for a neurosurgical unit, and chest physiotherapy takes priority over most things in the care of the comatose patient.

Pressure areas

Lying on one area of skin for more than 2 h causes local

05

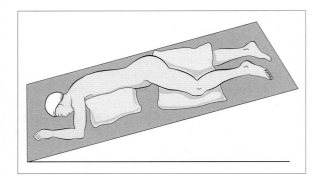

Figure 40.2 Position for nursing the unconscious patient. Note the feet-up, head-down position.

ischaemia and breakdown of the skin. This can deteriorate to form a deep intractable ulcer, sometimes called a decubitus ulcer. The most common site is the buttock, but pressure sores are also common on the heels, elbow and occiput. Pressure sores reflect a failure of care and should never occur. They are prevented by regular turning and the use of sheepskins and water bags.

Hygiene and sphincters
Scrupulous attention to hygiene, including mouth care, is essential. Urinary catheters should be used only if absolutely essential, although when the alternative is permanent wetness a catheter may be the only option. Regular laxatives or enemas are necessary to prevent constipation.

Eyes
An exposed cornea will rapidly ulcerate and this may lead to blindness. The eyes of an unconscious patient must always be closed but also inspected regularly to exclude ulceration; any redness should be treated aggressively. Gelatin pads are the most effective compromise.

Feeding
Most comatose patients, especially those with head injuries, have high calorific needs and if not fed adequately become rapidly malnourished. Feeding needs to be established as soon as possible, if necessary intravenously. When the gut is working, nasogastric feeds should be introduced carefully. Reflux can readily occur and lead to aspiration into a poorly protected airway. The use of metoclopramide to improve gastric emptying and, if necessary, a percutaneous jejunostomy can reduce this risk. Diarrhoea is common with feeding but usually resolves if the osmolarity of the feed is altered. Regular electrolyte checks are necessary and abnormalities should be corrected as they may prolong or worsen coma.

Movement
Early, regular, passive movement of the limbs is necessary to prevent contractures. Eventually, as the coma lightens, the patient will begin to move spontaneously and the movements may be powerful enough to result in falls from the bed or chair. At this stage it is best to place the patient on the floor on a couple of mattresses or in a padded cot so that he or she can move around without injury.

General care
Keep alert to other conditions that can occur when a patient is unconscious and unable to complain. Myocardial infarction, pulmonary embolus, meningitis and pneumonia may all present at first as an unexplained fever, tachycardia and tachypnoea in a comatose patient. Hyponatraemia may gradually develop and worsen the coma, and the use of steroids may predispose to gastric haemorrhage or silent perforation. Permanent vigilance is necessary, but when discussing the patient's condition at the bedside remember that the patient in coma may be able to hear every word that is said and attendants must behave accordingly.

Relatives
Handling the relatives of comatose patients is usually difficult. As well as coming to terms with the illness and its implications, most relatives expect their loved one to wake up suddenly and say 'Where am I?' and be back to normal within minutes. When this does not happen they become frustrated and may take it out on the attendants – 5 min late with a turn becomes a major crisis. Frequent explanation is important and unhurried time set aside to answer questions is time well spent.

You may find it easiest to liken waking from a coma to the feelings we all have on waking in the morning, except that everything is in slow motion, lasting days or weeks rather than minutes. Many relatives, especially of children, like to become involved in the care by feeding, washing and turning. This is to be encouraged as it helps both relatives and hard-pressed nursing staff. Also encourage the relatives to talk to the patient. Nobody knows for certain whether a comatose patient is aware of voices – most who recover cannot remember – but it will not cause any harm.

Brain death
Brain death exists when there is no demonstrable brain-stem function in the presence of a diagnosis compatible with irreversible structural brain damage. On establishing brain death the patient may be considered for organ donation. If organ donation is not to be performed, then the patient is disconnected from the ventilator (Table 40.5).

05

Table 40.5 Establishing brain death.

Tests for the absence of brainstem function
Do the pupils react to light?
Are there corneal reflexes?
Is there eye movement on caloric testing? (Ensure that the ears are clear of wax)
Are there motor responses in the cranial nerve distribution in response to stimulation of face, limbs or trunk?
Is there a gag reflex?
Is there a cough reflex?
Is the patient apnoeic (in the presence of normocapnia)?

The following guidelines are important
There should be no doubt that severe irremediable structural brain damage has occurred. Reversible causes, including poisoning, prolonged response to drugs, hypothermia (< 35°C), metabolic and chronic endocrinological disorders, must have been excluded
Two doctors are needed to certify brain death. The first should be the consultant in charge of the patient or his or her deputy (who must have been registered for 5 years or more and be adequately experienced). The second doctor must be suitably experienced and clinically independent of the first. Neither doctor must be a member of the transplant team
The tests should be recorded on a suitable form
The diagnostic tests should be recorded on at least two occasions, separated by several hours. The exact time interval will depend on the patient's condition
The time of the patient's death is the time of completion of the second set of brain death tests. It is important that this is the time of death which is both recorded in the notes and written on the death certificate
If organ transplantation is not to be carried out, on completion of the second set of tests the patient may be left disconnected from the ventilator
Caring for the relatives at this time requires tact and understanding. If organ transplantation is not to take place, they may wish to remain in the room until the heart stops beating

Care of the paraplegic and quadriplegic patient

Paraplegic and quadriplegic patients retain consciousness and higher mental functions. However, they have lost a large portion of their function and with it many everyday protective mechanisms. As with an unconscious patient, considerable time and effort coupled with psychological support are needed to care for these patients.

Chest
The higher the level of spinal damage, the greater the extent of chest involvement; midthoracic spinal lesions will result in paralysis of the intercostal muscles, cervical lesions may affect the diaphragm (remember 'C3, 4 and 5, keep the diaphragm alive') and higher lesions may involve the respiratory centres. Ventilation will be necessary if the respiratory centres or diaphragm are damaged. Good respiratory function can be maintained with a functioning diaphragm and paralysed intercostal muscles, but respiratory reserve will be less than normal and chest infections must be treated aggressively.

Homeostasis
The higher the spinal injury, the greater the dilatation of the blood vessels resulting from loss of sympathetic tone. Blood pressure falls and heat is lost, and both must be reversed in the acute phase. Never leave spinal patients in casualty or the X-ray department uncovered. Space blankets and heating pads must be used.

Pressure areas
The same attention to pressure areas must be given as for the unconscious patient (see earlier). In particular, watch the shoulder blades and occiput in those on cervical traction.

Hygiene and sphincters
Most spinal patients will have disturbed bladder and bowel function. Before the availability of good spinal injury care, the most common cause of death in paraplegics was pyelonephritis. Early catheterization to prevent overflow incontinence is required, but as soon as possible the patient should be taught to express urine by suprapubic pressure or to self-catheterize intermittently. Urological evaluation to measure residual urine and other urodynamic parameters is advisable. Constipation must be prevented by laxative use and enemas.

Feeding
Like comatose patients, paraplegic patients should be fed as soon as possible to prevent malnutrition and its complications. Paralytic ileus is common in the first few days after a spinal cord injury and should be treated conservatively with a 'drip-and-suck' regimen, and intravenous feeding if necessary.

Movement
Early mobilization is indicated if the spine is stable, although postural hypotension may delay this. The development of functioning muscle groups to compensate for non-functioning ones is a goal. Rapid learning of the use of any aids, e.g. a wheelchair or a computer for quadriplegics, is another goal and should not be delayed by unrealistic hopes for recovery, either on the part of the doctor or the patient.

Spasticity may be a problem and should be treated with an antispastic drug such as baclofen. Spinal patients are at considerable risk of developing deep vein thrombosis and pulmonary embolus. Prophylactic measures should therefore be taken for all patients. Some specialists of spinal injuries advocate full anticoagulation, while others use compression stockings (TED stockings) accompanied by low-dose subcutaneous heparin. Care of the paraplegic patient should be standard practice in all units where neurosurgery is practised, but spinal injury units are so well developed in this area that most patients should be transferred to one as soon as possible.

Common neurosurgical disorders

Head injury (see Chapter 18)

Central nervous system tumours

Central nervous system (CNS) tumours arise from all tissues associated with the brain and spinal cord: bone, neurones, glia, meninges, pituitary and germ cells. In addition, metastatic disease commonly manifests itself in the CNS (Fig. 40.3). Tumours usually present with epilepsy, raised intracranial pressure (ICP) or a neurological deficit.
- Late-onset epilepsy is commonly caused by the presence of a tumour.
- Increased ICP: the presence of a tumour within the skull will cause ICP to rise. Early morning headache made worse by coughing and straining is a typical symptom.

Papilloedema may be evident and may cause blindness. If untreated, the level of consciousness will fall and lead to coma and death.
- A neurological deficit and its rate of progression will depend on the type and position of the tumour.
A benign acoustic neuroma may cause deafness for many years before it begins to compress the brainstem, leading to ataxia and pressure effects from hydrocephalus. A malignant glioma in the motor strip may progress from mild contralateral weakness to hemiplegia within weeks. Pituitary tumours may have endocrine effects and, if growing upwards out of the pituitary fossa, may compress the optic nerves and lead to visual failure (classically, bitemporal hemianopia).

Classification

While the terms 'primary', 'secondary', 'benign' and 'malignant' are relevant in the CNS, the tissue of origin and its anatomical position are more important. For example, a colloid cyst of the third ventricle is completely benign histologically but may present with sudden death because its position at the foramen of Munro can cause acute hydrocephalus.

Tumours found in the CNS include the following (Fig. 40.3).
- Gliomas: astrocytomas, oligodendrogliomas, ependymomas.
- Meningiomas.
- Lymphomas (previously known as microgliomas).
- Neuromas.

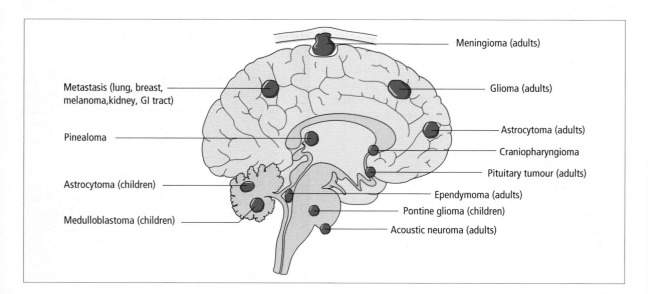

Figure 40.3 Distribution of common primary and secondary brain tumours.

- Pituitary tumours.
- Primitive tumours: primitive neuroectodermal tumours (PNETs), medulloblastomas.
- Pineal tumours: pineocytomas, pineoblastomas.
- Choroid plexus tumours.
- Malformations: hamartomas, colloid cyst of the third ventricle, craniopharyngiomas, chordomas.
- Metastatic tumours.

Specific CNS tumours

Glioma

Gliomas are the most common primary brain tumours arising from the supporting tissues of the CNS. They vary in their degree of malignancy, but are locally invasive and rarely metastasize outside the CNS. Gliomas are graded according to their histological appearance. For example, an astrocytic tumour may be graded as an astrocytoma (slow-growing with a good prognosis), an anaplastic astrocytoma (more rapidly growing) or a glioblastoma (aggressive, with a survival usually less than 1 year after diagnosis, whatever treatment is given). Treatment includes surgery, radiotherapy and chemotherapy, either alone or in combination. As yet, nothing has been shown to be very effective. Most gliomas occur in the cerebral hemisphere in adults (Fig. 40.4). Grade 1 cystic astrocytomas occur in children and carry a good prognosis. Cerebral lymphoma used to be included with the gliomas and was called microglioma. It tends to be more radiosensitive but its prognosis is still very poor, especially if associated with human immunodeficiency virus (HIV) infection.

Meningioma

Meningiomas are usually benign but there are malignant variants (Fig. 40.5). They arise from the dura and can occur anywhere within the skull or spinal canal but are most common in the cerebral hemispheres. If allowed by their anatomical position, removal is usually curative; however, some meningiomas may be incurable by virtue of their anatomical location (e.g. those arising from the clivus).

Neuroma

A neuroma is a benign tumour arising from nerves. The most common are the eighth-nerve acoustic neuroma and the spinal neurofibroma. Removal is usually curative.

Pituitary tumours (see also Chapter 34)

A pituitary tumour can present with:
- pituitary overactivity or underactivity;
- visual failure due to chiasmatic compression (characteristically a bitemporal hemianopia);
- pituitary apoplexy.

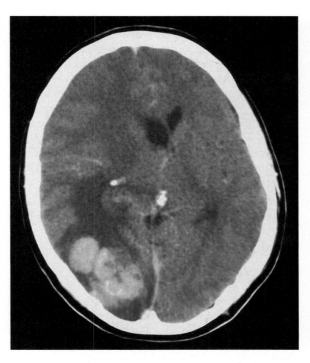

Figure 40.4 Computed tomographic scan showing glioblastoma in the left cerebral cortex. Note the deviation of the pineal, compression of the ventricles and presence of oedema.

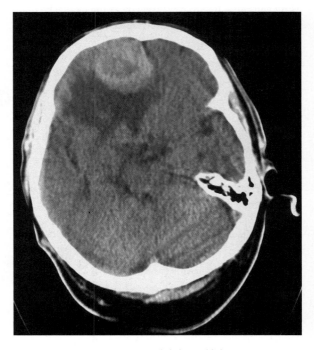

Figure 40.5 Meningioma over left frontal lobe.

05

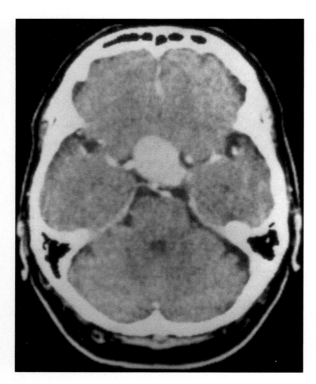

Figure 40.6 Computed tomographic scan showing a large pituitary adenoma.

Surgery is now less commonly performed for pituitary tumours than in the past because prolactin-secreting tumours can be controlled with bromocriptine. The trans-sphenoidal route is the fashionable approach to the gland but if the optic nerves are compressed, the trans-cranial route is still used (Fig. 40.6).

Metastatic tumour

Metastatic tumour (e.g. from a bronchial primary) is the most common tumour in the CNS but is uncommon in neurosurgical practice. Surgery is used where a diagnosis is in doubt or where there is a solitary secondary from a known, relatively slow-growing, treated primary, e.g. the kidney. For certain types of chemosensitive tumour, such as trophoblastic tumours or testicular teratoma, a reduction of tumour bulk is essential for a cure; it is then worth being aggressive and removing all secondaries, even if multiple.

Other tumours

Tumours other than those discussed above form only a small percentage of CNS tumours. In childhood, CNS tumours are the second most common malignancy after leukaemia and are most common in the posterior fossa.

The commonest childhood CNS tumours are cystic astrocytoma, which has a good prognosis, and medulloblastoma, which has a poor one. Overall, however, CNS tumours in children carry a better prognosis than in adults, with 50% surviving 10 years.

Management

If a tumour is suspected, diagnostic tests need to be carried out urgently. Direct imaging is the investigation of choice. CT usually confirms the diagnosis, followed by MRI to refine the imaging and help stage the disease.

If the tumour is thought to be benign, surgical excision is the usual treatment. However, in certain situations, e.g. if the patient is elderly and has no symptoms other than fits that are easily controlled by drugs, it may be safer to observe the tumour with serial CT scans rather than attempt excision. If the tumour has the appearance of malignancy, it is essential to establish the diagnosis. Rarely, such appearances may be mimicked by an abscess. If the tumour is easily accessible and not in a vital area (such as the speech area or the motor strip), a craniotomy may be performed to debulk the lesion. Computer-guided surgery, fusing images from CT and MRI, is becoming common and is likely to be standard practice in the next decade. If the tumour is deep or in a dangerous position, a needle biopsy under stereotaxic guidance is more appropriate. Further treatment of a malignant tumour usually involves neuro-oncologists and radiotherapists. The prognosis of childhood paediatric tumours is improved by complete resection of the tumour followed by adjuvant treatment.

Intracranial haemorrhage

Haemorrhage can occur into any of the spaces (extra-dural, subdural or subarachnoid) within the skull, as well as into the brain itself.

Extradural haemorrhage

An extradural haemorrhage is almost invariably caused by trauma and is discussed fully in Chapter 18.

Subdural haemorrhage

A subdural haemorrhage may develop following a severe head injury, or chronically following a minor head injury that is often unnoticed. The discovery of a chronic subdural haemorrhage in infancy should raise suspicion of non-accidental injury but is not diagnostic of the cause. Further investigation is essential. This condition is also discussed in Chapter 18.

05

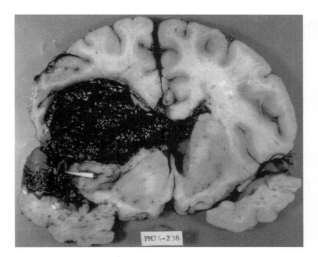

Figure 40.7 Intracerebral haemorrhage.

Intracerebral haemorrhage

Intracerebral haemorrhages occur spontaneously in elderly hypertensive patients and also in association with clotting defects or a pre-existing tumour. In young patients, an AVM or aneurysm may be the underlying cause. An intracerebral haemorrhage presents with sudden severe headache, which is followed by a rapidly progressive coma or focal neurological signs. Diagnosis is made by CT, which is followed by angiography if an AVM or an aneurysm is suspected and surgery is contemplated.

If a clot is seen it is tempting to remove it, although surgery is often not worthwhile except when:
- the clot is in the posterior fossa;
- its removal can alter the outcome considerably;
- a previously alert patient becomes progressively drowsier over a few hours due to the secondary effect of the size of the clot.

Comatose patients with a clot do badly and their outlook is not improved by its removal. Fully alert but hemiplegic patients with a clot usually improve, although their recovery is rarely accelerated by surgery (Fig. 40.7).

Subarachnoid haemorrhage

Acute haemorrhage into the subarachnoid space is caused by a ruptured aneurysm (usually a congenital berry aneurysm of the circle of Willis) in 70% of cases (Fig. 40.8) and an AVM in 10% of cases. No cause is ever found for 20% of patients. It is then presumed that a microaneurysm or AVM is the cause and destroys itself in the bleed.

Presentation

Subarachnoid haemorrhage (SAH) presents as sudden death (40% of cases) or as a severe sudden headache that

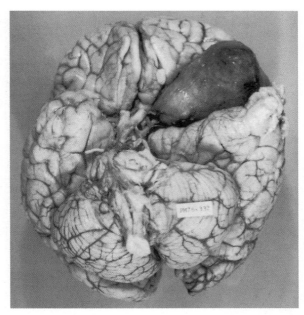

Figure 40.8 Cerebral aneurysm.

may be associated with nausea, vomiting, coma or the development of focal neurology. Clinical examination will reveal an ill patient with neck stiffness and, possibly, neurological signs. A diagnosis of SAH (blood in the subarachnoid space) is made by CT or lumbar puncture, which will reveal uniformly blood-stained CSF. The breakdown products of haemoglobin impart a yellow tinge to the supernatant (xanthochromia). SAH carries a poor prognosis: 30% of survivors of the initial event die within 6 weeks from the effects of the bleed, a further bleed or from delayed cerebral ischaemia in response to the initial bleed.

Delayed cerebral ischaemia

This is related to the severity of the initial SAH. It develops about 5 days later and lasts for 7–10 days. It may be asymptomatic, mild or very severe, leading to infarction and death. Angiography shows diffuse spasm of the cerebral arteries and cerebral blood flow falls. No treatment is known to reverse delayed cerebral ischaemia but its severity can be reduced by prophylactic treatment with the calcium channel blocker nimodipine. When cerebral ischaemia is established it is managed by nursing care, fluid loading to avoid a rise in blood viscosity and, if the source of bleeding has been secured, artificial hypertension using pressor agents to increase cerebral blood flow.

Rebleeding

Rebleeding is prevented by surgery to seal off the source of an SAH. Angiography will demonstrate the source and, if

an aneurysm is seen, it is exposed by craniotomy and isolated from the circulation using a small metal clip. The timing of surgery is controversial. Many advocate early treatment, within the first 5 days of haemorrhage, to prevent rebleeding and then treat cerebral ischaemia if it arises. Others advocate treatment after 2 weeks (the main risk period for rebleeding and ischaemia), the risks of treatment being lower at this stage. Overall management mortality is the same whichever approach is used, although the individual likely to rebleed is better having an early procedure, while the patient who will develop ischaemia should have a delayed one. Unfortunately, there is no way of predicting with any accuracy which patients will rebleed and which will develop ischaemia. Endovascular radiological embolization of berry aneurysms, using small coils to embolize the aneurysm, is now being performed with good results and is likely to become the treatment of choice in the next decade.

If an AVM is found, the risks of a fatal rebleed are less and a more leisurely approach can be taken. If the lesion is small and near the surface it can be surgically excised, but if it is deep or in a dangerous position it is best treated by non-operative measures. Intravascular embolization or stereotactically guided radiotherapy are alternative treatment methods.

Intracranial infection

Infection can involve the bones of the skull (osteomyelitis), the extradural or subdural spaces (empyema), the meninges (meningitis) or the brain itself, where an area of cerebritis can progress to abscess formation (Fig. 40.9). The source of an infection is either systemic (commonly associated with congenital heart disease, diabetes or septicaemia) or local (from middle-ear disease or sinusitis). Unless adequately treated, penetrating head trauma is a potent source of sepsis. A number of rare infections,

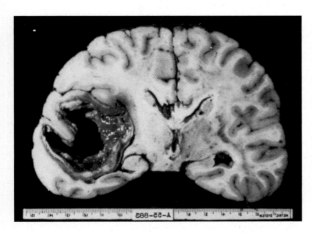

Figure 40.9 Postmortem specimen of pyogenic brain abscess.

especially toxoplasmosis, are now seen in immunocompromise associated with HIV infection, chemotherapy and transplantation.

Diagnosis of an intracranial infection is often difficult until it is well advanced. A history of a source of infection such as sinusitis followed by headaches often precedes rapid deterioration accompanied by epilepsy, meningism and coma. CT or MRI will reveal an empyema, area of cerebritis or abscess and is the investigation of choice.

Treatment follows the usual lines of drainage of pus and antibiotics. Areas of cerebritis or small early abscesses may be cured by antibiotics alone, but close follow-up is needed with this regimen. If tuberculosis is suspected with reasonable certainty, surgery is best avoided; however, if the lesions do not respond to treatment, biopsy is essential. Surgical drainage has the advantage of allowing an organism to be identified. It is important to treat the source of the infection at the same time as treating the intracranial problem. Appropriate antibiotics must be given in high doses for long periods, at least 3 months.

Hydrocephalus

Hydrocephalus is the accumulation of an excessive volume of CSF within the ventricular system and subarachnoid spaces. CSF is produced mainly by the choroid plexus of the lateral and fourth ventricles, although a small amount is produced by the whole neuraxis. Most is produced in the lateral ventricles at a rate of 0.3 mL/min. CSF then flows via the foramen of Munro to the third ventricle and thence down the aqueduct to the fourth ventricle and out into the subarachnoid space. In this space it is absorbed by the arachnoid granulations over the surface of the hemispheres. The average adult CSF volume is 150 mL. CSF is therefore renewed three times every 24 h.

Pathology

Hydrocephalus may result from overproduction of CSF, obstruction to its circulation or failure of its absorption. Whatever the cause, if CSF can leave the fourth ventricle and communicate with the subarachnoid space, it is called communicating hydrocephalus. When CSF is trapped within the ventricles and cannot reach this space, it is called a non-communicating hydrocephalus.

CSF overproduction
Hydrocephalus due to CSF overproduction is the least common cause of hydrocephalus and is caused by a CSF-secreting tumour, a choroid plexus papilloma. These are usually benign tumours of childhood although malignant carcinomas can occur, and hydrocephalus is the presenting symptom. CSF production may be four times normal and because the tumours tend to have minor

haemorrhages, there is often an element of absorption failure as well. Fourth ventricular choroid plexus papillomas may block the fourth ventricle and also cause an obstructive hydrocephalus.

Obstruction to CSF flow

Any obstruction to the flow of CSF within the ventricular system will cause an obstructive hydrocephalus. This results in non-communicating hydrocephalus and usually occurs at the narrowest points of the CSF circulation.
- In the lateral ventricles, when an intraventricular haemorrhage fills the ventricles.
- At the foramen of Munro, which can be obstructed by intraventricular tumours, most commonly colloid cyst, hypothalamic glioma, craniopharyngioma and, rarely, pituitary adenoma.
- In the aqueduct, which can be obstructed by pineal region tumour, brainstem glioma, congenital aqueduct stenosis or neonatal intraventricular haemorrhage (commonly blocks the aqueduct).
- In the fourth ventricle, which can be obstructed by congenital fourth ventricular (Dandy–Walker) cyst, fourth ventricular tumour (e.g. glioma, medulloblastoma, ependymoma) or any cause of cerebellar swelling (e.g. infarction, haemorrhage, tumour).

Failure of CSF absorption

Any process that raises the protein content of the CSF in the subarachnoid space and blocks the arachnoid granulations will cause a communicating absorptive hydrocephalus. These are the most common causes of hydrocephalus and include head injury, SAH and meningitis. Likewise, any process that obliterates the subarachnoid space (e.g. tuberculous meningitis, sarcoidosis and carcinomatous meningitis) will prevent CSF absorption.

Clinical manifestations

The symptoms and signs of hydrocephalus depend mainly on the speed of onset and age of the patient. Hydrocephalus should be confirmed or excluded in any patient with a head injury, haemorrhage or meningitis who reaches an unexpected plateau of recovery or deteriorates.

Infancy

Before suture fusion at 18 months, a child's head is elastic. The main feature of hydrocephalus is therefore rapid head growth, as measured by the occipitofrontal circumference. This growth rate will exceed the rate of length and weight gain on a growth chart. If the rate of ventricular enlargement exceeds the ability of the head to expand, the anterior fontanelle will become tense and the sutures splayed. The scalp veins will distend and the baby will lose

the ability to look upwards ('setting-sun' sign). These signs indicate a sick baby who needs urgent intervention.

Childhood/adult

Within a closed skull, hydrocephalus causes the signs of raised ICP (headache and a falling level of consciousness). With very rapidly developing hydrocephalus, usually due to a colloid cyst completely occluding the foramen of Munro, the rise in ICP may be so fast that coma and death rapidly ensue.

Old age

A syndrome that can affect the elderly is normal-pressure hydrocephalus, which is probably a variant of absorptive failure. The characteristic symptoms and signs are those of Adam's triad: dementia, ataxia and incontinence. There may be a history of head injury, meningitis or cerebral haemorrhage. It is difficult to differentiate normal-pressure hydrocephalus from senile dementia and often they may coexist.

Investigations

- Ultrasound: in the infant with an open fontanelle, an ultrasound probe can be used to measure ventricular size and plot the rate of growth.
- CT is the most useful screening investigation of hydrocephalus as it shows ventricular size and is easily available to assess changes over time (Fig. 40.10).
- MRI is now the investigation of choice for showing the cause of hydrocephalus and to aid decisions about the best form of treatment.
- Lumbar puncture must *not* be performed if there is a definite or suspected non-communicating hydrocephalus. However, if it is clearly established that the hydrocephalus communicates with the subarachnoid space, lumbar puncture may be used to measure pressure and to test the effect of draining a volume of CSF.

Treatment

At first, treatment must be aimed at removing the cause if possible, e.g. removing an underlying tumour. If this is not possible, treatment is directed at reducing the production of CSF, bypassing an obstruction, intermittently removing excess CSF or permanently diverting the CSF to a place where it can be absorbed.

Reduce production of CSF

The carbonic anhydrase inhibitor acetazolamide and some diuretics can reduce CSF production. This tends to be a temporary effect and electrolyte balance must be carefully maintained. The choroid plexus can be destroyed by

either open operation or using an endoscope. This is popular with some neurosurgeons but is not widely performed.

Bypass an obstruction
In certain types of obstructive hydrocephalus, e.g. aqueduct stenosis or fourth ventricular tumour, a new route for CSF to exit the ventricles may be made with an endoscope through the floor of the third ventricle (third ventriculostomy).

Remove excess CSF
Ventricular tapping (in infants), ventricular drainage and lumbar puncture and drainage can all be used as temporary measures to remove excess CSF where appropriate. These methods are particularly useful after a haemorrhage or meningitis when high CSF protein makes shunting liable to failure.

Permanently divert CSF (shunt)
Permanently diverted CSF is drained via a silicone tube passing through a one-way pressure-regulated valve into the right atrium, pleura or, most commonly, peritoneum, where it is absorbed back into the circulation. This is the most effective and permanent treatment of hydrocephalus. Once inserted, modern shunts are very reliable but are prone to complications arising from overdrainage, blockage or infections.

- Overdrainage in infants leads to overriding of the skull sutures and scaphycephaly and in adults causes subdural hygromas. Some of the latest shunts allow pressure settings to be altered by an external magnet to reduce the risk of these complications.
- Blockage usually occurs when the CSF is too thick because it contains too much protein. Hydrocephalus should be controlled by other means until the CSF protein content is reduced to prevent this complication. A late blockage arises when debris from the ventricles accumulates within the shunt, or when the choroid plexus or omentum occludes the shunt from the outside.
- Infected shunts can cause meningitis and chronic peritonitis and, if inserted into the right atrium, septicaemia, endocarditis, pulmonary hypertension and glomerulonephritis. Infected shunts need to be removed and the CSF sterilized by antibiotics. The shunt can then be replaced.

Spinal surgery

Neurosurgeons and orthopaedic surgeons who operate on the spine must have a thorough understanding of both the neurology and biomechanics of the spine and be conversant with spinal stabilization techniques. The spinal surgeon must also be able to approach the spine from

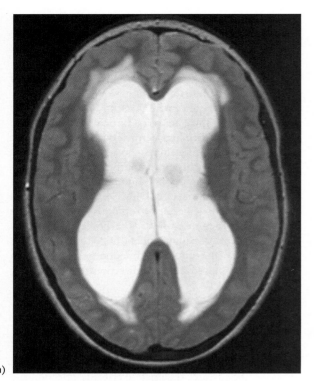

(a)

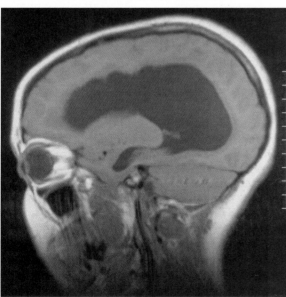

(b)

Figure 40.10 (a) Transverse and (b) sagittal MRI scans showing hydrocephalus in a young girl with a congenital cyst in the fourth ventricle (Dandy–Walker cyst).

many directions, should be comfortable operating through the mouth, neck, chest and abdomen if necessary, and be able to use an operating microscope.

Special considerations

Radiography, myelography, CT, MRI and electrophysiology are used to answer the following fundamental questions.
● What is the diagnosis?
● What level of the spine is involved?
● Is the spine stable?
● Will treatment affect spine stability?
● What approach should be used?

Spine stability is maintained by the strength of the vertebral body, the lateral masses and the laminae. Destruction of one element does not usually affect stability, whereas loss of two is likely to cause instability, which is guaranteed if all three elements are destroyed. A typical example of this is malignant cord compression. If this is posterior and erodes the lamina, a laminectomy to decompress the spine will not affect stability. However, if the tumour is anterior and has eroded the vertebral body and lateral masses, a laminectomy will remove the only element giving stability and the spine will become unstable with disastrous consequences. In these circumstances the operative approach has to be from the front, via the neck, chest or abdomen. The vertebral body is removed and replaced by a bone graft, metal or cement.

Spine stabilization

The spine can be stabilized either externally or internally.

External stabilization

External stabilization is most effective for the neck, either by traction or a halo device.
● Traction is applied by callipers fixed to the skull. Weights are applied until the cervical vertebrae are correctly aligned and the alignment is then held by the weight of the traction. This is the first treatment used for neck fractures, and may be used for 6–8 weeks until fusion has occurred.
● A halo is a metal ring fixed to the skull from which four metal rods pass to a strong plastic or plaster jacket worn over the chest and abdomen. It holds the neck rigid until fusion occurs, which usually takes 3 months.

Internal stabilization

Internal stabilization is performed at operation and a wide variety of techniques are used, sometimes in combination or with external fixation. There are three broad categories: bone grafting, cement and prosthetics.

● *Bone grafting*: bone grafts can be employed to stabilize the spine using either the patient's bone, usually from the iliac crest, or a commercial preparation of dried animal bone. Bone grafts are rarely sufficient by themselves for immediate stabilization, but when incorporated are the most effective method for providing long-term stability.
● *Cement*: biological cement is useful for replacing vertebral bodies but there are risks, particularly of infection. It is most useful when long-term survival is unlikely, e.g. malignant cord compression.
● *Prosthetics*: replacing or supporting bone with prosthetic material is a common technique and can be accompanied by bone grafting or cement. Techniques vary from a simple wiring together of two spinous processes to the replacement of a number of vertebral bodies with a tailor-made metal or porcelain prosthetic body.

Most parts of the spine from the odontoid to the sacrum can now be stabilized from one direction or another.

Spinal disorders

Care of the paraplegic patient is discussed on pp. 626–7. Other common spinal conditions are spinal injury, spinal tumours and malignant cord compression, disc prolapse, spondylosis, rheumatoid arthritis, infection and haemorrhage.

Spinal injury (see Chapter 17)

Malignant cord compression
Pathology
Metastatic compression of the spinal cord is common in advanced cancer, particularly with tumours of the bronchus, breast, prostate and kidney and myeloproliferative disorders. Spread is usually haematogenous, but can result from direct extension from a bronchial carcinoma. Malignant cord compression is usually extradural, although intradural compression does occur, and destruction of surrounding bone is common. The thoracic spine is the most common site, but any level of the spine can be involved. Although metastatic spread often involves multiple levels of the spine, usually only one is symptomatic at any one time.

Clinical features
Malignant cord compression presents with pain in the affected dermatome, followed by progressive spastic paraparesis below the level of the lesion. The rate of deterioration depends on the rate of compression, but sudden deterioration is commonly precipitated by bony collapse. Cord compression must be considered in any patient with known or suspected cancer who develops pain, especially girdle pain, followed by leg stiffness or difficulty walking.

If compression develops to the point of paraplegia, the patient will never walk again; however, if dealt with when there is only pain or slight weakness, full recovery is possible. It is not uncommon for patients in bed to deteriorate gradually without their doctors realizing it, the diagnosis only being considered when urinary retention develops. This should not happen and the patient's complaints must be taken seriously. Investigation of malignant compression is by plain radiography to reveal any bony erosion or collapse, followed by myelography, preferably with CT or MRI. These investigations confirm cord compression, establish single- or multiple-level involvement and allow for planning of appropriate treatment.

Management

Treatment should start as soon as the diagnosis of malignant compression is suspected. Dexamethasone is commenced to slow further deterioration and the patient should be transferred rapidly to neurosurgical care for investigation. Further treatment will include either surgery or radiotherapy or both. If there is no established diagnosis, histology must be obtained by open operation or needle biopsy. If the diagnosis is known, the first line of treatment is radiotherapy as this is as effective as an operation without the risks of surgery.

Surgery is reserved for those patients in whom the diagnosis is not established and needle biopsy is impractical or fails, and for those who do not respond to radiotherapy. The aim of surgery is to decompress the spine without making it unstable. If the compression is purely posterior and there is no destruction of the vertebral bodies, laminectomy is appropriate. If the vertebral bodies are involved, the anterior approach is required; this is more demanding for both patient and surgeon. The patient's expected survival from cancer must be considered before embarking on major surgery.

Disc prolapse (see also Chapter 21)
Pathology

The intervertebral discs are the shock absorbers between the vertebral bodies. They consist of a tough outer ring, the annulus fibrosis, which surrounds a gelatinous centre, the nucleus pulposus. With ageing the disc dehydrates and the collagen weakens. This can lead to rupture of the annulus fibrosis and extrusion of the nucleus pulposus into the spinal canal, where it sets up an inflammatory response and hardens. The hardened extrusion causes pain by both inflammation and stretching of the spinal nerves. Large prolapses may stretch the spinal nerves causing numbness and weakness in their distribution, and if large enough may even cause spinal cord or cauda equina compression.

Disc prolapses usually occur spontaneously, either acutely or gradually, but may also be precipitated by trauma and complicate spinal cord injury. The most common sites of disc prolapse are the lower lumbar region, especially L4/5 and L5/S1, and the lower cervical region, especially C5/6 and C6/7, probably because these are the most mobile areas of the spine. Less mobile segments are less often involved; the relatively immobile thoracic spine is rarely affected. However, because of the narrowness of the thoracic spinal canal, disc prolapse in this region may have serious consequences.

Clinical features

Disc prolapse usually presents with pain in the affected dermatome and area of the spine; lumbosacral prolapses present with low back pain associated with pain in the leg (sciatica), while cervical prolapses cause neck pain and pain in the affected arm (brachialgia). There may be signs of root tension, such as limited straight-leg raising, and neurological signs, including weakness in the affected myotome and reflex changes (e.g. footdrop and an absent ankle jerk in an L4/5 prolapse). Sensory changes may occur but are often inconsistent. A large central lumbar disc prolapse may cause bilateral sciatica, saddle anaesthesia and urinary retention (cauda equina syndrome). This is an emergency and warrants immediate referral to a neurosurgical unit as delay may lead to persisting urinary problems. A central cervical prolapse may cause quadriparesis or quadriplegia and is also a major emergency.

Management

At first a disc prolapse is treated with rest, adequate analgesia and sedation. A patient with lumbar prolapse requires strict bedrest, rising only to go to the toilet, whereas a cervical collar is necessary for cervical prolapse (a firm collar is more useful than a soft one). On these regimens 95% of prolapses settle spontaneously within 2 weeks.

Surgical intervention is required only if:
- the prolapse does not settle acutely;
- symptoms relapse within a short time;
- symptoms improve but never settle completely and become chronic; or
- there is an associated neurological deficit, such as footdrop.

Surgery is usually undertaken after appropriate investigation to confirm the clinical level. Plain CT, myelography, CT myelography or MRI may all be used, although MRI is now the investigation of choice. The surgical options include percutaneous discectomy under radiological control, chymopapain injection into the disc prolapse to dissolve it, or open discectomy. The first two options have not gained widespread popularity and can only be used in the lumbar region. Open discectomy is the most widely used surgical procedure. Only the prolapse is excised and the centre of the disc is cleared of as much of the nucleus pulposus as possible to reduce pressure within

05

it and allow healing of the tear in the annulus fibrosis. The disc itself is not removed. It is now common practice to make the incision as small as possible and to use a microscope in order to cause minimal disturbance to the normal tissues (microdiscectomy). Early mobilization is encouraged to prevent back stiffness.

Spondylosis

Pathology

Spondylosis is the response of the spine to ageing, although some individuals may develop the condition prematurely, especially if they have a history of trauma. Wear and tear of the spine causes bulging of the intervertebral discs, new bone (osteophyte) formation within the spinal canal, usually at the intervertebral joints, and calcification of the ligaments, especially the ligamentum flavum. As a result the spinal canal and the root-exit foramina gradually narrow. This may cause progressive spinal ischaemia (the blood supply of the spinal cord is via radicular arteries passing through the root-exit foramina) and direct compression of the spinal cord and its roots. As with disc prolapse, the more mobile areas of the spine are most commonly affected, and the disease is most prominent in lumbar and cervical regions.

Clinical features

The symptoms of spondylosis are usually progressive and are most common in old age. They include pain in the affected part of the spine and radicular pain due to root irritation. Interference with the blood supply and direct cord compression due to cervical spondylosis may result in spastic quadriparesis, while a syndrome of leg numbness and weakness on exercise, which is relieved by rest, results from cauda equina ischaemia due to lumbar canal stenosis. An acute event such as a fall may cause an acute deterioration against a background of chronic spondylosis, particularly if it involves the cervical spine.

Management

Spondylosis is very common in the population but only a few people require treatment. The indications for surgery are not clear-cut and good clinical judgement is necessary. Essentially, severe symptoms or a progressive neurological deficit are the main reasons for surgery. Operations for spondylosis prevent further deterioration rather than reverse changes that have already occurred. Surgery may not be indicated for mild numbness of the fingers in cervical spondylosis, but waiting for the symptoms to progress to a stage where the hands are too weak to be of any use is too late. Age is no bar to surgery if the patient's general health is good. At operation the area of entrapment is released. As spondylosis is usually diffuse, long cervical or lumbar laminectomies are often necessary, although in

the neck single- or two-level anterior decompressions may be appropriate.

Rheumatoid arthritis

Although the spine may be affected by rheumatoid arthritis at any level, the atlantoaxial junction is most commonly involved. Atlantoaxial subluxation may result and may be asymptomatic or associated with pain (especially occipital pain) or cord compression from a translocated odontoid peg. Atlantoaxial subluxation makes endotracheal intubation of patients with rheumatoid arthritis very hazardous. The atlantoaxial junction may be fixed to the occiput using wires or screws, but if there is anterior compression it may be necessary to remove the odontoid peg via the mouth and carry out posterior fusion at the same time.

Infection

The spine may be affected by metastatic pyogenic infection or tuberculosis, which usually presents with spinal cord compression (Pott's spine). Severe local pain and tenderness are features of pyogenic infection. To exclude infection, histological confirmation of the cause of a compression is mandatory before any treatment is undertaken. If pyogenic infection is suspected, open drainage, usually by laminectomy, and high-dose antibiotic treatment is given. If a diagnosis of tuberculosis is certain, antituberculous chemotherapy without surgery is acceptable; however, if there is doubt about the nature of the compression or the patient's condition deteriorates despite adequate treatment, surgical exploration is necessary.

Haemorrhage

Spinal haemorrhage is relatively rare and when it does occur is commonly missed. Haemorrhage may occur within the cord or in the subarachnoid or extradural space. Spontaneous cord or extradural haemorrhage is most common in anticoagulated patients, while SAH is usually associated with a spinal AVM. Spinal haemorrhage should be suspected if there is a sudden onset of spinal pain associated with a spinal cord syndrome. Such a suspicion warrants urgent investigation by myelography or MRI. Cord haemorrhages are not usually helped by surgery, although early evacuation of an extradural haemorrhage can lead to recovery, even when severe. Spinal AVMs can be treated by embolization or surgery.

Peripheral nerve disorders

Like spinal surgery, peripheral nerve surgery may be performed by neurosurgeons, orthopaedic surgeons and

plastic surgeons. Peripheral nerve problems tend to be due to trauma, tumour or entrapment.

Trauma

Traumatic nerve injuries usually result from penetrating wounds (often caused by a knife or bullet) or from fractures. The most common example of a fracture-induced nerve injury is radial nerve palsy following a humeral shaft fracture. Another common injury is trauma to the brachial plexus after a fall on to the shoulder. When peripheral nerve trauma is suspected, the wound should be explored. If possible the nerve ends are sutured together by the perineurium. If there is infection or a loss of length preventing tension-free apposition of the divided nerve ends, the nerve ends should be marked and delayed repair is performed. The nerves recover by regrowing down the neural tube, although this is slow and often associated with aberrant reinnervation. Specific nerve injuries are discussed in Chapter 22.

Tumour

Significant peripheral neurofibromas are common in von Recklinghausen's syndrome but rarely cause a serious neurological deficit, any problem being cosmetic. Brachial plexus neurofibromas can affect upper limb function and should be excised. Peripheral neuromas are a rare cause of severe pain.

Entrapment neuropathies

Peripheral nerves can be compressed by anatomical variants, the most common being:
- cervical rib, causing weakness and wasting of small hand muscles;
- ulnar nerve entrapment at the elbow, causing numbness of the little and ring fingers;
- median nerve entrapment in the carpal tunnel at the wrist, causing numbness of the radial three fingers.

Diagnosis of an entrapment neuropathy is confirmed by EMG studies. It is treated by surgical exploration of the nerve and decompression.

Miscellaneous neurosurgical problems

Congenital anomalies

There is a wide range of development anomalies of the CNS, some of which are amenable to surgery. Often the abnormalities are complex, particularly with some craniofacial anomalies. Surgical correction of such complex abnormalities requires a multidisciplinary approach involving neurosurgeons, plastic surgeons, faciomaxillary surgeons, orthodontists, ear, nose and throat surgeons, ophthalmic surgeons, paediatricians, anaesthetists and psychologists, as well as dedicated nurses and physiotherapists. Care of these children may continue into adult life and the neurosurgeon undertaking this work should have a special interest and expertise in the type of surgery required and appropriate back-up facilities. Spina bifida is also a multidisciplinary problem requiring neurosurgical, orthopaedic and urological expertise along with general paediatric care.

Pain

Neurosurgery may be of value in the treatment of pain in conjunction with a pain clinic. Surgery may cure pain caused by a mechanical problem, such as disc prolapse, spinal instability or trigeminal neuralgia. When the disease cannot be cured, pain control may be achieved by implanting electrical stimulators or injection catheters into appropriate areas of the CNS. As a final option when all else fails and life expectancy is limited, destructive operations such as rhizotomy or cordotomy may be appropriate.

Neurosurgical disorders at a glance

Definitions

Neurosurgery: a discipline concerned with disorders of the brain, spinal cord, peripheral nerves and their surrounding structures

Brain tumour: an abnormal mass of tissue that results from the excessive multiplication of cells within the cranial cavity

Primary brain tumour: one that arises from the tissues of the brain or pituitary gland or their coverings. They may be benign or malignant. In children primary brain tumours tend to occur below the tentorium, in adults above the tentorium

Secondary or metastatic brain tumour: arises from cells elsewhere in the body that spread to the brain. They are always malignant

Hydrocephalus: accumulation of an excessive volume of CSF within the ventricular system

Communicating hydrocephalus: CSF flows freely between the ventricles and the subarachnoid space

Non-communicating hydrocephalus: CSF is trapped within the ventricles

05

Evaluation of patients with neurosurgical disorders

History-taking
- Chronological
- General history
- Family history
- Collateral

Symptoms
Headache
- Stress/tension: chronic, relieved by rest
- Migraine: prodromal visual symptoms, severe, nausea, prostration
- Giant-cell arteritis: unilateral ± visual loss
- ICP: intermittent, worse in morning
- SAH: sudden 'thunderclap' onset
- Supratentorial lesion: frontal
- Cerebellar lesion: occipital

Weakness
- General
- Specific

Numbness
- Peripheral nerve lesion
- Neuropathies

Dizziness
- Rotational: vertigo
- Veering to one side: cerebellar lesion
- On looking up: vertibrobasilar

Visual disturbance
Blackouts

Physical examination
Central nervous system
- Check higher cerebral function by talking to patient
- Cranial nerves I–XII

Peripheral nervous system (upper and lower limbs)

Member	Muscle tone and power
Royal	Reflexes
College	Coordination
Surgeons	Sensation
Glasgow	Gait

Unconscious patient
- Check ABC, primary and secondary survey
- Calculate Glasgow Coma Scale

Investigations
General
- Haematology:
  (a) Full blood count: baseline investigation
  (b) Clotting screen: if abnormal promotes intracranial bleeding

- Biochemistry: if the following are abnormal, they may cause or exacerbate coma:
  (a) Urea, sodium, calcium
  (b) Glucose
  (c) Blood gas analysis
- Chest X-ray: cerebral secondaries are frequent from a primary lung tumour

Specific

Lumbar puncture
Measure CSF pressure
Useful in diagnosis of subarachnoid haemorrhage, meningitis, encephalitis, Guillain–Barré syndrome, multiple sclerosis

Imaging
Skull radiography: diagnosis of skull fracture
CT: diagnosis of intracranial lesions, e.g. tumour, haemorrhage, infarct, hydrocephalus
MRI: more sensitive than CT, imaging of choice for most neurosurgical conditions
Myelography: invasive method of assessing spinal cord, now rarely used
Angiography, MRA: used to demonstrate intracerebral circulation and therapeutic embolization
PET: dynamic scan of brain function

Neurophysiological studies
EEG: used in diagnosis of epilepsy
SSEP: assess sensory pathways
Nerve conduction studies: assess peripheral nerves
EMG: assess peripheral nerves

Managing the unconscious patient
Many of the tasks of daily living have to be performed for the patient:
- Chest care
- Pressure areas
- Hygiene and sphincters
- Eyes
- Feeding
- Movement
- General care
- Relatives

CNS tumours
Secondary brain tumours
- Most common tumours of the CNS and account for 20–30% of all intracranial tumours
- Generally spread via the bloodstream
- Common tissues of origin are lung (35%), breast (20%), skin (malignant melanoma) (10%), kidney (10%), gastrointestinal tract (5%)

Primary brain tumour

	Frequency (%)	Age at diagnosis (years)	Frequent location	Malignant or benign	5-year survival (%)
Intraparenchymal					
Glioma					
Astrocytoma	20	30–50	Cerebrum	Malignant	30
Oligodendroglioma	10	40–50	Cerebrum	Malignant	60
Ependymomas	5	Childhood	Fourth ventricle	Malignant	50
Medulloblastoma	5	0–12	Cerebellum	Malignant	60
Primary lymphoma*	2	30–40	Cerebrum	Malignant	0
Extraparenchymal					
Meningioma	20	40–50	Diverse	Benign	90
Schwannoma	5	30–50	VIII nerve	Benign	95

* Occurs in immunosuppressed patients (post organ transplantation, AIDS) and with treatment has a median survival of 2 years.

Clinical features

Intracranial tumours can present in several different ways depending on location and aggressiveness of the tumour
• Raised ICP caused by mass effect of tumour, haemorrhage into tumour or obstruction of CSF flow producing hydrocephalus:
  (a) Symptoms include headaches (especially in the morning and worse on straining or dependent head position), nausea, vomiting and eventually decreased level of consciousness
  (b) Signs include papilloedema or paralysis of the lateral rectus muscle
• Loss of brain function, e.g. ataxia with cerebellar tumours, unilateral deafness with VIII nerve lesion
• Hyperactive function: a tumour may initiate seizures by compressing or infiltrating adjacent brain tissue

Investigations

• General:
  (a) CT with iodinated contrast enhancement: demonstrates bone of base of skull very well
  (b) MRI: excellent imaging of brain tissue (T_1-weighted images)
• Specific:
  (a) Cerebral angiography: demonstrates vascularity of tumours
  (b) EEG: useful in analysis of patients with seizures
  (c) Ophthalmological and audiometric examinations: for suspected lesions of visual or auditory pathways
• Lumbar puncture should be *avoided* in patients with a suspected brain tumour as removal of CSF could precipitate fatal brain herniation

Treatment

• Surgery: mainstay of treatment of intracranial tumours:

  (a) CT- or MRI-guided stereotactic techniques make tumour biopsy relatively easy
  (b) Preoperative planning, computer guidance, stereotaxis, operative microscopy and microsurgical techniques permit resection of deep-seated tumours
  (c) Meningiomas, schwannomas and pituitary adenomas can be resected surgically but gliomas cannot be cured by surgical resection
• Radiotherapy: some tumours (e.g. medulloblastoma. ependymoma) are highly sensitive to radiotherapy
• Chemotherapy: used only as an adjunct to surgery and radiotherapy

Prognosis

• Prognosis depends not only on the type but also on the histological grading of the tumour

Intracranial haemorrhage

Extradural haemorrhage
• Tear in middle meningeal artery
• Haematoma between skull and dura
• Often a 'lucid interval' before signs of raised ICP ensue (falling pulse, rising blood pressure, ipsilateral pupillary dilatation, contralateral paresis or paralysis)
• Treatment: evacuation of haematoma via craniotomy

Acute subdural haemorrhage
• Tearing of veins between arachnoid and dura mater
• Usually seen in the elderly
• Progressive neurological deterioration
• Treatment: evacuation by craniotomy but even then recovery may be incomplete

Chronic subdural haematoma
• Tear in vein leads to subdural haematoma that enlarges slowly by absorption of CSF

- Often the precipitating injury is trivial
- Drowsiness and confusion, headache, hemiplegia
- Treatment: evacuation of the clot

Intracerebral haemorrhage
- Haemorrhage into brain substance causes irreversible damage
- Efforts are made to avoid secondary injury by ensuring adequate oxygenation and nutrition

Subarachnoid haemorrhage
- Caused by rupture of berry aneurysm (70%) or AVM (10%), unknown (20%)
- Haemorrhage into subarachnoid space
- Sudden severe headache + nausea, vomiting, coma (death in 40%)
- Diagnosis by CT or lumbar puncture
- Treatment: surgical clipping or endovascular embolization. Risk of rebleeding and delayed cerebral ischaemia

Hydrocephalus
Causes
Overproduction of CSF
- CSF-secreting tumour

Obstruction to CSF flow
- Lateral ventricle: intraventricular haemorrhage
- Foramen of Munro: intraventricular tumours
- Aqueduct:
  (a) Tumour
  (b) Congenital stenosis
  (c) Intraventricular haemorrhage
- Fourth ventricle:
  (a) Congenital cyst
  (b) Tumour
  (c) Cerebellar swelling

Failure of absorption of CSF
- Head injury
- Subarachnoid haemorrhage
- Meningitis

Clinical features
- Infant: rapid head growth
- Child/adult: features of raised ICP
- Old age: dementia/ataxia/incontinence

Investigations
- CT/MRI: most useful investigation

- Lumbar puncture: *contraindicated with non-communicating hydrocephalus*

Treatment
- Treat cause, e.g. remove tumour
- Reduce CSF production: acetazolamide, destruction of choroid plexus
- Bypass blockage: endoscopic third ventriculostomy
- Remove excess CSF:
  (a) Temporary: ventricular tapping, lumbar drainage
  (b) Permanent shunts: ventriculoperitoneum, ventriculopleural, ventriculoatrial
- Shunt complications: overdrainage, blockage, infection

Spinal surgery
Special considerations in spinal surgery
- What is the diagnosis?
- What level of the spine is involved?
- Is the spine stable?
- Will treatment affect stability?
- What approach should be used?

Spine stabilization
- External: effective for neck, e.g. halo traction
- Internal: bone grafting, cement, prostheses

Spinal disorders
Malignant cord compression
- Caused by metastatic tumour
- Treatment: dexamethasone, radiotherapy, surgery

Disc prolapse
- Herniation of annulus fibrosis
- Treatment: analgesia and rest (rarely surgery)

Spondylosis
- Narrowing of spinal canal and foramina
- Treatment: symptomatic (rarely surgery)

Rheumatoid arthritis
- Atlantoaxial subluxation
- Treatment: may need surgery

Infection
- Pyogenic (metastatic): treated by drainage + antibiotics
- Tuberculosis: treated with antituberculous drugs ± exploration

Haemorrhage
- Caused by anticoagulants or AVM

Evidence-based medicine

http://www.cancerbacup.org.uk Website of the Cancer-BACUP group, which provides a national cancer information service in the UK.

http://www.neurosurgery.mgh.harvard.edu/abta/primer.htm Website of American Brain Tumor Association.

http://www.neurosurgery.medsch.ucla.edu UCLA nuerosurgery website.

Musculoskeletal Disorders

41

Must know Must do

Must know

Core knowledge of common orthopaedic conditions
Understand the causes and consequences of the
    various types of arthritis
Differentiate between acute and chronic arthritis
How to detect nerve lesions
Pathophysiology and principles of management of
    major connective tissue disorders
Clinical features of the potentially serious conditions in
    childhood and understand their consequences in
    broad outline, in particular be able to deal with the
    natural questions and anxieties raised by parents

Must do

Link the examination of the joints described in
    Chapter 1 to the conditions described here
Attend an orthopaedic outpatient clinic
Attend a rheumatology clinic
Examine patients with osteoarthritis and rheumatoid
    arthritis
Examine a patient with one of the nerve entrapment
    syndromes
Clerk a patient with a septic arthritis
Examine a child with a slipped femoral epiphysis
Observe a hip joint replacement operation

Introduction

The word 'orthopaedics', which comes from Greek and
literally means 'straight child' (ορθοσ, straight; παισ,
child), reflects the history of the subject, which was based
around developmental musculoskeletal conditions in
childhood. The subject now spans all musculoskeletal disorders throughout life. With few exceptions, these disorders are non-fatal and cause pain and disturbance or
loss of function. Dealing with non-fatal conditions
requires a special kind of balanced clinical judgement to
ensure that the potential benefits of a particular treatment
outweigh inevitable risks from surgery. In order to reach

such a judgement we must know our patients well as
individuals and understand their goals of treatment. If the
patient's perceptions of outcome differ significantly from
the clinician's, then a satisfactory result is unlikely. The
making of a diagnosis in the musculoskeletal system generally is not difficult, although exceptions to this observation are indicated in the text where appropriate. The real
difficulty is not in diagnosis but in management and for
good management we must have accurate assessment.

Evaluation of the patient with orthopaedic disorders

Clinical assessment

Symptoms

The general principles of history-taking have already been
discussed, but there are a number of points worthy of
particular attention when considering orthopaedics.

Pain

Assessment of pain concentrates on severity rather than
location. With a few exceptions, musculoskeletal disorders are easy to localize. Pain is generally related to the
activities being carried out by the subject and so a
pain–function relationship should be established. This
may be summarized as a spectrum:

No pain → Pain on → Pain at → Pain →
            vigorous   work   walking
            activity   outside

Pain → Pain → Night pain
walking   at rest
inside

In general terms, pain occurring at night is an absolute
indication to do something for the patient, although the
threshold for action will vary from individual to individual. For example, a 45-year-old man who gets knee pain
playing football for his pub team may be advised to retire

05

from the game, but a young and otherwise fit man who plays the game for his county will have different priorities.

Drugs

The above system works extremely well in practice but it is useful to have other information and much can be learnt from finding out what drugs the patient takes for the pain. The type, dose, frequency and efficacy of analgesics give the clinician a valuable insight into the level of a person's discomfort. The severity of the pain in practice is roughly reflected in the potency of analgesics, as shown below:

No drugs → Proprietary   → Non-steroid
             over-the-counter   anti-inflammatory
             agents   drugs (NSAIDs)

→ Non-opiate → Opiates
   agents   centrally acting

This spectrum is not designed to decry simple analgesia, which includes aspirin and paracetamol, as such drugs can be very effective in the treatment of inflammatory conditions and this should be borne in mind.

How does the patient function?

Having established the level of pain and loss of function or disability, this must be offset against the lifestyle, age and outlook of the patient. The general physical and medical state of the patient will also need assessment, particularly if a surgical solution is contemplated.

Risk balance

With all this information it is possible to construct a risk–benefit balance as outlined in the box below. Essentially, the benefits must outweigh the risks before embarking on treatment.

Physical examination

It is important to examine the bones, soft tissues and skin, and an assessment of peripheral neurological and circulatory function should also be made. The examination of patients with orthopaedic problems is largely concerned with the examination of joints. Remember that the spine is a collection of segments joined by joints! Alan Apley was the doyen of teachers in orthopaedics and it was he who coined the notion that joints should be examined in three stages: (i) look, (ii) feel and (iii) move.

Looking

Inspect the joint to exclude scars, muscle wasting and obvious swelling. The general posture provides insight and any obvious deformity or shortening is noted.

Constructing a risk balance

1 Mrs Smith is 75 years old and has been troubled by right hip pain during walking outdoors for some 2 years. In the last few months she has had pain nearly all the time when in the house and occasionally has been woken at night. Initially she obtained benefit from analgesia and NSAIDs but recently had to stop taking the latter because of indigestion. She is generally well and is on an angiotensin-converting enzyme inhibitor and thiazide diuretic for well-controlled hypertension.
2 Mr Jones is 40 years old and has been known to have a bad right hip since childhood when he had Perthes disease. He is a farm worker and has three children and lives in a tied cottage. His hip is now niggling him and he occasionally takes codeine and paracetamol, on average one or two days a week, especially during busy times. He is very fit and well but is just getting worried about the future.

Balance 1
Mrs Smith will obtain great benefit from a hip replacement. She is old enough to have low functional demands and the hip is likely to outlast her (90% last at least 10 years). She now has night pain and will risk her independence if she waits too long. Pain-controlling drugs are exposing her to risk of gastrointestinal bleeding, which has a significant mortality. Although she has a heart condition, it is well controlled and her drugs can continue during surgery. Her risk balance greatly favours a good outcome from surgery.

Balance 2
Mr Jones is a young heavy-demand patient who would wear out a false hip in less than 10 years. He is otherwise well and so surgery as such carries low risk. However, in the long run he would be better to wait or consider alternative operations such as hip fusion. As yet his symptoms, although worrying, are controllable. His main priority is to keep working and support his young family. He must not be abandoned, however, and his progress should be carefully monitored and alternative strategies kept under constant review.

Feeling

The key is to know what one is feeling and to ask oneself 'What is happening underneath?' Lumps, bony or otherwise, swellings and joint effusions can be well appreciated in certain joints but not so easily in other situations. For example, the hip is covered by thick muscle and so is not easy to feel, but the knee is largely crossed by tendons, especially at the front and sides, and so a more direct examination of the joint may be made.

Moving

Start by obeying some simple rules.
- Know what movements the joint can do.
- Appreciate that loss of certain movements is more significant than others.
- Place the joint in its anatomically neutral position.
- Break the movements into their simple anatomical components (see box below).

Investigations

The investigations frequently performed in assessment of musculoskeletal disorders are given in Table 41.1.

Problems with joints

Of all the conditions treated by orthopaedic surgeons, arthritis takes up much of the clinic and operating theatre time. This reflects the high prevalence of arthritis in the western world and it is therefore important to understand this condition above all others. In general terms, arthritis is a painful and distressing disorder that has profound effects on how well people live. There is no specific treatment and all our strategies are based around symptom relief.

Assessment of movement of the hip joint

Know what movements the joint can do
The movements of the hip joint are:
- Flexion and extension
- Abduction and adduction
- Internal and external rotation
- Circumduction

Appreciate that loss of certain movements is more significant than others
Losses of major functional significance to the hip are extension, rotation in extension and abduction. Of course loss of any movement may matter but movements are relative and in day-to-day activity loss of key movements in walking are of most significance

Loss of extension
When we walk we do so in a way that minimizes energy consumption. Loss of energy-conserving movements makes walking literally hard work. To go forward we shift our centre of gravity in front of our feet so that we must fall forwards. To stop ourselves falling we put out the leading leg, leaving the trailing leg behind. In this manoeuvre we flex the leading leg a little and also extend the trailing leg. In relative terms we would have to lose an awful lot of our range of flexion before this affected walking, but the loss of only some of our rather limited extending ability would be highly significant. Loss of the ability to leave the trailing leg behind, through loss of extension, is an early feature in hip disease

Loss of rotation
Another mechanism we use to conserve energy in walking is to make maximum use of our bodies in generating forward momentum through twisting. We are all familiar with soldiers who swing their arms as they march and all of us when our hands are free and we are in a hurry tend to do the same subconsciously. Arm swinging and twisting of the upper limb girdle travels down the trunk and into the pelvis and lower limbs. The twisting is converted into forward movement as the legs swing. Most of the swinging occurs as the legs are in neutral or extended as the centre of gravity passes from one leg to the next, with the weight just on the extended trailing leg. Loss of rotation of the hips in the neutral or extended position is therefore very important. Loss of this ability again makes walking difficult and hard work. Loss of rotation in extension is not uncommon in early hip disease, particularly degenerative disease

Place the joint in its anatomically neutral position
When a patient lies on an examination couch the hip joints are not in the anatomically neutral position. Because the lumbar spine is lordotic, the pelvis is tilted as it rests on the couch. The hip is flexed, as are the knees, such that the calves make contact with the couch. In order to remove this overt hip flexion the contralateral hip should be fully flexed, so tilting the pelvis backwards and straightening the lordosis. The manoeuvre is known as Thomas' test, after Hugh Owen Thomas who devised it. The significance is that it puts the pelvis in the neutral position and so any fixed flexion deformity will be revealed. The importance of showing fixed flexion is that it means there must be loss of extension, which we now understand is highly significant in assessing the hip. Loss of extension means profound disturbance of walking

Break the movements into their simple anatomical components
Some of the movements that take place in the hip also take place in adjacent joints, particularly in the lumbar spine, resulting in pelvic tilt and twist. If Thomas' test is taken too far, the lumbar spine and the pelvis flex; equally if abduction is taken too far, the pelvis tilts laterally due to spinal movement. It is therefore important not only to neutralize the joint but to fix the pelvis to ensure only pure hip movement is being measured

05

Table 41.1 Investigations for assessment of musculoskeletal disorders.

Blood investigations
Haematology
Full blood count: baseline investigation, may be anaemia in arthritis
Erythrocyte sedimentation rate: simple test to perform, may be elevated in rheumatoid arthritis, osteomyelitis, multiple myeloma

Biochemistry
Calcium phosphate: will be abnormal in metabolic bone disease (e.g. hyperparathyroidism, rickets, osteomalacia)

Enzymes
Alkaline phosphatase: marker of bone turnover, raised in Paget's disease

Immunology
Rheumatoid factors: autoantibodies that react with patient's own IgG are present in rheumatoid arthritis

Imaging
Plain radiography
Look at bones in general for shape (deformity) and density
Look at cortex of the bone for breaks in continuity
Look at medulla of the bone for destruction or sclerosis (secondary deposits)
Look at joints for narrowing of joint space, erosion, irregularity or new bone formation (osteophytes)
Look at soft tissues for calcification, foreign body or gas

Contrast radiology
Myelography or radiculography is used to assess the spinal canal

Tomography
By moving the X-ray plate and tube in opposite directions a structure in the long axis of movement can be kept in focus while
  the surrounding tissues are blurred. Useful in exposing the spine but has been superseded by CT and MRI

CT and MRI
Very useful for detecting subtle changes in bone and (especially MRI) in soft tissues

Radioisotope scanning
Used for detecting skeletal metastases, primary bone tumours, bone and joint infections and stress fractures

Endoscopy
Arthroscopy
Used mostly for assessment of pathology in the knee (see Fig. 41.4) and shoulder joints

CT, computed tomography; MRI, magnetic resonance imaging.

Osteoarthritis

Osteoarthritis is a syndrome of pain and limitation of movement associated with a breakdown of the balance between the wear and repair processes in the joint. It occurs with increasing age, although it would be misleading to suggest that osteoarthritis is an inevitable accompaniment of old age, and almost certainly has a genetic basis.

Aetiology

It is convenient to classify osteoarthritis according to aetiology. The classification starts by grouping patients into those who have a known cause (secondary osteoarthritis) and those where the cause remains unknown (primary osteoarthritis). It is important to appreciate that the vast majority of patients fall into the primary category.

Primary osteoarthritis

This is a term of convenience and, despite much effort, there remains little insight into the cause of this very common condition. It is probably true that many cases of arthritis are in reality secondary to *mechanical stress*, e.g. congenital deformity, previous joint or bone injury, obesity. However, in the vast majority of patients with osteoarthritis the cause is obscure. It must be assumed that the primary cause is localized to the affected joints as a systemic disorder would be expected to affect most joints. There are a few cases who do appear to have generalized osteoarthritis but these are rare.

Table 41.2 Conditions that predispose to the development of secondary osteoarthritis.

Congenital: congenital dislocation of the hip
Childhood: Perthes disease, infection
Trauma: fracture into a joint, cartilage tear
Metabolic: gout, crystal arthropathy
Infection: tuberculosis
Chronic inflammation: rheumatoid arthritis

Another possible aetiological factor is that the mechanism of *cartilage nutrition*, which is mediated largely via the synovial fluid, is in some way abnormal. *Cartilage fragments* are found in worn joints and such minute fragments are known to initiate intense inflammatory reactions, which then lead to further cartilage damage. An initial event (such as trauma) might release a cartilage fragment into the joint, initiating a self-perpetuating cycle that leads ultimately to joint destruction.

Secondary osteoarthritis
In this minority group there are obvious causative factors that quite reasonably may be assumed to be responsible for the development of osteoarthritis. These are listed in Table 41.2 and discussed elsewhere in this chapter.

Clinical presentation

Osteoarthritis can present at any age but becomes increasingly common in later decades. In the younger patient there is more likely to be a recognizable predisposing cause but not always so. Both in history and examination it is essential to gain an overview of the patient's general health as not only is a diagnosis being reached but a plan of management which may include surgery is being assembled.

History
The patient presents with pain and associated loss of function. Stiffness is a feature but is nearly always secondary to pain. The onset may be insidious but occasionally the presentation can be quite dramatic and relatively short, making the diagnosis difficult. Initially, pain is associated with activity and if a lower limb joint is affected, the patient is often left with an indiscernible tiredness towards the end of the day. This latter feature is often caused by the gait modifications discussed earlier.

Help is sought when simple analgesia no longer relieves pain and specialist help is demanded by the primary carer when sleep is disturbed. The threshold for referral varies from patient to patient but, in general, younger patients tend to present earlier than the elderly who expect a degree of arthritis as they get older.

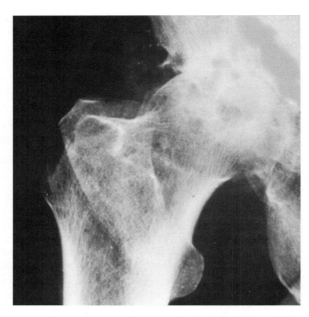

Figure 41.1 Advanced osteoarthritis of the hip showing osteophytes, sclerosis and joint space narrowing.

Management is heavily dependent on the clinician's ability to distinguish between many individuals and treat and offer surgery appropriately. It is important at this stage to have a clear concept of one's aim in treatment, which is to relieve pain.

Examination
The striking feature on physical examination is the limitation of movement by pain. It is important to appreciate that the perceived limitation of movement on routine examination is greater than any limitation observed during examination under anaesthesia. Once this is appreciated then the clinician will soon realize that results of surgery are related to pain relief rather than improvements in stiffness of the joint caused by the disease.

Investigations

In general, a plain anteroposterior and lateral radiograph is all that will be required (Fig. 41.1). Occasionally, in a very acute presentation a bone scan may be useful in order to isolate the occasional patient presenting with a metastatic deposit or bone death (also known as avascular necrosis; see p. 652).

The typical radiographic findings are as follows.
- Joint space narrowing: this indicates a loss of articular cartilage.
- Osteophyte formation: bony outgrowths at the joint margin (of obscure significance).

05

Table 41.3 Non-steroidal anti-inflammatory drugs available for treatment of arthritis.

Drug group	Name	Dose	Adverse effects
Salicylates	Aspirin	up to 4 g/day	Gastrointestinal upset*, tinnitus and deafness bruising and bleeding, hypersensitivity reactions†, drug interactions
Propionic acid derivatives	Ibuprofen Naproxen Fenprofen	400 mg t.d.s. 250–500 mg b.d. 300–600 mg q.d.s.	Gastrointestinal upset*, hypersensitivity reactions†
Indoleacetic acid derivatives	Indomethacin	25 mg b.d./q.d.s. 50 mg nocte	Gastrointestinal upset*, CNS symptoms (headache, vertigo, dizziness, depression, nightmares), hypersensitivity reactions†
Cox II inhibitors	Celoxib Meloxican	200 mg/day 15 mg/day	Less gastrointestinal upset, but otherwise side effects as above

* Gastrointestinal (GI) upset includes dyspepsia, nausea and vomiting, gastric erosions and bleeding and peptic ulceration.
† Hypersensitivity reactions are not uncommon and care should be taken in prescribing these drugs to patients with asthma.

● Cyst formation: around the subchondral region.
● Subchondral sclerosis: a thickening of bone induced by the loss of shock-absorbing cartilage.

The degree to which a joint is affected by these changes is not related to the severity of symptoms and it is on clinical rather than radiological grounds that decisions about surgical intervention are made.

Management

The key to management is to realize that there is no cure for osteoarthritis and that the clinical course is erratic. All management is aimed at pain relief and, through this, return of function. The ultimate way of relieving pain is surgery, although there are general measures that will alleviate symptoms and postpone the need for operation.

Non-surgical options

These include weight loss, use of a stick, rest and physiotherapy. Analgesia may be used subsequently or in parallel with these measures.

WEIGHT LOSS

Lower limb joints in particular are subject to large loads resulting from the leverage effects of muscles sited to good mechanical advantage. For example, the hip abductors arising from the pelvis are inserted on the trochanters well away from the centres of rotation of the hip joint. These leverage effects mean that quite modest changes in body weight will have useful effects on the total load being borne by the joint. Weight loss is usually accompanied by a general improvement in well-being, which often affects overall pain perception.

WALKING STICK

In lower limb joint disease, particularly in the hip, the use of a stick in the *contralateral* hand means that the shoulder girdle can help in tilting the pelvis and so assist in weight-bearing. This has the effect of reducing the work required of the weight-bearing abductors, which dramatically reduces muscle-induced loads on the hip.

PHYSIOTHERAPY

The role of physiotherapy and rest remains controversial and a balance is required. Overexercise cannot in the long term be beneficial but some exercise does relieve stiffness and spasm and pain. Young sufferers should be advised against excessive unnecessary activity and a change to a light job is useful, if practicable. However, total rest is equally counterproductive, especially in the elderly where maintenance of the activities of daily living is essential. Local heat and muscle-strengthening exercises are also useful, e.g. 'quad' exercises in osteoarthritis of the knee.

DRUG THERAPY

Drugs do not alter the course of osteoarthritis and there is no place for drug therapy in the absence of pain. However, in the presence of pain NSAIDs, analgesics and occasionally local corticosteroid injections may provide useful relief. Several different NSAIDs are available (Table 41.3) and individual patients respond differently to different agents. Thus a therapeutic trial is often necessary to find the drug most suited to the patient. It is very important to review NSAID drug use. If these drugs have no therapeutic benefit, they should be stopped because of the potentially very serious adverse effects on the gastrointestinal system. In later-stage arthritis pure analgesics,

especially codeine and paracetamol combinations, are often more appropriate.

Local steroid injection is useful for acute exacerbations or persistent pain and swelling in one or two joints. In general, it should reserved for patients who are older and unsuitable for surgery or as a temporary measure in patients awaiting a definitive operation. Steroid injections should be administered under aseptic techniques and should not be given if there is any suspicion of infection.

Hyaluronic acid is frequently prescribed by injection. This natural joint constituent has been subjected to clinical trials suggesting that a series of injections may be beneficial to symptoms of arthritis. Although statistically significant effects are reported, these are not to be guaranteed and the technique remains of doubtful long-term value except in patients unfit for surgery.

Surgical options

For most forms of arthritis there remain four options: nothing, arthroplasty, arthrodesis and osteotomy.

NOTHING

Nothing should always be borne in mind and the patient must appreciate that the benefits must outweigh the risks when surgery is being considered. Equally, for very disabled patients in a great deal of pain, the option to take risks must be considered. Provided patients have a good grasp of the risk–benefit equation as it affects them, then they may take the lion's share in the decision to have surgery. Patients should also understand the limitations of surgery: it can relieve pain but is not likely to alleviate disability due to intrinsic stiffness.

ARTHROPLASTY

Arthroplasty or joint replacement is probably one of the most successful surgical treatments ever devised. Hip and knee arthroplasties are now performed routinely with excellent results. However, there are some principles to be followed in selecting patients for arthroplasty and the procedures are not without complications. Arthroplasty is discussed more fully later.

ARTHRODESIS

Arthrodesis or surgical fusion in a position of function is an appropriate operation in a young person with a painful and limited range of motion. In the hip, for example, fusion in 30° of flexion and some abduction produces pain-free and functional gait while permitting sitting. It is more acceptable to the male than the female as any hip fusion is likely to interfere with female sexual activity.

Fusion is not a technically easy procedure and requires a prolonged recovery period of up to 6 months, often in a plaster splint. The long-term disadvantage of arthrodesis is that it puts stress on the adjacent joints. For example, in the hip this means extra stress on the lumbar spine and knee as well as the opposite hip. However, this problem may be anticipated by electing to fuse until the fifth decade and then performing a second operation to 'unpick' the arthrodesis and convert it to an arthroplasty. This latter operation has proved to be surprisingly effective for the hip, with good return to function of the temporarily defunct abductor muscles. Nevertheless, fusion is still a difficult option to 'sell' to patients, however logical the procedure.

Joints that are usefully fused are the ankle and the wrist. These are joints that at present are difficult to replace and which have a relatively limited range of functional movement in any case.

OSTEOTOMY

Osteotomy or surgical realignment of the joint is an option used widely in Europe and with varying degrees of popularity in the UK and the USA. This difference of attitude is traditional and otherwise impossible to explain. Accurate surgical realignment is technically difficult and very time-consuming. Perhaps the most likely reason for its varying popularity is the widely differing results of effectiveness and long-term outcome. Even in the best hands, osteotomy can only be viewed as a temporary measure lasting from 1–2 years to around 10 years.

Osteotomy may be used to realign any deformity in any bone. When used to treat arthritis, osteotomy is valuable in young patients who have maintained a good range of movement despite pain. The hip and the knee are suitable for osteotomy. In the hip joint, osteotomy may be performed on the pelvic side, either by forming a shelf or by total acetabular realignment. It may be performed on the femoral side by altering the angle of the femoral neck so as to change the attitude of the femoral head relative to the acetabulum.

In general, the effects of osteotomy are threefold.
● To alter the angle and so mechanical advantage of the muscles. For example, at the hip the action of the abductors may be modified. It may also be used to abolish flexion deformity (so-called extension osteotomy).
● To alter the contact area between surfaces. This may be particularly useful following a deformity leading to secondary osteoarthritis.
● To alter the dynamics of blood supply to the joint. It has been proposed that the pain of arthritis is due to subchondral venous tension and so osteotomy in crude terms may decompress the femoral head. This is very much a speculative idea but would in part explain the dramatic pain relief following this sort of surgery.

In general terms, osteotomy may be said to be a beneficial operation in young people who retain a good range of motion and have a reasonable preservation of articular cartilage.

05

Joint replacement (arthroplasty)

Strictly, the term 'arthroplasty' means the surgical re-shaping of a joint but it has become synonymous with joint replacement and is used in this accepted way here.

Principles of joint replacement

The same basic rules apply to all joints and provided they can be obeyed, then arthroplasty may be performed. The new joint must be:
- capable of a functional pain-free range of movement;
- able to withstand the forces placed upon it without undue wear and without working loose.

It must achieve all this while remaining stable.

Lower limb

Lower limb replacements are subject to high loads, although in the hip particularly and to a lesser degree the knee the required range of movement to provide reasonably normal gait is relatively small. Hip and knee arthroplasties are now very successful operations. The reason why arthroplasty of the hip is held in such high regard is due to the success of the operation; the current level of 80,000 cases per annum in the UK was achieved largely through the work of Sir John Charnley. For the majority, artificial joints work very well indeed, and well in excess of 90% will still be *in situ* after 10 years. However, most hip arthroplasties are carried out in older patients with a lower functional demand. Knee arthroplasty is also better carried out on older patients. In the UK, osteoarthritis of the knee is the most common disabling form of the disease and the emergence of a successful prosthetic joint now makes this a highly predictable operation, with long-term outcomes superior to that of hip replacement (Fig. 41.2).

Upper limb

In the upper limb, the relationship between pain relief and function is quite different to that observed in the lower limb. In the case of the arm the loads involved are quite low but the available range of motion required for normal function is large. Despite the low loads, the demanding range of movement seems to lead to early failure in many upper limb joint replacements through loosening. Remember that arthroplasty in particular tends to improve pain-related loss of function but does relatively little for intrinsic stiffness. In the upper limb this poses a problem if arthroplasty is contemplated. For example, the elbow must flex to 90° to permit eating (try reaching your mouth with an arm fixed at a greater angle!) and must extend more or less fully to reach the anus for cleansing. Therefore, any surgery must cater for these two fundamental activities of daily living. Slowly, elbow and shoulder replacements are approaching such high levels of function. Not

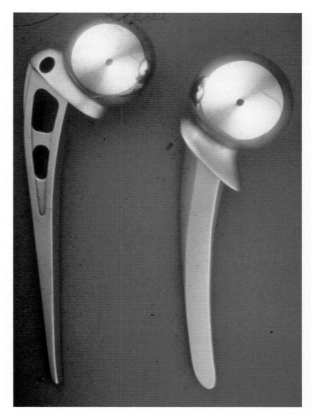

Figure 41.2 Hip hemiarthroplasties used in older patients with intracapsular fractures.

so the fingers and, to a much lesser degree, the wrist. Therefore, upper limb replacement cannot be regarded as routine but rather a highly specialized and gradually emerging specialty. Much progress is still to be made in this area.

Complications

Complications of arthroplasty may be divided into those general for any major surgery and those specific to the operation.

General complications

One must bear in mind that most patients undergoing surgery for arthritis are older: this is not to say that age *per se* is a risk factor. It is true that older people are more likely to have medical conditions predisposing to risk and if these are not recognized then problems may arise.

Patients undergoing major surgery are prone to problems such as respiratory and urinary tract infections. They may also develop pressure sores if they are not nursed adequately. Deep vein thrombosis and pulmonary embolism may follow any surgical procedure, although patients

undergoing hip surgery are especially at risk, as are patients who require any surgery in and around the pelvis.

Specific complications

These may be further classified into early and late.

EARLY COMPLICATIONS

Dislocation. In the immediate postoperative period the prosthesis will not be fully supported by the surrounding soft tissues. The muscles and their proprioceptors may be temporarily inactive because of surgical trauma and anaesthesia or analgesia and a secondary fibrotic capsule will not yet have formed around the prosthesis. The hip in this period is at risk from dislocation, particularly before the effects of anaesthesia wear off. The risk of dislocation is reduced as time passes but even after a long time an injudicious move (e.g. extreme flexion with adduction and internal rotation in the case of the hip) may result in a painful dislocation. For this reason the patient will need advice about dressing and may need aids to help in fitting stockings and also benefit from having a raised toilet seat.

Deep vein thrombosis. As stated above, patients undergoing arthroplasty are at risk from deep vein thrombosis and some sort of prophylaxis is probably justified. Each patient should be assessed for risk against a departmental policy that is clearly understood by all medical and nursing staff. People at high risk include obese patients, smokers, those relatively immobile and those who have a previous history of thrombosis. Minimum standards include admission to hospital as near the time of surgery as possible so optimizing mobility, the use of occlusive stockings, chemoprophylaxis and early postoperative mobilization. Further details can be found in Chapter 5. After surgery, all staff should regularly examine the limbs for swelling and any suspect cases investigated with ultrasound or phlebography.

Infection. Infection is always a risk following implantation of foreign material into the body. Infection may develop soon after surgery (early) or may be delayed for months or years (late). Many factors make an artificial agent prone to infection, not only from recognized hospital pathogens such as *Staphylococcus aureus* but also from organisms normally regarded as commensals, such as *Staph. epidermidis*, universally found in skin flora. It would appear that the presence of foreign material inhibits normal immune defences.

Infection of a prosthesis is such a disaster (see later) that every effort, including antibiotic prophylaxis and the provision of an ultra-clean environment, must be made to avoid this complication. If these precautions are taken, then immediate infections should be eliminated and long-term infections reduced to less than 0.1%. Unfortunately in the UK this figure is often exceeded, with rates of 1–3%

being not uncommon. Certainly anything greater than this is entirely unacceptable.

LATE COMPLICATIONS

Problems with joint replacement may occur as late as 10 years or longer following surgery. The principal problems are late infection, loosening and wear.

Infection. The causes of infection have already been discussed and it is probable that most cases of infection are caused at the time of insertion of the prosthesis. Why late infections occur is not fully understood. One suggestion is that infection may occur by other routes, e.g. blood-borne infection as a consequence of 'normal' bacteraemias. There is circumstantial evidence that some infections may follow tooth extraction, which is known to cause significant bacteraemias and may be a cause of endocarditis. However, there is agreement that this association is insufficient to warrant regular use of prophylactic antibiotics for dental work following joint arthroplasty.

Loosening and wear. Loosening is to some degree probably inevitable, though efforts are made to delay it as long as possible. The incidence of loosening increases with the age of the prosthesis. Because an implant inevitably suffers loosening and wear in the long term, replacement is best delayed as long as possible so that the joint may outlast the patient. It has been shown from careful long-term studies that loosening is far more likely to occur after wear and it is known that wear particles initiate inflammatory reactions that cause a cytokine response resulting in bone resorption. Bone resorption is associated with loosening. Therefore, joint bearings need to be improved to reduce wear and in consequence loosening. This relationship also explains why young patients wear and loosen their prostheses faster than older low-demand individuals.

Limitations of joint replacement

In the modern era of orthopaedics, the treatment of osteoarthritis is almost synonymous with joint replacement and in the hip joint this is very much the rule. However, it should not be regarded as the only treatment, although clinicians often come under strong pressure from patients, whatever their age, to offer them a 'new joint'. It is not always appreciated that the consequences of early prosthetic failure can be devastating. It is important to appreciate that a hip replacement is an artificial joint not a new transplant and that from the moment it is introduced it begins to wear out. The strategy of replacement should be to provide a joint that outlasts the likely lifespan of the patient. With our current level of knowledge this cannot be guaranteed for the younger patient and so alternatives (e.g. arthrodesis, osteotomy) are still required.

05

Table 41.4 Clinical features of rheumatoid arthritis.

Symptoms
Stiffness: early morning and after inactivity
Pain, tenderness and swelling of joints
Functional impairment, e.g. loss of hand grip strength
Constitutional symptoms, e.g. malaise, tiredness and
 depression

Physical signs
General
Symmetrical joint involvement
Joint swelling and deformity
Muscle wasting around involved joints

Hands (Fig. 41.3)
Matacarpophalangeal joint swelling and subluxation
Proximal interphalangeal joint swelling (spindling)
'Buttonhole' and 'swan neck' deformities of the fingers
Extensor tendon rupture, finger drop
Ulnar deviation of the fingers and hand
Carpal tunnel syndrome

Other joints
Wrists, knees, temporomandibular joint, cervical spine
Atlantoaxial subluxation is a potentially lethal problem

Non-articular manifestations
Skin: rheumatoid nodules
Cardiac: myocarditis, pericarditis
Vascular: vasculitis
Haemopoietic: anaemia, splenomegaly
Pulmonary: fibrosing alveolitis, pleural effusion
Neurological: entrapment neuropathy, e.g. carpal tunnel
 syndrome
Eye: keratoconjunctivitis, episcleritis

Rheumatoid arthritis

Aetiology

Rheumatoid arthritis (RA) is a multisystem disorder of unknown cause. It is a chronic inflammatory disease that predominantly affects synovium. It has some clear links with abnormalities of the immune system (autoantibodies reacting with the patient's own IgG are found in the serum of patients with RA) and there is growing evidence that there may be a genetic abnormality which causes an idiosyncratic reaction to certain infective agents (which is expressed as RA).

Clinical presentation

The most obvious clinical presentation of RA is severe pain, swelling and deformity of the joints (Table 41.4).

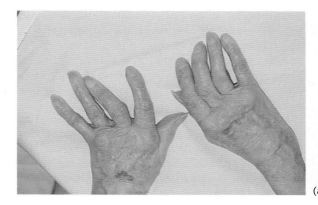
(a)

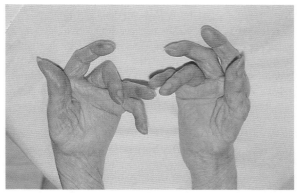
(b)

Figure 41.3 Severe rheumatoid arthritis of the hands: (a) swelling and subluxation of the metacarpophalangeal joints, spindling of the proximal interphalangeal joint and ulnar deviation; (b) joint swelling, muscle wasting and finger deformity.

The principal joints affected are the small joints of the hands and feet and, in a minority, the larger joints. The small joints are affected symmetrically but the larger joints are involved haphazardly. There is no known reason for this. RA may strike at any age and women are more affected than men. Classically it first presents with morning stiffness that improves through the day, in contrast to osteoarthritis.

The disease may also affect the cardiovascular system and can cause myopathies and small-vessel disease. It can also cause pulmonary fibrosis and treatment with steroids can make the skin thin and delicate.

Role of surgery

The role of the surgeon is to make the patient as comfortable as possible while retaining function. Patients with RA are best seen in conjunction with a rheumatologist, who will be responsible for therapeutic care. This is a disease to be tackled by a team.

05

Soft tissues

The rheumatoid process may result in pannus tissue invading tendon sheaths and the tendons themselves. Damage may be limited by removing excessive synovial swelling by synovectomy. This is a good operation at the wrist for extensor tendons. Sometimes tendons about the wrist actually rupture and some sort of repair is needed.

Joints

In early disease it is sometimes possible to reduce pain and stiffness by removing the joint synovium (synovectomy). This is of value in the younger patient who retains movement but who has pain. It is useful at the elbow and wrist, where it may be combined with a limited excision of the joint (excision arthroplasty). This relieves pain but because some joint has been removed there can never be a full return of function.

The surgeon's main role in the management of RA is salvaging function. The goals of surgery are pain relief and return of function. The surgeon must be sure that the chemotherapeutic control of the rheumatoid process is adequate or otherwise doctor and patient may be disappointed. The surgeon should also be sure that the aim of improvement is function and not deformity. This is particularly true in the hands, where even impossibly distorted hands often belie excellent function.

Osteoarthritis and rheumatoid arthritis at a glance

Osteoarthritis

Aetiology
- Largely unknown
- Small proportion can be attributed to primary causes, such as congenital deformities (e.g. developmental hip dysplasia), acquired conditions (Perthes disease) or infection (infective arthritis), or trauma

Presentation
- Degenerative disorder presenting with pain and related loss of function
- Any joint (single, bilateral or multilpe) may be involved
- Clinicians must make a careful assessment of history and examination to assess severity of symptoms

Radiographic changes
- Loss of joint space
- Osteophyte and cyst formation
- Subchondral sclerosis

Management
Conservative
- Correct use of drugs, including NSAIDS and purer analgesics
- Weight loss
- Use of stick (lower limb)
- Physiotherapy to maintain mobility and muscle fitness

Surgery
- Operative measures are preceded by a historical, physical and sociological assessment to ensure patients gain maximum benefit from any surgery
- Optimal results are obtained in older less active patients
- In most cases surgery means joint replacement
- Clinicians must be aware of alternatives, including osteotomy and fusion, especially in younger and higher-demand patients

Rheumatoid arthritis

Aetiology
- Chronic inflammatory disorder with a genetically linked immuno-incompetence element

Presentation
- Symmetrical disease primarily affecting the small joints of hands and feet
- Occasionally affects major joints such as hip and knee
- Early symptoms associated with morning stiffness and pain

Radiographic changes
- Normally first seen in the small joints of the hands and feet
- Associated with narrow joint spaces, osteopenia and periarticular joint erosions

Management
Conservative
- Rest and heat for acute episodes associated with carefully planned physiotherapy and remedial therapy to maintain residual function

Surgery
- Surgery is reserved for end-stage disease and appropriate strategic repair (e.g. ruptured tendons, entrapment neuropathies)
- Surgery consists of either repair or ultimately joint arthroplasty
- Arthroplasty, though suitable for RA, is associated with significant short-term morbidity and complications, but in the long term is as effective in lower-demand patients with significant disease

05

Avascular necrosis

Aetiology

Bone tissue death through loss of blood supply is found in certain circumstances throughout the body. In some cases the cause is clearly traceable to an anatomical source on which a secondary event is superimposed. Quite often avascular necrosis occurs spontaneously for no apparent reason. Studies using magnetic resonance imaging (MRI) have shown that bone oedema is associated with increased metaplasia of cells in the bone, forming fat rather than bone, and this in turn leads to mechanical failure of the weakened bone.

Post-traumatic avascular necrosis

Certain sites where the anatomical blood supply is unusual are at risk following trauma. These include the femoral head, the proximal part of the scaphoid in the wrist and the proximal part of the talus. In these situations, trauma cuts an otherwise good if rather awkward blood supply. In femoral neck fractures, the damage to the capsular blood vessels puts the head at risk; in the other two sites, a distal blood supply is severed from the proximal part of the bone.

Idiopathic avascular necrosis

In other areas, such as the lunate, avascular necrosis occurs in less obvious circumstances. Avascular necrosis of the head of the femur is seen following chronic alcohol abuse, high-dose steroid therapy and in deep-sea divers (decompression sickness). Cause and effect in these diverse associations remain a mystery but is associated with increased fat deposition in bone as described above. The patient presents with acute and often severe joint pain that is exacerbated by movement and to some degree relieved by rest. With the passage of time, symptoms become indistinguishable from osteoarthritis.

Investigations

Avascular necrosis may be reversed if a blood supply can be re-established. However, in the revascularizing phase the bone is very soft and prone to distortion, with secondary arthritic changes. Diagnosis can be very difficult. Initially there are no radiological changes but later the bone appears dense, reflecting the absence of blood vessels. Technetium bone scanning shows a reduction in uptake of isotope. However, with the advent of MRI avascular necrosis can be diagnosed sooner and monitored more closely.

Management

Treatment is non-specific. The spectrum of severity of the disease is now understood to be wide due to the value of MRI as a monitoring tool. The natural cycle is for the bone to eventually revascularize and remodel. In the revascularization phase the bone is very soft and susceptible to distortion, resulting in joint incongruity and onset of secondary arthritis. If possible, the affected joint should be rested. Surgery is of no value in treating the underlying condition and often the surgeon is left to salvage the situation with a joint replacement. As such patients are usually very young this is highly problematical.

Crystal arthropathies

In these conditions crystals of body products are deposited in the joints on the surface of the articular cartilage and within the synovial fluid. They cause chronic degenerative change in the joint and may be a cause of secondary arthritis. They also cause acute inflammatory episodes, which are generally self-limiting.

Gout

Gout is caused by urate crystal deposition. Urate is a product of nucleic acid metabolism. It becomes deposited in circumstances such as dehydration (particularly post surgery) and after chemotherapy with antimetabolites for malignancy. The most common cause in western societies is probably the injudicious overuse of diuretics.

Gout presents with a hot, tender and swollen joint. Any joint can be affected but it is seen commonly in the knee and the hallux. It is important to exclude infection early in the differential diagnosis. Diagnosis is made by the presence of a high uric acid in the blood and more accurately by the presence of birefringence urate crystals in joint fluid aspirated on admission. It may be treated using indomethacin in the relatively high dose of 50 mg three times a day. Chronic gout may be controlled with allopurinol.

Pseudogout

Pseudogout may mimic gout but usually has a less acute presentation. In this case the cause is the deposition of pyrophosphate, the origin of which is obscure. Chronic crystal arthropathy of this kind classically causes calcification of joint surfaces and the menisci in the knee. Symptoms may be controlled with anti-inflammatory drugs but long-term degeneration is likely.

Septic arthritis

Acute septic arthritis
Aetiology
Acute septic arthritis is usually blood-borne in origin, often originating from a distal site of trivial infection. It may come from an adjacent infected bone, especially in children where a metaphyseal site may be within a joint capsule; this is notably so at the hip. Very rarely it may occur from direct penetration of the joint. Three groups are at risk:
- children;
- immunosuppressed adults;
- anyone with chronic degenerative joint disorders.

Clinical presentation
In children, septic arthritis usually presents with a nasty acute illness and the child is unwell with a high fever. The affected joint is held stiff and is hot and tender. The most frequent causative organism in this group is *Staph. aureus*. In contrast, the other patient groups often present with a much less florid picture. The immunosuppressed or the chronically abnormal joint may give a false impression of a minor upset. The patient remains unwell for many days before presenting with a septicaemia, which is often difficult to ascribe to any source. Many of these patients die because of the delay in recognizing the condition. Beware also of the child on an intercurrent antibiotic as symptoms may also be blunted. In the relatively rare instance of a young adult presenting with septic arthritis, often with little constitutional upset, the most likely cause is gonococcus.

Management
Treatment consists of surgery and intravenous antibiotics. The joint should be opened and all loculated compartments broken down and irrigated. Antibiotics should be given according to culture. In children, the first-guess antibiotic should be an antistaphylococcal agent as this is still the most likely infecting organism. In adults, penicillin should be given intravenously to cover the risk of gonococcal infection. If treatment is not instigated immediately, apart from the risk of septicaemia, the articular cartilage is at great risk and may undergo lysis, leading to fibrous or even bony fusion of the joint.

Chronic septic arthritis
Aetiology
Tuberculosis is still an important cause of joint infection worldwide and recently has seen a resurgence in patients with acquired immunodeficiency syndrome (AIDS). Joint tuberculosis is acquired from blood-borne spread and there is a strong relationship between urinary and joint tuberculosis.

Clinical presentation
The clinical picture is of chronic malaise, weight loss and marked muscle wasting around the affected joint. The radiographs show highly characteristic loss of bone density.

Management
Treatment is by chemotherapy and only rarely is surgery necessary. Combinations of drugs such as ethambutol and rifampicin are given for many months.

Knee problems

Clinical presentation

Knee problems may present as chronic discomfort or as acute lesions, which commonly have a background of chronic trouble or a previous injury. The cardinal symptoms of knee pathology are:
- swelling;
- locking;
- giving way;
- pain.

All these features may be elicited as physical signs. A useful sign of significant knee pathology is wasting of the quadriceps muscle, which may be seen easily if the patient is asked to actively extend the leg.

Swelling

Information regarding the onset of swelling relative to an episode of pain or an accident is valuable. A rapid accumulation of fluid suggests bleeding, while a less dramatic and slower build-up of fluid (over hours or days) suggests an effusion of synovial fluid. A chronic and boggy swelling that never changes indicates a synovitis.

Locking

This is a symptom which must always be probed. Most patients use the term when they mean painful stiffness, often occurring on movement after rest in a sitting position. True locking is an inability to extend the knee fully due to a painful mechanical block, commonly caused by a torn meniscus, a loose body or, more rarely, a torn cruciate ligament. In contrast to painful stiffness, flexion is nearly always possible without pain in the locked knee.

Giving way

This means that the patient is unable to maintain the knee in extension and when weight is applied to the leg, the knee simply flexes and the patient may fall. This is similar to locking in that it suggests a painful block to movement that causes reciprocal quadriceps inhibition and so loss of active extension in the flexed knee. A slight jerk on descending stairs is suggestive of an internal ligamentous injury to the cruciates.

Pain

Pain may be linked to any of the above symptoms. Unremitting pain, worse on exercise and eventually causing loss of sleep, may indicate a degenerative knee disorder.

Meniscal lesions

Aetiology and patterns

The medial meniscus is generally more frequently torn than the lateral. The meniscus may be torn at its peripheral attachment to the joint capsule or within its substance. The meniscus may split horizontally (so-called cleavage lesion), which is very common in old age and may not generally be important. Occasionally, these cleavage lesions act like flap valves and allow build-up of synovial fluid within the meniscus; this forms a cyst. Common pathological tears within the substance of the meniscus are in the vertical plane and can be either a split off one end of the meniscus ('parrot beak') or a vertical split anchored at both ends ('bucket handle').

Clinical presentation

Although seen in both sexes, meniscal lesions are relatively rare in women. Although not common, it is well to remember that they can occur in adolescents. Occasionally, children are born with an abnormal discoid lateral meniscus. They present with pain, effusion, sometimes with locking and/or giving way. Their tenderness is poorly localized on examination, although generalized discomfort may be elicited by gently but forcibly extending the knee.

Management

The meniscus is an important structure and as much of it as possible should be preserved to help in distributing the load between femur and tibia. Peripheral tears can be reattached with sutures. Substance tears have no apparent

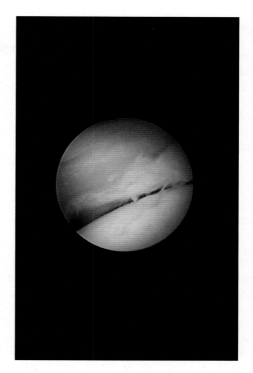

Figure 41.4 Arthroscopic view of a knee joint.

capacity to repair and so the torn peripheral part should be removed, usually by arthroscopy. Once there is strong clinical suspicion of a meniscal tear the patient should undergo arthroscopy. This usually means that a combination of all or most of the cardinal features of knee pathology, especially locking with effusion, should be present. If only one or two features are present but clinical suspicion remains high, MRI will exclude significant pathology. Arthroscopy should be reserved for cases with high expectation of a need for surgical intervention and not used simply as a diagnostic tool (Fig. 41.4).

Most meniscal lesions can now be removed via an arthroscope, although some require a small arthrotomy. The principal advantage of arthroscopic meniscectomy is that most patients recover from it within a few days or weeks. Open meniscectomy has a much more prolonged period of rehabilitation.

Loose bodies

Aetiology

In a knee injury small fragments of cartilage and bone (osteochondral fragments) may be sheared off into the

joint space to become loose bodies. The original injury may be remembered by the patient because the knee probably became swollen from associated bleeding (haemarthrosis). The osteochondral fragment is often not resorbed but survives floating free in the joint, obtaining its nutrition from the synovial fluid. The bulk, if not all, of the loose body is cartilage and so it may be radiolucent.

Clinical presentation

Months or years after a knee injury the patient presents with locking, pain and giving way. Often there is a knee effusion.

Management

Loose bodies are a nuisance and should be removed, preferably via the arthroscope. Very rarely in adolescents osteochondral fragments occur spontaneously, a condition known as osteochondritis dissecans. Such a condition tends to settle spontaneously but loose bodies may require removal.

Cruciate ligament injury

Aetiology

The cruciate ligaments are not capable of spontaneous healing because their nutrient vessels pass within their substance and are damaged at the time of the tear, except in rare circumstances when they are pulled off with a fragment of bone. Even then the fragment must be replaced surgically. The cruciate ligament is commonly injured by either hyperextension or a twist, often in association with a foot being anchored by a studded boot or a ski.

Clinical presentation

In the acute injury the knee swells quickly, indicating a haemarthrosis brought on by active bleeding from the end-artery in the cruciate ligament. Sometimes the patient reports feeling a 'pop', which is the ligament tearing. The swelling eventually resolves and it is only after a few weeks that the chronic problems arise. Loss of a cruciate leads to loss of anteroposterior stability, particularly in flexion. Thus, difficulty in going up or coming down stairs is a common symptom. There is also loss of rotatory stability when twisting and turning, making cruciate injury particularly disabling for athletes. Interestingly, however, not all patients have symptoms, a fact for which there is no explanation at present. Many patients only experience symptoms when involved in the sort of activities described above.

Management

In general, cruciate ligament injuries should be left untreated for a while and the knee muscles rehabilitated. Only if symptoms interfere with daily life or the patient demands it should treatment be offered. This consists of replacement of the torn ligament with a prosthesis or tendon transfer using part of the patella tendon or the biceps. The prosthetic ligaments have a dubious lifespan. Certainly, if patients persist in vigorous activity, the insensitive prosthetic ligament is likely to fail. At the moment most surgeons favour tendon transfer as a substitute for a deficient cruciate ligament.

Soft-tissue injuries to the collateral ligaments of the knee heal spontaneously and are treated by limiting motion through the use of braces. These prevent flexion but also prevent full extension when collateral ligaments are maximally loaded. In general, there is no need to openly repair ligaments and controlled active motion stimulates good collagen-based natural repair.

Dislocation of the patella

Aetiology

This condition is usually associated with a malformation of either the patella or the lateral femoral condyle. This leads to lateral maltracking, which is itself painful.

Clinical presentation

In some patients spontaneous dislocation of the patella and failure of the extensor apparatus occur. The net result is that the patient falls to the ground. This is usually associated with a haemarthrosis or effusion. Once it has occurred then recurrence, especially where the knee is not normally formed, is likely.

Management

A single dislocation may be treated by rest and splintage. Recurrence is more problematic and sometimes a medial refining of the vastus medialis may be required and, once growth has ceased, the patellar tendon may be resited more medially on the tibia. This condition should not be confused with anterior knee pain, often seen in adolescence particularly in girls. This condition is poorly understood and best left alone, as most cases settle spontaneously.

05

Knee problems at a glance

Clinical presentation
- Elicit by history and examination
- Cardinal signs and symptoms: locking, wasting, swelling and giving way
- Remember that history will give a clear report of likely recent or not so recent trauma

Meniscal lesions
- Commoner in men than women
- Associated with most of the cardinal signs and symptoms
- Usually related to trauma but can be associated with degeneration
- Requires early attention if causing locking and giving way
- Investigate by MRI if moderate suspicion
- Arthroscopy reserved for high suspicion where the procedure results in surgical intervention as well as confirming diagnosis

Cruciate ligament injuries
- Seen in trauma caused by skiing or football for example
- Complete tears result in loss of ligament because blood supply is within the substance of the ligament
- Reconstruction through substitution reserved for symptomatic patients
- Most common method of substitution is with patellar tendon graft

Anterior knee pain
- Common in adolescent girls
- Not amenable to surgical solutions
- Vast majority (but not all) settle with time

Patellar dislocation
- Usually associated with congenital dysplasia of patella and/or lateral femoral condyle
- Single dislocation managed by splintage and rest
- Multiple dislocations often follow and may require reconstructive surgery

Backache and neckache

It is no exaggeration to suggest that everyone will get backache or neckache at some time during their lives. This is often attributed to the fact that humans walk upright. However, we know that quadrupeds also get backache and so there must be an alternative explanation. Although common, most backache is usually self-limiting and so in that sense is not serious. Unfortunately, it is difficult to tell the small number of patients with serious back problems from the majority of minor aches and sprains; the result is that all are often extensively investigated in order to identify the minority with serious pathology.

Inappropriate investigation and management of back pain may create a new category of back sufferer: those who think they have a serious problem. Consider the scenario in which a patient presents with backache which lasts for a few weeks. The patient is referred to a hospital, thus reinforcing in his or her mind the possibility that the condition may be serious. The hospital doctor arranges a whole gamut of investigations, confirming the patient's worst fears. On a return visit the patient sees another doctor who orders more tests or even institutes empirical treatment. Now the cycle is almost complete: pain, some tests, treatment, more tests, more treatment, and so on. In this situation the patient concludes that the pain must be significant and it grows in importance; as the patient does not 'respond to treatment', all is reinforced and unwittingly doctor and patient collude in what is known as illness behaviour. This section is about learning to distinguish significant from insignificant back pain and so prevent the onset of illness behaviour.

Anatomical considerations

The vertebral column consists of bony, muscular and ligamentous elements and neurological tissue that takes advantage of the bony protection afforded by the vertebrae. The non-neurological tissues are termed 'spondylitides' and abnormalities of these tissues are rather crudely termed 'spondylitis'. Abnormalities can occur only in the spondylitides or, very rarely, only in the nerve tissue. Not uncommonly, structural abnormalities may lead to abnormalities in the nerve tissue due to compression, which may affect the spinal cord itself or, more commonly, the nerve roots.

Pain in spinal disorders

Pain may occur locally or be referred or may occur along the distribution of nerves.

Local pain

In general, pain is fairly poorly localized in the back. It tends to be related to a whole region, such as the lumbar or dorsal regions, and it is unusual to be any more specific.

Referred pain

The picture may be further complicated by referred pain from the back to the buttock and leg, or from the neck to the shoulder and arm. Other chapters have shown that

abdominal pain can represent referred pain from other parts of the body and this is of use in reaching a diagnosis. In contrast, when considering pain in the vertebral column, referred pain can be confusing and difficult to discern from root pain (see later). Leg pain occurring in the buttock and thigh and descending to the mid-calf is usually referred pain and is associated with a mechanical and poorly localized spondylitic disorder. Neck pain that radiates to the shoulder and upper arm is usually referred in a similar way, although this feature is less specific in the neck compared with the lumbar spine.

Nerve root pain

The nerve roots emerge from the vertebral foramina, which are in part bordered by the facet joints behind and the disc in front. Diseases of these structures may affect the nerve roots by direct pressure, inflammation or oedema. The brain interprets such disturbances as pain in the distribution of the affected spinal nerve. This commonly happens in lower lumbar foramina and so the nerve distribution of pain perception follows the sciatic nerve and hence gives origin to the term 'sciatica'. Sciatica is characterized by pain in the leg, mainly down the back but almost always into the foot. It may be exacerbated by coughing as this activity increases intrathecal pressure.

In the cervical spine, the mid to lower foramina are commonly affected and so hand and forearm pain, often associated with tingling, is characteristic. Both in the lumbar and cervical spines it is easy to see how referred pain and root pain may be confused. It should be noted that, in general, root pain is much rarer than referred pain. If the nerve root is significantly compromised, then localizing signs may be elicited and these may be sensory or motor.

Cauda equina syndrome

Cauda equina syndrome is rare but very important. It is due to central pressure on the cauda equina. This is commonly associated with a prolapsed disc, although tumours, particularly secondary neoplasms, may also cause this problem. The pressure on the cauda causes bowel and bladder disturbances, usually urinary retention, often with overflow incontinence. These symptoms should be positively excluded by direct questioning and whenever root entrapment is suspected a rectal examination should be routine in order to test anal tone. This condition is a real emergency and urgent investigation and surgery are mandatory if these important visceral functions are to be preserved.

Common causes of back pain

The common causes of back pain are listed in Table 41.5.

Table 41.5 Common causes of back pain.

Related to the spondylitides
  Aches and sprains
  Mechanical back pain
  Spondylolisthesis
  Ankylosing spondylitis
Entrapment neuropathies
  Discogenic
  Bony root entrapment
Neurological and support tissues
Tumours and space-occupying lesions
Arachnoiditis
Other visceral causes
  Urinary tract infection
  Leaking aortic aneurysm
  Duodenal ulcers
  Pancreatic lesions

Many of the visceral disorders can be excluded by taking a good history and by examining the patient. Some of the rarer pathologies, particularly tumours, are relatively easy to miss, often because they are not considered. Progressive signs and unremitting symptoms should alert the clinician to a neoplastic pathology.

Back sprains
Aetiology
As mentioned earlier, almost everyone will suffer from an episode of back pain at some time in their lives. Most are associated with ill-advised manoeuvres or poor lifting, which causes muscle or ligament injuries. These conditions should be separated from neurological causes by the absence of signs of nerve tension or compression.

Management
Back sprains require a brief period of rest followed by a gradual return to normal activities. NSAIDs aid in the relief of symptoms, although simple analgesia is usually sufficient. These conditions are common but must not be taken lightly should the doctor be consulted. A careful exclusion of significant pathology should be followed by a proper explanation in order to prevent the development of an illness cycle. Only one or at the most two visits to a clinic should be encouraged.

Mechanical backache

This is often difficult to discern from acute sprain episodes, except that mechanical backache is chronic or often consists of a series of acute exacerbations against a background of less significant chronic discomfort.

05

Aetiology

The cause of mechanical back problems is unknown, although as the name implies it is a non-neurological entity. Confusion may arise if referred leg pain is one of the presenting symptoms; difficulty may also arise in middle-aged patients, a minority of whom develop genuine root signs. Suggested causes include disc degeneration leading to increased loading and secondary osteoarthritis of facet joints. Primary arthritis of the facet joints has been implicated but there are probably many other factors, such as ligament or muscle pathology, that have yet to be determined.

Management

Recurring episodes of back pain are the norm for this condition. It is important to explain this to patients and reassure them that though the condition is chronic it does not deteriorate. There is no known cure for mechanical back pain and judicious use of rest, physiotherapy and medication will help the patient through a bad episode.

Most patients learn to live with their bad back and how to prevent recurrences. Support should be provided by general practitioners, with occasional interjections by specialists. Regular hospital review is to be discouraged, provided the general practitioner has access to support services. Physiotherapists may be of great value in providing such support. Alternative medical practitioners such as osteopaths and chiropractors can provide both time to listen and some ease by manipulation. However, it is important that everyone concerned, including the patient, understands the pathology and that the uncertain nature of the condition is kept in perspective.

Spondylolisthesis

This is a not uncommon finding on radiographs of patients presenting with back pain. The term refers to the slippage of one vertebra relative to another and is commonly seen in the lumbar spine. It is caused by an abnormality in the posterior complex of the spine that interferes with the stability of the facet joints and their associated bony and ligamentous elements.

Aetiology

Spondylolisthesis may be congenital or acquired and it is important to realize that it may present at any age, including infancy. Adult spondylolisthesis is thought to be acquired, although some may be late-presenting and mild congenital abnormalities. The mechanism of acquisition appears to be an acute, or more likely a fatigue, fracture of the pars interarticularis, which is that part of the neural arch linking the superior and inferior facets of any vertebrae.

Clinical presentation

The patient presents with low back pain almost identical to mechanical back pain. Diagnosis is nearly always made on X-ray, although in severe slippage a step may be felt at the affected level. Oblique films should be requested if spondylolisthesis is suspected, as these more clearly show the facets and their connecting bony bridges. Very rarely will the patient present with neurological deficit. Congenital spondylolisthesis is an exception and the stability may be so insecure as to threaten neurological structures.

Management

Surprisingly, most patients do not require surgery and decisions to operate depend almost entirely on the severity of the symptoms. A spinal support that offloads the spine by increasing intra-abdominal pressure may help. Otherwise the patient may be managed conservatively, rather like the sufferer of mechanical back pain.

The pars defect may be seen on the radiograph without a slip. This is known as *spondylolysis*. The significance of this finding should be viewed with caution as it may not be the cause of the pain. Such patients will usually respond to conservative measures, but severe pain may require spinal fusion.

Ankylosing spondylitis

This is a rare disease affecting men in early adulthood and usually presenting before 30 years of age. The spine is predominantly affected but major joints, particularly the hips, may also be affected. The patient presents with general back pain, tiredness and malaise. Early morning stiffness is common. Investigations show a high erythrocyte sedimentation rate and the presence of HLA-B27 in most patients. The natural history is of progressive stiffness and ultimately bony fusion of the whole of the spine. Patients need to be kept mobile and with good posture. Symptoms respond to NSAIDs. The major joints may require replacement.

Entrapment neuropathies
Prolapsed intervertebral disc (Fig. 41.5)

It is essential from the outset to allay the commonly held view in the general population that most back and leg ache is caused by a 'slipped disc'. This is a relatively rare condition and in any case the disc does not 'slip' but rather the disc contents prolapse.

Disc prolapse was first described in the late 1940s but first became a popular diagnosis in the early 1960s. It is true to say that since then the diagnosis has become somewhat overused. Disc prolapse may occur in the lumbar or cervical spine but the description below assumes that the condition is in the lumbar spine.

AETIOLOGY

The cause of symptoms is an abnormality in the interver-

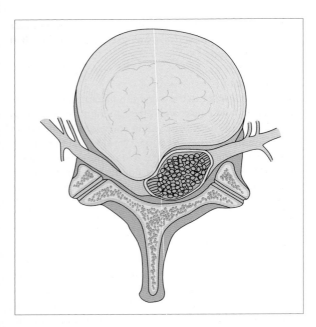

Figure 41.5 Schematic drawing illustrating disc tissue displacement (protrusion) resulting in nerve root compression and displacement of the spinal cord.

tebral disc that leads to prolapse of the nucleus pulposus through the surrounding annulus fibrosus with impingement on the spinal contents. If the prolapsed material passes backwards and laterally it impinges on the nerve roots, while posterior prolapse results in cord or cauda equina compression. The discs between the sacrum and the fifth lumbar vertebra are most commonly affected and the condition occurs with decreasing frequency further up the lumbar spine. Disc prolapse often presents with 'sciatica' as the nerve roots most frequently compressed are those forming the sciatic nerve. However, prolapse may occur at higher lumbar levels and may be perceived as pain in the distribution of the femoral nerve. Large centrally prolapsing discs can lead to the cauda equina syndrome (see earlier) and the patient may present with bowel or bladder incontinence.

CLINICAL PRESENTATION

The classical symptoms occur in people under 40 years old in either sex. The condition presents acutely with backache and leg ache or sometimes with leg ache alone, with backache developing later. Patients may describe a single event of lifting or strain, although there is no known correlation between cause and condition; it may arise spontaneously. The characteristic symptom is of leg ache passing down the back of the thigh and leg to the foot. This is in contrast to referred backache, which usually goes no further than the knee or upper calf.

On examination, the features of nerve root irritation may be present; straight-leg raising will be restricted and there may be tenderness on compressing the nerve (see Fig. 41.5). There may or may not be localizing signs. A rectal examination is essential to assess sphincter tone if there is any history of bowel or bladder abnormalities.

MANAGEMENT

First, central disc compression has to be excluded. The patient may then be treated by a combination of rest and gentle progressive mobilization. Analgesics and anti-inflammatory drugs may aid in symptom relief. Bedrest should be for a minimum period and traction only used to enforce rest – it will not materially alter the condition. It should be emphasized that with time most disc prolapses will resolve spontaneously. If symptoms do not relapse after about 6 weeks, pain is uncontrolled or localizing neurological signs progress, then the patient should be investigated with a view to surgery. A radiculogram is a contrast study where radiopaque contrast medium is injected into the thecal space and any occupying lesion will be highlighted. Computed tomography (CT) at the same time also gives useful information. However, MRI has replaced CT and radiculography as investigation of first choice, with CT being seen as complementary when there is thought to be a bony problem (see later).

Bony root entrapment neuropathy

In contrast to disc prolapse, this condition has been ignored until fairly recently. It has come to significance through the improved imaging techniques described above.

AETIOLOGY

The cause of the condition is commonly due to bony overgrowth around the vertebral foramina where the nerve roots emerge. The cause of the bony overgrowth would appear to be secondary to degenerative changes in the adjacent facet joints. These may degenerate from primary osteoarthritis or secondarily subsequent to disc degeneration (not prolapse!).

CLINICAL PRESENTATION

The clinical syndrome consists of a previous history of backache of a mechanical type occurring in a person of either sex, usually aged over 40 years. These patients are usually known back sufferers but develop new symptoms of leg pain radiating to the foot, usually exacerbated by exercise. Such a syndrome is rather poorly named 'spinal claudication', although it may indeed be confused with vascular disease. Episodes are usually acute and recurrent against a chronic history of back pain. The episodes may remain mild or may progress to affect the patient's lifestyle. Remedial therapy is unlikely to help and, should symptoms be severe, they should then be referred for surgery.

05

MANAGEMENT
Removal of the disc in such patients may make the condition worse and removal of bone is needed to free trapped nerve roots. This may destabilize the spine and lead to a need to fuse it. The decision to operate is entirely determined by the severity of the patient's symptoms.

Cervical spine disorders

The cervical spine is a very mobile part of the vertebral column and it is no surprise to find it prone to disease and injury. Most conditions are exactly analogous to those found in the lumbar spine.

Cervical spondylosis

This is very like the degenerative disc and joint disease seen in the lumbar spine and the aetiology, as far as any is understood, is the same.

Clinical presentation
The patient is usually over 40 years old and is more frequently female than male. The patient presents with dull neckache and this is often referred to the shoulders and upper arms. The tingling in the arms is often assumed to be an entrapment of nerve roots but this is not always confirmed on investigation. However, the spondylitic process can be progressive and bony root entrapment may occur, with localizing neurological signs. These signs may be confused with local nerve entrapments. Nerve conduction studies or even cervical myelography may be useful in making the diagnosis.

Management
Without localizing nerve signs the patient simply needs NSAIDs, a soft collar and physiotherapy, which helps spasm. Patients need counselling and a good explanation of the condition. They need to be warned that the natural history, as in the lumbar spine, is for acute episodic recurrence. If root entrapment is confirmed, then surgical intervention with anterior fusion and decompression may be indicated if symptoms cannot otherwise be controlled.

Cervical disc prolapse

Although not as frequent, cervical disc disease presents with a similar pattern to that of the lumbar spine. The lower cervical discs are most likely to cause the problem. Pain and referral are similar to spondylitic pain. The differential diagnosis can be difficult, although disc sufferers tend to have no previous history of neck trouble and characteristically the neck muscles are in more spasm following disc prolapse and the associated stiffness is severe. Most patients recover with a cervical collar or gentle traction. If localizing signs are marked or symptoms do not regress, then surgery and fusion of the affected segment may be necessary.

Back pain at a glance

Aetiology
- Back pain is extremely common
- Caused by local mechanical problems in ligaments, muscles, joints and through disc degeneration
- In a minority, back pain involves associated spinal tissue especially nerve roots
- Disc prolapse as a cause of nerve root entrapment is commoner in younger and early middle-aged people
- Nerve root problems in later life are associated with disc degeneration and bony outgrowths from degenerate facet joints

Symptoms
- Key to diagnosis is to elicit careful history and examination to differentiate between mechanical back pain and associated nerve root involvement
- Symptoms of low back pain can be felt in the back or the leg as far as the knee
- Similar referred pain from the neck can be felt in the shoulder and upper arm
- Leg pain below the knee going into the foot is likely to be nerve root pain
- Similarly, hand pain is likely to be either local nerve or neck root entrapment pain

Investigations
- MRI is the investigation of first choice in spinal problems suspected of involving nerve roots
- CT is complementary when the predominant problem is bony
- Plain radiography is of limited value

Management
- Most back pain will resolve spontaneously
- In nerve root conditions caused by prolapsed discs, the vast majority resolve without the need for surgery
- Surgery is reserved for intractable pain and increasing signs of sensory change and weakness
- Presence of urinary tract or bowel signs and symptoms require urgent investigation and surgical intervention if indicated

Minor adult disorders

In many ways the term 'minor' does some injustice to the conditions discussed here. It is important to appreciate that these conditions are common and will be of sufficient severity to cause considerable inconvenience and discomfort to the patient and may have important social and economic consequences. They are minor in the sense that many are self-limiting in their natural history and many have non-surgical solutions. They all need care in assessment and management, as it is possible to make people worse by casual or inaccurate management.

Enthesopathies

'Enthesis' is the term given to the short fibrous origin of a muscle and so 'enthesopathy' refers to an inflammation of a muscle origin. Common sites of enthesopathies include:
● common flexor muscle origin of the forearm (*golfer's elbow*);
● common extensor origin of the forearm (*tennis elbow*). The patient often complains of quite severe discomfort on using the affected muscle. It is possible that many entheses may be inflamed at one time, giving rise to many aches and pains. The common enthesopathies around the elbow may arise spontaneously, although they are commonly associated with repetitive movements or overuse. The prognosis is generally favourable, especially if there is a clear cause and rest will result in spontaneous recovery.

Occasionally, the condition may become chronic or be severe enough to warrant intervention. Recovery may be speeded up with a course of anti-inflammatory agents. Local steroid injections into the point of maximum tenderness can also be of value. Care must be taken to ensure that the steroid is injected into the enthesis, with no leakage into the subcutaneous fat or skin as otherwise the pain may be exacerbated and the patient left with an unsightly atrophic dimple. A very small number of patients require surgery, which consists of scraping the origin of the muscle from the bone, permitting it to slide distally and so decompress the area. If possible, patients should be encouraged to wait, as the long-term chance of spontaneous recovery is high.

Nerve entrapment syndromes

All nerves are sensitive to compression. Continued pressure will lead to *neuropraxia* and, if not relieved, atrophy of the nerve. At best such injury takes a very long time to recover and usually recovery is not complete. Therefore early diagnosis and management are likely to give the best results.

Nerve entrapments may be extrinsic to the body or intrinsic. Extrinsic causes include accidents where consciousness is lost and the victim inadvertently presses on a nerve (e.g. compression of the radial nerve between the humerus and the arm or back of a chair during inebriated sleep). Patients in bed, on the operating table and in plaster casts are at risk from pressure on nerves in exposed sites. The most common site at risk is the common peroneal nerve as it winds around the head of the fibula.

Most nerve entrapments, however, are intrinsic and common sites include:
● median nerve at the wrist (carpal tunnel syndrome);
● ulnar nerve at the elbow (ulnar neuritis);
● ulnar nerve at the wrist;
● posterior tibial nerve at the ankle (tarsal tunnel syndrome).

Carpal tunnel syndrome (median nerve entrapment at the wrist)
Aetiology
The median nerve supplies the intrinsic muscles of the thumb and sensory fibres to the volar surface of the hand and radial three-and-a-half fingers. The sensation to the palm is provided by a small branch passing over the flexor retinaculum at the wrist but the bulk of the nerve passes under the retinaculum through the carpal tunnel. Anything that limits the space in the carpal tunnel will compress the nerve and give rise to symptoms. Most causes of carpal tunnel syndrome remain obscure but a number of specific aetiologies are recognized.
● Trauma: following wrist fractures and dislocations.
● Pregnancy: associated with fluid retention.
● RA: linked to space occupation by granulation tissue.

Clinical presentation
Classical symptoms include numbness and tingling in the sensory distribution of the nerve, associated with certain positions of the wrist, worse at night. Patients are often woken and have to dangle the wrist and shake it to relieve the discomfort. The cause of this classical symptom is unknown. In later stages patients also complain of weakness of grip, clumsiness and a tendency to drop objects. Examination can be normal, although the symptoms may be reproduced by flexing the wrist and holding it for a few seconds. In 25% of cases the reverse manoeuvre may be required to reproduce the phenomenon. In more advanced cases the thenar eminence may be seen to be wasted and sensory changes associated with dry skin may be observed. Remember that sensation to the palmar branch will be preserved and this will distinguish compression at the wrist from compression from a more proximal source.

Nerve conduction studies
Generally, investigations are not necessary; occasionally, however, the clinician may be confused by symptoms of

05

discomfort more proximal to the wrist that occur for obscure reasons. In these cases nerve conduction studies tend to be unequivocal and will distinguish between nerve root and peripheral nerve problems.

Management

Management will depend on the cause. In the case of trauma, fractures require reduction but the nerve may still have to be decompressed by dividing the flexor retinaculum. In the case of pregnancy this is a self-limiting condition that may be relieved temporarily by conservative measures (described below). In RA, the compression of the nerve is but one feature of a complex problem that may need a radical solution, including synovectomy and wrist joint fusion.

In most cases where a cause is not apparent, surgery will be the treatment of choice if there are signs of nerve dysfunction. Surgery consists of decompressing the nerve by dividing the flexor retinaculum at the wrist and into the palm. In less severe cases, temporary splintage of the wrist in a 'cock-up' position is often adequate and certainly helps confirm the diagnosis. Some advocate steroid injections, although the results are mixed. Surgery consists of division of the flexor retinaculum but one should be aware that a significant percentage are not completely relieved and patients should be warned of this possibility.

Ulnar neuritis (ulnar nerve entrapment at the elbow)

Aetiology

The nerve is compromised by stretching and/or compression for a number of reasons. The nerve may be irritated by repeated trauma, as is sometimes seen in those using crutches. It may also be stretched by abnormal growth or malunion following elbow fractures. The nerve can be entrapped by a tough fibrous band as it passes between the two origins of flexor carpi ulnaris. Generally, however, most cases are of unknown cause.

Clinical presentation

Symptoms reflect the course and function of the ulnar nerve distally. Tingling in the little finger is common and loss of intrinsic muscle function in the hand ensues, with consequent lack of fine finger movement. Examination reveals tenderness, often quite exquisite, of the nerve on the medial side of the elbow. Dryness of the skin on the medial (ulnar) border of the hand and sensory changes are early features. Small-muscle wasting is a serious sign and is indicative of a poor prognosis. Once present, this condition tends to persist and once signs are elicited it is unlikely that they will be completely reversed, even with treatment. Decompression transposition of the nerve to

the front of the elbow is always recommended as this will usually halt the progress but, as implied above, rarely reverses it. It is important to distinguish ulnar neuritis from an enthesopathy and although this is usually easy with a proper history and examination, nerve conduction studies will be definitive.

Ulnar entrapment at the wrist

Although less common than median nerve compression, this condition may occur often in combination with median nerve entrapment. This is particularly so in RA and trauma. The nerve passes through its own tunnel at the wrist and so will require particular attention at surgery.

Tarsal tunnel syndrome (posterior tibial nerve entrapment at the ankle)

This is a rare condition and generally overdiagnosed. The posterior tibial nerve becomes entrapped as it passes beneath the retinaculum behind the medial malleolus. This causes foot pain, particularly at the heel, and can be confused with plantar fasciitis. It may be differentiated by testing sensation of the heel and is commonly accompanied by fasciculation of the medial plantar muscles. Nerve conduction studies are not reliable and surgery should be reserved for patients with the clinical signs described above.

Neuropathy at a glance

- Nerves are squashed rather than stretched and if treated appropriately have the capacity to fully recover
- Common neuropathies:
  - (a) median nerve at the wrist (carpal tunnel syndrome)
  - (b) ulnar nerve at the elbow (ulnar neuritis)
  - (c) ulnar nerve at the wrist
  - (d) posterior tibial nerve at the ankle (tarsal tunnel syndrome)
- History is important and clinical signs may be minimal but if present indicate significant problems
- Nerve conduction studies should be performed to confirm diagnosis and plan management
- Extrinsic causes should be avoided while intrinsic causes may need surgery

---

Tenosynovitis

Inflammation of tendons and their associated synovial sheaths is a common problem. It is of course associated with RA, where it is part of a multisystem disease. In other

situations it may arise spontaneously, often with no known cause, but is usually precipitated by unusual levels of activity or overuse. It is an important condition to be aware of, as it is often associated with worker compensation and litigation.

Bursitis

Bursae are synovial-lined structures adjacent to joints that act as a natural form of bearing aimed at improving muscle and joint function. They are prone to inflammation as a result of repetitive movement or strain or because of abnormal loads. Bursae around the shoulder are commonly affected and these are dealt with in the next section on shoulder discomfort. The common sites of bursitis are around the knee and the elbow, although the greater trochanter is not uncommonly affected at the hip.

Patients generally complain of chronic discomfort over the bursa, usually associated with the causative element, such as movement or pressure. They may present because of swelling of the bursa, as seen in *housemaid's knee*, when the prepatellar bursa swells. Occasionally a bursa becomes infected, resulting in a tense swelling associated with cellulitis and general malaise. Infected bursae should be incised and drained and often this leads to spontaneous recovery through scarring and fibrosis.

Chronic bursal swelling with no symptoms is benign and needs no treatment unless the patient demands it, either for convenience or cosmesis. If tender, bursae may be excised, although the patient should be encouraged to address the underlying cause (e.g. by using a kneeling mat). Bursae are sometimes seen in children around the hamstrings at the knee (so-called semimembranosus bursa). This is naturally a cause of parental anxiety but most disappear as the child develops.

Shoulder discomfort

The shoulder girdle consists of an articulation between scapula and chest wall as well as between scapula and humerus. There are of course other joints to consider, particularly the acromioclavicular joint. Good shoulder function relies on healthy ligaments, muscles and tendons. All these structures are frequently injured, particularly those involved in heavy repetitive work and contact sports.

Clinical presentation

Symptoms include pain, particularly on movement, and the pain may be limited to a particular range of movement. Symptoms are quite frequently associated with a recent incident such as a pull or a period of unusual activity (e.g. DIY).

The following structures are commonly involved in pathological conditions causing shoulder discomfort:

- subacromial bursa;
- supraspinatus tendon;
- acromioclavicular joint;
- biceps tendon;
- rotator cuff.

Unfortunately, it may be difficult or impossible to localize which of these structures gives rise to the symptoms. Fortunately, most of the minor conditions settle with rest and time. To resolve the differential diagnosis may require specialist examination, including arthrography or arthroscopy.

Management

If rest, gentle exercise and anti-inflammatory drugs do not help, then a careful examination may reveal a point of tenderness. Tenderness under active movement within a painful arc is suggestive of supraspinatus tendon inflammation or subacromial bursitis (Fig. 41.6). Injection of steroid into the bursa or around the tendon, but not into it, can be very effective. It remains controversial whether this is reasonable and certainly should only be done with care. Occasionally, the patient may present with very severe pain and a radiograph will show calcific material within the supraspinatus tendon. Injection or even surgery in this case is well justified for the pain relief achieved.

Unfortunately, many patients only respond temporarily to the injection. Repetitive injection is not indicated and further investigation often shows degenerative change in the acromioclavicular joint, with osteophytic impingement on the supraspinatus tendon. This may lead to attrition rupture of the supraspinatus, which is part of the rotator cuff. Such rotator cuff tears can become large rents and even small ones cause a lot of discomfort and pain. Surgery to relieve the cause and repair the cuff will bring effective pain relief and some return of function. Repetitive injections in such patients can result in further degeneration of the cuff and should not be practised.

Frozen shoulder

Most so-called frozen shoulders are sore shoulders and fit into the collection of conditions outlined earlier. True frozen shoulder is a condition where there is little or no glenohumeral movement. It occurs rarely, often in those who have had a specific trauma incident, particularly an epileptic fit or an electric shock. Often the cause is obscure. Such patients eventually recover in 18 months to 2 years. They require a lot of psychological and physiotherapy support. The condition may be helped by manipulation under anaesthetic.

05

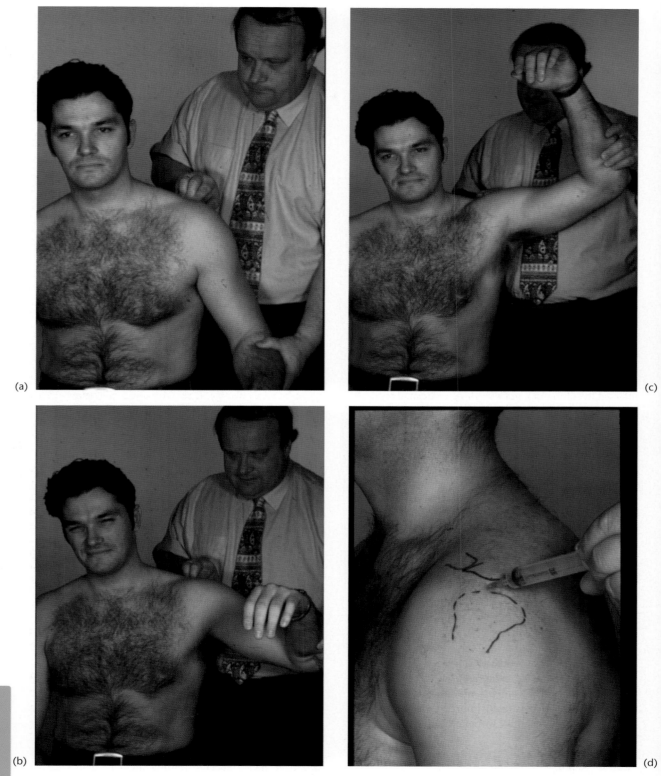

(a)

(c)

(b)

(d)

05

Figure 41.6 (a)–(c) Elicit the painful arc by inviting the patient to perform abduction and external rotations. (d) The area of point tenderness is injected with Glucocorticoid and local anaesthetic.

Adult foot disorders

Abnormalities of the feet are relatively common in the western world and this must relate in many ways to our shodden state. Also our perception of abnormality is very varied, as varied in fact as our feet. The only foot abnormalities that matter are those which cause symptoms and usually pain is the principal problem. Treatment or surgery is seldom if ever justified in the absence of functional abnormality and disaster will likely follow if operations are done to allow people to wear their preferred footwear. Foot-shaped shoes are the order of the day, not shoe-shaped feet.

Flat foot

The painful flat foot is a rare entity. Symptom-free flat feet are a variation on normal and are very common in certain races. The problem usually presents in childhood (see later) or in adolescence around the final growth spurt. Rarely, a very painful spasmodic flat foot may be associated with infection or chronic inflammatory disease. Occasionally, it may present acutely in middle age and examination reveals a painful and tender swelling over the insertion of tibialis posterior. This may indicate acute or impending degenerative rupture and warrants early intervention. Mostly the condition is benign and, if pain-free, should be ignored. If associated with pain, a medial heel lift will correct the deformity of the hind part of the foot and stabilize the medial arch. If pain is a persistent problem, fusion of the subtalar joint will help, although this is not something to contemplate lightly as it disturbs foot and ankle function profoundly.

Bunions and corns

Bunions are fluid-filled bursae found around bony prominences, commonly over the distal part of the first metatarsal and occasionally over the fifth (Fig. 41.7a). They are a natural response to pressure and indicate an underlying abnormality that should be treated rather than the bunion. Occasionally they become infected and need drainage, followed a few weeks later by treatment of the cause or a review of the footwear.

Corns are another way in which the body reacts to areas of high pressure. The painful excessive corny skin may be superficially removed but in the long term it will recur unless the underlying abnormality causing the excessive pressure is removed.

Hallux valgus and hallux rigidus

The hallux refers to the big toe and really these conditions

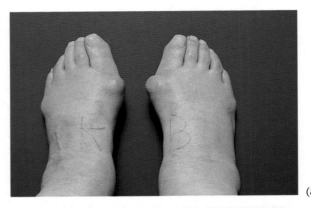
(a)

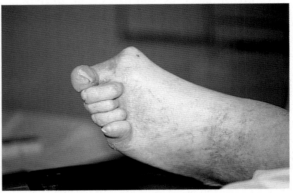
(b)

Figure 41.7 (a) Bunions are fluid-filled bursae found around bony prominences, commonly over the distal part of the first metatarsal. Occasionally, they become infected and need drainage, followed a few weeks later by treatment of the cause or review of the footwear. (b) Hallux valgus is a deformity of the big toe with turning away of the phalanges from the midline, usually because of a deformity at the joint line. It is usually associated with an exostosis of the head of the first metatarsal and an overlying bursa may be present.

are disorders of the first metatarsophalangeal joint. *Hallux valgus* is a deformity of the big toe with turning away of the phalanges from the midline, usually because of a deformity at the joint line. It is usually associated with an exostosis of the head of the first metatarsal and an overlying bursa may be present (Fig. 41.7b). *Hallux rigidus* is a poor term indicating osteoarthritis of the metatarsophalangeal joint. The two conditions may occur separately or together and treatment depends upon this and the age of the patient.

Hallux rigidus alone

Hallux rigidus in isolation can occur in adolescents and adults. In adolescents it is said to be a result of

05

osteochondral fracture, although this is not always easy to prove. Conservative treatment includes the use of a metatarsal bar to provide a rocker at the front of the foot so that the toe need not bend in normal walking. This usually fails because youngsters do not accept the cosmetic consequences on their shoes and so the same surgery as practised in adults is required. In adults the condition may present at any age, although in the elderly it rarely occurs without hallux valgus. Conservative measures are rarely sufficient and surgery is required. Removal of osteophytes with an osteotomy of the proximal phalanx for minor cases is often sufficient. Fusion is most reliable in a neutral position. Despite much folklore, this rarely gives women problems with heel height. Interposition arthroplasty with a Silastic spacer is an alternative that gives mixed results.

Hallux valgus alone

Hallux valgus alone may occur at any age. It gives more problems in women than men because of fashion in shoes. There is no evidence that shoes cause the condition. Many but not all sufferers have a short, often varus, first metatarsal. The cause of this common and troublesome condition is unknown. Management depends on age. Realignment of the first metatarsal to a more lateral position and excision of the exostosis over the first metatarsal head give satisfactory results at almost any age. Excision of the metatarsophalangeal joint (Keller's operation) is to be avoided in the young and is probably unnecessary if the joint is not painful.

Hallux valgus with hallux rigidus

This combination is seen in older patients where joint degeneration is usually secondary to the valgus deformity. These older patients may well be satisfied by having their pain relieved by well-fitting, extra-depth shoes. If this fails, then Keller's arthroplasty is a safe and rapid way of giving some relief. However, this operation is not benign and severely disrupts normal foot mechanics and so should be reserved for the older, less active patient.

Claw and hammer toes

These common abnormalities are almost a normal variant (Fig. 41.8). Clawing suggests intrinsic muscle weakness or deficiency. Indeed, on close analysis, many of these patients do indeed have weak or denervated small muscles of the feet. This is often associated with minor spinal abnormality such as spina bifida occulta. This means that claw toes should be approached with caution as far as surgery is concerned and only limited goals sought.

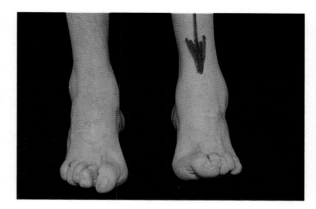

Figure 41.8 Claw and hammer toes.

Hammer toes are secondary to disruption of the metatarsophalangeal joints. Abnormalities of the foot leading to prolapse of metatarsal heads and joint disruption are not understood. The patients may present with generally sore forefeet, often called, rather grandly, metatarsalgia. The cause of the primary lesion is unknown and treatment is often unsatisfactory. Surgery to the secondary hammering of the toes includes fusion of the interphalangeal joints in a straight position so that they do not rub on the shoes. Often a good pair of soft and comfortable shoes is all that is required.

Neuromas

The cutaneous nerves to the toes may become trapped or irritated between the metatarsal heads, giving rise to a neuroma (*Morton's neuroma*). The cause is uncertain, except that it is almost certainly secondary to repetitive trauma and may therefore be associated with metatarsal head prolapse, as described above. The condition is difficult to diagnose with certainty, although the pain is characteristically dull and throbbing, often with sharp exacerbations accompanied by tingling of the toes. It is equally difficult to localize, although it is most frequently seen in the lateral two spaces. Classically, sideways compression of the foot produces a palpable click, reproducing the symptoms. Treatment by excision may be accompanied by subsequent sensory disturbance to the affected toes. Recurrence is common even with care, and patients should be warned about this.

Ingrowing toenails (Fig. 41.9) (see Chapter 36)

Plantar fasciitis

This often includes a number of vague but nevertheless

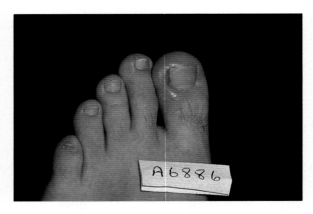

Figure 41.9 Infected ingrowing toenail.

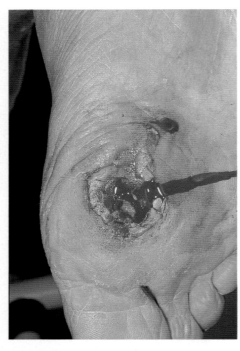

Figure 41.10 Neuropathic ulcer in a patient with diabetes mellitus.

very incapacitating painful disorders of the foot. Its cause is entirely obscure and it originates spontaneously with a fairly sudden onset. Patients characteristically complain of soreness of the instep, often worse first thing on rising or after sitting for a few hours. The symptoms are minimally relieved by walking but then persist as a debilitating ache, often exacerbated by a change of direction or rough ground. Most cases are self-limiting, although the symptoms may last a few months and some go on for years. On examination point tenderness may be elicited on the hindfoot at the origin of the plantar fascia medially. Discomfort is often more diffuse and care must be taken to exclude tarsal tunnel syndrome.

There is no specific cure and methods of relieving symptoms are various and less than satisfactory. Patients should be reassured that the condition will tend to get better. Insoles that are hollowed out over the tender area may help but may cause discomfort around the edge of the hollow. Soft shoes and insoles, particularly modern sports trainers, can be of considerable value. If there is marked point tenderness, then a local injection of steroids and long-acting local anaesthetic can be very effective, albeit rather painful to administer. Some demand a surgical solution and stripping of the fascia from the os calcis is practised. Results are entirely unpredictable, illustrating the highly uncertain nature of this otherwise self-limiting condition.

Neuropathic feet

Feet without sensation (i.e. sensory neuropathy) are prone to developing sores caused by the inability to perceive minor trauma from rubbing or treading on objects. Such problems are seen most commonly in the world where leprosy is endemic, particularly in the Far East. In the western world the most common cause of neuropathy

is diabetes mellitus and all diabetics need to be aware of the potential risk that may creep up on them gradually (see Chapter 37; Fig. 41.10). Such patients should regularly inspect their feet and be sure the nails are tidy. Footwear must be chosen with care and, if necessary, extra-depth shoes with very soft uppers may be prescribed. Once established, ulcers are difficult to heal and secondary infection may lead to amputation.

Achilles tendonitis and rupture

Pain around the tendo Achilles where it inserts into the os calcis is seen in two groups. In the younger athlete it may signify overuse. The area may be tender or even swollen. Rest is usually adequate. If it is recurrent, then surgical decompression of the paratenon tissue will often eradicate symptoms. Steroidal injection is to be avoided as penetration of the tendon may lead to rupture.

In the middle-aged man, a phase of discomfort may precede rupture of the tendo Achilles and this indicates degeneration within the tendon tissue. The cause is little understood, although it is known that the lower part of the tendo Achilles has a poor blood supply and is often a point of weakness in some people who keep particularly active into middle age.

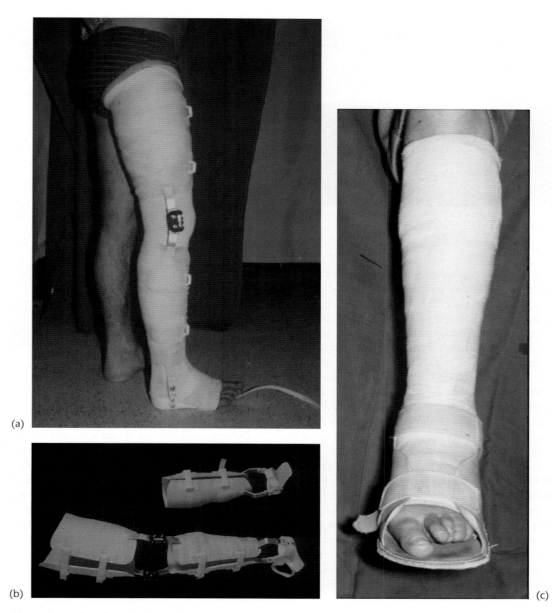

(a)

(b)

(c)

Figure 41.11 Types of equinus plaster.

05

If the tendon ruptures, it will heal without surgery if the ankle is kept in an equinus plaster for a minimum of 8 weeks (Fig. 41.11). The tendon can be sutured by either a closed technique or open suture. The latter technique has a high risk of complication. Whatever method is chosen, there is a significant risk of rerupture which decreases with time. Patients should be encouraged to wear a felt raise inside the heel of their shoes for as long as they will tolerate it.

Orthopaedic conditions of childhood

Some childhood musculoskeletal problems are common and minor, while others are rare and important and have major consequences for the child and the family. It is important to understand the nature of the minor conditions and treat them appropriately and have a more general understanding of the rarer major ones which need specialist, often multidisciplinary care.

Adult foot disorders at a glance

Problems affecting the hallux

Hallux valgus
- Deviation of great toe away from the midline
- Associated with sesamoid subluxation in severe cases
- If the deformity is > 15°, then progression is likely
- Treat according to symptoms
- Operations are designed to narrow the forefoot through osteotomy if there is no arthritis
- Osteotomy can be proximal or distal on the first metatarsal depending on the severity of the deformity

Hallux rigidus
- Osteoarthritis of the first metatarsophalangeal joint
- Seen in young without deformity and in old in association with hallux valgus
- Manage according to symptoms
- In the young without deformity, fusion is first-choice procedure
- In the elderly, fusion or excision arthroplasty may be used depending on the level of demand of the patient
- Toe joint replacement has a limited role as there is as yet no truly reliable prosthesis

Problems in the toes and rest of the foot

Claw and hammer toes
- Usually associated with poor intrinsic muscle function
- Commonly seen in older and middle-aged people
- Treat according to symptoms
- Where possible, avoid surgery by using adapted or special off-the-shelf footwear

Neuromas
- Usually affect second and third intermetatarsal regions
- Associated with poor intrinsic muscle function
- May require surgical excision plus or minus insoles
- Surgery may be associated with recurrence

Neuropathic feet
- In UK usually associated with diabetes mellitus
- May result in skin ulceration with or without secondary infection
- Can lead to very serious consequences such as amputation
- Best management is prevention by recognition of problem and then multidisciplinary approach

---

Key points in childhood orthopaedic disorders
- Appreciate the difference between major and minor childhood conditions
- Appreciate most children grow out of many minor disorders and careful explanations to parents are better than unnecessary interventions
- Differentiate the serious conditions that will respond to early interventions and potentially restore normal potential

The orthopaedic conditions of childhood are summarized in Table 41.6.

Minor conditions

Walking and posture problems

Children are often sent to an orthopaedic clinic because of parental anxiety about how or when they walk and stand. Normally children reach developmental milestones at certain times; children normally sit independently at 6 months, stand at a year and walk at about 18 months. These are averages and parents should be reassured that failure to achieve these goals by the specified age is not a sinister sign. When children start to walk their gait takes many months to mature and so minor variations are to be expected. Very occasionally, failure to achieve milestones will portend a serious problem but these are rare cases and are described in the next section (Major conditions).

All children referred should be examined carefully to exclude serious pathology. Ask the parents or grandparents about their own milestones, which is often reassuring as these tend to be strongly familial in pattern. Common minor problems associated with gait and stance are given in Table 41.7.

Knee deformity

Knock knees (genu valgum; Fig. 41.12a) and *bow legs* (genu varum; Fig. 41.12b) are frequently seen. These conditions are rarely, if ever, serious. The normal alignment of the knee is in valgus and when a child stands to attention there is normally a gap of 4 cm or so between the feet. If the gap is diminished, the knees are in varus; if it is increased, they are in valgus. If the children are followed until 7 years nearly all will have normal knee alignment.

Very rare serious causes of knee deformity are rickets and epiphyseal growth disorders. The child should not require an X-ray initially to exclude these conditions but should be seen again on one or two occasions and only investigated further if the condition gets worse or does not correct with the passage of time.

05

Table 41.6 Common orthopaedic conditions of childhood.

Minor conditions

Walking and posture problems
Knee deformities
    Knock knees (genu valgum)
    Bow legs (genu varum)
Intoeing
    Femoral neck angle variation
    Tibial torsion
    Abnormal forefeet
Flat feet
Curly toes

Pain around the knee
Osgood–Schlatter disease
Adolescent knee pain

Major conditions

Congenital dislocation of the hip (CDH)

Club foot (talipes equinovarus)

Neurological conditions
Spina bifida
    Spina bifida occulta
    Spina bifida cystica (meningocele, meningomyelocele,
      Arnold–Chiari lesion)
Cerebral palsy

Scoliosis

Limp in childhood
From birth: CDH, infection of the hip
1–4 years: infection of the hip
4–10 years: Perthes disease
10–15 years: Slipped upper femoral epiphysis

Table 41.7 Common causes of poor standing or walking in children.

Knee deformity
    Knock knees (genu valgum)
    Bow legs (genu varum)
Intoeing
    Femoral neck angle variation
    Tibial torsion
    Abnormal forefeet
Flat feet
Curly toes

Intoeing

A frequent cause of parental anxiety is when a child stands pigeon-toed, which is often exaggerated during running. The child is often referred with clumsiness but a careful enquiry suggests that the child is no more prone to falling than other children. Parents also often complain bitterly about shoe wear.

FEMORAL NECK ANGLE VARIATION

In the normal development of the fetus in its later stages, the leg rotates on the pelvis so that the acetabulum points almost backwards and the femoral head on the neck is orientated forwards. Sometimes the rotatory process is not completed by birth and so the femoral neck is more anteriorly orientated, i.e. it is anteverted. This means children born like this can internally rotate their femur a lot and externally rotate a little. This is reflected in their posture and they have an intoed gait. All will correct this delayed development by the time they are 10 years old, although some are left with residual deformity. This is seldom, if ever, severe enough to warrant surgery.

TIBIAL TORSION

Tibial torsion is a normal variation and should be ignored.

ABNORMAL FOREFEET

Abnormal feet, particularly the hooked or adducted forefoot, are commonly seen. They are a variation on normal. It is dubious whether surgery is ever justified and certainly should not be considered before 7 years. The vast majority correct spontaneously by then and any residual hooking rarely causes functional difficulties. There is no evidence that special shoes make any difference.

Flat feet

Flat feet is an abnormality in the minds of the public of the western world. In some races a flat foot is normal; indeed universally a flat foot is a normal variation that very rarely causes functional abnormalities, apart from uneven shoe wear. There are two kinds of flat foot, rigid and mobile. The vast majority are *mobile* and entirely innocuous. All children's feet are flat at birth and indeed the normal arch may not form until the child is 7 years old. In the infant the flatness of the medial arch is often exaggerated by a fat pad in the vicinity, which is normal. The essence of any child's deformity is that if it may be corrected passively it will correct spontaneously. Reassurance is required and all pressure to intervene should be resisted. Referral to hospital for mobile flat foot is not really required.

A *rigid* flat foot is rare at any age. It may be due to a tarsal coalition, which can be bony or fibrous. Even a tarsal coalition rarely needs surgery unless the foot remains stiff and painful.

A NOTE ON SHOES

Children should be kept out of shoes until walking is established. Then they require well-fitting shoes that leave

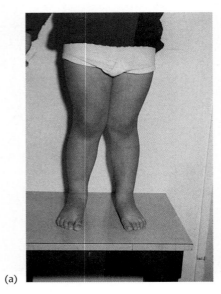
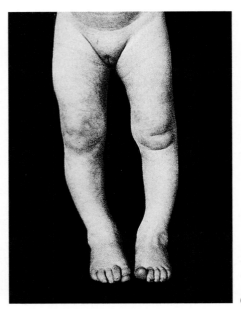

(a)   (b)

Figure 41.12 (a) Knock knees and (b) bow legs.

room for growth. They also need well-fitting socks which do not constrict the foot. There are no other rules and certainly young and healthy feet need no extra support from shoes or manufacturers. If the feet are more valgus than normal, then a heel seat may prevent excessive wear on the sole, but you must be clear you are treating the shoes and the parents' purse not the child's foot.

Curly toes
Minor overlapping, excess webbing or hooking, particularly of the fifth toe, are common. Most correct passively and should be left. Occasionally the fixed and hooked fifth toe causes discomfort in shoes. If fixed it requires surgical correction. Surgery on other curly toes should be discouraged despite often heavy parental pressure.

Pain around the knee

A very common cause of children's referral is pain around the knee. This is seen in both sexes from about 10–12 years of age and then far more commonly in older girls as they develop secondary sexual characteristics.

Osgood–Schlatter disease
Osgood–Schlatter disease is a traction epiphysitis of the patellar tendon insertion in the tibia. It accounts for the younger age of referral in both sexes. The cause is unknown but it is commoner in very active children, often associated with organized sport, and so may be an overuse

injury. The condition causes localized tenderness and discomfort, worse after exercise. It may be associated with a swelling and radiographs are characteristic.

The condition is episodic and usually can be treated by rest. Rarely, it is necessary to enforce rest with a plaster cast and occasionally in late adolescence sequestrated calcific bumps may be so uncomfortable as to require excision. Most important is to explain that the condition will settle with rest and that the child will cease to have symptoms in middle adolescence when the epiphysis fuses.

Adolescent knee pain and chondromalacia
Adolescent knee pain is seen mostly in girls and is of unknown cause. It is not the same as dislocation of the patella. Rarely, on arthroscopy an area of patellar cartilage is seen to be eroded (chondromalacia patellae). Most but not all girls grow out of the condition and a watching brief should be kept. Only if symptoms persist should arthroscopy be offered. Speculative surgery is to be avoided and often is psychologically harmful, reinforcing the condition and leaving scars which are often resented later.

Major conditions

Congenital dislocation of the hip

Congenital dislocation of the hip (CDH) occurs in 1 or 2 live births per 1000. It is a badly named condition because

05

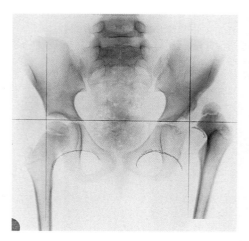

Figure 41.13 Congenital dislocation of the hip can be diagnosed radiologically by drawing Perkins' lines on the radiograph. The normally sited head of the femur lies below a line drawn horizontally through the triradiate cartilages and medial to a vertical line drawn from the outer edge of the acetabulum. In this radiograph, the right femoral head is normal but the left is congenitally dislocated.

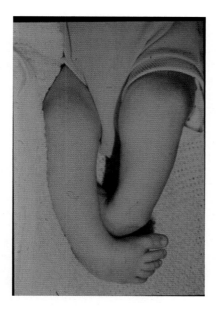

Figure 41.14 Bilateral talipes equinovarus or club feet.

the hip is rarely completely dislocated at birth but is abnormal and is likely to become troublesome if ignored. A better name would be 'congenital hip dysplasia', reflecting the underlying abnormality of the femoral head, the acetabulum or both (Fig. 41.13). The condition is more frequent in girls than boys, there are familial and racial tendencies and a significant number are bilateral.

Clinical presentation

All children should be screened for CDH at birth and rechecked at 3, 6 and 12 months. At birth it is diagnosed using a technique that either attempts to dislocate the hip or relocates it if dislocated. The test often produces a slight click or, more seriously, a 'clunk' as the hip dislocates or relocates. Sometimes, the test will fail to detect a dislocation if the hip cannot be reduced. The hip is often stiff and abduction is limited. Occasionally, CDH goes unrecognized at birth and presents late, in which case the condition may be diagnosed before weight-bearing (i.e. sitting), after weight-bearing (i.e. standing) or even when walking has been established. In the later cases clinical signs include shortening, asymmetrical skin creases, limited abduction and later a limp.

Management

All infants with hips that click should be re-examined in a specialist clinic at 3 months and radiography is usually then justified. All 'clunks' should be treated from birth.

If the head is reduced and maintained in the acetabulum, then the vast majority will settle and give no further trouble as the hip starts to develop normally.

The position of reduction at birth is in abduction at 45°, flexion at 90° and slight internal rotation. This is held using a metal splint or harness. Radiography of the splint is essential to ensure that the hip is being held in reduction. If there is any doubt, an arthrogram should be taken in the operating theatre. Reduction may be prevented by an infolding of the capsule into the joint (the limbus) or by a tight psoas tendon.

If discovered late but before weight-bearing, the hip may be reduced by a period of gentle traction followed by open or closed manipulation. It is then splinted in plaster for 3 months. If discovered late and walking has commenced, then major surgery is required to deepen the developed acetabulum and reangulate the femoral neck to stabilize the hip. The results of this are at best moderate and secondary arthritis is highly likely. This is why early diagnosis is so important.

Club foot (talipes equinovarus)

Talipes equinovarus is a deformity of the foot which makes it look like a golf club. It is important to recognize because, if treated early, mild cases can be fully corrected and major cases much improved to give an acceptably functioning foot (Fig. 41.14).

05

Aetiology

The condition is common and is seen in a mild postural form and a fixed form. The milder forms are often seen after breech presentation and are probably related to intrauterine posture, while the severe forms are associated with developmental abnormalities of nerves and muscles of the leg and back.

Management

The mild form is usually easily corrected at birth. The severe forms can also be corrected at birth, but with great difficulty; there are usually fixed skin creases and the whole leg seems smaller than the unaffected side. In both cases the condition can be bilateral. Initial treatment is gentle stretching, which should consist of two phases: (i) correct the hindfoot equinus and (ii) correct the mid and forefoot varus. In the mild cases, 6 weeks of stretching and strapping in a corrected or overcorrected position is all that is required. In severe cases, after 6 weeks the deformity should be reassessed and if correction is incomplete or cannot be maintained, then surgery is necessary. The children all need follow-up and special firm shoes until the feet stop growing at age 14 as late relapse requiring further surgery is possible. The affected foot is often always significantly smaller than the normal one, which can give difficulties in shoe fitting.

Neurological conditions

Conditions affecting the neurological structures at birth lead to abnormalities of the muscular and skeletal system during growth and development.

Spina bifida and meningomyelocele

Abnormal developments of the neural plate during the first 3 months may result in failure of closure of the spinal cord and vertebrae.

SPINA BIFIDA OCCULTA

This is a minor bony abnormality with failure of formation of vertebral spines that affects 2% of the population. This is usually of no significance, although some progress to mechanical backache and a very small number may suffer spinal cord tethering during growth (diastematomyelia).

SPINA BIFIDA CYSTICA

A small and decreasing number of babies are born with the neural plate tissues open and little or no skin or bony cover. This is spina bifida cystica. The condition can be recognized during prenatal routine blood screening for α-fetoprotein. The nerve tissue may be covered by a cyst (meningocele; Fig. 41.15) or the nerve tissue may be

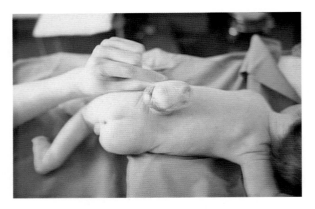

Figure 41.15 Spina bifida and meningocele.

incorporated in the cyst wall (meningomyelocele). Many children also have a malformation of the brain, leading to hydrocephalus (Arnold–Chiari lesion).

Many children die at or soon after birth. Some survive and have surgery to close the lesion on their back. Many of these children have formidable problems, including paralysis (which may be flaccid or spastic), flexion contractures of the knees and dislocation of the hips, secondary growth deformities through muscle imbalance and incontinence. Many, but by no means all, are mentally retarded. All this is a major burden for the child and the family, who need support from a team consisting of surgeons, therapists and social workers. Many children with spina bifida need early surgery to their feet to maintain a reasonable shape.

Every effort should be made to keep the child mobile until adolescence so that they grow to a reasonable size. Many children manage to walk aided by splints and hand-held aids until then. As they reach adolescence many go into a wheelchair as they find this socially and cosmetically easier for themselves. The care of such children and adults is a specialized area that requires an ability to work with other team members who often have much more to contribute than the doctor. All must support the family as a whole.

Cerebral palsy

Cerebral palsy consists of a birth abnormality of the brain resulting in delayed or arrested neuromuscular development. The spinal tissue develops normally and so such children have uninhibited spinal reflexes but lack higher-centre control and purpose. This results in a spastic type of paralysis. Some muscles are very spastic while others are very weak and flaccid, and this imbalance leads to abnormal muscle and bone growth with secondary deformities of joints. Some patterns are common, such as one arm and ipsilateral leg (hemiparesis). Two legs are often affected

05

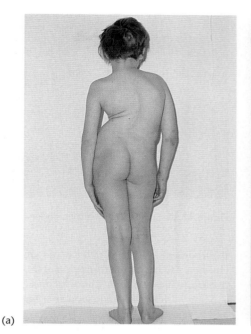
(a)

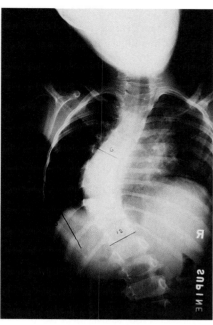
(b)

Figure 41.16 (a) Clinical and (b) radiographic appearances of severe scoliosis.

(paraparesis) and not uncommonly all limbs are affected (quadriparesis). Most, but not all, spastic children are mentally retarded and are often blind and/or deaf as well. Occasionally, children are spared mental and sensory impairment and such tragic cases are often unrecognized, to the utter frustration of the individual.

It is important to recognize that some people have very minor degrees of spasticity that may only affect one muscle group. These people commonly present with toe walking in adolescence. Examination reveals calf muscle spasticity and some may need tendo Achilles lengthening before growth ceases. Orthopaedic problems with growth are similar to those found in spina bifida but often much more severe. Deformities can be minimized by careful physiotherapy. Splintage should be used with caution as overzealous splintage can lead to increased spasm and ultimately deformity. Careful use of surgery to lengthen tight muscles, denervate them or occasionally to move them may maintain acceptable posture and help maintain some function. There is a need to recognize the importance of being part of a much wider supportive team who will provide regular day-to-day contact.

Scoliosis

Curvature of the spine with a rotatory abnormality of the vertebrae is known as scoliosis. It is a three-dimensional deformity based on abnormal lordosis of the spine, which leads to buckling and twisting of the vertebral column through muscle action and gravity (Fig. 41.16).

Aetiology

Scoliosis may be caused by congenital abnormalities of the vertebrae or neuromuscular imbalance but most cases have no known cause. Idiopathic scoliosis occurs in adolescence, although it may occur in infants and, rarely, in adults. It is far commoner in girls than boys. Its principal effects are cosmetic, which is not to be underrated as a cause of distress. It rarely causes physiological disturbances in the common idiopathic group.

Clinical presentation

The child usually presents because of twisting of the ribs, which causes a hump at the shoulder on one side. Girls also complain that their skirts hang crookedly. It may be painful but this is usually secondary to the anxiety and distress of what is commonly known as a sinister condition.

Management

Treatment is dictated by cosmetic problems. Not all curves progress and this should be emphasized to parents. If the curve is progressive or is causing distress, treatment should be offered early. Braces have no benefit and should

05

Table 41.8 Serious causes of limp in childhood.

Age	Cause
From birth	Congenital dislocation of the hip
	Infection of the hip
In infancy	Infection of the hip
4–10 years	Perthes disease
10–15 years	Slipped upper femoral epiphysis

not be used as they add to the stigma of the disease. If treatment is demanded due to distress or progress, then surgical correction is essential. The rotatory element of the deformity must be corrected as otherwise the hump remains, which is what distresses the patient. This is very complex surgery that is only carried out in a handful of regional spinal centres. All children with scoliosis should be referred for a specialist opinion if treatment is demanded or the curve is progressive. The earlier the referral the better.

Limp in childhood

A limp at any age must be taken seriously. Quite often the cause will be obscure and the condition will settle. However, when there is a serious cause it demands treatment and so the conditions listed in Table 41.8, which occur within characteristic age bands, must be excluded.

Perthes disease

This is an osteochondritis of the femoral head epiphysis. It is commoner in boys than girls and in 20% is bilateral. The cause is unknown but it has an incidence of up to 5 per 1000 children.

Clinical presentation

The natural history is for the child to present with a painful limp, which is followed by a slow recovery. Radiologically, the femoral head may be normal on first presentation but it later fragments to a greater or lesser degree. The condition is felt to have a vascular component and the condition is an avascular necrosis of the growing femoral head (Fig. 41.17). Nevertheless, the cause is obscure. Eventually the head will revascularize and reossify but the head may be enlarged and deformed.

Diagnosis is made from a high index of suspicion. Radiography repeated at a month may show previously unrecorded changes. Ultrasound reveals fluid in the hip joint and a bone scan is positive.

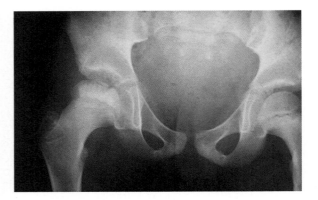

Figure 41.17 Perthes disease affecting the right femoral head. Note the increase in the joint space on the affected side.

Management

The strategy of treatment is to maintain the head concentrically within the acetabulum until the natural process of the disease runs its course. Minor degrees (involvement of up to half of the head) need no treatment as the prognosis in such children is good. In older children with full head involvement the prognosis is less good, although the child will return to normal in the short term but will be prone to secondary osteoarthritis in early middle age. In these severe cases splintage to achieve containment may help and some believe that osteotomy, either to enlarge the acetabulum or to redirect the femoral head, helps. All these treatments are of dubious value and careful follow-up with periods on traction to alleviate symptoms is probably all we can do to help these patients.

Slipped upper femoral epiphysis

This is a condition seen in boys in their early teens who are sexually immature for their age (Fig. 41.18) and in girls who are a little older and who have recently undergone an adolescent growth spurt. It consists of slippage of the capital femoral epiphysis on the neck. The neck comes to lie anteriorly and the head is tilted off behind. The cause is unclear but affected children appear to have an abnormal hormonal balance, which must be associated in some way.

Clinical presentation

The child presents with a limp, which may not be particularly uncomfortable or may be associated with pain that sometimes radiates to the knee in the sensory distribution of the obturator nerve. Any child with knee pain must have the hip examined. The slip may occur acutely or it

05

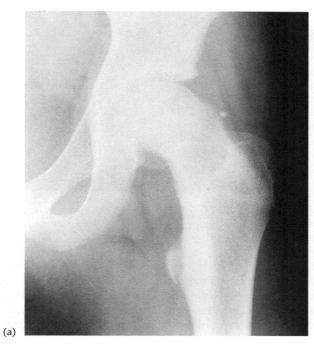

(a)

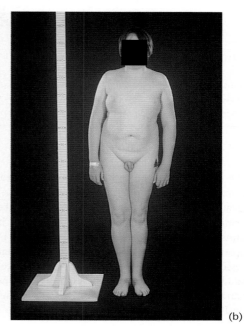

(b)

Figure 41.18 (a) Radiological and (b) clinical appearances in a patient with a left slipped upper femoral epiphysis.

may be preceded by many months of discomfort without clinical or radiological signs. All young adolescents with a painful hip must be regarded as having this condition until it is clinically and radiologically excluded. On examination there is limitation of abduction in flexion with loss of internal rotation because of the distorted femoral head on the neck. Radiography must include a lateral view or minor degrees of slippage may be missed.

Management
Treatment is surgical. If the slippage is minor or moderate, the hip should be pinned in its new deformed position. If the slippage is major a gentle reduction may be attempted, although the risk of avascular necrosis is high. The other side should be watched radiologically and pinned if any suspicion of slippage arises. The pins are best removed at fusion of the epiphysis around the age of 18 years.

Plastic and Reconstructive Surgery

42

Must know Must do

Must know
Wound healing and wound management
Complications of wound healing
Common congenital disorders requiring plastic surgical correction
Core knowledge of skin grafts and flaps
Assessment of hand function
Principles of management of facial injuries
Pressure sores
Compartment syndromes
Complex regional pain syndrome

Must do
Suture a skin wound in casualty (under supervision)
Follow healing of a patient with a surgical site infection treated by the exposure/packing method
Follow the management of a patient with a major compartment syndrome
Observe a skin grafting operation
Observe a plastic reconstructive operation

Introduction

The word 'plastic' comes from the Greek word *plastikos*, meaning to mould or to shape, and has been used in the English language since the 16th century. The first textbook to include a comprehensive account of plastic and reconstructive surgical operations was written by the French surgeon Velpeau in 1839. The forefathers of modern-day plastic surgery emerged out of the First World War, most famously the New Zealander Gillies. Since then the specialty has expanded at such a rate that it would be impossible to cover it all in this chapter. We have therefore concentrated on the fundamentals of the specialty and tried to provide a comprehensive overview.

Wound healing and management

Normal wound healing

This can be considered in four distinct stages, which are not mutually exclusive and show considerable overlap.

● *Coagulation (immediate).* Following wounding, the clotting cascade is initiated, local vasoconstriction occurs and a platelet clot forms. Platelet-derived growth factor (PDGF) is released.

● *Inflammation (0–4 days).* Vasodilation then ensues and inflammatory cells are attracted to the site of injury, initially neutrophils then macrophages, which remove tissue debris. Lymphocytes are recruited later and persist in chronic inflammation.

● *Fibroplasia (4 days to 3 weeks).* Fibroblasts are attracted by PDGF and leukocyte growth factors. They lay down type III collagen and ground substance. Vascular buds appear and this neovascularized tissue is known as granulation tissue.

● *Remodelling (3 weeks to 18 months).* Fibroblasts differentiate into myofibroblasts, which are responsible for wound contraction. Type III collagen is replaced by type I collagen and blood vessels atrophy. These processes result in wound healing by an epithelialized white scar. Maximal wound tensile strength is achieved at about day 60, when it is 80% of normal.

Abnormal wound healing

Many factors can delay wound healing, some of which are outlined in Table 42.1.

Hypertrophic scars

Hypertrophic scarring is characterized by an excessive build-up of scar tissue confined to the initial boundary of the wound. It tends to reach a maximum prominence about 3 months after the injury and then regresses over time. Hypertrophic scarring is related to excessive wound tension and delayed wound healing.

05

Table 42.1 Factors that impair wound healing.

Local
Nutritional
   Zinc deficiency
   Hypoproteinaemia
   Vitamin C deficiency
Wound infection
Foreign bodies

General
Collagen synthesis disorders
   Marfan's syndrome
   Ehlers–Danlos syndrome
Peripheral vascular disease
Steroids
Cytotoxic drugs
Radiotherapy
Diabetes mellitus

Keloid scars

Keloid scarring is characterized by an excessive build-up of scar tissue that invades the normal skin beyond the original boundary of the wound. It is 15 times more common in pigmented skin and has a familial tendency. It occurs gradually after the injury and shows no signs of regression over time. The ear lobe is the most commonly affected site.

Wound closure

Closure by first intention

If staples or sutures close a wound, healing is said to be by primary intention.

● *Primary closure.* When the wound is closed at the time of surgery. Primary closure is used in the majority of elective surgical cases and clean trauma wounds.

● *Delayed primary closure.* When a wound is contaminated or devitalized tissues have been débrided, it is left open and packed with suitable dressings, such as Jelonet or proflavine-soaked gauze. Wound closure is undertaken 2–3 days later, providing the wound is clean.

Closure by second intention

If a wound is left alone to heal, granulation tissue forms and healing is said to be by second intention. Grossly contaminated or infected wounds are débrided and left to heal in this manner. Pilonidal disease and hidradenitis are also often treated in this way.

Grafts

A graft refers to total detachment of tissue from one part of the body and transferral to another part, where it must establish its own blood supply.

● Autograft: transferral within the same individual.
● Allograft: transferral between individuals of the same species.
● Xenograft: transferral between different species.

Skin grafts

Various types of tissue may be grafted (skin, bone, nerve, cartilage). The majority are skin grafts, either split or full thickness (Fig. 42.1). Only tissues that heal by forming granulation tissue can be grafted onto and therefore cortical bone, bare tendons and cartilage are inappropriate sites.

Split-thickness skin graft (partial-thickness or Tiersch graft)

In this type of skin graft all of the epidermis and a variable portion of the dermis is included. This is the most common type of skin graft and is taken with a hand-held knife (Fig. 42.2) or a mechanical dermatome. Common donor sites include the thigh and buttocks (in children); however, in exceptional circumstances (burns) any area of the skin can be used. The graft can be meshed allowing it to be

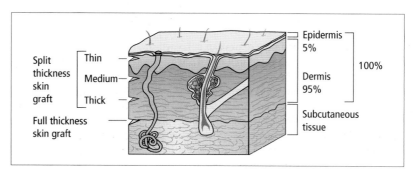

Figure 42.1 Thickness of skin grafts relative to thickness of skin.

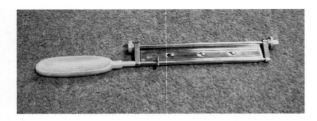

Figure 42.2 Hand-held knife.

Table 42.2 Differences between full- and split-thickness skin grafts.

Split-thickness skin grafts	Full-thickness skin grafts
Reliable take	Require well-vascularized bed
Shrink considerably	Less shrinkage
Abnormal pigmentation and contour	Better colour and contour match can be achieved
Susceptible to trauma	Adenexal structures maintained

expanded. This also prevents any accumulation of blood or serous fluid under the graft. Donor sites can be excised and closed directly if small or, more commonly, left to re-epithelialize.

Full-thickness skin graft (Wolfe graft)
In this type of skin graft all of the epidermis and dermis is taken but no subcutaneous fat. The donor site limits the size of the graft. No dermis is left on the donor site and therefore it cannot be left to re-epithelialize and must be closed directly.

Close approximation, which helps prevent seroma and haematoma formation and also maintains immobilization of the graft, is achieved by the application of appropriate dressings. β-Haemolytic streptococci dissolve skin grafts while *Pseudomonas* produce so much pus that the graft floats off. The differences between split- and full-thickness skin grafts are listed in Table 42.2.

Skin graft take
- *Adhesion*: initially a fibrin bond forms adhering the graft to its bed.
- *Plasmic imbibition*: the graft swells as interstitial fluid permeates into it from the recipient bed.
- *Inosculation*: ingrowth of vascular tissue starts to occur around day 3 and in thinner grafts revascularization is complete between days 5 and 7. Lymphatic circulation is restored after 1 week. Reinnervation occurs over many months.

Flaps

A flap refers to tissue transferred to an adjacent or distal site while retaining a functional vascular attachment. Flaps transferred to a local site while maintaining their original arterial and venous connections are known as pedicled flaps. Flaps transferred to a distant site with microvascular anastomosis of their native arterial and venous connections to vessels in the recipient bed are known as free flaps.

Blood supply of skin

Three types of artery supply blood to the skin.
- Direct cutaneous arteries and veins emerge from deeper vessels. Many of these arise in the axillae and groin (e.g. superficial thoracic artery, superficial epigastric artery) but also at other sites, such as the anterior chest wall (Fig. 42.3a).
- Musculocutaneous perforating arteries emerge from the surface of muscles. Generally, these muscles are broad and flat ones that largely exist on the trunk (Fig. 42.3b).
- Fasciocutaneous perforating arteries pass along an intermuscular or intercompartmental fascia septum. Generally, these vessels are found on the limbs (Fig. 42.3c).

The vessels ascend and anastomose at all levels to form horizontal plexuses that run in the skin subcutaneous tissue and fascia. The three-dimensional area of tissue supplied by a single vessel and its venae commitantes is known as an angiosome (Fig. 42.4).

Skin flaps
Random pattern flaps
These local flaps have no specifically identified vessels and rely on vessels in the subdermal and dermal plexuses. Because of the random nature of their pedicles, the distal circulation of these skin flaps is unreliable and they can only be safely raised using a length to width ratio of 2 : 1. These flaps are commonly used for small defects and are categorized according to their direction of movement (advancement, rotation, transposition) (Fig. 42.5). A Z-plasty is an example of a transposition flap.

Axial pattern flaps
These flaps have a defined single vascular pedicle running longitudinally within them (Fig. 42.6). This axial arrangement allows a flap to be raised with a length to breadth ratio greater than 2 : 1. Examples of this type of flap include the groin flap based on the superficial circumflex artery, the deltopectoral flap based on the internal mammary branches, and the median forehead flap based on the supratrochlear artery.

05

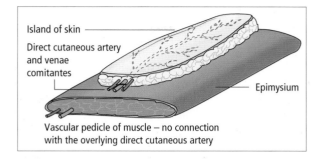

Island of skin

Direct cutaneous artery and venae comitantes

Epimysium

Vascular pedicle of muscle – no connection with the overlying direct cutaneous artery

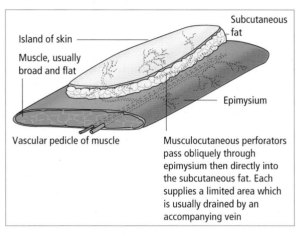

Subcutaneous fat

Island of skin

Muscle, usually broad and flat

Epimysium

Vascular pedicle of muscle

Musculocutaneous perforators pass obliquely through epimysium then directly into the subcutaneous fat. Each supplies a limited area which is usually drained by an accompanying vein

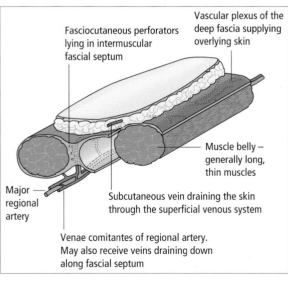

Fasciocutaneous perforators lying in intermuscular fascial septum

Vascular plexus of the deep fascia supplying overlying skin

Muscle belly – generally long, thin muscles

Major regional artery

Subcutaneous vein draining the skin through the superficial venous system

Venae comitantes of regional artery. May also receive veins draining down along fascial septum

Figure 42.3 Schematic representation of the principles of the blood supply to the skin from (a) direct cutaneous arteries, (b) musculocutaneous perforators and (c) perforators of the fasciocutaneous system.

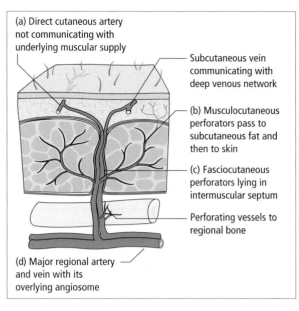

(a) Direct cutaneous artery not communicating with underlying muscular supply

Subcutaneous vein communicating with deep venous network

(b) Musculocutaneous perforators pass to subcutaneous fat and then to skin

(c) Fasciocutaneous perforators lying in intermuscular septum

Perforating vessels to regional bone

(d) Major regional artery and vein with its overlying angiosome

Figure 42.4 Diagram demonstrating the concept of an angiosome, with the various types of cutaneous blood supply.

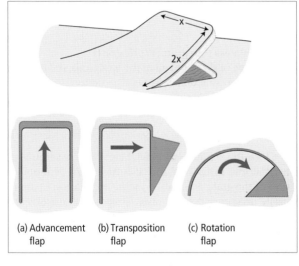

(a) Advancement flap

(b) Transposition flap

(c) Rotation flap

Figure 42.5 Random pattern skin flap and its variations: (a) advancement; (b) transposition; (c) rotation.

Muscle flaps

Muscle can be transferred either on its own as a muscle flap, usually covered with a split-thickness skin graft, or with a paddle of subcutaneous tissue and skin as a myocutaneous flap. Muscles are classified according to the nature of their vascular pedicle(s). They can be transposed locally (e.g. gastrocnemius flap in lower-limb reconstruction) or

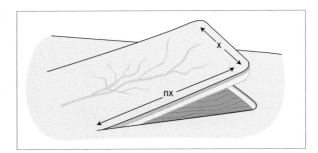

Figure 42.6 Axial pattern flaps.

completely detached from their origins and insertions and transferred as free flaps (e.g. free transverse rectus abdominis flap in breast reconstruction).

Fascial flaps

Fascia can also be transferred alone or with its overlying subcutaneous tissue and skin as a fasciocutaneous flap. These flaps are less bulky and avoid the need to sacrifice underlying muscle. A facial plexus exists and these flaps can either be transposed locally in random pattern or elevated on identifiable perforators.

Wound healing, grafts and flaps at a glance

Definitions

Wound: any injury involving a break in the surface of the skin or an organ by any means, including a surgical incision

Graft: a tissue (e.g. skin, bone, nerve) that is removed from one part of a body and transferred to another part of the same or different body, where it must establish its own blood supply. *Autograft*, transferral within the same individual; *allograft*, transferral between individuals of the same species; *xenograft*, transferral between different species

Flap: a tissue (skin, muscle) transferred to an adjacent or distal site but retaining a functional vascular attachment

Angiosome: three-dimensional area of tissue supplied by a single vessel and its venae commitantes

Wound healing
Phases of normal wound healing
- Coagulation (immediate)
- Inflammation (0–4 days)
- Fibroplasia (4 days to 3 weeks)
- Remodelling (3 weeks to 18 months)
- Maximal wound tensile strength at about day 60

Abnormal wound healing
- Hypertrophic scarring: excessive build-up of scar tissue confined to the initial boundary of the wound
- Keloid scarring: excessive build-up of scar tissue that invades the normal skin beyond the original boundary of the wound

Wound closure
Closure by first intention
- Primary closure: closed at time of surgery
- Delayed primary closure: closed at 2–3 days

Closure by second intention
- Wound closes by granulation

Grafts
- Split-thickness skin graft (Tiersch graft): epidermis +

portion of dermis. Not suitable for cortical bone, bare tendon, cartilage and cavities
- Full-thickness skin graft (Wolfe graft): epidermis + dermis. Small grafts
- Skin grafts take by adhesion, plasmic imbibition and inosculation

Flaps
Blood supply of skin
- Direct cutaneous arteries and veins emerge from deeper vessels
- Musculocutaneous perforating arteries emerge from the surface of muscles
- Fasciocutaneous perforating arteries pass along an intermuscular or intercompartmental fascia septum

Skin flaps
Random pattern flaps
- No specifically identified vessels
- Rely on vessels in the subdermal and dermal plexuses
- Length to width ratio of 2 : 1
- Types: advancement, rotation, transposition

Axial pattern flaps
- Single vascular pedicle running longitudinally within them
- Length to width ratio of > 2 : 1

Muscle flaps
- Muscle only
- Muscle + split-thickness skin graft
- Myocutaneous flap
- Muscle flaps can be transposed as:
  (a) Local flaps (retain local blood supply)
  (b) Free flaps (new blood supply has to be provided by microvascular anastomosis)

Fascial flaps
- Fascia only
- Fascia + subcutaneous tissue + skin (fasciocutaneous)

05

Hand surgery

Hand trauma is one of the most frequent reasons for attendance at casualty departments. It is also a major cause of lost working days because the specialized functions of the hand can be severely affected by even quite minor trauma. Despite the use of modern reconstructive techniques, a severe injury may lead to long-term unemployment or require the patient to seek retraining in less skilled work.

When managing hand trauma it is important to consider the five principal requirements for good function:
- good blood supply;
- a stable skeleton;
- soft pliable skin cover (which does not restrict mobility);
- innervation (both motor and sensory);
- motion (provided by smoothly gliding tendons).

Assessment of the injured hand

The key questions are as follows.
- When did the injury occur and how much time has since elapsed?
- Where did the injury occur and was the environment clean or dirty?
- What was the mechanism of injury and can you predict which structures are likely to have been damaged?

It is imperative to obtain the patient's age, hand dominance, occupation and hobbies. These factors together with the patient's general health are vital in determining the most appropriate treatment.

Examination must be thorough but at the same time avoid unnecessary discomfort to the patient. It should follow a standard scheme as detailed in the box.

Normal anatomy of the hand

Two groups of muscles power the hand: extrinsic and intrinsic muscles. The extrinsics have their muscle bellies in the forearm and tendinous insertions in the hand: flexor muscles are located on the volar or palmar surface of the forearm and flex the wrist and digits; extensor muscles are located on the dorsal surface of the forearm and extend the wrist and digits. The intrinsics have their origins and insertions within the hand.

Extrinsic muscles
Flexors
The extrinsic flexors are the flexor digitorum superficialis and flexor digitorum profundus to the fingers and flexor pollicis longus to the thumb.

Examination of the injured hand

Look
- Inspect volar and dorsal surfaces of the hand and note the site of any soft-tissue injury
- Colour: assess perfusion
- Swelling: underlying bone or ligament injury
- Wasting: nerve injury
- Position of hand: is there normal flexion cascade of fingers, clawing in ulnar nerve injury, subluxation of metacarpophalangeal (MCP) joints with ulnar drift in rheumatoid arthritis?

Feel
- Tenderness
- Joint stability
- Temperature: assess perfusion
- Sensation: specific nerves (see below)

Move
- Passive range of movement
- Active range of movement
- Motor function of specific nerves (see below)

The flexor digitorum superficialis arises from all three bones of the elbow joint, the common flexor origin on the medial epicondyle of the humerus and the ulnar and radial heads. Its belly passes down the volar surface of the forearm splitting into four distinct tendons, to each finger, above the wrist. The flexor digitorum profundus arises similarly from the common flexor origin and ulnar as well as the interosseous membrane. This bulky muscle lies deep to the flexor digitorum superficialis and similarly splits into four distinct tendons. All these tendons pass through the carpal tunnel and at the level of the distal palmar crease in the hand they enter the flexor sheaths of their destined fingers. In the flexor sheath the flexor digitorum superficialis lies superficially and splits into two slips. These slips then insert into either side of the middle phalanx base. The flexor digitorum profundus emerges through this divarification in the flexor digitorum superficialis tendon to insert into the base of the distal phalanx.

In the digits, the flexor tendons are bound to the skeleton by a system of five annular pulleys, which prevent them from bow-stringing when the fingers are flexed (Fig. 42.7). These pulleys, with the insertions of the long flexor tendons and the carpal tunnel, divide the hand into five distinct zones (Fig. 42.8).

The flexor pollicis longus arises from the anterior border of the radius and inserts into the base of the thumb's distal phalanx, thus flexing the interphalangeal (IP) joint

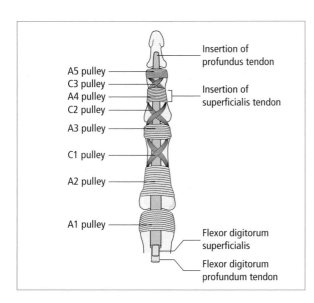

Figure 42.7 Flexor tendon sheath with the five annular pulleys.

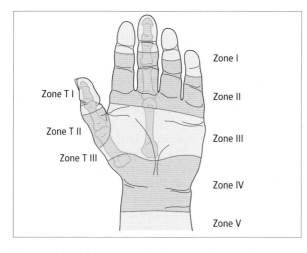

Figure 42.8 The five anatomical zones of the hand.

of the thumb. The thumb has two annular pulleys and one oblique pulley and is divided into three zones.

Extensors

The extrinsic extensors are the extensor digitorum communis, extensor indicis, extensor digiti minimi, extensor pollicis longus and extensor pollicis brevis. Also in this compartment is abductor pollicis longus.

The extensor digitorum communis arises from the common extensor origin on the lateral epicondyle of the humerus with extensor digiti minimi. Extensor indicis arises distal to this from the shaft of the ulna and travels

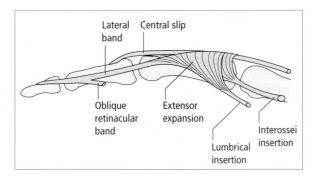

Figure 42.9 The extensor apparatus.

deep to it. Extensor digitorum communis separates into four distinct tendons and passes under the extensor retinaculum with the tendons of extensor digiti minimi and extensor indicis. As the extensor digitorum communis tendons pass over the MCP joints of the digits, the deeper fibres blend with the dorsal joint capsule. As the tendon passes over the dorsum of the proximal phalanx, it flattens out and divides into a central and two lateral slips. The central slip passes onto the base of the middle phalanx. The lateral slips diverge around this and receive the insertions of the interossei and lumbricals, forming a broad extensor expansion. The two lateral slips pass distally across the middle phalanx and then converge to be inserted together into the base of the distal phalanx (Fig. 42.9). The tendons of extensor indicis and extensor digiti minimi pass on the ulnar side of the extensor digitorum communis tendon to insert into the extensor expansion of the index and little finger respectively.

The extensor pollicis longus arises from the ulna while the extensor pollicis brevis arises lower down from the radius. The extensor pollicis longus has a long tendon that hooks around the dorsal tubercle on the distal radius (Lister's tubercle), where it forms the ulnar border of the radial snuffbox. It then passes over the MCP joint to insert into the base of the distal phalanx. There is no extensor expansion on the thumb but the tendon receives insertions from the adductor pollicis and abductor pollicis brevis. The extensor pollicis brevis forms the radial border of the radial snuffbox (with the abductor pollicis longus tendon) and inserts into the base of the proximal phalanx of the thumb.

Intrinsic muscles

The four groups of intrinsic muscles in the hand are the thenar, hypothenar, interossei and lumbricals.

Thenar

These are the short muscles to the thumb.

05

Flexor pollicis brevis
- Origin: flexor retinaculum and trapezius.
- Insertion: base of the thumb's proximal phalanx.
- Action: flexes the MCP joint of the thumb.

Opponens pollicis
- Origin: flexor retinaculum and trapezius.
- Insertion: radial border of first metacarpal.
- Action: opposes (medially rotates and flexes) the thumb.

Abductor pollicis brevis
- Origin: flexor retinaculum and scaphoid.
- Insertion: radial side of proximal phalanx of thumb and tendon of extensor pollicis longus.
- Action: abducts the thumb.

Adductor pollicis
- Origin: oblique head from second and third metacarpals and trapezoid and capitate. Transverse head from palmar shaft of third metacarpal.
- Insertion: ulnar side of thumb's proximal phalanx and tendon of extensor pollicis longus.
- Action: adducts thumb.

Hypothenar
These are the short muscles to the little finger.

Flexor digiti minimi brevis
- Origin: flexor retinaculum and hamate.
- Insertion: ulnar side of little finger's proximal phalanx.
- Action: flexes MCP joint of little finger.

Opponens digiti minimi
- Origin: flexor retinaculum and hamate.
- Insertion: ulnar border of fifth metacarpal shaft.
- Action: opposes little finger.

Abductor digiti minimi
- Origin: flexor retinaculum and pisiform.
- Insertion: ulnar side of proximal phalanx of little finger and extensor expansion.
- Action: abducts little finger.

Interossei
There are two groups of interossei, palmar and dorsal.

The four palmar muscles arise from the anterior shafts of the first, second, fourth and fifth metacarpal shafts and insert into the proximal phalanx and extensor expansion on the ulnar side of the thumb and index finger and the radial side of the ring and little finger. They adduct to the axis of the middle finger and flex the MCP joints while extending the IP joints. The palmar muscles cause adduction.

The four dorsal muscles arise as bipennate muscles from the inner aspects of all the metacarpal shafts (i.e. one for each web space). These insert into the proximal phalanges and dorsal extensor expansion on the radial side of the index and middle fingers and the ulnar side of the middle and ring fingers. They abduct from the axis of the middle finger and flex the MCP joints while extending the IP joints.

Lumbricals
These four muscles arise from each of the flexor digitorum profundus tendons. They insert into the dorsal extensor expansions on the radial side of the index, ring, middle and little fingers. They flex the MCP joints and extend the IP joints.

Tendon injury

Flexor tendon injury
Assessment
Flexion of the distal IP joint is assessed by holding the fingers, and the proximal IP joint of the finger being assessed, in full extension. If the distal IP joint of the finger being assessed can be actively flexed, then the flexor digitorum profundus of that finger is intact.

Flexion of the proximal IP joint is assessed by holding the fingers, and the MCP joint of the finger being assessed, in extension. If the proximal IP joint of the finger being assessed can be actively flexed, then the flexor digitorum superficialis of that finger is intact.

Note that flexor digitorum profundus can flex both interphalangeal joints, so it is important to ensure that the distal IP joint is lax while the proximal IP joint flexes to isolate the action of flexor digitorum superficialis. Remember that the lumbricals and interossei can also flex the MCP joints, so this is not an indication of the integrity of flexor digitorum profundus or flexor digitorum superficialis.

Repair
Flexor tendon lacerations are repaired under tourniquet control using magnification. Soft-tissue lacerations are extended in a manner that will expose the zone of injury but at the same time minimize contractures from healing scars. Normally, this is achieved in a zigzag pattern along the volar surface of the digits known as Brunner's incisions (Fig. 42.10).

Flexor tendons are traditionally repaired with a core suture to relieve tension and a continuous peripheral suture to align the ends so it can continue to glide in the narrow space of the tendon sheath (Fig. 42.11). Where possible pulleys and sheath are also repaired. Easy excursion

05

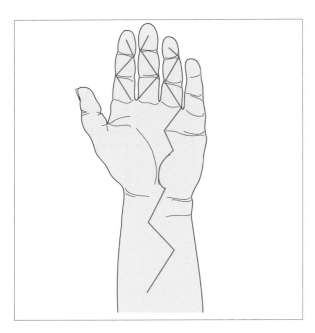

Figure 42.10 Brunner incision of the fingers and palm.

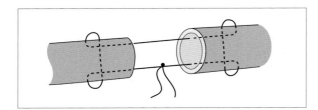

Figure 42.11 Modified Kessler core suture.

of the tendon should be visible post repair prior to skin closure. Strength of the repair is said to be proportional to the number of core suture strands crossing the repair site.

Extensor tendon injury

The extrinsic extensor tendons are located very superficially and are therefore susceptible to trauma. They are also thinner with less tendon substance compared with the flexor tendons.

Mallet finger

Division of the conjoined lateral bands at the distal IP joint leads to a characteristic deformity with drooping at the distal IP joint known as mallet finger (Fig. 42.12a). This type of injury can be open or closed. Open injuries occur when the overlying skin is also lacerated. Closed injuries are the result of forced flexion at the distal IP joint

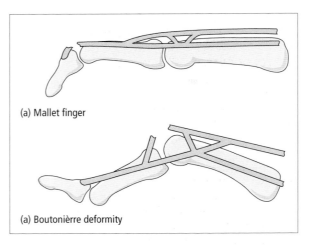

(a) Mallet finger

(a) Boutonièrre deformity

Figure 42.12 Disruption of the extensor apparatus leads to various deformities depending on the position of the lesion: (a) mallet finger; (b) boutonnière deformity.

and the tendon is avulsed from its insertion but the skin remains intact. The avulsion can also incorporate a flake fracture of the distal phalanx where the tendon inserts; this can be seen on X-ray. There are many ways to treat this type of deformity. Surgical repair is indicated if the injury is open but conservative splinting may be the treatment of choice if the injury is closed.

Boutonnière deformity

This occurs when the central slip of the extensor tendon is disrupted from its insertion into the base of the middle phalanx. The proximal IP joint then flexes. This allows the lateral bands to slip down the sides of the proximal IP joint. Contraction along this axis now hyperextends the distal IP joint. This results in the characteristic boutonnière or button-hole deformity (Fig. 42.12b). Again these injuries can be treated conservatively with splinting or by surgery.

Rehabilitation

Following tendon repair, healing occurs by the processes of inflammation, fibroplasia and remodelling. Strength of healing and rate of healing are maximal in a tendon that is moving and stressed, although overstressing a tendon repair may lead to rupture (this is most likely at about day 14 during a period of collagen lysis). However, complete immobility following tendon repair will lead to the formation of extratendinous adhesions, which greatly limits tendon gliding. Therefore a careful balance must be achieved. Several postoperative regimens exist: dynamic mobilization, passive mobilization and active mobilization.

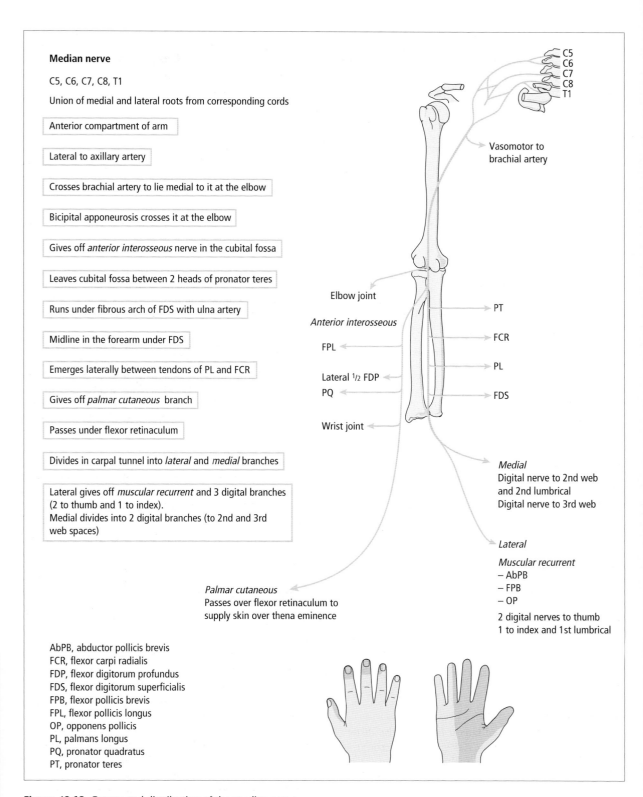

Median nerve

C5, C6, C7, C8, T1

Union of medial and lateral roots from corresponding cords

Anterior compartment of arm

Lateral to axillary artery

Crosses brachial artery to lie medial to it at the elbow

Bicipital apponeurosis crosses it at the elbow

Gives off *anterior interosseous* nerve in the cubital fossa

Leaves cubital fossa between 2 heads of pronator teres

Runs under fibrous arch of FDS with ulna artery

Midline in the forearm under FDS

Emerges laterally between tendons of PL and FCR

Gives off *palmar cutaneous* branch

Passes under flexor retinaculum

Divides in carpal tunnel into *lateral* and *medial* branches

Lateral gives off *muscular recurrent* and 3 digital branches
(2 to thumb and 1 to index).
Medial divides into 2 digital branches (to 2nd and 3rd
web spaces)

AbPB, abductor pollicis brevis
FCR, flexor carpi radialis
FDP, flexor digitorum profundus
FDS, flexor digitorum superficialis
FPB, flexor pollicis brevis
FPL, flexor pollicis longus
OP, opponens pollicis
PL, palmans longus
PQ, pronator quadratus
PT, pronator teres

Vasomotor to
brachial artery

Elbow joint

Anterior interosseous

FPL

Lateral ½ FDP

PQ

Wrist joint

PT

FCR

PL

FDS

Medial
Digital nerve to 2nd web
and 2nd lumbrical
Digital nerve to 3rd web

Lateral

Muscular recurrent
– AbPB
– FPB
– OP

2 digital nerves to thumb
1 to index and 1st lumbrical

Palmar cutaneous
Passes over flexor retinaculum to
supply skin over thena eminence

C5
C6
C7
C8
T1

05

Figure 42.13 Course and distribution of the median nerve.

Each has its merits but they all require regular hand therapy and review in outpatients to achieve satisfactory results. If a repair ruptures it is possible to resuture it, providing it is identified at an early stage; otherwise later tendon grafting is necessary, and this is performed in two stages. If adhesions occur that cannot be corrected by hand therapy, they are divided surgically (tenolysis).

Nerve injury

The three major nerves innervating the hand are the median, ulnar and radial. Their anatomical courses and motor and sensory functions in the hand are shown in Figs 42.13–42.15.

Assessment

Median nerve
- Observe wasting of the thenar muscles.
- Anterior interosseous: inability to make an 'O' sign with the thumb and index finger due to denervation of the flexor pollicis longus and index flexor digitorum profundus.
- Motor branch:
  (a) Weakness of thumb abduction due to denervation of abductor pollicis brevis.
  (b) Weakness of pulp-to-pulp opposition between thumb and little finger due to denervation of the opponens pollicis.
- Sensory: moving two-point discrimination over the index finger pulp.

Ulnar nerve
- Observe interosseous wasting (guttering) on the dorsum of the hand and hypothenar wasting.
- *Ulnar claw hand*: this is more marked if the ulnar nerve is divided after it gives a twig to the ulnar half of the flexor digitorum profundus. All the interossei are paralysed along with the ulnar lumbricals. This results in unopposed extension of the MCP joints by the intrinsic extensors and unopposed flexion of the IP joints by the extrinsic flexors. If the injury is more proximal, flexor digitorum profundus to the ring and little fingers is also paralysed, which obliterates flexion at the distal IP joint and makes the deformity appear less severe.
- *Froment's sign*: this is a test of adductor pollicis. The patient is required to grasp a piece of paper between thumb and index finger with the IP joints extended. If the ulnar nerve is paralysed, the adductor pollicis and first dorsal interossei are weak and cannot hold this position. In order to hold on to the piece of paper the patient compensates by flexing the thumb IP joint and index distal IP joint, thus using flexor pollicis longus and flexor digitorum profundus of the index finger to maintain a grip.

- Interossei: these can be tested by asking the patient to grip a piece of paper between the web spaces of their fingers. If the ulnar is paralysed, you will easily be able to pull the paper out of the web space.
- Sensory: moving two-point discrimination over the little finger pulp.

Radial nerve
- Observe wrist drop.
- Posterior interosseous nerve: with the palm flat the patient is unable to elevate the thumb off the table as the extensor pollicis longus is paralysed. The patient is unable to forcibly extend the wrist.
- Sensory: moving two-point discrimination over the dorsum of the hand.

Nerve repair

The cross-sectional anatomy of a typical myelinated peripheral nerve is shown in Fig. 42.16. Following division of a peripheral nerve, the axons in the distal segment undergo Wallerian degeneration, ultimately to the end receptor. This occurs over a period of about 6 weeks. There is also retrograde degeneration of the axons proximally back to the next most proximal branch. Regenerative sprouting of axons then commences in the proximal segment, providing the cell body has not been damaged. Nerve injury is classified according to the degree of anatomical damage (Table 42.3).

The principle of nerve repair is to obtain good fascicular alignment with minimal tension to enable the sprouting axons to bridge the gap of injury. If this cannot be achieved primarily, nerve grafting should be considered. This usually involves the sacrifice of a nerve from another site (e.g. sural), although vessels and synthetic tubes have been used.

Once they have crossed the repair, axons advance at a rate of about 1 mm/day. Tinel's sign is used to monitor their movement. The line of the affected nerve is percussed with the fingertip, commencing distally. Percussion over regenerating axon sprouts induces tingling.

Outcome of nerve repair is better if:
- the patient is young;
- less than 10 h has elapsed since the injury;
- sharp transection not avulsion has occurred;
- division is distal not proximal.

Neuroma formation can be a complication of nerve injury. Neuromas present as discrete areas of pain and exquisite tenderness on pressure or movement of adjacent joints. They are due to sprouting nerve endings, which grow into the surrounding tissues in a disorganized fashion forming a subcutaneous nodule. They are best treated

05

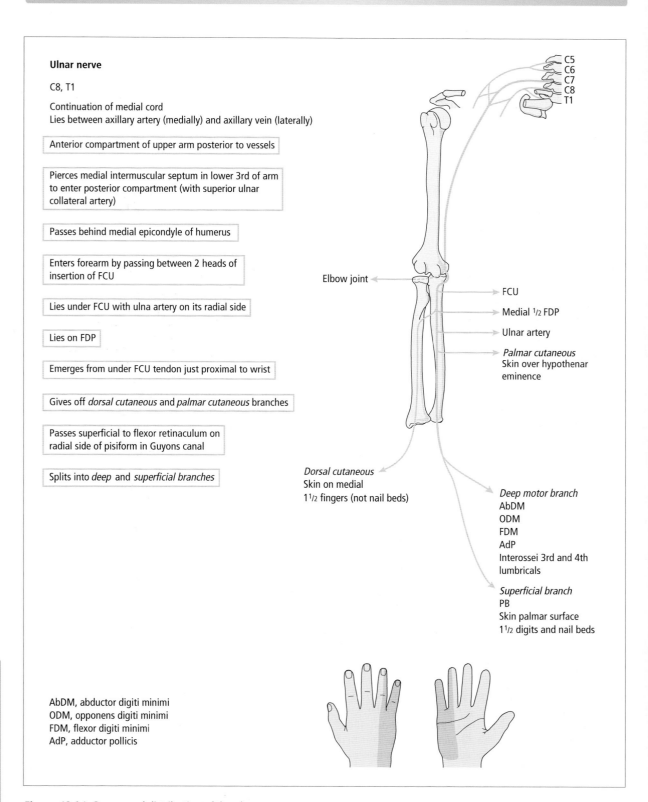

Ulnar nerve

C8, T1

Continuation of medial cord
Lies between axillary artery (medially) and axillary vein (laterally)

Anterior compartment of upper arm posterior to vessels

Pierces medial intermuscular septum in lower 3rd of arm to enter posterior compartment (with superior ulnar collateral artery)

Passes behind medial epicondyle of humerus

Enters forearm by passing between 2 heads of insertion of FCU

Lies under FCU with ulna artery on its radial side

Lies on FDP

Emerges from under FCU tendon just proximal to wrist

Gives off *dorsal cutaneous* and *palmar cutaneous* branches

Passes superficial to flexor retinaculum on radial side of pisiform in Guyons canal

Splits into *deep* and *superficial* branches

C5
C6
C7
C8
T1

Elbow joint

FCU
Medial 1/2 FDP
Ulnar artery
Palmar cutaneous
Skin over hypothenar eminence

Dorsal cutaneous
Skin on medial
1 1/2 fingers (not nail beds)

Deep motor branch
AbDM
ODM
FDM
AdP
Interossei 3rd and 4th
lumbricals

Superficial branch
PB
Skin palmar surface
1 1/2 digits and nail beds

AbDM, abductor digiti minimi
ODM, opponens digiti minimi
FDM, flexor digiti minimi
AdP, adductor pollicis

Figure 42.14 Course and distribution of the ulnar nerve.

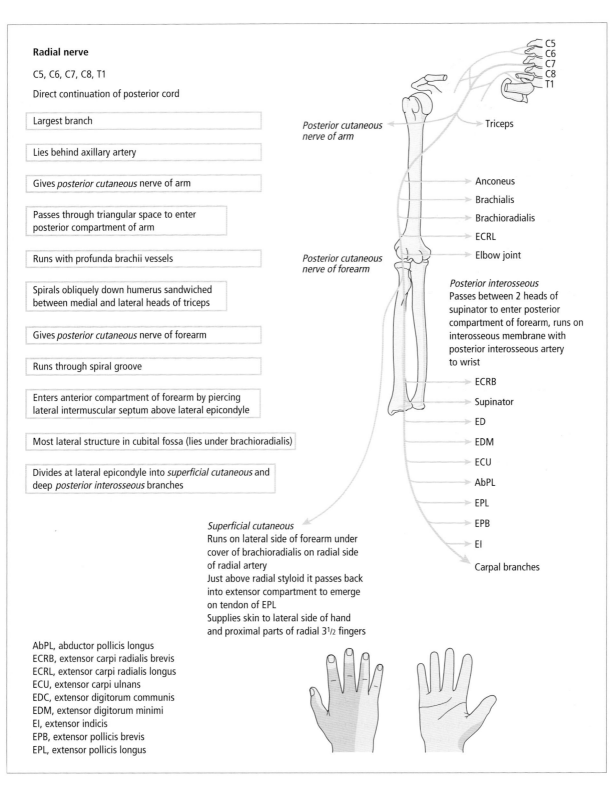

Radial nerve

C5, C6, C7, C8, T1

Direct continuation of posterior cord

Largest branch

Lies behind axillary artery

Gives *posterior cutaneous* nerve of arm

Passes through triangular space to enter posterior compartment of arm

Runs with profunda brachii vessels

Spirals obliquely down humerus sandwiched between medial and lateral heads of triceps

Gives *posterior cutaneous* nerve of forearm

Runs through spiral groove

Enters anterior compartment of forearm by piercing lateral intermuscular septum above lateral epicondyle

Most lateral structure in cubital fossa (lies under brachioradialis)

Divides at lateral epicondyle into *superficial cutaneous* and deep *posterior interosseous* branches

Posterior cutaneous nerve of arm

Posterior cutaneous nerve of forearm

Triceps

Anconeus
Brachialis
Brachioradialis
ECRL
Elbow joint

Posterior interosseous
Passes between 2 heads of supinator to enter posterior compartment of forearm, runs on interosseous membrane with posterior interosseous artery to wrist

ECRB
Supinator
ED
EDM
ECU
AbPL
EPL
EPB
EI
Carpal branches

C5
C6
C7
C8
T1

Superficial cutaneous
Runs on lateral side of forearm under cover of brachioradialis on radial side of radial artery
Just above radial styloid it passes back into extensor compartment to emerge on tendon of EPL
Supplies skin to lateral side of hand and proximal parts of radial 3½ fingers

AbPL, abductor pollicis longus
ECRB, extensor carpi radialis brevis
ECRL, extensor carpi radialis longus
ECU, extensor carpi ulnans
EDC, extensor digitorum communis
EDM, extensor digitorum minimi
EI, extensor indicis
EPB, extensor pollicis brevis
EPL, extensor pollicis longus

05

Figure 42.15 Course and distribution of the radial nerve.

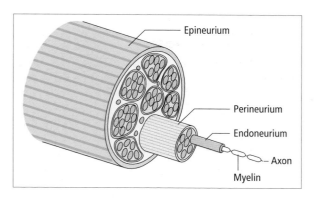

Figure 42.16 Cross-sectional anatomy of a myelinated peripheral nerve.

by prevention, although symptomatic neuromas can be excised.

Evaluation of peripheral nerve injuries and repairs can be performed by electromyography (EMG) and nerve conduction velocity studies.

Fracture management

Fractures can occur at multiple sites in all hand bones. The specific management of each is beyond the scope of this text. Accurate description of the injury is vital to make a management decision:

- open or closed;
- intra-articular or extra-articular;
- displaced or non-displaced;
- rotational deformity;
- shortening;
- stable or unstable.

As a general rule, all open or unstable injuries require surgical intervention. Splintage can be employed to treat most stable closed injuries. Ligamentous injuries must also be assessed. Unstable joints may require open repair or a period of immobilization.

Amputation

Anastomosis of small blood vessels can be performed under the operating microscope and these techniques are used to reperfuse the hand. Replantation is technically possible for amputations from the distal fingertips to amputation of the entire upper limb. However, each case must be assessed individually as there are many factors to consider in deciding if replantation is appropriate.

Time delay until surgery must be minimized because prolonged ischaemia causes permanent tissue damage. However, the permissible ischaemia time is longer for parts that do not contain muscle and can be lengthened by cooling the amputated part. This should be done by wrapping the amputated part in a saline-soaked swab and then sealing it in a dry polythene bag. The ideal storage temperature is 4°C, and placing the amputated part *on* ice is satisfactory. It should not be placed *in* ice as this will freeze the tissues and cause irreversible damage.

Pulp amputation can often be left to heal conservatively with dressings, particularly if the distal phalanx is not exposed. The defect will contract and heal, leaving only a small area of altered sensibility.

Complex regional pain syndrome (reflex sympathetic dystrophy or Sudek's disease)

This encompasses a variety of non-specific painful symptoms that occur following injury. They exceed, both in magnitude and duration, the expected clinical course of the inciting event. Signs and symptoms can include:

- pain (constant and burning);
- swelling;
- stiffness;
- vasomotor instability (vasoconstriction with cold intolerance);
- discoloration (erythema, cyanosis or pallor);

Table 42.3 Classification of nerve injury.

	Insult	Prognosis
Neuropraxia	Segmental demyelination: axons intact, normal conduction proximal and distal to the site of injury	Full recovery 1–4 months
Axonotmesis	Axon severed but epineurium, endoneurium and perineurium intact. Degeneration of axons distally	Full recovery 4–18 months
Neurotmesis	Entire nerve (axons, epineurium, endoneurium and perineurium) severed. Degeneration of axons distally and proximally. Needs surgical repair	No recovery if not repaired Variable recovery post surgical repair

- increased sweating;
- osteoporosis.

The aetiology of this condition is uncertain but it is considered to be a prolonged and exaggerated sympathetic response to injury. It often develops early in the postoperative period, when the diagnosis can be delayed because the physician believes the patient to have a low pain threshold. Initial treatment is physiotherapy, which can incorporate both mobilization and splinting. Drugs such as carbamazepine and amitriptyline are also useful. Sympatholytic drugs like phentolamine and local anaesthetics also have a place in the treatment of this condition. Resistant cases may require surgical sympathectomy.

Infections

Most suppurative hand infections follow penetrating trauma and the causative organism is usually *Staphylococcus aureus*. Human bites are commonly the result of punching someone in the mouth. They usually lead to infection over the metacarpal where the tooth laceration occurs. The causative organism is *Eikenella corrodens* and treatment involves débridment in conjunction with a penicillinase-resistant penicillin. Animal bites also lead to local infection. Here the causative organism is usually *Pasteurella multocida*. Again, débridment is indicated as well as appropriate antibiotic therapy.

Specific sites of infection

- Paronychia: this refers to infection of the soft tissue adjacent to the nail. It is probably the most common site of infection in the hand and is usually caused by *Staph. aureus*. Treatment is surgical incision and drainage, which involves deroofing the abscess and removing a segment (or all) of the neighbouring nail to allow adequate drainage through the lateral nail fold.
- Pulp space infections are also known as felons. Again, they require surgical drainage by opening the pulp.
- Tendon sheath infections are rare but serious. Pus tracks along the flexor sheath and if untreated the tendons can rupture. The finger involved becomes swollen and assumes a flexed position. There is exquisite pain on passive extension of the finger. The treatment involves opening the flexor sheath and irrigation with a feeding catheter.
- Palmar bursae infections can also occur. Two palmar bursae exist in the hand (Fig. 42.17): the radial bursa encloses the flexor pollicis longus tendon and the ulnar bursa encloses the long flexor tendons of the index to little fingers. This latter space is continuous with the flexor sheath of the little finger and thus infection in this sheath can spread into the palm. Again, treatment involves surgical incision and evacuation of the pus.
- Thenar space infections arise in the space under the thenar muscles and above the adductor pollicis muscle. This space is limited radially by the first metacarpal, while on the ulnar side it is limited by a fibrous septum attached to the third metacarpal. These infections are commonly drained through an incision on the dorsum of the hand.
- Midpalmar space infections occur deep to the flexor tendons of the ulnar three fingers. The space is bounded by the fifth metacarpal and the ulnar limit of the thenar space. Purulent infections in this space points in the third and fourth web spaces where incisions for drainage can be made.

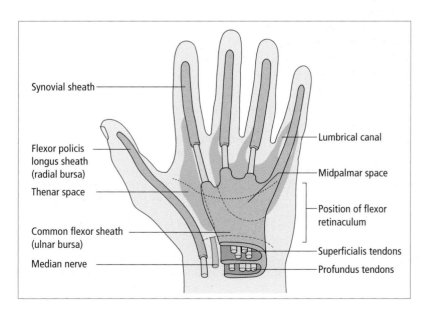

Figure 42.17 Palmar spaces/bursae and synovial sheaths.

05

Hand surgery at a glance

Requirements for good hand function
- Good blood supply
- A stable skeleton
- Soft pliable skin cover (which does not restrict mobility)
- Innervation, motor and sensory
- Motion (provided by smoothly gliding tendons)

Assessment of the injured hand
- When did the injury occur and how much time has since elapsed?
- Where did the injury occur and was the environment clean or dirty?
- What was the mechanism of injury and can you predict which structures are likely to have been damaged?
- Determine patient's age, hand dominance, occupation and hobbies

Examination
Look
- Volar and dorsal surfaces: any soft-tissue injury
- Colour: assess perfusion
- Swelling: underlying bone or ligament injury
- Wasting: nerve injury
- Position of hand: is there a normal flexion cascade of fingers, clawing in ulnar nerve injury, subluxation of MCP joints with ulnar drift in rheumatoid arthritis?

Feel
- Tenderness
- Joint stability
- Temperature: assess perfusion
- Sensation: specific nerves (see below)

Move
- Passive range of movement
- Active range of movement
- Motor function of specific nerves

Tendon injury
Flexor tendon injuries are more serious than extensor tendon injuries

Tendon	Clinical	Treatment	Rehabilitation
Flexor	Inability to flex distal IP joint or proximal IP joint with hand and fingers in extension	Brunner's incision, core suture	Most important after hand injury: dynamic, passive and active mobilization
Extensor	Mallett finger: inability to extend distal phalanx Boutonnière deformity: flexion of proximal IP and hyperextension of distal IP joints	Conservative treatment by splinting or surgery for open injury	

IP, interphalangeal.

Nerve injury
Classification
- Neurotmesis: complete anatomical division of a nerve with Wallerian degeneration
- Axonotmesis: nerve axons are damaged, with Wallerian degeneration, but connective tissues survive. Better prognosis than neurotmesis
- Neuropraxia: minimal damage without Wallerian degerneration

Evaluation
- Clinical
- EMG
- Nerve conduction studies

Principles of nerve repair
- Good fascicular alignment with minimal tension
- If this cannot be achieved primarily, nerve grafting should be considered
- Regeneration occurs at 1 mm/day
- Tinel's sign: a tingling sensation induced on percussion or pressure over the point to which regeneration of a peripheral nerve has advanced
- Good prognostic features:
  (a) Young patient
  (b) Injury for < 10 h
  (c) Sharp transection not avulsion
  (d) Site of injury is distal
- Complication: neuroma

05

Specific nerve injuries

Nerve	Motor	Sensory	Trophic
Median (at elbow)	'Pointing' index finger and 'simian hand' (loss of abduction and opposition of the thumb)	Sensory loss over all palmar aspect and distal dorsal aspect of radial $3^1/2$ fingers	Wasting of thenar eminence muscles
Median (at wrist)	Simian hand		
Ulnar (at elbow)	Claw hand (*main en griffe*)	Palmar and dorsal medial $1^1/2$ fingers	Interosseus (dorsum of hand) and hypothenar wasting
Ulnar (at wrist)	Marked claw hand		
Radial	Wrist drop	Anaesthesia of a small area at the base of the thumb and index finger	Wasting of long wrist extensors

Fractures
- Open or closed
- Intra-articular or extra-articular
- Displaced or non-displaced
- Rotational deformity
- Shortening
- Stable or unstable

Treatment
- Open or unstable injuries: surgical intervention
- Stable closed injuries: splints
- Unstable joints: open repair or immobilization

Amputation
- Pulp amputation: will heal with dressings, particularly if the distal phalanx is not exposed
- From distal finger to proximal arm: reimplantation is possible. Arteries, veins, nerves, tendons (muscle) and skin have to be repaired
- Time delay until surgery must be minimized
- Store amputated part in saline-soaked swab at 4°C
- Place part *on* ice not in ice

Reflex sympathetic dystrophy (Sudek's disease)
Definition
A variety of non-specific painful symptoms of unknown aetiology that occur following injury. Possibly due to prolonged and exaggerated sympathetic response to injury

Clinical features
- Pain: constant and burning
- Swelling
- Stiffness
- Vasomotor instability: vasoconstriction with cold intolerance
- Discoloration: erythema, cyanosis or pallor
- Increased sweating
- Osteoporosis

Treatment
- Physiotherapy (mobilization and splinting)
- Carbamezepine and amitriptyline
- Sympatholytic drugs (phentolamine and local anaesthetics)
- Surgical sympathectomy

Infections
- Paronychia: staphylococcal infection of the soft tissue adjacent to the nail. Treatment is incision and drainage
- Pulp space infection (felons): incision and drainage
- Tendon sheath infection: open flexor sheath and irrigate with catheter
- Palmar bursae infection: surgical incision and evacuation of pus
- Thenar space infection: drained through an incision on the dorsum of the hand
- Midpalmar space: drained through the third and fourth web spaces
- Human bites: infection over metacarpal heads where tooth laceration occurs. Organism involved is *Eikenella corrodens*. Treatment is débridment + penicillinase-resistant penicillin + metronidazole
- Animal bites: local infection. Organism involved is *Pasteurella multocida*. Treatment is débridment + appropriate antibiotic

05

Pressure sores

Pressure sores (decubitus ulcers or bed sores) are a common source of referral to the plastic surgical team. They are due to prolonged unrelieved pressure over bony prominences and are common in patients who are bedridden or have restrictive casts or appliances and in those who have large insensate areas.

Aetiology

If tissue pressure is greater than perfusion pressure, then the blood supply to the tissue will be compromised and ischaemia with eventual necrosis occurs. Muscle is more susceptible to ischaemia than skin. A cone-shaped area of tissue breakdown results, with its apex at the skin surface and its base overlying the bony prominence. The size of the resultant pressure sore is proportional to the pressure exerted and its duration.

Predisposing factors include the following.
- Infection of the pressure sore can increase its depth.
- Shearing forces lead to degloving of the subcutaneous tissues, impairing their blood supply.
- Excessive moisture worsens the situation by macerating or eroding the skin. If this is due to faecal or urinary incontinence, there is the added risk of infection.
- Malnutrition, anaemia and immunosuppression, from concomitant illness or pharmacotherapy, not only predispose to pressure sores but also impair healing once the ulcer is established. Unfortunately, these factors are common in debilitated individuals.
- Insensitivity, caused by peripheral or central nervous system damage, allows sores to develop unnoticed from minor trauma. Infection can also go undetected until the sore reaches a considerable size.

Risk assessment and grading

The Waterlow score was established to predict those patients most likely to develop pressure sores so that preventive measures can be taken. It involves scoring the patient on the following factors:
- body mass index;
- age;
- sex;
- continence;
- mobility;
- nutrition;
- skin changes;
- adverse wound healing factors;
- neurological deficit;
- surgical interventions;
- drugs.

Once a sore has developed it is graded according to depth as follows:
- erythema;
- blister;
- full-thickness skin loss into subcutaneous tissue;
- muscle breakdown;
- bone/joint involvement.

Sites

The site of the sore depends on the position the patient has been lying in.

Common
- Sacral: from lying supine.
- Ischial: from sitting, particularly in wheelchair-bound patients.
- Trochanteric: from lying on one side.
- Malleolar: from tight-fitting lower-limb plaster casts.
- Heel: from lying supine.

Rare
- Occipital: lying supine, particularly in neurosurgical patients.
- Ears: lying on one side or tight-fitting bandages.
- Elbow.
- Scapula.

Management

Prevention is the best treatment and so Waterlow scores should be recorded in debilitated or bedridden patients and appropriate preventive measures instituted in those deemed at risk. Once a pressure sore is established, treatment first addresses general factors, then relieves pressure and then involves specific management of the ulcer.

General factors

- Nutrition: malnutrition and hypoproteinaemia should be addressed. The patient should be considered for nasogastric or parenteral feeding if oral intake is insufficient or not possible.
- Anaemia should be assessed and corrected with dietary supplements or transfusion according to severity.
- Incontinence: catheterization is necessary for urinary incontinence. If faecal incontinence is causing recurrent infection or considerable deterioration of the pressure sore, faecal diversion should be considered.
- Infection should be assessed with regular swabs or tissue biopsy. Appropriate antibiotic therapy should be instituted and surgical débridement may be necessary.

05

Relief of pressure

- Turning is vital to eliminate prolonged pressure.
- Specific beds are available to eliminate continued localized pressure and decrease shearing forces. These include low air loss mattresses, Clinitron bed (fluidized by warm air), Pegasus bed (alternating pressure) and Nimbus bed (dynamic floatation).
- Padding of pressure areas with specific appliances can prevent sores developing and progressing. These include heel pads, horseshoe head rings and a variety of pressure-relieving cushions for wheelchairs.

Dressings

It has been famously quoted that you can put anything on a pressure sore, except the patient. A variety of dressings are available. These range from antisloughing dressings (to remove cellular debris) to foam-padded dressings (to protect areas at risk). In a clean pressure sore or following surgical débridement, the vacuum-assisted closure (VAC) system can be used. This is a sponge dressing which is made to measure and placed snugly into the cavity of the sore. Via a sealed tubing system it is connected to a free-standing vacuum device. An airtight seal is created with an occlusive dressing and negative pressure is then exerted over the wound. This removes oedema and wound effluent, which delays healing, as well as reducing the bacterial load. It is thought to actually increase local blood flow to the wound, although the exact mechanisms of this are unclear. Its main use in pressure sore management is to reduce the size of the wound, which it does by encouraging granulation and wound contraction.

Specific management

Firstly, the pressure sore needs to be accurately assessed. Microbiological evaluation should be obtained with wound swabs or tissue biopsies. The presence of more than 100,000 organisms per gram of tissue is usually indicative of infection and appropriate antibiotics should be instituted. The size and extent of the wound should be examined. This involves probing any cavity and obtaining radiographs of the underlying bone to detect osteomyelitis. Contrast studies are useful to delineate sinus tracts leading away from the ulcer.

The aims of surgical intervention are:
- thorough débridement of the ulcer, all necrotic tissue and the underlying bursa;
- resection of the underlying bone, which is often unhealthy or frankly osteomyelitic;
- coverage of the defect with well-vascularized tissue.

In general, large regional skin or myocutaneous flaps are used as rotation or advancement flaps to cover the defect.

Examples include gluteus maximus flap for sacral or ischial pressure sores and tensor fascia lata flap for trochanteric sores. Occasionally, it is possible to provide sensation by the use of innervated flaps, e.g. tensor fascia lata flap incorporating the lateral femoral cutaneous nerve. Postoperatively, it is important to avoid pressure on the flap for 3–4 weeks.

Since recurrence of pressure sores is common and progressively more difficult to treat, prevention is vital in these patients.

Lower limb trauma surgery

Lower limb trauma encompasses a wide range of injuries. As well as fracture management the integrity of vessels, nerves and soft tissues must be addressed. In most plastic surgery units a lower limb trauma team exists. This includes orthopaedic and plastic surgeons, occupational therapists and physiotherapists, as well as pain management and prosthetic services.

Anatomy

Compartments and muscles (Table 42.4)

The tibia and fibula are the bones of the lower leg. The tibia bears 85% of the weight and lies medially. It is bound to the laterally lying fibula by the interosseous membrane. The lower leg is enclosed in deep fascia like a stocking. This is a continuation of the popliteal fascia. It encloses the calf and lateral lower leg, attaching to the anterior and posterior borders of the tibia. Anterior and posterior

Table 42.4 Compartments and muscles of the lower limb.

Anterior compartment (dorsiflexes the foot)
Extensor hallucis longus
Extensor digitorum longus
Tibialis anterior
Peroneus tertius

Lateral compartment (everts the foot)
Peroneus longus
Peroneus brevis

Posterior compartment (plantar flexes the foot)
Superficial
  Gastrocnemius
  Soleus
  Planaris
Deep
  Flexor hallucis longus
  Flexor digitorum longus
  Tibialis posterior

05

Pressure sores at a glance

Definition

Pressure sores: ulcers over bony prominences caused by prolonged unrelieved pressure leading to ischaemic necrosis

Local predisposing factors
- Infection
- Shearing forces
- Excessive moisture
- Malnutrition, anaemia and immunosuppression
- Insensitivity

Risk assessment and grading
Waterlow score
Risk assessment score based on following:
- Body mass index
- Age
- Sex
- Continence
- Mobility
- Nutrition
- Skin changes
- Adverse wound healing factors
- Neurological deficit
- Surgical interventions
- Drugs

Grading (according to depth)
- Erythema
- Blister
- Full-thickness skin loss into subcutaneous tissue
- Muscle breakdown
- Bone/joint involvement

Sites
Common
- Sacral: from lying supine
- Ischial: from sitting, particularly in wheelchair-bound patients
- Trochanteric: from lying on one side
- Malleolar: from tight-fitting lower-limb plaster casts
- Heel: from lying supine

Rare
- Occipital: lying supine, particularly in neurosurgical patients
- Ears: lying on one side or tight-fitting bandages
- Elbow
- Scapula

Management
Preventive measures instituted in those deemed at risk based on Waterlow score

General
- Nutrition: make sure patient is fed (enterally or parenterally)
- Anaemia: correct
- Incontinence: catheter for urine, consider diversion for faeces
- Infection: treat appropriately

Pressure
- Turn patient frequently
- Use special beds:
    (a) Clinitron (fluidized by warm air)
    (b) Pegasus (alternating pressure)
    (c) Nimbus (dynamic floatation).
- Padding: heel pads, horseshoe head rings, pressure-relieving cushions
- Dressings: antisloughing dressings, foam padded dressings, VAC system

Specific management
Accurate assessment
- Swabs/tissue biopsies for microbiology (> 100,000 organisms/g of tissue means infection is present)
- Measure size and extent of wound by probing any cavity and obtaining radiographs

Aims of surgery
- Débridement of the ulcer
- Resection of the underlying bone
- Cover defect with well-vascularized tissue: probably a myocutaneous flap
- Recurrence is common

intermuscular septa are attached to the peroneal surface of the fibula and these, with the tibia and interosseous membrane, divide the lower leg into three compartments (Fig. 42.18). The anterior extensor compartment is bounded medially by the subcutaneous border of the tibia, laterally by the anterior intermuscular septum and behind by the interosseous membrane. The lateral peroneal compart- ment lies between the anterior and posterior intermuscular septa. The posterior flexor compartment is commonly called the calf. It is separated from the peroneal compartment by the posterior intermuscular septum and from the anterior compartment by the interosseous membrane. Its muscles lie in two groups, superficial and deep, subdividing it into two compartments.

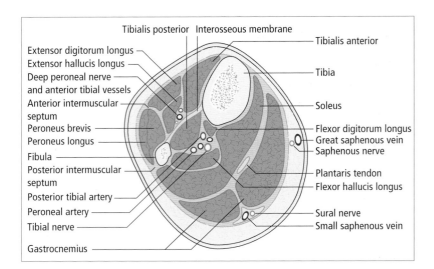

Figure 42.18 Cross-section of the right lower leg.

Arteries

● *Anterior tibial artery*: supplies the anterior (extensor) compartment of the lower leg. It starts at the bifurcation of the popliteal artery under the fibrous arch of the soleus muscle. It lies medial to the neck of the fibula. It passes forwards above the upper border of the interosseous membrane and then descends in front of it. It lies between the malleoli at the ankle joint and there becomes the dorsalis pedis artery, which can be easily palpated. It passes under the extensor retinacula with the deep peroneal nerve lying laterally.

● *Posterior tibial artery*: supplies the posterior (flexor) compartment of the lower leg. It also starts at the bifurcation of the popliteal artery under the fibrous arch of soleus. It runs deep to gastrocnemius and soleus on the tibialis posterior, flexor digitorum longus and tibia. At the ankle joint it lies behind the medial malleolus where it can be easily palpated. Here it is between the tendon of flexor digitorum longus and the tibial nerve.

● *Peroneal artery*: supplies the lateral compartment of the lower leg. It is a branch of the posterior tibial artery arising just after it commences. It runs medial to the fibula between tibialis posterior and flexor hallucis longus.

Nerves

About a hand's breadth above the knee the sciatic nerve divides into the tibial and common peroneal nerves. The common peroneal nerve divides under peroneus longus into the deep and superficial peroneal nerves. The nerve of the anterior compartment of the lower leg is the deep peroneal. The nerve to the lateral compartment is the superficial peroneal and the nerve to the posterior compartment is the tibial nerve.

The course and functions of these nerves are shown in Figs 42.19 & 42.20.

Lower limb injuries

Pretibial lacerations

These are flap lacerations of the thin skin overlying the subcutaneous tibial border. They are common in the elderly population, who tend to have thin fragile skin, and are often the result of minimal trauma.

Any haematoma should be evacuated to avoid pressure necrosis of the overlying skin. Broad-based skin flaps with a proximally based pedicle may be viable and can be relaid and secured with Steri-strips. Thin distally based flaps will have unreliable blood flow and are often not viable. This type of injury should be débrided and resurfaced with a split-thickness skin graft. This may be feasible under local anaesthetic.

Open fractures

These injuries are often the result of high-velocity trauma. Concomitant injury to other sites, including the head, chest and abdomen, are common. Therefore the initial management of these patients should be thorough assessment as per the ATLS protocol. The lower limb should then be carefully evaluated once the patient is stable.

Evaluation
● *Vascularity*: palpate the posterior tibial and dorsalis pedis arteries. If they cannot be felt manually, use handheld Doppler ultrasound. If there is any uncertainty or if revascularization may be needed, then angiography of the lower limb is indicated.

05

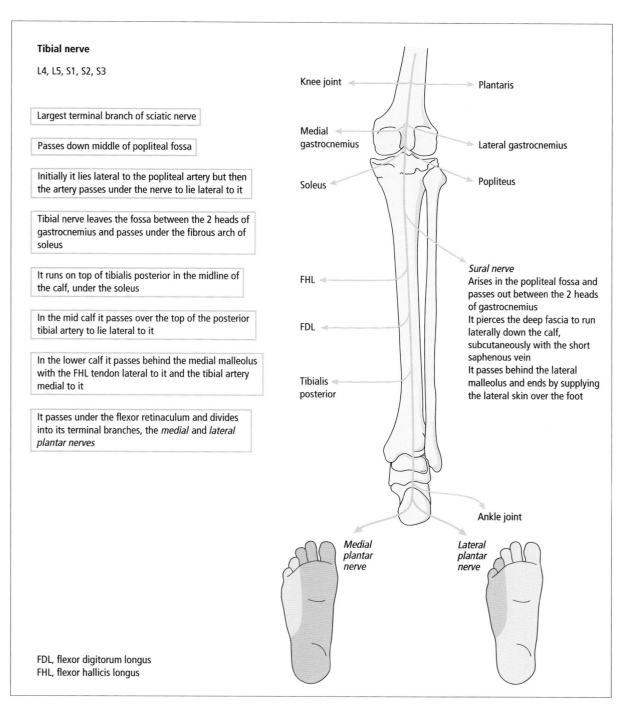

Tibial nerve

L4, L5, S1, S2, S3

Largest terminal branch of sciatic nerve

Passes down middle of popliteal fossa

Initially it lies lateral to the popliteal artery but then the artery passes under the nerve to lie lateral to it

Tibial nerve leaves the fossa between the 2 heads of gastrocnemius and passes under the fibrous arch of soleus

It runs on top of tibialis posterior in the midline of the calf, under the soleus

In the mid calf it passes over the top of the posterior tibial artery to lie lateral to it

In the lower calf it passes behind the medial malleolus with the FHL tendon lateral to it and the tibial artery medial to it

It passes under the flexor retinaculum and divides into its terminal branches, the *medial* and *lateral plantar nerves*

Knee joint → Plantaris

Medial gastrocnemius → Lateral gastrocnemius

Soleus → Popliteus

Sural nerve
Arises in the popliteal fossa and passes out between the 2 heads of gastrocnemius
It pierces the deep fascia to run laterally down the calf, subcutaneously with the short saphenous vein
It passes behind the lateral malleolus and ends by supplying the lateral skin over the foot

FHL ←

FDL ←

Tibialis posterior ←

Ankle joint

Medial plantar nerve

Lateral plantar nerve

FDL, flexor digitorum longus
FHL, flexor hallicis longus

Figure 42.19 Course and distribution of the tibial nerve.

- *Bony injury*: X-ray of the fracture should provide a clear description of fracture site, displacement and stability.
- *Soft-tissue damage*: the size and site of soft-tissue damage are important. They give a clue as to what underlying structures have been damaged and determine how the soft-tissue defect can be reconstructed.
- *Nerves*: motor and sensory function of each nerve must be assessed and documented (Table 42.5).

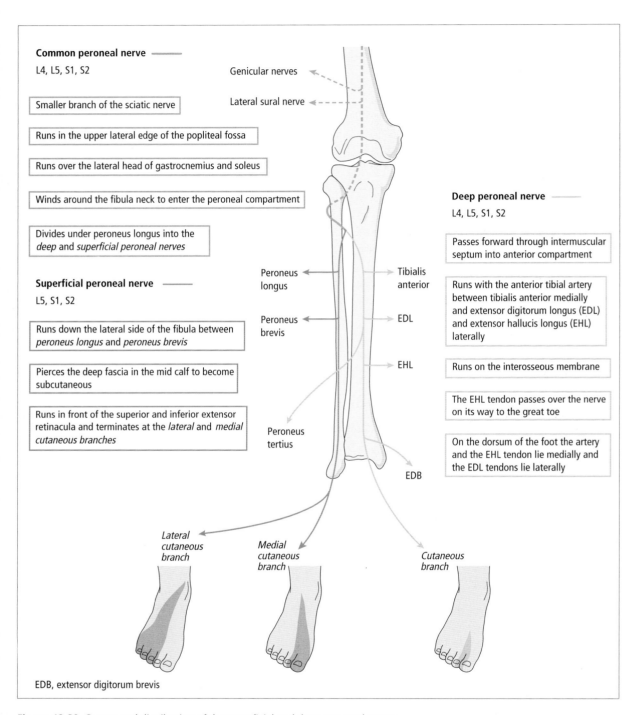

Common peroneal nerve ———
L4, L5, S1, S2

Genicular nerves ←--

Lateral sural nerve ←---

Smaller branch of the sciatic nerve

Runs in the upper lateral edge of the popliteal fossa

Runs over the lateral head of gastrocnemius and soleus

Winds around the fibula neck to enter the peroneal compartment

Divides under peroneus longus into the
deep and *superficial peroneal nerves*

Superficial peroneal nerve ———
L5, S1, S2

Runs down the lateral side of the fibula between
peroneus longus and *peroneus brevis*

Pierces the deep fascia in the mid calf to become
subcutaneous

Runs in front of the superior and inferior extensor
retinacula and terminates at the *lateral* and *medial
cutaneous branches*

Peroneus ←
longus

Peroneus ←
brevis

Peroneus
tertius

Deep peroneal nerve ———
L4, L5, S1, S2

Passes forward through intermuscular
septum into anterior compartment

Runs with the anterior tibial artery
between tibialis anterior medially
and extensor digitorum longus (EDL)
and extensor hallucis longus (EHL)
laterally

Runs on the interosseous membrane

The EHL tendon passes over the nerve
on its way to the great toe

On the dorsum of the foot the artery
and the EHL tendon lie medially and
the EDL tendons lie laterally

Tibialis
anterior

EDL

EHL

EDB

*Lateral
cutaneous
branch*

*Medial
cutaneous
branch*

*Cutaneous
branch*

EDB, extensor digitorum brevis

Figure 42.20 Course and distribution of the superficial and deep peroneal nerves.

Classification

There are a variety of classifications available for describing open fractures of the lower limb. The Gustillo classification is commonly used for open tibial injuries (Table 42.6). Not only is it useful for aiding management plans but it can also be a rough guide to prognosis. For example, approximately 4% of grade IIIC injuries often proceed to amputation and approximately 70% of grade IIIB injuries require flap cover.

05

Table 42.5 Assessment of motor and sensory function of lower limb nerves.

Tibial nerve
Motor
Inability to plantar flex the foot at the ankle indicates proximal lesions and paralysis of the gastrocnemius and soleus muscles

Sensory
Loss of sensation over the lower posterior calf, lateral foot and little toe (sural nerve)

Deep peroneal nerve
Motor
The patient has footdrop with inability to dorsiflex the foot and great toe due to paralysis of the extensor hallucis longus and tibialis anterior

Sensory
Loss of sensation over the first web space

Superficial peroneal nerve
Motor
Inability to evert the foot at the ankle due to paralysis of peroneus longus and peroneus brevis

Sensory
Loss of sensation over anterolateral calf and second and third web spaces

---

Table 42.6 Gustillo classification of open tibial fractures.

Grade	Tissue injury
I	Clean wound < 1 cm
II	Wound 1–5 cm but no significant tissue disruption
IIIA	Wound > 5 cm but adequate soft-tissue coverage with local tissues
IIIB	Extensive soft-tissue loss, contamination, periosteal stripping
IIIC	Arterial injury requiring repair

Management

Once the patient has been appropriately resuscitated, wound swabs should be taken and broad-spectrum antibiotics started. Tetanus prophylaxis should be assessed and immunoglobulin given if required. The wound should be dressed with a non-absorbent dressing and Betadine-soaked gauze and then wrapped and splinted. Manipulation of fractures at this stage should only be performed if they are impinging on the vascularity of the lower leg.

The patient is then transferred to theatre and further assessment of the injury is performed under general anaesthesia. The specific management is then dictated by the nature of the injury. As a rule all grossly contaminated and devitalized skin, muscle and free bone fragments are removed during this procedure and copious irrigation is performed. If possible the fracture is also stabilized at this time, with external or internal fixation as appropriate. If vascular injury is present it must be repaired as a priority. Often no attempt is made to close the wound at this stage and it is left open and packed with suitable dressings.

Quite often the zone of injury in these wounds is not demarcated on presentation. Tissues of marginal viability may become non-viable. Therefore re-exploration and further débridement may be necessary 48–72 h later. Once the viability of the remaining tissue is beyond doubt and the fracture has been appropriately fixed, the method of soft-tissue reconstruction can be addressed.

Soft-tissue reconstruction
This is dictated by the site and extent of the soft-tissue loss.
- *Split skin grafting.* This is appropriate for defects with a suitably clean and graftable bed. Therefore it is usually precluded if the fracture is exposed, as the periosteum will have been stripped.
- *Local muscle flaps.* These are ideal to cover small areas of exposed fracture site. The medial head of gastrocnemius is most commonly used. The muscle can be split in its midline through a longitudinal posterior calf incision. The medial half is then detached from its insertion into the Achilles tendon and tunnelled through to fill the defect. A split skin graft is then placed over the exposed muscle.
- *Local fasciocutaneous flaps.* Again these are useful for smaller defects. They can also be used to cover fracture sites. The donor site can be closed directly if small or split skin grafted.
- *Free tissue transfer.* This is necessary for larger defects and a variety of muscles can be employed. Microvascular anastomosis is necessary usually to the posterior or anterior tibial vessels.

Bone reconstruction
The problem of bony loss can also be addressed.
- Small defects can be bridged with cancellous bone grafts as long as there is a well-vascularized bed. It is advisable to wait 6–8 weeks after injury before doing this, as non-vascularized bone is susceptible to infection.
- Larger defects require vascularized bone as free tissue transfer.
- Intermediate-sized defects can be treated using the Ilizarov technique. An external fixator is used that encourages distraction osteogenesis.

Degloving injury

This is an avulsion of the skin, with or without underlying tissues from deeper planes. Degloving injuries are commonly the result of road traffic accidents. Those that result from being run over by a bus or truck are most serious, as the broad tyres of these vehicles distribute the shearing forces over a wide area, which can result in circumferential degloving of the entire skin and subcutaneous tissue of the leg.

The plane through which the skin is detached can be superficial, involving just skin and subcutaneous fat. However it can also incorporate the deep fascia. The skin may tear, creating a flap, or there may be no detectable skin breach, just bruising and swelling. The perforator blood supply from the muscles to the skin and subcutaneous fat is destroyed. So too is the vascular network in the superficial fascia. This results in ischaemic necrosis of the detached skin. There are two types of degloving injury.

● *Type I*: open wound due to degloving of the skin and subcutaneous fat with a narrow zone of undermined tissue around the periphery of the wound.
● *Type II*: extensive undermining of soft tissues with no or a relatively small open wound. The initial assessment of these wounds frequently underestimates the extent of damage, as most of the leg appears normal, apart from the presence of tyre marks and patches of ecchymosis. Unless treated early, the full extent of soft-tissue loss is apparent only a few days later, and gives rise to systemic sepsis due to necrosis of large areas of subcutaneous fat underneath the normal-looking skin. Fluoroscein injected intravenously circulates only to viable tissue and is a method of defining all non-viable tissue (that which does not fluoresce) at an early stage.

The clinical picture initially is less dramatic than expected, but the skin does not show blanching on pressure or capillary refill and skin edges do not bleed. All non-viable skin and underlying fat should be excised and the defect resurfaced with a split-thickness skin graft. There can be a delay in graft application, allowing a 'second look' at 48 h and further débridement if necessary. The non-viable areas excised can be used as donor sites if the defect requiring grafting is extensive. This should be performed early.

Compartment syndrome

Oedema is a sequela of trauma. If this occurs in a limited anatomical space, such as one of the four compartments of the lower limb, tissue pressure will rise. As tissue pressure rises, the pressure on and within the local venous system also rises. Arterial resistance subsequently increases and inflow is reduced. If left untreated there is vascular compromise and the enclosed muscles become ischaemic. Prolonged ischaemia will result in necrosis and, ultimately, fibrosis of the muscles and surrounding soft-tissue structures. Compartment syndrome in the lower limb is defined as intercompartmental pressures exceeding 35 mmHg. These can be measured at the bedside using a special manometer.

Clinically, the patient complains of pain out of proportion to the injury and this is exacerbated by stretching of the involved compartment muscles. As pressure increases there is loss of sensation in the distribution of the involved nerves and ultimately the local pulses are lost, although the latter is not necessary to make the diagnosis. The 'four Ps' of compartment syndrome that aid diagnosis comprise:
● pain;
● paraesthesia;
● paralysis;
● pulselessness.

Treatment involves immediate decompression. This is performed under general anaesthesia by incising all four muscle compartments (fasciotomy). The wounds are left open, allowing swelling to occur unrestricted, and dressed with appropriate sterile dressings. The wounds are closed at a later time once the acute episode has resolved. Sometimes this is not possible directly and split skin grafts are used.

Surgery for congenital deformities

Congenital head and neck problems

Embryology

The embryology of the head and neck is complicated. The normal skull develops from a membranous capsule that encloses a growing brain and then ossifies, whereas the base undergoes mainly cartilaginous ossification. In the third week of embryonic life these processes develop around the primitive mouth (Fig. 42.21).
● The *frontonasal process* projects down from the skull. The nostrils develop from two olfactory pits within it. This projection finally forms the nose, nasal septum, nostrils, philtrum (central upper lip depression) and the premaxilla.
● The two *maxillary processes*, one on each side, come to the midline and fuse with the frontonasal process. These form the cheeks, upper lip (excluding the philtrum), upper jaw and palate (excluding the premaxilla).
● The two *mandibular processes* meet in the midline to form the mandible.
Abnormalities of this complex fusion process result in one of the most common congenital deformities, cleft lip and palate.

05

Table 42.7 Embryology of the branchial arches.

Arch	Cartilage/bone structure	Cranial nerve	Muscles (mesoderm)	Soft tissue (endoderm and ectoderm)	Artery	Abnormality
First	Mandible, maxilla, incus, malleus	V, including chorda tympani	Muscles of mastication, mylohyoid, anterior belly digastric, tensor palati and tensor tympani	Anterior two-thirds tongue glands and mucous membranes	Maxillary	Cleft lip and palate, preauricular skin tags, Treacher–Collins syndrome, Pierre Robin syndrome
Second*	Stapes, styloid process, stylohyoid ligament, lesser horn and superior part hyoid bone	VII	Muscles of facial expression, buccinator, platysma, stapedius, stylohyoid, posterior belly of digastric			
Third	Greater horn and caudal part of hyoid	IX	Stylopharyngeus, upper pharyngeal constrictors		Carotid	
Fourth	Thyroid cartilage	X: superior laryngeal	Lower pharyngeal constrictors, levator paliti		Right: subclavian Left: aortic arch	
Sixth	Cricoid, epiglottic and arytenoid cartilages	X: recurrent laryngeal	Intrinsic laryngeal/pharyngeal muscles		Pulmonary arteries and ductus arteriosus on left	This explains why the recurrent laryngeal nerve is looped under the ductus arteriosus on the left

* The second arch grows down over the other arches, leaving a space known as a *cervical sinus*. This normally disappears but if it persists it may form a *branchial cyst or sinus* (filled with glairy fluid saturated with cholesterol crystals) or a *branchial fistula*. The fistula extends from the anterior border of the junction of lower and middle thirds of the sternocleidomastoid to between the external and internal carotid arteries and then opens into the tonsillar fossa.

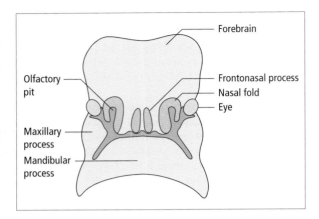

Figure 42.21 Fetal head (ventral aspect) showing the embryological development of the face.

Around the same time a series of *branchial arches* (or pharyngeal arches) develop, eventually fusing in the midline (Table 42.7). The external depressions between these arches are known as the ectodermal *branchial clefts*, whereas the internal grooves are known as the endodermal *branchial pouches* (Table 42.8).

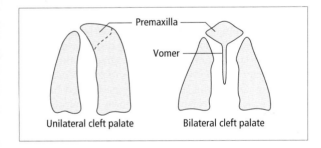

Figure 42.22

Cleft lip and palate

Cleft lip and/or palate is one of the most common congenital abnormalities, occurring in approximately 1 in 700 live births. There is a definite genetic influence. Subsequent siblings of an affected child have a risk of developing a cleft of between 1 in 10 and 1 in 50. When both parents have a cleft the risk of involvement of their offspring is 1 in 2 to 1 in 3.

Cleft lip and palate may occur separately or together and may be unilateral or bilateral:
- cleft lip and palate (50%) (Fig. 42.23a);
- cleft lip alone (25%) (Fig. 42.23b);
- cleft palate alone (25%).

Submucous cleft palate is one of the mildest forms. The palatal mucosa is intact but the muscular layers are not; it should be suspected in a child with a bifid uvula. It may not become apparent until the child has difficulty in phonation.

Management
- *Multidisciplinary teams* are necessary to treat this complex problem. Members include plastic, ENT and maxillofacial or orthodontic surgeons, speech therapists, nutritionists, paediatricians and psychologists.
- *Feeding* can be difficult with cleft palates and the baby will have difficulty in suckling but not swallowing. Breast-feeding may not be possible. Special teats have been developed to help bottle-feeding.
- *Surgical repair* is carried out in stages. Timing varies greatly between surgeons but the trend is now towards early (neonatal) repair of the lip and repair of the palate at 6 months.
- *Orthodontic treatment* is carried out in parallel with other procedures. Emphasis is placed on the early phase of permanent dentition. Bone grafting to the alveolar cleft defect at 10–12 years of age will allow teeth to migrate into the correct position.

Table 42.8 Embryology of the branchial clefts and branchial pouches.

Pouch	Structure (endoderm ± mesoderm)	Cleft	Structure (endoderm)
First	Middle ear, mastoid antrum, tympanic membrane	First	External auditory meatus, tympanic membrane
Second	Tympanic cavity, palatine tonsils	Second	
Third	Thymus gland, inferior parathyroid (III)	Third	Thymus gland descends, pulling parathyroid III below parathyroid IV
Fourth	Superior parathyroid (IV)	Fourth	Attached to the thyroid gland, therefore prevents parathyroid IV going below parathyroid III
Fifth	Ultimobranchial body, which develops into parafollicular (C) cells of thyroid gland		

05

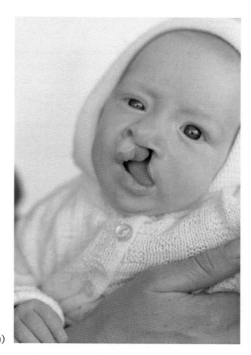

(a)

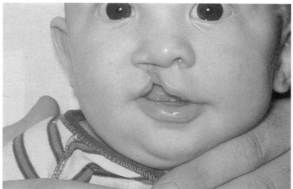

(b)

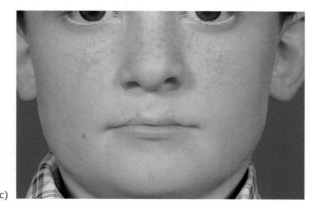

(c)

Figure 42.23 (a) Unilateral cleft lip and palate in an infant; 50% of cleft lip deformities are of this type. (b) Unilateral right-sided incomplete cleft lip. (c) Several operations later, the appearance of the repaired lip is satisfactory.

• *Rhinoplasty and submucous resection* to correct the deformity of the nasal bone and septum may be necessary when growth is complete at 18 years old.

• *ENT review* is necessary as patients have an increased risk of otitis media (glue ear) and frequently require myringotomy.

• *Speech therapy* is essential from the outset in order to assess and correct any problems in phonation. Shortness of the palate, either alone or combined with an inadequate nasopharyngeal sphincter, results in a characteristic cleft palate speech in which there is nasal escape of air. With successful intervention approximately 80% of children can be expected to talk normally.

• *Counselling* of parents and family is essential as soon as the defect is diagnosed. It can be unexpectedly discovered in routine antenatal scanning. Full discussion of the problems of cleft lip and palate, treatment options and the favourable results achieved with surgery should be emphasized.

Miscellaneous congenital head and neck disorders

Prominent (bat) ears

This is a relatively common problem in which the ear stands away from the side of the head, producing the typical jug-handled appearance (Figs 42.24 & 42.25). There are various types of surgical correction but all involve reshaping the cartilaginous underlying structure in some way. Solely excising posterior auricular skin is not sufficient to permanently correct the shape of the ears, as the elasticity of skin eventually leads to recurrence of the deformity. Operations are generally performed between 3 years (when the ears have reached 85% of adult size) and school age in order to avoid the psychological trauma of ridicule by classmates.

Accessory auricles

Accessory auricles represent abnormalities in development in the first branchial arch. They are ectopic ear tissue that has not been incorporated into the pinna during development (Fig. 42.26). The problem ranges from a simple narrow-based skin tag to a large wide-based pedunculated lesion, which contains cartilage. The cartilaginous 'root' should always be excised as deeply as possible in order to prevent residual palpable lumps under the operative scar.

Dermoid cyst

Dermoid cysts occur most frequently at the outer end of the eyebrow, where they are called *external angular dermoids*, but can occur at any point along the lines of fusion of the facial processes (Fig. 42.27). Those situated over skull sutures, such as the base of the nose or in the

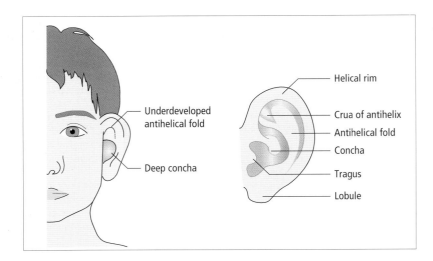

Figure 42.24 A normal ear compared with a prominent ear.

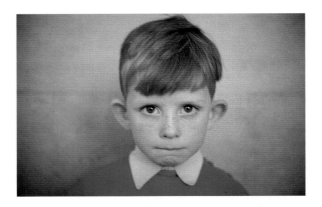

Figure 42.25 A young boy with prominent (bat) ears.

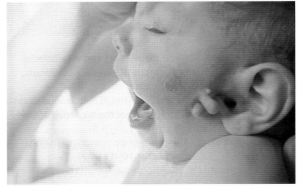

Figure 42.26 An infant with accessory auricles. Note the ectopic ear tissue anterior to the external auditory meatus.

midline of the skull, may have a dumb-bell type of intracranial extension. They represent developmental inclusion dermoids of skin elements occurring at the time of facial fusion. Treatment is by complete excision of the epithelial-lined cyst.

Congenital ptosis

Congenital ptosis results from deficient formation of the levator oculi muscle. There is an obvious droop of the upper lid and children will tilt their head backwards to enable them to see. Treatment is by shortening the levator muscle sufficiently to bring the lid margin to the correct level.

Facial clefts

Facial clefts result from failure of fusion of any of the facial processes previously described. They can occur in any position and can be multiple and bilateral. These deformities are rare. An example of a large lateral facial cleft resulting in an abnormally large mouth (macrostomia) is shown in Fig. 42.28.

Facial injuries

The main causes of facial injuries include road traffic accidents, altercations, athletic injuries, falls and home accidents. The main concern is treatment of the life-threatening complications of these injuries; functional repair is the next priority while the aesthetic significance of the injuries usually plays a small role in the early management of the patient. Fortunately, however, the management of each of these goes hand in hand with the others and early definitive treatment maximizes function and aesthetics and minimizes complications.

05

excessive flank adipose tissue. The umbilicus is then resutured into its new location, with care to ensure it is in the midline. Drains are placed and the skin flap is sutured to the inferior margin.

Complications include

- skin necrosis;
- wound dehiscence;
- wound infection;
- haematoma;
- seroma;
- umbilical necrosis;
- altered sensation;
- revisional surgery to lateral dog ears.

Aesthetic surgery at a glance

Definition

Cosmetic or aesthetic surgery: the correction of problems that patients perceive as making them look different or abnormal

Cosmetic procedures

Rhytidectomy (face-lift)
- Addresses the gravitational effects on the face
- Complications include facial nerve injury, skin necrosis, haematoma, infection, salivary fistula

Blepharoplasty (eyelid tuck)
- Modifies the appearance of the eyelids
- Complications include infection, inadequate correction, ptosis, injury to extraocular muscles, difficulty in wearing contact lenses, retrobulbar haematoma leading to blindness

Rhinoplasty (nose-job)
- Improves appearance of nose
- Complications include numbness to the upper teeth, asymmetry

Liposuction
- Surgical removal of adipose tissue through a small blunt-tipped metal cannula attached to a vacuum
- Complications include blood loss, fluid shifts, asymmetries, contour defects, skin necrosis, haematoma, altered sensation

Abdominoplasty (tummy tuck)
- Correction of a contour abnormality of the abdomen
- Complications include skin necrosis, wound dehiscence, wound infection, haematoma, umbilical necrosis, altered sensation

Ear, Nose and Throat Disorders

43

Must know Must do

Must know

Principles of management of upper airway obstruction

Clinical ENT and neck examination

Management of epistaxis

Management of patients with sore throat

Assessment and management of patients with neck lumps

Pathology of common malignancies of the head and neck

Assessment of patients who develop hoarseness

Assessment of patients with deafness and tinnitus

Tumours of the salivary glands

Must do

Examine patients with common ENT and neck disorders and learn how to diagnose specific disorders

Perform indirect laryngoscopy

Perform tests of auditory function

Perform otoscopy to learn what the normal eardrum looks like

Attend ENT outpatient clinics

Observe an operation to remove a parotid tumour

Introduction

It is probably not an exaggeration to say that ENT disorders are more or less ubiquitous. They affect all ages including the extremes of life, and account for 20–30% of a family doctor's workload. This chapter approaches these multifarious disorders by classifying them as emergency, urgent (suspected cancer), adult and childhood. The adult disorders may be conveniently subdivided topographically. Reading this chapter may be usefully supplemented not only by reference to the wealth of online information but also by browsing one of the many excellent atlases of otolaryngology and head and neck surgery.

ENT emergencies: diagnosis and first-line management

Stridor

Pathophysiology

Stridor is a noise caused by obstruction to the upper respiratory tract. Upper airway obstruction causes a noise during inspiration. If the obstruction is in the trachea, the noise is heard in both inspiration and expiration. It is important to note that obstruction of the lower airways causes a noise on expiration (wheeze). The distinction might appear simple but many expert clinicians have been embarrassed by failing to diagnose stridor and treating the patient for asthma.

Overall, stridor is commoner in children than adults. Children have narrower upper airways and are thus more vulnerable to occlusion. It is fairly common for children to exhibit mild stridor during an upper respiratory tract infection. Even with severe laryngitis, adults rarely develop stridor during an upper respiratory tract infection.

Congenital

Congenital infantile stridor is extremely worrying for the parents. The numerous rare causes of congenital stridor are nowadays diagnosed by flexible fibreoptic examination of the awake baby in the outpatient clinic. The most common cause is laryngomalacia, in which unusually floppy laryngeal cartilages collapse on respiration. The more active the baby, the louder the noise becomes. Laryngeal examination may reveal one of the following less common causes: laryngeal web, cyst, vocal cord paralysis, vascular abnormalities or a variety of benign tumours (including haemangiomas). The baby may also have a skin haemangioma, which suggests the diagnosis.

Acquired

Acquired stridor is either inflammatory or structural in origin. Inflammatory causes of stridor include acute

05

epiglottitis, which is often caused by *Haemophilus influenzae* and is commoner in children, although it can occur in adults. Never attempt examination or radiography of an acutely stridulous child. The associated stress can precipitate respiratory arrest. The treatment of acute epiglottitis is with chloramphenicol and steroids, with upper airway protection (see later). Epiglottitis occurs largely in children and the diagnosis in adults tends as a result to be rather delayed. Such delay can be catastrophic (George Washington died within 24 h of the onset of what was almost certainly acute epiglottitis).

A much commoner and less sinister cause of upper airway inflammation in children is acute laryngotracheobronchitis or croup. This viral infection may often be adequately managed by placing the child in the moist air of a croupette. Infectious mononucleosis can cause fatal upper airway obstruction in both children and adults if the tonsillar and pharyngeal swelling becomes sufficiently marked.

Inhaled foreign bodies in children are a well-known source of upper respiratory obstruction. A large sweet or a coin put into the child's mouth may be inhaled and lodge at the level of the vocal cords. The object may be swallowed, lodge at the cricopharyngeus and compress the upper trachea or laryngeal inlet. Sometimes this obstruction can be relieved by the Heimlich manoeuvre or by tilting the child and giving a sharp slap between the shoulder blades. Failing this, laryngotomy may be necessary or the child may die before being hospitalized.

Laryngeal trauma, either mechanical or due to thermal injury, may also cause stridor. Children not infrequently ride bicycles into low-lying ropes or tree branches. Blunt laryngeal trauma in adults as a result of road traffic accidents is much less common now that seat-belts are compulsory. A few cases are due to failed attempted strangulation, at times self-inflicted in a failed suicide attempt by hanging.

Cancer of the larynx may cause stridor, either by mechanical obstruction or by involvement of the recurrent laryngeal nerves. Bilateral recurrent laryngeal nerve palsy can cause stridor. If the cords come to rest close to the midline, the loss of normal inspiratory abduction causes stridor, especially on exertion. The problem may result from thyroid disease or surgery.

First-line management

In children with acute upper airway obstruction, primary treatment may be conservative with systemic steroids and antibiotics. If this appears inadequate, endotracheal intubation by a paediatric anaesthetist may be possible. The anaesthetist may request that an ENT surgeon be ready to intervene if necessary. In adults with acute respiratory obstruction, surgery is usually the treatment of choice. For the non-specialist, the relief of acute upper airway obstruction at the bedside, or indeed on the top of a bus, is best effected by inserting a penknife through the cricothyroid membrane (laryngotomy), a frequent procedure in the days of endemic diphtheria.

Laryngotomy

Extend the patient's neck and feel the ridge of the cricoid. The cricothyroid membrane is just above this. Keeping strictly in the midline, make an incision through the cricothyroid membrane. There are no intervening vessels. The vocal cords are very much higher, behind the midpoint of the thyroid cartilage. The scalpel, penknife blade or biro tubing may be used to hold the membrane open. An alternative is to insert one or two large-bore intravenous cannulae through this avascular superficial structure.

Tracheostomy

In contrast, an incision on the front of the trachea encounters not only the thyroid isthmus but also the anterior jugular veins and strap muscles. Even an ENT surgeon has difficulties in performing an emergency tracheostomy, although this is the only way to relieve airway obstruction at the level of the cricoid cartilage or below.

The time to arrange a tracheostomy is the time you first think of it. Unlike respiratory failure due to lower airway obstruction, there is no gradual change in blood gases. The patient will struggle through a period of compensatory hyperventilation, which postpones hypoxia until respiratory arrest is imminent. It is misleading to use a pulse oximeter because the readings may remain more or less normal until the patient arrests. Do not let any patient go to sleep with impending airway obstruction. Respiratory failure may supervene overnight and pass unnoticed. Consult your ENT surgeon early and the procedure can be carried out much more safely in an atmosphere of relative calm.

Pathophysiology of stridor

- Upper airway collapse is greater in inspiration
- Commoner in children: small high larynx
- Bilateral vocal cord paralysis:
  (a) Loss of normal inspiratory abduction
  (b) Congenital or acquired
- Congenital:
  (a) Collapsing laryngeal framework (laryngomalacia)
  (b) Obstructive lesion
- Acquired:
  (a) Inflammatory
  (b) Tumour
  (c) Neck trauma

Note that percutaneous tracheostomy is now quite commonly performed in intensive care units. There are advantages and disadvantages but one thing is certain: it is not recommended in a patient with upper airway obstruction. Its use by intensivists in sedated patients with indwelling endotracheal tubes and where the position of the tube can be checked by flexible endoscopy is quite a different situation. Percutaneous tracheostomy kits should *never* be used in acute upper airway obstruction.

Management of upper airway obstruction

- Remember that SaO_2 falls late
- Intervene sooner rather than later
- Steroids/endotracheal intubation
- Laryngotomy
- Tracheostomy
- *Never* use percutaneous tracheostomy kit

Epistaxis

Most of us can recall a childhood nose-bleed. Sadly, another peak of epistaxis incidence awaits us in the later years of life. Risk factors for epistaxis include:
- drying out of nasal mucosa (age, infection, septal deviation);
- seasonal (winter months);
- anticoagulation, possibly including aspirin therapy;
- alcohol consumption;
- hypertension;
- nasal fracture.

Causes

Most nasal bleeding follows microtrauma to Little's area on the anteroinferior aspect of the septum (insert your right index finger into the right vestibule and the pad of the distal phalanx rests on Little's area). Bleeding may be more likely when there is mild chronic infection; low-grade vestibulitis is almost universal in children. In older people, the nasal mucosa, like other body surfaces, tends to dry out and a dry crusty nasal vestibule is more likely to bleed. Further, if the nasal septum is bent, the unequal nasal airflow further exacerbates the dry friable lining. In some older people, however, the bleeding originates from much further back on the septum.

It is hard to assess the role of hypertension in epistaxis. Attendance at hospital tends to elevate blood pressure while the blood loss of epistaxis tends to reduce it. Coagulation defects, anticoagulation therapy and increased alcohol consumption, with or without measurable changes in coagulation, are all predisposing factors. The role of low-dose aspirin is harder to evaluate: it is difficult

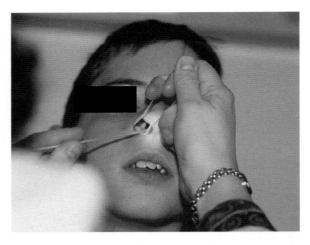

Figure 43.1 Silver nitrate cautery of Little's area on the anterior nasal septum.

to find a properly matched group of subjects who are not themselves on aspirin.

First-line management

The simplest treatment is to press hard on the anterior soft tip of the nose over Little's area. The patient leans forward and spits out any oral blood and sucks ice cubes. If this fails after 10 min of constant pressure, then intervention is necessary. Good vasoconstriction and local anaesthesia are achieved by application of Cophenylcaine on wool pledgets or ribbon gauze. After 10 min this will have reduced most bleeding and partially anaesthetized the nasal cavity. Cautery of Little's area may then be performed with commercially available silver nitrate sticks (Fig. 43.1). Failing this, a nasal pack is inserted. Despite the topical mucosal anaesthesia, nasal pack insertion is uncomfortable or even frankly painful for the patient due to pressure on the septum. Modern expanding packs, such as Merocel, are thus much more acceptable than the old-fashioned ribbon layers soaked in bismuth iodoform paraffin paste. Once the slim sponge of Merocel is inserted, it absorbs blood, expands and thus applies a compression force to the bleeding points.

If first-line measures fail

If the bleeding is more brisk or more posterior, consider an epistaxis balloon. Most have two channels, one to inflate in the nasal cavity and a smaller second balloon for the postnasal space. Some ENT specialists use a Foley bladder catheter balloon passed into the postnasal space and inflated with 8–10 mL of air, combined with an anterior Merocel pack. The last resort is to carry out a ligation or clipping operation to one of the major feeding vessels

05

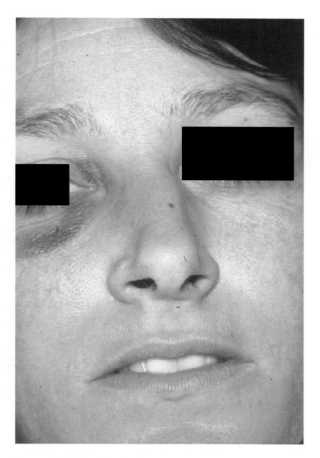

Figure 43.2 Nasal fracture.

on the affected side. The sphenopalatine artery may be clipped by a transnasal endoscopic approach. Ligation of the ethmoid, maxillary or even external carotid arteries requires a more invasive approach.

Nasal fracture

The most common causes of nasal fracture in countries with seat-belt legislation are body contact sports and fighting. Thus, more men than women fracture their noses. The diagnosis of a broken nose is clinical (Fig. 43.2). There is no value in X-ray, and the evidence is sufficiently strong that there is no medicolegal requirement for X-ray either.

The signs of nasal fracture include:
- deviation of the vault;
- gross swelling;
- epistaxis;
- periorbital bruising.

It is important to exclude a facial bone fracture, the signs of which include:

- palpable step in infraorbital ridge;
- subconjunctival haemorrhage;
- altered sensation in midface;
- ophthalmoplegia.

The most common ophthalmoplegia is limitation of upward gaze. This suggests that the inferior rectus is trapped in a fracture of the orbital floor (orbital blow-out fracture). Not all patients with a nasal fracture wish to seek the services of an ENT surgeon, but in suspected facial fractures specialist assessment is necessary by an ENT or oromaxillofacial surgeon.

First-line management

Manipulation under local anaesthetic in the outpatient clinic or under general anaesthesia in theatre may be used to manually reposition the nasal bones. The outcome of each method seems similar, i.e. about two-thirds of patients feel that their nose is more or less as straight as it was before the injury. The optimum time for manipulation is within 7–10 days after injury. By 14 days healing has become established and after 3 weeks a full refracture is necessary to mobilize the nasal bones. If manipulation fails, then a formal rhinoplasty will be required at a later date. The massively deviated nose may require open reduction with septoplasty under general anaesthesia to straighten the central nasal partition.

Quinsy (peritonsillar abscess)

Aggressive or undertreated tonsillitis may result in suppuration in the plane lateral to the tonsil. An abscess forms in the potential space between the tonsil and the pharyngeal wall. This is peritonsillar abscess or quinsy. It is one of the commoner indications for emergency admission to an ENT ward. Most quinsies occur in adults. It is fortunately rare in childhood, as quinsy is very painful. The principal differential diagnoses are severe tonsillitis and glandular fever and, in developing countries, diphtheria.

The features of quinsy include:
- severe sore throat;
- painful dysphagia;
- drooling;
- muffled speech;
- fever;
- trismus (makes pharyngeal examination difficult);
- unilateral tonsillar swelling, extending onto the soft palate;
- jugulodigastric lymphadenopathy.

The pus is aspirated or drained by a small incision in the awake patient, sitting up. Unfortunately, topical anaesthetic application is usually not very effective. However, the patient with a true abscess is very grateful, despite the

pain, because the relief is great and immediate. A small number of patients have failed aspiration or drainage if full-blown suppuration has not yet occurred.

Foreign bodies

Small children have a tendency to insert foreign bodies (e.g. pieces of sponge, Lego or rolled-up tissue) into the nose. Over the age of 4 years, the ear becomes the favoured site. If the insertion of a nasal foreign body is not apparent, it may present late with chronic, infected, unilateral nasal discharge, often with an offensive smell. All nasal foreign bodies should be removed with a reasonable degree of urgency: there is at least a theoretical risk of them passing into the postnasal space and being aspirated (in practice many are quite firmly lodged in the nasal cavity).

Attempted removal of ear or nasal foreign bodies is best avoided by the inexperienced, as the attempt often serves only to frighten the child and push the object deeper into the nose. The first attempt at removal of a foreign body in an unanaesthetized child is the best one. The ENT doctor may try to mildly vasoconstrict the nasal mucosa, thus loosening the object, prior to removal. Use of a fine aural sucker in the nose or ear canal is less traumatic than attempts to grasp with forceps. Not infrequently, a general anaesthetic is required.

Inhaled or swallowed foreign bodies (Fig. 43.3) may lodge in the upper airway and give rise to stridor or dysphagia. If an inhaled object such a peanut passes through the vocal cords, the effects may be less obvious and the diagnosis delayed.

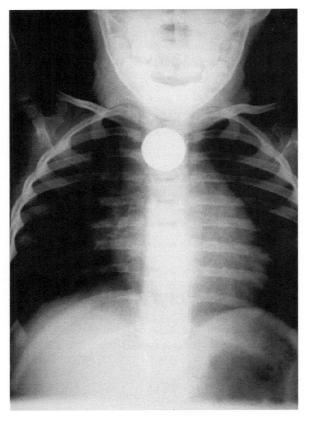

Figure 43.3 Chest radiograph showing swallowed coin lodged in upper thoracic oesophagus of a 2-year-old child.

ENT emergencies at a glance

Definitions

Stridor: a noise caused by obstruction to the upper respiratory tract, commoner in children

Epistaxis: another name for nose-bleed

Quinsy (peritonsillar abscess): a painful abscess in the potential space between the tonsil and the pharyngeal wall usually in adults

Stridor
Causes
Bilateral vocal cord paralysis
- Loss of normal inspiratory abduction
- Congenital or acquired (thyroid disease/surgery)

Congenital
- Collapsing laryngeal framework (laryngomalacia)

- Obstructive lesion:
  (a) Laryngeal web
  (b) Cyst
  (c) Benign tumour, e.g. haemangioma

Acquired
- Inflammatory:
  (a) Acute epiglottitis (*Haemophilus influenzae*)
  (b) Acute laryngotracheobronchitis or croup
  (c) Infectious mononucleosis
- Neck trauma:
  (a) Mechanical or thermal injury
  (b) Inhaled foreign bodies in children
- Tumour (laryngeal cancer):
  (a) Direct spread
  (b) Nerve involvement

05

First-line management
- Intervene sooner rather than later
- Remember that SaO_2 falls late
- Steroids and antibiotics in children
- Endotracheal intubation
- Laryngotomy
- Tracheostomy
- *Never* percutaneous tracheostomy

Epistaxis
Risk factors
- Drying out of nasal mucosa: age, infection, septal deviation
- Seasonal (winter months)
- Anticoagulation, possibly including aspirin therapy
- Alcohol consumption
- Hypertension
- Nasal fracture

Causes
- Microtrauma of Little's area on the anteroinferior aspect of the septum:
  (a) Low-grade vestibulitis in children
  (b) Dried-out nasal mucosa in elderly
- Hypertension
- Coagulation defects:
  (a) Anticoagulation therapy
  (b) Increased alcohol consumption
  (c) ? Aspirin

First-line management
- Pressure to the nasal tip
- Vasoconstrictor pledgets
- Silver nitrate cautery
- Merocel pack

If first-line measures fail
- Consider epistaxis balloon
- Ligation or clipping of one of the major arteries on the affected side:
  (a) Sphenopalatine artery
  (b) Ethmoid artery
  (c) Maxillary artery
  (d) External carotid arteries

Nasal fracture
Causes
- Body contact sports and fighting
- Road traffic accidents

Signs
- Deviation of the vault
- Gross swelling
- Epistaxis
- Periorbital bruising

Exclude facial bone fracture
- Palpable step in infraorbital ridge
- Subconjunctival haemorrhage
- Altered sensation in midface
- Ophthalmoplegia

First-line management
- Do not X-ray
- Timely assessment:
  (a) Not while massively swollen
  (b) Refer to specialist within 5 days
- Manipulation within 7–10 days after injury
- Formal osteotomies after 3 weeks

Quinsy (peritonsillar abscess)
Features
- Severe sore throat
- Painful dysphagia
- Drooling
- Muffled speech
- Fever
- Trismus: makes pharyngeal examination difficult
- Unilateral tonsillar swelling, extending onto the soft palate
- Jugulodigastric lymphadenopathy

First-line management
- Aspirate or incise pus in the awake sitting-up patient
- Relief is great and immediate

Foreign bodies
In nose
- Under 4 years of age
- Late presentation
- Chronic, infected, offensive, unilateral nasal discharge
- Treatment: remove foreign body often under general anaesthesia (theoretical risk of aspiration)

In ear
- Over 4 years of age
- Otitis externa ± ear discharge
- Treatment: remove foreign body often under general anaesthesia

05

Head and neck cancer: requirements for urgent referral

Risk factors

Over 95% of head and neck cancers are squamous cell carcinomas. Over 95% of head and neck squamous cell carcinomas occur in present or past cigarette smokers. Smoking has a synergistic carcinogenic effect with alcohol. The relative risks are greatest for those smoking continental (black) tobacco rather than American-style cigarettes and drinking brown spirits such as whisky, rum or brandy. Thus the highest European incidence is in the south-west, notably the Calvados region of France. Suspected cancer referrals should therefore include a current and past smoking and alcohol history. Male sex and age over 50 years are further risk factors.

Symptoms

Persistent symptoms that may be due to head and neck cancer include:
- hoarseness;
- oral ulcer/white or red patch;
- sore throat;
- dysphagia;
- cervical swelling.

Non-malignant causes of these symptoms are considered later in the chapter where relevant.

Sore throat

The cardinal suspicious features in sore throat are duration and referred otalgia. Self-limiting sore throat is almost ubiquitous in the UK as part of seasonal upper respiratory tract infections. It is very rare for such an infective condition to last for more than 2–3 weeks. Longer-lasting episodes should arouse suspicion. Non-endoscopic examination by the non-specialist may be unhelpful, e.g. the lesion may be tucked out of sight near the tongue base.

Hoarseness

If hoarseness persists for more than 3 weeks, the patient should be referred for exclusion of cancer. The risk of cancer is minimal in a non-smoker; nonetheless, occasional cancers do arise in lifelong non-smokers and thus every patient needs a laryngeal examination. Cancer of the larynx, as elsewhere in the head and neck, is usually squamous cell carcinoma. Fortunately, the glottis is the most common site as this tends to present early because of the hoarseness due to incomplete closure of the vocal cords. T1 tumours of the glottis have a greater than 95% cure

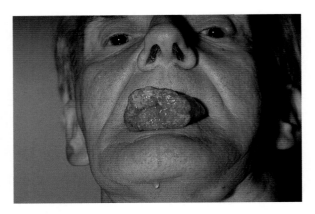

Figure 43.4 Carcinoma of the tongue.

rate. T3 tumours (fixed vocal cords) or T4 tumours (spread outside the larynx) are more likely to require resection, often total laryngectomy. The voice can be well rehabilitated using an oesophageal valve. Benign tumours of the larynx include viral papillomas, which occur predominantly in childhood or adolescence.

Oral ulcer/white or red patch

Oral tumours may present as an ulcer or exophytic lesion of the oral mucosa (Fig. 43.4). Some are preceded by a white patch (leucoplakia), which has a 15% incidence of malignant transformation, or by a red patch (erythroplakia), which has a very high malignant potential. Simple aphthous ulcers are essentially of unknown aetiology, although they appear to be increased by stress. Some are herpetic or traumatic, e.g. from ill-fitting dentures. In recurrent oral ulceration, consider vitamin B_{12} or folate deficiency. Rare causes of oral ulceration include leukaemia and acquired immunodeficiency syndrome (AIDS).

Dysphagia

Obstructive or painful dysphagia above the level of the suprasternal notch may be due to a tumour in the pharynx. Remember that the level of perceived block is always above the level of obstruction. Lesions in the lower or mid oesophagus may also therefore cause a sense of blockage in the neck.

Cervical swelling

This may be the only presenting feature, for example in 20% of tonsil carcinomas the only symptom will be of a metastatic lymph node in the neck. The extensive lymphatic drainage of the base of the tongue and hypopharynx (piriform fossa) gives cancer in these sites a greater risk

05

of nodes at presentation and a correspondingly poorer prognosis. Thyroid and salivary gland cancers also present as cervical swellings. Fine-needle aspiration cytology is often valuable for primary or nodal swellings. The differential diagnosis is discussed below.

Clinical assessment in suspected head and neck cancer

Neck examination

After inspection for obvious swellings, systematic bilateral palpation of the neck from behind should be performed. Palpate down along the trapezius muscles, up over the posterior triangles to the mastoid processes and down again anterior to the sternomastoids. Come up the central structures (thyroid, larynx, hyoid) to the submental triangle and finally the submandibular area.

Physical examination of the oral cavity and oropharynx

First, ask the patient to remove any dentures. Systematic examination with a light or torch and tongue depressor should include the following.
● Outer ring: lips, gums, buccal surfaces, buccoalveolar recesses.
● Inner ring: floor of mouth, lateral surfaces of tongue, dorsum of tongue.
● Area behind anterior pillars of fauces (oropharynx): medial displacement of the tonsil may be due to a deep parotid tumour or another mass deep in the neck in the parapharyngeal space.
● Parotid duct orifices: opposite second upper molar.
● Tongue: look for fasciculation (motor neurone disease), impaired movement (hypoglossal paresis), mucosa.
● Put on a glove and palpate the floor of the mouth bimanually (suspected submandibular duct calculus).
● Palpate tongue base if suspect occult cancer.
● Bite: if the lower alveolar teeth are not within the upper alveolar ring, there is bite overclosure.
● Relevant cranial nerves:
    (a) vagus/recurrent laryngeal nerve (voice quality, palatal movement, gag reflex);
    (b) facial nerve in parotid lesions;
    (c) third to sixth nerves in postnasal space cancers.

Common (non-malignant) throat and neck presentations

The common symptoms of throat disorders are sore throat, hoarseness, cervical swelling, high dysphagia, globus sensation, chronic cough, catarrh and habitual snoring.

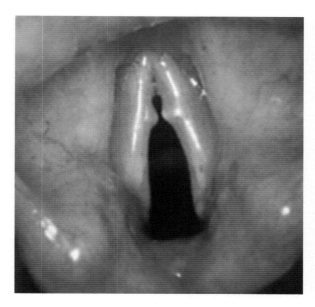

Figure 43.5 Endoscopic photograph showing vocal cord nodules.

Sore throat

In viral sore throat in children look for Koplik's spots, a prodromal sign of measles. Tonsillitis is now considered to justify tonsillectomy if it occurs as six mild or three to four severe attacks annually for at least 2 years, or if the patient has an extraordinarily severe attack typically requiring hospitalization. The patient has a high temperature, white spots on the tonsil and painful dysphagia. The principal hazards of tonsillectomy are haemorrhage and having to reanaesthetize a patient whose pharynx is full of blood in the event of persistent haemorrhage. Although fortunately rare, there are still occasionally recorded fatalities following tonsil dissection.

Hoarseness

The first priority is to assess the smoking habit and the presence or absence of other features suggestive of laryngeal cancer. The most common cause of hoarseness is acute laryngitis, which is suggested by a preceding upper respiratory tract infection. Voice strain is common in teachers or club and pub singers, particularly those singing at too high a pitch with tense laryngeal muscles and air escape. Untreated voice strain in adults and children can lead to vocal nodules ('screamer's nodes') (Fig. 43.5). Risk factors for chronic laryngitis are smoking, vocal abuse, pulmonary inhalers and gastro-oesophageal reflux. Vocal cord paralysis is commoner on the left because of the longer course of the left recurrent laryngeal

nerve. Recurrent nerve palsy is caused by lung cancer (at the left hilum or right lung apex), thyroid surgery or cancer, oesophageal cancer and left atrial hypertrophy, or may be idiopathic or viral. The vagal trunk is affected by base-of-skull disease or by bulbar palsy due to vascular or motor neurone disease. If one vocal cord is abducted, it can be medialized by an injection of Teflon or collagen or by insertion of a Silastic strut (thyroplasty).

Cervical swelling

The causes of cervical swelling are legion (Table 43.1; Fig. 43.6). Half of all neck masses seen in a general hospital are of thyroid origin. The most common neck swelling in children is an enlarged jugulodigastric lymph node secondary to pharyngeal inflammation. In adults (and some older children) the differential diagnosis has been greatly simplified by the advent of fine-needle aspiration cytology, which has a high level of accuracy (over 90%) in the head and neck. Also, because of the wide variety of anatomical structures and pathologies that can occur in the head and neck area, the early use of fine-needle aspiration allows subsequent investigations to be efficiently targeted. Thus if a lesion is found at an early stage to be lymphoma, the subsequent investigation is quite different than if it were of thyroid origin or a metastatic adenocarcinoma from some distant site.

Table 43.1 Neck masses.

Congenital cysts
  Thyroglossal duct cysts
  Branchial cysts
Nodal (infective)
  Bacterial: *Brucella*, tuberculosis
  Viral: glandular fever
  Toxoplasma
  Parapharyngeal abscess
Neoplastic
  Lymphoma
  Carcinoma
Thyroid disease
Salivary gland
  Inflammatory
  Neoplastic
Carotid body tumour

Congenital neck masses

Thyroglossal cysts are the most common midline neck cyst. The thyroid gland originates in the floor of the embryonic pharynx and moves down to the lower neck. If the linking stalk fails to atrophy, it becomes the thyroglossal duct in which cysts can develop. Treatment is by excision.

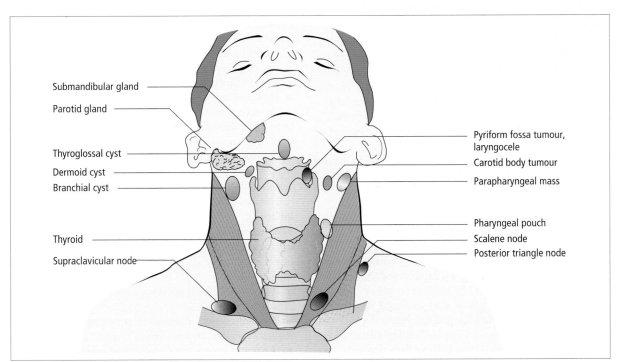

Figure 43.6 Cervical swellings.

05

The features of thyroglossal cysts include:
- mean age 5 years (range 4 months to 70 years);
- 90% occur in midline;
- mostly painless, mobile on swallowing or protruding the tongue;
- 75% arise prehyoid;
- 25% arise at the thyroid cartilage, cricoid cartilage or above the hyoid;
- mobile in all directions;
- can usually be transilluminated;
- may present with infection or fistula.

Branchial cysts may be the remains of pharyngeal pouches or branchial clefts, most often the latter. They contain straw-coloured fluid in which cholesterol crystals are found. Treatment is by excision. The features of branchial cysts include:
- peak incidence in third decade (range 1–70 years);
- two-thirds left side, two-thirds lie anterior to the upper third sternomastoid;
- one-third present with pain or infection.

Infective neck masses

Enquire about animal contact as both brucellosis and toxoplasmosis may present as cervical nodes. Lymph node involvement by *Mycobacterium tuberculosis* or *M. bovis* (tuberculous cervical adenitis) remains a very common manifestation in some areas of the world such as Asia. Diagnosis is by positive skin test, demonstration of acid-fast bacilli in lymph node biopsy and growth of *M. tuberculosis* from the biopsy. The patient should be treated by antituberculous chemotherapy followed by excision of any residual disease. More recently in the UK, atypical tuberculosis is regularly seen in children, most often in the submandibular area. Many such nodes will resolve with time but surgical excision is the mainstay of treatment.

The parapharyngeal space extends from the skull base to the level of the hyoid bone and a parapharyngeal abscess may develop following tonsillitis or tooth extraction.

Salivary gland disease
History
Benign tumours grow slowly over a period of years, but malignant ones usually grow rapidly and may exhibit pain and facial weakness. In inflammatory or calculus disease there is fluctuation in size, pain and tenderness, worse after eating. Consider general medical causes of sialomegaly: myxoedema, diabetes, Cushing's disease, cirrhosis, gout, bulimia, AIDS and alcoholism. Sarcoidosis is usually bilateral and diffuse. Sjögren's (sicca) syndrome

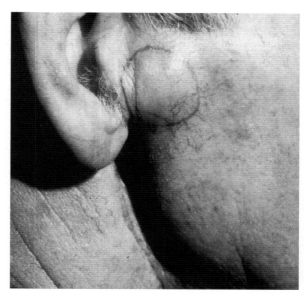

Figure 43.7 Neoplastic lesion within the parotid gland: the whole gland is not enlarged.

comprises xerophthalmia and xerostomia with or without a connective tissue disorder. Half of the patients have rheumatoid arthritis.

Examination of a salivary swelling
Conditions that mimic swelling of the parotid gland include:
- parotid nodes;
- sebaceous cysts;
- mandibular cyst/tumour;
- branchial cysts;
- masseter muscle swelling.

Having established that the swelling is truly salivary, compare its margins with the anatomical limits of the gland. Inflammatory processes enlarge the whole gland, whereas neoplasia, at least in the early stages, presents as a discrete swelling within the gland (Fig. 43.7).

The assessment of a salivary gland should include the following.
- Salivary or extraglandular?
- Does the swelling involve the whole gland or just part of it?
- Is it cystic?
- If the whole gland is enlarged, the process is probably inflammatory.
- If inflammatory, discover if one or more than one of the salivary glands is involved.
- If parotid, check the facial nerve, parotid duct orifice and pharynx (deep lobe).

05

- If submandibular, perform bimanual palpation of the gland and duct (for calculus).
- Remember that 90% of salivary tumours are parotid, 90% of parotid tumours are benign, and 90% of benign parotid tumours are pleomorphic adenomas.
- Check for nodes, especially if suspect malignancy.

Pleomorphic adenomas are slow-growing and found typically in the parotid tail. The average age at presentation is 40 years. On palpation, the tumour is usually smooth, superficial, round and mobile. Treatment is a superficial parotid lobectomy rather than local excision as the lesion has a tendency to recur.

Investigation
- Laboratory tests: blood glucose, thyroid function, angiotensin-converting enzyme (sarcoidosis).
- Plain X-ray of floor of mouth: submandibular stones are nearly always radiopaque.
- Chest X-ray: suspected sarcoidosis or in malignant lesions such as adenoid cystic tumours.
- Sialography: diagnostic of sialadenitis.
- Ultrasound: cysts.
- Computed tomography (CT)/magnetic resonance imaging (MRI): assess deep lobe extension of a parotid tumour.
- Fine-needle aspiration cytology/open biopsy: in recent years, fine-needle aspiration biopsy has become widely used in the diagnosis of salivary gland masses. However, sensitivity and specificity in salivary gland diagnosis depends on access to a cytopathologist who is both skilled and interested in the technique. Open biopsy is used if there is unexplained generalized enlargement or suspected malignancy.

Malignancy of the major salivary glands
The salivary glands give rise to a great many different histological tumour types, with corresponding variation in prognosis. A small percentage of unoperated pleomorphic adenomas will eventually become malignant. Pulmonary metastasis is not uncommon in salivary gland malignancies. Fewer than 50% of patients survive 10 years. Lymphomas may arise in an intraparotid lymph node or affect the general substance of the gland.

Carotid body tumour

The features of carotid body tumours include the following.
- High incidence in Peru, i.e. at high altitude chronic hypoxia leads to carotid body hyperplasia.
- Positive family history in 10% (autosomal dominant).
- Slow-growing tumour: history of over 5 years.
- Pulsatile, rubbery ('potato tumour').
- Bruit may be present.

Whenever a carotid body tumour is suspected, biopsy is contraindicated, although careful fine-needle aspiration cytology with a very narrow gauge needle has been described. Carotid angiography will demonstrate a tumour circulation, determine the extent of the tumour and whether there is a cross-circulation.

Cervical dysphagia

Any lower oesophageal cause of dysphagia may be falsely localized by the patient to the neck. The converse, i.e. misinterpretation of high blockage, does not occur. Thus a patient with a sense of cervical obstruction may have a lesion at or at any point below the perceived block. Pharyngeal pouch is an acquired pulsion diverticulum of the median posterior wall of the upper oesophageal sphincter and typically presents with dysphagia. A barium swallow demonstrates the pouch in all cases. Some are now treated by transoral endoscopic stapling, thus avoiding an external approach.

The clinical features of pharyngeal diverticula include:
- peak incidence in seventh and eighth decades;
- dysphagia almost universal;
- halitosis and regurgitation of undigested food;
- weight loss, cough, recurrent chest infection due to aspiration.

Upper oesophageal webs are seen on barium swallow as fine anterior indentations at the pharyngo-oesophageal junction, mostly in women and probably increased by iron deficiency. Treatment is by oesophageal dilatation and iron supplementation.

Globus sensation

The symptom of a feeling of something in the throat is known as globus hystericus (Latin *globus*, ball; Greek *hysteros*, womb) because the ancients thought it was due to a migrant uterus. However, the condition occurs more frequently in men (male/female ratio 3 : 1). In middle-aged females, the population prevalence can be as high as 6%. Therefore factors in addition to the mere presence of the sensation drive the patient to seek medical care. Patients with globus sensation have a tendency to minor affective disturbance: anxiety, borderline depression, and an excess of minor adverse life events and of major threatening life events around the time of onset. Patients give a history of an excess of previously unexplained medical symptoms, suggesting that in some patients at least the globus sensation is just one manifestation of an underlying tendency to somatize distress.

05

Pathological levels of gastro-oesophageal reflux occur in around one-third, although not all of these will respond to proton pump inhibitors. However, many of those with reflux do not have globus and so the link between reflux and globus is a complex one.

Patients with long-standing globus should be referred for specialist reassurance, which can itself have a therapeutic effect on the patient and allows detection of any associated structural lesion. Any patient who has atypical features (such as pain, true dysphagia or weight loss) should be referred as a matter of urgency. Even if no serious lesion is found by the specialist, the patient may be reassured by being shown the flexible laryngoscopic images on the camera monitor in the outpatient clinic.

Chronic cough

Patients may be seen with non-pulmonary cough. Associated upper respiratory tract factors are gastro-oesophageal reflux, chronic rhinosinusitis, non-specific catarrh and habit throat clearing. Focal trigger lesions in the laryngopharynx such as vocal polyp require to be excluded by flexible nasendoscopy.

Catarrh

A persistent and irritating sense of postnasal drip is one of the most common pharyngeal presenting symptoms. It is different from the true infected postnasal discharge of chronic rhinosinusitis, which the patient coughs up and which causes engorgement of the posterior pharyngeal wall lymphoid tissue (granular pharyngitis). Look for granular pharyngitis in your own oropharynx next time you have an upper respiratory tract infection.

In otherwise unspecified 'catarrh', the cardinal feature is that the patient cannot cough anything up whatsoever, unless it is an insignificant smudge of clear or white mucus. It can be hard to appreciate the degree of devastation that this apparently trivial symptom inflicts on the patient's quality of life. Worse, the patient must be told that there is no cure, unless perhaps emigration to a climate near a warm seashore or at high altitude. It is an accepted but poorly understood phenomenon that dairy product consumption tends to thicken mucous secretions.

The following are some non-specific approaches to catarrh reduction.
- Stop smoking.
- Avoid eating late at night.
- Eliminate associated gastro-oesophageal reflux.
- Empirical 4-month trial of a steroid nasal spray.
- Reduce dairy product intake.

Snoring

Ask about relevant risk factors and enquire about the degree of apnoea. Also ask whether any apnoeas have been witnessed. Snoring is the cardinal symptom of sleep apnoea: it is almost impossible to have sleep apnoea and not to snore. At the other end of the spectrum of sleep disorders is occasional light snoring, almost ubiquitous in the middle-aged western population. Thus a key point of the consultation is clinical assessment of the likelihood of sleep apnoea.

Risk factors for habitual snoring include:
- obesity;
- collar size > 16 inches (males);
- excess alcohol intake;
- recessed mandible;
- enlarged tonsils.
  Features suggestive of sleep apnoea syndrome include:
- excessive diurnal sleepiness;
- lethargy on waking, persisting throughout much of the morning;
- witnessed apnoeas on a regular basis;
- nocturia/headache/depression.

Management

The effects of many snoring treatments are short-lived. Thus there is little point referring for treatment an inveterate chip shop habitué who drinks 4 pints a night. Where sleep apnoea is suspected, an overnight sleep study in the respiratory medicine department will quantify the number of episodes of suspended or very shallow breathing per hour (apnoea–hypopnoea index). If high, the respiratory physician may recommend a trial of continuous positive airway pressure delivered by a mask worn overnight. If the tonsils are substantially enlarged, there is a place for consideration of tonsil dissection in simple snorers and those with less severe sleep apnoea. The range of treatments for snoring reflect the fact that it is a multifactorial condition in many patients, and the difficulty in assessing clinical outcomes (except in the most rigorous of research studies). Usually the outcome depends on the report of a single witness, who is for the most part asleep. Most single treatments can claim only a 65% success rate at best.

Treatments for habitual snoring include:
- weight reduction and abstinence from alcohol;
- nasal splints (as worn by sportsmen);
- mandibular advancement device to increase retrolingual airspace;
- palatal surgery to shorten and stiffen the vibrating soft palate;
- tonsillectomy.

Head and neck problems at a glance

Neck examination
External
- Inspection
- Systematic bilateral palpation of the neck from behind:
  (a) Trapezius muscles
  (b) Posterior triangles to the mastoid processes
  (c) Anterior to the sternomastoids
  (d) Central structures (thyroid, larynx, hyoid)
  (e) Submental triangle
  (f) Submandibular area
- Cranial nerves: III, IV, V, VI, VII, X, recurrent laryngeal

Internal
- Outer ring: lips, gums, buccal surfaces, buccoalveolar recesses
- Inner ring: floor of mouth, lateral surfaces of tongue, dorsum of tongue
- Area behind anterior pillars of fauces (oropharynx)
- Parotid duct orifices: opposite second upper molar
- Tongue:
  (a) Fasciculation (motor neurone disease)
  (b) Impaired movement (hypoglossal paresis)
  (c) Mucosa
- Floor of the mouth bimanually if suspected submandibular duct calculus
- Tongue base
- Bite

Head and neck cancer
Risk factors
- Cigarette smoking
- Smoking and alcohol are synergistic
- Male sex
- > 50 years of age
- Squamous cell carcinomas (95%)

Clinical features
- Sore throat > 3 weeks/referred otalgia
- Hoarseness > 3 weeks
- Oral ulcer/white (leucoplakia) or red (erythroplakia) patch
- Dysphagia
- Cervical swelling: metastatic lymph node in the neck

Common presentations of head and neck disease
Sore throat
- Viral sore: Koplik's spots in measles
- Tonsillitis: tonsillectomy for six mild or four severe attacks per annum for at least 2 years or severe attack requiring hospitalization

Hoarseness
- Exclude laryngeal cancer

- Acute laryngitis
- Voice strain: can lead to vocal nodules ('screamer's nodes')
- Chronic laryngitis: smoking, vocal abuse, pulmonary inhalers and gastro-oesophageal reflux
- Vocal cord paralysis:
  (a) Recurrent laryngeal nerve palsy: lung cancer, thyroid surgery or cancer, oesophageal cancer, left atrial hypertrophy, idiopathic or viral
  (b) Vagal trunk palsy: base-of-skull disease, bulbar palsy

Cervical swelling
- Congenital cysts:
  (a) Thyroglossal duct cysts
  (b) Branchial cysts
- Nodal (infective):
  (a) Bacterial (*Brucella*, tuberculosis)
  (b) Viral (glandular fever)
  (c) *Toxoplasma*
  (d) Parapharyngeal abscess
- Neoplastic:
  (a) Lymphoma
  (b) Carcinoma
- Thyroid disease
- Salivary gland:
  (a) Inflammatory
  (b) Neoplastic
- Carotid body tumour

Cervical dysphagia
- Pharyngeal pouch: acquired pulsion diverticulum of the median posterior wall of the upper oesophageal sphincter
- Upper oesophageal webs: occur at the pharyngo-oesophageal junction, iron deficiency in women

Globus sensation (a feeling of something in the throat)
- Male/female ratio 3 : 1
- No obvious cause in 60–70%
- Pathological levels of gastro-oesophageal reflux occur in 30–40%

Chronic non-pulmonary cough
- Gastro-oesophageal reflux
- Chronic rhinosinusitis
- Non-specific catarrh
- Habit throat clearing
- Focal trigger lesions, e.g. vocal polyp

Catarrh
- Persistent and irritating sense of postnasal drip
- Patient cannot cough anything up

05

- There is no cure
- Reduction in dairy product consumption may help

Snoring
Risk factors for habitual snoring
- Obesity
- Collar size > 42 cm (males)
- Excess alcohol intake
- Recessed mandible
- Enlarged tonsils

Features suggestive of sleep apnoea syndrome
- Excessive diurnal sleepiness

- Lethargy on waking, persisting throughout much of the morning
- Witnessed apnoeas on a regular basis
- Nocturia/headache/depression

Treatments for habitual snoring
- Weight reduction, abstinence from alcohol
- Nasal splints (as worn by sportsmen)
- Mandibular advancement device to increase retrolingual airspace
- Palatal surgery to shorten and stiffen vibrating soft palate
- Tonsillectomy

The ear

Symptoms

Deafness and tinnitus

Hearing impairment is the most common symptom of ear disease and the most common cause is age-related loss (presbyacusis). Enquiry should be made about excessive noise exposure, both at work (e.g. shipyards, weaving, factories) and recreational (e.g. shooting).

Risk factors for bilateral sensorineural hearing loss include:

- ageing;
- familial;
- noise induced;
- trauma;
- drug induced, e.g. aminoglycoside antibiotic.

Tinnitus is a subjective sensation of sound in the absence of any external noise in the environment. It is usually thought to be caused by spontaneous discharge in the cochlea. It is usually more troublesome in the absence of background noise and is exacerbated by caffeine, quinine, aspirin and, in some patients, smoking or drinking.

Discharge

Discharge from the ear has many causes. The most common cause in adults is otitis externa, a localized dermatitis of the ear canal characterized by itching. The middle ear mucosa may discharge through a perforation. A scanty, offensively smelling discharge gives more cause for concern than a copious mucoid one. A scanty discharge may indicate cholesteatoma.

Otalgia

The ear is richly innervated and thus many conditions in the ear and ear canal are very painful. The skin of the canal wall is tethered to the cartilage and so even the swelling of otitis externa can be extremely painful. The eardrum is also exquisitely sensitive. Stretching of the drum (by infection in the middle ear or due to pressure changes when flying) can be almost unbearable. However, more chronic pain in the ear or mastoid region can present a diagnostic problem. Because of the rich innervation (local cervical plexus sensory innervation, vagal and glossopharyngeal), referred pain in the ear is very common.

Sources of referred pain to the ear include:

- teeth;
- temporomandibular joint;
- oropharynx;
- larynx or hypopharynx;
- cervical spine;
- sinuses.

Non-specific dizziness can be caused by a multitude of diseases, from agoraphobia to uncontrolled diabetes. True vertigo is a very distressing symptom of movement relative to the surroundings. It usually indicates a lesion in the vestibular system. Usually the patient complains of a sensation of rotation but a history of staggering to one side may also indicate vertigo of peripheral (vestibular) or cerebellar origin.

Facial nerve palsy (Table 43.2)

The facial nerve has the longest bony canal of any cranial nerve. When it eventually emerges from the skull it has to make a further hazardous trip through the parotid gland, where it may be affected by tumour or the surgeon's knife. Thus there are many causes of facial palsy that must be considered and pursued appropriately before it can be safely concluded that the patient does indeed have the common idiopathic (Bell's) palsy and that most will have a spontaneous recovery. There is no specific treatment. Steroids may be tried in patients with no general medical

Table 43.2 Causes of facial nerve palsy.

Bell's palsy
Vascular: stroke
Trauma: head injury
Surgical
   Parotidectomy
   Mastoidectomy
Infective
   Herpes zoster
   Mastoiditis
Neoplastic
   Cerebellopontine angle
   Parotid
Degenerative
   Sarcoid
   Multiple sclerosis

contraindication but hard evidence of their benefit remains lacking.

For the non-specialist, perhaps most important is to refer the patient if there is any doubt about the diagnosis. Central causes of facial nerve palsy, e.g. a stroke, may spare the forehead muscles because both hemisphere areas for the forehead distribution project onto both facial nerve nuclei.

Physical examination and investigations

Inspect the shape and set of the pinna (outer ear). Look for scars of previous surgery, skin disease or mastoid swelling.

Otoscopy

Much the best way to learn how to use an auroscope is to examine as many normal eardrums as possible, starting with your colleagues. The external auditory canal slopes downwards and forwards in the adult. Gently pull the pinna upwards and backwards with the left hand while the right hand holds the auroscope to look in the right ear. Use the auroscope in the left hand to look in the left ear. Always insert the speculum under direct vision to avoid tympanic membrane trauma; this is a particular hazard in children where the eardrum lies much more superficially. Note the colour of the tympanic membrane. Are the blood vessels unduly prominent? A very common finding is of white patches on the drum (tympanosclerosis), usually a sign of burnt-out infection or previous surgery. A red bulging eardrum suggests acute infection, a golden or blue eardrum otitis media with effusion.

Is there a perforation? If so, what is the size (as a percentage of drum area) and condition (dry, moist, frankly discharging)? It can be surprisingly difficult to assess the integrity of the eardrum. If you cannot see an actual hole but there is a pulsatile discharge in the deep canal, there will almost certainly be an underlying perforation. Some commercially available hand-held aurosopes have a pneumatic attachment. The principle of pneumatic otoscopy is that if there is a hole in the tympanic membrane, it will not move when a puff of air is gently directed towards it, because the air goes down the hole and escapes via the eustachian tube (which connects the middle ear cleft to the postnasal space). If there is no hole, the light reflex of the eardrum moves.

Auditory function

The assessment starts with a clinical test of hearing. Stand behind the subject, gently massaging the tragus of one ear. Ask the patient to repeat back a series of numbers, preferably numbers greater than 10, which are harder to guess. The volume of a whispered voice at 1 m is about 30 dB. A conversational voice is about 60 dB.

The 512-Hz tuning-fork tests

In Rinne's test, air conduction is compared with bone conduction. Hit the tuning fork on a padded surface, i.e. the back of a chair or your elbow. Hold the vibrating tuning fork near the ear and ask the patient 'Can you hear that?' Then, while still vibrating, the base of the tuning fork is applied to the mastoid process and the patient asked 'Which is louder, the one at the front or this one at the back?' In a normal person, air conduction ('at the front') should be better than bone conduction, i.e. the Rinne test is positive (normal). It is normal to hear through the air: the telephone receiver is applied to your ear canal not plastered on to the mastoid process! Air conduction is naturally amplified by:
1 the lever system of the three ossicles (malleus moulded to the drum, stapes sitting in the oval window and incus between them);
2 relative size of the eardrum and oval window; and
3 separation of sound between the oval and round windows.

If these mechanisms for sound amplification are disturbed (conductive hearing loss), then bone conduction becomes better than air conduction (negative Rinne test).

In the Weber test, the tuning fork is placed centrally on the head and the patient asked 'Do you hear that in the middle or in one ear?' You would expect this sound to be heard better in the better ear. And so it is, provided any deficit is of a sensorineural type. Confusingly, however, if airborne sounds are not conducted properly, then the fork is heard in the worse ear. You can test this by placing the fork centrally on your own forehead and putting a finger

05

in one ear. The fork is heard in the occluded ear. This is because natural background noises are not being conducted into the bad ear, there is less interference on that side and the 'internal' bone-conducted sound of the tuning fork is dominant.

Assessment of the dizzy patient

Many clinicians find the assessment of the dizzy patient daunting. In fact, the essentials for evaluation, listed in the box below, can be completed in about 10 min. Some of the difficulty probably arises because of the presence of multiple causes in a fair number of patients, particularly older subjects. The initial tests are carried out with the patient seated. Once the patient is standing for the Romberg test, he or she is then asked to walk to a couch for erect and supine blood pressure measurement, while gait is observed en route. Finally, the positional provocation tests for benign paroxysmal positional nystagmus are performed.

Examination of dizzy patients

- Eyes: nystagmus, fundoscopy
- Cerebellar signs
- Tympanic membranes
- Romberg's test
- Gait
- Cardiovascular:
  (a) Erect and supine blood pressure
  (b) Neck bruits
- Positional testing

Vestibular nystagmus is fine-amplitude horizontal jerk nystagmus. Cerebellar hemisphere lesions may also give horizontal jerk nystagmus but typically of a more coarse amplitude. Also, a patient with central nystagmus may not be unduly dizzy. In contrast, a patient with vestibular nystagmus will usually be confined to bed. Nystagmus that changes direction or is more marked in the abducting eye indicates a central disorder. Fundoscopy can reveal signs of hypertension, papilloedema or optic atrophy (multiple sclerosis can present with isolated vertigo). The key cerebellar signs to elucidate are dysdiadochokinesis and past-pointing. The lower limbs may also be examined (heel–shin test). Romberg's test, especially with the eyes closed, can be non-specific: a patient moderately dizzy from whatever cause at the time of testing will be fairly unsteady standing with the eyes closed. The cardiovascular examination is vital, especially in older people.

Investigations of ear or balance disorders

Audiometry hearing tests

Hearing is tested by pure-tone audiometry at octave steps from 125 to 8000 Hz in patients of 4 years of age and older (Fig. 43.8). The sounds are presented to each ear in turn via headphones (air conduction) and by a probe applied to the mastoid process (bone conduction) while the other ear is masked.

Conductive deafness can be further defined by tympanometry. A probe is placed in the ear canal while the pressure in the canal is changed above and below normal

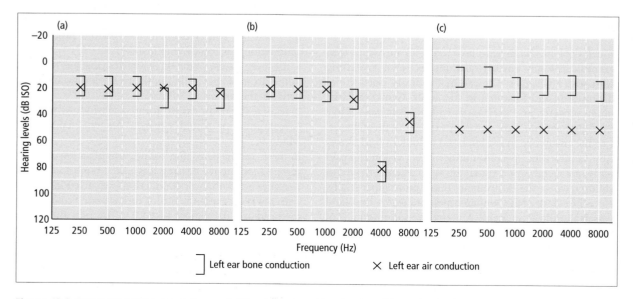

Figure 43.8 Pure-tone audiogram: (a) normal; (b) noise-induced hearing loss; (c) conductive hearing loss.

atmospheric pressure. The tympanogram traces the subsequent movement of the tympanic membrane. Reduced pressure in the middle ear implies eustachian tube dysfunction. Fluid in the middle ear is incompressible and generates a flat tympanogram (Fig. 43.9).

Electrophysiological tests of hearing such as evoked-response audiometry can be used, with sedation as needed, to establish thresholds, e.g. in infants and very young children. Electrical impulses that occur in the region of the brainstem in response to a click stimulus are averaged from skull surface electrodes.

Vestibular function

In caloric tests, the lateral semicircular canals are subjected to stimulation by irrigation of the ear canals with warm and cool water. The normal response is for the subject to feel dizzy and for horizontal nystagmus to be recorded. If there is depression of vestibular function on one side, the response to cold and hot irrigation is reduced on that side ('canal paresis').

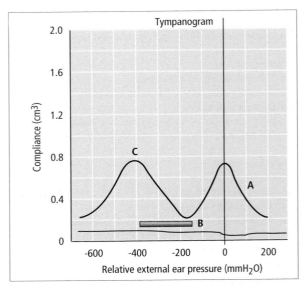

Figure 43.9 Tympanometry: A, normal; B, secretory otitis media (flat trace as fluid is incompressible); C, reduced middle ear pressure.

Ear assessment at a glance

Clinical presentations
Deafness
Risk factors for bilateral sensorineural hearing loss:
- Ageing
- Familial
- Noise induced
- Trauma
- Drug induced, e.g. aminoglycoside antibiotics

Tinnitus
- Subjective sensation of sound in the absence of any external noise

Discharge from ear
- Otitis externa
- Perforation
- Cholesteatoma.

Otalgia
- Local pathology in the ear or ear canal
- Referred pain:
  (a) Teeth
  (b) Temporomandibular joint
  (c) Oropharynx
  (d) Larynx or hypopharynx
  (e) Cervical spine
  (f) Sinuses

Dizziness
- A sensation of light-headedness
- Non-specific, has a multitude of causes

Vertigo
- Feeling that the environment or the body is moving
- Lesion in the vestibular system or cerebellum

Nystagmus
- Persistent rapid rhythmical movements of the eye

Facial (seventh) nerve palsy
- Bell's palsy
- Vascular: stroke
- Trauma: head injury
- Surgical: parotidectomy, mastoidectomy
- Infective: herpes zoster, mastoiditis
- Neoplastic: cerebellopontine angle, parotid
- Degenerative: sarcoid, multiple sclerosis

Physical examination
Inspect
- Pinna, ostium and mastoid

Otoscopy (pneumatic otoscopy)
Colour of the tympanic membrane
- White patches (tympanosclerosis): previous infection or surgery

05

- Red bulging drum: acute infection
- Golden or blue drum: otitis media + effusion

Perforation
- Size: percentage of drum area
- Condition: dry, moist, frankly discharging
- Effect of puff of air:
  (a) Perforation: no movement of membrane
  (b) No perforation: light reflex moves on drum

Auditory function
Clinical test of hearing
- Stand behind the subject
- Massage the tragus of one ear
- Ask the patient to repeat a series of numbers

512-Hz tuning-fork tests
Rinne's test (vibrating fork on mastoid and then by ostium)
- Compares air conduction to bone conduction
- Positive Rinne test (air conduction better than bone conduction) is normal
- Negative Rinne test indicates conductive hearing loss

Weber test (vibrating fork on forehead)
- With unilateral sensorineural deafness (and normal airborne sound) sound best heard in contralateral ear

Audiometry hearing tests
- Pure-tone audiometry at octave steps from 125 to 8000 Hz in patients aged 4 years or older

Tympanometry
- Conductive deafness can be further defined
- Measures movement of tympanic membrane in response to changes in canal pressure

Electrophysiological tests
- Evoked-response audiometry

Vestibular function
Clinical testing of patient with dizziness
Eyes
- Nystagmus:
  (a) Vestibular nystagmus: fine-amplitude horizontal jerky movements + dizziness
  (b) Cerebellar nystagmus: coarse-amplitude horizontal jerky movements ± dizziness
- Fundoscopy: signs of hypertension, papilloedema, optic atrophy

Cerebellar signs
- Dysdiadochokinesis
- Past-pointing
- Heel–shin test

Romberg's sign
- Tendency to fall or sway while standing with feet together, arms outstretched and eyes closed

Cardiovascular
- Erect and supine blood pressure
- Neck bruits

Other tests
- Positional testing
- Gait
- Tympanic membranes

Caloric tests
- Irrigation of ear canals with warm and cool water
- Normal response is a feeling of dizziness and horizontal nystagmus
- Response reduced on abnormal side

Disorders of the ear

Sensorineural deafness

Sensorineural deafness presents with reduced and distorted sound levels. The most common cause by far is presbyacusis, i.e. hearing loss due to ageing. The sensory (cochlear) components of sensorineural deafness give a high-tone loss while the neural component affects discrimination. Thus the patient experiences difficulty in unravelling complex speech sounds, especially in the presence of background noise, even when the volume of sound is increased. Sudden sensorineural deafness is a medical emergency and should be referred within 24 h to an ENT department, as some cases may be reversible by the use of vasodilators and steroids.

Noise-induced deafness may be occupational (e.g. boiler-making, riveting, weaving) or recreational (e.g. motor cycles, guns, music). The initial temporary threshold shift later becomes permanent and is maximum at 4 kHz. Ultimately, all frequencies are affected. Some people are more sensitive to noise than others. The maximum safe level for the workplace remains at 85 dB for a working week. The most effective form of ear protectors are ear-muffs but even these provide attenuation of only 30 dB at the lower frequencies. Acute noise trauma can occur during blast injuries.

Temporal bone fracture can be missed on X-ray but may produce bruising over the mastoid process. The range of possible effects include conductive deafness due to involvement of the middle ear, cerebrospinal fluid (CSF) otorrhoea, and inner ear damage with vertigo,

sensorineural deafness or facial nerve weakness. Inner ear trauma also results from labyrinthine window rupture, either explosive (sneezing or straining) or implosive (blast or barotrauma). There is fluctuating hearing loss, tinnitus and vertigo.

Ototoxicity is less common than formerly due to awareness of the main culprits, the aminoglycoside antibiotics such as gentamicin and the diuretic furosemide. Many drugs are only occasionally ototoxic and almost any medication may be responsible for a hearing defect.

A great deal of ENT time is expended on looking for acoustic neuroma, a rare neurilemmoma of the vestibular part of the eighth nerve. Despite its origin from the vestibular division, vertigo is rare because the very slow expansion is accompanied by central compensation of balance. Subjects present with unilateral deafness or tinnitus. The current investigation of choice is MRI.

Non-organic hearing loss may relate to possible compensation for industrial or military noise exposure, or occur in isolation. The tester may find low thresholds but discover that the subject responds promptly to a quiet question while still wearing the headphones.

Conductive deafness

In conductive deafness, bone conduction (nerve function) is preserved but the vibrations of a noise stimulus are prevented from reaching the cochlear hair cells. On rare occasions this is due to an exceptional wax plug or foreign body in the ear canal. The most common cause of adult conductive deafness is otosclerosis, although infection and trauma are also quite frequent. Congenital and childhood conductive deafness (secretory otitis media) are discussed later.

In otosclerosis, the formation of spongy new bone around the stapes footplate leads to fixation of the footplate and to a conductive or mixed deafness, with onset in young adulthood. There is a female preponderance and a positive family history in 50% of cases. In 10% of cases, otoscopy shows a flamingo-pink blush due to the vascular bone but most have normal tympanic membranes. Beethoven suffered from otosclerosis and was rendered profoundly deaf. Nowadays, results of intervention are good with either conservative treatment (hearing aid) or microsurgery to bypass the immobile footplate (stapedotomy).

Hearing aids

Hearing aids comprise a microphone to pick up sound, a small amplifier and a receiver. A poorly fitting or inadequately inserted mould produces feedback (squealing). Most hearing aids have a T (Telecoil) position in addition to the M (microphone) position. Users in public places with an electromagnetic induction loop, e.g. theatres and cinemas, can switch to the T position. An improved quality of sound is then transmitted by electromagnetic induction of the coil rather than via the microphone. Ancillary aids include loud telephone bells, flashing door bells and fittings for television sets.

Tinnitus

Tinnitus is the sensation of sound that is entirely subjective, i.e. it is not caused by a noise in the environment. When a patient is asked to match noise intensity with tinnitus, the volume is only about 10–20 dB, much quieter than a conversational voice. However, because it is a noise over which the patient has no control it is extremely annoying. (This is analogous to the irritation caused by a neighbour's machine while no such annoyance is caused by the much louder sounds emanating from one's own appliances.) Minor degrees of non-intrusive tinnitus are extremely common and often idiopathic. The National Study of Hearing showed that 7% of adults have consulted a doctor about tinnitus lasting over 5 min. At the extreme end, 1 in 100 adults has tinnitus that severely affects their quality of life, while 1 in 200 experiences tinnitus that has a severe effect on their ability to lead a normal life. Pseudotinnitus is a noise caused by a true environmental sound, e.g. the hum of electricity pylons or of a refrigerator.

Causes

Sometimes tinnitus is caused by inner ear disease or by wax impinging on the eardrum or debris from otitis externa. Pulsatile tinnitus may be of vascular origin: check the patient's blood pressure and listen to the neck for a cervical bruit. More rarely, pulsatile tinnitus is caused by a vascular tumour (chemodectoma) such as a glomus tympanicum or glomus jugulare. General precipitating factors of non-pulsatile tinnitus include excessive coffee, aspirin or cigarette consumption, which should be eliminated.

Management

No drug treatment is effective but a hearing aid, by increasing the volume of ambient noise, will act as a masker, i.e. drown out the noise and distract the patient's attention. The hours before sleeping are often the worst as there is little ambient noise, and a radio played quietly may help the patient get to sleep. A more sophisticated device is a tinnitus masker, which looks like a hearing aid but generates a sound that can be matched to the patient's tinnitus. Because this is a sound over which the patient has complete control, it is much less annoying. As an added bonus, patients occasionally have residual inhibition, i.e. for a very short period of time after use the tinnitus is abolished. Patients may also be referred to the Royal National Institute for the Deaf website, which has a very helpful resource for patients and healthcare workers.

05

As people gradually come to terms with their tinnitus, they are less alarmed by it. Through habituation, the brain 'registers' the noise much less. This is analogous to the situation where people who live near a busy road over time do not hear the traffic noise. A fairly new approach for treating troublesome tinnitus is called tinnitus retraining therapy, which speeds up the habituation process.

Discharge from the ear

Otitis externa

This localized dermatitis is the most common cause of ear discharge in adults. The ear canal is the only blind-ending skin-lined tract in the body and normally is self-cleansing, with a complex system of wax formation and skin migration. This may be interrupted by the ingress of water, chemicals, cotton buds or an allergenic hearing aid mould. Bacteriology swabs usually show a mixed growth, including *Pseudomonas*.

The cornerstone of treatment is keeping the ears dry. Patients seem to have difficulty accepting this, even if the condition is recurrent. The situation is not helped by the current fashion for frequent, even daily, hair-washing. The hair must not be washed in a shower or bath because it is totally impossible to keep water out of the ears. Hair-washing must be done in the wash-hand basin.

The ears should be plugged with cotton wool generously covered in petroleum jelly or with well-fitting ear plugs or commercial malleable wax plugs. Swimming is contraindicated in the active stages of the disease. For chronic sufferers who wish to swim, plugs can be worn with a cap and the patient advised not to dive or submerse the head. Useful preparations include:

- aluminium acetate drops or spray (which create an acid microenvironment and prevent the growth of *Pseudomonas*);
- Betnesol drops, which counteract the itch;
- 1% hydrocortisone or Vioform-Hydrocortisone ointment (an antiseptic–steroid combination) if the pinna itself is heavily involved.

Chronic suppurative otitis media

This disease is conveniently subdivided into cases with and without cholesteatoma. Cholesteatoma is a sac of keratinizing squamous epithelium rather like an aggressive sebaceous cyst surrounded by granulation tissue and enzymes that erode bone, particularly when infected. The sac grows slowly into the mastoid bone. Cholesteatoma is easily missed: the perforation may be quite small. The discharge is scanty with an offensive smell. Treatment is surgical (mastoidectomy).

The complications of cholesteatoma include:

- conductive deafness (erosion of ossicles);
- facial nerve weakness (erosion of bony canal);
- vertigo (erosion of semicircular canal);
- extradural or brain abscess.

Chronic suppurative otitis media without cholesteatoma is less aggressive. There is usually a central perforation with a copious mucoid discharge. The treatment may be conservative, e.g. drops and advice to keep the ear dry. Surgery may be used to clear the mastoid or graft the drum.

Vertigo

Viral labyrinthitis is the most common cause in young adults. There is a short history of rotatory dizziness, usually following an upper respiratory infection. Initially the patient may be confined to bed but, as central compensation and recovery of the affected labyrinth occur, balance gradually improves. In middle-aged subjects, there may be a recurrent form of vestibular neuronitis.

In older subjects, especially smokers, vertebrobasilar ischaemia is probably the most common cause of rotatory dizziness. There may be associated features of cervical spondylosis. Rotatory vertigo appears to be a greater risk factor for subsequent stroke in the elderly than generalized unsteadiness.

In benign paroxysmal positional nystagmus, short bursts of rotatory vertigo are provoked by head position and can be reproduced by clinical positional testing.

Ménière's disease is among the rarest causes of dizziness. It presents with a triad of dizziness, tinnitus and deafness. It is caused by a build-up of excessive endolymph within the inner ear. The inner ear membrane ruptures episodically, causing acute dizziness that confines the patient to bed for a few hours. This rare diagnosis requires specialist confirmation.

> **Dizziness in older people**
>
> - Dizziness is very common over the age of 65 years
> - Most have multiple causes
> - Central vascular insufficiency
> - Eyesight poor
> - Poor proprioception
> - Cervical spondylosis
> - Degenerative changes in the inner ear

Ear wax

Wax is a natural secretion. It provides a natural waterproof coating for the sensitive skin of the ear canal and also has immune components that counter infection. Yet many patients, and quite a few healthcare professionals, regard the presence of wax in the ear as a disease. The ear canal is the only blind-ending skin-lined tract in the body. Thus the ear canal has had to develop a unique system of

skin migration in order to counter the lack of surface desquamation found elsewhere on the body surface. Sometimes the migration process fails. This may be spontaneous or it may be due to overuse of cotton buds, determinedly impacting the wax deep into the canal. It may also be due to syringing on so frequent a basis that the ear skin effectively loses the natural self-cleansing pattern. Thus patients become caught in a vicious cycle of repeated syringing. This cycle can sometimes be broken by the use of sodium bicarbonate ear drops, preferably a week at a time, on a regular basis. This allows the patient to stop

using cotton buds and obviates the need for syringing. Syringing is the most common source of iatrogenic ear disease in general practice. The complications of syringing include some which are mild but frequent, such as otitis externa or a flare-up of discharge from a pre-existing perforation. Others are less common but more serious, e.g. traumatic perforation of the drum, acute vertigo. Only once in every thousand or more ENT patients does wax accumulate to the extent of a disease process. Indeed this situation is so rare that very few clinicians other than ENT specialists will ever see it.

Disorders of the ear at a glance

Definitions

Sensorineural deafness: hearing loss arising from pathological changes affecting the biochemistry, electrical potential, vascular supply and end-organ structure of the cochlea or its neural connections with the brainstem

Conductive deafness: hearing loss arising from pathology located in the external ear canal or middle ear structures. Bone conduction (nerve function) is preserved

Tinnitus: a subjective sensation of sound, i.e. not caused by a noise in the environment. The sound is described as whistling, ringing, hissing or clicking but the most distressing aspect is the patient's inability to control it

Sensorineural deafness
Causes
Presbyacusis
- Hearing loss due to ageing
- Sensory (cochlear) component: high tone loss
- Neural component: discrimination loss

Noise-induced
- Maximum loss at 4 kHz
- Occupational: boiler-making, riveting or weaving
- Recreational: motor cycles, guns or music

Traumatic deafness
- Temporal bone fracture
- Inner ear trauma due to labyrinthine window rupture:
  (a) Explosive causes (sneezing or straining)
  (b) Implosive causes (blast or barotrauma)

Ototoxicity
- Aminoglycoside antibiotics

Acoustic neuroma
- Rare neurilemmoma of vestibular part of the eighth nerve

Non-organic hearing loss
- Compensation for industrial or military noise exposure

Conductive deafness
Causes
- Wax plug or foreign body in the ear canal (rare)
- Otosclerosis: formation of spongy new bone around the stapes footplate leads to fixation of the footplate and conductive or mixed deafness
- Infection
- Trauma
- Congenital
- Childhood conductive deafness (secretory otitis media)

Hearing aid
- A device comprising a microphone, amplifier and receiver capable of increasing sound intensity at the ear
- Many include an electromagnetic pick-up for use in buildings or with special telephones
- Hearing aids are useful in conductive deafness
- Ancillary aids include loud telephone bells, flashing door bells and fittings for television sets

Tinnitus
Causes
- Inner ear disease
- Wax impinging on the eardrum
- Debris from otitis externa
- Vascular:
  (a) Carotid bruit
  (b) Vascular tumour (chemodectoma)
- 'Drug' induced: coffee, aspirin, cigarettes

Management
- Hearing aid may mask noise
- Radio played quietly especially before sleep
- Tinnitus masker
- Support groups: Royal National Institute for the Deaf
- Tinnitus retraining therapy

05

Discharge from the ear
Causes
Otitis externa
- Localized dermatitis of the ear canal

Chronic suppurative otitis media with *cholesteatoma*
- Cholesteatoma is a sac of keratinizing squamous epithelium surrounded by granulation tissue and enzymes that erode into bone, especially the mastoid bone. The discharge is scanty with an offensive smell. Treatment is surgical (mastoidectomy)
- Complications of cholesteatoma:
    (a) Conductive deafness: erosion of ossicles
    (b) Facial nerve weakness: erosion of bony canal

(c) Vertigo: erosion of semicircular canal
(d) Extradural or brain abscess

Chronic suppurative otitis media without *cholesteatoma*
- Central perforation with a copious mucoid discharge
- Treatment is conservative initially

Vertigo
Causes
- Viral labyrinthitis: young adults
- Vestibular neuronitis: middle-aged
- Vertebrobasilar ischaemia: elderly smokers
- Benign paroxysmal positional nystagmus
- Ménière's disease (rare): triad of dizziness, tinnitus and deafness

The nose and sinuses

Symptoms

The main symptoms of nasal disorders are nasal blockage, nasal deformity, sneezing, rhinorrhoea, postnasal drip, epistaxis, disordered sense of smell and facial pain. Alternating right and left nasal obstruction may indicate a deviated nasal septum. The nasal history should encompass relevant precipitating factors.
- Smoking.
- Occupation.
- Allergies, notably inhaled allergens.
- Family history of atopy: asthma, eczema, hay fever.
- Asthma, bronchiectasis and other major lower respiratory tract disease.
- Nasal trauma.
- General medical history: antihypertensive medication, inflammatory disorders (e.g. sarcoid), gastro-oephageal reflux.

Smoking makes nasal discharge more apparent: the mucus is thicker and the mucociliary clearance mechanism is impaired. Patients with polyps or other forms of chronic rhinosinusitis may give a history of excessive exposure to dusts or chemicals in the workplace, although a true diagnosis of occupational rhinitis may be hard to substantiate. Patients may be aware of suffering from hay fever but in fact also have perennial rhinitis due to a related dust allergy. Conversely, in the absence of a personal or family history, skin-prick testing will yield few surprises.

Many rhinologists and chest physicians now regard the nose and lungs as parts of the same functional unit, the 'United Airways'. Certainly there is a clear link between nasal polyps and asthma in at least 30% of sufferers. If a patient with chronic rhinosinusitis has bronchiectasis, then the prospects of achieving long-term therapeutic success are much lower. A number of rare chronic inflammatory processes, like Wegener's granulomatosis, may present with aggressive and destructive nasal inflammation, with severe associated malaise. The role of gastro-oesophageal reflux in nasal disease is controversial. There is some intuitive appeal in the concept that high reflux in the supine position may reach the postnasal space but little evidence.

Physical examination and investigation of the nose

First, look at the shape of the nose. Is there any deviation and, if so, is it worse high up in the nasal bones or lower down in the cartilage? If the bones are bent as well as the cartilage vault, then surgical correction implies rhinoplasty rather than simple cartilage repositioning (septoplasty). Sometimes skin discoloration will signal systemic disease, e.g. lupus vulgaris (cutaneous tuberculosis), sarcoid or systemic lupus erythematosus. There may be evidence of tumour or the much commoner rhinophyma, a bulbous nasal tip due to excessive seborrhoeic tissue (Fig. 43.10).

Now inspect the nostrils by asking the patient to tilt up the chin. Gently elevate the columella and see if the end of the septal cartilage tends to protrude into one vestibule, suggesting that there is septal deviation posteriorly. Then assess the nasal airway. In a child, hold a mirror or metal tongue depressor under the nostrils and inspect the two steam marks. In the adult, each nostril should be gently occluded by applying the pad of the (gloved) thumb, taking care not to push the septum into the test nostril, and asking the patient to sniff.

The tip of the nose should then be pushed gently up by the thumb and the interior illuminated by either a

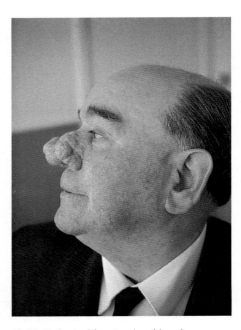

Figure 43.10 Patient with extensive rhinophyma.

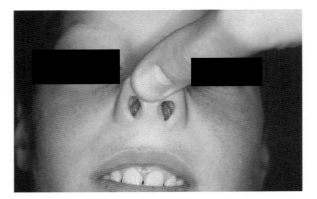

Figure 43.11 Engorged inferior nasal turbinates in a child with allergic rhinitis.

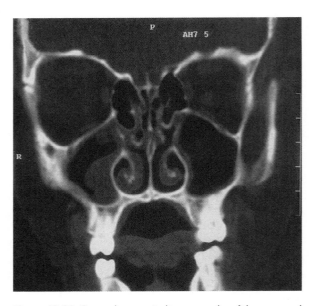

Figure 43.12 Coronal computed tomography of the nose and paranasal sinuses.

torch or, preferably, an auroscope with a wide aural speculum, which gives a greater depth of field. The septum is examined for deviation and bleeding points. Examine the cavity for discharge, polyps, tumour and, in children, foreign bodies. The side walls carry three lateral swellings (conchae), known in clinical practice as the superior, middle and inferior turbinates (Fig. 43.11). The superior turbinate is hidden, but the middle turbinate may be swollen and, if in contact with the septum high up, may be a source of pain. The distinction of grey polyps from pink swollen turbinates is usually straightforward, although confusion can arise. Occasionally, large postnasal lesions (polyps, adenoids or tumours) hang down into the mouth.

Differentiation of turbinates and polyps

- Turbinates normally the same colour as the septum (salmon pink)
- Very allergic turbinates can be pale grey
- Many children have large turbinates
- Polyps are usually pale shiny grey
- Big polyps near the vestibule may be pinker than usual (squamous metaplasia)
- Peak age for polyps is in the fifth to seventh decades
- Polyps are extremely rare in children without cystic fibrosis

Specialist examination includes use of the rigid nasendoscope. This allows a much better view of the middle turbinate area and an excellent view of the postnasal space. Plain radiography has essentially no part to play in nasal assessment. CT is sensitive to mucosal changes and shows the bony boundaries of the nose and sinuses, separating them from the orbit and cranial cavity (Fig. 43.12). However, it is expensive and involves not inconsiderable radiation exposure to the eye (enhances cataract development). Thus sinus CT is reserved for those with proven or suspected tumours or with positive endoscopic findings in whom surgery is planned.

05

Disorders of the nose

Nasal obstruction and rhinorrhoea

Simple inflammatory nasal polyps are prolapsed sinus mucosa and are related to intrinsic asthma and aspirin sensitivity. They tend to recur after surgical removal. Medical management is now the treatment of choice, typically a short course of oral steroids with nasal steroid drops or a spray. Surgery is reserved for uncontrollable disease.

Allergic rhinitis often starts in childhood and is discussed later. The healthy nasal lining is surprisingly dynamic, constantly adjusting itself to changes in temperature and humidity, e.g. the runny nose of the winter morning or following a highly spiced meal. In vasomotor rhinitis, the autonomic control of these adaptive changes can break down. This is particularly frequent in older people (senile rhinorrhoea). There may be a brisk response to nasal ipratropium. Failing this, surgery is used to reduce the bulk of the turbinate tissue.

A deviated nasal septum may also cause nasal obstruction. This may be present from birth or be caused later by trauma or facial growth asymmetry. The nasal blockage may be alternating due to the effect of the deviation on the turbinates. If symptoms warrant, the treatment is surgical (septoplasty). If the nasal bones are also bent, rhinoplasty may also be performed.

Nasal and sinus tumours are very rare. The early symptoms are unfortunately non-specific. Only when more advanced symptoms occur, such as epistaxis, chronic pain or loosening of dentition, is the diagnosis suspected. Thus the overall survival rate for sinus tumours is only 25%.

Fracture of the cribriform plate following nasal or head trauma may lead to CSF rhinorrhoea.

Mucopurulent nasal discharge

Bacterial superinfection frequently follows a common cold. The nasal lining may be damaged by addiction to topical pseudoephedrine preparation (rhinitis medicamentosa), best treated by topical nasal steroids. Discharge may also follow the presence of a foreign body or rhinolith, or primary ciliary dyskinesia with bronchiectasis and sometimes situs inversus (Kartagener's syndrome).

Sinusitis most often affects the maxillary and ethmoid sinuses. It follows mechanical or inflammatory obstruction of the natural ostium of the sinus. The discharge may be scanty and is accompanied by pain, increased by bending and peaking in the afternoon. Treatment of the acute phase is medical: steam, analgesia, decongestants and antibiotics.

Chronic rhinosinusitis is diagnosed once the symptoms have been present for 3 months. There are few if any external physical signs. Diagnostic nasendoscopy is used to inspect the areas close to the sinus openings for pus or inflammation. The treatment of chronic rhinosinusitis involves the following measures:
- underlying cause (e.g. allergy, septal deviation);
- prolonged course of antibiotics;
- topical nasal steroids;
- steam, douching;
- where all else fails, endoscopic sinus surgery;
- complementary medicine such as homeopathy may have a place.

The complications of sinusitis include orbital cellulitis, meningitis and intracranial abscess.

Differential diagnosis of facial pain

Nasal or sinus disease very rarely presents as primary facial pain. There is nearly always some other major symptom, such as postnasal discharge, nasal blockage or rhinorrhoea. Yet many patients automatically attribute facial pain to 'the sinuses'. The following are but a few of the myriad alternative diagnoses.
- Dental disease is much the most common cause of facial pain.
- Temporomandibular joint dysfunction.
- Neuralgia: important in its own right and as a presenting feature of multiple sclerosis. Trigeminal neuralgia is the most common primary neuralgia. Glossopharyngeal neuralgia is focused on the tongue base or the ear and is worse on chewing. Postherpetic neuralgia follows severe shingles (herpes zoster).
- Giant-cell arteritis affects older people and may lead to blindness. Diagnosed by high erythrocyte sedimentation rate and temporal artery biopsy.
- Atypical facial pain typically affects middle-aged women. Complex aetiology but psychological factors undoubtedly contribute.
- Periodic migrainous neuralgia wakes the patient with unilateral pain, flushing, lacrimation, nasal blockage and rhinorrhoea.

Common presentations in childhood

The management of recurrent sore throat in childhood is very similar to that in adults, except that the condition may have a slightly greater tendency to be self-limiting in childhood. The following are common childhood conditions with specific concerns relating to the age of the patient.

The nose and sinuses at a glance

Clinical features

Nasal symptoms
- Nasal blockage
- Nasal deformity
- Sneezing
- Rhinorrhoea
- Postnasal drip
- Epistaxis
- Disordered sense of smell
- Facial pain

Factors relevant to a nasal history
- Smoking
- Occupation
- Allergies, notably inhaled allergens
- Family history of atopy: asthma, eczema, hay fever
- Asthma, bronchiectasis, other major lower respiratory tract disease
- Nasal trauma
- General medical history:
  - (a) Antihypertensive medication
  - (b) Inflammatory disorders, e.g. sarcoid
  - (c) ?Gastro-oeophageal reflux

Physical examination and investigation of the nose
Inspection
- Shape of the nose
- Nasal skin discoloration
  - (a) Lupus vulgaris (cutaneous tuberculosis)
  - (b) Sarcoidosis
  - (c) Systemic lupus erythematosus
  - (d) Tumour (basal cell carcinoma/squamous cell carcinoma)
  - (e) Rhinophyma
- Nostrils: septal deviation, nasal airways

Ausoscopy
- Septum: deviation, bleeding
- Nasal cavity:
  - (a) Discharge
  - (b) Polyps
  - (c) Tumour
  - (d) Foreign body (children)
- Side walls:
  - (a) Superior, middle and inferior turbinates (pink)
  - (b) Polyps (grey)
- Rigid nasendoscopy:
  - (a) Middle turbinate
  - (b) Postnasal space
- Radiology: CT for proven or suspected tumours or before surgery

Disorders of the nose
Nasal obstruction and rhinorrhoea
- Simple inflammatory nasal polyps: oral steroids + nasal steroid drops or a spray
- Allergic rhinitis
- Vasomotor rhinitis: treat with ipratropium

- Nasal septal deviation (may be alternating):
  - (a) Congenital
  - (b) Post trauma
  - (c) Facial growth asymmetry: correction with septoplasty/rhinoplasty
- Nasal and sinus tumours (rare): epistaxis, chronic pain and loosening of dentition
- CSF rhinorrhoea: post cribriform plate fracture

Mucopurulent nasal discharge
- Bacterial superinfection post common cold
- Addiction to topical pseudoephedrine
- Foreign body
- Rhinolith
- Primary ciliary dyskinesia + bronchiectasis (+ situs inversus in Kartagener's syndrome)

Sinusitis
Acute
- Most often affects the maxillary and ethmoid sinuses
- Mechanical or inflammatory obstruction of the natural ostium of the sinus
- Scanty discharge + pain, increased by bending, and peaking in the afternoon
- Treatment: steam, analgesia, decongestants and antibiotics

Chronic rhinosinusitis
- Symptoms for 3 months or longer
- Treat underlying cause (allergy, septal deviation):
  - (a) Prolonged antibiotics
  - (b) Topical nasal steroids
  - (c) Steam, douching
  - (d) Endoscopic sinus surgery

Complications of sinusitis
- Orbital cellulitis
- Meningitis
- Intracranial abscess

Causes of facial pain
- Dental disease
- Temporomandibular joint dysfunction
- Neuralgia (single nerve or as part of multiple sclerosis):
  - (a) Trigeminal neuralgia: most common primary neuralgia
  - (b) Glossopharyngeal neuralgia: focused on the tongue base or the ear, worse on chewing
  - (c) Postherpetic neuralgia: follows severe shingles (herpes zoster)
- Giant-cell arteritis affects older people
- Atypical facial pain typically affects middle-aged women
- Periodic migrainous neuralgia wakes the patient with unilateral pain, flushing, lacrimation, nasal blockage and rhinorrhoea
- Nasal or sinus disease: usually additional symptoms of discharge, obstruction, rhinorrhoea

Hearing impairment

Congenital deafness

Congenital sensorineural deafness is significant and bilateral in 1 per 1000 live births. There is increasing use of neonatal screening for hearing impairment. This is tending to replace the use of the 8-month health visitor hearing check. Hearing impairment should be identified under 9 months of age. However, hearing aids can be fitted as young as 6 months. For the most profound losses, cochlear implants provide the potential for oral communication in children who might otherwise have had to rely on sign language for communication.

Dominant syndromes include Waardenburg's syndrome (deafness, white forelock and bushy eyebrows) and Treacher–Collins syndrome (deafness, hypoplasia of the mandible). Non-hereditary prenatal deafness arises from maternal infection with rubella, cytomegalovirus or infectious mononucleosis in the first trimester. Perinatal risk factors for congenital deafness include:

- family history;
- infection in pregnancy (rubella);
- prematurity;
- low birth weight;
- hypoxia;
- hyperbilirubinaemia.

Postnatal deafness

Postnatal deafness is specifically associated with meningitis, mumps and measles. Mumps tends to cause unilateral deafness. When deafness in a child is suspected, it is worth remembering that by the age of 1 year most children have two or three words and by 18 months about 18 words. By 2 years of age, words are beginning to be strung together into phrases and short sentences.

Audiometry

In distraction audiometry, the child (aged 6–12 months) is tested by inducing a head-turning response to sounds presented behind its line of vision. Somewhat older children (1–3 years) are tested by visual reinforcement audiometry. The sounds are generated from speakers at the side of the room. When the child turns to the speaker, a novel visual stimulus is delivered, e.g. teddy bear whose eyes flash. The child's interest is then re-engaged by the tester in a small toy directly in front. The novel visual stimulus prevents boredom and maintains the child's visual response to a series of stimuli at different pitches and intensities. From the age of 4 years most children can cooperate with simple pure-tone audiometry.

Middle ear disease

Middle ear disease is much commoner in childhood than in adult life. Reasons include the generally smaller eustachian tube and the presence of adenoids in the postnasal space, further reducing middle ear ventilation. Also, the average young child will experience up to 11 upper respratory tract infections per annum, almost one every 6 weeks. Rates are probably higher in settings where large numbers of children spend considerable periods in care or school groups. There are two very common childhood middle ear disorders: acute suppurative otitis media and otitis media with effusion. Children can also suffer from chronic suppuration or cholesteatoma but these are much rarer.

Acute suppurative otitis media

This usually follows a cold. It is all too clear in some children that the problem is in an ear because there may be complaints of severe otalgia or a tendency to pull at the ear. In infants, presentation may be much less specific: there may be a pyrexia of unknown origin or even a febrile convulsion as the middle ear begins to develop an exudate. As the pus accumulates, the eardrum bulges and ultimately perforates. The pain subsides, the ear discharges and, in most cases, heals spontaneously.

The disease can be arrested by the early use of antibiotics and decongestants (topical pseudoephedrine or Otrivine nose drops) together with steam and possibly systemic decongestant elixir such as pseudoephedrine. The antibiotic should be active against *Haemophilus influenzae* (amoxicillin, Augmentin). The rare complication of acute mastoiditis, which was once very common, gives a velvety feel to the periosteum over the mastoid bone, sometimes a subperiosteal abscess and the ear tends to protrude on the affected side. There may be swelling of the posterosuperior canal wall. If there is no response to systemic antibiotic therapy within 48 h, the mastoid is explored and a cortical mastoidectomy carried out by drilling all the air sinuses into continuity.

Otitis media with effusion

This is the most common cause of conductive deafness in children. If it occurs in a persistent form under the age of 2 years, it may interfere with expressive language development. In older children the modest conductive deafness may pass relatively unnoticed in the home but can have a major impact on education. The eardrum may have an obvious yellow or bluish colour, or be slightly dull or even look fairly normal. In other words, otoscopy is an unreliable form of diagnosis. Many cases resolve spontaneously.

The process may be enhanced by a 6-week continuous course of antibiotics or by the use of balloon inflation to encourage reventilation of the middle ear. Where the effusion persists, grommet insertion may be required, with or without removal of the adenoids.

The indications for surgical treatment of glue ear include:

- two failed hearing tests at least 2 months apart;
- bilateral effusions (20 dB or worse in better ear);
- evidence of some impact on performance.

Nasal obstruction

This may be considered chronologically. In preschool children the most common cause is adenoid hypertrophy while in schoolchildren it is allergic rhinitis or a congenitally deviated septum. Adenoid tissue is very scanty under the age of 2 years and usually regresses before the age of 10 years. Children have polyps extremely rarely and usually only if they have a disorder like cystic fibrosis. Even rarer are the neoplastic or congenital intranasal malformations such as encephaloceles, which can also present with nasal obstruction.

Adenoids

The adenoid pad of postnasal space lymphoid tissue may give rise to snoring, mouth-breathing and hyponasal speech. It is evident that these symptoms bother adults more than the children themselves. The hazards of adenoid removal include general anaesthesia and bleeding in 1–2% of cases. As adenoid tissue usually involutes, expectant management is often preferable, except where sleep apnoea syndrome is suspected (see later). Adenoid removal may increase the efficacy of surgical intervention for glue ear and is more commonly performed now in this context.

Allergic rhinitis

Allergic nasal problems may affect as many as 1 in 10 children. The most common inhaled allergens are dust, house-dust mite protein, pollen, spores and animal dander. There may be associated sneezing and a history of eczema or extrinsic asthma in the subject or family. The diagnosis may be made clinically, on the basis of radioallergosorbent testing or, in those over 7 years old, by skin-prick testing (the most sensitive method and the one preferred in adults).

Allergens are often multiple and thus allergen avoidance is often quite impractical. In adults, therapy often centres on topical nasal steroids, but there are concerns that these might retard growth if overused in childhood.

Thus more emphasis is placed on the use of systemic or topical nasal antihistamines.

Snoring/aleep apnoea

Children as young as 18 months may present with nocturnal obstructive symptoms. Their parents will give a history of frequent episodes of interrupted breathing at night, which can be very alarming. On examination, there may be obviously enlarged tonsils. If the history is in doubt, an overnight sleep study may be performed in hospital. However, if the tonsils are huge and the history clear-cut, the child may proceed directly to adenotonsillectomy. The parents must be informed, however, that tonsillectomy in the under 4 year old is proportionately more hazardous and also that special postanaesthetic monitoring will be required overnight following the surgery. At least 30% of childhood tonsillectomy procedures are now performed for obstructive symptoms rather than for recurrent sore throat.

Key points

- Otitis externa is the main cause of adult ear discharge and the mainstay of treatment is keeping the ear dry
- Adults with an unexplained onset of asymmetrical hearing loss have an acoustic neuroma until proved otherwise
- First-line treatment for a discharging perforation of the eardrum is topical drops or spray including antibiotic and steroid
- It is safe to fly with a perforation or grommet in the tympanic membrane. Decongestant therapy is helpful for those who wish to fly with a blocked eustachian tube to prevent the severe pain on descent of the aeroplane
- It is not safe to syringe cavities, perforations or grommets. When in doubt, refer to a specialist
- Nasal manipulation is best performed within 7–10 days of fracture, otherwise the bones begin to set
- First aid management of epistaxis is to pinch the nose on the soft part and to tip the head forward
- Cardinal symptoms of head and neck cancer are persistent hoarseness, oral ulcer or white patch, cervical dysphagia or lump in the neck in a current or past smoker
- The major risk factors for hoarseness in non-smokers are reflux, voice abuse or overuse, stress and use of inhalers
- In young children with stridor, consider epiglottitis. Never upset, attempt to examine or lie down such children until full facilities are available to support the airway (intubation, tracheostomy)

05

Common ENT presentations in childhood at a glance

Hearing impairment

Congenital deafness
- 1 per 1000 live births
- Should be identified under 9 months of age
- Hearing aids
- Cochlear implants

Syndromes
- Waardenburg's syndrome: deafness, white forelock and bushy eyebrows
- Treacher–Collins syndrome: deafness, hypoplasia of the mandible
- Non-hereditary prenatal deafness: first-trimester maternal infection with rubella, cytomegalovirus or infectious mononucleosis

Risk factors for congenital deafness
- Family history
- Infection in pregnancy (rubella)
- Prematurity
- Low birth weight
- Hypoxia
- Hyperbilirubinaemia

Postnatal deafness
- Post meningitis, mumps, measles

Audiometry
- Distraction audiometry (6 and 12 months): head-turning response to sounds behind line of vision
- Visual reinforcement audiometry (1–3 years): head-turning response to speakers and visual stimulus at the side of the room
- Pure-tone audiometry (4 years and older)

Middle ear disease

Risk factors
Poor middle ear ventilation due to:
- Small eustachian tube
- Presence of adenoids in the postnasal space
- Frequent upper respiratory tract infections

Acute suppurative otitis media
- Usually follows a cold
- Otalgia
- Tendency to pull at the ear
- Pyrexia of unknown origin
- Febrile convulsion
- Eardrum bulges and perforates
- Pain subsides, the ear discharges, heals spontaneously
- Treatment:
  (a) Early use of antibiotics and decongestants
  (b) Steam + systemic decongestant elixir (pseudoephedrine)

Otitis media with effusion
- Most common cause of conductive deafness in children
- Diagnosis is difficult
- Treatment:
  (a) 6 weeks of continuous antibiotics
  (b) Balloon inflation to encourage reventilation of middle ear
  (c) Grommet insertion ± adenoidectomy for persistent infection
- Indications for surgical treatment of glue ear:
  (a) Two failed hearing tests at least 2 months apart
  (b) Bilateral effusions (20 dB or worse in better ear)
  (c) Evidence of some impact on performance

Nasal obstruction

Adenoids
- Adenoid tissue is very scanty under the age of 2 years and regresses before the age of 10 years
- Symptoms: snoring, mouth-breathing, hyponasal speech
- Expectant management preferable
- Adenoidectomy may be beneficial when grommets inserted for glue ear
- Tonsiladenoidectomy for sleep apnoea

Allergic rhinitis
- 1 in 10 children
- Allergens: dust, house-dust mite protein, pollen spores, animal dander
- Associated with sneezing, history of eczema, extrinsic asthma
- Treatment: topical nasal antihistamines, systemic antihistamines, topical nasal steroid

Snoring/sleep apnoea
- Nocturnal obstructive symptoms
- Frequent episodes of interrupted breathing at night
- May be obviously enlarged tonsils (treat by adenotonsillectomy)
- Overnight sleep study if diagnosis in doubt

Evidence-based medicine

Books

Browning, G.G. (1998) *Clinical Otology and Audiology*, 2nd edn. Arnold, London.

Bull, P.D. (1996) *Lecture Notes on Diseases of the Ear, Nose and Throat*, 8th edn. Blackwell Science, Oxford.

Jones, A.S., Philips, D.E. & Hilgers, F.J.M. (eds) (1997) *Diseases of the Head and Neck, Nose and Throat*. Arnold, London.

Kerr, A. (ed.) (1997) *Scott Brown's Otolaryngology*, 6th edn. Butterworth Heinemann, Oxford.

McGarry, G.W. & Browning, G.G. (1999) *ENT*. Churchill Livingstone, London.

Watkinson, J.C., Gaze, M.N. & Wilson, J.A. (2000) *Stell and Maran's Head and Neck Surgery*, 4th edn. Butterworth Heinemann, London.

Journals

Archives of Otolaryngology Head and Neck Surgery. One of the strongest all-round journals (affiliated to the American Medical Society).

ENT News. Widely distributed free of charge due to the level of advertising revenue. Partly a professional journal, but includes 100-word summaries of key papers in a wide range of relevant journals. The abstracts are written by interested clinicians rather than professional academics or reviewers, but the salient features of the papers reviewed are usually incorporated.

Otolaryngologic Clinics of North America

Yearbook of Otolaryngology Head and Neck Surgery (Mosby)

Websites

http://www.entgroup.demon.co.uk Cochrane ENT Group.

http://www.NOTO.org National Otolaryngology Trials Office. Includes abstracts of Annual UK Head and Neck Cancer EBM Day abstracts.

http://www.orl-baohns.org British Association of Otorhinolaryngologists Head and Neck Surgeons. Includes access to nationally agreed UK guidelines for management of common conditions.

http://www.rnid.org.uk Royal National Institute for the Deaf.

http://www.ndcs.org.uk National Deaf Children's Society.

http://www.entnet.org American Academy of Otolaryngology Head and Neck Surgery.

http://www.aro.org Association of Research in Otolaryngology.

http://www.bcm.tmc.edu/oto Bobby Alford Department of Otorhinolaryngology, Baylor College of Medicine, Houston, Texas.

http://cancernet.nci.nih.gov/index.html Head and neck cancer website of the National Cancer Institute, USA.

http://www.laparoscopy.com Includes a number of ENT procedures, such as endoscopic stapling of pharyngeal diverticulum.

http://www.vesalius.com For access to surgical images for presentations; head and neck page is http://www.vesalius.com/foli2_headneck.asp

http://www.medinfo.ufl.edu/year1/trigem/home.html For a site that brings trigeminal nerve anatomy to life.

Ophthalmic Disorders

44

Must know Must do

Must know

Gradual visual field loss occurring over a period of many months may go unnoticed by an individual, often until there is extensive loss of visual field. This can occur in both glaucoma and chiasmal compression from pituitary tumour

Diabetics may have normal visual acuity with no visual symptoms in the presence of serious sight-threatening retinopathy

Inflammatory eye disease may be a manifestation of systemic disease, e.g. sarcoidosis causing uveitis

Symptoms of acute glaucoma may mimic the systemic illness in the elderly population, e.g. influenza or acute abdomen

Sudden onset of floaters in the vision may herald a retinal tear and subsequent retinal detachment

Topical eye medication (eye drops) can result in systemic effects, e.g. β-blockers can result in an acute fatal asthma attack

Corneal ulceration can result from bacterial contamination of soft contact lenses, e.g. *Pseudomonas aeruginosa*

Macular degeneration is the most common cause of poor vision in the elderly population. The visual loss is central and often associated with distortion

Prolonged use of steroid eye drops can result in raised intraocular pressure and subsequent glaucoma

Pupil response/swinging flashlight test is very important for detecting unilateral optic nerve disease, e.g. optic neuritis

Must do

Examine visual fields of patients

Examine visual acuity by Snellen's charts

Perform direct and consensual light reflexes

Become proficient in ophthalmoscopic examination

Attend a cataract surgery operation and ask the patient about the benefits of operation several weeks later

Introduction

The medical student traditionally worries about ocular disease. Sight is such an important faculty and the eye seems to be small and difficult to examine It is not surprising then that students are apprehensive about ocular signs. In fact, things are relatively uncomplicated, for the symptoms are usually confined to pain or blurring of vision, just occasionally double vision. A basic understanding of the anatomy of the eye and visual pathways is mandatory and can be found in any student's anatomy textbook. The following chapter attempts to give a résumé of the important ocular conditions that will allow a sufficient ophthalmic knowledge to carry students through their examinations and then hopefully on the wards as a house officer in casualty departments or in general practice.

Evaluation of the patient

Clinical assessment

Symptoms

Most ophthalmic problems can be diagnosed with a good history and careful clinical examination. As many systemic diseases affect the eye, a good general history needs to be obtained first. General points to consider include the following.

- Medical history: hypertension, diabetes mellitus, sarcoidosis, inflammatory bowel disease.
- Family history: squint and some types of glaucoma may be familial.
- Drug history: some drugs affect the eye, e.g. chloroquine, ethambutol, systemic steroids.

The specific points to consider in eye disease include the following.

- Ocular history: short- or long-sightedness, history of trauma, previous eye surgery.
- Eye pain: mode of onset, severity, gritty feeling, associated discharge/redness, photophobia.

05

● Visual symptoms: monocular or binocular blurring or loss of vision, related to posture, rate of onset, flashing lights, field loss, double vision, amaurosis fugax (see Chapter 37).

Physical examination

For the purpose of physical examination, the eye includes the following elements: eyelids, conjunctiva, cornea, sclera, orbits and eyeball. An assessment of eye function is made by examining visual acuity, visual fields, pupillary reflexes and eye movements. The fundi may be examined with the ophthalmoscope.

The elements
● Eyelids: look for ptosis, xanthelasma, exophthalmos (lid lag), ectropion, basal cell carcinoma, stye (chalazion).
● Conjunctiva: pallor, injection, chemosis.
● Cornea: ulcer, arcus senilis.
● Anterior chamber: check for blood (hyphaema) or pus.
● Sclera: yellow in jaundice, blue in osteogenesis imperfecta.
● Orbit: palpate for tenderness, anaesthesia or hypoaesthesia of the cheek indicates inferior orbital nerve damage.
● Eyeball: palpate to get an impression of intraorbital pressure.

Eye function
● *Visual acuity*: this is usually checked using a standard Snellen chart at 6 m with glasses if worn or pinhole.
● *Visual fields*: the patient sits facing the examiner and both examiner and patient cover their respective eyes not being tested, e.g. the patient covers the right eye and the examiner covers the left eye. The patient looks at the examiner's face while the examiner moves a red-headed pin into the visual field from the periphery. The patient indicates when he or she first sees red.
● *Pupillary reflexes*: the direct and consensual light reflex and the accommodation reflex are a simple way of checking the integrity of the anterior visual pathways.
● *Swinging light reflex*: the symmetry of pupil responses should be checked by the swinging light test, which will detect a relative defect in the afferent input in one eye compared with the other, e.g. an optic nerve lesion on one side. As the light moves from the normal to the defective eye, the pupil response is to dilate rather than to constrict. This difference is made more obvious if the light is moved repeatedly from one eye to the other.
● *Eye movements*: the eyes should be assessed for movement in all directions to check the function of third, fourth and sixth cranial nerves. Fatiguability of eye muscles should be tested by continuous upward gaze. In myasthenia gravis the muscles tire and ptosis occurs. In Horner's syndrome the pupil is small but reactive (miosis); there is also ptosis and lack of sweating (anhidrosis). In third-nerve palsy, the pupil may be large, with ptosis and sometimes abnormal eye movement.
● *Corneal reflex*: the patient blinks when the cornea is stimulated. This checks the integrity of cranial nerve V.

Investigations

The general investigations depend on the clinical evaluation and the need to identify an underlying cause for the eye signs. For example, a brain scan would be indicated in someone with bitemporal hemianopia to confirm the presence of a pituitary lesion, whereas carotid Doppler studies would be indicated in a patient with a history of amaurosis fugax. However, simple specific eye investigations include fluorescein testing and ophthalmoscopy. More sophisticated investigation requires referral to an ophthalmologist.

Ophthalmoscopy
The 'red reflex' should be elicited first. The ophthalmoscope is set at the 0 lens and the eye is viewed from about 60 cm away. The reflection from the fundus is seen as red; this is the red reflex. (It is also seen in photographs of people taken with a flash.) Any opacity between the cornea and the fundus will disrupt the reflex, the most common cause being a cataract. The ophthalmoscope is then brought close to the patient's eye and the lens setting is altered until a clear view of the retina can be obtained (Fig. 44.1). The optic disc is sought and the edges of the disc are examined (a blurred edge may indicate a cerebral tumour). The retina should be scanned for exudates, haemorrhage or new vessel formation. Finally the macula should be examined (macular exudates may be seen in diabetes; see Fig. 44.6).

Fluorescein testing
A few drops of fluorescein are instilled on to the cornea and the cornea is examined with a blue light. Any abrasion or ulceration will easily be seen as a green lesion on the cornea.

Dilating the pupil
Most optic discs are visible through a normal pupil but dilating drops should be used if the pupils are too small, if there is a cataract or if the retina in general (particularly the fovea) needs to be inspected. Tropicamide 1%, available as a single-dose 'minim', dilates the pupil within 20 min and wanes after about 2 h. Do not dilate if acute neurological observation is needed. Using this agent the risk of precipitating acute glaucoma is extremely low.

05

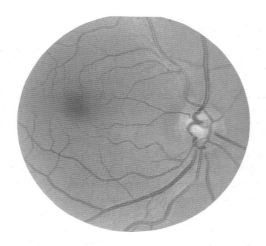

Figure 44.1 Normal fundus showing optic nerve head (disc) and macula, which surrounds the central fovea.

Table 44.1 Causes of an acute red eye.

Conjunctivitis
  Bacterial
  Viral
  Chlamydial
  Allergic
  Foreign body
Acute anterior uveitis (iritis, iridocyclitis)
Acute glaucoma
Episcleritis and scleritis

The acute red eye

For the medical student the acute red eye is the principal ocular emergency. The categories that need to be considered are given in Table 44.1.

Acute conjunctivitis

Bacterial

The common bacterial invasions are usually from *Staphylococcus aureus*, although *Haemophilus influenzae* may occur in epidemics. Pneumococcal conjunctivitis may be unpleasant, particularly in children, and *Pseudomonas* may invade the conjunctiva in debilitated patients, especially those in intensive care units. The eyes generally are very red with a sticky discharge. Patients usually describe a gritty sensation rather than pain in the eyes. The lids may be stuck together on waking in the morning. Unless the

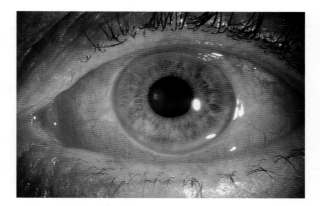

Figure 44.2 Red eye due to adenovirus conjunctivitis. Note the swelling of conjunctiva and scanty discharge.

cornea is involved, photophobia is rare and generally the vision is good and unimpaired by the condition beyond minor blurring. The pupil reaction is always normal. The treatment of bacterial conjunctivitis is generally intensive topical antibiotics, with chloramphenicol being most commonly used. It is important to instil the drops on a 2-hourly basis for at least 24 h before tailing off the treatment, otherwise insufficient application will produce relatively little improvement.

Viral

Viral conjunctivitis is more common and may accompany a flu-like illness, particularly that due to the adenovirus. Type 8 adenovirus may be responsible for epidemics of keratoconjunctivitis If the cornea is involved, there may be quite acute photophobia and pain. Viral conjunctivitis tends to settle spontaneously but topical antibiotics will do no harm (Fig. 44.2).

Chlamydial

An increasingly common form of conjunctivitis is due to *Chlamydia trachomatis*, which is often found in young people and may be sexually transmitted, such that there is chlamydial infection in the genitourinary tract as well as the eye (see Chapter 39). Chlamydial conjunctivitis is best treated with tetracycline or erythromycin orally unless there is some contraindication, such as pregnancy. If the disease is found in a young child or pregnant adult, he or she should not be given tetracycline as it causes staining in developing teeth. Tetracycline ointment used five times daily is also necessary.

Ophthalmia neonatorum is contracted at birth from an infected cervix or vagina and used to be due to the

gonococcus (see box below). Now it is far more commonly due to *Chlamydia*. It is a notifiable disease: any eye discharge occurring within 3 weeks of birth is considered notifiable. Treatment is as described for chlamydial conjunctivitis after swabs have been taken. Systemic treatment with antibiotics is indicated as the infant may also develop pneumonitis.

Elizabeth Blackwell

Elizabeth Blackwell (1821–1910) graduated from Geneva Medical College, New York in 1849, the first woman to become a medical doctor. She wanted to be a gynaecological surgeon but being a woman in a male-dominated profession she could only obtain training as a midwife in La Maternite Hospital in Paris. One night she was syringing the eyes of a baby with ophthalmia neonatorum when the water splashed up into her own eyes. She rapidly developed a purulent conjunctivitis that left her completely blind in one eye and partially blind in the other. Undaunted she abandoned her surgical ambitions, applied herself to medicine and eventually established a medical practice in New York. She also opened a hospital and founded a medical school for training women doctors in the USA and eventually returned to her native England, where she became professor of gynaecology at the London School of Medicine for Women.

Allergic

Atopic patients are often susceptible to outbreaks of allergic disease of the conjunctiva, particularly during the pollen season, when the eye may become acutely congested and extremely itchy. Sticky discharge is generally described as white, in contrast to the yellow pus associated with infective conjunctivitis, and is stringy in texture.

Allergy may be seen with a form of contact sensitivity in the eye due to the application of make-up or the use of astringent drops purchased without prescription from a pharmacist, when the skin takes on a typical look of contact dermatitis.

The treatment for acute allergic conjunctivitis in the atopic patient is topical anti-inflammatory drops combined with a mast-cell stabilizer drug, e.g. Opticrom drops. Steroid eye drops may be necessary particularly when there is corneal involvement. The use of Opticrom may prevent or reduce the frequency of further attacks. Steroid eye drops must be used with caution due to their potential to cause raised intraocular pressure and glaucoma.

Foreign body

A conjunctival or corneal foreign body may induce a painful red eye and this is a problem commonly seen in casualty departments. Usually there is a history of trauma, but sometimes patients have no recollection of injury. It is important to recognize and remove foreign bodies as soon as possible. Local anaesthetic eye drops will be required to examine the eye properly. The upper lid should be everted to exclude or remove a subtarsal foreign body. A superficial foreign body may be washed out of the eye or removed with a cotton-wool bud, but foreign bodies embedded in the cornea may have to be removed with a needle tip or special drill under local anaesthetic. Following removal, chloramphenicol ointment and a pad should be applied to the eye for 24–48 h. More serious eye injuries require expert management by eye surgeons.

Acute anterior uveitis, iritis, iridocyclitis

The uveal tract is made up of the iris, ciliary body and choroid; if the inflammation is mainly anterior it is termed anterior uveitis, iritis or iridocyclitis.

Anterior uveitis/iritis is a serious cause of the acute red eye. Classically, the eye redness is most marked adjacent to the corneal margin. This is unlike conjunctivitis, where the whole eye tends to be red. A small pupil is common with spasm of the iris sphincter due to inflammation. There will be cells in the anterior chamber but this is often only seen on examination with a slit lamp. In severe cases the inflammation may build up as a hypopyon if the outflow from the eye is obstructed and intraocular pressure rises. Adhesions between the iris and the lens are known as posterior synechiae and cause distortion of the pupil, which is most obvious when the pupil is dilated. If the posterior synechiae are confluent all the way round the pupil margin, aqueous cannot drain through the pupil; this causes an iris bombe, with severe secondary glaucoma.

Anterior uveitis/iritis is painful and, unlike conjunctivitis, this pain is aching rather than 'gritty'. Closing the eyes or bathing does nor relieve any of the symptoms. The eye is often excessively light-sensitive (photophobia). Acute iritis often takes 2 or 3 days to develop into a painful red eye. Patients who have previous attacks sense that things are building up again and they confusingly present themselves at casualty departments with a white eye and relatively little to find. However, the experienced practitioner will ensure that careful slit-lamp examination is carried out.

In practical terms most anterior uveitis/iritis is of unknown aetiology and is treated using topical steroids

and pupillary dilators to prevent synechiae forming between the lens and the posterior iris. Moreover, dilatation paralyses the muscles of the iris and ciliary body and relieves painful spasm. It is therefore particularly important when treating a patient with a red eye to distinguish between anterior uveitis/iritis (sometimes with a small pupil that requires pupillary dilatation) and acute glaucoma (with a large oval pupil that requires pupillary constriction).

Acute glaucoma

Acute glaucoma is a rare condition. To understand it, a basic knowledge of the anatomy of aqueous production and drainage within the eye is required (Fig. 44.3). Aqueous is normally produced in the ciliary body by a process of ultrafiltration and active secretion. The aqueous passes into the posterior chamber, circulates through the pupil into the anterior chamber and is able to escape from the eye through the trabecular meshwork. This links up with the canal of Schlemm and then into the episcleral veins and main circulation. The angle between the iris and the trabecular meshwork is called the drainage angle.

Most drainage angles are wide open, with easy access from the anterior chamber to the trabecular meshwork. Some eyes, however, have very narrow drainage channels. These are usually small eyes and patients with small eyes tend to be long-sighted, for the optical power of the eye cannot overcome the short axial length If for some reason the drainage channel between the iris and cornea narrows in patients with already narrow drainage angles, complete closure of the angle may take place, leading to acute obstruction to the circulation of aqueous. This process is called *acute-angle closure glaucoma*. This can be provoked by the pupillary dilating effects of topical mydriatics or the anticholinergic effect of many medications, e.g. tricyclic antidepressants, antiemetics and antispasmodics. Similarly, the drainage angle may narrow with age or an increase in lens size due to a cataract will result in the lens pushing forwards to obliterate the angle.

The sudden rise in intraocular pressure provoked by acute-angle closure may cause corneal oedema due to interference with normal corneal endothelial cell function. This produces the visual symptoms of haloes with a rainbow pattern around white lights. This is very striking and may cause the patient some consternation. It is different from the haloes produced by cataracts, which tend not to be coloured. The patient may have intermittent symptoms of glaucoma, with spontaneous resolution for months prior to an acute attack.

Once the pressure has risen and the cornea becomes oedematous, the eye rapidly becomes ischaemic. The iris becomes enlarged and oval. The pain is intense; it is described as an aching pain and is often severe enough to provoke vomiting. Sight is lost because the high pressure affects the ocular circulation and it is only a matter of hours before irreversible blindness occurs. Elderly patients with acute glaucoma may be misdiagnosed as having

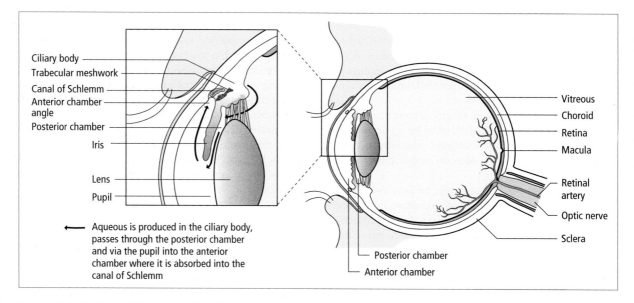

Ciliary body
Trabecular meshwork
Canal of Schlemm
Anterior chamber angle
Posterior chamber
Iris
Lens
Pupil

← Aqueous is produced in the ciliary body, passes through the posterior chamber and via the pupil into the anterior chamber where it is absorbed into the canal of Schlemm

Vitreous
Choroid
Retina
Macula
Retinal artery
Optic nerve
Sclera

Posterior chamber
Anterior chamber

Figure 44.3 Anatomy of the eye and (inset) the aqueous circulation.

a flu-like illness or even acute abdomen if they have profound symptoms with vomiting. The acutely inflamed eye may be overlooked during the clinical examination. The difference between acute glaucoma and other causes of a red eye is the degree of visual deterioration and the irregular, oval, dilated pupil. The pain tends to be far worse than that produced by other forms of acute red eye, except perhaps intense scleritis, in which there is also a mixture of ischaemia and inflammation.

Treatment is a matter of urgency and the first-line treatment is to administer intravenous acetazolamide (Diamox) 500 mg. This will reduce aqueous production in the eye. Pilocarpine drops are then instilled; this may constrict the pupil and pull the iris away from the closed angle. Topical β-blocking agents may also be used to bring the pressure down. Sometimes these measures are ineffective and intravenous mannitol is required. Surgery as a means of treating acute glaucoma is hazardous unless the pressure is brought down medically first. Laser iridotomy with a YAG laser is undertaken to create an opening in the peripheral iris. This creates an alternative route for aqueous flow and relieves the pressure build-up behind the pupil. Laser iridotomy is not always possible, particularly in a darkly pigmented iris. Surgical removal of a small piece of iris tissue is undertaken via an incision in the peripheral cornea.

The use of potent agents such as intravenous acetazolamide or mannitol must be measured against the patient's general health. They can be detrimental in diabetics (where intense dehydration or acidosis may be produced) or in patients with chronic renal failure.

In suspected cases of acute glaucoma it is generally best to commence therapy with acetazolamide tablets immediately if there may be a delay in referring the patient to an ophthalmologist, by which time severe damage may have occurred in the eye. It is always possible to diagnose angle-closure glaucoma in retrospect, so there is no need to fear that medication will interfere with later assessment.

Corneal ulcers

Corneal ulceration is most commonly viral, bacterial or traumatic. An ulcer characteristically causes pain, watering and photophobia. Ulcers are highlighted with fluorescein, especially if viewed with a blue light. Herpes simplex often produces a dendritic or branching pattern in the acute stage; herpes zoster may cause a similar appearance. Traumatic ulcers may become secondarily infected with bacteria, especially with contact lens wear. Hypersensitivity to chronic staphylococcal infection of the eyelids (blepharitis) may cause marginal ulcers at the edge of the cornea, which tend to be recurrent. Each type of ulcer needs specific treatment so patients should be referred without delay to an ophthalmic specialist, otherwise a permanent corneal scar may result.

Episcleritis and scleritis

The inflammatory causes of a red eye include episcleritis and scleritis. Scleritis may or may not be associated with systemic diseases, particularly rheumatoid arthritis, polyarteritis nodosa and Wegener's granulomatosis.

Episcleritis presents classically as an uncomfortable red eye or sometimes the eye may simply be red with no other features at all. The pupil is not involved and vision is unimpaired. The condition is generally not associated with systemic illness and is often self-limiting.

Scleritis can be very severe and is a potentially blinding disease. There is a distinction between scleritis which simply forms inflammatory painful nodules and a form where a vasculitis leads to painful ischaemia. These conditions are termed either nodular scleritis, which is relatively benign, or severe necrotizing scleritis.

Treatment of episcleritis is confined to the use of weak topical steroid or non-steroidal anti-inflammatory drops. In addition, scleritis requires oral treatment with either non-steroidal anti-inflammatory drugs or in severe cases high-dose systemic steroids.

Topical steroids and the red eye

Steroid eye drops must be used with caution. For example, if herpes simplex virus is responsible for the initial redness, corneal ulceration will be exacerbated due to reduction in the local corneal immune response. Serious corneal scarring with loss of vision may result. Allergic eye disease will improve dramatically with steroids, but the problem is weaning patients off the medication. If used for a prolonged period, topical steroids may cause a rise in intraocular pressure, with irreversible damage to the optic nerve (glaucoma). Topical steroids may be used in patients with iritis if the diagnosis is established, but supervision by an ophthalmologist is necessary. Generally, the red eye should not be treated with topical steroids unless the diagnosis is certain and the treatment appropriate.

Conclusion

The acute red eye is one of the most important topics for the medical student. A detailed history and a careful but simple examination should differentiate between the various causes and the patient can be directed towards the appropriate management or expert.

05

The acute red eye at a glance

Definition

Acute red eye: a physical sign characterized by redness of all or part of the conjunctiva or sclera ± discomfort in the eye

Causes
- Conjunctivitis
- Foreign body
- Anterior uveitis, iritis, iridocyclitis
- Corneal ulcer
- Acute glaucoma
- Episcleritis and scleritis
- Subconjunctival haemorrhage

Conjunctivitis
Clinical features
- Inflammation of the conjunctiva
- Red eye with sticky discharge, especially after sleep
- Pupil is normal and vision is not impaired

Causes and treatment
- *Staphylococcus aureus*, *Haemophilus influenzae*, *Pseudomonas*: topical antibiotics 2-hourly
- Virus: settles spontaneously
- *Chlamydia trachomatis*: systemic or topical tetracycline
- Herpes simplex: idoxuridine, aciclovir
- Allergic reaction: topical steroids, but only under expert supervision

Foreign body
A conjunctival or corneal foreign body is a common cause of red eye. May or may not be history of trauma

Clinical features
- Painful 'gritty' eye
- Pupil normal and vision not impaired

Treatment
- Topical anaesthesia to examine eye properly
- Evert upper lid to exclude subtarsal foreign body
- Irrigate superficial foreign body or remove with cotton-wool
- Foreign body embedded in cornea has to be removed with needle tip or drill
- Topical antibiotics and eye pad for 24–48 h following removal

Uveitis, iritis, iridocyclitis
Inflammation of all or part of the uveal tract

Clinical features
- Red eye with circumcorneal injection
- Constant 'aching' pain in eye and photophobia

- Pupil is *small* and fixed and the anterior chamber may be turgid
- Intraocular pressure is normal

Causes
- Ankylosing spondylitis
- Psoriasis
- Sarcoidosis
- Crohn's disease
- Ulcerative colitis
- Syphilis, tuberculosis

Treatment
- Treat underlying cause
- Topical steroids
- Pupillary dilators

Corneal ulcer
Ulcer of the cornea caused by viruses, bacteria or trauma

Clinical features
- Pain, watering and photophobia
- Highlighted with fluorescein in blue light

Treatment
- Identify and treat cause
- Neglected ulcers lead to corneal scarring

Acute glaucoma
Precipitated by narrowing of the drainage angle between iris and cornea. This is a medical emergency, as blindness will ensue if not treated promptly

Clinical features
- Red eye with injected conjunctiva and iris
- Severe 'aching' pain
- Patient sees haloes with rainbow pattern around white light
- Pupil is dilated, fixed and oval
- Intraocular pressure is very high

Treatment
- Acetazolamide 500 mg i.v. to reduce aqueous production
- Pilocarpine drops to constrict the pupil and widen the drainage angle
- Topical steroids and β-blockers to reduce intraocular pressure
- Occasionally, intravenous mannitol is required

Episcleritis and scleritis
Clinical features
- Localized inflammation of the sclera

- Small oval, slightly raised red area on the sclera
- May be 'aching' pain or not

Causes
- Allergic
- Rheumatoid arthritis
- Polyarteritis nodosa
- Wegener's granulomatosis

Treatment
- Treat underlying cause, if any is identified
- Topical steroids

Conjunctival and subconjunctival haemorrhage
- A conjunctival haemorrhage is in the conjunctiva and is usually due to trauma
- A subconjunctival haemorrhage is a painless collection of blood under the conjunctiva. It is associated with anterior cranial fossa fracture and the posterior limit of the haematoma cannot be defined
- Neither requires specific treatment

Table 44.2 Causes of sudden loss of vision.

Bilateral visual loss
Cerebrovascular accident
Toxic substances, e.g. methyl alcohol
Bilateral ocular disease

Unilateral visual loss
Arterial occlusion
    Retinal artery occlusion
    Ciliary artery occlusion (giant-cell arteritis)
Venous occlusion
Inflammatory conditions
    Optic neuritis
    Leber's optic neuropathy
    Optic nerve compression
Vitreous haemorrhage

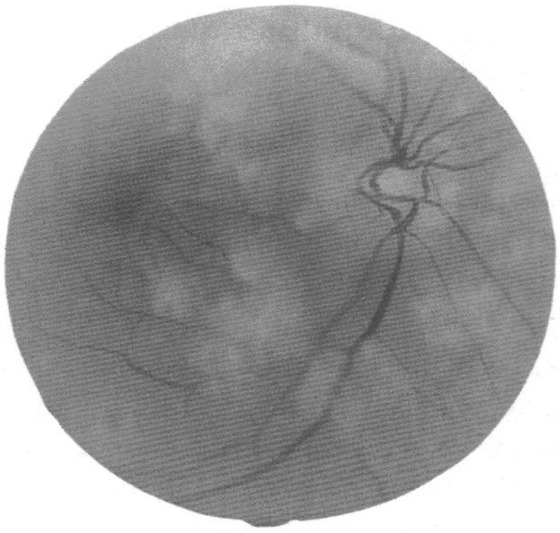

Figure 44.4 Central retinal artery occlusion responsible for acute loss of vision. There is pallor of the retina and narrowed branch arteries without haemorrhage.

Sudden loss of vision (Table 44.2)

Bilateral visual loss

Bilateral visual loss of sudden onset is very uncommon and usually caused by disease of the visual pathways or visual cortex.
- The most common cause of sudden bilateral visual loss is cerebrovascular accident affecting the visual cortex. In these circumstances the pupil reactions remain normal because they do not require an intact visual cortex but merely depend on the pupillary pathway, which passes through the upper midbrain.
- Occasionally, visual loss occurs due to ingestion of toxic substance, e.g. methyl alcohol.
- Rarely, causes of unilateral visual loss affect both eyes simultaneously, e.g. acute bilateral optic neuritis, although this is a very unusual form of demyelination. Giant-cell arteritis can also result in bilateral visual loss.

Unilateral visual loss

Sudden loss of vision occurring in one eye can occur due to a number of causes, including disturbance of the vascular supply to the eye, bleeding into the vitreous (vitreous haemorrhage) and optic nerve demyelination.

Arterial occlusion

Arterial occlusions may affect either the circulation in the retina or the optic nerve.

Retinal artery occlusion
Occlusion of the retinal artery may be transient, with episodes of visual loss lasting 15–20 min. It is often called amaurosis fugax and is usually described by the patient as 'like a black shutter across half or all the vision'. Vision returns gradually. Permanent occlusion of the central retinal artery results in complete loss of vision. (Fig. 44.4). The cause may be embolism from the carotid arteries or,

05

less commonly, be cardiac in origin. The embolism lodges in the small retinal arterial tree, commonly at a bifurcation. Management is directed towards locating the source of emboli and then the appropriate medical or surgical treatment. Simply listening to the carotid arteries or heart may reveal a murmur or bruit and further investigations include echocardiography, 24-h electrocardiogram and carotid Doppler studies. Low-dose aspirin therapy is indicated if carotid platelet embolism is suspected.

Posterior ciliary artery occlusion

The optic nerve may be damaged by occlusion of the ciliary circulation. This is separate to the retinal circulation and, if occluded, results in ischaemic optic neuropathy due to infarction of the head of the optic nerve. The symptoms are of sudden disturbance of vision and commonly there is loss of half the visual field (altitudinal visual field defect).

Giant-cell arteritis

In elderly patients the most important underlying disease to consider is giant-cell (temporal or cranial) arteritis. In this case the visual disturbance may be preceded by headache, particularly in the temporal area, and symptoms of polymyalgia rheumatica with stiffness around the shoulder girdle and pelvis. Whenever optic neuropathy is suspected, blood must be taken for erythrocyte sedimentation rate (ESR). Classically, ESR is significantly elevated, often > 80 mm/h. However, giant-cell arteritis can occur without a high ESR and if symptoms are suggestive then a temporal artery biopsy should be taken. Temporal artery biopsy should also be done in typical cases to confirm the diagnosis but treatment must start immediately. It is rare to see temporal arteritis in patients under 60 years old. The treatment of giant-cell arteritis is high-dose systemic steroids, i.e. methylprednisolone 500 mg i.v. initially followed by oral prednisolone 60 mg daily. Urgent treatment is imperative otherwise bilateral permanent visual loss will occur.

Retinal venous occlusion

Retinal venous occlusion is generally not as devastating as arterial occlusion. Visual loss is mostly confined to blurring of vision, although if the central retinal vein is involved symptoms may be more severe. Predisposing factors for retinal venous occlusion are smoking, diabetes mellitus, myeloma, hyperlipidaemia and glaucoma. Patients are usually hypertensive and as a consequence the thickened retinal arteries impinge on the retinal veins at arteriovenous crossings, impairing venous flow. Flame haemorrhages and cotton-wool spots may be seen on ophthalmoscopy, the latter indicating an ischaemic retina

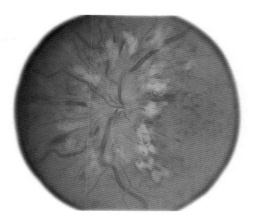

Figure 44.5 Central retinal vein occlusion responsible for acute loss of vision. There are retinal haemorrhages, a swollen disc, dilated veins and pale cotton-wool spots.

and a bad prognosis (Fig. 44.5). Retinal ischaemia induces neovascularization, which may lead to glaucoma. Fluorescein angiography further delineates the diseased retina, which can be ablated by panretinal photocoagulation to prevent neovascularization and bleeding.

Inflammatory conditions

Inflammatory conditions that provoke sudden visual loss are less common.

Optic neuritis

Optic neuritis as part of demyelination is the most common inflammatory cause of unilateral visual loss. The patients are usually young and may have other symptoms suggesting demyelinating disease. The visual loss is very variable and at least in the first attack tends to recover subjectively, although there are objective signs that the optic nerve has been damaged. These signs include failure of the afferent pupil defect to resolve and a colour vision deficit. A careful visual field test generally shows central loss. There is no good treatment for optic neuritis, although high doses of systemic steroids relieve the pain and possibly accelerate recovery. The condition may be mimicked by sarcoidosis or indeed any other inflammatory cause of optic nerve disease. Syphilis must never be forgotten and just occasionally there can be metastatic malignant infiltration of the nerve that may mimic optic neuritis.

Compression of the optic nerve

Compression of the optic nerve is rare. Haemorrhage into a pituitary tumour may compress the optic chiasm acutely leading to bilateral visual loss. This 'pituitary apoplexy' is a rare condition, where there are symptoms and signs of

hypopituitarism accompanied by bilateral visual loss. Very high doses of systemic steroids and urgent neurosurgical consultation are required. Meningioma arising from the sphenoid ridge may result in gradual unilateral visual loss due to progressive compression of the optic nerve.

Vitreous haemorrhage

Vitreous haemorrhage results from surface retinal capillaries bleeding into the vitreous cavity. These may be normal vessels that tear when the vitreous gel separates from the retinal surface. This may occur spontaneously in middle life (vitreous detachment) or as a result of severe blunt trauma. Alternatively, the bleeding occurs from abnormal vessels called new vessels that form on the retinal surface as a result of retinal ischaemia. This occurs in severe diabetic retinopathy in sickle cell disease and following extensive retinal vein occlusion. Rarely, generalized bleeding diathesis may be associated with vitreous haemorrhage. The most common cause of vitreous haemorrhage is vitreous detachment, tearing the peripheral capillaries and sometimes the retina as well. The ageing process allows vitreous jelly to move into the centre of the eye, but if the peripheral attachments are firm then structures may be pulled along with the vitreous. Premonitory symptoms of flashing lights accompanied by floaters may herald this.

This main problem with vitreous haemorrhage is identifying the cause because the view of the retina is obscured. There may be a tear in the retina with impending retinal detachment that needs urgent surgical treatment. Ultrasound is done to exclude detachment of the retina. When the haemorrhage is due to diabetic retinopathy, gradual clearing of the vitreous may occur that allows appropriate laser treatment. Surgery to remove the vitreous is necessary if the blood fails to clear or if there is an associated retinal detachment.

From the student's point of view, patients with flashing lights and floaters must be assumed to have vitreoretinal pathology until proved otherwise and an urgent consultation is sought, requiring dilatation of the pupil and examination of the peripheral retina. Ophthalmological referral is therefore mandatory.

Diabetes mellitus

Blindness is a feared complication for many diabetics. It remains the most common cause of blindness in the UK for patients between the ages of 30 and 64 years. Screening of diabetic patients to identify early sight-threatening retinopathy is of paramount importance. A hospital clinician or general practitioner has the responsibility to include a careful retinal examination in the assessment of a diabetic patient. Serious retinopathy may be present without the patient having any untoward symptoms in the early stages. Laser treatment is effective in controlling the two main categories of sight-threatening retinopathy: diabetic maculopathy and proliferative retinopathy. Unfortunately, good diabetic control does not protect an individual from developing serious retinopathy. Indeed, there is not a close relationship between control and the development of diabetic retinopathy. However, early treatment yields better results than late treatment.

Classification of retinopathy
Background retinopathy
This is characterized by the presence of microaneurysms and haemorrhages scattered over the posterior fundus, i.e. within the arcades of major vessels. There may also be scattered exudates but to fit within this classification they must not involve the macular area. Background retinopathy may progress to maculopathy or proliferative retinopathy or a combination of both.

Diabetic maculopathy
This is the most common cause of visual loss in diabetes. It is due to the accumulation of oedema fluid or lipoprotein that has leaked from abnormal capillaries. The underlying problem is abnormal permeability of the retinal capillaries. The lipoprotein collects as exudates, often in a circinate (or circular) pattern. These are easily seen with the ophthalmoscope as yellow/white collections (Fig. 44.6). Macular oedema may also occur due to leakage of fluid, producing blurring or distortion of vision.

Proliferative retinopathy
Proliferation refers to the development of abnormal blood vessels on the surface of the retina or on the optic disc.

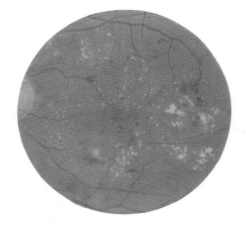

Figure 44.6 Diabetic macular changes showing pale hard exudates and blot haemorrhages.

05

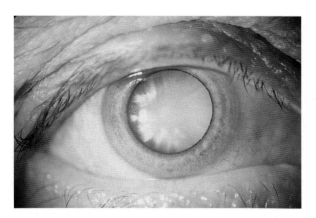

Figure 44.7 Cataract (lens opacity) causes whitening of the pupil.

This proliferation of new vessels may lead to the serious complication of vitreous haemorrhage. Neovascularization occurs in response to retinal ischaemia. The new blood vessels grow forwards from the retinal surface into the vitreous gel. These vessels are friable and bleed easily, often resulting in profound and sudden loss of vision when the vitreous gel fills with blood. Repeated bleeding produces a fibrotic process that may result in retinal detachment by bands, and blindness if treatment is neglected.

Preproliferative retinopathy

Before the development of true neovascularization, changes in the retina can be identified that indicate significant ischaemia. The changes to be noted are multiple cotton-wool spots, retinal venous dilatation, large dark haemorrhages and intraretinal vascular abnormalities. These patients require regular assessment as they are very likely to develop proliferative retinopathy.

Cataract

Opacification of the intraocular lens occurs earlier in diabetic patients; indeed a patient presenting with cataract in mid-life must be tested to exclude diabetes mellitus. The cataract may develop quite suddenly in young patients (so-called 'snow-storm' cataract) (Fig. 44.7).

Treatment

● *Photocoagulation.* The main treatment for diabetic retinopathy is photocoagulation with the argon laser. Treatment is delivered via a contact lens with local anaesthesia. Maculopathy is treated by directing the laser at the areas of leakage, allowing the exudate to absorb. Prolifer-

ative retinopathy is treated with panretinal photocoagulation. With this treatment the more peripheral retina is covered with laser burns, leaving only untreated the central retina consisting of the macula and the neuroretina extending from the macula to the optic disc. This treatment alters the perfusion of the retina and in the majority of cases results in resolution of neovascularization.

● *Vitrectomy.* Vitrectomy is necessary in advanced cases of proliferative retinopathy when there has been recurrent vitreous haemorrhage and/or detachment of the retina. The vitreous is removed by microsurgery using a vitreous cutting instrument passed into the eye immediately behind the lens.

● *Education.* As with all aspects of diabetes, the patient must be educated as to the seriousness of the complications that may develop and must attend for regular assessment, reporting any visual disturbance early.

Macula

The macula is the central critical area of retina that serves detailed acuity and colour vision. The macular receptors are exclusively cones. The paramacular area consists of a combination of cones and rods, while the remaining retina is made of rod photoreceptors. Sensitivity of the macula is increased at the fovea as the transmission layers of the retina are shelved, forming a central pit. A normal macula may be identified with the ophthalmoscope by the light reflex (foveal reflex), in which the viewing light is reflected out from the foveal pit. The macular area is free of retinal capillaries and receives its principal blood supply from the underlying choroidal vessels. Symptoms of macular disease are early reduction of central vision, which may be associated with distortion.

Macular degeneration

Degeneration of the macula with loss of central vision is common in the elderly and is the principal cause of registered blindness in the over 64-year-old age group. The degenerative process results in disruption of the normal retinal architecture, with loss of support for the photoreceptors. The process is principally an age-related degenerative process. Exposure to excessive ultraviolet light may be a risk factor in patients with presenile macular degeneration.

Classification
Atrophic degeneration

In this condition, vision gradually deteriorates over a number of years. Clumps of pigment with areas of depigmentation at the macula are seen on the retina. Visual acuity is generally in the range 6/36. Affected individuals

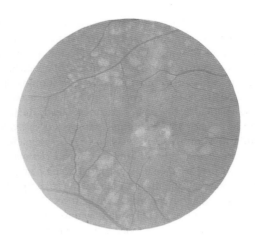

Figure 44.8 Age-related macular change with scattered pale retinal drusen.

therefore remain independent, with preservation of peripheral vision.

Haemorrhagic macular disease
This is a serious condition characterized by disruption of the retinal layer, including a break in the membrane separating the choroidal layer from the pigment epithelial layer. Blood vessels then grow through the break in this membrane and may bleed under the retinal surface, causing acute disruption and eventual destruction of cones due to scarring. The loss of vision is more abrupt, usually associated with distortion, and is generally more profound than that occurring in atrophic macular disease. Retinal examination in an established case reveals an irregular grey area of scarring covering the macula. In the acute phase there is an elevated central area with surrounding retinal haemorrhage.

Drusen (colloid bodies)
Drusen appear as collections of yellow/white round bodies in the retina. They are collections of material at the level of Bruch's membrane of the retina and are associated with macular degeneration. They are commonly seen in the macular and paramacular area of elderly patients. They may be difficult to distinguish from collections of exudate for the inexperienced ophthalmoscopist. However, exudates usually collect in a focal, sometimes circinate pattern in the retina. Drusen are spread more randomly and do not collect in circles (Fig. 44.8).

Hereditary macular disease
There are a number of rare macular degenerative conditions that result in visual deterioration in childhood or early adult life.

Drug-induced macular problems
Certain drugs specifically affect the retina, chloroquine being the principal example. This drug binds to the retinal pigment epithelium, resulting in disturbance of macular function.

Treatment

No effective treatment is known for atrophic macular degeneration. In a small number of cases of haemorrhagic macular degeneration, laser photocoagulation directed at the abnormal collections of blood vessels may be effective in preventing progression of the condition. Magnifying and telescopic low-vision aids are very valuable for maximizing the limited vision for patients with macular degeneration. Good lighting conditions are important when using these aids.

Chronic glaucoma

Chronic open-angle glaucoma is a condition that affects the optic nerve. It is much more common than acute-angle closure glaucoma and affects up to 1% of the population over the age of 40 years. The condition is familial but does not follow a definite Mendelian pattern. In the usual form, intraocular pressure is elevated above normal, often greater than 30 mmHg (normal eye pressure 10–21 mmHg). The chronic elevation of pressure over a period of many months or years results in ischaemic damage to the optic nerve, resulting in progressive atrophy and loss of function. Screening for the condition (measurement of intraocular pressure by an optometrist) is of great importance because the condition does not generally cause any symptoms until significant optic nerve damage has occurred. Glaucoma results in gradual paracentral visual field loss and affected individuals do not generally become aware of the condition until it is quite advanced. When the condition is advanced, the optic nerve has a characteristic appearance of pallor with 'cupping'. Normal-tension glaucoma is less common but results in similar visual field loss. Intraocular pressure is within the normal range and optic nerve damage is due to localized optic nerve head ischaemia.

Treatment for chronic glaucoma is generally to reduce intraocular pressure. This can be achieved by reducing aqueous production and/or increasing outflow of aqueous from the eye. This can be achieved with β-blocker eye drops, which reduce aqueous production, and prostaglandin analogues, which increase outflow. Surgery in the form of trabeculectomy is a good method of permanently reducing pressure in glaucoma. However, like all operations there are risks involved. A small flat of sclera is created and a fistula made by removing a block of tissue of

05

the trabecular meshwork. Fluid then drains through the opening under the conjunctival lining to create a bleb under the upper eyelid. Antimetabolites (e.g. 5-fluorouracil) are often used to prevent scar tissue forming that may obstruct the fistula.

Cataract

Cataract is opacification or loss of clarity of the crystalline lens of the eye. The human lens becomes progressively larger with increasing age and also becomes coloured, initially yellow and eventually dark brown (brunescent). Nuclear cataract affecting the central part of the lens often results in the eye becoming progressively myopic, allowing older individuals to read easily without reading spectacles. However, change in the cortical part of the cataract results in significant disturbance of clarity due to local areas of opacity within the lens structure. Cataract is part of ageing, although presenile cataract is seen in a number of medical conditions, particularly diabetes. Myotonic dystrophy is another example. Galactosaemia results in infantile cataract. Cataract that is inherited usually runs in families as a dominant condition. Chronic steroid medication, e.g. in the long-term treatment of asthma, may result in cataract formation. Blunt eye trauma may result in early or late development of cataract. Early cataract is best detected with the ophthalmoscope by setting the focusing down to +10 and viewing the red reflex. The cataract appears as black spokes or opacity against the reflex.

Treatment for cataract is surgical and the operation is usually undertaken nowadays under local anaesthesia. A combination of bupivacaine and lidocaine are injected around the eye to anaesthetize and also to block the movement of extraocular muscle. However, simple topical anaesthesia in the form of eye drops can also be used for suitable patients who can hold their eye steady during the procedure. The usual technique employed is called phacoemulsification. A small incision (3 mm) is made into clear cornea and a rim of anterior capsule removed. An ultrasonic probe is then inserted into the lens. This has the result of fragmenting the hard central nucleus, allowing it to be aspirated by a vacuum system connected to the same probe. The ultrasonic energy and vacuum are controlled by the surgeon via a foot pedal, rather like the accelerator pedal of a car. With the lens material removed, a 'capsular bag' remains in which the prosthetic intraocular lens is inserted. Intraocular lenses are designed to be folded prior to insertion, allowing them to be inserted through the same small corneal opening. The lens then unfolds within the eye, reverting to its normal diameter (usually 6 mm). The materials used include acrylic, silicone and polymethylmethacrylate. The intraocular lens is held in place by flexible arms called 'haptics', which open up into the sulcus of the capsular bag. Intraocular lenses are graded according to dioptre. The correct dioptric power for an individual eye is assessed preoperatively by ultrasonic examination to determine the length of the eye and by examination of the cornea to establish its curvature and hence its refractive power.

Visual loss at a glance

Definitions

Blindness: inability to see or the lack of the power of sight

Amaurosis fugax: a fleeting or temporary loss of sight usually caused by transient retinal ischaemia

Drusen: hyaline deposits found on the fundus as a result of degenerative changes

Normal intraocular pressure: 10–21 mmHg

Sudden loss of vision
Bilateral visual loss
- Cerebrovascular accident affecting the visual cortex: pupil reactions remain normal
- Ingestion of toxic agents, e.g. methyl alcohol
- Simultaneous unilateral visual loss:
  (a) Acute bilateral optic neuritis
  (b) Giant-cell arteritis

Unilateral visual loss
Arterial occlusion
- Retinal artery: amaurosis fugax or complete visual loss from carotid or cardiac embolus
- Posterior ciliary artery: ischaemic optic neuropathy
- Giant-cell arteritis: inflammation of temporal artery associated with optic neuropathy

Venous occlusion
- Retinal vein: blurring of vision due to retinal arteries impinging on retinal veins at arteriovenous crossings, impairing venous flow

Inflammatory conditions
- Optic neuritis: demyelinating disease. (Optic neuritis may be mimicked by sarcoidosis, syphilis, metastatic malignant infiltration)
- Optic nerve compression:

(a) Haemorrhage into a pituitary tumour
(b) Meningioma arising from the sphenoid ridge

Vitreous haemorrhage
- Spontaneous (vitreous detachment)
- Severe blunt trauma
- Neovascularization as a result of retinal ischaemia:
    (a) Diabetic retinopathy
    (b) Sickle cell disease
    (c) Following extensive retinal vein occlusion.
- Generalized bleeding diathesis

Gradual loss of vision
Diabetes mellitus
Classification of diabetic retinopathy
- Background retinopathy: microaneurysms and haemorrhages scattered over the posterior fundus
- Diabetic maculopathy:
    (a) Most common cause of visual loss in diabetes
    (b) Accumulation of oedema fluid or lipoprotein
    (c) Abnormal permeability of the retinal capillaries
- Proliferative retinopathy: development of abnormal blood vessels on the surface of the retina/optic disc, response to retinal ischaemia
- Preproliferative retinopathy: changes indicating significant ischaemia (cotton-wool spots, retinal venous dilatation, large dark haemorrhages, intraretinal vascular abnormalities)
- Cataract: opacification of the intraocular lens

Treatment of diabetic retinopathy
- Photocoagulation: argon laser for maculopathy and proliferative retinopathy
- Vitrectomy: advanced proliferative retinopathy, recurrent vitreous haemorrhage, detachment of the retina
- Education: patient must know the complications, attend for regular assessment, report any visual disturbance early

Macula
Macular degeneration
- Atrophic degeneration: vision gradually deteriorates over a number of years, no effective treatment

- Haemorrhagic macular disease: abrupt loss of vision with distortion
- Drusen (colloid bodies): collections of hyaline material at the level of Bruch's membrane of the retina associated with macular degeneration
- Hereditary macular disease: visual deterioration in childhood or early adult life
- Drug-induced macular problems: chloroquine binds to retinal pigment epithelium causing disturbance of macular function

Chronic glaucoma
- Affects the optic nerve
- Affects ~ 1% of the population > 40 years
- Familial but not definite Mendelian pattern
- Intraocular pressure > 30 mmHg
- Ischaemic damage to optic nerve
- Progressive atrophy and loss of function
- No symptoms until significant optic nerve damage has occurred

Treatment
- Reduce intraocular pressure
- Reduce aqueous production: β-blocker eye drops
- Increase outflow of aqueous from the eye: prostaglandin analogues
- Surgery: trabeculectomy

Cataract
- Opacification or loss of clarity of the crystalline lens of the eye
- Cataract is part of ageing
- Presenile cataract:
    (a) Diabetes
    (b) Myotonic dystrophy
    (c) Galactosaemia
    (d) Familial
    (e) Chronic steroid medication
    (f) Blunt eye trauma

Treatment
- Surgical removal of the cataract (phacoemulsification) and insertion of prosthetic lens

05

Squint (strabismus)

Squint or strabismus is the term applied to misalignment of the visual axis of the eyes. The visual system is arranged to achieve binocular single vision. Both eyes must therefore be aligned to allow an object of view to project onto the fovea of both eyes simultaneously. The convergence reflex provides the mechanism for continued binocular vision when the object of view becomes progressively

closer to the eye. The visual cortex has cells that receive an input from each eye (binocular cells). During infancy and early childhood the visual system continues to develop and the normal adult state of binocular single vision is achieved only if the eyes are aligned and if each eye is projecting a focused image to the cortex. Amblyopia or lazy eye develops when this system fails. The child's visual system is 'plastic' up to the age of approximately 8 years and therefore lazy eye may be reversible up to this age.

However, the results of treatment are much better the earlier the defect is corrected.

Types of squint

Concomitant squint

The angle of misalignment does not alter in different positions of gaze. This is the classical squint of childhood. An infant may be born with squint or develop it within a few months of life. The cause is not known but there is often a family history of a similar condition in siblings or the parents. When examining the infant, full abduction of the squinting eye must be demonstrated to exclude a lateral rectus palsy.

The infant's visual system has the capacity to suppress the image from the squinting eye to prevent double vision. Treatment of the condition is initially to induce free alternation of the squint by patching the non-squinting eye. This will prevent the squinting eye from becoming amblyopic (lazy). Uncorrected, the child will have permanently reduced vision in the affected eye. Corrective surgery is generally performed at the age of 18 months.

Paralytic or inconcomitant squint

The deviation alters in different gaze positions, e.g. sixth nerve palsy, as there is weakness of particular eye muscles.

Accommodation and convergent squint

Children who have a high degree of hypermetropia (longsightedness) may develop convergent squint due to the increased accommodative effort required to see clearly. There is an accommodation convergence reflex that normally results in convergence when viewing close objects. A child with a high degree of hypermetropia has to employ a significant amount of accommodation even to see in the near distance.

Correction of the hypermetropia with spectacles will in many cases correct the squint. Surgery for many of these children is therefore unnecessary. This type of squint generally develops at the age of 3 or 4 years.

Divergent squint

Divergent squint may be present at birth but this is uncommon. Divergence is usually intermittent and occurs in childhood. It tends to become gradually less intermittent and more permanent. Corrective surgery is then necessary.

Retinal disease causing squint

Poor central vision in a child will result in a squint. It is therefore very important to exclude a retinal condition as the cause. Retinoblastoma, a rare tumour of childhood, is an example where the child may present initially with a squint and possibly whitening of the pupil. All children who are squinting or suspected of squinting should be referred for assessment by an ophthalmologist.

Pseudosquint

Many infants have a broad bridge to the nose with a large epicanthus. This results in the appearance of a convergent squint. The corneal reflections are seen to be symmetrical on the cornea of each eye, thus excluding a true squint. With normal growth of the face the appearance of pseudosquint due to epicanthus gradually disappears.

Strabismus (squint) at a glance

Definitions

Squint (strabismus): misalignment of the visual axis of the eyes

Amblyopia (lazy eye): visual defect resulting from failure to form sharp central images in early life

Binocular single vision
Depends on:
● Correct eye alignment to allow an image to project onto the fovea of both eyes simultaneously
● Convergence reflex
● Amblyopia (lazy eye) develops when this system fails. The child's visual system is 'plastic' up to the age of ~ 8 years and therefore lazy eye may be reversible up to this age. Results of treatment are much better the earlier the defect is corrected

Types of squint
Concomitant squint
● Angle of misalignment does not alter in different positions of gaze
● Classical squint of childhood
● Treatment: patching the non-squinting eye, corrective surgery at 18 months

Paralytic or inconcomitant squint
● Angle of misalignment alters in different positions of gaze, e.g. sixth nerve palsy

Accommodation and convergent squint
- Children who have hypermetropia (long-sightedness)
- Significant amount of accommodation required to see in the near distance
- Age of 3 or 4 years
- Treatment: correct hypermetropia with spectacles

Divergent squint
- Intermittent in childhood
- Treatment: corrective surgery

Retinal disease causing squint
- Poor central vision in a child, e.g. retinoblastoma

Pseudosquint
- Broad bridge to the nose with a large epicanthus
- Gives appearance of a convergent squint
- Disappears with time

Diseases of the eyelid

Blepharitis

Eyelid inflammation is a common condition. The underlying problem is abnormal secretion from the meibomian glands of the lid. This results in secondary bacterial infection with commensal staphylococci (*Staphylococcus epidermidis*). There may be an associated skin condition of rosacea. Blepharitis results in conjunctivitis with ocular irritation and redness. Treatment consists of regular cleansing of the lid margins and the use of appropriate topical or oral antibiotics.

Stye

This is a common condition and is simply an infection of the lash follicles. A stye generally resolves without specific antibiotic treatment. However, recurrent styes in childhood may require topical or oral antibiotics.

Meibomian cyst (chalazion)

This is a retention cyst of a meibomian gland due to obstruction of the outlet duct in the lid margin. The cyst may rupture into the lid tissue, causing an acute reaction and the development of a foreign-body granuloma. Meibomian cysts are removed by incision through the conjunctiva, but only if they persist.

Ectropion and entropion

Ectropion is an out-turning of the eyelid, generally the lower lid. This usually occurs in the elderly due to the loss of normal muscle tone of the lid. It results in watering of the eye and discomfort due to drying of the exposed conjunctiva. Ectropion may also result from scarring of the eyelid skin following trauma.

Entropion is an inturning of the lid, again generally of the lower eyelid. This also occurs as a senile change due to loss of muscle tone. Irritation occurs due to the eyelashes turning in and abrading the cornea (trichiasis). Senile entropion and ectropion are corrected surgically, generally with local anaesthesia.

Eyelid malignancy

Basal cell carcinoma (rodent ulcer) is the most common malignant eyelid tumour. It is more common in fair-skinned individuals who have had excessive exposure to sunlight. The typical appearances are of a pearl-like appearance with rolled edges. Treatment is by wide excision or by radiotherapy. *Squamous cell carcinoma* is rare but a serious condition as it may metastasize.

Ptosis

The position of the eyelid is controlled principally by the levator muscle. This is composed mainly of striated muscles supplied by the third nerve but also has a smooth muscle portion (Müller's) supplied by the sympathetic nerve supply. The eyelid position is also influenced by the action of the frontalis muscles.
- *Third-nerve palsy* results in ptosis but there may also be interruption of the supply to the extraocular muscles, resulting in outward and downward deviation of the eye, sometimes with dilated pupil.
- *Horner's syndrome* occurs when there is disruption of the sympathetic nerve supply. This results in a small degree of ptosis, generally 2 mm, and also pupillary miosis. Miosis is due to unopposed action of the parasympathetic supply to the sphincter pupillae muscle. Horner's syndrome is caused by damage to the sympathetic pathway. Surgical injury and malignant injury from lymph nodes or an apical lung tumour are common causes.

Thyroid eye disease

Upper eyelid retraction occurs due to abnormal stimulation of the smooth muscle part of the levator due to circulating sympathomimetic agents (see also exophthalmus in Chapter 34).

05

Diseases of the eyelid at a glance

Definitions

Blepharitis: abnormal secretion from the meibomian glands of the lid with secondary bacterial infection

Stye: infection of the lash follicles

Meibomian cyst (chalazion): retention cyst of a meibomian gland due to obstruction of the outlet duct in the lid margin

Ectropion: out-turning of the eyelid, generally the lower lid

Entropion: inturning of the eyelid, generally the lower lid

Ptosis: drooping of the upper eyelid

Eyelid malignancy
- Basal cell carcinoma (rodent ulcer) is the most common malignant eyelid tumour

- Squamous cell carcinoma is rare but serious condition as it may metastasize

Ptosis
- Third nerve palsy
- Horner's syndrome (ptosis, miosis, enophthalmos, hemianhidrosis)

Thyroid eye disease
- Exophthalmos: protrusion of the eyeball
- Upper eyelid lag: failure of the normal downward following movement of the upper lids on looking down
- Upper eyelid retraction: upper eyelid is retracted, exposing the sclera above the pupil. Due to abnormal stimulation of the smooth muscle part of the levator

Principles of Transplantation

45

Must know Must do

Must know
Types of organ grafts
Pathology and immunology of organ graft rejection
Core knowledge of immunosuppressive therapies used
in transplantation of organs
Organ donation

Must do
See patients before renal transplantation and follow
their progress, attending the operation and
observing their recovery
Make an attempt to contact at least one patient 1
month after discharge from hospital to find out the
improvement in the quality of life of the patient

Introduction

The field of clinical transplantation is one of the youngest surgical subspecialties, developing entirely during the 20th century. It was in 1902 that the first experimental transplants were performed. These were done by Emerich Ullmann using kidneys in a canine model. In 1951, human kidney transplants were started in Paris, Boston and Chicago. A decade later, the 1960s saw massive progression in the development of transplantation of extrarenal organs. Thomas Starzl, then at the University of Colorado, started performing human liver transplants in 1963. However, after a series of five failures, further attempts were ceased until 1967, when the programme was reinitiated. Liver transplants were also beginning in the UK at that time with the efforts of Sir Roy Calne in Cambridge. The first pancreas transplant was performed in 1966 at the University of Minnesota. In 1967, Christiaan Barnard performed the first cardiac transplant in Cape Town, South Africa.

The technical surgical aspects of transplantation can be quite demanding, and they continue to be developed and refined today. However, the surgery of transplantation was not, and never has been, the limitation to maximizing clinical success in this field. Therefore, it should be recognized that the most substantial contribution to the development of transplantation was made in 1943 by Sir Peter Brian Medawar when he documented that rejection of transplanted organs is an immunological phenomenon. This discovery initiated the cascade of research that continues today as scientists and doctors around the world attempt to manipulate the immune system to a degree that will allow recipients to accept a foreign organ while minimizing total immunosuppression and drug toxicity. Research in transplantation and immunology has accounted for 23 Nobel prizes in the past century.

Terminology

The type of graft used for transplantation can be described as an autograft, allograft or xenograft. An *autograft* is transplanted into the same organism, while an *allograft* is an organ transplanted into a different organism of the same species. An organ transplanted across species is termed a *xenograft.*

The placement of the graft is described as orthotopic or heterotopic. *Orthotopic tranplantation* describes a graft that is placed in its normal anatomical position, as for clinical liver or heart transplants. In these instances, the native (diseased) organ is removed and replaced with an allograft. *Heterotopic transplantation* describes surgical placement of the graft in a non-anatomic location. This is the type performed in clinical renal transplants where the allograft is placed in the iliac fossa, inferior to the native kidneys, which are left in place.

Immunology

The compatibility between a donor organ and the immune system of the recipient remains the most important barrier to the field of transplant science. The cellular recognition of self by immunological components of the recipient allows for the assault on tissues that possess foreign antigens.

This process of recognition of cells as either self or *foreign* starts with cell-surface antigens, such as the ABO

05

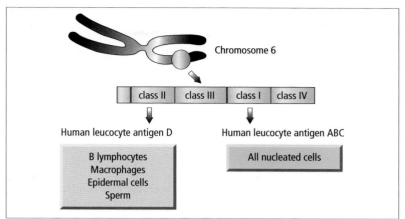

Figure 45.1 Components of the major histocompatibility complex.

blood antigen system. In humans, A and B antigens protrude from erythrocyte membranes. Simplistically stated, patients who do not express either the A or B antigen on erythrocyte surfaces possess antibodies specific to the non-expressed antigen (haemagglutinins) and are therefore unable to tolerate tissues that do express that antigen.

More specific antigen recognition exists in the major histocompatibility complex (MHC) antigens (Fig. 45.1). As these were first discovered on leukocytes, they were termed human leukocyte antigens (HLA). These transmembrane glycoproteins are divided into two major classes, class I and class II. Class I antigens, labelled A, B and C, are expressed on the surface of all nucleated cells and platelets. This class of molecules is recognized by CD8$^+$ cytotoxic T cells, initiating lysis of the target cells. Class II antigens are found on specific immunologically active cells such as macrophages, monocytes, B lymphocytes, dendritic cells, Kupffer cells and activated T cells. They are labelled 'D-related' (Dr) antigens and are thought to be the most important for cross-matching purposes because of their vital role in immune attacks. This class is recognized by CD4$^+$ T helper cells, which leads to T-cell activation and the mounting of a full immune response. Both CD4 and CD8 complexes on T cells are associated with CD3.

Rejection

Allograft damage as a product of attack by the recipient immune system is termed rejection. The three general types, differentiated by both timing and mechanism, are hyperacute, acute and chronic rejection.

Hyperacute rejection occurs immediately upon reperfusion because preformed antibodies exist in the serum of the recipient against antigens expressed on the donor organ. This is usually due to ABO incompatibility, and results in an immediate and massive inflammatory

response against the vascular endothelium of the donor organ. Hyperacute rejection is not reversible and should be treated by graft removal.

Acute rejection is a cell-mediated response whereby antigen-presenting cells recognize the donor organ as foreign and present those antigens to T cells. This results in T-cell activation and immune attacks against the organ. The purpose of immunosuppressive regimens is to avoid this normal physiological response and, even after acute rejection begins, it can be treated medically by increasing the dose of immunosuppression and/or the use of additional agents.

Chronic rejection occurs over the course of months to years. It is the product of antibody response, cell-mediated response or a combination thereof. This type of rejection is characterized by vascular obliteration with replacement by fibrotic tissue and is not reversed with immunosuppressives.

Immunosuppression

The immune system of the recipient needs to be pharmacologically manipulated for the remainder of the recipient's life to prevent the immune system from recognizing the graft as foreign and mounting a destructive attack. There are many different regimens used but listed below are some of the most common immunosuppressive agents currently used clinically.

Corticosteroids

These drugs block membrane phospholipase, preventing the production of arachidonic acid, which is the substrate for the creation of prostaglandins, kinins, leukotrienes and thromboxanes. This is not a specific mechanism of immunosuppression but this class of medication is currently part of most immunosuppressive regimens.

Metabolic inhibitors

These cytotoxic agents are antiproliferative, preventing efficient mitosis, a process upon which the immune response is highly dependent.

Azathioprine is metabolized by the liver to become 6-mercaptopurine, which is a purine analogue and thus a competitive inhibitor of DNA and RNA synthesis. In addition to being hepatotoxic and nephrotoxic, all cell lines are affected by azathioprine, leading to anaemia, leukopenia and thrombocytopenia.

Mycophenolate mofetil, a new agent, selectively inhibits proliferation of leukocytes. It has been shown to effectively reduce rejection rates and is not associated with the toxicities of azathioprine; its adverse effects are mainly gastrointestinal.

Calcineurin inhibitors

This very important class of immunosuppressive agents inhibit the production of interleukin-2 (IL-2). IL-2 is a key messenger that is released by T cells after recognition of an antigen and the complete cell-mediated immune response occurs subsequent to its release. Calcineurin is a serine phosphatase enzyme activated by the secondary messenger calcium, which leads to cytokine gene transcription.

Cyclosporin and tacrolimus (FK 506) are the two main calcineurin inhibitors. Cyclosporin, an 11 amino acid peptide, has the adverse effects of hyperglycaemia, hypertension, hyperuricaemia, hyperkalaemia, hypertrichosis, tremors and gingival hyperplasia. However, the most significant disadvantage of cyclosporin is nephrotoxicity, which can be confused with acute rejection.

Tacrolimus, a macrolide antibiotic, is also nephrotoxic but is more neurotoxic and diabetogenic than cyclosporin. Most immunosuppressive regimens utilize a calcineurin inhibitor.

Sirolimus (rapamycin) is structurally very similar to tacrolimus, even binding the same cytoplasmic proteins, but mechanistically distinct. Sirolimus is not calcineurin dependent in its action. It causes substantial dyslipidaemia but is not as nephrotoxic or diabetogenic as cyclosporin.

Polyclonal antibodies

This class of drugs is composed of a heterogeneous population of antibodies directed against multiple sites on the surface of T cells, leading to depletion of circulating T cells by complement-mediated lysis and reticuloendothelial trapping.

Antithymocyte globulin (ATG) is the most commonly used polyclonal antibody. Fever and chills typically occur with infusion, necessitating pretreatment with antihistamines and steroids. Other adverse effects include leukopenia, thrombocytopenia, serum sickness, skin rashes and phlebitis. There is batch-to-batch variation in potency so it is prudent to track biological activity by measuring peripheral blood lymphocyte counts. Directed antibody medications, both monoclonal and polyclonal, are used for the treatment of acute rejection. Antibody medications are effective in this task because they transiently destroy leukocyte colonies.

Monoclonal antibodies

As the name implies, these drugs are a homogeneous mixture of antibodies directed against a single target. OKT3, a commonly used monoclonal antibody, binds the CD3 receptor, which is present on all leukocytes. The adverse effect of infusion is massive release of inflammatory cytokines, resulting in nausea, vomiting, diarrhoea, fever, chills, myalgia and, in severe cases, bronchospasm and hypotension. Pretreatment with antihistamines, steroids and non-steroidal anti-inflammatory medications (indomethacin) is important. Monitoring of $CD3^+$ lymphocytes during treatment is recommended.

Other monoclonal antibodies include basiliximab and daclizumab. Both agents bind the α-chain of IL-2, causing selective inhibition of this important cytokine.

Immunosuppressive considerations

While patients receiving organ transplants are freed from terminal disease, the commitment to lifelong immunosuppression is in itself a burden. These patients will be at increased risk of infection of all types, including those opportunistic infections not otherwise seen. Whenever a transplant patient presents with even a mild fever, infection must be excluded with consideration to viral, bacterial, fungal and parasitic aetiologies.

These patients also have a clearly increased risk of developing skin cancer, leukaemia, lymphoma and solid tumours associated with viral infections (e.g. Kaposi's sarcoma, cervical carcinoma and nasopharyngeal carcinoma).

Organ donation

Definition of death

In order for an organ to be retrieved for the purpose of transplantation, the donor must be legally defined as dead. The Uniform Determination of Death Act states that a patient is dead when there is *irreversible* cessation of either cardiopulmonary activity or entire brain function. Entire brain function death is defined by specific legislation in most countries with transplant programmes. In the UK, declaration of brain death, which legally equals actual

05

complete physiological death, depends on complete apnoea and the absence of brainstem reflexes.

Apnoea is determined when, on withdrawal of all sedation and with no delivered mechanical ventilation, the patient fails to initiate a breath until $Paco_2$ reaches 6.55 kPa (50 mmHg), which is proven by arterial blood gas analysis.

Absence of brainstem reflexes requires a ventilated comatosed patient with no known reversible causes present who displays the following:
- no pupillary response to light;
- no corneal reflex;
- no vestibulo-ocular reflex;
- no motor response within the cranial nerve distribution (i.e. grimace to somatosensory stimuli);
- no gag reflex to bronchial stimulation.

With family consent, patients who have irreversible brainstem death as defined above can be considered candidates for donation, and they provide excellent quality organs because the heart continues to beat and thus keeps the organs viable. The other definition of death, i.e. complete and irreversible loss of cardiorespiratory activity, provides donors known as non-heart-beating donors. However, cardiac death subjects the organs to harmful warm ischaemia. These organs are being used by some programmes and are a topic of current debate in the field of transplantation.

Living donation

Organs may be retrieved from living patients as well, particularly kidneys where a patient can donate one without substantial physiological compromise. Currently many centres are also beginning living donor programmes for livers, which is technically demanding surgery involving full hepatic lobectomy of the donor. This surgery itself poses substantially more risk to the healthy donor than living donation for kidneys. Living donation offers considerable advantages over cadaveric donation.
- *Donor quality.* The profound and widespread effects of brain death on the entire physiology of the donor are well documented. These patients are in the intensive care unit (ICU) on a multitude of medications, with sometimes severe metabolic disturbances. The age, backround diseases and periods of hypotension are often suboptimal in cadaveric donors. However, living donors are usually in excellent health.
- *Timing.* The operation can be planned on an elective basis and thus the patient can be optimally medically managed prior to the surgery. This is particularly advantageous in liver transplantation, where the recipients who receive cadaveric organs are very ill, in some cases within hours of dying, and the sicker the patient, the worse the outcome after transplant.
- *Ischaemic time.* The operations for donor and recipient are performed simultaneously in the same hospital, limiting the ischaemic time to a minimum.
- *Tissue compatibility.* The living donor is usually an immediate family member of the donor and thus shares a large amount of genetic and antigenic expression.

These advantages have translated clinically into superior graft survival rates, superior patient survival rates, fewer rejection episodes, fewer infectious episodes and shorter hospital stays.

Organ retrieval

The retrieval of visceral organs is performed by complete dissection of the respective organs until only the vascular attachments remain. Then the organs are flushed with cold preservation solution until the procedure is completed. If the heart is retrieved simultaneously, then the abdominal retrieval teams wait until the cardiac surgeon is ready to cross-clamp the major vessels of the heart before flushing. This method of retrieval minimizes the ischaemic period before the temperature of the organ is decreased to slow metabolism and minimize ischaemic damage.

After being flushed and filled with preservation solution, the organs are placed in sterile bags, free of air, and placed in an icebox. The length of effective preservation allowable is organ dependent. The following organs are listed in decreasing order of preservation time: kidney, pancreas, liver, heart and lung.

Living donor operations for kidneys are beginning to be performed laparoscopically at many centres.

05

General transplantation at a glance

Definitions

Graft: any tissue or organ that is totally detached from the body and implanted in another site of the same body (*autograft*) or into another body of the same species (*allograft*) or a different species (*xenograft*)

Donor: the person from whom the graft is taken

Recipient (host): the person receiving a graft

Orthotopic transplantation: graft is placed in its normal anatomical position

Heterotopic transplantation: graft is placed in a non-anatomic location

Host vs. graft reaction (rejection): when the host's immune system attacks and destroys the allograft or xenograft

Graft vs. host reaction: when immunologically competent transplanted cells attack the host

Immunosuppression: any process that acts on any part of the immune system to interfere with the normal reaction to the presence of an antigen

Antigen: any substance, organism or foreign material recognized by the immune system as 'non-self' that provokes the production of an antibody

Antibody: a protein (immunoglobulin) produced by B lymphocytes in response to the presence of an antigen

Immunology

- Recognition of cells as either *self* or *foreign* starts with cell-surface antigens, e.g. ABO blood group antigens
- Specific antigen recognition exists in the MHC antigens:
  (a) Class I antigens (HLA-A, HLA-B and HLA-C) are expressed on the surface of all nucleated cells and platelets and are recognized by recipient CD8+ cytotoxic T cells, initiating lysis of the transplanted cells
  (b) Class II antigens (Dr antigens) are found on specific immunologically active cells and are recognized by recipient CD4+ T-helper cells, leading to T-cell activation and a full immune response
- Minor histocompatibility complex consists of a series of genes scattered across the chromosomes that generate proteins that can initiate an allograft reaction
- Implantation of foreign proteins elicits both cellular and humoral (antibody) responses

Rejection

Type of rejection	Timing	Cause	Outcome
Hyperacute	Minutes to hours	Humoral	Graft destruction
Acute	First month	Cell mediated	Prevented with immunosuppression
Chronic	Months to years	Humoral and cellular	Vascular obliteration and fibrosis

Immunosuppression
Patients receiving organ transplants:
- are committed to lifelong immunosuppression
- are at increased risk and must maintain vigilance of infection
- are at increased risk of developing malignancies

Immunosuppressive agents

Drug	Action	Adverse effects
Corticosteroids	Block membrane phospholipase, inhibit inflammatory mediators	Cushing's syndrome
Metabolic inhibitors: azathioprine, mycophenolate mofetil	Antiproliferative cytotoxic agents: prevent efficient mitosis, inhibit complete cell-mediated immune response	Hepatic, renal, haematological, gastrointestinal
Calcineurin inhibitors: cyclosporin, tacrolimus (FK506), sirolimus (rapamycin)	T-cell suppression, block release of IL-2	Nephrotoxicity (cyclosporin and tacrolimus), dyslipidaemia (sirolimus)
Polyclonal antibodies: ATG	Heterogeneous population of antibodies to T cells	Fever and chills, leukopenia, thrombocytopenia
Monoclonal antibodies: OKT3, basiliximab, daclizumab	Homogeneous mixture of antibodies directed against a single target	Nausea, vomiting, diarrhoea, fever, chills, myalgia, bronchospasm, hypotension

Organ donation
- Living: better grafts but major surgery for donor
- Cadaveric: patients declared dead can be considered candidates for donation upon family consent
- Definition of death: irreversible cessation of either cardiopulmonary activity or entire brain function
- Diagnosis of death: complete apnoea and the absence of brainstem reflexes

05

Renal transplantation

Indications

The goal of renal transplantation is to cure patients with end-stage renal disease (ESRD) and allow them to live free from dialysis. Most diseases resulting in isolated ESRD are amenable to transplantation as long as the other organ systems are intact. The diseases that leave a patient with dysfunctional kidneys and place them on the transplant waiting list include diabetes mellitus, chronic hypertension, glomerulopathies, cystic renal disease, interstitial renal disease, obstructive uropathy, congenital disorders, metabolic diseases (amyloidosis, oxalosis, etc.), trauma, haemolytic–uraemic syndrome and even malignancy (Wilms' tumour, renal cell carcinoma).

The standard contraindications to transplantation that apply to all organs are active infection, malignancy and unstable disease in another organ system. In particular, renal transplant candidates must be assessed for vascular disease since the most common reason for ESRD requiring transplant is diabetes, which is a major risk factor for arteriosclerosis. Most units require a coronary angiogram on prospective patients, with treatment of any significant disease prior to transplant. In fact, even after transplantation, 55% of deaths in this population are secondary to coronary artery disease. While old age is a consideration, there is no absolute age limit to transplantation; it is the physiological status of the patient that determines their candidacy.

Operative procedure

The kidney retrieved from a cadaveric donor generally comes with a generous amount of renal artery and vein, usually including a cuff of aorta and vena cava, respectively. The implantation is performed in the heterotopic position of the iliac fossa. The cuff of aorta and vena cava allow renal artery and vein to be sewn into the external iliac vessels using end-to-side anastomosis (Fig. 45.2). When the kidney is retrieved from a living donor, an end-to-end anastomosis with the internal iliac artery is preferred. Some surgeons prefer to use the internal iliac artery for cadaveric donors as well, although this requires more technical expertise. The ureter is attached to the recipient bladder using a submucosal tunnel to prevent reflux.

Complications

Early

In addition to hyperacute rejection, there are several complications of concern that may occur soon after transplantation.

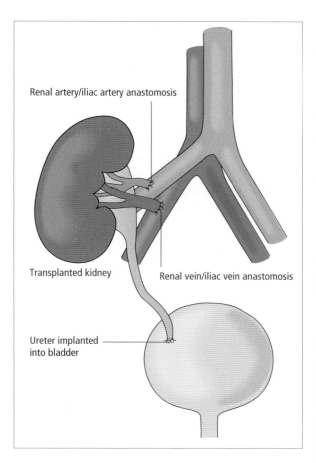

Renal artery/iliac artery anastomosis

Transplanted kidney

Renal vein/iliac vein anastomosis

Ureter implanted into bladder

Figure 45.2 Renal transplantation. The donor kidney is transplanted into an extraperitoneal site in the pelvis. The patient's own kidney is left *in situ*. The donor renal vessels are anastomosed to the recipient's iliac vessels and the ureter is implanted into the bladder.

Renal artery or vein thrombosis, which occurs relatively infrequently, represents a surgical emergency and requires a high index of suspicion. It presents with sudden drop in urine output and can usually be confirmed by renal Doppler ultrasound, although the diagnosis is often too late for intervention, necessitating graft removal to prevent systemic illness.

Urine leak occurs early as a technical complication. The presentation includes decreased urine output, local pain and increased creatinine (peritoneal absorption). Ultrasound shows fluid around the kidney and radionuclide scan shows extravasation. Treatment involves repairing the anastomosis.

A further complication is lymphocele. These can cause compression resulting in decreased urine output, local pain and mass effect. Particularly suggestive of this

05

diagnosis is unilateral leg swelling and should raise suspicion. Ultrasound confirms its presence. Aspiration is worth attempting but usually fails so it is best treated by surgically opening fenestrations to allow communication with the peritoneal cavity, which can easily be done laparoscopically.

Late

Again, acute and chronic rejection are always threats to the transplant patient who makes it through the early period after transplantation.

Renal artery stenosis is a complication presenting later in the course. It may be suggested by marked sensitivity to cyclosporin or tacrolimus, with spiking creatinine levels when these drugs are used. Renal artery stenosis can be managed by balloon dilatation or surgical reconstruction.

Graft toxicity from the immunosuppressive regimens used can also be a source of late graft failure. All transplant procedures are associated with risks of infection, bleeding, wound complications and other standard surgical complications. Infectious complications are more common in transplant patients and they must be taken more seriously as these patients will be immunosuppressed after surgery.

Outcomes

Renal transplantation has seen a steady rise in graft success over the past decade. Patients at most centres can expect a 1-year graft survival rate approaching 90%. Even at 5 years, about two-thirds of patients can expect to have functioning grafts. The increased use of living related donors will continue to bolster the number of successful outcomes, and hopefully improvements in preservation and the utilization of non-heart-beating donors will allow more patients to live free of dialysis.

Liver transplantation

Indications

The most common reason for liver transplant is end-stage disease from cirrhosis. Alcohol abuse and viral hepatitis (B and C) are the most common aetiologies of cirrhosis. Those with a history of alcohol abuse have to display long-term abstinence (at least 6 months) in order to be listed and any evidence of recidivism results in their removal from the waiting list. Other reasons for transplantation include acute fulminant disease, primary biliary cirrhosis, primary sclerosing cholangitis, biliary atresia, metabolic disorders, Budd–Chiari syndrome and primary liver tumours.

Operative procedure

The operation can be divided into three phases. The first is hepatectomy of the diseased liver in the recipient. Because of the massive portal congestion and large collateral vessels that have developed secondary to cirrhosis, this portion of the operation can be associated with large volumes of blood loss. The second phase is the anhepatic phase, which can be handled in several ways. Originally, survival of the recipient through this phase depended on the use of venovenous bypass; however, many institutions are replacing this with rapid surgical anastomosis or by beginning revascularization with the native liver still in place. The final phase is revascularization, requiring five anastomoses to be performed with the suprahepatic vena cava, infrahepatic vena cava, hepatic artery, portal vein and common bile duct. A cholecystectomy is generally performed to prevent biliary stasis. This surgery is technically demanding and requires skilled surgical and anaesthetic teams in order to be successful (Fig. 45.3).

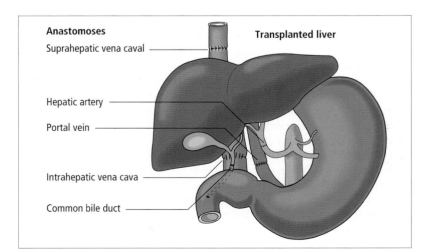

Figure 45.3 Liver transplantation. The recipient's liver is removed. The donor liver is implanted using the following sequence of anastomoses: superior vena cava, inferior vena cava, portal vein, hepatic artery and bile duct.

Anastomoses
Suprahepatic vena caval
Transplanted liver
Hepatic artery
Portal vein
Intrahepatic vena cava
Common bile duct

05

Complications

Primary non-function

The most important adverse outcome in liver transplantation is the graft that fails to function upon implantation. Most patients receiving a liver are seriously ill from hepatic insufficiency and will therefore tolerate very little time with no liver function. These patients will usually expire within 48–72 h unless they can receive another liver.

Biliary complications

Biliary tract complications were once considered the Achilles heel of liver transplantation. While improved techniques have reduced problems substantially, they are still a continuing source of complications. Bile leaks present with bile in peritoneal drains, increased bilirubin levels and bile ascites. They are due to anastomotic failure, cut surface of split liver grafts or the site of a T tube. Once considered standard, many centres are abandoning the use of T tubes for common duct drainage. Bile duct strictures typically present later with elevated transaminases, alkaline phosphatase and bilirubin (direct). If ultrasound does not reveal dilated ducts, then cholangiography is the standard technique for identifying the stricture, the location and its severity. When anastomotic strictures present within the first month, they represent technical failure and prompt surgical revision provides the best long-term results.

Vascular complications

Hepatic artery thrombosis is the most common and most threatening complication of a liver transplant. It is reported to occur in up to 5% of adults and 25% of children. Its presentation can vary greatly, from a picture of fulminant hepatic necrosis to bile leaks and even subclinical acidosis. Doppler ultrasound examination of the hepatic vessels may make the diagnosis but false positives are possible from non-arterial vascular flow in nearby vessels. Angiography remains the definitive investigation. Thrombectomy and anastomotic revision can be attempted, although most patients will need to be retransplanted for long-term survival. Portal vein thrombosis and caval complications are relatively rare and can be diagnosed by Doppler ultrasound. Reoperation with vascular repair is possible in early cases, while late presentations can often be managed by interventional radiology.

Liver transplants pose a higher threat of haemorrhagic complications and are associated with more blood loss than the transplantation of other organs.

Outcomes

Most centres currently achieve 1-year patient survival rates in excess of 80%, which is an enormous improvement over the 1-year survival rates of 30–40% just 20 years ago. Many centres demonstrate 5-year survival rates approaching 70%. Patients receiving transplants for primary hepatic malignancies do much worse than all other indications, with 5-year survival rates around 35%.

Pancreas transplantation

Indications

The indication for pancreatic replacement is diabetes. In other words, the pancreas is replaced in patients almost entirely for the single purpose of restoring endogenous production of insulin. The candidates for this surgery fall into three groups.
1 Patients with severe diabetes and a functional renal transplant at risk for recurrent ESRD in their graft.
2 Patients with ESRD and diabetes: these patients can particularly benefit from combined pancreas/kidney transplant.
3 Non-uremic diabetics with substantial extrarenal complications of diabetes.

Operative details

Procurement

Special care must be taken during pancreatic procurement, with very delicate dissection and handling to avoid post-reperfusion pancreatitis. Harvesting usually entails preserving the entire arterial supply from both the coeliac and superior mesenteric artery on an aortic patch. If the liver is also harvested, the gastroduodenal artery is ligated, leaving blood supply to the head to come from the inferior pancreaticoduodenal off the superior mesenteric artery. Venous outflow is preserved with a segment of portal vein, tied inferiorly, open superiorly. The second portion of the duodenum is usually taken as well, along with the head to preserve blood flow and protect the ampulla of Vater, which is the exocrine outflow tract of the pancreas.

Implantation

As with the kidneys, reimplantation is carried out in the heterotopic location of the iliac fossa, leaving the native organ in place (Fig. 45.4). After vascular anastomosis with the iliac vessels, the graft produces insulin in its functional endocrine portion (islets of Langerhans), which only

05

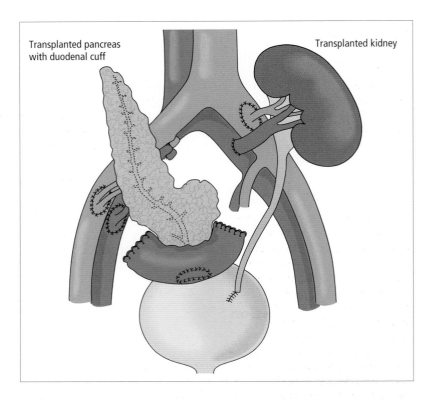

Figure 45.4 Combined kidney and pancreas transplantation.

needs access to the systemic circulation. However, the exocrine pancreas, the producer of every enzyme required to digest all biological macronutrients, must be adequately drained. This can be done through the bladder or enterically into a loop of small bowel.

Complications

Pancreatitis

Graft pancreatitis is a common concern after transplantation and can occur early or late. The treatment is the same as for normal pancreatitis. The potential complications of pancreatitis include systemic inflammatory response syndrome, pancreatic necrosis/abscess, peritonitis, pancreatic fistula, anastomotic leak and vascular thrombosis, which requires graft removal.

Rejection

Rejection is a common concern for all grafted organs but deserves special mention in the case of the pancreas because the diagnosis is such a difficult one. Hyperglycaemia is insufficient because by the time this occurs, 90% of the islets have been destroyed. Urinary diversion of exocrine drainage allows some surveillance by sequen-

tial measurement of urinary amylase. A drop in urinary amylase by 30–50% is suggestive of rejection.

Vascular complications

Vascular thrombosis with subsequent graft necrosis is a relatively common and severe complication of pancreatic transplantation, reported to occur in 6–12% in the largest series.

Outcomes

Patients with a successful pancreatic transplant enjoy good glucose control free of insulin. Currently, 1-year graft survival is usually in excess of 75%.

Future

As evident from the discussion, an entire pancreatic transplant is a tremendous undertaking when only a very small portion of the cell lines present in a pancreas are necessary for the intended cure of diabetes. It is for this reason that islet cell transplantation is an aggressively pursued research field at centres around the world. Recent reports suggest this may be the future hope for researchers and diabetics everywhere.

05

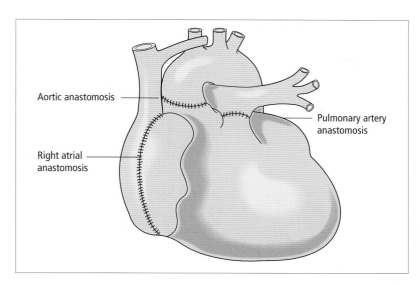

Figure 45.5 Heart transplantation. The recipient's atria are left *in situ*. The donor heart is anastomosed to the atria, the pulmonary artery and the aorta.

Cardiac transplantation

Indications

Three-quarters of the patients listed for cardiac transplantation have cardiomyopathy of either ischaemic or idiopathic origin. The other one-quarter have congenital disorders, valvular disease, restrictive cardiomyopathy, viral cardiomyopathy or a failing previous transplant.

Operative details

The pulmonary artery and aorta are anastomosed end to end in the recipient. The pulmonary veins are usually handled by leaving a patch of left atrium with all the pulmonary vein ostia included to be anastomosed to the donor left atrium. The right atrium can be handled the same way, with a patch including both superior and inferior vena cava, or these vessels can be each anastomosed end to end (Fig. 45.5).

Complications

Graft atherosclerosis

Once patients complete the acute phase of cardiac instability by avoiding acute rejection, the natural history of a heart transplant is accelerated atherosclerosis. It is felt to be, at least in part, a manifestation of chronic vascular rejection. Risk factors for this complication include two or more episodes of acute rejection, cytomegalovirus infection, high serum lipid levels and an elderly donor heart.

Outcome

Cumulative data from 251 centres reveals a 1-year survival rate of 80% and an actuarial 5-year survival rate of 65%. This is impressive as patients listed are those with heart disease severe enough that life expectancy is limited to 6–12 months.

Other organs

Lung

Patients are considered for transplantation who have less than 1 year expected survival due to end-stage pulmonary disease that is not malignant in origin. Diseases requiring transplant include chronic obstructive pulmonary disease, emphysema, idiopathic pulmonary fibrosis, cystic fibrosis, α_1-antitrypsin deficiency, primary pulmonary hypertension, retransplantation and secondary pulmonary hypertension due to congenital cardiac shunts. Lung transplants can be either single-lung or double-lung procedures.

Since pathology of the lungs will adversely affect the heart, and vice versa, patients are considered for combined heart–lung transplant when they display right ventricular diastolic dysfunction, severe intrinsic left ventricular dysfunction, severe coronary artery disease not amenable to repair and Eisenmenger's syndrome with inoperable shunts. The combined procedure is technically straightforward, with only caval, aortic and tracheal connections to consider.

Infection is the leading cause of early mortality, accounting for 30–50% of deaths. The 1-year survival rate is 70–80%. Patients with functioning grafts generally experience dramatic improvements in lifestyle since they are so limited in activity preoperatively.

Small bowel

Intestinal transplantation is an attempt to save the unfortunate few who suffer from the irreversible inability to absorb enough nutrients to support their needs. This is limited to patients with short-gut syndrome due to resection and rare functional disorders. The incidence of intestinal failure is only about 2 per million. While total parenteral nutrition is a life-preserving alternative for this population and can be used long term, there are substantial limitations, including extraordinary expense, complications associated with central lines and progressive liver failure.

Rejection is a particular issue with small-bowel transplants as there is no effective way to monitor for its presence and it is very common with this organ. Most patients will experience at least one episode of rejection, and the diagnosis must be suspected on clinical signs (bloating, abdominal pain, fever, bloody stool, diarrhoea, sepsis, etc.).

The results have been rapidly improving and the most recently published series from a large volume centre reports nearly 75% 1-year survival rates.

Specific transplantation at a glance

Transplantation of kidneys, liver, heart and pancreas are routine now. Lung and small-bowel transplantation are less common. Difficulty in obtaining donors remains a problem for all transplants

Renal transplantation
Indications
- ESRD
- Diabetes mellitus
- Chronic hypertension
- Glomerulopathies
- Cystic and interstitial renal disease
- Obstructive uropathy
- Congenital disorders
- Metabolic diseases (amyloidosis, oxalosis, etc.)
- Trauma
- Haemolytic–uraemic syndrome
- Malignancy (Wilms' tumour, renal cell carcinoma)

Contraindications
- Active infection
- Malignancy
- Unstable disease elsewhere
- Coronary artery disease

Operative procedure
- Heterotopic transplant to iliac fossa
- Arterial and venous anastomoses to iliac vessels
- Ureter attached to bladder via submucosal tunnel to prevent reflux

Complications
Early
- Hyperacute rejection
- Renal artery or vein thrombosis
- Urine leak
- Lymphocele
- Graft toxicity from immunosuppressive treatment
- Infection, bleeding, wound complications

Late
- Acute and chronic rejection
- Renal artery stenosis

Outcomes
- 1-year graft survival rate 90%
- 5-year graft survival rate 65%

Liver transplantation
Indications
- End-stage liver disease from cirrhosis (alcoholic or viral)
- Acute fulminant disease
- Primary biliary cirrhosis
- Primary sclerosing cholangitis
- Biliary atresia
- Metabolic disorders
- Budd–Chiari syndrome
- Primary liver tumours

Contraindications
- Continuing alcohol abuse
- Secondary malignant deposits

Operative procedure
- Hepatectomy of the diseased liver in the recipient
- Anhepatic phase: venovenous bypass or rapid surgical anastomosis or revascularization with the native liver still in place
- Orthotopic transplantation of donated liver: five anastomoses (suprahepatic vena cava, infrahepatic vena cava, hepatic artery, portal vein, common bile duct) + cholecystectomy

Complications
Primary non-function
- Usually fatal unless another transplant can be performed immediately

Biliary complications
- Bile leak from:
  (a) Anastomotic failure

05

(b) Cut surface of split liver grafts
(c) Site of a T tube
- Bile duct strictures: usually late complication

Vascular complications
- Hepatic artery thrombosis: 5% of adults and 25% of children
- Portal vein thrombosis
- Caval complications

Haemorrhagic complications
- More blood loss than other transplantations

Outcomes
- 1-year survival rate > 80%, 5-year survival rate ~ 70%
- Primary hepatic malignancy, 5-year survival rate ~ 35%

Pancreatic transplantation
Indications
- Severe diabetes mellitus + functional renal transplant at risk for recurrent ESRD in the graft
- ESRD + diabetes mellitus
- Non-uremic diabetes mellitus + substantial extrarenal complications of diabetes mellitus

Operative details
Procurement
- Careful handling of organ
- Preserve arterial supply and venous outflow
- Second portion of the duodenum is included in specimen

Implantation
- Heterotopic in iliac fossa leaving the native organ in place
- Vascular anastomoses (arterial + venous) to iliac vessels
- Exocrine drainage to bladder or small bowel

Complications
- Pancreatitis
- Rejection: a decrease in urinary amylase of 30–50% is suggestive of rejection
- Vascular: thrombosis and graft necrosis occurs in 6–12% of patients

Outcomes
- 1-year graft survival rate 75%
- Good glucose control free of insulin

Cardiac transplantation
Indications
- Cardiomyopathy: ischaemic or idiopathic
- Congenital disorders
- Valvular disease
- Restrictive cardiomyopathy
- Viral cardiomyopathy
- Failing previous transplant

Operative details
- Orthotopic transplant after removal of native heart

Anastomoses
- Donor pulmonary artery and aorta to recipient counterparts
- Donor left atrium attached to patch of recipient left atrium containing ostia of pulmonary veins
- Donor right atrium attached to patch of recipient right atrium containing ostia of inferior vena cava (IVC) and superior vena cava (SVC). Alternatively, direct donor–recipient IVC and SVC anastomoses

Complications
- Cardiac instability
- Acute rejection
- Accelerated graft atherosclerosis

Outcome
- 1-year survival rate 80%
- 5-year survival rate 65%

Lung transplantation
Indications
Non-malignant end-stage pulmonary disease with less than 1 year expected survival, including:
- Chronic obstructive pulmonary disease
- Emphysema
- Idiopathic pulmonary fibrosis
- Cystic fibrosis
- α_1-Antitrypsin deficiency
- Primary pulmonary hypertension
- Retransplantation
- Pulmonary hypertension secondary to congenital cardiac shunts

Operative details
- Orthotopic single- or double-lung transplantation
- Combined heart–lung transplant

Complications
- Infection (30–50% mortality)

Outcomes
- 1-year survival rate 70–80%
- Dramatic improvements in lifestyle

Small-bowel transplantation
Indications
- Short-gut syndrome (occurs in 2 per million of population) due to resection or rare functional disorders

Complications
- Rejection: most patients will experience at least one episode of rejection

Outcome
- 1-year survival rate 75%

05

Surgical Conditions in Neonates, Infants and Children

46

Must know Must do

Must know

Core knowledge of congenital abnormalities and their management

Core knowledge of abnormalities presenting in the paediatric age group and their management

How to obtain a history of a child's condition from parents

Normal growth parameters of infants and children

Principles of intravenous fluid therapy in children

How to detect surface/joint abnormalities in a child

How to diagnose an inguinal hernia in a child

Clinical features of acute appendicitis and mesenteric adenitis in children

Must do

See a child with acute appendicitis

See an infant with pyloric stenosis

Attend a paediatric operating list

Visit a paediatric ward

Visit the neonatal intensive care unit

Introduction

Surgery in the neonate, infant and child covers all surgical specialities. Unlike much of adult surgical practice, which deals mainly with the consequences of degenerative and malignant disease, paediatric surgery, in its broadest context, is the surgery of the growing and developing human organism. This adds an important extra dimension to dealing with surgical problems in this age group. Treatment outcomes, both successful and unsuccessful, last a lifetime and many may impact on future growth and development.

The scope of the speciality of general paediatric surgery (which this chapter addresses) is too wide to cover completely. Readers are referred to the Evidence-based medicine section for further, more detailed reading.

History

The basis of all good surgical practice rests on a comprehensive history. In children this may come from a variety of sources. For the newborn, the history of the pregnancy and the obstetric and general medical history of the mother may be very important. For infants and older children, the parents or carers will be the main source of such information. Parents are remarkably good at detecting when their child is unwell. Changes in behaviour, temperament, sleep patterns, play routines and many other normal day-to-day activities may herald the onset of ill health. Consequently, time spent obtaining a good history from parents or carers is time well spent.

Physical examination

The rules for physical examination in neonates, infants and children are essentially the same as for adults, with one or two minor differences. In neonates, a head to toe examination is probably the best way of ensuring that nothing is missed, as often the history will not necessarily point to the affected body system. It is also useful to perform any auscultation while the baby is quiet and before removing all clothing.

In older children, simple observation may provide much useful clinical information. Does the child walk with a limp? Does he avoid using one arm? Is the respiratory pattern normal? Distraction techniques may be required to allow an objective evaluation of abdominal and other physical signs. Asking the child to distend and retract the abdominal wall and to cough is a very sensitive test for peritonism. Rebound tenderness should never be elicited in children. Gentle tapping with the percussing finger will elicit the same information (tap tenderness) in a much less cruel way.

In all children, knowledge of normal physiological parameters for different age groups is essential before an evaluation of the abnormal is possible (Table 46.1).

05

Table 46.1 Normal physiological parameters in neonates, infants and children.

Age	Respiratory rate (breaths/min)	Heart rate (beats/min)
Neonate (0–1 month)	40–60	140–160
Infant (1–12 months)	25–35	90–120
Preschool child (under 5 years)	20–30	80–100
Preadolescent (under 13 years)	15–20	70–90

Fluid management

The percentage water content of newborn babies and children is higher than in adults. As a consequence, the maintenance fluid requirements of the neonatal and paediatric surgical patient are higher than in adults. In the first few days of life, in relative terms, the newborn is waterlogged and the kidneys immature. Maintenance fluid requirement at birth is about 75 mL/kg body weight per day. This increases to 150 mL/kg daily at 7 days; premature infants can require as much as 200 mL/kg daily at 7 days.

After the first month, fluid requirements decrease. The first 10 kg of body weight requires approximately 100 mL/kg per day (equates to approximately 4 mL/kg per h); the next 10 kg of body weight requires approximately 50 mL/kg per day (equates to 2 mL/kg per h); every kilogram of body weight thereafter requires approximately 25 mL/kg per day (equates to 1 mL/kg per h). From these values, the '4/2/1' formula has been developed (excludes neonates in the first month of life). Using this formula a 35-kg child would require:

$$(10 \times 4 \text{ mL}) + (10 \times 2 \text{ mL}) + (15 \times 1 \text{ mL}) = 40 + 20 + 15$$
$$= 75 \text{ mL/h of maintenance fluids}$$

Electrolyte and mineral requirements are also calculated by body weight, e.g. children require approximately 2–3 mmol of sodium and potassium per kilogram body weight daily. A 3-kg neonate who requires 450 mL/day (150 mL/kg per day) of maintenance fluid will need approximately 9 mmol of sodium per day; 450 mL of normal (0.9%) saline contains 67.5 mmol of sodium (150 mmol/L), whereas the same volume of fifth-strength (0.18%) saline contains 13.5 mmol of sodium, which is much closer to the baby's sodium requirement. This is the reason that the maintenance intravenous fluid used in children is not normal saline.

Neonatal conditions

Abdominal wall and inguinoscrotal abnormalities

Umbilical hernia

An umbilical hernia is a common finding in neonates. It is more common in the negroid races, in premature neonates and in some rare syndromes and chromosomal abnormalities. The hernia protrudes through a defect in the fascia at the umbilical ring but may only be apparent when the baby cries or strains; a small defect may allow a large amount of bowel to enter the hernial sac causing a significant and, for the parents, a worrying swelling. Over 90% close spontaneously during the first 3 years of life.

The risk of incarceration or strangulation in infancy is negligible. Although umbilical herniae are more prominent when the baby cries, they rarely cause pain and rupture of the overlying skin is exceedingly uncommon. For these reasons, observation alone is appropriate until the third birthday. Persistence beyond that age dictates that surgical closure should be considered. This is most commonly done as a day case under general anaesthesia. The results of repair are good.

Inguinal hernia and hydrocele

Inguinal herniae are the most common condition requiring surgery during childhood (Fig. 46.1). Bowel or omentum in boys and the ovary or fallopian tube in girls can protrude into a patent processus vaginalis (PPV) along the inguinal canal. Indirect inguinal herniae, where the sac originates at the level of the deep inguinal ring lateral to the inferior epigastric vessels, are far more common in children than direct herniae, which are usually only seen in teenagers.

Inguinal herniae are six to ten times more common in boys than in girls. The incidence is approximately 1 in 50–100 live male births and is up to 30 times higher in premature infants; 60% affect the right side, 25% the left and 15% are bilateral.

In complete herniae the contents of the sac extend down to the scrotum, whereas in incomplete herniae the contents extend only partway along the cord. Incarceration can occur with either type and the treatment is the same.

The history provided by the parents is important in determining whether an inguinal hernia exists. They describe an intermittent groin swelling, extending towards or into the scrotum that often appears when the baby cries or strains. There is often no apparent discomfort associated with the presence of the bulge.

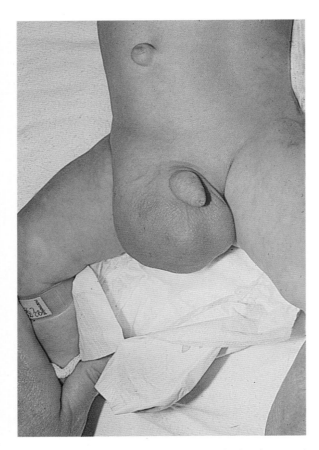

Figure 46.1 Male infant with a large right inguinoscrotal hernia.

To confirm the diagnosis you need to see and feel the herniated viscus or fluid in the sac and to feel its reduction by gentle taxis. The 'silk glove' sign (the feeling elicited by rolling your fingers across the hernial sac) and thickening of the cord detected by palpation are useful if unreliable diagnostic signs, but when taken together with a reliable and consistent parental history may allow you to recommend surgery. The differential diagnosis includes hydrocele, femoral hernia, an undescended testis in the inguinal canal (always check the position of the ipsilateral testicle when examining for a hernia) and groin lymphadenopathy. The contralateral groin should always be examined.

The treatment of an inguinal hernia is herniotomy under general anaesthesia. Given the high risk of incarceration in early infancy, there is no reason to delay operation even in the first few weeks of life. The operation can be performed on a day-case basis in children over 6 months of age. The only exceptions to this are patients with other medical conditions, including extreme prematurity and severe cardiac or respiratory disease. In such patients, repair of an asymptomatic hernia may be delayed. Exploration of the opposite groin is not recommended unless there is clinical evidence of a hernia on that side.

The symptoms of incarceration include irritability, loss of appetite, abdominal pain and vomiting. On examination, there is a tender mass in the inguinal canal with oedema of the distal spermatic cord and testis. On rectal examination, the herniated viscus may be palpable entering the inguinal canal at the deep inguinal ring. In most infants, an incarcerated hernia can strangulate in a matter of hours, leading to infarction of the ipsilateral testis and the contained viscus. In girls, the ovary may be chronically incarcerated but the risk of ischaemic injury is low.

The initial treatment of an incarcerated hernia is reduction by taxis after a period of carefully monitored analgesia or sedation. If reduction is successful, the hernia should be repaired in 48 h to allow oedema to subside. If reduction is unsuccessful, the hernia should be repaired immediately.

The incidence of infantile hydrocele is much higher than inguinal hernia. If the channel is too narrow to allow bowel or other structures to pass through, fluid can trickle down the PPV resulting in a hydrocele of the tunica vaginalis testis or of the spermatic cord. Classically, the parents will report that the swelling is absent in the morning but most obvious just before bedtime. The swelling is usually restricted to the scrotum but hydroceles of spermatic cord can occur. Treatment is essentially the same as for an inguinal hernia. Surgery to ligate the PPV is undertaken as a day case under general anaesthesia.

Exomphalos

Exomphalos is an abnormality where the abdominal wall has failed to develop properly around the umbilical stalk. The exact cause for the abnormality is unclear. It may relate to the process of physiological herniation of the intestine into the umbilical cord at about 10 weeks of fetal life. Alternatively, it may relate to a failure of migration of mesodermal tissue (which ultimately forms the myotomes of the abdominal wall) into the primitive body wall.

This condition is often detected antenatally. An elevated level of maternal serum α-fetoprotein at about 16 weeks' gestation prompts a more detailed fetal ultrasound scan. The abnormality is usually easily recognized at this gestational age. A large sac is seen covering the anterior abdominal wall and the umbilical cord root sits in the middle of this sac. The contents of the sac will depend on the size of the defect. Exomphalos major, in particular, is associated with other serious abnormalities. Approximately 30% of affected fetuses will have an associated cardiac anomaly (often fatal) and 30% will have a chromosomal abnormality. Pulmonary hypoplasia is also seen

05

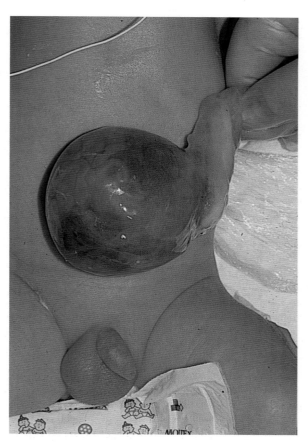

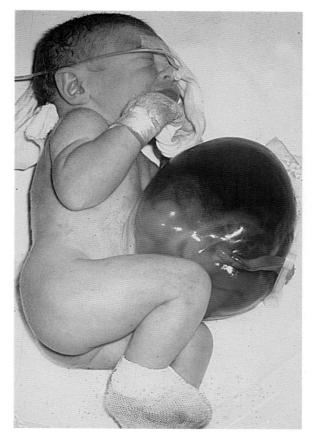

Figure 46.2 Neonate with exomphalos minor: frontal view. The sac contains intestine only and the umbilical cord is seen coming from the apex of the sac.

Figure 46.3 Neonate with exomphalos major. Sac contains liver, spleen, small and large intestine.

in exomphalos major. The absence of abdominal contents within the abdominal cavity results in a failure of outward growth of the ribcage. This limits pulmonary growth and can, in itself, be the critical factor that limits outcome.

Postnatally, exomphalos is divided into minor and major varieties. In exomphalos minor (Fig. 46.2), the neck of the defect is arbitrarily defined as being less than 4 cm in diameter. The sac contains only intestine and the defect is relatively easy to repair surgically. Exomphalos major is a severe abnormality. The sac can be massive and contain liver, spleen, small and large intestine and stomach (Fig. 46.3).

Delivery of an affected fetus should be carefully planned. Caesarean section is usually preferred to ensure that the exomphalos sac remains intact during the birthing process. Where the defect is small, primary closure may be possible, although if the closure is tight, abdominal organ ischaemia can occur. Staged closure using a Silastic silo may be possible for moderate-sized lesions. The sac is excised and a Silastic pouch attached to the abdominal wall to contain the abdominal organs. Over a period of time, the abdominal contents are gradually returned to the abdominal cavity and the defect in the abdominal wall is closed secondarily at a second operation. The final option available is to apply an astringent 'paint' to the sac. In the past, mercurochrome was widely used, but this caused mercury toxicity and has been abandoned in favour of other less toxic substances, e.g. Flamazine. The 'paint' dries out the sac, which then granulates and epithelializes. Skin cover is thus achieved, although future surgery to repair the residual gap between the abdominal wall muscles is usually necessary later in life.

The outcome for treatment for exomphalos minor is good. This is not the case for more major forms of this abnormality. Associated cardiac, chromosomal and other anomalies and pulmonary hypoplasia have an adverse effect on survival, which varies between 30 and 80% in different published series.

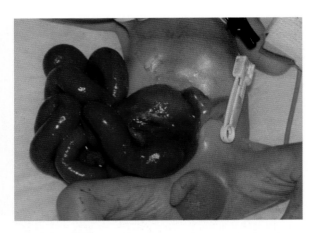

Figure 46.4 Neonate with gastroschisis and marked intrauterine growth retardation. The defect is to the right of the umbilical cord root. The protruding intestine is oedematous and matted.

Gastroschisis

Gastroschisis (Fig. 46.4) is an abnormality where the intestine is seen to protrude through the abdominal wall, usually to the right of the umbilicus. Unlike exomphalos, where the protruding viscera are covered by a membrane, in gastroschisis the protruding bowel floats freely and as such is prone to direct injury.

Most cases of gastroschisis are detected antenatally. Maternal serum α-fetoprotein level is elevated, prompting a detailed ultrasound scan to be performed. Normal vaginal delivery close to term is preferred, but one-third of those affected will require a Caesarian section for obstetric indications and a further one-third require an emergency Caesarian section for fetal distress during labour.

Following delivery, the neonate with gastroschisis is resuscitated and the exposed intestine is covered with sandwich wrap or similar. This has the benefits of keeping the bowel moist and limiting heat loss. As soon as is practical (and preferably within 4–6 h of birth), the baby is taken to the operating theatre where the intestine is replaced in the abdominal cavity. This is achievable in over 80% of cases. In the remainder, a Silastic silo is fashioned and sutured to the abdominal wall. In the following week or so, the intestinal contents are gradually eased into the abdominal cavity and the abdominal wall is closed at a second operation.

Approximately 25% of neonates with gastroschisis have associated bowel injury (e.g. atresia, stenosis or ischaemia). Other associated congenital anomalies are uncommon. The most important postsurgical problem facing these babies is that they suffer from a protracted ileus. Parenteral nutrition is required to allow the baby to grow and to help the abdominal wall heal. As a consequence of improvements in neonatal critical care and nutrition, over 90% of neonates with gastroschisis survive after treatment.

Head and neck abnormalities

Cleft lip and palate

Cleft lip and palate (Fig. 46.5) affects approximately 1 in 600 live births and is more common in boys than girls. Lip clefts are more common than palate clefts and both genetic and non-genetic factors have been implicated in their aetiology. Environmental factors have also been implicated, including drugs, diet, excess alcohol, viral infection *in utero* and irradiation during pregnancy. Nearly half of clefts are associated with other congenital abnormalities.

Clefts usually present at birth and can have a devastating impact on the new parents; a specialist nurse counsellor is an essential member of any cleft team. Pictures of other children taken before and after corrective surgery can be of considerable help in calming parental anxiety. Some cleft lips are now being diagnosed antenatally.

The diagnosis of a cleft lip is usually obvious at birth. Incomplete clefts may only become obvious when the infant starts to smile and a gap in the muscle of the upper lip is seen. Clefts of the lip and palate are also usually obvious. Isolated palate clefts are best diagnosed by direct inspection using a tongue depressor and a small torch. Passing a finger along the palate may miss a minor submucous cleft (palatal mucosa intact but palatal muscles not fused in the midline); a bifid uvula might be seen in this form of cleft.

Initial respiratory difficulties may necessitate urgent intervention with oropharyngeal suction, placement of an airway adjunct and, in a few cases, tracheostomy. Initial attention is directed towards feeding. Attempts at breast- or bottle-feeding using a normal teat should be encouraged; a variety of special teats have been developed to assist with bottle-feeding. Early orthodontic assessment is essential to determine the relative position of the alveolar margins; a wide gap will prevent good closure of the cleft lip. An orthodontic appliance to realign the premaxillary and lateral segments may be necessary.

Cleft lip repair is usually undertaken at about 3 months of age. Palatal closure is usually performed between 6 and 12 months. Surgery to prevent nasal escape of air due to a short palate may be required when the child is older. Grommets may be required if the child develops significant middle ear effusion secondary to eustachian tube obstruction (glue ear). Lip scar revision and major maxillofacial surgery may be required later in life.

05

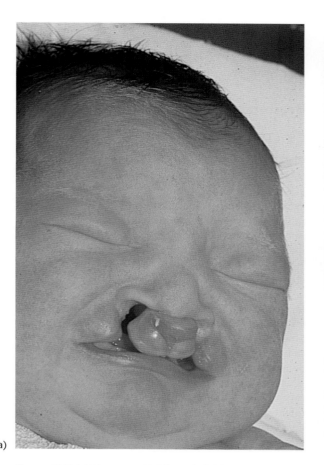

(a)

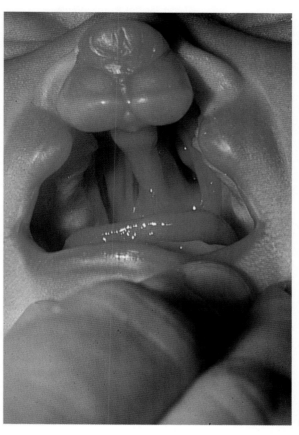

(b)

Figure 46.5 (a) Neonate with bilateral cleft lip and palate. The nose is flattened and the nasal alae spread. The premaxillary segment is displaced anteriorly. (b) Close-up view of neonate shown in (a). The palate is cleft and the vomer can be seen in the nasal cavity. The premaxillary segment is displaced anteriorly. Reproduced with permission from Walker *et al.* (2000).

A multidisciplinary team best achieves the management of a child with a cleft. This team should include paediatric/plastic surgeons, orthodontists, otorhinolaryngologists, maxillofacial surgeons, specialist nurses/nurse counsellors, audiologists, speech therapists, geneticists and educational psychologists.

Cystic hygroma

A cystic hygroma is a benign lymphangiomatous lesion characterized histologically by the presence of fluid-filled spaces lined by endothelium. The head and neck are the most common sites presenting during childhood (Fig. 46.6a). It can be a feature of Turner's syndrome and other chromosomal abnormalities. The lesion has a tendency to infiltrate tissue planes, including the tongue and floor of the mouth (Fig. 46.6b). This can lead to life-threatening airway compromise; intubation is often impossible and emergency tracheostomy may be necessary.

Prenatal diagnosis offers the best chance of a planned delivery and consequent good outcome, with the appropriate surgical personnel available in the delivery room for particularly large lesions.

Complete surgical excision is the optimal treatment of a cystic hygroma; this is often technically difficult (Fig. 46.6c). Many vital structures in the neck are at risk of injury or division during surgery and careful preoperative imaging is essential. Injection of the lesion with OK432 (a lyophilized mixture of group A *Streptococcus pyogenes*) has proven to be useful in shrinking these types of lesion in some cases. Recurrence following treatment is common, particularly if initial excision was not complete.

05

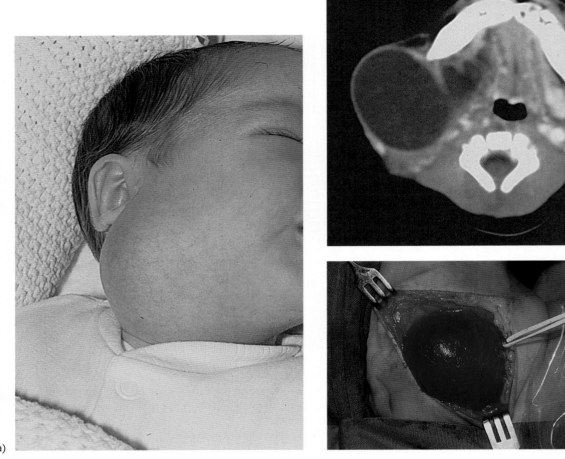

(a)

(b)

(c)

Figure 46.6 (a) Infant with cystic hygroma affecting the right side of the neck. (b) Computed tomography of the infant shown in (a). The cystic swelling is seen to extend into the root of the tongue and has displaced the airway slightly to the opposite side. (c) Operative photograph of cystic hygroma shown in (a) and (b). Care needs to be taken at operation to avoid damage to underlying nerves and blood vessels.

Gastrointestinal abnormalities

Oesophageal atresia and tracheo-oesophagal fistula

Oesophageal atresia (OA), with or without an associated tracheo-oesophageal fistula (TOF), is one of the most common conditions requiring surgical correction in the first few days of life. It affects between 1 in 2000 and 1 in 5000 live births.

Oesophageal atresia occurs in a number of forms. The most common abnormality, which occurs in 85%, comprises a blind-ending proximal oesophageal pouch with a fistula from the trachea to the distal oesophagus (Fig. 46.7(a)). Isolated OA without TOF, isolated TOF without OA (H-type fistula), OA with fistula to the upper and lower oesophageal pouches, and OA with fistulae to upper pouch only are less common (Fig. 46.7(b)–(e)).

Maternal polyhydramnios is seen in 50% of affected pregnancies but antenatal diagnosis is uncommon. Affected neonates have symptoms of frothing of saliva at the mouth and nose, episodes of coughing, cyanosis and respiratory distress shortly after birth. Feeding worsens these symptoms and may cause aspiration and respiratory collapse. Infants who have an isolated TOF in the absence of OA may present later in life with chronic respiratory

05

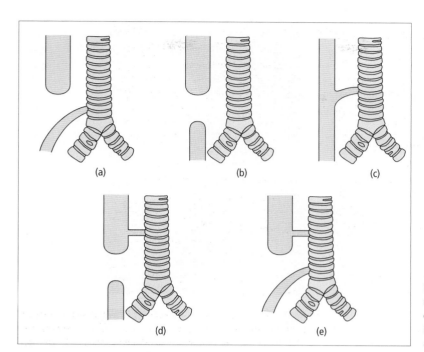

Figure 46.7 Diagrammatic representation of the five most common forms of oesophageal atresia. Reproduced with permission from Walker *et al.* (2000).

symptoms, including bronchospasm and recurrent chest infections.

Associated congenital anomalies are common. The VACTERL or VATER associations are the most frequent findings (*v*ertebral anomalies, *a*norectal malformations, *c*ardiac abnormalities, *t*racheo-*e*sophageal fistula, *r*enal or radial anomalies, and *l*imb malformations).

The diagnosis of OA is essentially clinical; the inability to pass a large-bore orogastric or nasogastric tube into the stomach is diagnostic. The presence of gas in the abdomen on an abdominal radiograph indicates the presence of a coexisting TOF (Fig. 46.8). Associated skeletal abnormalities can be detected on plain films. Ultrasound examination should be performed to identify any renal anomalies and echocardiography should be considered to exclude cardiac lesions, particularly if a murmur is heard or the infant's oxygen saturation is low. In isolated TOF, a pull-back oesophagogram of the patient in the prone or lateral position is necessary to detect the isolated fistula.

Initial management should be to maintain a patent airway and prevent aspiration of saliva. The baby should be nursed prone with a sump suction tube in the upper pouch set on continuous aspiration. This tube should be injected regularly with air to prevent blockage. Intubation should be avoided where possible; gas forced into the gastrointestinal tract under pressure through the TOF can result in splinting of the diaphragm and gastric rupture.

The surgical treatment of OA and TOF is ligation of the TOF and end-to-end anastomosis of the oesophagus,

through a right lateral thoracotomy. In cases where the gap between the ends of the oesophagus is too long for a primary anastomosis, an alternative approach is required. These include:

- ligation of the fistula, creation of a gastrostomy and long-term suction of the upper pouch with later definitive repair;
- delayed primary repair;
- oesophageal replacement using stomach or colon.

Complications of surgery include anastomotic leak, refistulation, oesophageal stricture and gastro-oesophageal reflux. Thankfully, most of these are rare except for gastro-oesophageal reflux; nearly 25% of patients with OA require a fundoplication at a later date.

Duodenal atresia and stenosis

The duodenum is the most common site of gastrointestinal atresia after the oesophagus, with a reported incidence of 1 in 10 000 births. There are three subtypes (Fig. 46.9):

- type I is a complete membrane or mucosal diaphragm causing obstruction without any break in the duodenal serosal or muscle coats;
- in type II, proximal and distal blind-ending duodenal segments are joined by a fibrous cord;
- type III is a complete discontinuity of the duodenum with a gap between the ends. Most occur in the region of the ampulla of Vater.

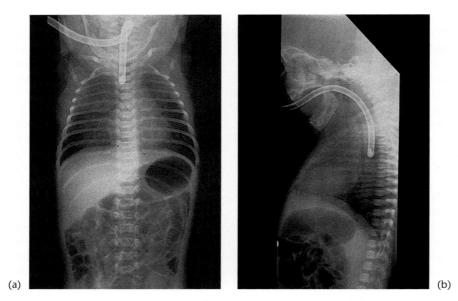

(a)   (b)

Figure 46.8 (a) Anteroposterior radiograph of chest and abdomen in a neonate with oesophageal atresia and a tracheo-oesophageal fistula. A large-bore radiopaque oral tube has been passed to delineate the distal level of the atretic oesophageal segment (with permission). (b) Lateral view of (a). The distal level of the atretic segment is seen. Reproduced with permission from Walker *et al.* (2000).

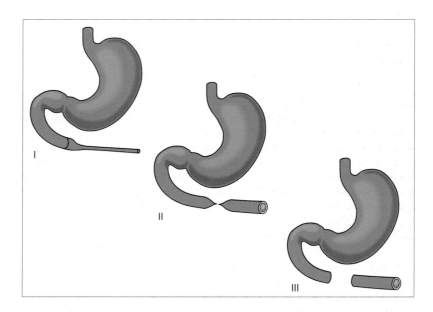

Figure 46.9 Diagrammatic representation of the three types of duodenal atresia.

Duodenal atresia is associated with a number of common anomalies including OA, anorectal malformations and cardiac, urinary tract and vertebral abnormalities. Malrotation is common and approximately one-third have trisomy 21.

Duodenal atresia presents during the first few days of life. The newborn infant vomits all feeds. The vomitus may or may not contain bile depending on the level of the atresia; most atretic segments occur beyond the ampulla and, as a consequence, most present with bilious vomiting. Abdominal distension is rare, although epigastric fullness, which disappears on nasogastric aspiration, can be a feature. Visible gastric peristalsis may be obvious on abdominal inspection.

The diagnosis is usually obvious on a plain abdominal radiograph. The stomach is massively dilated and the

typical double gas–fluid level in the stomach and proximal duodenum, with absent distal intestinal gas, is diagnostic (so-called 'double bubble'). Antenatal diagnosis by ultrasound is also possible. If the stomach is empty at the time of the X-ray, injection of air down the nasogastric tube will reveal the duodenal obstruction. Rarely is radiopaque contrast necessary, except to exclude a diagnosis of malrotation and volvulus.

After a period of preoperative intravenous fluids and nasogastric decompression, laparotomy is necessary. The dilated proximal duodenum is opened transversely to avoid damage to the biliary tree. The distal duodenum is opened vertically. An end-to-end duodenoduodenostomy is fashioned. A transgastric transanastomotic tube or nasojejunal tube is passed to allow early enteral feeding while the anastomosis is healing.

If the duodenal atresia is type I, the external surface of the duodenum will not exhibit an obvious gap but there is usually a change in duodenal calibre at the site of the membrane. Treatment can either be by duodenoduodenostomy or by excision of the membrane. The ampulla should be identified and care taken to avoid damage to the bile duct.

Incomplete duodenal obstruction occurs when a type I membrane has a centrally or eccentrically placed hole through it. Affected children may not present until much later in life. Recurrent episodes of vomiting and failure to thrive are common. The diagnosis may not be possible on plain abdominal X-ray and contrast studies may be similarly unhelpful. Endoscopic examination of the duodenum may provide the diagnosis.

Treatment involves resection of the membrane through a duodenotomy incision or, as in duodenal atresia, a duodenoduodenostomy. A change in the calibre of the duodenum may indicate the site of the perforate membrane, although where the membrane has become stretched distally by passing gut content, the attachment of the membrane may be found more proximal to the calibre change.

Malrotation

During embryological development, the intestine outgrows the abdomen resulting in herniation of the intestine into the umbilical stalk. As the abdomen grows to 'catch up', the intestine returns to the abdominal cavity at about 10 weeks of fetal life. At this stage the intestine undergoes a process of rotation. The first phase rotates the c-loop of duodenum 90° so that the third part of the duodenum comes to lie under the superior mesenteric vessels. In the second phase, the caecum rotates a further 180° to come to lie in the right iliac fossa. This results in a broad base for the small-bowel mesentery, which runs from the right iliac fossa to the site of the duodenojejunal flexure to the left of

the first lumbar vertebra. Failure of this process results in the condition known as malrotation of the intestine.

In malrotation, the duodenum comes to lie to the right of the vertebral column and the caecum usually lies in the right hypochondrium. This results in a very short small-bowel mesentery, which is prone to twist. Such a twist, or volvulus, cuts off the blood supply to the intestine and ischaemia and gangrene result. In addition, a condensation of tissue from the caecal pole to the right hypochondrium comes to lie across the duodenum, causing a degree of obstruction. Most cases of malrotation present in the neonatal period with bilious vomiting.

Any neonate that presents with bile-stained vomiting must be considered to have malrotation until proven otherwise. The abdomen may be distended (in the presence of a volvulus) or scaphoid. Plain abdominal radiographs are often misleading. The diagnosis of malrotation relies on the location of the duodenojejunal flexure to the right of the midline on upper gastrointestinal contrast study (Fig. 46.10). On a lower gastrointestinal contrast

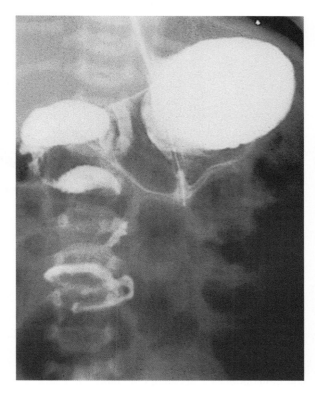

Figure 46.10 Upper gastrointestinal contrast study showing a malrotation and volvulus. The contrast has left the stomach and has entered the duodenum and the first loop of jejunum. Contrast has failed to reach to the left side of the vertebral column to the level of the pylorus and is seen spiralling down along the line of the vertebral column.

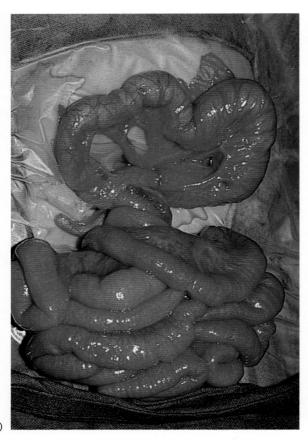
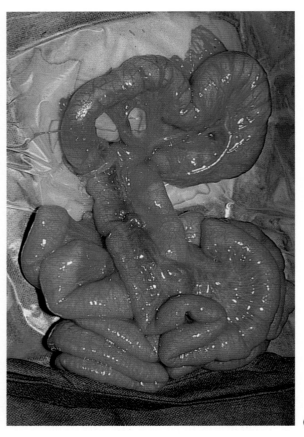

(a)   (b)

Figure 46.11 (a) Operative photograph showing malrotation and small-bowel volvulus. The colon is seen at the top of the picture. The small bowel is seen to have twisted around the root of the mesentery. (b) The small bowel in (a) has now been untwisted. The root of the mesentery is seen to be very narrow. The colon and terminal ileum are seen running down the left centre of the picture with the duodenum running down the right. The gap between the two needs to be widened to broaden the small bowel mesentery.

study, the caecum may be seen to lie in an abnormal position. Abdominal ultrasound may reveal an abnormal relationship of the superior mesenteric artery and vein.

After a period of intravenous fluid resuscitation and antibiotics and nasogastric aspiration, urgent laparotomy is required. At operation, the Ladd's bands are divided and the small-bowel mesentery is widened. Bringing the duodenum down the right side of the abdomen and moving the caecum across to the left iliac fossa achieve this (Fig. 46.11).

Intestinal atresia

Intestinal atresia presents early in the newborn period. The atretic segment(s) can affect any part of the gastrointestinal tract; the proximal small bowel is more commonly affected than distal small bowel and the colon is the least commonly affected.

The neonate will present with the signs and symptoms of intestinal obstruction: vomiting (usually bilious), abdominal distension, constipation and colicky abdominal pain. The level of the atresia will determine which symptoms and signs predominate; a high small-bowel atresia will present early with vomiting but abdominal distension, colicky pain and constipation may not be prominent features. The passage of meconium after birth does not exclude the diagnosis of intestinal atresia, as the atretic event, usually caused by impairment of the blood supply to the affected segment of intestine, can occur relatively late in fetal life, after meconium has passed into the distal bowel.

Abdominal films aid the diagnosis. Fluid-filled loops of distended obstructed intestine with or without fluid levels are usually diagnostic in a proximal atresia. More distal obstructions are less easy to diagnose and contrast enema may be helpful; it may reveal a microcolon or the site of

05

the obstruction if present in the colon or terminal ileum. In some cases, laparotomy is required to make the final diagnosis.

At laparotomy, the atretic segment is usually obvious. There are four subtypes of intestinal atresia.

● Type 1: mucosal atresia with no interruption to the serosal surface of the intestine.
● Type 2: the continuity of the intestine is completely interrupted but a fibrous cord joins the ends of the atretic segment and there is no gap in the bowel mesentery.
● Type 3: similar to type 2 but the ends of the atretic segment are not joined in any way and there is a wedge-shaped gap in the mesentery.
● Type 4: describes a situation where there is more than one atretic segment. It is important to realize that mutiple atretic segments can coexist and for this reason, at operation, the distal intestine should be irrigated through a small tube to ensure that there is no occult atresia distally.

Surgical treatment involves resection of the ends of the atretic segments and anastomosis of the ends. Preservation of as much intestine as possible is essential to avoid the problems of short-gut syndrome.

Hirschsprung's disease

Hirschsprung's disease is a condition where the ganglion cells found in the various layers of the intestine fail to migrate from the neural crest. Absence of these ganglion cells results in hypertrophy of associated nerve fibres, features which are used to diagnose the condition histologically. The length of affected segment, which is contiguous from the rectum proximally, can vary tremendously. Most commonly the aganglionic segment runs to the sigmoid colon (short-segment disease); however, long-segment disease or total colonic aganglionosis are not uncommon.

The newborn affected by Hirschsprung's disease is usually large and postdates at birth. There is a strong association with Down's syndrome. The baby usually presents in the first few days of life having failed to pass meconium. The baby stops feeding, develops abdominal distension and vomits, often bilious fluid. Plain abdominal X-ray will reveal gas down to the distal colon but no gas in the rectum.

Investigations include contrast enema to determine the level of the transition zone where aganglionic intestine becomes normal. This is seen as a narrow rectum or sigmoid colon with an area of dilated colon more proximally. The definitive diagnosis requires histological examination of a suction rectal biopsy. Staining with haematoxylin and eosin and immunostaining for acetylcholinesterase demonstrates absence of ganglion cells and hypertrophy of nerve fibres, which clinches the diagnosis.

Current best practice involves a period of rectal washout until the newborn regains his or her birth weight.

A neonatal pull-through operation is then performed where the aganglionic segment is resected and normally innervated bowel is anastomosed to the anal canal. A number of different pull-through operations are in general use. The results of surgery are good, although some patients suffer from constipation and some are prone to intestinal infection as a consequence of an associated deficiency in intestinal IgA.

Other abnormalities

Congenital diaphragmatic hernia

Congenital diaphragmatic hernia is a serious anomaly where the diaphragm has not developed properly. The majority affect the left side and develop following failure of the embryological foramen of Bochdalek to close. The consequences of this failure are significant. Abdominal contents, including small bowel, colon, stomach, spleen and part of the liver, migrate into the thoracic cavity through the defect. This impairs development of the ipsilateral lung and, depending on the amount of abdominal content in the chest, can also impair development of the opposite lung. This pulmonary hypoplasia and associated pulmonary hypertension are responsible for the high mortality (in excess of 50%) seen in this condition.

The neonate presents with acute respiratory failure in the first few minutes or hours of life. Antenatal diagnosis by ultrasound is becoming more common. Congenital diaphragmatic hernia that presents later in childhood may have been asymptomatic for many years; in this situation it can present with dyspnoea, intermittent abdominal pain, or vomiting if the bowel becomes obstructed at the site of herniation. It may be identified as an unexpected finding on chest X-ray.

Physical examination may reveal decreased breath sounds over the involved thorax and dullness to percussion. A chest X-ray usually suggests the diagnosis (Fig. 46.12).

In all cases of congenital diaphragmatic hernia, the treatment is surgical repair, usually through an abdominal incision after a period of stabilization, which includes endotracheal intubation, administration of surfactant, neuromuscular paralysis and positive-pressure ventilation with high concentrations of oxygen. In some cases more sophisticated measures are required, such as high-frequency oscillatory ventilation, administration of inhaled nitric oxide or extracorporeal membrane oxygenation. Strategies to treat the condition *in utero* are currently under evaluation.

At surgery the viscera are reduced into the abdomen and the diaphragm is repaired with non-absorbable sutures. In cases of complete agenesis of the hemidiaphragm, a prosthetic patch may be required. In the post-

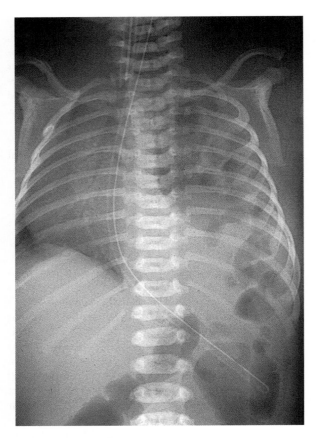

Figure 46.12 Chest X-ray of a neonate with a left-sided congenital diaphragmatic hernia. The left hemithorax contains loops of intestine and no lung is visible on that side. The mediastinum (including the heart and the oesophagus containing a nasogastric tube) has been pushed to the right. The tracheobronchial tree (containing the endotracheal tube) has also been pushed to the right.

operative period, supportive measures are maintained as further cardiovascular and respiratory instability are both common.

The survival rate following treatment for congenital diaphragmatic hernia has slowly improved in the last 20 years. Survival figures of 70–80% have been reported in some centres, although comparison is difficult, given differing referral patterns in different places.

Other conditions

There are a number of other conditions seen in neonatal surgical practice that are not covered in this chapter:
- neonatal necrotizing enterocolitis;
- meconium disease (meconium ileus, meconium plug syndrome);
- anorectal malformations;
- vitello-intestinal duct remnants;
- biliary atresia;
- hydronephrosis;
- posterior urethral valves;
- neurogenic bladder;
- extrophy of the bladder;
- cloacal anomalies;
- neural tube defects and hydrocephalus.

The reader is referred to the Evidence-based medicine section for further reading resources covering these conditions.

Infant conditions

Tongue tie

This minor but common abnormality is caused by an excessively short frenulum between the floor of the mouth and the underside of the tongue. The mobility of the tip of the tongue is impaired. It does not interfere with speech development, although it can interfere with articulation if the tie is tight.

Many tongue ties will release themselves during feeding and sucking. Tight ties should be released under a short general anaesthetic as a day case.

Pyloric stenosis

Hypertrophic pyloric stenosis is a common cause of vomiting in the first 8 weeks of life. Male first-born infants are most frequently affected and there is a higher incidence in the presence of an affected male relative (twin, sibling, father, grandfather). The infant vomits increasing amounts of milk, until vomiting after every feed becomes established; this is a more important observation than the description of the vomit as being 'projectile'. The child cries with hunger after vomiting but further feeds will result in further vomiting, which ultimately results in dehydration, loss of gastric acid and the classical picture of a hypokalaemic hypochloraemic metabolic alkalosis. The child may have paradoxical aciduria as the kidneys retain potassium at the expense of hydrogen ions.

The diagnosis can be made clinically if the child is examined during a 'test' feed. Visible gastric peristalsis and the palpation of the hypertrophied pyloris establish the diagnosis in 60–75% of cases. In the rest, a pyloric ultrasound scan will usually reveal thickening and lengthening of the pyloric canal.

After a period of careful rehydration using half-strength (0.45%) sodium chloride solution containing potassium to correct any biochemical imbalances, the child is taken to the operating theatre. A pyloromyotomy

05

is performed using an open or, in a few centres, a laparoscopic technique. The serosa of the pyloris is incised and the thick hypertrophied muscle of the pylorus is split down to the mucosa using an artery forceps (Ramstedt's operation).

Complications following Ramstedt's operation are rare but include haemorrhage, inadequate myotomy, wound infection and wound dehiscence.

Gastro-oesophageal reflux disease

Vomiting is a common symptom of many conditions seen in paediatric practice. Bile-stained vomiting in the neonatal period has to be regarded as being due to malrotation of the intestine, until proven otherwise. It can also be seen in duodenal and intestinal atresia, Hirschsprung's disease, meconium ileus, meconium plug syndrome and necrotizing enterocolitis. In infants, vomiting is seen in urinary tract and other infections, pyloric stenosis and many other acute surgical conditions. Perhaps the most frequent explanation for persistent vomiting in infancy is gastro-oesophageal reflux.

The normal gastro-oesophageal sphincter mechanism is complex and not fully understood. The length of intra-abdominal oesophagus, the angle between the cardia of the stomach and the oesophagus, the oesophageal mucosa, the oesophageal stripping wave, the right crus of the diaphragm and the effects of various enteric hormones all have a role to play in maintaining the integrity of the gastro-oesophageal sphincter. Gastro-oesophageal reflux is a common condition in infants where this mechanism fails and the infant vomits feeds.

The presentation of gastro-oesophageal reflux can be very variable. Vomiting often starts in early infancy as the volume of milk feeds administered increases. The infant vomits after some, but not all, feeds. Weight gain and growth may be impaired in more severe cases. Crying at night is common and is thought to be due to the irritant effect of refluxing acid on the lower oesophagus. In the early stages, oesophagitis is rare and the complications of oesophagitis, including stricture and haemorrhage even rarer.

In the vast majority of cases, the condition is self-limiting. Medical therapy is employed to tide things over until spontaneous resolution occurs. Feeds can be thickened with a number of additives and the baby sat up after feeds (a car seat is useful for this purpose). The alginate/antacid Gaviscon is a useful addition to treatment at this stage, but if this fails the addition of a histamine H_2-receptor antagonist (cimetidine or ranitidine) or a proton pump inhibitor (omeprazole) may be helpful. Careful monitoring of growth and development is essential at this stage.

In the initial stages of the condition, investigations may not be required and a trial of therapy (thickening feeds, postural changes) may be appropriate. Thereafter, contrast swallow examination, oesophageal pH study and/or upper gastrointestinal endoscopy and biopsy may be useful. Contrast study is prone to false-negative results and pH study, particularly in those under 3 months of age, may be inaccurate.

The indications for surgical intervention include failure to thrive despite optimal medical treatment, recurrent respiratory infections due to reflux and aspiration, oesophagitis resistant to medical therapy, oesophageal stricture and oesophageal haemorrhage. The operative approach used is the same as described below for hiatus hernia.

Intussusception

Intussusception is a common cause of intestinal obstruction in the first year of life. This most commonly occurs after a viral illness, which causes enlargement of Peyer's patches in the terminal ileum. The terminal ileum is peristalsed into the caecum and ascending colon, thus causing intestinal obstruction (ileocolic intussusception) (Fig. 46.13a). In older children, small-bowel polyps, tumours, Meckel's diverticulum and the intestinal wall haematomas seen in Henoch–Schönlein purpura can act as lead points in an intussusception (ileocolic, ileoileal or ileo-ileocolic).

The affected infant presents with a short history of screaming attacks, often associated with pallor and drawing up of the knees. Anorexia and vomiting are common and the normal stooling pattern is lost. The abdomen becomes distended and tender, especially in the right hypochondrium over the intussusception, and the child may pass a 'redcurrant jelly' stool. The symptoms are sometimes difficult to distinguish from gastroenteritis. Severe dehydration is common and affected infants can become drowsy and unrousable.

Initial assessment and treatment must address the problem of dehydration. Intravenous access is essential (and often very difficult to obtain) and resuscitation with crystalloid or colloid solutions initiated. Abdominal examination may reveal an 'empty' right iliac fossa and a sausage-shaped mass may be palpable in the right hypochondrium. Abdominal radiography may help make the diagnosis (Fig. 46.13b) but is often unhelpful. Abdominal ultrasound is now the main investigative tool used to confirm the diagnosis. A 'target sign' is seen when the intussusception is scanned transversely (the rings of the target represent the various layers of the bowel wall).

After a short period of rehydration, an attempt is made to reduce the intussusception pneumatically using an air enema. Air is pumped into the rectum via a small tube

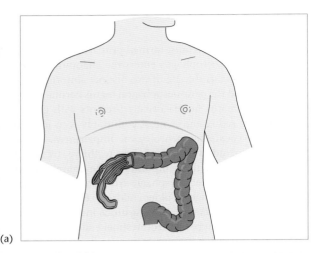

(a)

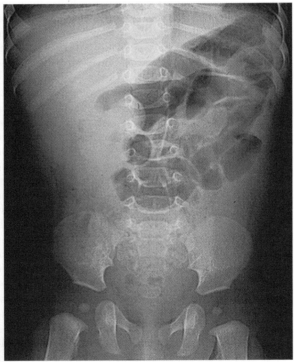

(b)

Figure 46.13 (a) Diagrammatic representation of an ileocolic intussusception. (b) Plain abdominal radiograph demonstrating some of the features of an intussusception. There is a paucity of bowel gas in the right iliac fossa and a suggestion of the lead point of the intussusception seen in the gas-filled transverse colon. There are also some distended loops of small intestine.

using a pressure-limited valve under X-ray screening. Reduction of the intussusception is successful in about 60–70% of cases. Further attempts after a delay of an hour or so may succeed where the initial attempt fails,

increasing the overall reduction rate to 80–90%. Failure of pneumatic reduction requires a laparotomy and reduction or resection of the affected intestine.

Paediatric conditions

Trauma in children

Trauma is a common cause of death and morbidity in children; after the first year of life it is the most common cause of death. The most frequent causes of serious injury in children are road traffic accidents and falls. Non-accidental injury accounts for a significant number of the remainder, particularly in infants. There are often significant psychological sequelae to major trauma in children; as many as 60% are left with behavioural or learning difficulties.

The pattern of injury seen in children differs from adults. The small mass of the child is less able to disperse the kinetic energy of impact and, consequently, multisystem injury is more common. The child's head is large (in proportion to the rest of the body) and, as a result, head injuries are also common. A relatively larger body surface area results in heat loss; this is particularly important to recognize during resuscitation and warmed fluids in a warm resuscitation room are essential.

The effective resuscitation of the injured child requires knowledge of normal cardiovascular and respiratory parameters, which vary with age – knowledge of the normal is required to appreciate the abnormal (see Table 46.1).

Suitable paediatric equipment is essential to resuscitate children of different ages and sizes. Uncuffed endotracheal tubes are used in small children. Small intravenous cannulae may be necessary and intraosseous needles can be used for intravenous fluid administration in children under 6 years of age. Different-sized cervical collars, oxygen masks, laryngoscopes and other equipment are also necessary.

The sequence of resuscitation that is followed in the child is the same as that followed in the adult: *Airway* with cervical spine control, *Breathing* with oxygen, *Circulation* with control of bleeding, *Disability* (neurological evaluation) and *Exposure* (exposure of the whole patient) and *Environment* (making sure the resuscitation room is warm). When the child is stable and cardiorespiratory parameters have returned to normal, a thorough secondary head-to-toe survey is undertaken to detect other injuries.

Appendicitis

Appendicitis is the most common acute surgical

05

emergency encountered by the children's surgeon. The aetiology and disease process are similar to those seen in adults. Unfortunately, the presentation can be quite variable and can mislead the unwary clinician. The classical history of central colicky abdominal pain radiating to the right iliac fossa may, or may not, be present. The history may be particularly vague in very young infants and children. Non-specific associated symptoms such as anorexia, nausea, vomiting and diarrhoea and signs such as fever, fetor, pallor and abdominal distension can lead to diagnostic confusion. The finding of tenderness and guarding in the right iliac fossa usually makes the diagnosis without the need for other investigations. Fever is usually low grade in appendicitis unless the appendix has ruptured and an abscess or more general peritonitis has developed.

The differential diagnosis of appendicitis in children includes mesenteric adenitis, urinary tract infection, testicular torsion, Henoch–Schönlein purpura, constipation, non-specific abdominal pain and intestinal volvulus. Urine should be sent for culture in all such cases. Abdominal radiography may reveal distended loops of intestine with or without fluid levels and, in approximately 10%, a faecolith may be identified. Abdominal ultrasound scan may be helpful in difficult cases, especially in girls. This investigation is very operator dependent and misdiagnosis is not uncommon. The visualization of the appendix usually means that it is pathological and should be removed.

After a period of vigorous intravenous fluid resuscitation and antibiotics, treatment is appendicectomy. This can be done using an open or, more recently, a laparoscopic technique.

Mesenteric adenitis

Mesenteric adenitis commonly affects children during the school years. It is often confused with appendicitis and is the most common finding at appendicectomy when the appendix is found to be normal.

Children often experience a prodromal viral illness, often weeks before their presentation with abdominal pain. Such pain is often diffuse and not localized, although maximal abdominal tenderness can be found in the right iliac fossa, overlying inflamed lymph nodes in the terminal small-bowel mesentery. Affected children can have an extremely high temperature. They have a facial flush but often have a degree of circumoral pallor.

Investigations are unhelpful in this condition. White cell count may or may not be elevated, although a lymphocytosis is more common than a neutrophilia. Treatment involves repeated observation, rehydration (either enteral or intravenous) and bedrest.

Hiatus hernia

The diaphragmatic hiatus, formed primarily by the right crus, where the oesophagus enters the abdominal cavity from the thorax, is the site of two distinct abnormalities: the sliding and the para-oesophageal hiatus hernia.

A sliding hiatus hernia usually presents with gastro-oesophageal reflux and is most commonly seen in children with coexisting neurological impairment. These symptoms include vomiting, failure to thrive, recurrent chest infections or the symptoms of the complications of acid reflux, namely dysphagia from stricture formation and haemorrhage. In older children, retrosternal discomfort can be a feature. Investigations include contrast radiography and upper gastrointestinal endoscopy. Contrast will reveal the proximal stomach to be present in the lower thorax (sometimes intermittently, hence the name 'sliding'), often with associated gastro-oesophageal reflux. Endoscopy reveals a portion of the stomach entering the lower chest, with the indentation of the diaphragm appearing distal to the gastro-oesophageal junction in the gastric wall. There may also be evidence of oesophagitis.

Treatment of an asymptomatic sliding hiatus hernia may not be necessary. Symptomatic reflux should be treated on its merits. In severe cases, particularly those associated with bleeding or oesophageal stricture or where optimal medical therapy has failed, surgery may be indicated. This involves tightening the right crus of the diaphragm and a partial or complete oesophageal wrap using the fundus of the stomach. In recent years the laparoscopic approach to this operation has been developed and practised in children, particularly in those with neurological problems and compromised respiration.

Complications are rare during the operation but are common postoperatively. Major complications include death (1% in neurologically impaired and 0.1% in neurologically normal children), operative failure (7%), chest infection, gas bloat syndrome and dysphagia. Postoperative retching can be a difficult problem to treat.

A para-oesophageal hiatus hernia is often a coincidental finding during investigation for other problems. Dysphagia can be a prominent symptom and pain is often a feature while gastro-oesophageal reflux is rare. Surgery is always indicated because of the significant risk of incarceration of the stomach in the hernial sac, gastric volvulus or gastric perforation.

Paediatric tumours

Wilms' tumour (nephroblastoma)

Wilms' tumour is the most common solid tumour of childhood, affecting 5–10 per 100,000 children. More

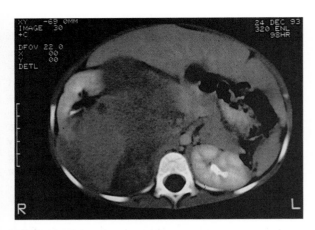

Figure 46.14 Computed tomography of a right-sided nephroblastoma. The remains of the normal right kidney have been displaced laterally and forwards by the tumour mass.

than 70% present before the age of 5 years, with a median at 3 years.

Macroscopically, the tumour is large and encapsulated and occupies all or most of the affected kidney. It contains areas of haemorrhage, necrosis and large and small pseudocysts. Extension of tumour into the renal vein, inferior vena cava and right atrium is not uncommon. The histological appearance falls into two broad subtypes: favourable or unfavourable. Favourable tumours exhibit multicystic, tubular or fibroadenomatous histology and have a better prognosis than unfavourable tumours, which exhibit anaplastic changes.

The usual presentation is of a large abdominal mass, often felt by the parents, or an increase in abdominal girth. Pain is uncommon but may occur when the tumour increases rapidly in size or there is bleeding. Frank haematuria is rare (but microscopic haematuria is reported in 40%), hypertension occurs in 25% and fever, anorexia and vomiting are also common.

The diagnosis is often made on the clinical presentation alone. Ultrasound examination is essential to determine the origin and nature of the mass, to evaluate the opposite kidney and to look for tumour extension. A chest X-ray is performed to detect pulmonary metastases. Computed tomography (CT) of the abdomen (Fig. 46.14) and chest will clarify the extent of disease but may be unnecessary.

Imaging investigations are performed to define preoperative stage. If surgery is the preferred mode of initial treatment, accurate operative staging is performed. A radical transperitoneal nephrectomy is undertaken in unilateral disease followed by chemotherapy, depending on operative stage and histology. Preoperative chemotherapy is used only in cases of bilateral disease, those found to be inoperable at surgery and patients with intravascular tumour extension beyond the level of the hepatic veins. Other centres recommend preoperative chemotherapy to shrink the tumour prior to excision in all cases. Bilateral tumours (5%) should be confirmed at open biopsy and treated by preoperative chemotherapy followed by excision of residual tumour.

The outcome following treatment has improved since the introduction of the first multidisciplinary multicentre studies. Survival figures of 95% in stage I disease with favourable histology have been reported.

Neuroblastoma

Neuroblastoma accounts for 7–10% of all malignant disease in childhood. It originates from the neural crest (adrenal medulla or sympathetic chain). Neuroblasts are small round cells with little cytoplasm and neuroblastoma can be difficult to distinguish from other small round-cell tumours. Neuroblastoma is extremely invasive and local and metastatic spread occurs in the majority. Spontaneous resolution can occur, particularly in children under 1 year old. The median age of onset is 2 years and over 90% of cases occur in the first 8 years.

Up to 80% of cases exhibit genetic abnormalities, the most consistent of these being deletions or translocations affecting the short arm of chromosome 1. Amplification of the N-*myc* oncogene (on chromosome 2) is a poor prognostic sign. Histological examination is important to determine prognosis and response to therapy. Tumours rich in stromal tissue have a better prognosis.

Clinical features depend on tumour site, the presence of metastases and the effects of secreted humoral agents. The tumour arises in the abdomen in 60% (the majority from the adrenal gland); over half of all patients present with a mass but abdominal pain is variable. Pelvic tumours may cause symptoms of bowel or bladder dysfunction. Diarrhoea is prominent if the tumour secretes vasoactive intestinal polypeptide. Thoracic tumours are the next most common and may cause respiratory distress, dysphagia or venous obstruction. Intraspinal extension may occur causing spinal cord compression, which may require urgent surgery. Head and neck tumours may cause compression of adjacent structures and may present with Horner's syndrome or with a palpable neck mass.

Non-specific symptoms include weight loss, failure to thrive, pallor, anaemia, metastatic bone pain, fever and sweating. Many of these features can be attributed to the effects of high circulating levels of catecholamines. Myoclonic encephalopathy ('dancing eye' syndrome) is another feature and hypertension occurs in 25%.

Three-quarters of patients have metastases at diagnosis. Distant spread is via lymphatics or blood and metastases

05

are frequently seen in bone, bone marrow and lymph nodes; spread to liver and skin is less common and to brain and lungs is rare. In infants, the development of an enlarging liver due to tumour infiltration is often the first sign of disease.

Investigations seek to image the primary tumour, establish a tissue diagnosis, assess the degree of spread (staging) and determine whether the tumour is secreting any tumour markers. Abdominal X-ray may reveal fine stippled calcification. Ultrasound and CT will define the site of tumour origin and the presence of metastases. Magnetic resonance imaging (MRI) has the advantage of detecting intraspinal extension. Radioisotope studies are useful to detect bone spread and technetium-labelled meta-iodobenzylguanidine (MIBG), if it is taken up by tumour tissue, is useful in diagnosis, therapy and follow-up. Lumbar puncture, bone marrow aspiration and trephine are performed to detect spread to central nervous system and bone marrow. Urinary and serum catecholamine levels are measured and are useful markers of disease progression and response to therapy.

In early stages of the disease, surgical resection aims to achieve complete eradication of disease. In more advanced disease, biopsy will confirm the diagnosis and tumour debulking may be indicated. Combination chemotherapy is the subject of many collaborative trials, and intensive treatment, which results in bone marrow ablation and requires rescue with bone marrow transplantation, has also been the subject of recent study. Radiotherapy has been used in residual or recurrent disease and for palliation of bone pain.

The prognosis has improved with multimodality treatment. In stage I, disease-free survival in excess of 90% has been reported with surgery alone but this figure falls such that survival in stage IV following bone marrow ablation and bone marrow transplantation rescue is between 15 and 40% (and much less without rescue).

Liver tumours

One-third of childhood liver tumours are benign. Metastatic disease from other tumours, notably neuroblastoma, is more common than primary hepatic malignancy. Resection is the mainstay of therapy, often after chemotherapy has downstaged a malignant tumour.

The benign liver tumours most commonly reported are haemangioma and haemangioendothelioma. Most present within the first 6 months of life with abdominal distension, hepatomegaly and high-output cardiac failure. Platelet consumption by the tumour may result in disseminated intravascular coagulopathy (Kasabach–Merritt syndrome). In many patients, these tumours regress spontaneously but where cardiac failure cannot be controlled medically, other therapies may be helpful (e.g. steroid administration, radiotherapy and hepatic artery embolization or ligation). Resection may be life-saving but carries a high risk. Interferon alfa-2a has been shown to accelerate tumour regression in some patients.

Over 90% of primary malignant liver tumours in children are either hepatoblastoma or hepatocellular carcinoma. Most present with painless, massive hepatomegaly or upper abdominal distension. Jaundice is unusual in hepatoblastoma but occurs more frequently in hepatocellular carcinoma because of underlying cirrhosis. Anorexia, weight loss, lethargy and pallor are common. Ultrasound, CT and MRI provide the likely differential diagnoses. Estimation of serum α-fetoprotein is useful in monitoring response to therapy.

In hepatoblastoma, 80% of patients present in the first 3 years of life; serum α-fetoprotein is elevated in 70% of cases. Over 50% are deemed to be unresectable and 10% have pulmonary metastases at presentation. Complete resection offers the best outcome. In unresectable cases, biopsy followed by chemotherapy to shrink the tumour and subsequent resection is the next best option. Following complete resection and subsequent chemotherapy, the survival rate is almost 90%. Equivalent cure rates have been reported in children subjected to chemotherapy prior to resection in the early-stage groups. Children with advanced disease have a better survival with combination therapy (median 3-year survival 50–60%) but this falls dramatically if the tumour is not resected.

Hepatocellular carcinoma is a disease of older children (median age 9 years) with the same aetiology and clinical features as adult disease, including the presence of cirrhosis. Hepatitis B status is positive in a significant number of older children. Serum α-fetoprotein is elevated in 50% of cases. The outlook for children with hepatocellular carcinoma is poor except where complete tumour resection is performed. This tumour is much less responsive to chemotherapy than hepatoblastoma and survival is at best 40%.

Key points

- In all children, knowledge of normal physiological parameters for different age groups is essential before an evaluation of the abnormal is possible
- The percentage water content of newborn babies and children is higher than in adults
- The first 10 kg body weight requires approximately 100 mL/kg per day of intravenous fluids (equates to 4 mL/kg per h); the next 10 kg body weight requires approximately 50 mL/kg per day (2 mL/kg per h); every kilogram of body weight thereafter requires ~ 25 mL/kg per day (1 mL/kg per h). A 35-kg child would therefore require 40 mL + 20 mL + 15 mL = 75 mL/h of intravenous fluids
- Over 90% of umbilical herniae close spontaneously during the first 3 years of life
- Inguinal herniae in children:
  (a) are more common in boys than girls
  (b) are more common on the right side
  (c) are almost always indirect
  (d) always require surgical repair
- Exomphalos major is frequently associated with other serious congenital abnormalities
- Gastroschisis is rarely associated with other congenital abnormalities except injury to the protruding intestine
- The most common form of oesophageal atresia also involves a fistula between the trachea and the distal oesophagus
- Oesphageal atresia is frequently associated with other congenital abnormalities (VATER or VACTERL associations)
- Bile-stained vomiting in a neonate should be considered due to malrotation of the intestine until proven otherwise
- Passage of meconium at birth does not exclude a diagnosis of intestinal atresia in a newborn
- Hirschsprung's disease is a condition where ganglion cells have failed to migrate into the distal intestine
- Congenital diaphragmatic hernia has a high mortality
- Pyloric stenosis causes a hypokalaemic hypochloraemic metabolic alkalosis
- Gastro-oesophageal reflux is the most common cause of persistent vomiting in infancy
- Gastro-oesophageal reflux is, in most cases, a self-limiting condition
- Intussusception is a common cause of intestinal obstruction in the first year of life
- After the first year of life, trauma is the leading cause of death in childhood
- Clinical presentation of appendicitis in children can be very variable
- Nephroblastoma is the most common solid tumour seen in childhood

Paediatric 'general' surgery at a glance

Surgery through the ages
Neonatal surgery
- Defined as surgery up to 1 month of age corrected for gestation at birth
- Largely the surgery of congenital anomalies which are rare
- Neonatal surgery is only undertaken in highly specialized units

Surgery in infancy
- Infancy is usually defined as the first year of life
- Much of the surgery undertaken during this part of life is required because of problems with the gastrointestinal tract
- Three most common conditions that require surgery are:
  (a) Pyloric stenosis
  (b) Gastro-oesophageal reflux disease
  (c) Intussusception

Surgery in the childhood years
- As children, grow many other conditions seen in adult practice are encountered
- Trauma in children can be devastating, not just from the high fatality rate but also because of the impact of sublethal injury on growth, behaviour and development
- Cancer: while most solid tumours are rare, treatment can be complex and requires close cooperation between many disciplines. Many childhood cancers can be effectively treated and outright cure is possible in some

Gastro-oesophageal reflux disease
Definition and aetiology
- Common condition characterized by incompetence of the lower oesophageal sphincter, resulting in retrograde passage of gastric contents into the oesophagus resulting in vomiting
- Aetiology: immaturity of lower oesophageal sphincter, short intra-abdominal oesophagus

Clinical features
- Vomiting, often related to feeds, may contain blood and rarely is projectile

Investigation
If oesophagitis, stricture, anaemia or aspiration is suspected the following are indicated:
- Barium swallow
- Oesophagoscopy and biopsy
- 24-h pH monitoring

05

Treatment
- As there is a natural tendency towards spontaneous improvement with age, a conservative approach is adopted initially: thickening of feeds, positioning infant in 30° head-up position after feeds, antacids (e.g. Gaviscon), drugs to increase gastric emptying and increase lower oesophageal sphincter tone
- Surgery (Nissen fundoplication) is reserved for failure for respond to conservative treatment with oesophageal stricture or severe pulmonary aspiration

Infantile hypertrophic pyloric stenosis
Definition and aetiology
- Condition characterized by hypertrophy of the circular muscle of the gastric pylorus that obstructs gastric outflow
- Aetiology unknown but affects 1 in 450 children, 85% male, often first-born, 20% have family history

Clinical features
- Non-bile-stained projectile vomiting (after feeds) beginning at 2–6 weeks of age
- Baby is hungry, constipated and dehydrated. Loss of H^+ and Cl^- from stomach and K^+ from kidney causes *hypochloraemic hypokalaemic metabolic alkalosis*
- Palpable pyloric 'tumour' during a test feed or after vomiting.
- Gastric peristalsis may be seen, ultrasound I if diagnosis is uncertain

Management
- Correct dehydration and electrolyte imbalance with 0.45% saline in dextrose 5% with added K^+. May take 24–48 h to become normal
- Ramstedt's pyloromyotomy via transverse right upper quadrant or per umbilical incision. Normal feeding can commence within 24 h

Malrotation of the gut
Definition and aetiology
- Malrotation describes a number of conditions caused by failure of the intestine to rotate into the correct anatomical position during embryological development
- Midgut volvulus, internal herniae and duodenal obstruction may occur

Clinical features
- Bile-stained vomiting in the newborn period is most common presentation but older children may present with recurrent abdominal pain, abdominal distension and vomiting

Management
- Surgery is required to release the obstructions and to broaden the small bowel mesentery

Intussusception
Definition
- Invagination of one segment of bowel into an adjacent distal segment
- The segment that invaginates is called the *intussusceptum* and the segment into which it invaginates the *intussuscepiens*. The tip of the intussusceptum is called the *apex* or *lead point*

Aetiology
- 90% are idiopathic
- Viral infection can lead to hyperplasia of Peyer's patches, which become the apex of an intussusception
- Other lead points include Meckel's diverticulum, a polyp or a duplication cyst

Clinical features
- Most common cause of intestinal obstruction in infants 3–12 months of age, M > F
- Presents with pain (attacks of colicky pain every 15–20 min, lasting 2–3 min with screaming and drawing up of legs), pallor, vomiting and lethargy between attacks
- Sausage-shaped mass in right upper quadrant, empty right iliac fossa
- Passage of blood and mucus ('redcurrant jelly' stool)
- Tachycardia and dehydration

Diagnosis
- Plain X-ray may show intestinal obstruction and sometimes the outline of the intussusception
- Ultrasonography may help showing right upper quadrant mass and the diagnostic target sign
- Definite diagnosis by air or (less commonly) barium enema

Management
- Intravenous fluids to resuscitate infant (shock is frequent because of fluid sequestration in the bowel)
- Air or barium reduction of intussusception if no peritonitis (75% of cases)
- Remainder require surgical reduction

Inguinoscrotal conditions
Acute scrotum
Definition
- Red, swollen, painful scrotum caused by torsion of the hydatid of Morgagni (60%), torsion of the testis (30%), epididymo-orchitis (10%) and idiopathic scrotal oedema (10%)

Management
- All cases of 'acute scrotum' should be explored
- If true testicular torsion, treatment is bilateral orchidopexy (orchidectomy of affected testis if gangrenous)

- If torsion of hydatid of Morgagni, treatment is removal of hydatid on affected side only

Inguinal hernia and hydrocele
Definition and aetiology
- During the seventh month of gestation the testis descends from the posterior abdominal wall into the scrotum through a peritoneal diverticulum called the processus vaginalis, which obliterates just before birth
- An *inguinal hernia* in an infant is a swelling in the inguinal area due to failure of obliteration of the processus vaginalis, allowing bowel (rarely omentum) to descend within the hernial sac below the external inguinal ring

- A *hydrocele* is a collection of fluid around the testis that has trickled down from the peritoneal cavity via a narrow but patent processus vaginalis

Diagnosis
- Diagnosis of hydrocele is usually obvious
- Diagnosis of a hernia may be entirely on the mother's given history or a lump may be obvious
- Strangulation is a serious complication as it may compromise bowel and/or the blood supply to the testis

Management
- Hernia should be treated by operation to obliterate the remaining processus vaginalis. Over 90% of hydroceles resolve spontaneously by age one year

Evidence-based medicine

Recommended textbooks

Ashcraft, K.W. & Holder, T.M. (1993) *Pediatric Surgery*, 2nd edn. W.B. Saunders, Philadelphia.

Freeman, N.V., Burge, D.M., Griffiths, D.M. & Malone, P.J. (eds) (1994) *Surgery of the Newborn*. Churchill Livingstone, Edinburgh.

Raine, P.A.M. & Azmy, A.A.F. (eds) (1994) *Surgical Emergencies in Children: A Practical Guide*. Butterworth Heinemann, Oxford.

Skandalakis, J.E. & Gray, S.W. (eds) (1994) *Embryology for Surgeons*, 2nd edn. Williams & Wilkins, Baltimore.

Spitz, L. & Coran, A.G. (eds) (1995) *Rob and Smith's Operative Surgery: Pediatric Surgery*, 5th edn. Chapman & Hall Medical, London.

Stringer, M.D., Oldham, K.T., Mouriquand, P.D.E. & Howard, E.R. (eds) (1998) *Pediatric Surgery and Urology: Long-term Outcomes*. W.B. Saunders, London.

Walker, W.A., Durie, P.R., Hamilton, J.R., Walker-Smith, J.A. & Watkins, J.B. (eds) (2000) *Pediatric Gastrointestinal Disease: Pathophysiology, Diagnosis, Management*, 3rd edn. B.C. Decker, Hamilton, Ontario.

Journals

Journal of Pediatric Surgery
Seminars in Pediatric Surgery
Pediatric Surgery International
European Journal of Pediatric Surgery
Archives of Diseases of Childhood
Journal of Pediatric Gastroenterology and Nutrition

Websites

http://www.baps.org.uk   Website of the British Association of Paediatric Surgeons with an extensive library and useful weblinks

http://www.eapsa.org   Website of the American Pediatric Surgical Association

http://www.aap.org/sections/surgery   Website of the section of Surgery of the American Academy of Pediatrics

http://www.cybermedicalcollege.com   Website of a large medical resource hosted by the Royal College of Physicians and Surgeons of Glasgow

05

Index

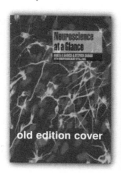

Clinical Surgery